Perinatal and Pediatric Respiratory Care

SECOND EDITION

Perinatal and Pediatric Respiratory Care

Editors

Michael P. Czervinske, BSRT, RRT
Clinical Instructor,
School of Allied Health,
Respiratory Care Education,
University of Kansas Medical Center,
Kansas City, Kansas

Sherry L. Barnhart, AS, RRT
Asthma Educator,
Arkansas Allergy and Asthma Clinic,
Little Rock, Arkansas

With 457 illustrations

SAUNDERS
An Imprint of Elsevier

SAUNDERS

An Imprint of Elsevier

11830 Westline Industrial Drive
St. Louis, Missouri 63146

Perinatal and Pediatric Respiratory Care

Notice

Respiratory Care is an ever-changing field. Standard safety precautions must be followed, but as new research and clinical experience broaden our knowledge, changes in treatment and drug therapy may become necessary or appropriate. Readers are advised to check the most current product information provided by the manufacturer of each drug to be administered to verify the recommended dose, the method and duration of administration, and contraindications. It is the responsibility of the licensed prescriber, relying on experience and knowledge of the patient, to determine dosages and the best treatment for each individual patient. Neither the publisher nor the editor assumes any liability for any injury and/or damage to persons or property arising from this publication.

Previous edition copyrighted 1995

ISBN-13: 978-0-7216-8231-0
ISBN-10: 0-7216-8231-6

Acquisitions Editor: Karen Fabiano
Developmental Editor: Mindy Copeland
Publishing Services Manager: Pat Joiner
Project Manager: David Stein
Designer: Mark Oberkrom
Cover Art: Meiklejohn, UK Gianelli/SIS

GW/MVY

Printed in the United States of America

Last digit is the print number: 9   8   7   6

CONTRIBUTORS

Robert G. Aucoin, RPh
Pediatric Clinical Pharmacist,
Children's Center,
Our Lady of the Lake Regional Medical Center,
Baton Rouge, Louisiana

Loren A. Bauman, MD
Associate Professor,
Pediatric Anesthesia and Pediatric Critical Care;
Director, Pediatric Critical Care Unit,
Brenner Children's Hospital,
Wake Forest University Baptist Medical Center,
Winston-Salem, North Carolina

Ronald E. Becker, MD
Assistant in Medicine,
Center for Pediatric Sleep Disorders,
Developmental Medicine Center,
Children's Hospital Boston;
Instructor in Pediatrics,
Harvard Medical School,
Boston, Massachusetts

Kathy Boyle, MS, RRT
Education Coordinator,
Respiratory Care Services,
Arkansas Children's Hospital,
Little Rock, Arkansas

Melissa K. Brown, RRT
Clinical Specialist,
Sharp Mary Birch Hospital for Women,
San Diego, California

Perry L. Clark, MD
Assistant Professor of Pediatrics,
Department of Pediatrics,
Division of Neonatology,
University of Missouri at Kansas City,
Kansas City, Missouri

Heidi J. Dalton, MD
Medical Director, Intensive Care Unit,
Department of Critical Care Medicine,
Children's National Medical Center,
Washington, District of Columbia

Kathy Davidson, RRT
Clinical Services Manager,
Respiratory Care Services,
Primary Children's Medical Center,
Salt Lake City, Utah

David L. Ellwanger, BS, RRT
Education Coordinator,
Respiratory Care Services,
Southern Regional Medical Center,
Riverdale, Georgia

James B. Fink, MS, RRT, FAARC
Fellow, Respiratory Science,
Aerogen, Inc.,
Mountain View, California

Debra Fiser, MD
Professor and Chairman, Critical Care Medicine,
Department of Pediatrics,
University of Arkansas for Medical Sciences,
Arkansas Children's Hospital,
Little Rock, Arkansas

Jerril Green, MD
Assistant Professor,
Critical Care and Emergency Medicine,
Department of Pediatrics,
University of Arkansas for Medical Sciences,
Arkansas Children's Hospital,
Little Rock, Arkansas

Debra Greene, RRT
Manager,
Allied Healthcare Systems,
Jamestown, New York

Jay S. Greenspan, MD
Professor and Vice Chairman,
Department of Pediatrics;
Director of Neonatology,
Thomas Jefferson University,
A.I. duPont Hospital for Children,
Philadelphia, Pennsylvania

Barry Grenier, BA, RRT
Education Coordinator,
Respiratory Care Department,
Children's Hospital,
Boston, Massachusetts

Douglas R. Hansell, BS, RRT
ECMO Program Coordinator,
Respiratory Care Services,
The North Carolina Baptist Hospitals, Inc.,
Wake Forest University Baptist Medical Center,
Winston-Salem, North Carolina

Robert L. Hopkins, MD
Associate Professor of Pediatrics,
Director, Section of Pediatric Critical Care,
Department of Pediatrics,
Tulane University School of Medicine,
New Orleans, Louisiana

J. David Ingram, MD
Associate Professor of Radiology,
University of Colorado Health Sciences Center,
Mae Boettcher Center for Pediatric Imaging,
The Children's Hospital,
Denver, Colorado

Ian N. Jacobs, MD
Assistant Professor,
Department of Otorhinolaryngology, Head and Neck
    Surgery,
Department of Pediatric Otolaryngology and Human
    Communication,
The Children's Hospital of Philadelphia,
Philadelphia, Pennsylvania

Karl Kalavantavanich, MD
Attending Physician,
Department of Pediatrics,
Ramathibodi Hospital,
Mahidol University,
Bangkok, Thailand

Thomas Kallstrom, RRT, FAARC
Director, Cardiopulmonary Services,
Fairview Hospital,
Cleveland, Ohio

James P. Keenan, BS, RRT, FAARC
Technical Manager,
Primary Children's Medical Center,
Salt Lake City, Utah

Antoun Y. Khabbaz, MD
Chief Resident,
Department of Obstetrics, Gynecology and
    Reproductive Medicine,
State University of New York at Stony Brook,
Stony Brook, New York

Scott Kirley, RRT
Respiratory Therapist,
Division of Pulmonology,
Department of Pediatrics,
University of South Florida College of Medicine,
Tampa, Florida

George B. Mallory, Jr., MD
Assistant Professor of Pediatrics,
Direct Lung Transplantation,
Washington University School of Medicine,
St. Louis Children's Hospital,
St. Louis, Missouri

Loretta Mathews, RN, BA, CEN, LNC
Staff Nurse, Emergency Department,
Menorah Medical Center,
Overland Park, Kansas;
Adjunct Assistant Professor,
School of Allied Health;
Adjunct Clinical Instructor,
School of Nursing,
University of Kansas Medical Center,
Kansas City, Kansas

Paul Mathews, PhD, RRT, FCCM, FCCP
Associate Professor,
Respiratory Care Education;
Associate Professor,
Physical Therapy and Rehabilitation Sciences,
School of Allied Health,
University of Kansas Medical Center,
Kansas City, Kansas

Keith S. Meredith, MD
Director of Phoenix Neonatal Operations,
Phoenix Perinatal Associates,
Phoenix, Arizona,

Ronald P. Mlcak, BA, RRT
Director, Respiratory Care,
Shriners Hospital for Children,
Galveston, Texas

Mary M. Pettignano, RRT, MMSc
Winter Park, Florida

Robert Pettignano, MD, FAAP, FCCM
Pediatric Intensivist,
Nemours Children's Clinic Orlando,
Arnold Palmer Hospital for Children and Women,
Division of Pediatric Critical Care,
Orlando, Florida

J. Gerald Quirk, MD, PhD
Professor and Chairman,
Department of Obstetrics, Gynecology and
    Reproductive Medicine,
State University of New York at Stony Brook,
Stony Brook, New York

Mark Rogers, BS, RRT
Pediatric Clinical Coordinator,
Loma Linda University Medical Center,
Loma Linda, California

Bruce K. Rubin, MD, FRCP(C), FCCP
Professor and Vice-Chair for Research,
Department of Pediatrics;
Professor of Biomedical Engineering, Physiology and
    Pharmacology,
Wake Forest University School of Medicine,
Winston-Salem, North Carolina

John W. Salyer, RRT, BS, MBA, FAARC
Director, Respiratory Care,
Children's Hospital and Regional Medical Center,
Seattle, Washington

Bruce Schnapf, DO
Chief, Division of Pulmonology,
Associate Professor, Department of Pediatrics,
University of South Florida College of Medicine,
Tampa, Florida

Craig M. Schramm, MD
Associate Professor of Pediatrics,
University of Connecticut Health Center;
Division Chief, Pediatric Pulmonology,
Connecticut Children's Medical Center,
Hartford, Connecticut

Adam Schwarz, MD
Clinical Associate Professor of Pediatrics,
University of Arizona School of Medicine,
Associate Director,
Pediatric Intensive Care Unit,
Phoenix Children's Hospital,
Phoenix, Arizona

Garry Sitler, RRT
Program Director, Intensive Care Transport Team,
Texas Children's Hospital,
Houston, Texas

Anthony D. Slonim, MD, MPH
Attending Physician and Fellowship Director,
Pediatric Critical Care Medicine,
Children's National Medical Center,
Washington, District of Columbia

Roberta E. Sonnino, MD, FACS, FAAP
Professor of Surgery and Pediatrics,
Chief, Section of Pediatric Surgery,
The University of Kansas Medical Center,
Kansas City, Kansas

Patrick Sorenson, MA, RPSGT
Sleep Lab Supervisor,
Department of Clinical Neurophysiology,
Center for Pediatric Sleep Disorders,
Children's Hospital Boston,
Boston, Massachusetts

Alex Stentzler, RPFT
Vice President, Advanced Technologies,
VIASYS Healthcare, Inc.,
Yorba Linda, California

Paul C. Stillwell, MD
Chief of Pediatric Pulmonology,
Department of Pulmonology,
Phoenix Children's Hospital,
Phoenix, Arizona

W. Gerald Teague, MD
Professor and Vice Chairman of Pediatrics;
Director, Division of Pulmonary Medicine,
Emory University School of Medicine,
Atlanta, Georgia

Donald W. Thibeault, MD
Professor of Pediatrics,
Section of Neonatology,
University of Missouri at Kansas City,
Children's Mercy Hospital,
Kansas City, Missouri

Brian K. Walsh, BS, RRT
Clinical Team Leader for Respiratory Care,
University of Virginia,
Children's Medical Center,
Charlottesville, Virginia

Lorilie A. Weber-Hardy, MEd, RRT
Director of Clinical Education, Respiratory Therapy,
Department of Cardiopulmonary and Diagnostic
    Sciences,
School of Health-Related Professions,
University of Missouri,
Columbia, Missouri

Douglas F. Willson, MD
Associate Professor of Pediatrics,
Division Chief, Pediatric Critical Care,
Department of Pediatrics,
University of Virginia Medical Center,
Charlottesville, Virginia

Marla Wolfson, PhD
Associate Professor of Physiology and Pediatrics,
Department of Physiology,
Temple University School of Medicine,
Philadelphia, Pennsylvania

PREFACE

Welcome to the second edition of *Perinatal and Pediatric Respiratory Care*. Since the first edition of this book was published in 1995, appreciation for the distinction between neonatal, pediatric, and adult respiratory care continues to grow. Today there is no doubt that the field of perinatal and pediatric care requires specialization. Over the past 2 decades, we have personally observed and experienced the evolution and increasing maturity of this area of patient care. As the field of perinatal and pediatric respiratory care has grown, so has the role of the respiratory care practitioner. Now more than ever, practitioners find that they must expand their assessment, decision-making, and technical skills. Furthermore, just as the practitioner's role has changed, so have clinical guidelines, protocols, medical devices, and our understanding of disease management. Along with these changes comes a tremendous need for the practitioner to have an informative source concerning the current developments in patient care.

Although principally designed as a textbook for the respiratory care student and practitioner new to the field, this book is also intended to be detailed enough to serve as a current reference for the experienced practitioner engaged in the respiratory care of infants and children, regardless of professional discipline. As with the first edition, the textbook may also serve as a study guide for the National Board for Respiratory Care's specialty examination concerning the respiratory care of neonatal and pediatric patients.

New to this edition, the text is divided into five major content sections: (I) Fetal Development, Assessment, and Delivery; (II) Assessment and Monitoring of the Neonatal and Pediatric Patient; (III) Therapeutic Procedures for Treatment of Neonatal and Pediatric Disorders; (IV) Neonatal and Pediatric Disorders: Presentation, Diagnosis, and Treatment; and (V) Neonatal and Pediatric Transient and Ambulatory Care.

In Section I, Chapters 1 through 4 cover the perinatal topics of fetal pulmonary development and physiology, circulation, and assessment. Discussion of high-risk delivery and neonatal resuscitation is also provided. Section II comprises Chapters 5 through 11, which cover the assessment, diagnostic, and monitoring techniques used in both neonatal and pediatric patients. Section III, consisting of Chapters 12 through 27, provides discussion of the current therapies and procedures used in the respiratory care of neonates, infants, and children. Disorders and disease states specific to neonatal and pediatric patients are covered in Section IV. This section, comprised of Chapters 28 through 44, includes discussion of the etiology, pathophysiology, diagnosis, clinical presentation, management, and outcome. In Section V, Chapters 45 and 46, information is provided concerning the respiratory care of the infant and child during transport and in the home setting.

We believe that *Perinatal and Pediatric Respiratory Care* will continue to be a reference source concerning the care of neonatal and pediatric patients with respiratory disorders. Although the changing medical environment was the major reason for the birth of this second edition, one thing has not changed: our hope that through the use of this text, practitioners are able to improve the respiratory care of neonates, infants, and children.

Michael P. Czervinske
Sherry L. Barnhart

ACKNOWLEDGMENTS

We thank and acknowledge the contributors of the first edition of *Perinatal and Pediatric Respiratory Care.* It was their work that laid the foundation for most of the chapters found in this edition. We also thank our current group of contributors for the many hours they gave toward this project and especially for the expertise they brought to each and every chapter.

Additionally we want to thank the publishing staff that has been so gracious to us throughout this project. To our developmental editor, Mindy Copeland; we are awed by her extraordinary atti-tude and never-ending supply of patience, in spite of the many interruptions and changes along the way. And to David Stein, who put the finishing touches on each page; we give him all the credit for the attention to detail and perfection that is required.

Last, but by no means least, we especially thank our spouses for their love, support, and encouragement to persevere through yet another book. We are blessed beyond words.

Michael P. Czervinske
Sherry L. Barnhart

CONTENTS

Fetal Development, Assessment, and Delivery

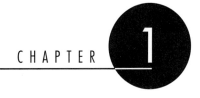

CHAPTER 1

Fetal Lung Development

Bruce Schnapf
Scott Kirley

This chapter is concerned with the structural development of the fetal human lung. At birth, the lung must abruptly supply oxygen for the infant. Fetal lung development is therefore programmed so that at this crucial moment, the organ reaches a functional degree of morphologic, physiologic, and biochemical maturity. This does not mean, however, that lung development is complete at birth. The newborn lung undergoes further differentiation and growth to reach maturity.[1] Functionally, fetal lung development is not complete until the alveoli possess an adequate gas-exchanging surface. The pulmonary vascular system must also have sufficient capacity to transport an adequate amount of blood through the lungs for carbon dioxide and oxygen exchange. The alveoli need to be structurally and functionally stable and elastic and resilient enough to undergo the stretching associated with tidal breathing and crying.

A great deal has been learned about the normal development of the human lung. In the 1960s, Reid formulated the laws of development of the human lung: (1) the bronchial tree develops by the sixteenth week of intrauterine life, (2) after birth the alveoli develop in increasing number until the age of 8 years and increase in size until growth of the chest wall is finished, and (3) blood vessels are remodeled and increased, certainly while new alveoli are forming and probably until growth of the chest is complete.[2]

Although these facts are known, we remain remarkably ignorant about the mechanics of structural development of the fetal lung. New interest is being kindled by the desire to understand and prevent chronic lung injury in premature infants. Much more information is needed about the mechanisms of cellular repair in the immature lung that permit recovery of injured lungs in premature infants. Improved knowledge concerning the complex process of geometric growth is also necessary.

As stated earlier, birth does not signal the end of lung development. There is a remarkably complex process of growth after birth, accommodating differing proportions of airway size, alveolar size, and surface area. The term infant, with approximately 50 million alveoli, has the potential to add another 250 million alveoli and increase the total alveolar surface area from approximately 3 m² to 70 m² at maturity. There are more than 40 different cell types in the lung, and they have many functions. There are also growth factors responsible for normal cell and structural development that affect various aspects of prenatal and postnatal lung function, growth, and structure.

STAGES OF LUNG DEVELOPMENT

In the human, there are five well-recognized stages of lung development: embryonal, pseudoglandular, canalicular, saccular, and alveolar (Table 1-1).[3,4]

EMBRYONAL STAGE

The first stage is the embryonal period, which covers primitive development and is generally regarded as encompassing the first 2 months of gestation. The lung begins to emerge as a bud from the pharynx at 26 days following conception (Fig. 1-1). This lung bud elongates and forms two bronchial buds and the trachea, which then become separate from the esophagus through the development of the tracheoesophageal septum. Further subdivisions occur in an irregularly dichotomous way at the end of the embryonal stage. By this time, the

TABLE 1-1	CLASSIFICATION OF STAGES OF HUMAN INTRAUTERINE LUNG GROWTH	
Stage	**Time of Occurrence**	**Significance**
Embryonal	Day 26–day 52	Development of trachea and major bronchi
Pseudoglandular	Day 52–week 16	Development of remaining conducting airways
Canalicular	Week 17–week 28	Development of vascular bed and framework of acinus
Saccular	Week 29–week 36	Increased complexity of saccules
Alveolar	Week 36–term	Development of alveoli

major airways are completely developed, resulting in 10 branches on the right and nine branches on the left. The left and right pulmonary arteries form plexuses even before the heart descends into the thorax. Left and right pulmonary veins start to develop around the fifth week as a single evagination in the sinoatrial portion of the heart.

During this phase, the respiratory epithelium also develops in the endodermal layer (the innermost layer of the three primary germ layers) foregut bud and interacts with the bronchial mesoderm (the middle layer). The mesenchyme will eventually give rise to the pulmonary interstitium, smooth muscle, blood vessels, and cartilage.[5] The mesenchyme determines the nature of the branching by a complex interaction of epithelial cells with the bronchial mesoderm.[6] The surrounding mesenchyme is cellular and composed of cells that have not differentiated into cartilage or other connective tissue cells. The mesenchyme and epithelium are separated from each other by a basal lamina that contains Type I collagen at the sites of branching. The diaphragm also develops during the embryonal stage of lung development. Complete development of the diaphragm occurs by approximately the seventh week of gestation.

PSEUDOGLANDULAR STAGE

The next stage is the pseudoglandular phase, in which the conducting airway system develops; this stage extends to the sixteenth week of gestation. During this stage, there is extensive subdivision of the airway system as well as development of the entire conducting airway system. The branching pattern that occurs in both lungs determines the pattern in the adult lung.[7] The subsequent growth of these airways is in size only. The most peripheral structures are terminal bronchioles, which likely undergo differentiation to later form the respiratory bronchioles and alveolar ducts.[8] Again, once the pattern is laid, the subsequent growth of these airways is in size only. The potential gas-exchanging part of the lung, the acinus—the part of the lung distal to the terminal bronchiole—may also be laid down completely during the pseudoglandular phase. The last several divisions of airways are destined to become the acinus. During the pseudoglandular phase, cilia appear on the surface of the epithelium of the trachea and the mainstem bronchi at 10 weeks of gestation and are present in the epithelial cells of the peripheral airways by 13 weeks of gestation. Goblet cells appear in the bronchial epithelium at 13 to 14 weeks' gestation, and submucosal glands arise as solid buds from basal layers of the surface epithelium at 15 to 16 weeks of gestation. Smooth muscle cells derived from the primitive mesenchyme surrounding the airways can be seen at the end of the seventh week of gestation and by the twelfth week form the posterior wall of the large bronchi. The development of cartilage has been documented at 24 weeks' gestation and may be present earlier. Cartilage may be present in about 10 to 14 airway generations at 24 weeks' gestation. The cartilage is immature at this stage. Lymphatics appear first in the hilar region of the lung during the eighth week of gestation and in the lung itself by the tenth week. This phase has been termed pseudoglandular because random histologic sections show the appearance of multiple, apparently round structures resembling glands. They are separated from each other by

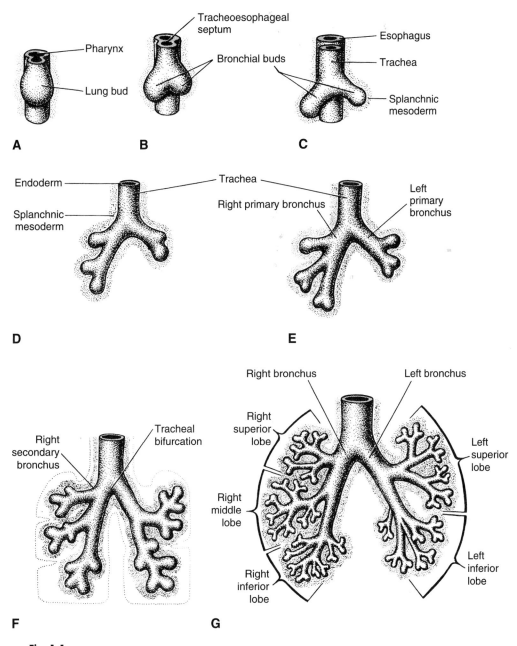

Fig. 1-1

Successive stages in the development of the bronchi and lungs. **A** to **C,** Four weeks. **D** and **E,** Five weeks. **F,** Six weeks. **G,** Eight weeks. (From Moore KL, Persaud TVN: *The developing human,* ed 5. Philadelphia, WB Saunders, 1993; p 230.)

mesenchyme and its derivatives. The cells lining the spaces are columnar and contain glycogen. By the end of this stage, airways, arteries, and veins have developed in the pattern corresponding to that found in the adult.

CANALICULAR STAGE

The canalicular phase follows the pseudoglandular stage and lasts from approximately 17 weeks to about 26 weeks of gestation. This stage is so named because of the appearance of vascular channels, or capillaries, which begin to approximate the air passages and form a capillary network around them.[9] Some of the capillaries extend into the epithelium. The capillaries develop at 20 weeks' gestation and increase in number by 22 weeks. Satisfactory gas exchange cannot occur until capillaries have sufficient surface area and are close enough to the airspaces for efficient gas transfer. This development, along with the appearance of surfactant, is therefore critical to the extrauterine survival of the immature fetus. The acinar units are also formed during the canalicular period (Fig. 1-2). The acinus is the gas exchange unit associated with a single terminal bronchiole. This unit will eventually contain three orders of respiratory bronchioles: alveolar ducts, alveolar sacs, and alveoli. It follows that primitive lobules will have formed by the beginning of the canalicular period. Each lobule will contain three to five terminal bronchioles; approximately 25,000 terminal bronchioles will be found in the adult lung. If the primitive acinar units are all formed by the end of the canalicular period, this would imply that the full complement of 25,000 terminal bronchioles should be present by 28 weeks of gestation. Thinning of the extracellular matrix, or mesenchyme, continues through the canalicular period. By 20 to 22 weeks of gestation, Type I and Type II epithelial cells can be differentiated in the human fetal lung. The Type II cells retain the cytoplasmic shape of their precursors. Lamellar bodies and glycogen begin to appear in the Type II cell cytoplasm. The Type I cells begin their flattening process and elongate. The conducting airways have now developed smooth muscle.

By the end of the canalicular period, the potential air-blood barrier is thin enough to support gas exchange. The vessels develop alongside conducting airways with muscularization to a peripheral position that is more distant than that present in the adult.[10] The bronchial artery system may be as critical for the lung's development as the pulmonary artery is, although the role of the bronchial artery in lung differentiation and growth is not clear.[11] It has been suggested that the most peripheral parts of the developing lung are supplied only by the pulmonary arterial vasculature.[10] The epithelial cells at this point are capable of producing fetal lung liquid.

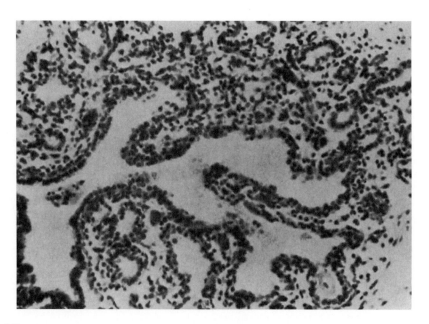

Fig. 1-2

Canalicular stage at 22 weeks of gestation. A terminal bronchiole *(bottom left)* leads into a prospective acinus. Note that branches are sparse. (From Langston C et al: Human lung growth in late gestation and in the neonate. *Am Rev Respir Dis* 1984; 129:607.)

SACCULAR STAGE

The saccular period was formerly thought to be the last stage of lung development prior to birth. However, because alveoli form before birth, the termination of this period is now arbitrarily set at 35 to 36 weeks of gestation. At the beginning of this phase, or 26 weeks of gestation, the terminal structures are referred to as saccules and are relatively smooth-walled, cylindrical structures. They then become subdivided by ridges known as secondary crests (Fig. 1-3). As the crests protrude into the saccules, part of the capillary net is drawn in with them, forming a double capillary layer.[12] Further subdivisions between the crests result in smaller spaces, which have been termed subsaccules. Exactly when these subsaccular structures can be termed alveoli is a matter of judgment (Fig. 1-4). Some have advocated that any structure bordered on three sides should be termed an alveolus. Alveoli can be seen as early as 32 weeks of gestation and are present at 36 weeks of gestation in all fetuses (Fig. 1-5). During this saccular phase, there is a marked increase in the potential gas-exchanging surface area.

ALVEOLAR STAGE

Clearly the distinction between the saccular and alveolar stages is difficult and arbitrary. Hislop and colleagues[13] claim that alveoli are present at 29 weeks of gestation; Langston and co-workers[3] feel that 36 weeks' gestation is the earliest that one can distinguish between subsaccules and alveoli.

At birth, the number of alveoli is highly variable, ranging from 20 to 150 million. The accepted mean of alveoli is also variable in the literature, given as 50 million by Langston and colleagues[3] and 150 million by Hislop and associates.[13] It has been estimated that only 15% to 20% of the adult number of alveoli are present at birth, and thus alveolar multiplication is largely a postnatal event. Hislop and co-workers[13] feel that almost half the total number of alveoli are present at birth. The important point is that alveolarization is rapidly progressing during the period of development from late fetal to early neonatal life and may be complete by a year or so after birth.

POSTNATAL LUNG GROWTH

Normal lung growth is a continuous process that begins early in gestation and extends through infancy and childhood. Major structural development occurs in late gestation and continues over the first years of postnatal life.[14,15] As stated earlier, estimates of alveolar number at birth vary widely, and the average of 50 million is generally accepted. These alveoli provide a total gas-exchanging surface of approximately 3 to 4 m^2. More than 80% of the eventual number of 300 million alveoli

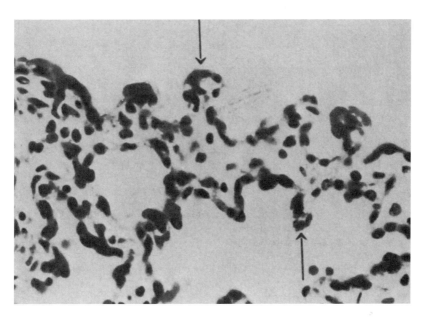

Fig. 1-3

Saccular stage at 29 weeks of gestation. Secondary crests *(arrows)* begin to divide saccules into smaller divisions. (From Langston C et al: Human lung growth in late gestation and in the neonate. *Am Rev Respir Dis* 1984; 129:607.)

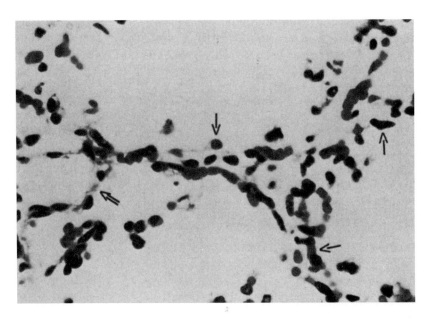

Fig. 1-4

Alveolar stage at 36 weeks of gestation. Note the double capillary network *(arrows with one tail)* and the single capillary layer *(arrow with double tail)*. (From Langston C et al: Human lung growth in late gestation and in the neonate. *Am Rev Respir Dis* 1984; 129:607.)

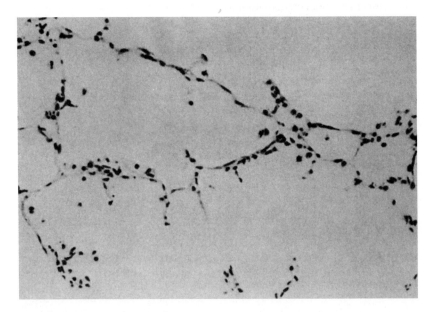

Fig. 1-5

Alveolar stage with thin-walled alveoli present. (From Langston C et al: Human lung growth in late gestation and in the neonate. *Am Rev Respir Dis* 1984; 129:607.)

will form after birth. Lung volume will increase 23-fold, alveolar number will increase 6-fold, alveolar surface area will increase 21-fold, and lung weight will increase 20-fold. Volume increases disproportionately to alveolar number. As body weight doubles in the human infant at 6 months and triples by 1 year, oxygen uptake will increase proportionally; this is matched by an increase in alveolar growth. The area of the air-tissue interface increases in a linear relationship to body surface area.[16] Alveolar volume and alveolar surface area increase in proportion to each other. However, alveolar number and alveolar diameter do not change proportionately. Most of the postnatal formation of alveoli in the infant occurs over the first 1.5 years of life.[17,18] Thereafter, the lung continues to grow in proportion to body growth. Boyden and Tompsett[19] described a mechanism of alveolar formation. They found a centripetal extension of the gas-exchange region with transformation of respiratory bronchioles into alveolar ducts and of terminal bronchioles into respiratory bronchioles. Lateral pouches from these transformed respiratory bronchioles formed new alveoli. It was proposed that new alveolar formation occurs in this manner into later childhood and that this is the likely mechanism for new alveolar formation throughout life. At 2 years of age, the number of alveoli varies substantially among individuals. After 2 years of age, boys have large numbers of alveoli than girls. After the end of alveolar multiplication, the alveoli continue to increase in size until thoracic growth is completed.[15]

FACTORS STIMULATING LUNG GROWTH

There are several factors that stimulate both normal and compensatory lung growth. It is generally accepted that a pneumonectomy results in compensatory changes in both size and weight in the remaining lung to nearly match that of the missing lung.[20] Both alveolar multiplication and lengthening of alveolar septa probably occur. Following pneumonectomy, a disproportionate growth of alveoli and airways takes place, although some compensation through increased length and conducting airway volume has been reported.[21] There is no evidence that new conducting airways can form once branching is completed by the beginning of the canalicular period or the sixteenth week of gestation.

Several studies have examined the effects of an altered metabolic rate on the growing lung. This occurs in hypoxia, starvation, and hyperoxia. Natives of high-altitude regions are known to have both an increased lung volume and an increased gas-exchanging surface. The effects of hypoxia on the growing lung have been studied in 3- to 4-week-old rat pups and fetal rats by exposing the mother to 10% oxygen.[22,23] Fetal exposure to hypoxia resulted in a decrease in body weight and a smaller lung that remained appropriate for body weight.

Prenatal and postnatal nutritional deprivation can affect various aspects of lung function, growth, and structures. Kerr and associates[24] produced emphysematous changes in the lungs of growing rats and postulated that connective tissue, specifically collagen, was altered in the alveolar septa. Starvation of adult humans results in emphysema-like lesions. The enlargement of airspaces that is found with starvation affects alveolar duct size as well as alveoli without apparent alveolar septal destruction.[25] Changes in connective tissue elements, pulmonary surfactant, ultrastructural features, and elastic recoil occur following caloric restriction in adult rats after a few weeks.[26,27] Structural alterations are not reversible after a short period of refeeding, whereas surfactant-associated functional changes are.

High concentrations of oxygen are toxic to pulmonary tissue. This damage is a causative factor in the development of bronchopulmonary dysplasia and associated abnormal lung repair following oxygen treatment in infants with hyaline membrane disease. The premature infant's antioxidant defense mechanisms are inadequate to prevent lung injury secondary to exposure to high concentrations of oxygen. In addition, young rats exposed to 40% oxygen have suppressed lung growth.[23,28,29] Also, DNA synthesis is suppressed by an increase in oxygen tension, and lung repair is adversely affected by oxygen.[30]

Pregnant rats exposed to cigarette smoke have been studied. These animals produced growth-retarded fetuses with a reduced lung to body weight ratio, decreased DNA content, and structural abnormalities.[31] The affected fetuses demonstrated a reduced lung volume, a decrease in the number of saccules, an increase in saccular size, and a decrease in surface area. These changes are thought to result in part from a decrease in lung elastic tissue.

There are other clinical factors that have been cited as causing diminished lung growth. These conditions can be divided into four categories. The first is chest wall compression as in diaphragmatic hernia, chest wall abnormalities, and probably hydrops fetalis (resulting from hydrothorax and ascites). The second category that may decrease lung growth is oligohydramnios. Reduced amniotic fluid for an extended period, with or without renal anomalies, is associated with lung hypoplasia.[32-34] The mechanisms by which amniotic fluid volume influences lung growth remain unclear. Possible explanations include mechanical restriction of the chest wall, interference with fetal breathing, or failure to produce fetal lung liquid. These clinical and experimental observations possibly point to a common denominator, lung stretch, as being a major growth stimulant. The third category, diminished respiration, has been shown to have a severe effect on lung growth. This effect could be mediated through a lack of stretch of the developing lung parenchyma.[35] The fourth category includes a variety of hormonal or metabolic abnormalities that may alter lung growth and structure. Leprechaunism, associated with abnormal carbohydrate metabolism, results in dysmorphic lungs with a decreased number of terminal bronchioles, dilated alveolar ducts and saccules, and enlarged airspaces.[36] Experimental diabetes produced by streptozotocin administration to 3-week-old rats resulted in diminished airspace and increased alveolar number and a marked effect on pulmonary connective tissue metabolism.[37,38]

An example of altered lung development is seen in children with Down syndrome. Although fetal lung growth is normal, postnatal lung growth is characterized by larger and fewer alveoli than normal.[39]

ABNORMAL DEVELOPMENT

Structural development of the lung may be altered by a number of conditions affecting the lungs in utero or by postnatal events.[40] Complex relationships exist among humoral, hormonal, and physical forces acting on the developing lung, altering its growth in ways that are poorly understood. Growth retardation of the fetal lung may affect size and weight but not maturation of airways and alveoli, whereas malnutrition may slow functional rather than structural maturation. Timing or dating of adverse events influencing fetal lung development is important in considering the approach to treatment and prognosis. Abnormalities occurring in the embryonic period are often associated with renal agenesis or dysplastic kidneys; branching of the lungs may also be affected. Abnormalities occurring later in development, such as diaphragmatic hernia, may affect the lungs during the pseudoglandular period, or prior to 16 weeks of gestation, and therefore decrease airway branching. If abnormalities occur during the second trimester of pregnancy, completion of pulmonary vascularization and acinar development may not proceed, and hypoplasia in the gas-exchanging area may result. Abnormal influences occurring during the last trimester of pregnancy, such as premature birth and hyaline membrane disease, may alter subsequent alveolar growth and differentiation, ultimately leading to a decrease in alveolar number.

PULMONARY HYPOPLASIA

Pulmonary hypoplasia is a relatively common abnormality of lung development with a number of clinical associations and anatomic correlates. Hypoplasia can be considered to be present when there are too few cells, too few alveoli, or too few airways. The incidence of pulmonary hypoplasia diagnosed at autopsy is between 10% and 25% of all cases.[41-43]

The best-studied condition associated with hypoplasia is diaphragmatic hernia. The incidence of diaphragmatic hernia is about 1 in 4000 births. The range of abnormalities reported is wide and is probably related to variations in the severity and timing of the onset of lung compression.[44] Compression of the lung before 16 weeks' gestation causes incomplete branching of the conducting or terminal airways or both. Early and severe compression results in severe hypoplasia, causing the lung to be less than half the weight of the contralateral lung. The ipsilateral lung demonstrates a decreased number and size of alveoli, a decreased gas-exchanging surface area, and a proportionate decrease in pulmonary vasculature.

Other forms of lung compression may result in hypoplasia. Causes include osteogenesis imperfecta, hypophosphatasia,[45] and thoracic dystrophies. In addition to chest wall anomalies, pleural effusion, ascites, intrathoracic tumors, and extralobular sequestration may cause lung compression.

Pulmonary hypoplasia occurs in oligohydramnios as a result of leakage of amniotic fluid. It was first described by Potter in association with renal agenesis.[32] There is experimental evidence to support the conclusion that the amount of lung liquid present in the fetus is a major determinant of lung growth because chronic tracheal drainage produces pulmonary hypoplasia, and tracheal ligation produces lungs with increased tissue mass.[46] It has been shown that experimental oligohydramnios causes pulmonary hypoplasia, which can be more or less severe depending on its timing.[41,47]

There are several experimental studies suggesting that lung growth alteration may be caused by various hormonal imbalances.[48-52] Changes caused by endocrine effects may cause lung compression or diminished lung liquid and respiration. Glucocorticoid administration has been shown to accelerate lung maturation but may also affect lung growth. Type II epithelial cell maturation is induced both functionally and anatomically by this drug. Depending on the dose, glucocorticoids may reduce the amount of DNA and thus produce hypoplasia. Thyroidectomy in fetal sheep produces pulmonary hypoplasia and diminished Type II cell differentiation. Maternal growth hormone apparently plays little role in fetal growth, but the effect of maternal administration of growth hormone on fetal lung growth has not been studied. Maternal experimental diabetes results in diminished tissue maturity in the fetus.[53]

ALVEOLAR CELL DEVELOPMENT AND SURFACTANT PRODUCTION

As the primordial epithelium evolves further, the epithelial lining undergoes cellular division and differentiation into the highly specialized Type I and Type II pneumocytes. Type I squamous cells serve as a thin, gas-permeable membrane for the diffusion of gases and as a barrier against water and solute leakage.[54] They account for more than 97% of the alveolar surface area, primarily as a result of their size, shape, and large cellular surface.[55]

Despite a smaller surface area, the cuboidal appearing Type II pneumocyte is the principal structure involved in surfactant production, storage, secretion, and reuse. Using the pulse-labeling technique [³H] utilizing thymidine, an additional function of the Type II cell is differentiation into Type I pneumocytes.[56] The Type II cells contain the precursors to surfactant[55] synthesis and the osmiophilic lamellar bodies that function as the storage apparatus for the synthesized surfactant. Through the continuous process of exocytosis, the lamellar bodies release their contents of tubular myelin into the alveolar hypophase. The now liberated tubular myelin unravels and disperses to form the monolayer at the air-liquid interface.[56]

The primary role of mammalian surfactant is to lower the surface tension within the alveolus, specifically at the air-liquid interface. This allows the delicate structure of the alveolus to expand when filled with air. Without surfactant, the alveolus remains collapsed because of the high surface tension of the moist alveolar surface. Surfactant is composed predominantly of an intricate blend of phospholipids, neutral lipids, and proteins. See Chapter 16 for more information on surfactant composition.

Various chemical and mechanical stimulatory mechanisms leading to increased surfactant precursor production have been identified and include, but are not limited to, β-adrenergic agonists, prostaglandins, epidermal growth factor, and mechanical ventilation. Late gestational analysis of phosphatidylglycerol was shown to be a sensitive indicator of lung maturity and is associated with a previous rise in phosphatidylcholine.[57]

FETAL LUNG LIQUID

Fetal lungs are secretory organs that make breathing-like movements but serve no respiratory function before birth. They secrete about 250 to 300 ml of liquid per day. Thus the fetal airways are not collapsed but filled with fluid from the canalic-ular period until delivery and the initiation of ventilation. This liquid flows from terminal respiratory units through conducting airways into the oropharynx, where it is either swallowed or expelled into the amniotic sac. The presence of fetal lung fluid is essential for normal lung development. This luminal fluid is high in chloride and low in bicarbonate, with a negligible concentration of protein.[59,60] Active transport of chloride ion across the fetal pulmonary epithelium generates an electric potential difference and causes liquid to flow from the lung microcirculation through the interstitium into the airspaces.[61] The pulmonary circulation, rather than the bronchial circulation, is the major source of this liquid. The balance between production and drainage of this liquid has an important effect on lung development. During fetal breathing, there is a small but steady movement of fluid outward from the trachea. The net movement of fluid away from the lungs has been measured at about 15 ml/h and was about five times higher during periods of fetal breathing than during apnea.[62] Prolonged outflow obstruction expands the lungs and leads to a decrease in Type II cells.[63] In contrast, unimpeded removal of lung liquid decreases lung size, increases apparent tissue density, and stimulates proliferation of Type II cells.[46]

The clearance of fetal lung fluid is essential for normal neonatal respiratory adaptation. However, several studies have shown that both the rate of liquid formation and the volume within the lumen of the fetal lung normally decrease before birth.[64-66] It is unknown what causes a reduction in fetal lung secretions prior to birth. Hormonal changes, which occur in the fetus just before and during labor, may have an important role in triggering this process. The influence of catecholamines on fetal lung liquid volume has been investigated. It has been shown that injecting β-adrenergic agonists into pregnant rabbits reduced the amount of water in the lungs of their pups.[67] Epinephrine has been shown to inhibit secretion of fetal lung liquid.[68] Other hormones, such as arginine vasopressin and prostaglandin E₂, which are secreted around the time of birth, may reduce production of lung luminal liquid.[69,70]

Removal of lung liquid continues following birth. When breathing begins, air inflation shifts residual liquid from the lumen into distensible perivascular spaces around large pulmonary blood vessels and bronchi. Accumulation of liquid in these connective tissue spaces, which are distant from the sites of respiratory gas exchange, allows time for small blood vessels and lymphatics to remove the displaced liquid with little or no impairment of neonatal lung function at this critical juncture.[71,72] The clearance of the fluid from the interstitial spaces occurs over many hours.

ACKNOWLEDGMENT

The authors wish to express their sincere gratitude to Mrs. Brenda Ham and Ms. Kathy Sullivan for their untiring energy in preparing this chapter.

REFERENCES

1. Boyden EA: Development and growth of the airways. In Hodson WA, editor: *Development of the lung.* New York, Marcel Dekker, 1977, pp 3-35.
2. Reid L: The embryology of the lung. In DeReuek AV, Porter R, editors: *Development of the lung.* Boston, Little, Brown, 1967, pp 109-130.
3. Langston C et al: Human lung growth in late gestation and in the neonate. *Am Rev Respir Dis* 1984; 129:607.
4. Liggins GC: Growth of the fetal lung. *J Dev Physiol* 1984; 97:237.
5. Loosli CG, Potter EL: Pre- and postnatal development of the respiratory portion on the human lung. *Am Rev Respir Dis* 1959; 80:5.
6. Spooner BS, Wessells MK: Mammalian lung development: interactions in primordium formation and bronchial morphogenesis. *J Exp Zool* 1970; 175:445.
7. Hislop AA, Reid L: Growth and development of the respiratory system: anatomical development. In Davies JA, Dobbing J, editors: *Scientific foundation of paediatrics.* London, Heinemann Medical Books, 1974, pp 214-254.
8. Hoh K, Hoh H: A study of cartilage development in pulmonary hypoplasia. *Pediatr Pulmonol* 1988; 8:65.
9. Thurlbeck WM: Prematurity and the developing lung. *Clin Perinatol* 1992; 19:497.
10. Hislop A, Reid L: Formation of the pulmonary vasculature. In Hodson WA, editor: *Development of the lung.* New York, Marcel Dekker, 1979, pp 37-86.
11. Boyden EA: The time lag in the development of bronchial arteries. *Anat Rec* 1970; 166:611.
12. Cooney TP, Thurlbeck WM: The radial alveolar count method of Emery and Methal—a reappraisal: II. Intrauterine and early post-natal lung growth. *Thorax* 1982; 37:580.
13. Hislop A, Wigglesworth JS, Desai R: Alveolar development in the human fetus and infant. *Early Hum Dev* 1986; 13:1.
14. Reid L: The lung: its growth and remodelling in health and disease. *Am J Roentgenol* 1977; 129:777.
15. Thurlbeck WM: The state of the art: postnatal growth and development of the lung. *Am Rev Respir Dis* 1975; 111:803.
16. Dunnill MS: Postnatal growth of the lung. *Thorax* 1962; 17:329.
17. Zeltner TB, Burri PH: The postnatal development and growth of the human lung. II. Morphology. *Respir Physiol* 1987; 67:269.
18. Zeltner TB, Burri PH: The postnatal development and growth of the human lung. I. Morphometry. *Respir Physiol* 1987; 67:247.
19. Boyden EA, Tompsett DH: The changing patterns in the developing lungs of infants. *Acta Anat (Basel)* 1965; 61:164.
20. Cagle PT, Thurlbeck WM: Postpneumonectomy and compensatory lung growth. *Am Rev Respir Dis* 1988; 138:1314.
21. Boatman ES: A morphometric and morphological study of the lungs of rabbits after unilateral pneumonectomy. *Thorax* 1977; 32:406.
22. Bartlett D, Remmers JE: Effects of high altitude exposure on the lungs of young rats. *Respir Physiol* 1971; 13:116.
23. Burri PH, Weibel ER: Morphometric estimation of pulmonary diffusion capacity. II. Effect of PO_2 on the growing lung. Adaptation of the growing rat to hypoxia and hyperoxia. *Respir Physiol* 1971; 11:247.
24. Kerr JS, Riley DJ, et al: Nutritional emphysema in the rat: influence of protein depletion and impaired lung growth. *Am Rev Respir Dis* 1985; 131:644.
25. Harkema JR et al: A comparison of starvation and elastase models of emphysema in the rat. *Am Rev Respir Dis* 1984; 129:584.
26. Sahebjami H, Vassallo CL: Effects of starvation and refeeding on lung mechanics and morphometry. *Am Rev Respir Dis* 1979; 119:443.
27. Sahebjami H et al: Lung mechanics and ultrastructure in prolonged starvation. *Am Rev Respir Dis* 1978; 117:77.
28. Bartlett D: Postnatal growth of the mammalian lung: influence of low and high oxygen tensions. *Respir Physiol* 1970; 9:58.
29. Butcher JR, Roberts RJ: The development of the newborn rat lung in hyperoxia: a dose-response study of lung growth, maturation, and changes in antioxidant enzyme activities. *Pediatr Res* 1981; 15:999.
30. Witschi HR et al: Potentiation of diffuse lung damage by oxygen: determining of variables. *Am Rev Respir Dis* 1981; 123:98.
31. Collins MH et al: Fetal lung hypoplasia associated with maternal smoking: a morphometric analysis. *Pediatr Res* 1985; 19:408.
32. Potter EL: Bilateral renal agenesis. *J Pediatr* 1946; 29:68.
33. King JC et al: Effect of induced oligohydramnios on fetal lung development. *Am J Obstet Gynecol* 1986; 154:823.
34. Perlman M, Williams J, et al: Neonatal pulmonary hypoplasia after prolonged leakage of amniotic fluid. *Arch Dis Child* 1976; 51:349.
35. Nagai A et al: The effects of maternal CO_2 breathing in lung development of fetuses in the rabbit. Morphologic and morphometric studies. *Am Rev Respir Dis* 1988; 135:130.
36. Thurlbeck WM, Cooney TP: Dysmorphic lungs in a case of leprechaunism: case report and review of literature. *Pediatr Pulmonol* 1988; 5:100.
37. Ofulue AF et al: Experimental diabetes and the lung: I. Changes in growth, morphometry, and biochemistry. *Am Rev Respir Dis* 1988; 137:162.
38. Ofulue AF, Thurlbeck WM: Experimental diabetes and the lung: II. In vivo connective tissue metabolism. *Am Rev Respir Dis* 1988; 138:284.
39. Cooney TP et al: Diminished radial count is found only postnatally in Down's syndrome. *Pediatr Pulmonol* 1988; 5:204.
40. Reale FR, Easterly JR: Pulmonary hypoplasia: a morphometric study of the lungs of infants with diaphragmatic hernia, anencephaly, and renal malformations. *Pediatrics* 1973; 52:91.
41. Moessinger AC et al: Pulmonary hypoplasia, a disorder on the rise? (Abstract) *Pediatr Res* 1983; 17:327A.
42. Moessinger AC et al: Oligohydramnios-induced lung hypoplasia: the influence of timing and duration. *Pediatr Res* 1986; 20:951.
43. Page DV, Stocker JT: Anomalies associated with pulmonary hypoplasia. *Am Rev Respir Dis* 1982; 125:216.
44. George DK et al: Hypoplasia and immaturity of the terminal lung unit (acinus) in congenital diaphragmatic hernia. *Am Rev Respir Dis* 1987; 136:947.
45. Silver MM, Vilos GA: Pulmonary hypoplasia in neonatal hypophosphatasia. *Pediatr Pathol* 1988; 84:83.

46. Alcorn D et al: Morphological effects of chronic tracheal ligation and drainage in fetal lamb lung. *J Anat* 1977; 123:649.

47. Blatchford KG, Thurlbeck WM: Lung growth and maturation in experimental oligohydramnios in the rat. *Pediatr Pulmonol* 1987; 3:328.

48. Crone RK et al: The effects of hypophysectomy, thyroidectomy, and postoperative infusion of cortisol or adrenocorticotrophin on the structure of the ovine fetal lung. *J Dev Physiol* 1983; 5:281.

49. Erenberg A et al: The effect of fetal thyroidectomy on ovine fetal lung maturation. *Pediatr Res* 1979; 13:230.

50. Liggins GC et al: Pulmonary maturation in the hypophysectomized ovine fetus. Differential responses to adrenocorticotrophin and cortisol. *J Dev Physiol* 1981; 3:1.

51. Morishige WK, John NS: Influence of glucocorticoids on postnatal lung development in the rat: possible modulation by thyroid hormone. *Endocrinology* 1982; 111:1587.

52. Pinkerton KE et al: Hypophysectomy and porcine fetal lung development. *Am J Respir Cell Mol Biol* 1989; 1:319.

53. Sosenko IRS et al: Morphologic disturbance of lung maturation in fetuses of alloxan diabetic rats. *Am Rev Respir Dis* 1980; 122:687.

54. Schneeberger EE: Alveolar type I cells. In Crystal RG, West JB, editors: *The Lung Scientific Foundations.* New York, Raven Press, 1991, pp 1677-1685.

55. Notter RH, Shapiro DL: Lung surfactants for replacement therapy; biochemical, biophysical, and clinical aspects. *Clin Perinatol* 1987; 433.

56. Adamson YR, Bowden DH: The type II cell as a progenitor of alveolar epithelial regeneration. *Lab Invest* 1974; 30:35-42.

57. Kresch MJ, Gross I: The biochemistry of fetal lung development. *Clin Perinatol* 1987; 481.

58. Reference deleted in proofs.

59. Mescher EJ et al: Ontogeny of tracheal fluid, pulmonary surfactant, and plasma corticoids in the fetal lamb. *J Appl Physiol* 1975; 39:1017.

60. Adams FH et al: The nature and origin of the fluid in the fetal lamb lung. *J Pediatr* 1963; 63:881.

61. Olver RE et al: Ion fluxes across the pulmonary epithelium and the secretion of lung liquid in the foetal lamb. *J Physiol* 1974; 241:327.

62. Harding R et al: The regulation of flow of pulmonary fluid in fetal sheep. *Respir Physiol* 1984; 57:47.

63. Carmal JA et al: Fetal tracheal ligation and lung development. *Am J Dis Child* 1965; 109:452.

64. Kitterman JA et al: Tracheal fluid in fetal lambs: spontaneous decrease prior to birth. *J Appl Physiol* 1979; 47:985.

65. Dickson KA et al: Decline in lung liquid volume before labor in fetal lambs. *J Appl Physiol* 1986; 61:2266.

66. Brown MJ et al: Effects of adrenaline and of spontaneous labour on the secretion and absorption of lung liquid in the foetal lamb. *J Physiol* 1983; 344:137.

67. Enhorning G et al: Isoxsuprine-induced release of pulmonary surfactant in the rabbit fetus. *Am J Obstet Gynecol* 1977; 129:197.

68. Lawson EE et al: The effect of epinephrine on tracheal fluid flow and surfactant efflux in fetal sheep. *Am Rev Respir Dis* 1978; 118:1023.

69. Bland RD et al: Vasopressin decreases lung water in fetal lambs. *Pediatr Res* 1985; 19:399A.

70. Kitterman JA: Fetal lung development. *J Dev Physiol* 1984; 6:67.

71. Bland RD et al: Lung fluid balance in lambs before and after birth. *J Appl Physiol* 1982; 53:992.

72. Bland RD et al: Clearance of liquid from lungs of newborn rabbits. *J Appl Physiol* 1980; 49:171.

CHAPTER 2

Fetal Gas Exchange and Circulation

Michael P. Czervinske

A network to supply nutrients and remove waste begins in the earliest stages of the rapidly developing human embryo. Fetal gas exchange must take place in an environment that does not require an alveolar-capillary interface.

MATERNAL-FETAL GAS EXCHANGE

Although the fetus depends on maternal circulation for nutrients and gas exchange, the maternal and fetal vascular networks are separate systems. No blood is shared between the two.

As the fertilized egg, or zygote, travels to the uterus, it undergoes various degrees of cell division, but has no nutrient source as in bird egg. So the developing cells, at this point termed the blastocyst, must implant into the uterine lining for nourishment. The outer surrounding layer is the trophoblast, which combines with tissues from the endometrium to form the chorionic membrane around the blastocyst.[1] Inside the blastocyst, a group of cells arrange on one side in the shape of a figure eight. The center portion is the embryonic disk, which forms the three embryonic germ layers: the ectoderm and the endoderm, followed by the mesoderm.[2] Box 2-1 lists the tissue systems that arise from the three germ layers.

The outer or top loop of the figure eight envelops the embryonic structure and forms the amniotic sac, while the inner or bottom loop forms the yolk sac. The yolk sac soon degenerates and incorporates into the embryo, giving way for the amniotic sac to grow. Suspended in the cavity of the blastocyst, the amniotic sac then surrounds the entire embryo. The embryo attaches to the outer layer through the umbilical stalk, and later the umbilical cord. The umbilical cord connects to the fingerlike projections in the outer lining of the chorion, or chorionic villi (Fig. 2-1). Within the chorionic villi a capillary network forms and connects to the umbilical stalk. The villi intertwine

---

BOX 2-1

ORIGIN OF DIFFERENT TISSUE SYSTEMS FROM THE THREE EMBRYONIC GERM LAYERS[2]

ECTODERM
Central nervous system
Cranial nerves, spine
Peripheral nervous system
Sensory epithelia
Eyes, ears, nose
Glandular tissues
Mammary, pituitary, subcutaneous
Epidermal tissues
Epidermis, hair, nails
Teeth

MESODERM
Cardiovascular system
Heart, blood and lymph vessels
Connective tissue
Bone, cartilage

MESODERM—cont'd
Muscle tissue
Striated and smooth
Kidney and spleen tissues
Reproductive tissues
Serous linings
Pericardium, pleura, peritoneum

ENDODERM
Epithelial tissue
Respiratory system
Digestive system
Urinary system
Liver and pancreatic tissues
Large gland parenchyma
Tonsils, thymus, thyroid
Auditory epithelial structures

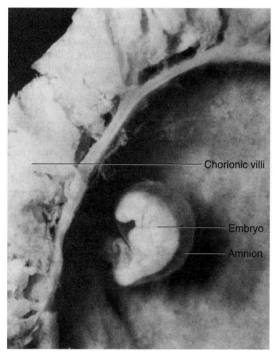

Chorionic villi

Embryo

Amnion

Fig. 2-1

Implanted human embryo showing the relationship of the chorion, amnion, and chorionic villi. (From Blechschmidt E, editor: *The stages of human development before birth.* Philadelphia, WB Saunders, 1961.)

into the blood-filled lacunae cavities of the endometrium of the maternal uterus.[1] Oxygen, carbon dioxide, and nutrients diffuse through the vast capillary surface area of this indirect connection between mother and fetus. As fetal development continues, the region of this interface becomes limited to the discus-shaped placenta, since the amniotic sac completely fills the chorionic cavity. The umbilical cord connects the placenta to the fetus with two smaller arteries and one large vein. As the cord grows, the vessels tend to spiral.[3] Wharton's jelly, a gelatinous substance inside the umbilical cord, helps protect the vessels and prevents the cord from kinking.

CARDIOVASCULAR DEVELOPMENT

During the third gestational week, the heart is the first organ formed during fetal development. By 8 weeks of gestation, the normal fetal heart is fully functional, complete with all chambers, valves, and major vessels. Additionally, the fetal heart must adapt to accommodate the circulatory configuration required while in the fluid-filled uterine environment. During the following description of the embryonic heart changes, note which of them may result in the anomalies discussed in Chapter 31.

The cardiovascular system forms from the mesoderm layer. During early embryonic development, small cellular pools, referred to as angiogenic clusters or "blood islands," supply nutrition to the growing embryo. These clusters combine to form two heart tubes lined with specialized myocardial tissue.[4] On approximately day 18, the heart tubes fold into what will become the thoracic cavity. At this point, they become close enough in proximity to fuse, and grow into a complete single-chamber tubular structure by day 21. By day 22

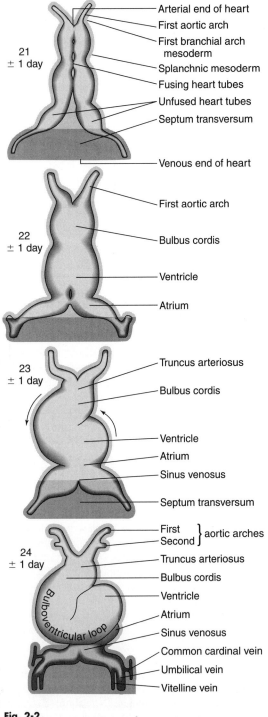

Fig. 2-2

Formation of the primordial heart chambers following fusion of the heart tubes at 3 weeks gestational age. (From Moore KL, editor: *The developing human: clinically oriented embryology,* ed 3. Philadelphia, WB Saunders, 1982.)

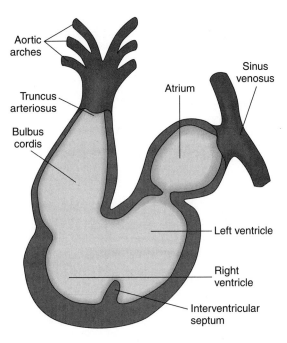

Fig. 2-3

Sagittal view of the developing heart at the beginning of week 5 showing the position of the atrium, bulbus cordis, ventricles, and budding ventricular septum. The ventricular septum continues to fold and grow upward between the ventricles. (Modified from Moore KL, editor: *The developing human: clinically oriented embryology,* ed 3. Philadelphia, WB Saunders, 1982.)

cardiac contractions are discerned, and bidirectional tidal blood flow begins.[3]

Dramatic changes begin to occur during the fourth week of gestation. The heart tubes continue to merge into three recognizable structures: the bulbus cordis, the ventricular bulge, and the atrial bulge, which empty into the sinus venosus (Fig. 2-2). These structures continue to bend and fold, and soon afterward, the truncus arteriosus becomes recognizable. Note that initially the atrial bulge is inferior to the ventricular bulge. Between days 25 and 28 the ventricular bulge expands into a D-shaped loop that pushes the atrial bulge in a superior direction. At this stage, the embryonic heart appears as a twisted S shape, and the ventricular structure merges with the bulbus cordis to form a one-ventricle structure known as the bulboventricular loop, which continues to dilate (Fig. 2-3).

Simultaneous with the external changes, the septum primum begins the separation of the common atrium, followed shortly by the growth of the endocardial cushion. During this time, the left atrium incorporates the primordial pulmonary veins as four pulmonary veins empty into the primordial left

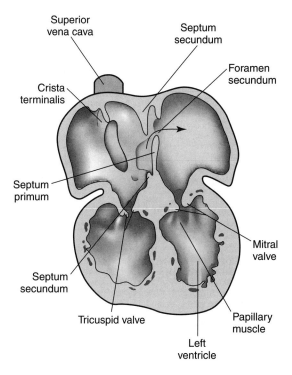

Superior
vena cava

Septum
secundum

Foramen
secundum

Crista
terminalis

Septum
primum

Mitral
valve

Septum
secundum

Tricuspid valve

Papillary
muscle

Left
ventricle

Fig. 2-4

Frontal view of the fetal heart showing the development of the four chambers nearing completion. The arrow shows the one-way path through the foramen ovale. (Modified from Moore KL, editor: *The developing human: clinically oriented embryology,* ed 3. Philadelphia, WB Saunders, 1982.)

atrium. The right horn of the sinus venosus grows in dominance and merges into the future right atrium from the inferior and superior vena cava. By the end of the fourth week, the dilating ventricular spaces fold into each other and force the ventricular septal bud upward at the base of the bulboventricular loop (see Fig. 2-3).[5] By this time, bloodflow begins a unidirectional path.[6]

During weeks 5 and 6 the internal and external structures continue to rapidly mature. Between the atria, the septum secundum begins to appear. By week 6, the septum secundum and a flap from the septum primum form the foramen ovale, one of the fetal shunts discussed later in this chapter (Fig. 2-4). The atrioventricular canal continues to mature, and the endocardial cushion separates the ventricular spaces from the atrium. The muscular portion of the ventricular septum continues to grow into the ventricular space as the two ventricles dilate. Ridges also appear opposite each other in the bulbus cordis and truncus. They grow toward each other and fuse into a spiraling aorticopulmonary septum.[6] A fetal heart rate around 95 beats

per minute becomes discernible during this period and increases approximately 4 beats per day until heart development is complete.[7]

Continuing maturation of the internal and external structures characterize weeks 7 and 8. The ventricles finish forcing the ventricular septum up from its base. A small intraventricular foramen remains, and blood flows between the two ventricles until the endocardial cushion fuses with the ventricular septum (see Fig. 2-4). At the end of the seventh week, tissue from remnants of the bulbus cordis and tissue from the endocardial cushion grow into the ventricular foramen, closing it as they merge with the muscular ventricular septum. The tricuspid and mitral valves form from specialized tissue surrounding the two atrioventricular openings. The aorticopulmonary septum divides the bulbus cordis and truncus into an aortic and pulmonary trunk. As these outflow tracts continue to mature, the semilunar valves form at the base of each structure. Early in the eighth week the outflow tracts and valves are completely developed. At this stage, development of the cardiac structures is complete, and blood flows through the fetal circulation pathway. The heart, however, continues to develop, increasing proportionately greater in length than width.[8]

FETAL CIRCULATION AND FETAL SHUNTS

Fetal circulation differs from circulation after the infant is born. Fig. 2-5 illustrates fetal circulation and the three fetal shunts that must close after birth. The mother's lungs and liver perform most of the functions required by the same organs in the fetus. The fetal circulation pathway allows for shunting of blood flow around the fetal liver and lungs. Shunting this blood volume also helps the heart pump large quantities of blood to the placenta, which is the interface between the maternal and fetal organ systems.

Oxygenated blood travels from the placenta to the fetus through the umbilical vein. The ductus venosus, which appears continuous with the umbilical vein, shunts approximately 30% to 50% of the oxygen-rich blood around the liver. The amount of shunting through the ductus venosus appears to decrease with gestational age.[9] The shunted oxygen-rich blood empties into the inferior vena cava (IVC) and mixes with venous blood as it flows to the right atrium (RA). Even though some admixture takes place, this volume of blood contains the highest oxygen saturations available to the fetus. In the RA most of the blood flowing from the IVC crosses through the foramen ovale, the second fetal shunt, and into

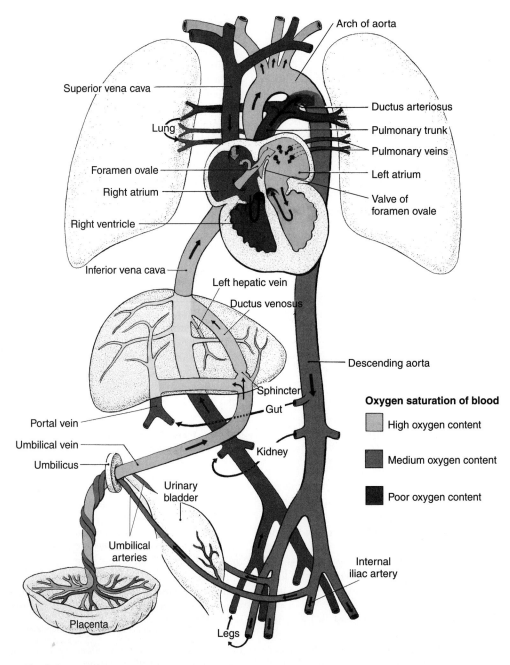

Fig. 2-5

A diagram of fetal circulation as blood containing oxygen and nourishment moves from the placenta to the fetal heart through the three fetal shunts, ductus venosus, foramen ovale, and ductus arteriosus. (Modified from Moore KL, Persaud TVN, editors: *The developing human: clinically oriented embryology,* ed 6. Philadelphia, WB Saunders, 1998.)

the left atrium (LA). The remainder of the blood in the RA mixes with desaturated blood from the superior vena cava (SVC) and empties into the right ventricle (RV). Blood flow in the RV contains slightly higher oxygen content than blood from the SVC, which is pumped into the pulmonary artery to the developing lungs.

The pulmonary vascular resistance (PVR) in utero remains very high. Likely mechanisms are physical compression of the vessels due to relatively low lung volumes and low oxygen concentrations, since the lungs are devoid of air. Both of these mechanisms help induce chemical mediators, which maintain a high resistive tone in the pulmonary vascular bed.[10] Approximately 10% of the fetal blood flow reaches the lungs.[11]

The high PVR causes most of the pulmonary artery blood flow to bypass the lungs by flowing through the ductus arteriosus into the aorta. Blood from the pulmonary veins empties into the LA and then flows into the left ventricle (LV), out the aortic valve, and into the ascending aorta, where it supplies blood with the highest oxygen content to the head, right arm, and coronary circulation. The deoxygenated blood from the upper torso returns to the RA via the SVC. Finally, a portion of the blood in the descending and abdominal aorta flows through the two umbilical arteries and back to the placenta for oxygenation.

TRANSITION TO EXTRAUTERINE LIFE

Clamping the umbilical vessels removes the low-pressure system of the placenta from fetal circulation. During the first breath, several factors drastically improve pulmonary blood flow and reduce the PVR.[12] Inflating the lungs initiates gas exchange, which increases and directly dilates pulmonary arterioles. Rising PaO_2 also stimulates the release of endogenous pulmonary vasodilating factors.[13] Stretching of the pulmonary units also physically stretches open vascular units as well as stimulates the release of other vasodilating compounds. Besides vasodilation, lung inflation results in the inhibition of vasoconstricting agents produced by the lung to facilitate fetal circulation.[12]

Once the PVR decreases and the cord is clamped, pressures in the right side of the heart decrease and pressures in the left side increase. Since the foramen ovale flap allows blood to flow only from right to left, it closes when the pressures in the LA become greater than those in the RA. Closing the foramen ovale further facilitates the increase of blood flow to the lungs during the transitional period, and is necessary to maintain normal extrauterine circulation.

Since the pressure in the aorta also increases and becomes greater than the pressure in the pulmonary artery, the amount of shunting through the ductus arteriosus decreases. The functional closure of the ductus arteriosus usually occurs rapidly as the result of sudden increases in oxygenation and changes in prostaglandin levels.[14] Normally, con-

striction starts to occur at birth, and 20% of the ductus closes within 24 hours, with 80% closed in 48 hours, and 100% by 96 hours following birth.[15] Anatomic closure of the ductus begins in the last trimester as endothelial tissue begins to proliferate into the lumen of the ductus, forming bulges known as *intimal mounds*. Initially assisted by vasoconstriction, the ductal lumen completely closes as gestational and postgestational age advances.[16] By 2 to 4 weeks of age, the anatomic closure is complete and blood flow normalizes to the adult pattern of circulation.[15]

REFERENCES

1. Kingdom JC, Kaufmann P: Oxygen and placental vascular development. *Adv Exp Med Biol* 1999; 474:259-275.
2. Moore KL, Persaud TVN, editors: *The developing human: clinically oriented embryology,* ed 6. Philadelphia, WB Saunders, 1998, pp 63-82.
3. England MA, editor: *Color atlas of life before birth: normal fetal development,* ed 2. Chicago, Year-Book Medical Publishers, 1996, pp 40-41.
4. Gourdie RG, Kubalak S, Mikawa T: Conducting the embryonic heart: orchestrating development of specialized cardiac tissues. *Trends Cardiovasc Med* 1999;9: 8-26.
5. England MA, editor: *Color atlas of life before birth: normal fetal development,* ed 2. Chicago, Year-Book Medical Publishers, 1996, p 102.
6. Moore KL, Persaud TVN, editors: *The developing human: clinically oriented embryology,* ed 6. Philadelphia, WB Saunders, 1998, pp 349-403.
7. Tezuka N et al: Embryonic heart rates: development in early first trimester and clinical evaluation. *Gynecol Obstet Invest* 1991; 32:210-212.
8. Marecki B: The formation of heart-proportion in fetal ontogenesis. *Z Morphol Anthropol* 1992; 79:197-202.
9. Kiserud T: Fetal venous circulation: an update on hemodynamics. *J Perinat Med* 2000; 28:90-96.
10. Heymann MA: Control of the pulmonary circulation in the fetus and during the transitional period to air breathing. *Eur J Obstet Gynecol Reprod Biol* 1999; 84:127-132.
11. Lakshminrusimha S, Steinhorn RH: Pulmonary vascular biology during neonatal transition. *Clin Perinatol* 1999; 26:333-336.
12. Rudolph AM: The development of concepts of the ontogeny of the pulmonary circulation. In Weir EK, Archer SL, Reeves JT, editors: *The fetal and neonatal pulmonary circulations.* Armonk, NY, Futura Publishing, 2000.
13. Hageman JR, Caplan MS: An introduction to the structure and function of inflammatory mediators for clinicians. *Clin Perinatol* 1995; 22:251-261.
14. Hammerman C: Patent ductus arteriosus: clinical relevance of prostaglandins and prostaglandin inhibitors in PDA pathophysiology and treatment. *Clin Perinatol* 1995; 22:457-479.
15. Lim MK et al: Intermittent ductal patency in healthy newborn infants: demonstration by coulour doppler flow mapping. *Arch Dis Chil* 1992; 67:1218-1230.
16. Mirro R, Gray P: Aortic and pulmonary blood velocities during the first 3 days of life. *Am J Perinatol* 1986; 3:333-336.

CHAPTER **3**

Antenatal Assessment and High-risk Delivery

Antoun Y. Khabbaz
J. Gerald Quirk

The transition from intrauterine life to the outside world is critical. It involves major physiologic changes and requires medical attention for an optimal outcome. Cooperation and communication among all members of the health care team are essential to identify potential problems and to intervene in a timely manner. Maternal history, antenatal assessment (as dictated by maternal-fetal risk factors), and intrapartum monitoring are all-important in identifying the fetus-newborn at risk of decompensation during the perinatal period. This chapter outlines the essentials of antenatal assessment and touches briefly on the management of some high-risk conditions: preterm delivery and postterm pregnancy.

MATERNAL HISTORY AND RISK FACTORS

At the initial prenatal visit, the obstetrician obtains a comprehensive maternal history and performs a physical examination. Risk factors are identified and included in an initial problem list that serves as a quick summary for future reference. Subsequent periodic visits serve the purpose of identifying new obstetrical risks that will necessitate special interventions. Following are discussions of commonly encountered maternal-fetal risk factors with their impact on obstetrical care and perinatal outcome.

PRETERM BIRTH

Other than major congenital anomalies, preterm birth (birth before 37 weeks of gestation) is the greatest cause of neonatal morbidity and mortality. Preterm birth can be the consequence of preterm labor, preterm premature rupture of the fetal membranes, or obstetrical intervention mandated by fetal jeopardy or maternal clinical status. Interestingly enough, prior preterm delivery is one of the most important risk factors for subsequent preterm labor. With one prior preterm birth, a woman carries a 15% risk of subsequent preterm delivery; this risk increases to 32% with a history of two previous preterm births. Risk factors, diagnosis, and treatment of preterm labor will be discussed in a subsequent section of this chapter.

INCOMPETENT CERVIX

Incompetent cervix is an obstetrical condition diagnosed most traditionally by a history of painless dilation of the cervix in the second or early third trimester, with prolapse of the membranes into the vagina. This is usually followed by rupture of the membranes and delivery of a premature infant. Cervical incompetence may result from previous cervical trauma such as vaginal delivery with cervical laceration, dilation and curettage procedure (D & C), or cone biopsy of the cervix. It might also be due to congenital weakness of the cervix. Of importance here is that once the correct diagnosis of cervical incompetence is made, intervention in the form of cervical cerclage (placing a suture around the cervical canal) can prevent a subsequent early pregnancy loss. This procedure is usually performed electively at around 14 weeks of gestation after confirmation of absence of gross congenital anomalies in the fetus by ultrasound. It can also be done emergently later in pregnancy in case of an unanticipated event of cervical incompetence.

TOXIC HABITS IN PREGNANCY

Maternal habits should be assessed early in the course of gestation. Smoking, alcohol use, and illicit drug use in pregnancy can cause welldescribed adverse effects on the fetus. The American College of Obstetricians and Gynecologists estimates that the prevalence of substance abuse in pregnant women is around 10%.[2]

Alcohol is a potent teratogen (an agent or factor that causes malformation in the fetus). The fetal alcohol syndrome associated with maternal use of alcohol in pregnancy was first described in 1973 by Jones and colleagues. It is usually seen among children of women who consume four to six drinks daily throughout pregnancy.[3] However, there is no safe range of drinking in pregnancy. The syndrome is characterized by mental retardation and prenatal and postnatal growth restriction, as well as by brain, cardiac, spinal, and craniofacial anomalies.[4]

Smoking during pregnancy can cause several adverse effects. Carbon monoxide and nicotine, the main ingredients responsible, mediate their effects by decreasing availability of oxygen to the fetus and placenta. There is a strong association between cigarette smoking and lower birth weight. The mean birth weight of infants of women who smoke during pregnancy is around 200 g less than that of infants of nonsmokers.[5] Smoking is also associated with a higher incidence of premature preterm rupture of membranes,[6] placental abruption and placenta previa,[7] and risk of infant death from sudden infant death syndrome.[8]

Cocaine has a potent sympathomimetic action and hence is a potent constrictor of blood vessels. It can cause numerous maternal medical complications that include myocardial infarction, stroke, seizures, bowel ischemia, and death. Cocaine is also associated with adverse pregnancy sequelae: placental abruption, preterm delivery, and growth restriction.[9] It is also thought to cause congenital malformations of the limbs, heart, brain, and genitourinary tract. Finally, infants born to women who abuse opiates or amphetamines in pregnancy tend to have significant withdrawal symptoms after birth and to be small for gestational age.

The obstetrician-gynecologist can have an impact on prevention of substance abuse in pregnancy by identifying the patient at risk, educating patients about the effects of drugs, and referring patients already abusing drugs.

HYPERTENSION AND DIABETES MELLITUS

The obstetrician frequently encounters patients with hypertension and diabetes mellitus presenting for prenatal care. Hypertensive disease complicates 6% to 8% of pregnancies in the United States and is second only to embolism as a cause of maternal mortality.[10] Perinatal morbidity and mortality are increased secondary to intrauterine growth restriction, placental abruption, and preterm delivery. Preeclampsia is traditionally described as a triad of hypertension, proteinuria, and generalized edema. It is commonly cited that preeclampsia complicates approximately 5% of pregnancies. Predisposing factors include nulliparity, advanced maternal age, chronic hypertension, chronic renal disease, diabetes mellitus, twin gestation, molar pregnancy, and hydrops fetalis.

Preeclampsia remains a poorly understood disease despite extensive research. Immunologic mechanisms, genetic predisposition, dietary deficiencies, vasoactive substances, and endothelial dysfunction have all been implicated in the pathophysiology of preeclampsia.[11] Severe preeclampsia is diagnosed in the presence of systolic blood pressure higher than 160 mm Hg, diastolic blood pressure higher than 110 mm Hg, proteinuria higher than 5 g per 24-hour urine collection, pulmonary edema, intrauterine growth restriction, oliguria (below 500 cc urine output in 24 hours), thrombocytopenia (platelet count below 100,000), headache, epigastric or right upper quadrant abdominal pain, hepatocellular dysfunction, or grand mal seizure (definition of eclampsia).

Treatment of preeclampsia is by delivery of the fetus. Magnesium sulfate is used to prevent seizures, and antihypertensive agents like hydralazine and labetalol are usually used to control severe hypertension. The recurrence rate of preeclampsia is around 25%.[12] Calcium, magnesium, and zinc supplementation and use of low-dose aspirin have been studied for prevention of pregnancy-induced hypertension, with conflicting results thus far.

Diabetes in pregnancy is classified broadly as pregestational or gestational. Women with pregestational diabetes are at increased risk for adverse maternal and fetal outcomes. Adverse maternal outcomes include increased risk of developing diabetic ketoacidosis, proliferative retinopathy, and preeclampsia/eclampsia. Close maternal metabolic surveillance focused on attaining normal blood glucose levels throughout pregnancy has significantly decreased the risk of these outcomes.

Adverse fetal outcomes include unexplained fetal death in the third trimester of pregnancy and major fetal structural malformations. Close maternal metabolic surveillance coupled with close fetal biophysical evaluation has significantly decreased the risk of fetal death as well as the necessity of delivering a fetus prematurely because of abnormal test results. The rate of fetal structural malformations in infants born to pregestational diabetic women can be as high as 10% to 15% compared with a rate of 1% to 2% for infants of otherwise normal women. The most frequently encountered defects include malformations of the cardiovascular system (including both the heart and great vessels) and the central nervous system (including the brain and spinal cord). No amount of maternal metabolic surveillance or fetal biophysical assessment after the period of fetal organogenesis will decrease this risk. Therefore it is recommended strongly that women with diabetes mellitus receive counseling and treatment with the goal of achieving optimal glycemic control before they become pregnant.

Gestational diabetes mellitus (GDM) is abnormal glucose tolerance that occurs or is first recognized during pregnancy. The frequency of this disorder varies according to the ethnic background of the woman but is said to complicate about 3% of pregnancies in the United States. Poor blood sugar control in these women is associated with an increased risk of macrosomia (birth weight greater than 4000 g), traumatic vaginal delivery, and preterm delivery, and with a small increased risk for fetal death in selected women. Following delivery, the infants are at increased risk for metabolic disturbances in the neonatal period; these include hypoglycemia, hypocalcemia, hyperkalemia, hyperbilirubinemia, and idiopathic respiratory distress syndrome. In the long term, women with GDM are at risk of developing Type 2, or adult-onset, diabetes; nearly 50% will be diagnosed with Type 2 diabetes within 10 years. Among pregnant women, selective screening based on risk factors identifies only one half. Thus, at the present time, it is recommended that all pregnant women should be screened for gestational diabetes with the 1-hour glucose challenge test administered between 24 and 28 weeks of gestation. For those with an abnormal screening result, the diagnosis of GDM is made when there are two abnormal values on a 3-hour, 100 g oral glucose tolerance test. Maternal glycemic control and fetal biophysical status are monitored in a manner similar to protocols for managing the pregnancy complicated by pregestational diabetes. With good maternal glycemic control, pregnancies complicated by GDM can proceed to full term with a normal delivery; cesarean delivery is reserved for traditional obstetric indications.

INFECTIOUS DISEASES

A number of infectious agents can affect pregnancy outcome. Among the most important in the United States are Group B streptococcus (GBS), herpes simplex virus (HSV), hepatitis B virus (HBV), and the human immunodeficiency virus (HIV). As many as 10% to 40% of pregnant women are colonized with GBS. Their infants are at risk for death or severe morbidity if they are born prematurely or after prolonged rupture of the fetal membranes. At present clinicians take one of two approaches to preventing these outcomes. One approach involves identifying women at risk based on vaginal/rectal cultures obtained near term. Another, recommended by the American College of Obstetricians and Gynecologists, involves identifying women at risk based on clinical factors that include preterm labor, premature rupture of the fetal membranes, prolonged rupture of the membranes for more than 18 hours, maternal fever in labor, or a previously affected child.[13] Women thus identified are treated with appropriate antibiotics from the time of membrane rupture or from the onset of labor. Using either screening method, the woman can deliver vaginally and expect to have a normal outcome.

Women who have primary or recurrent HSV outbreaks during pregnancy are at risk for infecting their baby if the outbreak occurs at the time of membrane rupture or the onset of labor. In this circumstance, the virus can ascend to infect the fetus; therefore cesarean delivery is undertaken as soon as possible following membrane rupture.

At this time, all pregnant women should be screened for HIV and HBV infection. Both viruses can cause disease in the fetus. In the general obstetric population in the United States, the frequency of HIV infection is around 1 per 1000. The prevalence is as high as 1% to 1.5% in inner-city populations.[14] Approximately 30% of the exposed fetuses will also acquire the infection.[15] Zidovudine (an antiretroviral drug) used in pregnancy, during labor, and as chemoprophylaxis for 6 weeks in exposed newborns is associated with a decrease in perinatal HIV transmission to 8.3%.[16] When care includes both zidovudine therapy and a scheduled cesarean delivery, the risk is approximately 2%.[17] Nursing should be discouraged in HIV-positive women because the virus is secreted in breast milk. Infants of women infected with HBV become infected at delivery. When these infants are treated with anti–hepatitis B immunoglobulin and are begun on vaccination within the first 12 hours of life, 95% of neonatal infections are prevented. There is no advantage to cesarean delivery of these newborns.[18] Cytomegalovirus, rubella, *Toxoplasma, Listeria,* mycobacteria, and *Treponema pallidum* (syphilis) can all affect the mother, fetus, and fetoplacental unit significantly. Early diagnosis and treatment of the pregnancy complicated by infection with *Listeria, Toxoplasma,* or syphilis can result in normal pregnancy outcomes.

PLACENTA, UMBILICAL CORD, AND FETAL MEMBRANES

In utero, the fetus is contained in the sterile fluid-filled amniotic sac. If the membranes that compose the external lining of the amniotic sac rupture before term (before 37 weeks of gestation) or before the onset of normal labor at term, the fetal environment is no longer sterile, increasing the risk of fetal infection. At the same time, the volume of fluid in the sac decreases. This may cause compression of the umbilical cord, resulting in compromised blood flow between the placenta and fetus. The causes of premature rupture of the fetal membranes are generally not known but are responsible for nearly 50% of preterm births in the United States. Preterm rupture of the fetal membranes can be seen as being responsible for all of the problems faced by most prematurely born infants.

Abnormalities of the umbilical cord and placenta can have profound effects on fetal development and pregnancy outcome. The umbilical cord has a mean length of 55 cm and contains three vessels: two arteries and one vein. The two arteries arising from the end of the fetal aorta bring relatively deoxygenated blood from the fetus to the placenta, while the single umbilical vein returns oxygenated blood from the placenta to the fetus. In 3% of pregnancies, the umbilical cord contains a single umbilical artery. A single artery umbilical cord is associated with an 18% incidence of major fetal malformations.[19]

The length of the umbilical cord has long been recognized to be of clinical significance. A short cord predisposes to placental abruption (separation of the placenta before birth of the newborn) and uterine inversion. A long cord is associated with cord prolapse (delivery of the cord before the infant, with compromise of blood flow from compression), cord knots, and nuchal cords (cord wrapped around the infant's neck). Marginal cord insertion (on the edge of the placenta) is of little clinical importance. Velamentous insertion of the cord (umbilical vessels cross the fetal membranes unsupported by placenta or cord structure) may be associated with risk of rupture of a fetal vessel at the time of rupture of membranes, resulting in fetal exsanguination. Placental abruption can cause fetal distress and death in addition to serious vaginal bleeding and coagulopathy. It is usually associated with hypertensive disease in pregnancy, advanced maternal age, multiparity, preterm premature rupture of membranes, trauma, cigarette smoking, cocaine abuse, and uterine leiomyoma behind the placental implantation site.[20] Placenta previa occurs when the placenta covers the cervical os. Cesarean delivery is usually required. Placenta previa is associated with advanced maternal age, multiparity, prior cesarean delivery, and multiple gestation.

DISORDERS OF AMNIOTIC FLUID VOLUME

Early in pregnancy, amniotic fluid is derived from the fetal membranes that compose the amniotic sac. Later on, the majority of amniotic fluid is the product of fetal urination, with little contribution from the fetal skin. Fetal swallowing is an important mechanism for absorption of amniotic fluid. The fetal lungs help in circulating the amniotic fluid. The amniotic fluid index (AFI) is calculated by measuring the largest vertical pockets of fluid in each of the four equal uterine quadrants at the time of ultrasound examination. It is the most commonly used method for quantification of amniotic fluid.

Oligohydramnios (too little amniotic fluid or AFI below 5 cm) is usually associated with congenital anomalies (especially renal agenesis or urinary tract obstruction), fetal growth restriction or demise, postterm pregnancy, ruptured membranes, uteroplacental insufficiency, and use of prostaglandin synthase inhibitors. When oligohydramnios occurs early in gestation, it can cause lung hypoplasia and limb deformities. When renal agenesis occurs in association with oligohydramnios, it is always fatal and is called Potter's syndrome. Later in gestation, oligohydramnios is usually associated with adverse perinatal outcomes secondary to compression of the umbilical cord. In labor, there is an increase in variable decelerations (due to cord compression) and an increase in cesarean delivery rates.[21]

Polyhydramnios (too much amniotic fluid or AFI higher than 24 cm) is frequently associated with fetal malformations that might affect swallowing of amniotic fluid (e.g., anencephaly, esophageal atresia, and tracheoesophageal fistula). It is also associated with hydrops fetalis, twin gestation (with twin-twin transfusion syndrome), and maternal diabetes. Polyhydramnios overdistends the uterus and can lead to premature rupture of membranes or preterm labor.

MODE OF DELIVERY

Most deliveries are spontaneous through the vaginal route. Typically, infants are delivered vaginally from vertex presentation (head first). However, there are times when assisted vaginal delivery (with forceps or vacuum) or abdominal delivery (cesarean) is needed. Breech presentation (legs or buttocks first) occurs in 3% to 4% of all births. The breech position creates a situation in which there is greater potential for complications at time of delivery. Predisposing factors for breech presentation include multiparity, previous breech delivery, uterine anomalies, fetal anomalies, multiple gestation, and polyhydramnios. The Term Breech Trial Collaborative Group conducted a multicenter randomized controlled trial of planned cesarean versus planned vaginal delivery for breech presentation at term. It concluded that planned cesarean delivery is preferred because of less risk for perinatal mortality or serious morbidity and no increase in serious maternal complications.[22] Two small randomized controlled trials published earlier have not found planned cesarean delivery of substantial benefit to the fetus.[23,24] Transverse lie, in which the fetus is oriented transversely inside the uterus, is another malpresentation that requires cesarean delivery.

Obstetrical forceps is an instrument used to cradle and guide the fetal head while applying traction to expedite delivery. The vacuum extractor is a suction device that holds the head tightly and allows traction to be applied. Indications for forceps or vacuum use include maternal cardiac, pulmonary, or neurologic diseases (contraindicating the pushing process); maternal exhaustion in labor; and nonreassuring fetal status.

Cesarean delivery is the operative delivery of the fetus through the abdominal wall. It accounts for approximately 22% of all births in the United States.[25]

Major indications for cesarean delivery include previous cesarean delivery, failure to progress in labor, malpresentation (breech or transverse), placenta previa, and fetal distress. Although cesarean delivery might be the least traumatic method of delivery of the fetus, for the mother it is associated with an increased risk of significant blood loss, anesthesia complications, intraoperative bladder or bowel injuries, postoperative wound infection, endomyometritis, and thromboembolic events. The syndrome of transient tachypnea of the newborn (wet lung or Type II respiratory distress syndrome), which includes the clinical features of cyanosis, grunting, and tachypnea during the first hours of life, is more commonly seen in infants delivered by cesarean. The preferred explanation for the clinical features is delayed absorption of fetal lung fluid.[26]

ANTENATAL ASSESSMENT

To ascertain the pregnancy at risk for an adverse outcome, one must begin with a thorough history and physical examination. Over the last 25 years, technologic advances have made it possible to make many assessments of fetal condition. Both invasive and noninvasive methods of evaluating fetal structure and function are used with regularity. It is possible to view fetal anatomy, measure fetal biochemical and genetic status, assess fetal biophysical status, and evaluate uteroplacental function and determine the ability of the fetus and placenta to function during the normal stresses of labor. Depending on the characteristics of any given pregnancy, most perinatal centers are capable of performing detailed antepartum assessment.[27]

ULTRASOUND

One of the most widely used methods of noninvasive assessment is ultrasonography (Fig. 3-1). Using ultrahigh frequency sound waves to obtain real-time images and with transabdominal or transvaginal transducers, the clinician can diagnose multifetal pregnancy and evaluate fetal anatomy, growth, and position. One can also localize the placenta within the uterus, measure amniotic fluid volume, estimate fetal growth over time, and assess fetal biophysical status. In addition, using Doppler flow studies, it is possible to measure blood flow to fetal organs. This permits identification of fetuses at risk who would benefit from early delivery or transport to sophisticated perinatal centers. Ultrasonography is also invaluable in guiding the physician while performing amniocentesis, umbilical blood sampling, and other invasive procedures.

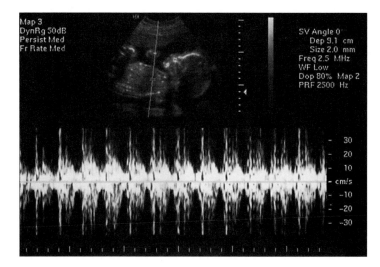

Fig. 3-1

Ultrasound picture of a fetus at 23 weeks' gestation with Doppler study of the fetal heart. (Courtesy Frank Fox, RDMS.)

AMNIOCENTESIS

The most commonly performed invasive procedure to assess fetal condition is amniocentesis. In this procedure, under sterile conditions, a needle is inserted through the skin and uterine wall to obtain a sample of fluid from the amniotic sac. Depending on the reason for performing the procedure, the concentration of many substances in the fluid can be measured. For example, as the fetal lung matures, pulmonary surfactant is secreted from the fetal lung into the amniotic fluid where its concentration can be measured. Women with Rh isoimmunization are at risk for delivering babies with severe anemia secondary to hemolysis. The degree of hemolysis is correlated with the concentration of bilirubin urinated by the fetus into amniotic fluid. If the concentration of bilirubin in amniotic fluid is markedly elevated, interventions to assist the fetus (preterm delivery or intrauterine fetal transfusion) can be undertaken. Fetal cells isolated from amniotic fluid can be used to assess for fetal chromosomal abnormalities (e.g., trisomy 21), fetal enzyme deficiencies (e.g., Tay-Sachs), and certain discrete genetic mutations (e.g., sickle cell disease).

NONSTRESS TEST AND CONTRACTION STRESS TEST

Fetal well being is highly dependent on placental function. Assessment of placental function is most commonly done by monitoring fetal heart rate (FHR) response when the fetus moves (nonstress test [NST]) or to induced uterine contractions (contraction stress test [CST]). For both tests, the FHR is monitored continuously. In the normally oxygenated fetus (as with a child or adult) cardiac output rises to support physical activity. This rise in cardiac output can be mediated by an increase in either heart rate or stroke volume. In the fetus, cardiac output rises by increasing the heart rate. A reactive NST (Fig. 3-2) is one that demonstrates a rise in FHR of at least 15 beats per minute lasting at least 15 seconds associated with maternal perception of fetal movement. A reactive NST is highly correlated with normal uteroplacental function; if there is no change in maternal clinical status, this result predicts normal fetal survival if performed within 1 week of delivery.[28] The CST is conducted most commonly by continuously monitoring the FHR while uterine contractions are stimulated by the intravenous infusion into the mother of a dilute solution of oxytocin. Even in a normal pregnancy, fetal Po_2 decreases with each uterine contraction, then rapidly returns to normal. When there is uteroplacental insufficiency, the fetal Po_2 can drop below 12 mm Hg, resulting in slowing of the FHR. This slowing of the FHR in response to uterine contractions is called a late deceleration. A negative CST is one in which there are no late decelerations of the FHR with contractions that occur with a frequency of three per 10 minutes. A positive CST is diagnosed when late decelerations are seen with every contraction; a suspicious CST is one in which some but not all of the contractions are accompanied by late decelerations. Assuming no change in maternal clinical status, a negative CST predicts fetal survival if performed within 1 week of delivery. An abnormal CST must prompt further evaluation or delivery.

FETAL BIOPHYSICAL PROFILE

More recently, the so-called fetal biophysical profile (BPP) (Table 3-1) has gained in popularity as a tool to assess placental function and fetal well being.[29]

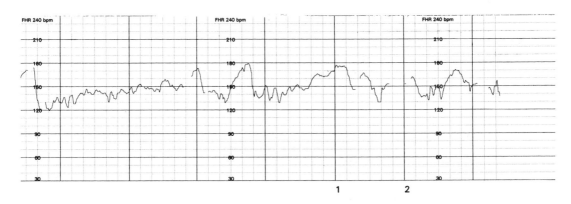

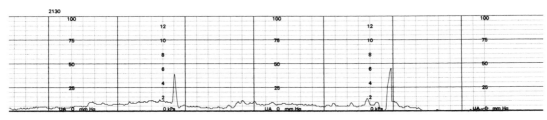

Fig. 3-2

Reactive nonstress test.

TABLE 3-1	BIOPHYSICAL PROFILE SCORING	
Biophysical Variable	**Normal (Score = 2)**	**Abnormal (Score = 0)**
Fetal breathing movements	At least one episode of FBM of at least 30 seconds' duration in 30-minute observation	No FBM or no episode of >30 seconds in 30 minutes
Gross body movements	At least three discrete body-limb movements in 30 minutes (episodes of active continuous movement, considered as a single movement)	Two or fewer episodes of body-limb movements in 30 minutes
Fetal tone	At least one episode of active extension with return to flexion of fetal limb or trunk; opening and closing of hand considered normal tone	Either slow extension with return to partial flexion or movement of limb in full extension or absent fetal movement
Reactive FHR	At least two episodes of FHR acceleration of >15 bpm and of at least 15 seconds' duration associated with fetal movement in 20 minutes	Less than two episodes of acceleration of FHR or acceleration of <15 bpm in 40 minutes
Qualitative AFV	At least one pocket of AF that measures at least 1 cm in two perpendicular planes	Either no AF pockets or a pocket <1 cm in two perpendicular planes

Modified from Manning FA et al: Fetal biophysical profile score and the nonstress test: a comparative trial. *Obstet Gynecol* 1984; 64:326.
FBM, Fetal breathing movements; *FHR,* fetal heart rate; *bpm,* beats per minute; *AFV,* amniotic fluid volume; *AF,* amniotic fluid.

The BPP has been likened to the Apgar score. Five determinants of fetal status are assessed and given a score of 0 to 2. The four assessed by ultrasonography are fetal breathing, fetal tone, fetal gross body movement, and amniotic fluid volume. The fifth determinant is the NST. A BPP score of 8 to 10 is considered normal and reassuring; a score of 6 is equivocal and is generally repeated within 24 hours; BPP scores of 0 to 4 are clearly abnormal and are associated with poor perinatal outcomes and

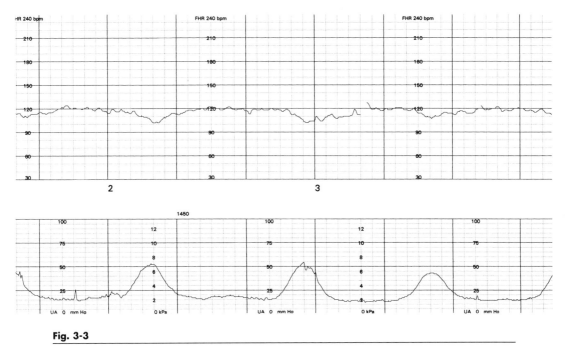

Fig. 3-3

Early decelerations (coinciding with uterine contraction) are usually due to fetal head compression and pose little threat to the fetus.

require careful evaluation and usually immediate delivery.[30]

INTRAPARTUM MONITORING

Available evidence suggests that the use of continuous FHR monitoring during labor in uncomplicated pregnancies has little to no impact on neonatal outcome.[31] Despite this, its use has become routine in the United States. Its utility in high-risk patients is of value. The response of the FHR to uterine contractions does provide information concerning the fetus' status during labor. FHR responses to uterine contractions and their likely etiologies are described in Figs. 3-3, 3-4, and 3-5. On many obstetric services, when persistent severe variable or late decelerations of the FHR are diagnosed, fetal scalp blood is obtained via transvaginal fetal scalp puncture, and blood gas measurements can be obtained. Scalp blood pH greater than 7.25 is considered reassuring; values of 7.15 or less signal high risk of fetal acidemia. Many clinicians feel that scalp blood gas assessment in the face of an abnormal FHR pattern more precisely defines the fetus at risk and can thus prevent unnecessary forceps and cesarean deliveries. An alternative to scalp blood gas assessment is fetal scalp stimulation. Using the underlying rationale of the NST, transvaginal stimulation of the fetal scalp to induce fetal movement results in acceleration of the fetal heart rate and reassures the clinician that the fetus is not hypoxemic or acidemic.[31] Table 3-2 lists normal values for fetal scalp blood and umbilical cord blood gases.

HIGH-RISK CONDITIONS

PRETERM LABOR

Preterm labor is defined as labor before 37 weeks of gestation. It complicates around 8% of pregnancies and is associated with significant neonatal morbidity, including sepsis, respiratory distress syndrome, intraventricular hemorrhage, retinopathy of prematurity, bronchopulmonary dysplasia, necrotizing enterocolitis, visual and hearing problems, and cerebral palsy. The smaller the infant is, the more the risks increase.

Risk factors for preterm delivery include previous preterm delivery, premature rupture of membranes, genital infections (*Chlamydia, Gardnerella vaginalis*), nongenital infections (pyelonephritis, pneumonia), chorioamnionitis (infection of fetal membranes and amniotic fluid), conditions that overdistend the uterus (multiple gestations, increased amount of amniotic fluid), placental conditions (placental abruption or placenta previa), abnormalities of the uterine cavity (uterine septum or fibroids), fetal anomalies, and incompetent cervix.

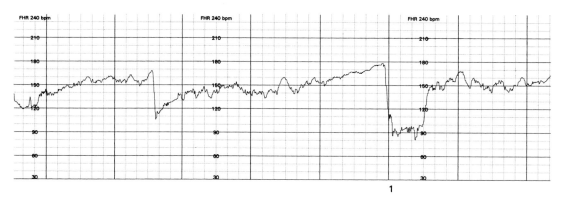

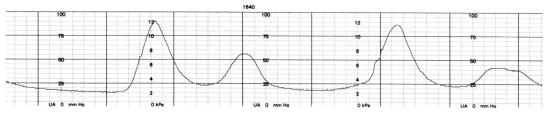

Fig. 3-4

Variable decelerations are the most common. They are due to cord compression and have different configurations. Repetitive severe variable decelerations are associated with increased risk of fetal hypoxia.

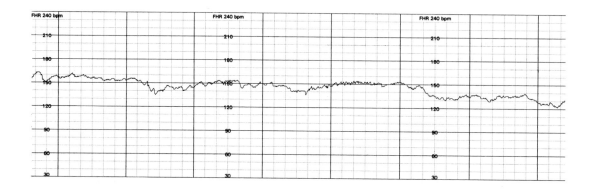

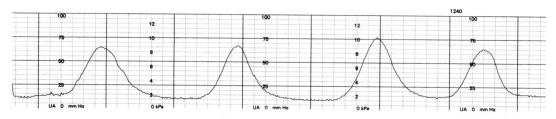

Fig. 3-5

Late decelerations are due to uteroplacental insufficiency. They usually begin at the peak of the contraction and are associated with fetal distress.

TABLE 3-2	BLOOD GAS VALUES						
	Fetal Scalp During Labor		Umbilical Cord at Birth		Arterial Sample After Birth		
	First-stage Labor	Second-stage Labor	Umbilical Artery	Umbilical Vein	5-10 Minutes	30 Minutes	60 Minutes
pH	7.33	7.29	7.24	7.32	7.21	7.30	7.33
P_{CO_2} (mm Hg)	44	46	49	38	46	38	36
P_{O_2} (mm Hg)	22	16	16	27	50	54	63
Bicarbonate (mEq/l)	20	17	19	20	17	18	19

Data from Beard RW, Nathanielsz PW: *Fetal physiology and medicine.* New York. Marcel Dekker, 1984; and Koch G, Wendel H: Adjustment of arterial blood gases and acid-base balance in the normal newborn infant during the first week of life. *Biol Neonate* 1968; 12:136.

Signs of preterm labor include back pain, menstrual-like pains, pelvic heaviness, vaginal discharge, and vaginal bleeding. Diagnosis of labor is based on having six contractions in a 1-hour period associated with cervical changes in dilation or effacement. Several approaches to prevention of preterm labor have been studied. These include serial cervical examinations, home uterine activity monitoring, prophylactic use of oral tocolytics (drugs used to stop labor), and bed rest. None has been shown to be clearly effective. Fetal fibronectin (a glycoprotein produced in the chorion) seems to be expressed in cervical and vaginal secretions in cases of preterm labor. It has been studied recently as a potential marker of preterm labor in symptomatic patients. The absence of fetal fibronectin is a strong predictor that preterm delivery is unlikely to happen within 1 to 2 weeks, with a negative predictive value exceeding 95% in some studies.[32] Its use may be beneficial in providing reassurance to asymptomatic women who have high-risk factors for preterm delivery.[33]

Once preterm labor is diagnosed, prompt measures should be taken to try to stop labor and prevent an early delivery. Intravenous hydration is commonly the first approach used. It does not seem to be of clinical significance in a well-hydrated patient.[34] Excessive hydration should be avoided, since it might potentiate the risk of pulmonary edema that is usually associated with tocolytic use. The most commonly used tocolytics are magnesium sulfate, β-mimetic agents, and indomethacin (a prostaglandin inhibitor). Less commonly used are nifedipine (calcium channel blocker), nitroglycerine (nitric oxide donor drug), atosiban (oxytocin antagonist), and combination therapy.

Magnesium sulfate is usually given as an initial intravenous bolus of 4 to 6 g followed by intravenous infusion at 2 to 4 g per hour. Its main mechanism of action seems to be by decreasing free intracellular calcium ion concentration, resulting in decreased electrical potential of the cell.

Magnesium sulfate is contraindicated in patients with hypocalcemia, renal failure, and myasthenia gravis. Potential toxic effects include pulmonary edema, respiratory depression, cardiac arrest, muscular paralysis, and profound hypotension.[35] Loss of deep tendon reflexes usually precedes the abovementioned complications. It is frequently used to monitor patients on magnesium sulfate therapy. Magnesium blood level can also be assessed. Toxic effects are rarely seen with levels less than 8 mg/dl.

β2-Mimetic drugs (terbutaline, ritodrine) can also cause uterine relaxation and are commonly used tocolytic agents. They decrease the electrical potential of the cell by increasing calcium binding to the intracellular sarcoplasmic reticulum, an effect mediated by cyclic adenosine monophosphate (AMP). They are contraindicated in patients with poorly controlled diabetes, thyrotoxicosis, and maternal cardiac disease. Potential side effects include hyperglycemia, hypokalemia, hypotension, pulmonary edema, dysrhythmias, and myocardial ischemia. β-Mimetic drugs are administered intravenously. The rate of infusion is slowly titrated upward until a clinical response is obtained. Maternal pulse rate correlates with the blood concentration of the drug. It is usually used to assess the adequacy of the dosage. A pulse rate higher than 120 per minute should be avoided. Indomethacin (a prostaglandin inhibitor) reduces synthesis of prostaglandins by inhibiting cyclooxygenase. It is contraindicated in patients with asthma, gastrointestinal bleeding, renal failure, coronary artery disease, and oligohydramnios. Its major potential complications include renal failure, gastrointestinal bleeding, and hepatitis (with chronic use). It can cause oligohydramnios, and when used after 32 weeks of gestation it may induce closure of the ductus arteriosus in the fetus, leading to heart failure and hydrops. Indomethacin is used orally or via the rectal route. Ultrasound is used to periodically assess the amniotic fluid volume when indomethacin is used. Tocolytics are widely used for treatment of preterm labor. Studies have failed to show much success beyond delaying delivery for 48 hours.[36,37] Adjunctive therapy with corticosteroids for induction of fetal lung maturity is beneficial and justifies use of tocolytics.

All women between 24 and 34 weeks of gestation with intact membranes and in preterm labor are candidates for antenatal corticosteroid therapy.[38] Most commonly used is betamethasone, two doses of 12 mg intramuscularly 24 hours apart. Maximum benefit occurs 48 hours after initiation of therapy and lasts for 7 days. Benefit of corticosteroids in preterm premature rupture of membranes awaits further research.[39] Corticosteroids reduce respiratory distress syndrome and neonatal mortality by 50%.[38] This effect is due to induction of proteins that regulate production of surfactant by Type II cells in the fetal lungs. Corticosteroids also decrease the incidence of intracranial hemorrhage, probably by promoting maturation of the germinal matrix in the fetal brain.

POSTTERM PREGNANCY

Postterm pregnancy occurs when pregnancy continues beyond 42 weeks from the first day of the pregnant woman's last menstrual period (more than 294 days). This condition complicates from 3% to 12% of pregnancies. The most frequent reason for a diagnosis of postdate gestation is inaccurate dating due to either irregular ovulation or inaccurate recall of last menstrual period. This is frequently encountered in patients who become pregnant after discontinuation of birth control pills. These patients tend to have 2 or more weeks' delay in ovulation. Less common causes of postterm pregnancy are fetal anencephaly, placental sulfatase deficiency, and abdominal pregnancy. Most postterm pregnancies are of unknown cause; deficiency of prostaglandin production or refractoriness of the cervix to endogenous prostaglandins could be the cause.[40]

Postterm pregnancy may be associated with maternal and neonatal problems. The woman may suffer from anxiety of being past her due date and still undelivered. She is at higher risk of obstetrical trauma (vaginal and cervical laceration) from delivery of a large infant. Physically, she is at increased risk of long-term sequelae of incontinence and pelvic relaxation. The infant may suffer from oligohydramnios, macrosomia, meconium aspiration, and placental insufficiency. After reaching a maximum of around 1 liter at 37 weeks' gestation, amniotic fluid volume decreases gradually. The decrease in amniotic fluid may result in cord compression, fetal hypoxia, and higher incidence of cesarean delivery for FHR abnormalities. Intrapartum amnioinfusion, the installation of fluid into the amniotic cavity, significantly improves the neonatal outcome and lessens the rate of cesarean section in the presence of oligohydramnios.[41]

Fetal macrosomia (weight more than 4000 g) increases the risk of cesarean delivery for dystocia and increases the risk of birth trauma during vaginal delivery due to shoulder dystocia, resulting in brachial plexus palsy. Meconium aspiration is another significant problem. Meconium passage in utero is very common after 42 weeks of gestation. It is frequently associated with fetal hypoxia. Meconium becomes more concentrated in the amniotic fluid when associated with oligohydramnios. Aspiration of meconium may lead to obstruction of the respiratory passages and interference with surfactant function.[40] The infant should be intubated after delivery and meconium should be aspirated from below the vocal cords for a better outcome. A recent meta-analysis of prospective clinical trials of intrapartum amnioinfusion for meconium-stained fluid revealed significant improvement in neonatal outcome and a lower cesarean delivery rate.[42] Placental insufficiency is another hazard to the fetus. When the placenta "ages," it fails to provide the fetus with substantial nutritional requirements. This may result in fetal intrauterine growth restriction. In labor, poor beat to beat variability, late decelerations, and bradycardia may be signs of fetal compromise due to placental insufficiency.

In order to decrease fetal risk of adverse outcome, two strategies are widely used: antenatal surveillance and induction of labor. There is a lack of evidence that antenatal testing improves neonatal outcome. However, it became standard practice due to its universal acceptance. Due to lack of evidence, it is not clear when to start antenatal surveillance. There are wide variations of practice regarding what method of testing to use (NST, CST, or BPP) and how often to perform testing. Furthermore, it is unclear whether labor induction results in a better outcome when compared with antenatal surveillance. The American College of Obstetricians and Gynecologists recommends labor induction for pregnancies at 42 weeks or more when the cervix is favorable. When the cervix is unfavorable, cervical ripening followed by labor induction and fetal antenatal surveillance are acceptable options.[44]

Labor induction can be achieved with different medications when the cervix is favorable for induction. Intravenous infusion of oxytocin is most commonly used. Oxytocin is started at a rate of 1 or 2 milliunits/min and increased periodically until an adequate pattern of uterine contractions is effected. Possible side effects include water retention with long use of high doses (usually more than

20 milliunits/min). This can result in hyponatremia with seizures and coma. Oxytocin also causes hypotension when administered rapidly as an intravenous bolus. Uterine rupture and amniotic fluid embolism have been cited with oxytocin use.

When the cervix is unfavorable for induction, its texture, dilation, and effacement can be improved by several modalities. Mechanical methods include placement of Foley catheter balloons or osmotic dilators (Laminaria tents) into the cervical canal. Laminaria are thought to act by absorbing water from the cervix, rendering it softer and more dilated. Their use for cervical ripening was associated with increased maternal and neonatal infection rate.[45] Pharmacologic agents have also been used for cervical ripening. Prostaglandin E_2 cervical gel (Prepidil) and vaginal insert (Cervidil) are widely used. They act by causing dissolution of collagen fibers in the cervix. The most common side effects include maternal fever, nausea, vomiting, and diarrhea. Misoprostol (Cytotec) is a prostaglandin E_1 analogue that is approved by the Food and Drug Administration for the prevention of ulcers that occur during long-term treatment with nonsteroidal antiinflammatory drugs. Due to its uterotonic effect, it has been increasingly used for cervical ripening and labor induction. Its popularity stems from its effectiveness, low cost, and stability at room temperature.[46] Safety concerns have been raised recently in view of reports of uterine rupture occurring after misoprostol induction in patients with previous uterine scars.[47]

REFERENCES

1. Carr-Hill RA, Hall MH: The repetition of spontaneous preterm labor. *Br J Obstet Gynaecol* 1985; 92:921.
2. American College of Obstetricians and Gynecologists: Substance abuse in pregnancy. *Technical Bulletin 195,* July 1994.
3. Jones KL et al: Patterns of malformation in offspring of chronic alcoholic mothers. *Lancet* 1973; 1:1267.
4. Committee on Substance Abuse and Committee on Children with Disabilities: Fetal alcohol syndrome and fetal alcohol effects. *Pediatrics* 1993; 91:1004-1006.
5. Haworth JC et al: Fetal growth retardation in cigarette smoking mothers is not due to decreased maternal food intake. *Am J Obstet Gynecol* 1980; 137:719-723.
6. Harfer JH et al: Risk factors for preterm premature rupture of membranes: a multicenter case control study. *Am J Obstet Gynecol* 1990; 163:130-137.
7. Naeye RL: Abruptio placentae and placenta previa: frequency, perinatal mortality, and cigarette smoking. *Obstet Gynecol* 1980; 55:701-704.
8. Taylor JA, Sanderson M: A reexamination of the risk factors for sudden infant death syndrome. *J Pediatr* 1995; 126:887-891.
9. Shiono PH et al: The impact of cocaine and marijuana use on low birth weight and preterm birth: a multicenter study. *Am J Obstet Gynecol* 1995; 172:19.
10. American College of Obstetricians and Gynecologists: Hypertension in pregnancy. *Technical Bulletin* 219, January 1996.
11. Cunningham FG et al: *Williams obstetrics,* ed 20. Norwalk, Conn, Appleton & Lange, 1997, pp 698-699.
12. Sibai BM, El-Nazer A, Gonzalez-Ruiz AR: Severe preeclampsia-eclampsia in young primigravida women: subsequent pregnancy outcome and remote prognosis. *Am J Obstet Gynecol* 1986; 155:1011.
13. American College of Obstetricians and Gynecologists: Prevention of early onset group B streptococcal disease in newborns. *Committee Opinion 173,* June 1996.
14. Guinan ME, Hardy A: Epidemiology of AIDS in women in the United States. *JAMA* 1987; 257:2039.
15. MacGregor SN: Human immunodeficiency virus infection in pregnancy. *Clin Perinatal* 1997; 18:33.
16. Connor EM et al: Reduction of maternal-infant transmission of HIV 1 with zidovudine treatment. Pediatric AIDS Clinical Trials Group Protocol 076 Study Group. *N Engl J Med* 1994; 331:1173-1180.
17. The European Mode of Delivery Collaboration: Elective caesarean section versus vaginal delivery in prevention of vertical HIV transmission: a randomized clinical trial. *Lancet* 1999; 353:1035-1039.
18. Duff P: Maternal and perinatal infection. In Gabbe SG, Niebyl JR, Simpson JL, editors: *Obstetrics: normal and problem pregnancies,* ed 3. New York, Churchill Livingstone, 1996, p 1218.
19. Bryan EM, Kohler HG: The missing umbilical artery, pediatric follow-up. *Arch Dis Child* 1975; 50:714.
20. Cunningham FG et al: *Williams obstetrics,* ed 20. Norwalk, Conn, Appleton & Lange, 1997, pp 748-749.
21. Baron C, Morgan MA, Garite TJ: The impact of amniotic fluid volume assessed intrapartum on perinatal outcome. *Am J Obstet Gynecol* 1995; 173:167.
22. Hannah ME et al: Planned caesarean section versus planned vaginal birth for breech presentation at term: a randomized multi centre trial. *Lancet* 2000; 356:1375-1383.
23. Collea JV, Chein C, Quilligan EJ: The randomized management of term frank breech presentation: a study of 208 cases. *Am J Obstet Gynecol* 1990; 137:235-244.
24. Gimovsky ML et al: Randomized management of the nonfrank breech presentation at term: a preliminary report. *Am J Obstet Gynecol* 1983; 146:34-40.
25. Clark SC, Taffel SM: Caesarean rates decreasing. *Ob Gyn News* 1996; 31:10.
26. Rosenberg AA: The neonate. In Gabbe SG, Niebyl JR, Simpson JL, editors: *Obstetrics: normal and problem pregnancies,* ed 3. New York, Churchill Livingstone, 1997, pp 663-664.
27. Blocking A: Observations of biophysical activities in the normal fetus. *Clin Perinatol* 1989; 16:583-594.
28. Druzin ML: Antepartum fetal heart rate monitoring —state of the art. *Clin Perinatol* 1989; 16:627-642.
29. Manning FA et al: Fetal biophysical profile score and the nonstress test: a comparative trial. *Obstet Gynecol* 1984; 64:326-331.
30. Vintzileos AM, Campbell WA: Fetal biophysical scoring: current status. *Clin Perinatol* 1989; 16:661-690.
31. American College of Obstetricians and Gynecologists: Antepartum fetal surveillance. *ACOG Practice Bulletin 9.* Washington, DC, 1999.
32. Lockwood CJ et al: Fetal fibronectin in cervical and vaginal secretions as a predictor of preterm delivery. *N Engl J Med* 1991; 325:669.
33. Andersen HF: Use of fetal fibronectin in women at risk for preterm delivery. *Clin Obstet Gynecol* 2000; 43(4): 746-758.

34. Pircon RA et al: Controlled trial of hydration and bed rest versus bed rest alone in the evaluation of preterm uterine contractions. *Am J Obstet Gynecol* 1989; 161: 775-779.

35. American College of Obstetricians and Gynecologists: Preterm labor. *ACOG Technical Bulletin 206*. 1995.

36. King JF et al: Betamimetics in preterm labor: an overview of the randomized controlled trials. *Br J Obstet Gynaecol* 1988; 95:211-222.

37. Cox SM, Sherman ML, Leveno KJ: Randomized investigation of magnesium sulfate for prevention of preterm birth. *Am J Obstet Gynecol* 1990; 163:767-772.

38. National Institutes of Health Consensus Development Conference: Effect of corticosteroids for fetal maturation on perinatal outcomes. *National Institutes of Health Consensus Development Conference Statement,* May 27, 1994, pp 1-18.

39. American College of Obstetricians and Gynecologists. Antenatal corticosteroid therapy for fetal maturation. *Committee Opinion 147*. 1994.

40. Spellacy WN: Postdate pregnancy. In Scott JR et al, editors: *Danforth's obstetrics and gynecology,* ed 8. Philadelphia, Lippincott, Williams and Wilkins, 1999, pp 287-292.

41. Pitt C et al: Prophylactic amnioinfusion for intrapartum oligohydramnios: a meta-analysis of randomized controlled trials. *Obstet Gynecol* 2000; 95(5 Pt 2):861-866.

42. Pierce J, Gaudier FL, Sanchez-Ramos L: Intrapartum amnioinfusion for meconium-stained fluid: meta-analysis of prospective clinical trials. *Obstet Gynecol* 2000; 95(6 Pt 2):1051-1056.

43. American College of Obstetricians and Gynecologists. Management of post-term pregnancy. *ACOG Practice Patterns, Number 6,* Washington, DC. 1997.

44. American College of Obstetricians and Gynecologists: Quality, evaluation and improvement in practice: post-term pregnancy. *Committee on Quality Assessment. Criteria set number 10.* Washington, DC. 1995.

45. Krammer J et al: Pre-induction cervical ripening: a randomized comparison of two methods. *Obstet Gynecol* 1995; 85:614.

46. Wing DA et al: Misoprostol: an effective agent for cervical ripening and labor induction. *Am J Obstet Gynecol* 1995; 172:4844-4846.

47. Wing DA, Lovett K, Paul RH: Disruption of prior uterine incision following misoprostol for labor induction in women with previous cesarean delivery. *Obstet Gynecol* 1998; 91:828-830.

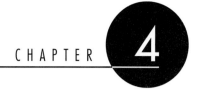

CHAPTER 4

Neonatal Assessment and Resuscitation

Melissa K. Brown

The first few moments of an infant's life are the most critical. At this time the newborn must make the transition from intrauterine to extrauterine life. Most infants enter extrauterine life with crying and vigorous activity. However, of the approximately 4 million babies born in the United States each year, 7.3% are *low birth weight* (LBW), or less than 2500 g, and 1.3% are *very low birth weight* (VLBW), or less than 1500 g.[1] Adverse maternal and fetal conditions contribute to the need to initiate resuscitative efforts in approximately 6% to 10% of all deliveries.[2]

Current resuscitation methods are directed toward (1) providing oxygen and removing carbon dioxide by positive-pressure ventilation, (2) maintaining the circulation by external cardiac massage, (3) using a volume expander to combat shock, and (4) infrequently, using a cardiotonic medication.[3] Proper care of the newborn can be divided into four phases: (1) preparation, (2) stabilization, (3) assessment, and (4) resuscitation.

PREPARATION

Neonatal resuscitation guidelines require skilled personnel to function as a team in an appropriately equipped delivery room. Successful resuscitation in the delivery room depends on advanced preparation, including the availability of equipment to (1) maintain warmth, (2) provide and maintain an airway, (3) obtain vascular access, and (4) provide resuscitative drugs.

As soon as it is evident that neonatal resuscitation may be necessary, put a prearranged plan into action. Assign personnel according to their area and level of competence.

There is usually a detailed history on perinatal problems associated with an infant who may require resuscitation (Box 4-1). If time is not available to obtain a detailed history, the neonatal resuscitation

PERINATAL FACTORS ASSOCIATED WITH INCREASED RISK OF NEONATAL DEPRESSION

ANTEPARTUM (FETOMATERNAL)
Diabetes
Postterm status
Hemorrhage
Substance abuse
No prenatal care
Age over 35 years
Multifetal gestation
Diminished fetal activity
Anemia or isoimmunization
Oligohydramnios or polyhydramnios
Small fetus for maternal dates
Previous fetal or neonatal death
Immature pulmonary maturity studies
Chronic or pregnancy-induced hypertension
Preterm labor or premature rupture of
    membranes
Other maternal illness (e.g., cardiovascular,
    thyroid, neurologic)
Drug therapy (e.g., magnesium, adrenergic
    blockers, lithium)
Congenital abnormalities

INTRAPARTUM
Infection
Prolapsed cord
Prolonged labor
Maternal sedation
Operative or device-assisted delivery
Meconium-stained delivery
Prolonged rupture of membranes
Breech or other abnormal presentation
Indices of fetal distress (e.g., abnormal heart rate)

team will be better prepared if they at least know (1) the mother is in premature labor, (2) the number of babies expected, and (3) if meconium is present in the amniotic fluid.

STABILIZING THE NEONATE

DRYING AND WARMING

Stabilizing the newborn starts with drying and warming the infant. Preventing heat loss is important when caring for a newborn. *Cold stress* increases oxygen consumption and impedes effective resuscitation.

Immediately place the infant in a preheated radiant warmer. If possible, deliver the infant in a warm, draft-free area.[4] Heat loss can be greatly reduced by rapidly drying the infant's skin, immediately removing wet linens, and wrapping the infant in prewarmed blankets.[5] If the infant is less than 1500 g, wrapping the newborn in a topical polyethylene film reduces evaporative heat loss but permits radiant heat transfer.[6] Using polyethylene wrapping on a VLBW infant at delivery reduces the risk of a decrease in postnatal temperature and may reduce the mortality rate.[7] Hyperthermia is also avoided because an increase in body temperature causes an increase in oxygen consumption.[8]

AIRWAY

Stabilizing the infant continues by stimulating and positioning the infant with the neck slightly flexed (Fig. 4-1). Placing a small roll under the shoulders often attains the correct position.

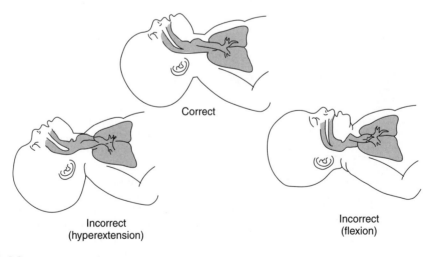

Correct

Incorrect
(hyperextension)

Incorrect
(flexion)

Fig. 4-1

Correct and incorrect head positions for resuscitation. (From American Academy of Pediatrics: *Textbook of neonatal resuscitation,* ed 4. Chicago, American Heart Association, 2000.)

Suspect airway obstruction if respiratory efforts are not effective. Immediately reposition the head and clear the airway of the obstruction.

Once positioned, suction the infant to clear secretions. Positioning the infant and clearing secretions open the infant's airway. Use either a bulb syringe or a suction catheter, and limit each pass to 3 or 5 seconds at a time. It is important to remember to monitor heart rate for possible bradycardia during suctioning.[9] Aggressive pharyngeal or stomach suctioning may cause laryngeal spasm and vagal stimulation with bradycardia and may delay the onset of spontaneous breathing.[5,9] Avoid excessive suctioning of clear fluid from the nasopharynx, which may cause injury or atelectasis and may interfere with the infant's ability to establish adequate ventilation.[2]

In the absence of meconium or blood, limit mechanical suctioning with a catheter to a depth of 5 cm from the lips for 5 seconds. Negative pressure of the suction apparatus should not exceed 90 to 100 mm Hg.[5]

If meconium has contaminated the amniotic fluid, suction the mouth, pharynx, and nose as the infant's head is delivered. Do not dry or stimulate the infant until the airway is cleared. If respirations are depressed or absent, if the heart rate is less than 100 beats per minute (beats/min), or if muscle tone is poor, the infant may require direct laryngotracheal suctioning of the meconium. Intubate the infant and apply suction directly to the endotracheal tube with the help of a special adapter (Fig. 4-2). Constantly apply suction while removing the tube

from the airway. Repeat the intubation and suctioning procedure until meconium is no longer visible in the airway or until resuscitation is required.

If positive pressure is required, reintubate with a clean endotracheal tube after meconium has been removed with repeated suctioning attempts. Perform subsequent suctioning by passing a suction catheter through the endotracheal tube. If the newborn is severely depressed, positive-pressure ventilation may be required, even if some meconium remains in the airway. Do not suction the stomach until vital signs are stable and the infant has been fully resuscitated.

STIMULATION

If the newborn does not respond to the extrauterine environment with a strong cry, respiratory effort, and the movement of all extremities, the infant requires stimulation. Flicking the bottoms of the feet, gently rubbing the back, and drying with a towel are all acceptable methods of stimulation. Slapping, shaking, spanking, and holding the newborn upside down are *contraindicated* and potentially dangerous to the infant.[10]

Basic or advanced life support should be initiated if the newborn does not establish effective, spontaneous respirations after brief stimulation. Tactile stimulation should stimulate spontaneous breathing in an infant who is in primary apnea. If the infant has already progressed to secondary apnea, the newborn will not resume spontaneous respirations without positive-pressure ventilation.

ASSESSING THE NEONATE

In addition to maternal history, make a thorough delivery room assessment of the newborn according to the American Heart Association/American Academy of Pediatrics (AHA/AAP) Neonatal Resuscitation Program (NRP) guidelines.[3] The assessment process includes evaluating the newborn's respirations, heart rate, and color; deciding what action to take; and then taking that action. Perform a quick visual assessment to detect external structural anomalies, lesions, or trauma.

RESPIRATIONS

An appropriate respiratory response to stimulation would be spontaneous crying with adequate respiratory rate and depth. If the respiratory response is appropriate, the heart rate is evaluated next.

An inadequate respiratory response with shallow, slow, or absent respirations necessitates the immediate initiation of positive-pressure ventilation (Fig. 4-3). It is important to remember, however, that the presence of respirations does not guarantee

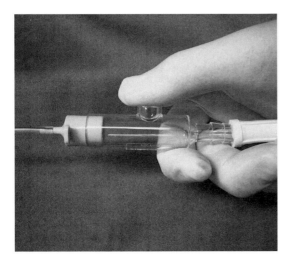

Fig. 4-2

Meconium aspirator attached to an endotracheal tube on one end and a suction source on the other end. (Courtesy Neotech Products, Chatsworth, Calif.)

an adequate pulse rate. Shallow respirations may primarily ventilate dead space and thus provide inadequate alveolar ventilation. Initiate positive-pressure ventilation if the infant is apneic or gasping or if respirations are ineffective.

HEART RATE

The heart rate can be evaluated by (1) feeling the pulse by lightly grasping the base of the umbilical cord, (2) listening to the apical beat with a stethoscope, or (3) feeling the brachial or femoral pulse. The heart rate is a critical determinant of the resus-

citation sequence. If the heart rate is greater than 100 beats/min and spontaneous respirations are present, the assessment is continued. If the heart rate is less than 100 beats/min, positive-pressure ventilation should be started immediately. If the heart rate is 60 beats/min or less and adequate ventilation is being provided, chest compressions should be initiated.

COLOR

Color is not as sensitive an indicator of the infant's condition as heart rate. Many infants demonstrate

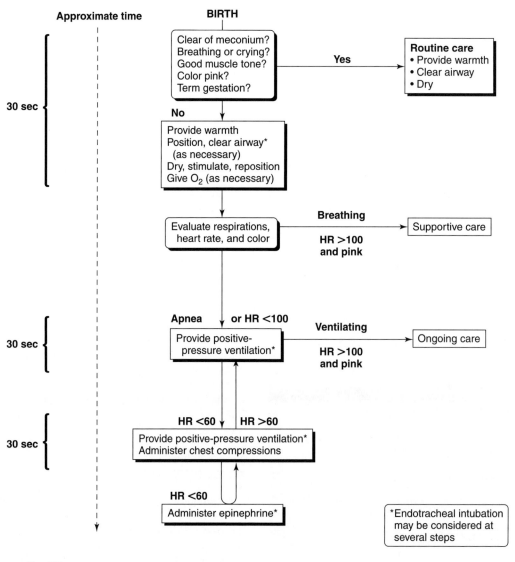

Fig. 4-3

Algorithm for resuscitation of the newborn. *HR,* Heart rate (beats per minute). (From American Academy of Pediatrics: *Textbook of neonatal resuscitation,* ed 4. Chicago, American Heart Association, 2000.)

peripheral cyanosis (blue extremities only) shortly after birth. This condition is common in the first few minutes of life because of sluggish peripheral circulation; oxygen therapy is unnecessary.

Occasionally, despite adequate ventilation and a heart rate greater than 100 beats/min, an infant may continue to be cyanotic. If central cyanosis is present in an infant with spontaneous respirations and a heart rate greater than 100 beats/min, free-flow oxygen should be given until the cause of the cyanosis is determined.

APGAR SCORE

Introduced in 1952 by Virginia Apgar, the Apgar score evaluates five factors: heart rate, respiratory effort, muscle tone, reflex irritability, and color[11] (Table 4-1). The scoring system provides a clinical picture of the infant's condition after delivery.

The Apgar score has encouraged clinicians to evaluate newborns immediately after birth and to observe several clinical signs simultaneously. The score has also been used as a predictive index of neonatal mortality and neurologic or developmental outcome. The Apgar score continues to be used as the best-established index of immediate postnatal heath.[12,13] More importantly, the Apgar score 1 minute after delivery provides an immediate evaluation of the infant and guides the appropriate clinical intervention.

Do not postpone immediate therapeutic interventions or resuscitation to assign an Apgar score at 1 minute. In infants significantly compromised at birth, begin appropriate resuscitative efforts immediately. Any delay in proper medical treatment to the newborn may prove disastrous.

Scoring again at 5 minutes of age gives information on the infant's ability to recover from the stress of birth and adapt to extrauterine life. When the 5-minute score is less than 7, additional scores

are usually obtained at 5-minute intervals until the score is greater than 7. Survival of the infant is unlikely if the score remains 0 after 10 minutes of resuscitation.[14]

APGAR SCORE IN THE VLBW INFANT

Three of the assessment criteria used in the Apgar score—muscle tone, respiratory effort, and reflex irritability—reflect the neonate's level of developmental maturity. Muscle tone is typically flaccid in the infant with less than 28 weeks' gestation. Respiratory effort and regulation of respiration also decrease with declining gestational age. Primitive reflexes that are present in the full-term infant, such as sucking and rooting, are variably present or absent as gestational age declines.[15]

The most important of the signs is heart rate, which indicates life or death. Failure of the heart rate to respond to resuscitation is an ominous prognostic sign.[12] Heart rate appears to be least affected by developmental maturity but may still be inadequate because of developmental difficulties in establishing cardiorespiratory function at birth.

In the immediate newborn period, skin color has the weakest correlation with the other four components of the Apgar score. Also, color does not reliably correlate with umbilical arterial pH, carbon dioxide pressure, and base excess.[15] Although the Apgar score may be limited in predicting morbidity and short-term mortality in preterm infants, it remains the best tool for the identification of preterm infants in need of cardiopulmonary resuscitation.[12]

RESUSCITATING THE NEONATE

Begin resuscitation immediately once the newborn has been assessed and the need for resuscitation determined. Ensure that the infant is dry and warm and that the airway is open. Resuscitation consists of administering oxygen, assisting ventilation, and initiating cardiopulmonary resuscitation and cardiotonic drugs as indicated.

OXYGEN ADMINISTRATION

If there is evidence of central cyanosis, as assessed by examining the lips and mucous membranes, but ventilation is adequate with a heart rate greater than 100 beats/min, administer 100% free-flow oxygen through a mask toward the infant's mouth and nose. If a mask is not available, use a funnel, or cup the hands around the oxygen tubing. Holding the oxygen $\frac{1}{2}$ inch from the nose at 6 to 8 L/min provides approximately 60% to 80% oxygen.[2] Gradually withdraw the oxygen source once the infant's color improves.

TABLE 4-1	APGAR SCORING		
Parameter	**0**	**1**	**2**
Heart rate	None	<100 beats/min	>100 beats/min
Respiratory rate	None	Weak, irregular	Strong cry
Color	Pale blue	Body pink, extremities blue	Completely pink
Reflex (irritability to suctioning)	No response	Grimace	Cry, cough, or sneeze
Muscle tone	Limp	Some flexion	Well flexed

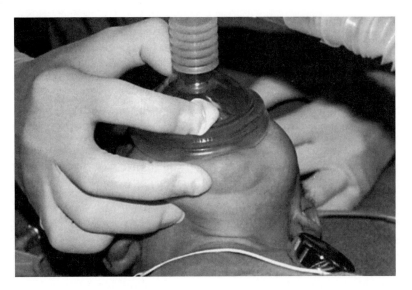

Fig. 4-4

Correct technique for holding a mask to the face of a newborn. Note that fingers do not touch the neck or soft tissue under the chin. (From Bahar PM, Todd NW: Resuscitation of the newborn with airway compromise. *Clin Perinatol* 1999; 26[3]:727.)

Research has raised questions concerning the routine use of 100% oxygen versus room air for neonatal resuscitation. It is now recognized that oxygen can be a toxic drug and has the potential to cause lung injury. Giving too much oxygen during the brief time needed for resuscitation should not be a cause for concern. Use oxygen judiciously, however, and avoid prolonged and unnecessary high concentrations.[16,17]

While in the delivery room, *continuous positive airway pressure* (CPAP) may provide benefit to an infant with mild to moderate respiratory distress. The mission of this form of early ventilatory support is to keep the lungs open, avoiding the potentially harmful collapse and reexpansion of terminal air spaces (see Chapter 18). CPAP may also prevent consumption of surfactant in newborns with a limited supply of this material in their lungs. CPAP also has a well-documented effect on apnea.[18] In some studies, early CPAP in the delivery room reduced the number of premature infants requiring mechanical ventilation.[18-20] To initiate CPAP in the delivery room, initially use a mask-bag setup, but place the infant on a nasal apparatus designed for CPAP administration as soon as practical.

VENTILATION

Indications for assisted ventilation include apnea (gasping) after stimulation or heart rate less than 100 beats/min. The recommended ventilation rate is from 30 to 60 breaths/min.[6] In the delivery room, ventilation is usually accomplished using a manual resuscitation bag and mask.

Appropriate-sized face masks for preterm, term, and large newborns must be available in the delivery room and at the bedside. A properly sized mask fits the contours of the face and has little dead space (less than 5 ml). The mask should be large enough to form a seal around the mouth and nose but should not cover the eyes or overlap the chin. For best results, the mask should be clear and should have a cushioned rim.[2,3,5]

Proper technique is essential when performing mask ventilation (Figs. 4-4 and 4-5). Place the fingers on the anterior margin of the mandible, and lift the face into the mask. Erroneously placing the fingers onto the soft tissue under the mandible will collapse the floor of the mouth and obstruct the airway by pushing the tongue against the roof of the mouth.[21] Even if the neonate is intubated, an appropriate-sized face mask must always be readily available, especially during transport.

The two types of resuscitation bags used in neonatal resuscitation are self-inflating bags and anesthesia bags. The *self-inflating bag* is a resuscitation bag that refills without supplementary gas flow. Because this type of bag uses an intake valve, room air dilutes the oxygen concentration delivered by the bag. To deliver high concentrations of oxygen, attach an oxygen reservoir. It is important to note that many self-inflating bags do not effectively deliver free-flow oxygen through the mask.[22]

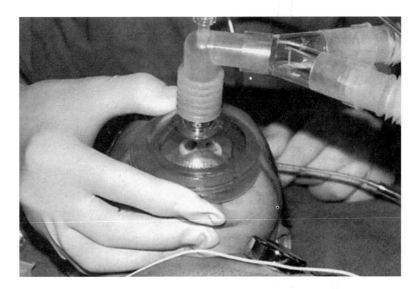

Fig. 4-5

Incorrect technique for holding a mask to the face of a newborn. Note that the fingers are touching the neck and soft tissue under the chin, causing airway obstruction. (From Bahar PM, Todd NW: Resuscitation of the newborn with airway compromise. *Clin Perinatol* 1999; 26[3]:727.)

The appropriate-sized bag for a neonate has a volume of at least 450 ml but does not exceed 750 ml. Some bags are equipped with a pressure-limited pop-off valve, usually preset at 30 to 35 cm H_2O. Because a neonate's lungs are not aerated at birth, high pressures are often required to initially inflate them. This pressure usually exceeds the preset pressure limit in bags equipped with a pop-off valve. Thus a bypass device is necessary with these self-inflating bags. Connect an in-line manometer to monitor constantly the pressure delivered with each breath.

The *anesthesia bag,* or non–self-inflating bag, inflates only from a compressed gas source of air, oxygen, or both. Successful use of this type of resuscitation bag requires an appropriate flow of gas, correct adjustment of the flow control valve, and careful attention to a tight seal at the face mask. To control all these factors, more training is required than with a self-inflating bag. Set flow at 8 to 10 L/min, and adjust it to maintain bag distention without causing overdistention, or allowing the bag to deflate with subsequent breaths. Using anesthesia bags requires constant monitoring of baseline and peak ventilation pressures through an adapter attached to a pressure manometer.

The anesthesia bag offers the advantage of being able to provide a more precise control of oxygen concentration, a greater range of peak inspiratory pressures, and the ability to deliver free-flow oxygen through the mask. Neither style

of resuscitation bag offers an advantage in terms of consistent ventilation.[23] Consistent ventilation with either type of bag improves only with practice and experience.

Bag-mask ventilation is adequate if there is bilateral expansion of the lungs with chest wall motion and auscultation of bilateral breath sounds. In addition to this assessment, the infant's condition must improve, heart rate must increase to more than 100 beats/min, and the infant's color must become pink. Failure to move the chest with bag-mask ventilation may indicate a poorly positioned or obstructed airway, inadequate inspiratory pressures, the presence of a pneumothorax, or some other respiratory compromise. Avoid overdistention and hyperventilation to minimize the risk of lung and brain injury.[2]

Once the heart rate reaches 100 beats/min, gradually reduce the rate and pressure of assisted ventilation. Observe the infant for signs of adequate spontaneous respiration and clinical stability before discontinuing ventilation.

Endotracheal intubation is indicated when (1) bag-mask ventilation is ineffective, (2) tracheal suctioning is required, especially of thick meconium in a respiratory depressed neonate, or (3) prolonged ventilation is anticipated. When suspecting a congenital diaphragmatic hernia, immediately perform endotracheal intubation to minimize overdistention of the stomach resulting from bag-mask ventilation. Additionally, place a nasogastric tube to decompress the bowel and allow the lungs to inflate.[4]

With the exception of diaphragmatic hernia, intubation is an elective procedure and should be performed in the preceding conditions only after preoxygenation and initial stabilization of the infant have been performed with bag-mask ventilation. Appropriate size of endotracheal tube, correct tube placement, verification, secure fastening, and monitoring are all essential in the successful resuscitation of the neonate. (See Chapter 15 for details on airway management and tube sizes.) Head position does affect the endotracheal tube position. Maintain a midline head position to avoid accidental extubation or mainstem intubation.

CHEST COMPRESSIONS

Cardiopulmonary resuscitation in the delivery room requiring chest compressions and medications is an infrequent occurrence. In one large study, chest compressions and medications were given to 39 (0.12%) of 30,839 infants delivered.[24]

Providing adequate ventilation is the primary factor in the effective resuscitation of a neonate. Most neonates will respond once ventilation is established. Chest compressions can impede the delivery of effective ventilations and should not be started until effective ventilation is established.[5] After 30 seconds of positive-pressure ventilation, if the heart rate is absent or less than 60 beats/min, begin chest compressions.

The NRP guidelines of the AHA/AAP provide recommendations for the decision-making process in the delivery room (see Fig. 4-3).[9] In the neonate, bradycardia is usually caused by inadequate oxygenation, and therefore positive-pressure ventilation with 100% oxygen should always accompany chest compressions.[3]

There are two accepted techniques for delivering chest compressions to the neonate, the thumb method and the two-finger technique. The *thumb technique* consists of holding the torso of the infant, with both hands encircling it. The thumbs are on the sternum, and the fingers are under the infant. The fingers are used to support the back, and the thumbs are used to compress the sternum. The advantage of the thumb technique is better coronary perfusion pressure.[2] The disadvantage is interference with access to the infant for umbilical catheter placement and medication delivery.[3]

In the second method, the *two-finger technique,* the index and middle fingers are used to compress the chest. The other hand supports the back if a firm surface is not available.

With both techniques the compressions should be applied on the lower third of the sternum. Com-press to approximately one third of the anteroposterior diameter of the chest to generate a palpable pulse.[5] Resuscitation should be a coordinated effort, with compressions and ventilation delivered in a 3:1 ratio, approximately 90 compressions to 30 ventilations.[3] Every 60 seconds the heart rate should be reassessed. When the heart rate is greater than 60 beats/min, chest compressions can be discontinued.

MEDICATIONS

Medications and the dosages recommended for neonatal resuscitation have been extrapolated mainly from adult and animal research.[24] Neonatal anatomy and physiology differs from animal and adult physiology, with the potential for unrecognized effects and hazards. More research is necessary on the effects of emergency medications in the neonate.

Epinephrine. Epinephrine is an endogenous catecholamine with both α-adrenergic and β-adrenergic stimulating properties; in cardiac arrest, α-adrenergic-mediated vasoconstriction may be the more important action. This vasoconstriction elevates the perfusion pressure during chest compression, enhancing delivery of oxygen to the heart and brain. In addition, epinephrine enhances the contractile state of the heart, stimulates spontaneous contractions, and increases heart rate. Epinephrine is indicated in asystole or with a spontaneous heart rate of 60 beats/min or less, after at least 30 seconds of ventilation with 100% oxygen and chest compressions.

An epinephrine dose of 0.01 to 0.03 mg/kg body weight (0.1 to 0.3 ml/kg of 1:10,000 solution) may be repeated every 3 to 5 minutes if required. Some children and adults who do not respond to standard doses of epinephrine may respond to doses as high as 0.2 mg/kg. However, the routine use of this dose in neonates is not recommended. Neonates most often have hemodynamically significant bradycardia, and scientific dose-response data are lacking for the use of epinephrine in neonates or in neonatal animal models for this rhythm. Further, this dose has been associated with prolonged periods of hypertension after administration. Because the newborn, especially the premature infant, has a very vascular germinal matrix (an area of the brain at high risk for the development of hemorrhage after hypertension), the risk of intracranial hemorrhage may be increased.[24]

Epinephrine is given intravenously or through an endotracheal tube. Although giving epinephrine by the endotracheal route is expeditious and the drug is absorbed systemically, low plasma concentrations result. Data from animal models and a single adult human study suggest that if the typical intravenous dose of epinephrine is administered by the endotracheal route, the resulting serum concentration will be approximately 10% of that achieved by the intravenous route.[16,24] Theoretically, and supported by limited research, a risk exists for increased incidence of intracranial hemorrhage in the neonate from acute hypertension that persists as a result of high-dose epinephrine.[2,5,16,24]

Because of the potential risks and limited scientific knowledge in this area, the current NRP guidelines recommend giving the same dose endotracheally as intravenously, and to quickly acquire intravenous access if there is no response to endotracheal epinephrine. Administer epinephrine every 3 to 5 minutes during the treatment of pulseless arrest.

Volume expanders. Volume expanders may be necessary to resuscitate a newborn with hypovolemia, which should be suspected in any neonate who fails to respond to resuscitation. Inappropriate intravascular volume expansion is a risk in an asphyxiated neonate, particularly if the newborn is significantly preterm. However, volume expanders are indicated when acute blood loss is suspected or indicated in a neonate with poor response to resuscitation.

Blood volume expansion may be accomplished with 10 ml/kg of normal saline or lactated Ringer's solution. Use of O-negative blood cross-matched with the mother's blood may be indicated with large-volume blood loss. Albumin solutions are less frequently used because of infection concerns and limited availability. The volume expander may be given as a rapid infusion over 5 to 10 minutes through an umbilical catheter.

Naloxone. Naloxone hydrochloride is a narcotic antagonist that does not possess direct respiratory depressant activity. Naloxone is indicated in the neonate for reversal of respiratory depression induced by narcotics given to the mother within 4 hours of delivery. Adequate ventilation should always be maintained before administration of naloxone. Because the duration of action of narcotics may exceed that of naloxone, continued monitoring of the neonate is necessary. Naloxone can induce a withdrawal reaction in a newborn with a narcotic-dependent mother and should be avoided in this situation.

The initial dose of 0.1 mg/kg of naloxone for infants of every gestational age may be repeated every 2 to 3 minutes as needed.[3,5] Recurrent doses may be necessary to prevent recurrent apnea in the neonate. Naloxone should be given intravenously or endotracheally. If perfusion is adequate, however, the subcutaneous or intramuscular route is an option.

Sodium Bicarbonate. Systemic acidosis decreases myocardial contractility, causes vasodilation resulting in lower blood pressure, and diminishes cardiac responsiveness to catecholamines and other inotropes. Sodium bicarbonate can reverse systemic acidosis and is recommended in neonatal cardiopulmonary resuscitation after ventilation has been established and metabolic acidosis is presumed or documented.[16] Although sodium bicarbonate may be useful in correcting a metabolic acidosis, its effects depend on the presence of adequate ventilation and perfusion. No evidence indicates that bicarbonate is useful in the acute phase of a neonatal resuscitation.

Other risks associated with bicarbonate administration are special concerns for the premature infant, including hypernatremia and intraventricular hemorrhage. Volume expanders to reverse metabolic acidosis may be more effective and less likely to cause hyperosmolarity than sodium bicarbonate.[16]

Sodium bicarbonate may be indicated when the newborn with prolonged respiratory arrest does not respond to other therapy.[3,24] A dose of 1 to 2 mEq/kg of 0.5 mEq/ml solution may be given by slow intravenous push after adequate ventilation and perfusion have been established. Higher concentrations have been associated with higher risks of intracranial hemorrhage.[2,3,5,16,24]

POSTRESUSCITATION CARE

Optimal care of the neonate after resuscitation requires frequent reassessment and careful monitoring, including appropriateness of therapy and determination of arterial pH and blood gas levels. Physiologic stability should be maintained by (1) treatment of hypotension with volume expanders or pressors, (2) appropriate fluid therapy, and (3) treatment of seizures. During the first hours after resuscitation, the patient must be monitored closely for hypoglycemia and hypocalcemia. Also, radiographic documentation of the appropriate placement of intravascular lines and the endotracheal tube should be obtained.[6,17]

ETHICAL CONSIDERATIONS

The issue of whether to initiate resuscitation arises with the birth of extremely premature infants or those with congenital birth defects. With advances in technology and improved medications, however, VLBW infants who previously would have died now can survive. Survival with normal neurodevelopmental outcome has been documented in infants weighing less than 1 pound (454 g).[16,25,26]

Initiating resuscitative efforts does not preclude withdrawing life support later. In fact, later withdrawal of support allows more time to gain better clinical information and to counsel a family on expected outcomes. Extremely premature infants or those with anencephaly may have no chance of survival, however, and they may be the exception to this recommendation. There is no advantage to delayed, graduated, or partial support if the infant survives. Worse outcomes may result because of this approach.[5]

REFERENCES

1. Bernstein S, Heimler R, Sasidharan P: Approaching the management of the neonatal intensive care unit graduate through history and physical assessment. *Pediatr Clin North Am* 1998; 45(1):97-105.
2. Wolkoff L, Davis J: Delivery room resuscitation of the newborn. *Clin Perinatol* 1999; 26(3):641-658.
3. Niermeyer S et al: International Guidelines for Neonatal Resuscitation: an excerpt from the *Guidelines 2000 for Cardiopulmonary Resuscitation and Emergency Cardiovascular Care*: International Consensus on Science. *Pediatrics* 2000; 106(3):E29.
4. Chahine A, Ricketts R: Resuscitation of the surgical neonate. *Clin Perinatol* 1999; 26(3):693-713.
5. Kattwinkel J et al: An advisory statement from the Pediatric Working Group of the International Liaison Committee on Resuscitation. *Pediatrics* 1999; 103(4):E56.
6. Narendran V, Hoath S: Thermal management of the low birth weight infant: a cornerstone of neonatology. *Pediatrics* 1999; 134(5):E547.
7. Vohra S et al: Effect of polyethylene occlusive skin wrapping on heat loss in very low birth weight infants at delivery: a randomized trial. *J Pediatr* 1999; 134(5):547-551.
8. Kattwinkel J, Niermeyer S, Denson SE: *Textbook of neonatal resuscitation,* ed 4. Dallas, American Heart Association, 2000.
9. Halbower A, Jones D: Physiologic reflexes and their impact on resuscitation of the newborn. *Clin Perinatol* 1999; 26(3):621-627.
10. Nadkarni V, Hazinski MF, Zideman D: Pediatric resuscitation: an advisory statement from the Pediatric Working Group of the International Liaison Committee on Resuscitation. *Circulation* 1997; 95:2185-2195.
11. Juretschke L: Apgar scoring: its use and meaning for today's newborn. *Neonatal Network* 2000; 19(1):17-19.
12. Hegyi T, Carbone T, Anwar M: The Apgar score and its components in the preterm infant. *Pediatrics* 1998; 101(1):77-81.
13. Weinberger B et al: Antecedents and neonatal consequences of low Apgar scores in preterm newborns: a population study. *Arch Pediatr Adolesc Med* 2000; 154(3):294-300.
14. Jain L et al: Cardiopulmonary resuscitation of apparently stillborn infants: survival and long-term outcome. *J Pediatr* 1991; 118(5):778-782.
15. Catlin E et al: The Apgar score revisited: influence of gestational age. *J Pediatr* 1986; 109(5):865-868.
16. Ginsberg H, Goldsmith J: Controversies in neonatal resuscitation. *Clin Perinatol* 1998; 25(1):1-15.
17. Piazza A: Postasphyxial management of the newborn. *Clin Perinatol* 1999; 26(3):749-765.
18. Verder H et al: Nasal continuous positive airway pressure and early surfactant therapy for respiratory distress syndrome in newborns of less than 30 weeks' gestation. *Pediatrics* 1999; 103(2):E24.
19. Lindner W et al: Delivery room management of extremely low birth weight infants: spontaneous breathing or intubation? *Pediatrics* 1999; 103(5):961-967.
20. Lacroze M et al: Early continuous positive pressure in the labor room (abstract). *Arch Pediatr* 1997; 4(1):15-20.
21. Behar P, Todd N: Resuscitation of the newborn with airway compromise. *Clin Perinatol* 1999; 26(3):717-732.
22. Martell RJ, Soder CM: Laerdal infant resuscitators are unreliable as free-flow oxygen delivery devices. *Am J Perinatol* 1997; 14(6):347-351.
23. Dockery WK et al: A comparison of manual and mechanical ventilation during pediatric transport. *Crit Care Med* 1999; 27(4):802-806.
24. Burchfield D: Medication use in neonatal resuscitation. *Clin Perinatol* 1999; 26(3):683-691.
25. Boyle R, Kattwinkel J: Ethical issues surrounding resuscitation. *Clin Perinatol* 1999; 26(3):779-793.
26. Clark R: Support of gas exchange in the delivery room and beyond: how do we avoid hurting the baby we seek to save? *Clin Perinatol* 1999; 26(3):669-681.

Assessment and Monitoring of the Neonatal and Pediatric Patient

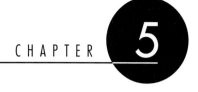

CHAPTER 5

Examination and Assessment of the Neonatal Patient

Melissa K. Brown

Many factors, including size, weight, and gestational age, influence neonatal outcome. Therefore it is important to perform a newborn assessment early in the admission process.

GESTATIONAL AGE AND SIZE ASSESSMENT

Ideally, gestational age assessment is performed before the neonate is 12 hours old to allow the greatest reliability for infants less than 26 weeks of gestational age.[1-3] Evaluating gestational age requires consideration of several factors. The three main factors are (1) gestational duration based on the last menstrual cycle, (2) prenatal ultrasound evaluation, and (3) postnatal findings based on physical and neurologic examinations. Postnatal examinations for determining gestational age include the *Ballard score,* which is based on external physical findings and neurologic criteria (Fig. 5-1).

Once gestational age is determined, weight, length, and head circumference are plotted on a standard newborn grid. Any infant whose birth weight is less than the 10th percentile for gestational age is *small for gestational age* (SGA); similarly, an infant whose birth weight is more than the 90th percentile is *large for gestational age* (LGA). When using intrauterine growth curves, it may be necessary to consider specific charts that are race and gender specific.[4]

PHYSICAL EXAMINATION

The physical examination of an adult is generally conducted in a rigid head-to-toe format. When examining an infant, however, the order of the examination is modified to establish critical information, such as auscultation of the heart and lungs,

Neuromuscular maturity

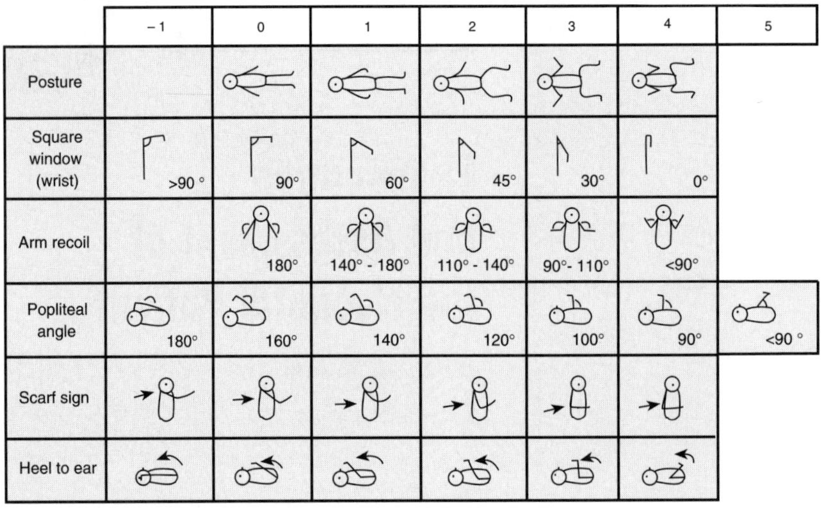

	−1	0	1	2	3	4	5
Posture							
Square window (wrist)	>90°	90°	60°	45°	30°	0°	
Arm recoil		180°	140° - 180°	110° - 140°	90°- 110°	<90°	
Popliteal angle	180°	160°	140°	120°	100°	90°	<90°
Scarf sign							
Heel to ear							

Physical maturity

Skin	Sticky Friable Transparent	Gelatinous red, translucent	Smooth pink, visible veins	Superficial peeling &/or rash, few veins	Cracking pale areas, rare veins	Parchment, deep cracking, no vessels	Leathery, cracked, wrinkled
Lanugo	None	Sparse	Abundant	Thinning	Bald areas	Mostly bald	
Plantar surface	Heel-toe 40 - 50 mm: −1 <40 mm: −2	>50 mm no crease	Faint red marks	Anterior transverse crease only	Creases anterior 2/3	Creases over entire sole	
Breast	Imperceptible	Barely perceptible	Flat areola, no bud	Stippled areola, 1 - 2 mm bud	Raised areola, 3 - 4 mm bud	Full areola, 5-10 mm bud	
Eye/ear	Lids fused loosely: −1 tightly: −2	Lids open; pinna flat, stays folded	Sl. curved pinna; soft, slow recoil	Well-curved pinna; soft but ready recoil	Formed & firm; instant recoil	Thick cartilage; ear stiff	
Genitals (male)	Scrotum flat, smooth	Scrotum empty, faint rugae	Testes in upper canal, rare rugae	Testes descending, few rugae	Testes down, good rugae	Testes pendulous, deep rugae	
Genitals (female)	Clitoris prominent, labia flat	Prominent clitoris, small labia minora	Prominent clitoris, enlarging minora	Majora & minora equally prominent	Majora large, minora small	Majora cover clitoris & minora	

Maturity rating

score	weeks
−10	20
−5	22
0	24
5	26
10	28
15	30
20	32
25	34
30	36
35	38
40	40
45	42
50	44

Fig. 5-1

Ballard score for estimating gestational age using scores derived from neurologic and physical signs. (From Ballard JL: New Ballard score, expanded to include extremely premature infants. *J Pediatr* 1991; 119:417-423.)

before the infant becomes agitated and begins to cry. However, the examiner must still completely examine the baby in an orderly and prioritized manner. As a general rule the following order works best, although this approach may require modification based on the clinical situation.

VITAL SIGNS

Quickly assess the vital signs of the infant. Table 5-1 lists normal ranges for neonatal vital signs. Absolute numbers are not as important as the relative ranges when considering the clinical situation. As an example, heart rate is normally 120 to 170 beats per

TABLE 5-1	NORMAL VALUES FOR VITAL SIGNS IN THE NEONATAL PATIENT	
Birth Weight (g)	Systolic/Diastolic Blood Pressure (mm Hg)*	Mean Blood Pressure (mm Hg)
>600	45/20	25
>1000	48/25	35
>2000	50/30	40
>3000	50/35	45
>4000	65/40	50
Newborn older than 12 hours	75/50	60

RESPIRATORY RATE

30-60 breaths/min

HEART RATE

120-170 beats/min

*From Versmold HT et al: Aortic blood pressure ranges during the first 12 hours of life in infants with birth weight 610 to 4220 grams. *Pediatrics* 1981; 67:607.

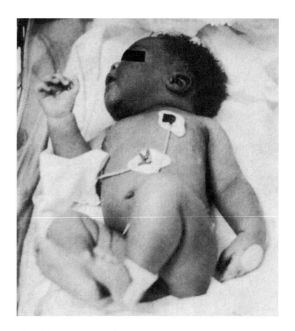

Fig. 5-2

"Waiter's tip" positioning of the left arm in an infant with brachial plexus injury from a traumatic delivery.

minute (beats/min). The heart rate of a term infant in deep sleep may decrease to 80 or 90 beats/min. An infant undergoing a painful procedure or who is hungry may have a transient heart rate greater than 200 beats/min. In comparison, a neonate older than 35 weeks' gestation has greater variability in heart rate than an infant born at 27 to 35 weeks' gestation. Presumably, in the younger infant, parasympathetic-sympathetic interaction and function are less developed.[5]

Similarly, normal values for temperature are 97.6° F ±1° axillary and 99.6° F ±1° rectally. Temperature on arrival in the nursery may be lower if the delivery room was cold. The temperature may also be higher if the radiant warmer was operating at a higher temperature due to incorrect probe position or warmer malfunction.

Record respiratory rate and blood pressure when performing vital signs (see later discussions).

GENERAL INSPECTION

Observing the infant's overall appearance is an important aspect of the physical examination. Ideally, examine the infant lying quietly and unclothed in a neutral thermal environment. Body position and symmetry, both at rest and during muscular activity, provide valuable information regarding possible birth trauma. For example, an infant who does not move the arms symmetrically could have a broken clavicle or an injury to the brachial plexus (Fig. 5-2).

The infant's skin is an indicator of intravascular volume, perfusion status, or both. Both perfusion and underlying skin color affect the appearance of the skin. Capillary refill time should be less than 3 seconds. Assess refill by pressing onto the sole of the foot or the palm of the hand with a finger. Perfusion should be good and skin color pink. Some infants have blue hands and feet with decreased perfusion, or *acrocyanosis,* in the immediate postnatal period. True cyanosis is associated with blue or dusky mucous membranes and circumoral area.

Observing skin and color often provides diagnostic clues. *Mottling* refers to irregular areas of dusky skin alternating with areas of pale skin. An extremely pale or mottled infant suggests hypotension or anemia. A ruddy, reddish blue appearance is frequently associated with a high hematocrit value or polycythemia. The yellow color associated with mild to moderate jaundice is common among newborns after the first day of life. Jaundice on the first day of life, however, is always an indication for an immediate evaluation.[6]

Often a gray-white cheeselike substance, called *vernix caseosa,* is present in the skin folds of a term infant. However, vernix is even more abundant on a preterm infant and suggests an earlier gestational age. The presence of *lanugo,* the fine hair that covers premature infants mostly over the shoulders, back, forehead, and cheeks, indicates an even

TABLE 5-2	COMMON DERMAL FINDINGS IN THE NEONATAL PATIENT	
Finding	**Description**	**Condition**
Jaundice	Yellowish skin	Hyperbilirubinemia
True cyanosis	Centrally blue or dusky skin	Hypoxia
Acrocyanosis	Bluish hands and feet	Cold stress, ↓ circulation—normal for first few hours
Petechiae	Pinpoint hemorrhagic areas	Birth trauma, thrombocytopenia
Telangiectatic nevi	"Stork bites": red, flat areas	Capillary dilation, benign
Subcutaneous fat necrosis	Discrete firm masses in subcutaneous tissue	Trauma
Lanugo	Fine hair	More noticeable in preterm infants, benign
Sclerema	Hardening of skin	Septicemia, shock, cold stress
Ruddy complexion	Deep reddish skin	Polycythemia or high hematocrit value
Ecchymoses	Bruising of various sizes	Birth trauma, disseminated intravascular coagulation
Mongolian spots	Irregular areas of pale blue over sacrum and buttocks	Benign, common in black and Asian infants
Strawberry hemangiomas	Bright red, flat spots 1-3 mm in diameter	Benign, usually resolve spontaneously
Milia	White papules <1 mm on forehead, chin, and nose	Distended sebaceous glands that disappear later
Erythema toxicum	Whitish pink papular rash	Cause unknown
Pallor	Pale or white skin	Blood loss or hypovolemia
Vernix caseosa	Whitish gray, cheeselike substance	More abundant on preterm infants
Mottled skin	Uneven color, blotchy	Decreased perfusion

younger gestational age. An infant exposed to meconium-stained amniotic fluid in utero for more than a few hours frequently presents with yellow-green staining of the skin, nails, and umbilical cord. Irregular areas of pale blue-black pigmentation over the sacrum and buttocks *(mongolian spots)* are often seen on black and Asian infants. These spots are frequently confused with bruising (Table 5-2).

RESPIRATORY FUNCTION

The normal newborn respiratory rate is 40 to 60 breaths/min but may vary depending on multiple factors. Watch respiratory effort closely and note irregular respirations. Respiratory rates that exceed 60 breaths/min but normalize over the next several hours may indicate transient tachypnea of the newborn. All newborns display an irregular breathing pattern. The neonate normally breathes in the range of 70 to 80 breaths/min for 10 to 20 seconds, then slows to a rate of 20 or 30 for a short time, and then breathes at a faster rate again. The average respiratory rate over several minutes is 40 to 60 breaths/min. *Periodic breathing,* a frequent finding among premature infants, is characterized by an irregular pattern of intermittent respiratory pauses longer than 5 seconds.

Apnea is a pathologic condition in which breathing ceases for longer than 20 seconds. Apnea may be associated with cyanosis, bradycardia, pallor, and hypotonia. Frequently, apnea is associated with nonspecific symptoms of diseases seen with many neonatal conditions. All episodes of apnea must be investigated to establish the cause.[7]

It is important to note signs of respiratory distress. The *Silverman scoring system* considers multiple factors to quantify the infant's distress (Fig. 5-3). Although not always recorded as a measure of distress, the Silverman system highlights important respiratory observations during a physical examination. Signs of distress include nasal flaring, expiratory grunting, tachypnea, and retractions. *Nasal flaring,* a sign of air hunger, occurs during inspiration as an effort to draw in more air through the nares. Partially closing the glottis during expiration causes *grunting,* apparently an attempt to maintain lung volume by increasing end-expiratory pressure.

Retractions of the chest wall during inspiration may occur in the suprasternal, substernal, subcostal, and intercostal regions. Retractions usually indicate reduced lung compliance but are also associated with obstructive airway processes with normal lung

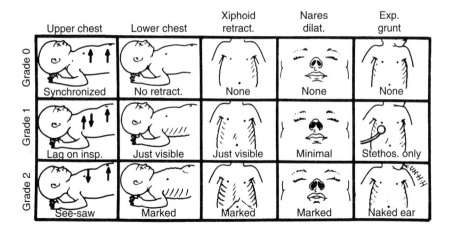

	Upper chest	Lower chest	Xiphoid retract.	Nares dilat.	Exp. grunt
Grade 0	Synchronized	No retract.	None	None	None
Grade 1	Lag on insp.	Just visible	Just visible	Minimal	Stethos. only
Grade 2	See-saw	Marked	Marked	Marked	Naked ear

Fig. 5-3

Silverman score for assessing the magnitude of respiratory distress. (From Silverman WA, Anderson DH: A controlled clinical trial of effects of water mist on obstructive respiratory signs, death rate and necropsy findings among premature infants. *Pediatrics* 1956; 17:1-6.)

compliance. Chest wall retractions are more prominent and easily observed in the neonate than in an older child or adult. The newborn musculature is relatively thin and weak, and the thoracic cage is not as rigid. The flexible chest wall and thoracic cage of the newborn exhibit noticeable retractions as lung compliance worsens. Abdominal and thoracic respiratory muscles normally move in parallel. *Paradoxical respirations* represent thoracic and abdominal respiratory efforts that are not synchronous. This "seesaw" effect frequently indicates severe respiratory distress (see Chapter 28).

Auscultation of the newborn can sometimes prove difficult. The newborn chest is small, and sounds easily transmit from one lung region to another. Localizing auscultation findings in a preterm infant is frequently difficult or impossible with single-head stethoscopes. Auscultation with a double-head stethoscope has proved useful in some situations.[8] Comparison of the breath sounds from the right and left sides helps distinguish asymmetries. Asymmetric sounds may indicate unilateral disease such as pneumothorax or a malpositioned endotracheal tube. Bowel sounds heard in the place of absent breath sounds are associated with a diaphragmatic hernia (see Chapter 29).

Diminished breath sounds occur in neonates with respiratory distress syndrome (RDS), atelectasis, pulmonary interstitial emphysema, and shallow respirations. *Rhonchi*, coarse sounds similar to snoring, emanate from large bronchi as air rushes through fluid contained within them. Suctioning with the endotracheal tube, if present, may eliminate the responsible secretions. *Wheezes* are commonly heard during expiration. Air rushing through fluid in the smaller airways and alveoli produce rales or crackles. *Rales* are heard in infants with RDS, pneumonia, and pulmonary edema, as well as in normal infants soon after birth. Frequently, infants with large upper airway obstruction generate *stridor*, a high-pitched creaking or squeaking and primarily an inspiratory sound. To distinguish stridor from wheezing, place the head of the stethoscope over the neck area, and isolate the noise to that region.

Other methods of respiratory assessment include chest radiography (see Chapter 8) and invasive or noninvasive blood gas analysis (see Chapters 10 and 11). Frequently, chest radiographs and blood gas analysis assist in the interpretation of physical examination findings. Many pathologic processes, including pneumothorax and pleural effusion, may cause symptoms but may be difficult to diagnose based on physical findings alone. Blood gas measurements supply additional information that facilitates the interpretation of physical findings. For example, an infant with severe tachypnea, normal chest examination, and normal chest radiograph has a blood gas diagnosis of a severe metabolic acidosis. The tachypnea is not caused by a cardiopulmonary problem but rather by an effort to blow off carbon dioxide and increase the blood pH.

Table 5-3 summarizes signs of respiratory distress associated with several neonatal disorders.

CHEST AND CARDIOVASCULAR SYSTEM

The circumference of a newborn's chest is equivalent to the head circumference. Inspection of the chest may reveal malformations such as *pectus*

TABLE 5-3	SIGNS OF RESPIRATORY DISTRESS IN THE NEONATAL PATIENT								
	Apnea	Tachypnea	Refractions	Grunting	Nasal Flaring	Stridor	Cyanosis	Breath Sounds	Other Clinical Findings
Respiratory distress syndrome		++	++	++	++		+	Decreased rales	Premature infants, infants of diabetic mothers
Pneumothorax		++	+	+	+		+	Decreased asymmetric	Asymmetry of the chest, PMI shifted
Pneumonia	+	++	++	++	++		+	Rales and rhonchi	
Upper airway obstruction	+	±		++		++			Gasping or labored breathing
Diaphragmatic hernia		++		+	++		++	Bowel sounds in chest	Scaphoid abdomen, often associated with pneumothorax
Meconium aspiration	+	++	++	+	+		+	Decreased	Hyperexpansion of chest, atelectasis, pneumothorax
Transient tachypnea		++	+	+	+			Fine rales	Resolves in <24 hr
Apnea of prematurity	+++		±				±	Normal	Bradycardia

+, Usually present; ++, significantly present; +++, predominantly present; ±, sometimes present; *PMI,* point of maximum cardiac impulse.

carinatum (protruding xiphisternum or xiphoid process) or *pectus excavatum* (funnel chest). Bulging or asymmetry of the chest wall usually indicates an important pathologic condition, such as enlargement of the heart, pneumothorax, phrenic nerve damage, or diaphragmatic hernia.

The *point of maximum cardiac impulse* (PMI) is the position on the chest wall at which the cardiac impulse can be maximally seen. The PMI is usually seen in newborns because of the relatively thin and flexible chest wall. Typically, the PMI is relatively close to the sternal border because of the predominance of the right ventricle in the fetal period. A mediastinal shift due to a pneumothorax will move the PMI away from the affected side of the chest.

With suspected pneumothorax, perform transillumination of the chest wall using a high-energy flashlight or fiberoptic device in a darkened room. Place the light source on the chest wall of the suspected side. A large pneumothorax will reveal an excessively pink and illuminated area of light, or "glowing" area, through the chest wall when compared to the contralateral side.

Heart rate variations from 120 to 170 beats/min may be normal depending on gestational age, as discussed earlier. The rapid rate and rhythm of heart sounds make them difficult to determine. Neonates have a high incidence of arrhythmias in the first few days of life. From 1% to 5% of all newborns exhibit some disturbance in heart rate or rhythm.[9] Many demonstrate "dropped beats," which on evaluation are premature atrial contractions. These episodes are usually benign, but any newborn with an irregular rhythm should have an electrocardiogram (ECG) performed to assess the arrhythmia.

Cardiac *murmurs* are described as a soft to loud, harsh sound similar to a forcible exhalation with the mouth open. Many heart murmurs are transient and not associated with anomalies. Murmurs may be normal after birth and associated with the acute angle at the pulmonary artery bifurcation, patent ductus arteriosus (PDA), or tricuspid regurgitation. However, some murmurs are associated with congenital heart malformations and must be evaluated by chest radiography and echocardiography.

The heart size, shape, and thoracic positioning on chest x-ray film are often helpful in assessing infants with congenital heart disease. Investigate any uncertainty in the variations from a normal radiograph by using other diagnostic radiographic techniques. Other examination procedures, such as a four-limb blood pressure determination, may help to identify anomalies.[10]

Palpating the pulses of the quiet infant often provides important diagnostic information. Weak pulses suggest low cardiac output states such as shock and hypoplastic left-sided heart syndrome. Bounding pulses are seen in infants with PDA and left-to-right shunt (see Chapter 31). The *bounding* characteristic of the pulse results from rapid runoff of the blood into the low-resistance pulmonary circulation. This lowers the systolic blood pressure and produces a wider pulse pressure. Brachial and femoral pulses should be equal in intensity and felt simultaneously. A delayed or weak femoral pulse can indicate coarctation of the aorta.

Comparison of upper and lower extremity blood pressures is frequently helpful in establishing this diagnosis. Normally, lower extremity blood pressure is slightly greater than the pressure in the upper extremities. The recognition and treatment of hypotension are particularly important to avoid complications, such as cerebral ischemic injury and intraventricular hemorrhage.[11] The range of normal blood pressures at various weights has been well established (see Table 5-1). In the absence of data, use Ackerman's law to calculate an adequate *mean blood pressure* (MBP) as follows:

$$\text{Adequate MBP} = \text{Gestational age} + 5$$

For example, an infant of 24 weeks' gestation should have a MBP of approximately 29 mm Hg, and a term newborn, 40 weeks' gestation, should have a MBP of approximately 45 mm Hg.

A pulse oximeter can provide valuable information in the evaluation of the cardiovascular system. Because the sensor of the pulse oximeter is applied to a distal extremity, the oximeter will display a low pulse rate and perfusion signal as peripheral pulses and perfusion decrease. The cause of this poor perfusion must be determined. However, if the oximeter suggests decreased perfusion while central blood pressure remains normal, the cause may be volume depletion with compensatory peripheral vasoconstriction. In addition, placing pulse oximeters on preductal and postductal sites allows for assessing right-to-left ductal level shunting, as seen with persistent pulmonary hypertension of the newborn. In this case the right arm, or *preductal* site, will have a high saturation. The *postductal* site, or left arm and lower extremities, will have a lower saturation because venous admixture occurs after the ductus.

ABDOMEN

Successful abdominal examination requires a calm and quiet infant. Observe the contour of the abdomen, and determine if it is scaphoid, flat, or distended. *Distention* is a significant finding characterized by tightly drawn skin through which you can easily see engorged subcutaneous vessels. Distention can suggest a variety of pathologic conditions, including sepsis, obstruction, tumors, ascites, pneumoperitoneum, or necrotizing enterocolitis. Enterocolitis is a bowel infection characterized by sepsis, peritonitis, bowel perforation, and significant mortality.[12,13] Any of these conditions may cause elevation of the diaphragm and therefore compromise lung expansion.

A scaphoid, hollowed, or unusually flattened abdomen may be associated with *congenital diaphragmatic hernia* (CDH), in which abdominal contents are displaced into the chest through a defect in the muscular diaphragm.[14] More noticeable abnormalities of the abdomen include *prune-belly syndrome,* which is a congenital lack of abdominal musculature (Fig. 5-4); *omphalocele,* a protrusion of the membranous sac that encloses abdominal contents through an opening in the abdominal wall into the umbilical cord; and *gastroschisis,* a defect in the abdominal wall lateral to the midline with protrusion of the intestines.[12,15]

When examining the abdomen, auscultate and palpate over all four quadrants. Bowel sounds are usually heard over the entire abdomen, generally described as a "tinkling" or "rumbling." Because bowel sounds are not continuous, it may take several seconds to hear them. Decreases or increases in the amount or changes in the characteristics of bowel sounds may indicate a pathologic abdominal condition.

The liver is usually felt as a rounded edge that rolls under the lightly palpating hand. Palpation should begin in the right lower quadrant so that an enlarged liver is not missed. The liver edge is

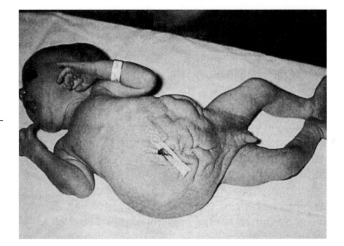

Fig. 5-4

Infant with prune-belly syndrome.

usually easily defined 1 to 2 cm below the right costal margin in newborns. Hepatomegaly may be associated with congenital heart disease, infection, or hemolytic disease.[16] The spleen tip can sometimes be felt overlying the stomach. An easily palpable spleen more than 1 cm below the costal margin may indicate infection and requires further investigation. Abnormalities of the renal system are the most common cause of palpable abdominal masses in the newborn period. Normally the kidneys are felt on deep palpation.

The umbilical cord is yellowish white with three blood vessels. The two small and thick-walled arteries and one large and thin-walled vein are easily visible on the end of a freshly cut cord. Wharton's jelly surrounds the vessels. A single umbilical artery suggests congenital anomalies, especially those of the urinary tract. The presence of meconium in the amniotic fluid causes a greenish yellow staining of the umbilical cord. The umbilical cord of an LGA infant born to a diabetic mother is frequently large and fat. Conversely, infants with intrauterine growth retardation often have thin cords with little Wharton's jelly. With an umbilical hernia the intestinal muscles do not close around the umbilicus, and the intestines protrude into this weakened tissue. Such a defect may require surgery or may resolve without intervention as the muscles become stronger.

HEAD AND NECK

The head is usually the presenting part and often shows evidence of bruising and molding as a result of pressures exerted during the birth process. Molding of the skull with overlapping cranial bones is common. In term infants the molding should resolve within a few days. In addition, edema of the scalp, *caput succedaneum,* may be present. Scalp edema is movable across suture lines and should be distinguished from subperiosteal bleeding, *cephalhematoma,* which does not cross suture lines. The fontanels are the nonossified areas between the cranial bones that make up the skull. The fontanels and suture lines should be soft and should not bulge.[17]

A previously healthy infant who experiences a spongy scalp with a rapidly enlarging head circumference, along with a decreasing hematocrit, has likely developed a *subgaleal bleed.* This serious problem occurs almost exclusively with instrument deliveries. Because blood collects in the scalp, subgaleal bleed is a potential medical emergency because of the potential for hemorrhagic shock. *Craniotabes* are soft skull areas that can be compressed like a Ping-Pong ball and may be a normal finding, especially in premature infants. However, congenital syphilis is also associated with craniotabes.

More than 150,000 children are born with notable birth defects and syndromes in the United States each year.[18] Congenital anomalies are the leading cause of infant mortality in the postneonatal period. Unusual facies may suggest a number of distinct dysmorphic genetic syndromes. *Smith's Recognizable Patterns of Human Malformation* is an invaluable resource in the evaluation of infants with an unusual facies.[19] It also provides standard measurements for the newborn. Facial paralysis or an asymmetric facies is frequently noticed in the otherwise normal-appearing infant. Facial paralysis may be readily apparent only when the infant cries.

The eyes are often swollen and edematous from the birth process. After resolution of the swelling, assess the eyes for excessive spacing and any unusual slant. Apply antibiotic ointment or silver nitrate to the eyes after delivery to prevent infection. In infants older than 28 weeks of gestation, the pupils should be round, regular, and should react to light. Examine the fundi of the eyes with an ophthalmoscope. In white infants the light ("cat's eye") reflex should be red. In Asian and black infants it is gray to yellow. A white reflex suggests cataracts or retinoblastoma, necessitating a complete ophthalmologic examination.

Examine the ears for placement and deformation. Deformed, posteriorly rotated, or low-set ears are associated with various anomalies. Consider ears low set when the upper insertion of the ear is below the level of a line drawn through the corner of the orbits of the eyes. The ears are abnormally rotated if the slope of the auricle is greater than 10 degrees. The preauricular area frequently has tags containing cartilage. Although these tags are benign, they are a minor embryonic branchial cleft malformation. However, infants with preauricular tags have a higher incidence of additional branchial cleft abnormalities.

Newborns breathe preferentially through the nose, so alternately occlude each side and listen to breath sounds to assess the patency of each nostril. If the infant appears to be breathing comfortably, many nurseries no longer attempt to pass catheters because nasal trauma, obstruction, and edema are serious risks. An oral airway or endotracheal tube is often required if bilateral choanal atresia, the incomplete opening into the nasopharynx due to membranous or bony structures, is present.

Abnormalities of the mouth, lips, and oral cavity are seen in many infants. *Microstomia,* small mouth, is commonly seen in infants with the chromosomal defect trisomy 18, whereas midfacial clefts, cleft lip and palate, are frequently seen with trisomy 13. Pierre Robin syndrome is characterized by a cleft palate, posteriorly displaced tongue, and *micrognathia,* a small lower jaw. An artificial airway may be required in this condition to ensure an unobstructed airway. In previous years these infants were all thought to be congenitally mentally impaired. However, chronic hypoxia from airway obstruction has been recognized as a significant contributor to the retardation in these infants.[20]

Examination of the oral cavity and pharynx for less obvious palatal clefts, mucous cysts, Epstein's pearls, or natal teeth can be performed with a flashlight or laryngoscope blade light. A bifid uvula or no uvula can occur in normal infants but is often associated with a hidden cleft of the soft palate. A high-arched or cleft palate is associated with many syndromes. Excessive oral secretions may indicate the presence of a tracheoesophageal fistula or esophageal atresia.

Examine the neck for obvious shortening, vertebral anomalies, or limitations in movement. A variety of cysts, hygromas, sinuses, and masses may be present laterally or in the midline. Large neck lesions may apply pressure to the trachea and impair breathing.

The clavicles are often broken during the delivery process of large infants with shoulder dystocias or in breech deliveries. Frequently the injury is noted when the infant refuses to move the affected shoulder. The break is usually easily palpable as an area of crepitus overlying the bone. Therapy is usually not necessary for fractured clavicles in the newborn because they heal without intervention.

MUSCULOSKELETAL SYSTEM, SPINE, AND EXTREMITIES

The intrauterine environment frequently affects the extremities and musculoskeletal system. Many limb and other deformations in the fetus result from intrinsic (fetal) or extrinsic (uterine) factors.[19]

Extra digits may be familial or may be associated with a number of syndromes. They can be present on hands or feet, or both. The digits can vary from fully formed and articulated to simple skin tags. Variations in dermatoglyphic patterns, such as skin folds, palm print, and fingerprint, are frequently noted. The most widely known is the *simian crease,* a single transverse crease across the palm instead of the usual two creases. Simian creases are seen in several disorders, including Down syndrome, but are also found in 5% to 10% of normal individuals.

Joint contractures or abnormal positioning of one or more limbs may result from a fetal problem or intrauterine compression. Clubfoot, *talipes equinovarus,* is a typical example.[21,22] An isolated joint-extremity malformation suggests extrinsic factors, whereas multiple deformations are more often seen with primary fetal neurologic or muscular diseases.

The symmetry and bony structure of the spine are easily examined in the newborn. Suspend the infant in a prone position with one hand, then visually and digitally evaluate the structures. Many infants have a small indentation (sacral dimple) near the end of the spine. If the bottom of the dimple is easily seen without associated bony defects, no further evaluation is required. However, if the defect cannot be fully visualized or if there are bony defects, associated tufts of hair, or drainage of clear fluid, further evaluation is required. A few infants have the congenital malformations collectively called *spina bifida* (Fig. 5-5). These defects result from failure of the embryonic neural tube to form correctly in the third to fifth week of gestation. The defects usually involve bone, skin, the covering of the central nervous system *(meninges)*, and nerve tissue. Defects that occur over the spine are called *myelomeningoceles,* and those involving the brain are called *encephaloceles* (Fig. 5-6).

It is important to evaluate the hips of all infants even if there is no evidence of asymmetry or other bone, joint, or muscular problems. Stabilize the pelvis on a flat surface while the joint is flexed and abducted to the surface. A telescoping feeling or the presence of a "clunk" suggests congenital laxity or dislocation of the hip.[22] Frequently, several days must pass before the hips of infants born in the breech position can be appropriately evaluated.

CRY

After the examiner has obtained some newborn experience, it is impressive how much information something as simple as a baby's cry can provide. A loud and vigorous cry is usually a sign of a healthy infant. A moaning, weak, or faint cry suggests serious illness. Frequently, an infant with RDS strains with a grunting cry. An infant with a piercing, high-pitched cry often has a neurologic injury, drug withdrawal, or increased intracranial pressure. Hoarse crying can be associated with laryngeal edema, as in recently extubated infants. However, a hoarse cry may also be heard with congenital hypothyroidism, cretinism, or hypocalcemia with laryngospasm. Perhaps the most distinctive cry is associated with a deletion of the short arm of the fifth chromosome. The catlike cry of these infants gives the syndrome the name *cri du chat,* French for "cry of the cat."

NEUROLOGIC ASSESSMENT

The general neurologic state of the infant is assessed during much of the physical examination.

Note whether the infant responds appropriately to the surroundings or if the neonate is lethargic or overly irritable. It is also important to determine if the infant moves all extremities and if the movements are symmetric and smooth or jittery and jerky. Infants with evidence of difficult delivery may manifest signs of extremity weakness associated with trauma to the brachial plexus.

Pick the neonate up under the arms to assess muscle tone in the term infant. A normal infant will suspend well. An infant with decreased tone will noodle through the hands. Infants with normal tone will maintain their extremities in a flexed position at rest.

A number of reflexes are present in the newborn. Everyone has observed the *grasp reflex,* in which the newborn infant grasps a finger placed in the palm of the hand. A similar downward curving of the toes occurs if a finger is pressed against the sole of the foot; this is referred to as the *plantar grasp reflex.* The startle reaction to sound or touch is similar to the *Moro reflex,* which occurs when the head is allowed to fall back slightly. The normal term infant's extremities will extend rapidly with open hands. The neonate will then slowly flex them back toward the body. Infants will respond to a bright light by shutting their eyelids tight. They will often turn toward unique sounds or sights and may focus on objects, especially faces. Suspending the infant and touching the top of the foot against a surface can demonstrate the *stepping reflex.* The infant should lift the leg and then place it flat on the surface.[23]

Significant hearing loss at birth is common and if undetected can interfere with the development of speech and language. The American Academy of Pediatrics endorses hearing evaluation in the newborn period using auditory-evoked brain wave responses or otoacoustic response.[24] Many physi-

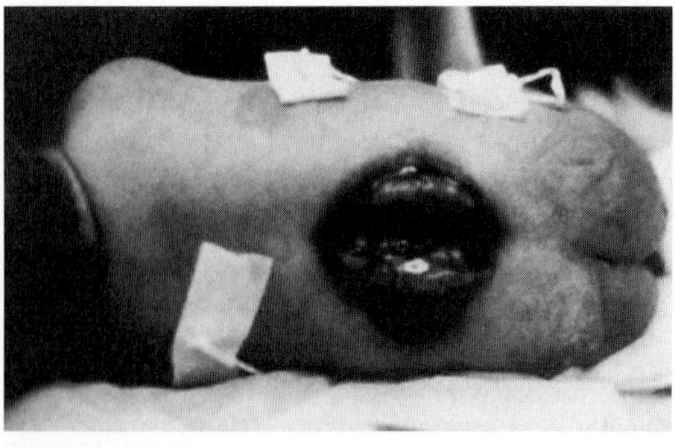

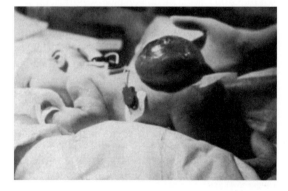

Fig. 5-5

Infant with an open spinal defect.

Fig. 5-6

Infant with myelomeningocele.

cians and hospitals routinely screen some or all infants before discharge.

LABORATORY ASSESSMENT

Routine laboratory studies play a limited but important role in the immediate newborn period. Most laboratory abnormalities seen in the first 24 hours of life result from sepsis, abnormally high or low levels of red blood cells (RBCs), RBC isoimmunization, or temporary derangement in the regulation of glucose metabolism.

Infection is one of the most common problems in newborns. The diagnosis and initial therapy of neonatal sepsis are frequently based on clinical presentation and are seldom delayed until laboratory test results are available. The septic baby is often pale, mottled, or floppy. Some may lose interest in feeding, be slightly irritable, or even unresponsive. A typical sepsis evaluation includes blood cultures and a complete blood count. Many physicians also include lumbar puncture for cerebrospinal fluid and suprapubic aspiration for urine.[25] The advisability or necessity of these last two tests in the typical newborn is not clear.

The white blood cell (WBC) count of the newborn is usually significantly higher than pediatric or adult values. *Leukopenia,* WBCs less than 3500/mm^3, and *leukocytosis,* WBCs greater than 25,000/mm^3, suggest infection. WBCs greater than 25,000/mm^3, however, are not unusual in the immediate newborn period. A number of investigators have studied ratios of immature to total granulocytes and have suggested that ratios greater than approximately 0.2:1 are predictive of infection. Similarly, the absolute number of platelets is associated with fetal/neonatal infection. A platelet count of less than 150,000 cells/mm^3 is abnormally low and usually seen with acute or chronic infections. Platelets are also decreased in a widespread disorder of the clotting system called *disseminated intravascular coagulation* (DIC). Overstimulation of the coagula-

tion system leads to depletion of many coagulation factors and a generalized coagulation abnormality.

The newborn infant tends to have increased *hemoglobin* and *hematocrit* levels at birth. The fetus requires extra hemoglobin to maintain appropriate oxygen transport in the relatively low oxygen pressure of the fetal environment. The newborn's hematocrit is affected by many factors, including gestational age, the presence of placental abnormalities, the speed and mode of delivery, and the length of time after delivery that the infant remains attached to the placenta (with or without cord stripping by the obstetrician). Table 5-4 lists the range of normal values for newborns.

A number of biochemical and metabolic evaluations are performed in neonates. Electrolyte determinations, renal function tests, and calcium levels are typically measured after the first 12 to 24 hours of life in sick or at-risk neonates. There is little value in performing these measurements earlier because the infant's serum levels reflect those of the mother at birth. Conversely, glucose measurements are important for many infants in the first minutes to hours of life. Many newborns are at risk for hypoglycemia, and screening is performed routinely in most nurseries. Bilirubin should be measured in infants who are significantly jaundiced. Some hospitals routinely perform blood typing on cord blood and Coombs' tests to determine if there is evidence of neonatal RBC hemolysis from maternal antibodies.

All states operate newborn programs that mandate mass screening of all newborns for uncommon metabolic diseases. These programs have proved effective in preventing mental retardation associated with unusual metabolic diseases such as congenital hypothyroidism.

Box 5-1 lists clinical symptoms, laboratory abnormalities, and physical signs that may be found in newborns. These "red flags" should alert the examiner and clinician to investigate further.

TABLE 5-4	LABORATORY VALUES IN THE NEONATAL PATIENT			
Age	Hgb (g/dl)	Hct (%)	WBCs*	Platelets*
28 weeks' gestation	14.5	45	—	275
32 weeks' gestation	15	47	—	290
Term newborn	16.5	51	18.1	310
1-3 days	18.5	56	18.9	300

Data from Oski FA, Naiman JL: *Hematological problems in the newborn infant.* Philadelphia, Saunders, 1981.
Hgb, Hemoglobin; *Hct,* hematocrit; *WBCs,* white blood cells.
*1000 cells/mm^3.

BOX 5-1

"RED FLAGS" IN NEONATAL PATIENTS

RESPIRATORY
Respiratory rate >60 breaths/min
Grunting or retractions
Cyanosis
Apnea

CARDIAC
Heart rate >170 or <90 beats/min
New heart murmur
Cyanosis
Hypotension
Decreased or no pulse

RENAL
Edema
Anuria (no urine)
Oliguria (decreased urine output)
No urine in first 24 hours

GASTROINTESTINAL
Abdominal distention
Bile-stained vomitus
Abdominal mass

GASTROINTESTINAL—cont'd
Bloody stools
Failure to pass stool in first 48 hours

METABOLIC
Vomiting
Diarrhea
Jitteriness
Seizures
Jaundice on first day
Hypoglycemia

GENERAL
Lethargy
Poor feeding
"Not acting right"
Floppy
Cord blood pH <7.2
Low Apgar score
Small for gestational age
Large for gestational age
Minor congenital anomalies

Modified from Ackerman NB, Curran JS: The newborn. In Kaye R, Oski FA, Bainars LA, editors: *Textbook of pediatrics.* Philadelphia, Lippincott, 1988.

REFERENCES

1. Donovan E et al: Inaccuracy of Ballard scores before 28 weeks' gestation. *J Pediatr* 1999; 135:147-152.
2. Sanders M et al: Gestational age assessment in preterm neonates weighing less than 1500 grams. *Pediatrics* 1991; 88(3):542-546.
3. Ballard JL et al: New Ballard score to include extremely premature infants. *J Pediatr* 1991; 199(3):417-423.
4. Thomas P et al: A new look at intrauterine growth and the impact of race, altitude, and gender. *Pediatrics* 2000; 106(2):e21.
5. Dunster K: Physiologic variability in the perinatal period. *Clin Perinatol* 1999; 26(4):801-809.
6. Bhutani V et al: Noninvasive measurement of total serum bilirubin in a multiracial predischarge newborn population to assess the risk of severe hyperbilirubinemia. *Pediatrics* 2000; 106(2):e17.
7. Rigatto H, Brady JP: Periodic breathing and apnea in preterm infants: hypoxia as a primary event. *Pediatrics* 1972; 50:219-228.
8. Ackerman NB, Bell RE, DeLemos RA: Differential pulmonary auscultation in neonates. *Clin Pediatr* 1982; 21:566-567.
9. Page J, Hosking M: An approach to the neonate with sudden dysrhythmia: diagnosis, mechanisms, and management. *Neonat Network* 1997; 16(6):7-18.
10. Monett ZJ, Moynihan PJ: Cardiovascular assessment of the neonatal heart. *J Perinat Neonat Nurs* 1991; 5:50-59.
11. Nuntnarumit P, Yang W, Bada-Ellzey H: Blood pressure measurements in the newborn. *Clin Perinatol* 1999; 26(4):981-996.
12. Chahine A, Ricketts R: Resuscitation of the surgical neonate. *Clin Perinatol* 1999; 26(3):693-713.
13. Reyes HM, Meller JL, Loeff D: Neonatal intestinal obstruction. *Clin Perinatol* 1989; 16:85-111.
14. Thebaud B, Mercier JC, Dinh-Xuan AT: Congenital diaphragmatic hernia: a cause of persistent pulmonary hypertension of the newborn which lacks an effective therapy. *Biol Neonate* 1998; 74(5):323-336.
15. Blakelock RT et al: Gastroschisis: can the mortality be avoided? *Pediatr Surg Int* 1997; 12(4):276-282.
16. Thureen P et al: *Assessment and care of the well newborn.* Philadelphia, Saunders, 1999.
17. Popich GA, Smith DW: Fontanels: range of normal size. *J Pediatr* 1972; 80:749-752.
18. Bodurtha J: Assessment of the newborn with dysmorphic features. *Neonat Network* 1999; 18(2):27-30.
19. Jones KL: *Smith's recognizable patterns of human malformation,* ed 4. Philadelphia, Saunders, 1988.
20. Dennison WM: The Pierre Robin syndrome. *Pediatrics* 1965; 36:336.
21. Hashimoto BE, Filly RA, Callen PW: Sonographic diagnosis of clubfoot in utero. *J Ultrasound Med* 1986; 5:81-83.
22. Fernach S: Common orthopedic problems of the newborn. *Nurs Clin North Am* 1998; 33(4):583-594.
23. Majnemer A et al: A comparison of neurobehavioral performance of healthy term and low risk pre-term infants at term. *Dev Med Child Neurol* 1992; 34:417-424.
24. Task Force on Newborn and Infant Screening, American Academy of Pediatrics: Newborn and infant hearing loss: detection and intervention. *Pediatrics* 1999; 103(2): 527-530.
25. Horns K: Neoteric, physiologic and immunologic methods for assessing early-onset neonatal sepsis. *J Perinat Neonat Nurs* 2000; 13(4):50-66.

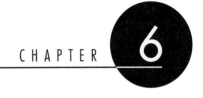

CHAPTER **6**

Examination and Assessment of the Pediatric Patient

Paul C. Stillwell

The respiratory care practitioner (RCP) has an ever-expanding role in the clinical practice of pediatrics and therefore must be prepared to contribute accurate historical and physical findings to the health care team.[1] This input can be valuable in the intensive care unit, hospital ward, laboratory setting, and outpatient clinic.

This chapter reviews key points in the patient history and physical examination that will prepare the RCP to provide appropriate information for the evaluation and treatment of children with respiratory disturbances. Because the history is the primary tool that provides diagnostic information in pulmonary medicine, the RCP will spend considerable effort enhancing history-taking skills.

PATIENT HISTORY

Although some patients have an established diagnosis when they encounter the RCP, others may be new patients who present with a specific complaint. An example of the diagnosed patient is the child admitted to the ward for treatment of a cystic fibrosis (CF) exacerbation. An example of the new patient is the child who comes to the office or clinic for evaluation of cough and chest pain. In either case, careful and detailed history taking can help select a form of treatment or change the course of treatment.[2,3]

CHIEF COMPLAINT

For the new patient the initial agenda item is establishment of a chief complaint or primary concern. Additional information is then sought, including duration of symptoms, intensity or severity, and improvement or deterioration. Aggravating or alleviating factors, including medication trials, may

---

BOX 6-1

STRUCTURE OF HISTORY TAKING FOR THE PEDIATRIC PATIENT

1. Chief complaint or primary reason for the visit
2. Details of the chief complaint
   a. Duration
   b. Diurnal variation
   c. Change over time: better, worse, same
3. Aggravating factors or triggers
4. Alleviating factors
   a. Avoidance
   b. Medicine trials (and failures)
5. Associations with the chief complaint
6. Prior evaluations (if any)

BOX 6-2

HISTORY TAKING IN THE PEDIATRIC PATIENT WITH ASTHMA

MANIFESTATIONS
Cough
Wheeze
Dyspnea

AGGRAVATING FACTORS
Upper respiratory tract infections
Exercise or activity
Allergens or exposures
Irritants
Emotions

ALLEVIATING FACTORS
Bronchodilators
Avoidance
Failed medication trials (antibiotics, decongestants, humidification)

ASSOCIATED CONDITIONS
Atopy: rhinitis, eczema, urticaria
Dysphagia, dyspepsia, emesis
Steatorrhea, growth parameters, recurrent pneumonia
Snoring
Tuberculosis exposure
Foreign body aspiration

FAMILY HISTORY
Atopic diseases: asthma, rhinitis, eczema, urticaria, food allergy
Cystic fibrosis
α_1-Antiprotease deficiency
Infertile males
Dextrocardia
Immunodeficiency states

ENVIRONMENTAL EXPOSURES
Pets
Tobacco smoke

---

help narrow the differential diagnosis. Identification of associated factors may help link the symptom to a generalized systemic disease[2,3] (Box 6-1). The following example clarifies the importance of this approach.

A 6-year-old girl is brought by her mother to the pulmonary office because of recurrent pneumonia. This establishes the chief complaint. With only this information the RCP faces an extensive differential diagnosis that might include CF, immunocompromise, aspiration, chronic infection, and asthma. Further questioning reveals that the child has had at least one episode of pneumonia in each of the last 4 years, usually in the winter months. Her symptoms during the acute illness include cough, fever, and dyspnea. Only one of the pneumonias resulted in hospitalization. The patient recovered completely between episodes.

At this point the RCP needs to pursue additional history. The girl's growth has been good, and she does not have frequent greasy bowel movements, making CF less likely. Her mother is healthy and has no acquired immunodeficiency syndrome (AIDS) risk factors, making AIDS less likely. Each of the pneumonia episodes started with a common cold, often accompanied by wheezing. The patient has had occasional coughing when exposed to irritating smells such as cigarette smoke and cold air. During one emergency department visit she received nebulized medication, which greatly relieved her respiratory distress. This finding suggests that her primary disease might be asthma (Box 6-2).

The child has had no recognized exposure to tuberculosis and no foreign body aspiration history. She denies swallowing difficulty, frequent emesis, or heartburn. She has had a red itchy rash in the elbow and knee regions in the past that her mother thinks is eczema, but the patient has not had urticaria. The associated atopic history also points to asthma as the underlying explanation for the pneumonias.

MEDICAL HISTORY

The past medical history is another important component of history taking. If the child was born prematurely and required ventilatory support, bronchopulmonary dysplasia or chronic lung disease might be a consideration. The immunization history, prior hospitalizations, and previous surgeries should be identified for potential contribution to diagnosis.

FAMILY HISTORY

The family history may also reveal valuable clues. For the 6-year-old girl in the case example, her older brother had suffered from asthma as a young child; there was no recognized CF, infertile males, dextrocardia, immunodeficiency, or α_1-antiprotease deficiency. This further supports asthma as a potential cause of her recurrent pneumonia.

ENVIRONMENTAL HISTORY

Environmental factors should be explored during the history taking. Environmental tobacco exposure and personal smoking can have enormous impact on pulmonary health during childhood.[4] The deleterious effects of tobacco smoke have led some to suggest that the question about tobacco exposure should be part of the routine assessment of vital signs.

The travel history may identify an unsuspected exposure risk. For example, travel to the Sonoran Desert of the southwestern United States may suggest coccidioidomycosis infection. Adult visitors to the child's home from areas endemic for tuberculosis place the child at risk. Exposure to pets in the child's environment may suggest an immunoglobulin E allergic reaction or similar immunologic response, such as hypersensitivity pneumonitis or extrinsic allergic alveolitis.

INTERVIEW AND FOLLOW-UP

For patients with an established diagnosis or prior visits, the history is still vital to maintaining lung health. Rather than focus on a diagnosis, the emphasis is on interim health. Questions are directed toward stability, improvement, or deterioration. Compliance with and understanding of the treatment plan should be reviewed carefully; this is also an excellent opportunity to provide reinforcement of patient and family education.

If the patient's symptoms are worse or less well controlled, the RCP should seek an explanation. Often the medications have been "forgotten" or used less frequently than originally prescribed. Occasionally an upper respiratory tract infection may have caused an exacerbation of the primary disease.[5] If an explanation is not easily forthcoming, the RCP should take a more detailed history similar to the initial history.

The specific series of questions at the interim visit is generally tailored to the primary disease. For example, an asthmatic follow-up visit might focus on exercise tolerance, nocturnal symptoms, and frequency of use of rescue medications.

BOX 6-3

STRUCTURE OF PULMONARY EXAMINATION FOR THE PEDIATRIC PATIENT

INSPECTION
Vital signs including respiratory rate and pulse oximetry
Color
Work of breathing
Retractions or head bobbing
Clubbing of digits
Perfusion
Chest wall shape and excursion with deep breathing
Allergic shiners

PALPATION
Anterior neck for masses and midline trachea
Quantity of muscle mass
Tactile fremitus

PERCUSSION
Dullness
Hyperresonance
Symmetry

AUSCULTATION
Intensity of breath sounds
Symmetry from homologous segment to segment
Adventitious sounds: stridor, wheezing, crackles (fine, coarse)
Phase delays: inspiration, expiration

PULMONARY EXAMINATION

The pulmonary examination consists of inspection, palpation, percussion, and auscultation[2,3] (Box 6-3). The "rush to the stethoscope" often bypasses important information that can be gleaned from inspection, palpation, and percussion. The inspection component starts almost subconsciously at the initiation of contact with the child.

INSPECTION

Inspection begins with determining if the patient is experiencing respiratory distress. Respiratory distress consists of one or more of the following: tachypnea, retractions, and cyanosis.

The respiratory rate is a sensitive indicator of underlying lung disease or health.[6-8] The respiratory rate varies widely by age and activity level; the best time to measure the rate is when the patient is asleep or resting quietly (Table 6-1).[9] Fever usually increases the respiratory rate, so the child with fever but no respiratory disturbance may appear to have respiratory distress.

Head bobbing, caused by sternocleidomastoid accessory muscle contraction, is a sign of increased respiratory distress in babies (Fig. 6-1). *Retractions* are the inward pulling of the soft tissue and skin between or below the ribs or above the sternum (Figs. 6-2 to 6-4). Paradoxical inward motion of the chest with concomitant outward movement of the abdominal wall indicates upper airway obstruction. With the sleeping patient, snoring and retractions may be the best clue to upper airway dysfunction. Fussiness, irritability, or somnolence may be signs of significant respiratory disturbance.

TABLE 6-1	NORMAL RESPIRATORY RATES IN SLEEPING AND AWAKE PEDIATRIC PATIENTS					
	Sleeping			**Awake**		
Age	**No. Studied**	**Mean**	**Range**	**No. Studied**	**Mean**	**Range**
6-12 mo	6	27	22-31	3	64	58-75
1-2 yr	6	19	17-23	4	35	30-40
2-4 yr	16	19	16-25	15	31	23-42
4-6 yr	23	18	14-23	22	26	19-36
6-8 yr	27	17	13-23	28	23	15-30
8-10 yr	19	18	14-23	19	21	15-31
10-12 yr	11	16	13-19	17	21	15-28
12-14 yr	6	16	15-18	7	22	18-26

From Iliff A, Lee VA: Pulse rate, respiratory rate, and body temperature of children between two months and eighteen years of age. *Child Dev* 1952; 23:237.

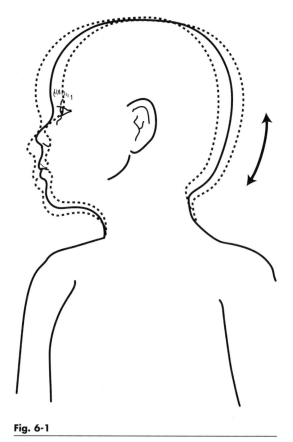

Fig. 6-1

Head bobbing.

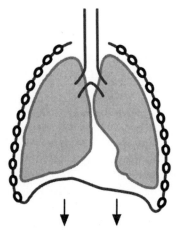

Intercostal muscles with normal negative pleural pressure during inhalation

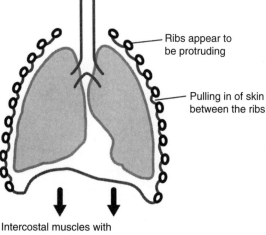

Ribs appear to be protruding

Pulling in of skin between the ribs

Intercostal muscles with abnormal negative pleural pressure during inhalation

Fig. 6-2

Intercostal retractions. Soft tissue between the ribs is pulled inward (retracted) because of the extremely high negative pleural pressure.

Examine the shape of the chest wall with the patient unclothed. Chronic obstructive diseases such as CF and bronchopulmonary dysplasia may produce an increase in the anteroposterior diameter of the chest wall. Note restrictive chest wall shapes, such as pectus carinatum or pectus excavatum (see Chapter 5). It is important to inspect the chest wall from the back as well as the front because scoliosis or kyphosis may also contribute to chest wall restriction. Assess the muscle mass of the chest wall and neck for weakness as a cause of the respiratory problems. Excessive adipose tissue around the neck, chest, and abdomen may contribute to restrictive disease.

Inspect the fingers and toes for evidence of clubbing with every patient in pulmonary clinic. *Digital clubbing* is associated with chronic, usually severe, respiratory diseases such as CF (Fig. 6-5). Clubbing may also be found with congenital heart disease and liver disease.[10] If a patient with asthma is noted to have digital clubbing, the diagnosis should be reevaluated.

Examine the skin for evidence of poor circulation, hemangiomas, and telangiectasias, which may suggest extrapulmonary diseases associated with respiratory dysfunction. Inspection of the ears, nose, and throat is part of the respiratory assessment and is usually performed by the physician with the aid of an otoscope or flashlight. Purulent nasal secretions, edematous dusky nasal mucosa, or postnasal drip may indicate significant upper airway disease contributing to the patient's symptoms, particularly cough.

PALPATION

Palpation of the respiratory system is becoming a less prominent diagnostic tool with the increased availability and use of imaging techniques. Palpating chest wall excursion with voluntary deep inspiration can help separate normal from restrictive defects. *Tactile fremitus,* the palpation of vocal sounds over the chest wall, may be increased over areas of the chest wall corresponding to underlying lung infiltrates.

Palpation of the tissues around the chest may lead to important findings. Palpate the anterior neck to ensure that the trachea is in the midline (Fig. 6-6) and that no masses or adenopathy are compressing the adjacent airway. The supraclavicular space, axillae, and inguinal regions are palpated for signs of adenopathy, malignancy, or infection.

PERCUSSION

Percussion, or the tapping over the chest wall, is also becoming a less common diagnostic tool. The percussion note will be hyperresonant over areas of

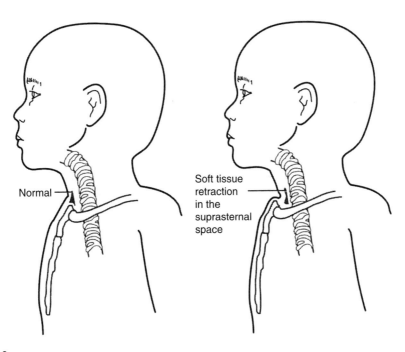

Fig. 6-3

Suprasternal retractions. Soft tissue in the suprasternal space is retracted because of high negative pressure, most often caused by the patient's attempt to breathe against an airway obstruction.

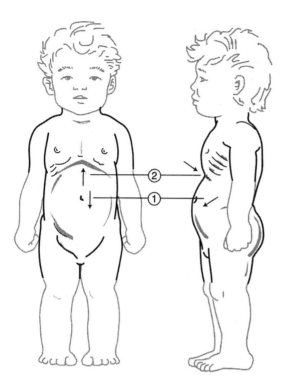

Fig. 6-4

Subcostal/substernal retractions. Airway obstruction results in a pulling inward of the lower costal margins. The abdomen is protruding (*1*), and there is a sunken substernal notch (*2*). Seesaw movement of the chest and stomach is also present.

air trapping and overinflation. This sound is usually diffuse in chronic obstructive disease such as CF, but it may be localized with segmental obstruction, as with foreign body aspiration. The percussion note is dull over infiltrates or effusions. The sound is a good noninvasive marker that can be done serially to assess an increase or decrease in the pleural fluid level.

AUSCULTATION

Auscultation is performed with the naked ear as well as the stethoscope. In general, abnormal sounds such as stridor or wheezing heard without the aid of the stethoscope signify more severe airflow obstruction than the same sounds heard only with the stethoscope. Because auscultation with the stethoscope may be frightening to small children, perform it early in the examination to avoid trying to listen with the child crying or screaming. Auscultate before any potentially painful examination is performed, such as examining the ears.

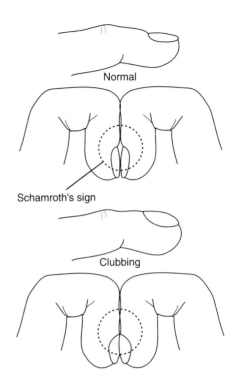

Fig. 6-5

Schamroth's sign is useful for bedside assessment of digital clubbing. The dorsal surfaces of the terminal phalanges of similar fingers are placed together. With clubbing the normal diamond-shaped "window" at the bases of the nailbeds disappears, and a prominent distal angle forms between the ends of the nails. This angle is minimal or nonexistent in normal children. (Redrawn from Pasterkamp H: The history and physical examination. In Chernick V, editor: *Kendig's disorders of the respiratory tract in children,* ed 5. Philadelphia, Saunders, 1990.)

During the auscultation with the stethoscope, intensity of breath sounds should be assessed and any asymmetry noted. If there are isolated areas of abnormal intensity (usually decreased), percussion should be performed over the same area. The duration of the inspiratory and expiratory phases should be assessed. Prolonged inspiration is associated with upper airway obstruction, and prolongation of the expiratory phase is associated with intrathoracic obstruction. Clinical examples of prolonged inspiration include infectious laryngotracheobronchitis and subglottic stenosis. Asthma is the most common illness that accounts for a prolonged expiratory phase.

Adventitious sounds include stridor, crackles, and wheezing.[11] *Stridor* is a low-pitched monophonic sound usually heard on inspiration and

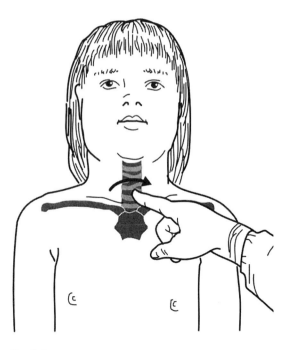

Fig. 6-6

Technique for determining tracheal position in the older child.

usually loudest over the neck and upper sternal region. Most often, stridor is caused by turbulent flow from upper airway obstruction. Stridor should be categorized as high or low pitched and present on inspiration, expiration, or both. High-pitched stridor heard on both inspiration and expiration and associated with retractions is an indication of severe airway obstruction that requires immediate attention.

The terminology describing crackles has been confusing.[11] Also called rales and rhonchi, *crackles* are now categorized as *fine* and *coarse*. Fine crackles (*rales*) are caused by distal airway or alveolar disease such as pneumonia or pulmonary edema. Coarse crackles (*rhonchi*) are caused by more central airway disease such as bronchitis. Fine crackles are most often heard on inspiration as the negative inspiratory pressure pulls open small airways. Coarse crackles can be heard on either inspiration or expiration or both. As acute severe asthma improves and wheezing begins to disappear, coarse crackles are often heard on expiration. Rubbing hair between fingers close to the ear can mimic the sound of fine crackles, which can help the student learn how to listen for crackles through a stethoscope. The part of the respiratory cycle where crackles are heard should be identified.

BOX 6-4
NONPULMONARY FINDINGS ASSOCIATED WITH PULMONARY DISEASE

INTEGUMENTARY SYSTEM
Eczema, urticaria
Telangiectasia, hemangioma

MUSCULOSKELETAL SYSTEM
Scoliosis, kyphosis
Muscle atrophy
Clubbing, arthritis
Edema

CARDIOPULMONARY SYSTEM
Murmurs
Abnormal rhythm
Augmented pulmonic component of the second heart sound

GASTROINTESTINAL SYSTEM
Abdominal distention
Bowel sounds

LYMPH NODE ENLARGEMENT

Wheezing is a polyphonic musical sound that is often high pitched. It is a hallmark sound associated with asthma. Although usually heard on expiration, wheezing can also be heard on inspiration. Wheezing on both inspiration and expiration in the asthmatic patient is an indication of severe obstruction. Wheezing over an isolated segment or lobe may be the cardinal finding with foreign body aspiration. Expiratory wheezing is often associated with prolongation of the expiratory phase.

NONPULMONARY EXAMINATION

Examination of nonpulmonary systems may reveal pertinent information that relates directly to the pulmonary dysfunction (Box 6-4). Eczema and urticaria suggest allergic diseases. Tachycardia, heart murmurs, gallop rhythm, peripheral edema, or an augmented pulmonic second heart sound may identify heart disease as the cause of respiratory difficulty. Abdominal distention can impair diaphragmatic excursion and cause tachypnea.

LABORATORY TESTING

After the history and examination are completed, laboratory tests are considered to corroborate the initial findings (Box 6-5). Pulse oximetry has become commonly available and is often obtained with the patient's vital signs.[12] Laboratory tests typically performed on respiratory disease patients include chest radiographs, pulmonary function testing, and blood gas analysis (arterial, venous, capillary).

More complex tests of potential benefit include bronchoscopy, computed tomography, and angiography. Rarely, lung biopsy is required, which can be done by the transbronchial approach, video-assisted thoracoscopy, or thoracotomy. Polysomnography is performed to evaluate obstructive sleep apnea or sleep-disordered breathing. Provocation testing (methacholine, histamine, exercise, cold air, inhaled allergen) may be performed to evaluate bronchial hyperreactivity.[13]

WORKING AS A TEAM MEMBER

The RCP often has an opportunity to interact with the patient in a different atmosphere than the nurse or physician. The practitioner may have several minutes for additional history taking during nebulized medication administration, while performing chest percussion, or during pulmonary function testing. The RCP is in a unique position to repeat physical examinations during contact with the patient, such as before and after bronchodilator therapy. Additional history or examination findings should be recorded in the medical record and communicated verbally to the appropriate health care members. This valuable information may help change the diagnosis or therapy.

The following examples demonstrate how the RCP's participation can have an important impact on the pulmonary health of children under their care.

CASE 1

A 6-year-old asthmatic patient was undergoing pulmonary function testing during a follow-up asthma clinic visit. She reported to the pulmonary nurse that her asthma had been under worse control over the past 2 months, especially during exercise and at night. The attending physician was prepared to prescribe a short course of oral prednisone and double the baseline dose of the inhaled corticosteroid. During the administration of the inhaled bronchodilator as part of the pulmonary function test, the RCP noticed that the metered-dose inhaler technique was quite poor (despite prior demonstration of correct technique). Further questioning identified that the spacing device prescribed to improve aerosol deposition had been "lost" several weeks ago. Neither the patient nor her family realized the significance of this "loss." After discovering this, the RCP told the asthma team about her concerns that neither the inhaled steroids nor the bronchodilators were likely to be optimally deposited in the lower airways. Rather than increase the patient's exposure to corticosteroids, inhaler technique was reviewed and another spacing device prescribed. Both the patient and her mother were reeducated about the importance of compliance.

In this example the RCP's participation with the health care team helped avoid unnecessary additional medications.

CASE 2

A 7-month-old infant was admitted to the intermediate care unit because of severe wheezing and respiratory distress, believed to be caused by respiratory syncytial virus (RSV) bronchiolitis. Albuterol nebulizations were ordered every 1 hour as well as supplemental oxygen to keep oxygen saturation on pulse oximetry greater than 93%. The RCP administering the albuterol nebulizations noted little or no improvement in the wheezing and found that 4 L/min were required to maintain oxygen saturation within the ordered parameter. The astute RCP called the admitting resident to obtain a suctioning order to clear nasal secretions, which allowed only 1 L/min to meet the saturation criteria. The RCP also asked the resident to consider racemic epinephrine rather than albuterol. The nebulized racemic epinephrine reduced the child's respiratory rate and decreased the wheezing.[14]

In this example the RCP's participation improved the treatment and outcome for the patient by sharing observations and knowledge with the health care team.

REFERENCES

1. Stoller JK: Why therapist driven protocols? A balanced view. *Respir Care* 1994; 39:706-707.
2. Pasterkamp H: The history and physical examination. In Chernick V, Boat TF, editors: *Kendig's disorders of the respiratory tract in children*. Philadelphia, Saunders, 1998, pp 85-106.
3. Brown MA, Morgan WJ: Clinical assessment and diagnostic approach to common problems. In Taussig LM, Landau LI, editors: *Pediatric respiratory medicine*. St Louis, Mosby, 1999, pp 136-152.
4. Committee on Environmental Health: Environmental tobacco smoke: a hazard to children. *Pediatrics* 1997; 99:639-642.
5. Glezen WP et al: Impact of respiratory virus infections on persons with chronic underlying conditions. *JAMA* 2000; 283:499-505.
6. Morley CJ et al: Respiratory rate and severity of illness in babies under 6 months old. *Arch Dis Child* 1990; 65: 834-842.
7. Harari M et al: Clinical signs of pneumonia in children. *Lancet* 1991; 338:928-930.
8. Margolis P, Gadomski A: Does this infant have pneumonia? *JAMA* 1998; 279:308-313.
9. Liff A, Lee VA: Pulse rate, respiratory rate, and body temperature of children between two months and eighteen years of age. *Child Dev* 1952; 23:237.
10. Alberts WM, Moser KM: A clinician's guide to clubbing. *J Respir Dis* 1981(November); pp 17-21.
11. Ward JJ. Lung sounds: easy to hear, hard to describe. *Respir Care* 1989; 34:17-19.
12. Mower WR et al: Pulse oximetry as a fifth pediatric vital sign. *Pediatrics* 1997; 99:681-686.
13. Crapo RO et al: Guidelines for methacholine and exercise challenge testing, 1999. *Am J Respir Crit Care Med* 2000; 161:309-329.
14. Menon K, Sutcliffe T, Klassen TP: A randomized trial comparing the efficacy of epinephrine with salbutamol in the treatment of acute bronchiolitis. *J Pediatr* 1995; 126:1004-1007.

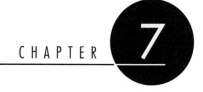

CHAPTER 7

Pulmonary Function Testing in Neonatal and Pediatric Patients

Alex Stentzler
Michael P. Czervinske

*P*ulmonary function testing (PFT) evaluates the respiratory system under various conditions of normal, disease, and stress states. Having an objective measurement of lung function at a given point in time is the primary purpose of PFT in children. Rather than a primary diagnostic tool, pulmonary function measurements usually act as a "yardstick" to compare previous or subsequent assessments. PFT results may help confirm a diagnosis that is suspected from the other components of the pulmonary assessment, mainly the patient history and physical examination.[1,2]

Because the absolute values of PFT measurements change with growth and development, using the percentage of predicted values best compares pulmonary function over the long term.[3-5] Ability to assess whether a specific measurement is "normal" may be clouded because of (1) the wide range of variability in normal children and (2) the relatively small number of children from whom the predicted norms have been gathered.[5-9] Despite these limitations, PFT measurements remain an integral component in evaluation and longitudinal follow-up of children with lung disease. PFT measurements evaluate the degree of illness and help determine the efficacy of various therapeutic interventions.

The full range of pulmonary function tests includes assessing lung, airway, and respiratory muscle performance, as well as gas exchange. Traditionally these tests have been conducted in a laboratory with patient cooperation to determine maximum capability, for example, with physical exercise. Laboratory testing includes controlled measurement of lung compliance, airway resistance, and lung volumes and capacities.[5,6]

Bedside *pulmonary mechanics* (PM) studies apply PFT systems in the intensive care unit at the bedside to aid in patient-ventilator management. PM studies conducted during mechanically assisted ventilation actually assess the interaction of the ventilator and the patient, which is not a true evaluation of the lungs or airway. Perform PM tests during resting ventilator-assisted breathing. Use these measurements to optimize ventilator support and reduce the hazards of positive-pressure ventilation. Changes in ventilator settings affect PM values. Because of the differences in purpose, test conditions, and clinical application, PM studies at the bedside are differentiated from standard laboratory PFT studies.

DEFINITIONS

Terminology used to describe which tests are required by which specific orders at individual institutions varies. "Complete pulmonary function testing" may mean an extensive testing protocol at one institution or a more select group of tests at another. Similar variations exist for "lung function survey" and "pulmonary screening." Therefore, clinicians need to be familiar with the specific testing protocols within their institution.

In this chapter the term *spirometry* denotes flow-volume or time-volume measurements. Spirometry measurements include forced vital capacity (FVC), forced expiratory volume in 1 second (FEV_1), the ratio of FEV_1 to FVC, forced expiratory flow at 25% to 75% of vital capacity, and forced expiratory flow at 50% of vital capacity. Lung volume describes the measurements of thoracic gas volume, functional residual capacity, residual volume (RV), total lung capacity (TLC), and the ratio of RV to TLC. Consider other measurements, such as carbon monoxide diffusing capacity, resistance or conductance, compliance, and maximum voluntary ventilation as separate tests. Sophisticated and seldom used tests are not addressed in this chapter, and more extensive texts for additional information are available.[1,2,9-13]

Bedside PFT refers to those tests often performed at the bedside, including tidal volume, vital capacity, minute ventilation, peak expiratory flow rate, and maximal inspiratory pressure. PM is the interaction of forces and physical principles that determine the characteristics of gas movement into and out of the lungs. Elasticity of the lung and chest wall, resistance to flow through the airways, and the action of the respiratory muscles (diaphragm, intercostal muscles, and accessory muscles) are measurable forces affecting ventilation. Volume, flow rate, duration, and frequency are characteristics of breathing. Most frequently, these are performed at the bedside in the neonatal (NICU) or pediatric (PICU) intensive care unit.

SPECIAL CONSIDERATIONS

NEONATAL TESTING

A laboratory offering PFT for infants must be prepared to meet the special needs of these patients.[14] Infants, unlike older children and adults, are unable to cooperate voluntarily during PFT procedures. They may be lightly sedated in the laboratory for the 2 or 3 hours needed to complete a full set of studies. Some drugs may alter PM or the normal characteristics of breathing. Chloral hydrate is preferred by many laboratories because a dose of 60 to 75 mg/kg does not affect PM or respiratory pattern.[15] Resistance to breathing and dead space of the measuring devices should be minimal. Using a face mask can cause trigeminal nerve stimulation and induce vagal reflexes that may alter the pattern of heart or respiratory rhythm. All emergency supplies and equipment for infant resuscitation must be available in the laboratory area.

PEDIATRIC TESTING

The greatest obstacle to satisfactory pulmonary function measurements in children is enlisting their cooperation and effort. Clinicians who work predominantly with children develop their own unique systems for making children comfortable and eliciting an appropriate testing effort. Conversely, pulmonary function laboratories that have limited experience with children frequently do not obtain satisfactory cooperation, and therefore the test results are inconclusive and the information is not used.

There are several key factors common to successful approaches in performing PFT on children. The testing environment or laboratory should have a warm and friendly atmosphere with pediatric-oriented pictures and toys. Each portion of the testing procedure should be carefully explained at an age-appropriate level, and the child's participation should be elicited in a playful rather than challenging fashion. For children undergoing their first PFT procedure, several efforts may be required before a satisfactory test is achieved. There is no substitute for patience and tolerance in this setting. Satisfactory performance can generally be achieved in the 5- or 6-year-old child, but some 8-, 9-, and 10-year-old children continue to have difficulty. Although uncommon, 3-year-old children may be able to do well, and good results have been reported more frequently among 4-year-old children. If the child is unable to perform satisfactorily at the first session, repeated attempts at subsequent visits should be encouraged, because most children learn quickly and frequently do much better at the next opportunity. Also, many software programs have visual aids to help make the breathing maneuvers a game, such as blowing out candles or blowing a boat across a lake.

Frequently, tests of younger children do not meet the American Thoracic Society (ATS) criteria for end of testing and are discarded as clinically irrelevant. Although they may not be able to complete a minimum expiratory time of 6 seconds, with less than 30 ml volume change in 1 second after that, small children can generate reproducible results over multiple test efforts.[16] Use caution when interpreting such results, but use these results to guide clinical judgments and interpret the effectiveness of therapies.

INSTRUMENTATION

Routine clinical application of pediatric and infant PFT requires overcoming certain technical complexities. The use of microcomputers and precision electronics overcomes many of these difficulties, which include high respiratory rates, the need for low dead space in the airway connection, and accurate measurements of very small gas volumes. Current instrumentation employs rapid-response gas flow sensors that are easily calibrated, remain stable, and are accurate in a measurement range that extends to the gas volumes of the smallest newborns.[1,17]

The primary PFT measurements are gas volume and flow rates into and out of the lungs. A *pneumotachometer,* or "pneumotach," is a device that measures the rate of gas flow. Several types of pneumotachs are available as part of neonatal PFT systems. The most common type is called a *Fleisch pneumotach.* This device has been in use for many years with several variations, such as a fixed or variable orifice. However, all variations are based on the principle that an obstruction within a gas stream will cause a drop in pressure that is directly proportional to gas flow. Comparing gas pressure on both sides of the obstruction with a differential pressure transducer electronically converts the value to gas flow. Gas flow measured over a known time is *volume.* Importantly, with a pneumotach that uses a differential pressure transducer, any additional obstruction within the gas stream will cause a falsely high reading. Frequently, pneumotachs are internally heated to prevent water condensation when used for longer durations (Fig. 7-1).

Another common type of flow measurement device is the *hot-wire anemometer.* This device incorporates a thin wire electrically heated to a high temperature, up to 400° F (204° C), placed within a gas flow stream. As gas moves past the wire, it cools in proportion to the amount of gas in the stream and produces a flow reading that is converted electronically to volume. Some anemometers have two wires to determine the direction of gas flow.

SELECTION OF DATA FOR ANALYSIS

Computerized infant PFT systems quickly provide an amazing amount of accurate data quickly. However, not all this information is clinically useful. The clinician is still responsible for the difficult task of deciding which information is valid and how to apply it to the care of the infant or child. Study results should be reproducible and consistent with other clinical data. Spontaneous and ventilator-assisted breaths have different mechanics and should not be included together in any study.

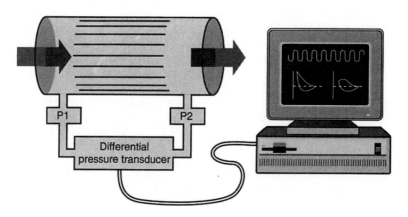

Fig. 7-1

Pneumotachometer and pulmonary function testing (PFT) computer. This system is used for neonatal PFT.

MECHANICS OF BREATHING IN NEWBORNS

With the first breaths of extrauterine life, a newborn must replace the in utero lung fluid with air. Surface tension forces in the fluid-filled lung require high negative pressure within the chest to establish normal air volume in the lungs. A newborn, particularly if born prematurely with respiratory distress syndrome (RDS), has low lung compliance. More pressure, or energy, is required to provide the normal amount of air volume brought into the baby's lungs with each breath. Because the newborn's ribs are mostly cartilage, the chest wall is flexible. With significant lung disease, the infant's chest wall may actually be more compliant than the lungs, causing retractions in which the ribs and sternum distort inward during inspiration instead of expanding the lungs. The lung-thorax mechanical relationship is less of the traditional "bag in a box" analogy and more like a "bag in a bag."

The combination of *lung compliance* (CL) and *airway resistance* (Raw) is the major force opposing inspiration, whereas *elastic recoil* is the force responsible for passive normal exhalation. When measured under static conditions, no gas flow into or out of the lungs, CL is an assessment of the *elasticity* (compliance) *of the total respiratory system* (Crs).[18]

Lung Inflation and Transpulmonary Pressure

For both spontaneous and mechanically assisted breaths, the change in pressure within the airways is the driving force for gas movement into and out of the lungs. During spontaneous inspiration, moving the diaphragm and other muscles of ventilation expands the chest volume, which creates subatmospheric pressure in the thorax. During mechanically assisted breathing the ventilator applies positive pressure to the airways. Expiration is usually considered passive, but in fact the elastic recoil of the lungs and chest wall that causes gas movement out of the lungs requires energy.

To assess PM, measure the change in pressure across the lung simultaneously with the flow and volume measurement. During mechanically assisted ventilation, measure pressure in the airway at the endotracheal tube. Measure gas flow and *airway pressure* with a sealed face mask for spontaneous-breathing studies. In some systems the same pressure transducer used for the pneumotach measures pressure as well. *Intrapleural pressure* may be approximated using a catheter placed in the thoracic esophagus.[18-20] The catheter is connected to a pressure transducer and either is filled with fluid or has an air-filled balloon at its tip.

Transpulmonary pressure is the pressure exerted on the lungs for gas movement; it is the difference between intrapleural and airway pressure. Intrapleural pressure measurements may not always be performed in assessing PM for ventilator-patient management. Generally, under these circumstances, it is assumed that the pressure in the large airways equalizes to the distal airways in the lungs. In this case the compliance measurements are actually of the respiratory system, including the chest wall, rather than of the lungs alone.

NEONATAL PULMONARY FUNCTION TESTING IN THE LABORATORY

MEASURING STATIC COMPLIANCE AND AIRWAY RESISTANCE

Static compliance (Crs) describes the elastic properties of the total respiratory system. Crs is measured during no airflow using the passive exhalation occlusion technique and assesses elasticity of the respiratory system.[5,18,21] Volume and pressure are measured with a pneumotachometer at two points of a passive resting exhalation.

The airway is momentarily occluded at end inspiration by a shutter placed between the face mask and the pneumotachometer. Stimulation of the Hering-Breuer reflex creates an apneic pause and relaxation of the respiratory muscles. Pressure is measured during the occlusion, and passive exhaled volume is measured after shutter opening. Crs is calculated by dividing the total passive expiratory volume by the corresponding pressure change at the airway opening.

Airway resistance (Raw) reflects the nonelastic airway and tissue forces resisting gas flow. Raw is calculated from the ratio of airway occlusion pressure to expiratory flow. Express Raw in centimeters of water per liter per second (cm H_2O/L/sec). Raw depends on the radius, length, and number of airways and varies with volume, flow, and respiratory frequency. The small diameters of an infant's tracheobronchial tree result in high resistance to gas flow. Airway irregularities; partial blocks caused by mucus, tumor, or foreign bodies; and partial closure of the glottis can also elevate Raw. The passive exhalation occlusion technique is noninvasive and can be performed with little disturbance to the infant.[22,23] However, infants with severe lung disease have an increased respiratory drive, and it may not be possible to induce a Hering-Breuer response.[5]

Raw measurements may be derived from body plethysmograph data, using a modified infant Isolette as the enclosure. Raw determined by this method also incorporates the acquisition of lung volume measurements described later.

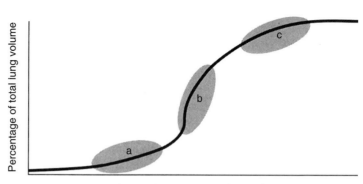

Fig. 7-2

Volume-pressure loops of tidal breathing at different levels of functional residual capacity (FRC): low FRC (*a*), normal FRC (*b*), elevated FRC (*c*).

Another method of determining Raw is to generate random noise signals at high frequencies at the mouth while the infant is breathing normal tidal breaths through a mouthpiece or mask. This technique is known as *forced oscillation* and measures the oscillation pressures compared with the flow and pressure measurements at the mouth. This technique is rapid, requires minimal patient cooperation, and helps optimize patient comfort.[23-25] As with the plethysmograph, forced oscillation also may be able to determine thoracic gas volume measurements described later, with minimal infant discomfort. This is now approved by the Food and Drug Administration.

Crs and Raw measurements may be useful in infants who (1) are receiving diuretics for chronic lung disease such as bronchopulmonary dysplasia, (2) have received high-frequency ventilation, (3) had meconium aspiration syndrome, (4) have had extracorporeal membrane oxygenation, (5) have respiratory syncytial virus infections and pneumonias, (6) have had diaphragmatic hernia, or (7) are receiving aerosolized bronchodilator therapy.

MEASURING FUNCTIONAL RESIDUAL CAPACITY

Functional residual capacity (FRC) is the resting volume of the lung at end expiration.[6] A newborn's chest wall is very compliant, and supine FRC values are lower than adult values, approximately 20% of total lung capacity. Preterm infants with RDS have an abnormally low FRC because of alveolar collapse. This results in low lung volume, low compliance, and increased work of breathing to achieve adequate tidal volume. Fig. 7-2 shows tidal volume-pressure loops at different FRC levels. Note that the slope of compliance is best, and thus work of breathing is least, at a normal FRC. Some infants maintain a dynamic FRC at this level by incorporating breathing strategies that limit the expiratory flow rate, such as expiratory grunting and increased postinspiratory diaphragmatic mus-

cle tone. Neonates with severe RDS need positive airway pressure during expiration to establish a normal FRC.

There are several methods for determining FRC.[26] Systems using helium dilution and nitrogen washout techniques are basically scaled-down versions of adult systems. Neonatal systems to determine FRC by plethysmography are also commercially available.

Helium Dilution Method. The helium dilution method of measuring FRC measures only the gas that is in direct communication with the central airways. This technique uses the principle that the concentration of a gas in one volume is proportional to the concentration of that same gas in another volume, provided there is no production or consumption of the measured gas. Therefore, knowing the concentration of the gas inside the lungs and outside, as well as knowing the external volume, allows calculation of the lung volume. The volume of gas in the lung at end expiration (FRC) mixes and equilibrates with a known amount and concentration of helium (usually 5% to 10%) in a closed breathing circuit. Apply petroleum jelly to the edges of a disposable mask for an airtight seal on the infant's face. Connect the mask to the helium-oxygen rebreathing circuit. Soda lime in the circuit absorbs exhaled carbon dioxide. The infant breathes the helium-oxygen mixture connected to a spirometer until the helium concentration equilibrates between the circuit and lungs. The reduction in measured helium concentration in the circuit is equated to the FRC. Any gas leak in the circuit, which is often seen in intubated infants, must be corrected in FRC calculations. The helium dilution method may be used for very sick infants with a fraction of inspired oxygen (FIO$_2$) as high as 0.95.[5,26]

Nitrogen Washout Method. The nitrogen washout method of measuring FRC also measures only

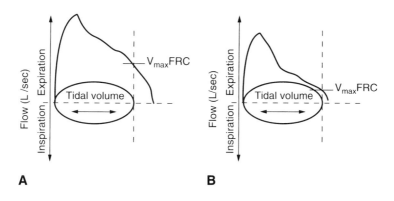

Fig. 7-3

Partial expiratory flow-volume (PEFV) curves with identification of maximal expiratory flow at FRC (V_{max} FRC) demonstrating a normal resting tidal breath and one with flow limitation. **A,** Normal. **B,** Abnormal: flow limited.

the gas that is in direct communication with the central airways. With a sealed face mask in place, the infant breathes 100% oxygen in an open circuit, which displaces nitrogen in the lung. The circuit must have no gas leak. The system measures the volume of nitrogen washed out of the lungs. Based on the starting alveolar concentration of nitrogen, the computer uses a regression equation to calculate the volume of air in the lungs at end expiration, which is FRC.[27] The nitrogen washout method cannot measure FRC if the infant's FIO_2 is greater than 0.65.[26] Atelectasis may result from washout of poorly ventilated and partially obstructed areas of the lung.

PLETHYSMOGRAPHY

The principle of body plethysmography is similar to the gas concentration techniques.[28] In a closed system the product of pressure and volume is constant (Boyle's law). The infant lies in an airtight Isolette. Only *thoracic gas volume* (TGV) is actually measured; the other values are calculated. TGV is the total gas in the thorax and is measured at FRC because it is the easiest volume for the subject to reproduce consistently. In addition to measuring lung volumes, body plethysmography is used mainly to measure resistance and conductance.[5,29]

MEASURING MAXIMAL EXPIRATORY FLOW BY RAPID THORACIC COMPRESSION TECHNIQUE

Measuring gas flow during a forced expiratory maneuver is the conventional procedure used to evaluate airway obstruction in a cooperative infant. A relatively noninvasive technique to generate a *partial expiratory flow volume* (PEFV) curve in infants allows one to measure expiratory flows during a forced maneuver in infants and small children.[28-30]

A rapid thoracic compression or "hug" is delivered to the sleeping infant's chest and abdomen with an inflatable jacket to produce a forced expiration. A pneumotachometer with sealed face mask measures exhaled gas flow. The flow at the end-expiratory point of a normal resting tidal breath (FRC) is measured on the PEFV curve. This flow value, *maximal expiratory flow at FRC,* is reported in liters per second (Fig. 7-3). Multiple tests at varying jacket inflation pressures are conducted for a "best test" assessment.

The maximal expiratory flow test can demonstrate flow limitation in airway disease and is valuable for evaluating the response to bronchodilator therapy in infants.[31,32] PEFV studies are frequently performed before and after aerosolizing a bronchodilator. An increase in maximal expiratory flow at FRC by at least 20% demonstrates a positive response to bronchodilator therapy. A significant number of infants with chronic lung disease have a *negative* bronchodilator response.[33]

Problems with the "hug technique" occur infrequently in experienced hands. The clinician must avoid collapsing the upper airway due to hyperextending the neck, resulting in a forced airflow limitation solely because of positioning. Other upper airway impedance may also affect the accuracy of the intrathoracic flow rates, and reflex glottic closure may complicate testing.[5]

PEDIATRIC PULMONARY FUNCTION TESTING IN THE LABORATORY

STANDARD SPIROMETRY

Standard spirometry is performed most often in PFT because of its relative ease and reproducibility.[5,13,34,35] It was traditionally carried out by time

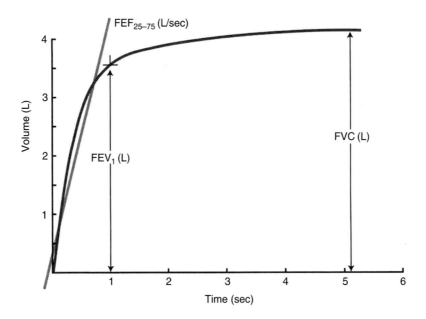

Calculation of FEF_{25-75}: 1. Determine 25% and 75% of FVC
2. Slope of line through 25% and 75% =

$$\frac{(V_{75}) - (V_{25})}{(T_{75}) - (T_{25})} \text{ (L/sec)}$$

Fig. 7-4

Demonstration of a normal standard time-volume spirometry graph depicting the forced vital capacity *(FVC)*, forced expiratory volume in 1 second *(FEV₁)*, and forced expiratory flow between 25% and 75% of vital capacity *(FEF₂₅₋₇₅)*.

and volume measurements using either a water seal spirometer or a wedge spirometer. This equipment required careful calibration, keen attention to technical detail during the performance of the test, and careful calculation of the reported values from the graph paper. Technologic advances in the measurement of flow with a pneumotachograph and microprocessing have greatly simplified spirometry. This allows the clinician to focus on eliciting optimal patient cooperation and effort while the computer reports the predicted and measured values. This technology does not, however, allow clinicians to be ignorant of the basis of spirometry; it is their responsibility to guarantee that the reported values accurately reflect the testing situation.[5]

Fig. 7-4 demonstrates traditional time-volume spirometry, indicating the various measurements available from this test. Integrating the flow signal with respect to time allows the computer to calculate volume and thus produce the time-volume curve.

Flow-Volume Loop. Fig. 7-5 demonstrates the flow-volume loop and its specific measurements.[20,36] Interestingly, no FEV_1 is clearly demonstrable on this visual representation, but the reported values include the FEV_1 as a key measurement. One advantage to the flow-volume representation is a clear depiction of whether subjects exhale to RV or whether they terminate their effort prematurely (Fig. 7-6). This is less evident when using the time-volume plot. It is frequently assessed by the duration of the effort, that is, "early termination." A disadvantage of the flow-volume method is that the computer automatically assigns the initiation of flow to TLC, whether or not subjects actually start with their lungs full (Fig. 7-7). This is a particular problem in

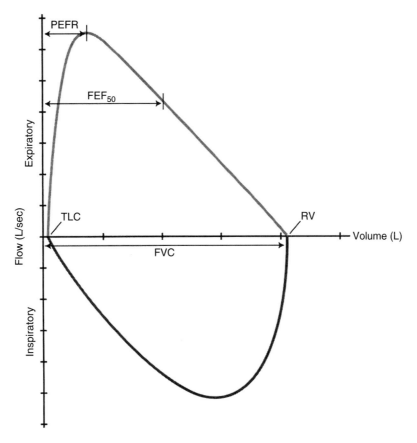

Fig. 7-5

Normal flow-volume loop showing both the expiratory and the inspiratory loops. The usual flow rates are identified. Note that no forced expiratory volume in 1 second (FEV_1) is evident because there is no time axis. *TLC,* Total lung capacity; *PEFR,* peak expiratory flow rate; *RV,* residual volume; *FEF_50,* forced expiratory flow at 50% of vital capacity; *FVC,* forced vital capacity.

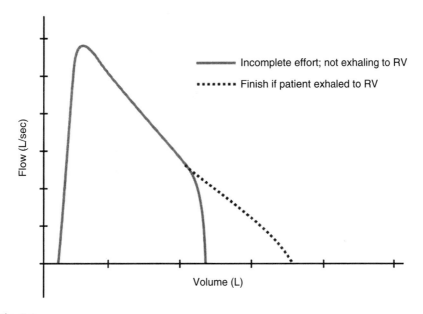

Fig. 7-6

This expiratory flow-volume loop demonstrates a failure to exhale completely to residual volume *(RV).* This will artificially decrease FVC and increase FEF_{50}.

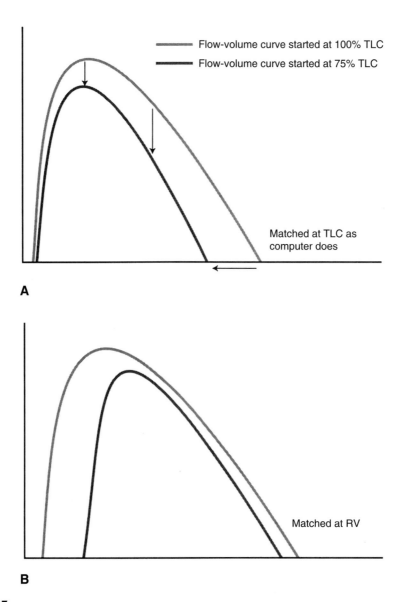

Fig. 7-7

Comparison of a maximal expiratory flow-volume curve started from 100% total lung capacity *(TLC)* with a curve started at 75% of TLC. The computer software will have no way of knowing that the smaller curve was not started at 100% TLC and will start the smaller curve at zero volume. This artificially decreases FVC, PEFR, and FEF_{50}. **A** matches the curve at TLC, as the computer does. **B** matches the curves at RV, which better reflects that the smaller curve was not started at full lung volume. Clinicians must do their best to ensure that the patient starts the expiratory maneuver at 100% TLC.

children, who may be apprehensive and therefore unable to fill their lungs completely before starting maximal exhalation. In this case the reported values will be artificially low, similar to those in restrictive disease.

Forced Vital Capacity, Forced Expiratory Volume, and Forced Expiratory Volume/Forced Vital Capacity. The most common measurements from spirometry include the FVC, FEV_1, and FEV_1:FVC ratio. These measurements are repro-

TABLE 7-1	PULMONARY FUNCTION MEASUREMENTS IN CHILDREN		
Measurement	**Variability (%)**	**Normal Range (% Predicted)**	**Important Change (%)**
FVC	5-7	80-120	>10
FEV	8	80-120	>15
FEV_1/FVC	—	*	—
FEF_{25-75}	15	60-140	>30
FEF_{50}	15	60-140	>30
TLC	7	80-120	>10
RV	7	80-120	>10
RV/TLC	7	†	—

*Absolute value is used; normal range for children is 82% to 95%.
†Absolute value is used; normal range for children is 20% to 30%.
FVC, Forced vital capacity; *FEV₁*, forced expiratory volume in 1 second; *FEF₂₅₋₇₅*, forced expiratory flow at 25% to 75% of vital capacity; *FEF₅₀*, forced expiratory flow at 50% of vital capacity; *TLC*, total lung capacity; *RV*, residual volume.

ducible for many disease states in adult patients, such as chronic obstructive pulmonary disease. Physiologists were concerned, however, that the FVC and FEV_1 might be relatively preserved despite the presence of moderately severe small airway disease, and thus significant lung disease might be missed by using only these measurements. Because small airways less than 2 mm in diameter contribute a very small part of the total lung resistance, 20% or less, these tiny airways have been described as the "silent zone" of the lung. In an effort to measure their function more independently, without the large airway functions obscuring the measurements, the "maximal midexpiratory flow rates" were calculated. In current terminology, this is the FEF_{25-75} or the FEF_{50}.[5,37]

Forced Expiratory Flow at 25% to 75% and at 50% of Vital Capacity. Although the FEF_{25-75} and FEF_{50} reflect primarily the function of smaller airways, their measurement is considerably more variable than that of the FEV_1 or FVC.[6,14,38] This decreases their usefulness in determining normal from abnormal and requires a considerably larger change to be considered physiologically significant, as opposed to just the normal variability found from one measurement to another.[39]

Table 7-1 demonstrates the variability, normal range, and clinically significant change for the most common spirometric and lung volume measurements in children. Furthermore, because many pulmonary diseases affect both the large and the small airways, the FEF_{25-75} and the FEV_1 often deteriorate in the same time frame, thus decreasing the usefulness of the FEF_{25-75} as an early detector of lung disease. However, because these measurements are often reported with standard spirometry, it makes no sense to ignore them. Also, many common childhood lung diseases, such as asthma and cystic fibrosis, have their roots in the tiny airways. Measurement of small airway function and attention to the results may enhance the overall interpretation of the tests. An abnormality isolated to the measurement of FEF_{25-75} or FEF_{50} is uncommon but more likely in children than adults. Therefore, most pediatric PFT centers pay careful attention to small airway function. Fig. 7-8 demonstrates the potential importance of these measurements in an asthmatic child.

Spirometry Values. Spirometric values are frequently used to determine whether the disease has a restrictive or an obstructive pattern. Table 7-2 demonstrates the expected changes with each pattern. The primary difference is whether the FEV_1:FVC ratio is decreased or preserved. The most common chronic diseases in children—asthma, cystic fibrosis, and bronchopulmonary dysplasia—are *obstructive*. Most *restrictive* defects in children are related to an abnormal chest wall configuration or neuromuscular weakness rather than to interstitial fibrosis, as seen in adults. Caution must be used in describing restrictive lung disease based on spirometry alone because complete lung volumes are not measured. If the child did not start the expiratory maneuver from TLC, the FVC will be artificially decreased, and the reported values may appear restricted. Similarly, in a patient with severe obstructive disease in which the RV has expanded to encroach significantly on the FVC, the spirometry values may suggest a restrictive pattern. Therefore, if restrictive lung disease is a concern, consider one of the lung volume studies. Figs. 7-6 and 7-7 show examples of incomplete exhalation to RV and not starting at TLC, both of which produce artificially low spirometry values.

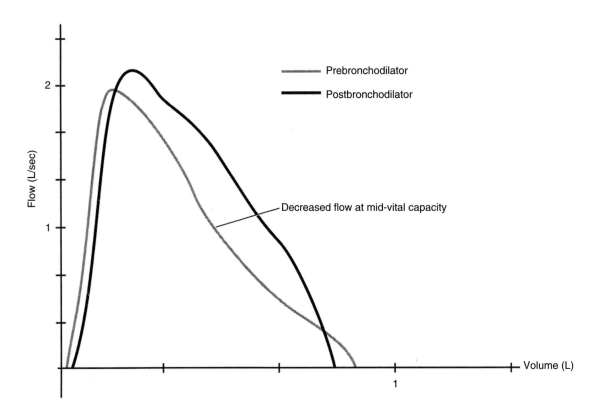

	Predicted	Prebronchodilator	Postbronchodilator	% Change
FVC (L)	0.89	0.81 (91)	0.78 (87)	−3
FEV$_1$ (L)	0.87	0.72 (83)	0.78 (89)	+8
FEV$_1$: FVC (%)	95	88	100	
PEFR (L/sec)	2.13	1.78 (83)	2.18 (102)	+22
FEF$_{50}$ (L/sec)	1.66	0.90 (54)	1.53 (92)	+70

Fig. 7-8

Prebronchodilator and postbronchodilator expiratory loops in a 5-year-old asthmatic patient. The prebronchodilator curve is slightly concave with respect to the volume axis, which is not evident on the postbronchodilator curve. The FEF$_{50}$ is the only prebronchodilator measurement below the expected normal range of variability; it increases by 70% after bronchodilator therapy. *FVC,* Forced vital capacity; *FEV$_1$,* forced expiratory volume in 1 second; *PEFR,* peak expiratory flow rate; *FEF$_{50}$,* forced expiratory flow at 50% of vital capacity.

LUNG VOLUMES

In contrast to the relative simplicity of spirometry, lung volume measurements are somewhat more involved and more difficult to perform. They include FRC, RV, TLC, RV:TLC ratio, and TGV. With the child sitting, the same techniques described earlier are used to measure lung volumes. These methods include helium dilution, nitrogen washout, body plethysmography, and forced oscillation.[24,40-42] Helium dilution or nitrogen washout techniques directly measure FRC.

Body plethysmography requires that the patient sit in an airtight box that looks similar to a telephone booth (Fig. 7-9).[42] During constant-volume

TABLE 7-2	CHARACTERIZATION OF OBSTRUCTIVE AND RESTRICTIVE PATTERNS IN PULMONARY FUNCTION TESTING	
Measurement	**Obstructive**	**Restrictive**
FVC	Normal or decreased	Decreased
FEV_1	Decreased	Decreased
FEV_1/FVC	Decreased	Normal or increased
TLC	Normal or increased	Decreased
RV	Increased	Normal or decreased
RV/TLC	Increased	Normal or increased

FVC, Forced vital capacity; *FEV_1,* forced expiratory volume in 1 second; *TLC,* total lung capacity; *RV,* residual volume.

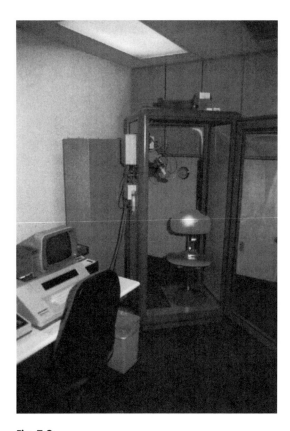

Fig. 7-9

Body plethysmography "box."

body plethysmography, the child voluntarily pants against a closed shutter. Using Boyle's law, the change in pressure against the closed shutter results in a volume measurement, the TGV. Unlike the infant box, voluntary spirometry measurements are usually determined as well. TGV is measured at a known FRC value rather than assumed values. TLC, the inspiratory capacity, is obtained from spirometry and added to the FRC. To calculate the RV, the expiratory reserve volume is subtracted from the FRC (Fig. 7-10). In addition to measuring lung volumes, body plethysmography measures resistance and specific conductance.

When children perform these tests, several potential errors are common. If they are uncomfortable and anxious, pediatric patients may not be able to find FRC and may breathe at a slightly higher lung volume. Likewise, if they are unable to start spirometry at TLC or exhale to RV, the values of inspiratory capacity and expiratory reserve volume will be incorrect. Therefore it is important to perform the test with the child completely relaxed and cooperative and to recognize if this is the case so that it is reflected in the interpretation.

Lung volume measurements are most useful in restrictive lung diseases, in which they are decreased. It is critical to determine if the lung volumes are smaller than expected because of a musculoskeletal problem (e.g., scoliosis, kyphosis), muscle weakness (e.g., Duchenne's muscular

dystrophy, spinal muscular atrophy), or lung parenchymal disease (e.g., idiopathic pulmonary fibrosis). If it can be established that the patient's FVC measured on spirometry correlates well with the TLC as measured by lung volumes, spirometry may be sufficient for most patients' follow-up.

Other measures of pulmonary function are seldom used in children for a variety of reasons. Some tests that have an invasive component, such as an esophageal balloon, are performed infrequently because of the perceived discomfort to the child. Other tests, such as diffusion capacity, are not often used because of uncertain predicted normal values and the infrequency of clinical diseases that make this a critical measurement in children. It is difficult persuading a young child to cooperate with the maximal voluntary ventilation test and to provide a consistent maximal effort throughout the testing period. This raises the uncertainty of whether the test is reliable in children.

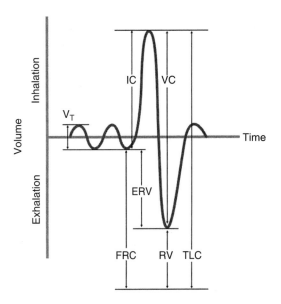

Fig. 7-10

Graphic display of the subdivisions of total lung capacity *(TLC),* from quiet tidal breathing on the left to maximal inhalation and exhalation on the right. V_T, Tidal volume; *VC,* vital capacity; *RV,* residual volume; *FRC,* functional residual capacity; *IC,* inspiratory capacity; *ERV,* expiratory reserve volume.

PROVOCATION TESTS

Challenge testing, also known as *bronchial provocation,* may be used in documenting bronchial hyperreactivity.[5,43-45] This can help solidify the diagnosis of hyperreactive airway disease, or asthma, in a patient whose symptoms may not be typical of asthma. Alternatively, for the patient who has symptoms that might mimic asthma, the lack of bronchial oversensitivity may help initiate the search for an alternative explanation. Because the challenge tests are somewhat involved and time-consuming, they are not routinely used to document bronchial hyperreactivity. However, they are frequently used for research purposes to document a reversal of bronchial hyperreactivity in response to specific therapies.

Various techniques exist for challenging the airways, including administration of aerosolized medications, exercise, and hypertonic saline administration. Each institution tends to develop expertise in one or two of these challenge techniques, choosing those that best fit patient needs. No standardized, universally acceptable protocol is in current use. Perhaps the most common testing is with aerosolized medication designed to induce bronchoconstriction. *Methacholine* and *carbachol* are two cholinergic medications that induce nonspecific bronchoconstriction. Histamine is a byproduct of mast cell degranulation and may play an important role in allergic responses. Histamine has also been used to induce bronchoconstriction during challenge testing. Antigen inhalation is infrequently used as a challenge because of the difficulty in quantifying the dose of antigen administered. Furthermore, antigen inhalation carries the risk of a late-phase reaction 6 to 8 hours after the challenge, at which time the patient is unlikely to be near a medical facility for therapeutic intervention.

Many laboratories have used *exercise* as a challenge. Unfortunately, because the primary driving forces for bronchoconstriction appear to be lack of humidity and low air temperature, an exercise challenge in a comfortable pulmonary function laboratory may not be provocative. This has led some investigators to use *hyperventilation* while having the patient breathe cold air, without exercise, as the provocation test.

Provocation testing is usually considered positive if the FEV_1 falls more than 20% from baseline.[39,44,45] The concentration of the challenge drug is used as a marker of the degree of bronchial reactivity and is called the PD_{20}, the provocative dose that produces a 20% fall in FEV_1. For example, a patient with highly reactive asthma may have a fall in FEV_1 of 20% with a methacholine concentration of 0.25 mg/ml. A patient with mild asthma may experience a 20% fall in the FEV_1 at 10 mg/ml.

Table 7-3 shows a positive methacholine challenge test in a 7-year-old girl evaluated for a chronic cough. This positive study led to therapy for asthma, and her cough resolved. Interestingly, her previous spirometry measurements were normal and showed no improvement after bronchodilator therapy. The responses to exercise and cold air are measured by the duration of the challenge as well as the work performed during the exercise test. If other test parameters are used, such as the peak expiratory flow rate or specific Raw, different critical levels of positivity are used.

MEASURING PULMONARY MECHANICS AT THE BEDSIDE

CALCULATED PARAMETERS

Tidal Volume. Tidal volume (V_T) is the gas volume (in milliliters) inhaled and exhaled during each resting breath. Frequently, V_T is indexed to body weight, and reported in milliliters per kilogram (ml/kg). Some PFT systems report inspired and expired V_T values separately, whereas some

TABLE 7-3	Positive Methacholine Challenge in 7-year-old Girl with Chronic Cough			
Methacholine		**Pulmonary Function**		
Concentration	**Cumulative Dose**	**FVC (L) (% Predicted)**	**FEV₁ (L) (% Predicted)**	**% Change FEV₁**
Saline	0	1.51 (83)	1.4 (82)	—
0.025	0.125	1.51	1.38	−1
0.25	1.375	1.64	1.53	+9
2.5	13.875	1.54	1.39	−1
10	63.875	1.33	1.07	−24
Albuterol	—	1.41	1.26	−10

FVC, Forced vital capacity; *FEV₁,* forced expiratory volume in 1 second.

combine the two values. Infants in an NICU may not normally inhale the same volume as they exhale for any given breath. This is visible as flow-volume (F-V) and pressure-volume (P-V) loops that are not closed. An average of at least 10 resting breaths is probably a better method of reporting V_T.[46] Infants receiving positive-pressure ventilation may have a gas leak around the endotracheal tube. In this case it is more accurate to report expired V_T. Some PFT systems report leakage as a percentage of exhaled to inhaled V_T, which is helpful in determining the delivered effective tidal volume. A system used for ventilator patient management should report V_T values for spontaneous and ventilator-delivered breaths separately.[47]

Respiratory Frequency. Most PFT systems report respiratory frequency, or rate, in breaths per minute. If the child or infant is intubated and on mechanical ventilation, the system should report spontaneous and ventilator breaths separately. Frequently, increased respiratory frequency is one of the first signs of reduced compliance, increased resistance, or fatigue.

Minute Ventilation. Minute ventilation (V_E) is the volume of gas inspired and expired each minute by the infant. It is reported in liters per minute (L/min) or liters per minute per kilogram (L/min/kg) of body weight and is the product of V_T and respiratory frequency. Viewing spontaneous and ventilator-delivered breathing separately or as a fraction of the total minute volume indicates the mechanical contribution of ventilation. This is helpful in assessing progress in weaning of the patient from assisted ventilation.

Rapid Shallow Breathing Index. The rapid shallow breathing index (RSBI) is a value that integrates two variables to determine the efficiency of tidal breathing. The RSBI is the ratio of spontaneous respiratory rate to V_T: divide respiratory rate by V_T (in liters) to calculate the index. A calculated value less than 100 to 105 is predictive of a successful extubation in adults.[48,49] The RSBI has less predictive value when applied to children and infants.[50-52] Factors such as age, endotracheal tube size, agitation, sedation, and duration of mechanical ventilation all contribute to the success of extubation and the usefulness of RSBI as a pediatric weaning tool. RSBI can be a useful tool in evaluating relative increases or decreases in work of breathing and monitoring an infant before and after extubation. For infants and pediatrics, normalize the RSBI equation for infant size by dividing the V_T by weight. The resulting unit of measure becomes breaths/ml/kg and allows easier comparison among the various measurements.[49,52] Due to the range of normal respiratory rates and tidal volumes, no single RSBI value will predict extubation success in the pediatric population.

Inspiratory and Expiratory Times. PFT systems measure inspiratory and expiratory times (T_i and T_e) by gas flow. The reported values will be different from the set, or duty cycle, times of a ventilator. Some systems also calculate the inspiratory/expiratory ratio (I:E) or inspiratory time percent (T_i/T_{total}) from measured time.

Lung Compliance. At the bedside, C_L measurements use the same technique as in the PFT laboratory.[18] When making bedside measurements, it is important to know the C_L test conditions to interpret the meaning of the reported value. *Specific* lung compliance describes C_L when it is measured at a known level of total lung volume. When measuring compliance under static conditions by airway occlusion, C_L is similar to the value derived in the laboratory and assesses Crs.[18] *Dynamic* lung compliance (CL_{dyn}) is measured during resting tidal breathing and is affected by Raw.

There are some limitations to CL_{dyn} measurement. This value reflects true CL only when measuring transpulmonary pressure during spontaneous breathing using an esophageal catheter. Some centers do not routinely place an esophageal catheter for ventilator management studies. Instead, if the scalar tracing demonstrates that gas flow reaches zero at the end of inspiration and expiration, it is assumed that pressure has equalized from the proximal airway to the lungs. CL varies at different points of total lung volume, which is usually unknown during dynamic testing.

Airway Resistance. During bedside testing the best evaluation of Raw also uses transpulmonary pressure measurements. A high Raw is visualized on the P-V loop, described later, as a bowing out of the curve from the line of idealized CL, or slope of the curve. The presence of an endotracheal tube with a small inner diameter is an airway obstruction, and Raw will be high. Changes in ventilator settings greatly affect Raw values, as do airway impairments such as secretions, bronchospasm, and edema. Bedside measurements of Raw usually preclude techniques used in the laboratory and are derived from the passive occlusion technique.

Time Constants. Respiratory time constants, tau (τ), are the mathematical product of compliance and resistance expressed in seconds, because all the units of pressure and volume measurement cancel out except time. A time constant is an interval over which a given change occurs, as a percentage of total change. Measured T_i, or inflation time, and T_e should be at least three respiratory time constants for 95%, which is optimal, for inspiration or expiration to occur.[53]

PRESSURE, FLOW, AND VOLUME OVER TIME

Most infant PFT systems graphically display measured airway (or transpulmonary) pressure, inspired and expired gas flow rates, and V_T on appropriate scales over a horizontal time axis "on screen" as the data are collected by the computer. This type of graphic display is also a component of some newer neonatal ventilators. Fig. 7-11 shows a scalar tracing of pressure, flow, and volume over time. Pressure (top tracing) is either transpulmonary pressure or airway pressure measured at the endotracheal tube connection with the ventilator circuit. Gas flow at the airway (middle tracing) shows inspiratory flow rate as a downward deflection and expiratory flow rate as an upward deflection, with the center line being zero flow. V_T (lower tracing) portrays inspiration as upward, with a return to the baseline as volume is exhaled. The vertical dashed lines delineate the change from inspiration to expiration for each breath. Breaths are numbered from left to right; *1, 2, 4,* and *5* are mechanically ventilated. Breath *3* is a spontaneous breath, with a lower V_T than the ventilator-delivered breaths.

FLOW-VOLUME LOOPS

During bedside testing, F-V loops are generally performed during tidal breathing.[6,54] Normally the peak of expiratory flow occurs within the first one third of expiratory volume. F-V loops that show decreased flow with relatively normal volume indicate an obstructive process in the airways; loops

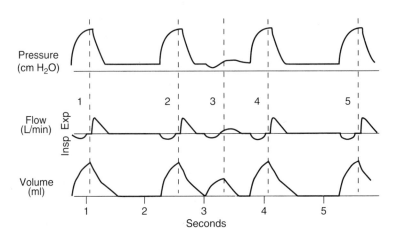

Fig. 7-11

Scalar tracing of pressure, flow, and volume over time (in seconds).

with decreased volume and normal flow suggest a restrictive disorder (Fig. 7-12).

F-V loops demonstrate fixed airway obstruction, with flow limited during both inspiration and expiration. Fig. 7-13 illustrates variable obstruction. Flow limitation on the inspiratory portion of the loop is characteristic of an extrathoracic obstruction. Flow limitation on the expiratory part of the loop demonstrates an intrathoracic obstruction.[55] Variable obstructions may also show a flutter or irregular flow pattern on either portion of the loop.

PRESSURE-VOLUME LOOPS

Graphically displaying a tidal breath with pressure change (airway or transpulmonary) on the horizontal axis and volume on the vertical axis also forms a loop. Spontaneous breathing is evidenced by a negative pressure change, and mechanical ventilator breaths display pressure in the positive direction. If the action of inhalation had only the elastic forces of lung tissue to overcome, the P-V graph would not be a loop but rather a straight line between the beginning and end points of inspiration (dashed line

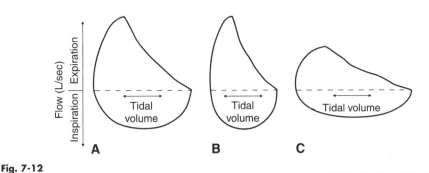

Fig. 7-12

Patterns of flow-volume loops. **A,** Normal. **B,** Restrictive. **C,** Obstructive.

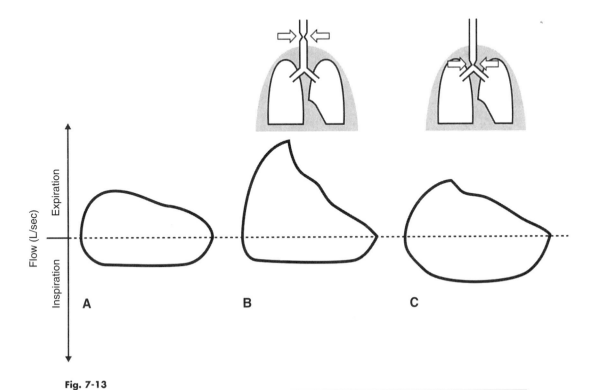

Fig. 7-13

Flow-volume loops showing various forms of airway obstruction. **A,** Fixed obstruction. **B,** Variable extrathoracic obstruction. **C,** Variable intrathoracic obstruction.

Fig. 7-14

Pressure-volume loops demonstrating normal and decreased lung compliance. **A,** Normal lung compliance. **B,** Decreased lung compliance.

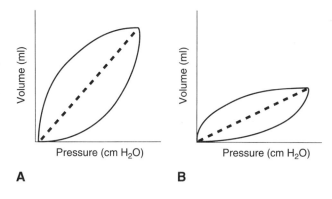

A B

in Fig. 7-14). The P-V loop bows out from that line of pure C_L mostly because of pressure needed for gas flow through narrow, resistive airways. The loop meets the line of ideal C_L at the end points of a tidal breath, where gas flow is zero. The slope of the line, and of the loop as a whole, depends on C_L. The more compliant the lung, meaning less pressure needed for normal V_T, the more vertical the P-V loop appears.

Lung Overdistention. Pulmonary barotrauma is a major complication of positive-pressure ventilation in neonates. Applying excessive distending airway pressures results in a characteristic distortion in appearance of the normal P-V loop (Fig. 7-15). To visualize this, imagine blowing up a balloon. At first you must blow hard (apply a large amount of pressure) to get any volume into the balloon. It then seems easier to push additional volume into the balloon as it expands. Finally, as the balloon reaches its expansion limit, that is, starts to overdistend, it again becomes more difficult to blow up. In other words, the compliance of the balloon or lung changes with total volume.

Applying additional pressure to an overdistended lung produces little or no increase in delivered volume and is hazardous to the infant. Lung overdistention is quantified by comparing compliance change in the last 20% of inspiratory pressure (C_{20}) with compliance change for the entire breath (C), in the ratio C_{20}:C (see Fig. 7-15). A C_{20}:C value less than 1.0 indicates lung overdistention during mechanical ventilation. Gas exchange can be improved in mechanically ventilated neonates with lung overdistention by reducing peak inspiratory pressure.[56]

Work of Breathing. The calculated resistive work of breathing is represented graphically as the area within the P-V loop. Work of breathing is usually indexed to body weight, reported in grams-centimeters per kilogram (g-cm/kg). Although work of breathing certainly exists in infants, the variables of elastic, resistive, and inertial forces and the influence of test conditions such as respiratory frequency are nonspecific. Changes in work of breathing with therapeutic intervention are probably more useful to clinicians than the absolute value reported by the computer. Work is being done during assisted ventilation, but not by the infant, and reported work of breathing has little meaning.

OTHER BEDSIDE TESTS

Other common pulmonary function measurements performed at the bedside are vital capacity (VC), peak expiratory flow rate (PEFR), and maximum inspiratory pressure (MIP), often referred to as negative inspiratory force (NIF). These measurements require a respirometer or pneumotachometer, a peak flowmeter, and an NIF meter. The values are helpful in a variety of clinical situations, including weaning from mechanical ventilation, evaluating neuromuscular disorders such as myasthenia gravis or muscular dystrophy, and evaluating treatment for reactive airways.

Each of these measurements depends on patient cooperation and effort, which makes it challenging with children and prevents their use for infants. Pediatric patients may need to be older than 4 or 5 years to perform some of these tests because of equipment limitations. Also, the child must be able to understand the instructions and use the correct technique to perform the tests. Thoroughly explain the technique for each maneuver and provide a chance for practice before actually collecting the data. It is imperative that clinicians record their impression of the child's understanding and effort with the actual measurements.

Vital Capacity. VC is the maximum amount of gas that can be expired after a full inspiration. The patient inhales to TLC and then exhales completely through a respirometer or other measuring device. VC values are effort dependent, and the child must cooperate completely when asked to perform the maneuver. Incomplete effort will result in an

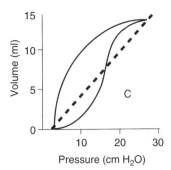

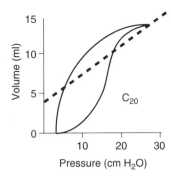

Fig. 7-15

Pressure-volume loops demonstrating overdistention. Note the "penguin" or "bird's beak" appearance in the shape of the loop. These loops demonstrate idealized slopes *(dashed lines)* for change in compliance for the entire breath *(C)* and change in compliance in the last 20% of inspiratory pressure (C_{20}). The C_{20}:C ratio identifies lung overdistention.

artificially low value, which may lead to misdiagnosis. Forced vital capacity (FVC) differs from VC in that during the FVC maneuver the patient exhales as forcefully and rapidly as possible after a maximal inspiration. FVC is usually the same as a slow VC except in patients who experience airway collapse with rapid, forceful expiration.

Peak Expiratory Flow Rate. PEFR is the maximum achievable flow during a rapid, forced expiration. The primary use of the PEFR is monitoring patients with hyperreactive airways. It is generally measured with hand-held devices that sense flow against a turbine, through a variable orifice, or against a spring-loaded diaphragm. With increasing flow rates an indicator advances linearly on a scale that reveals the PEFR, usually in liters per minute. Note that the PEFR on the F-V loop measures the same function as the peak flowmeter, air flow in the large airways, but reported in L/sec. The PEFR measurement made during a F-V loop is an actual measurement of air flow. Because the hand-held peak flowmeter measures only the inertia from the initial blast of air, the value is not identical to the value reported during F-V loop measurement.

Portable peak flowmeters are used extensively in the study and management of asthmatic patients. A significant decrease in the individual's baseline PEFR may indicate worsening asthma and the need for therapeutic interventions. In addition, measuring PEFR before and after bronchodilator administration evaluates the effectiveness of the therapy.[34]

Portable hand-held models are low cost and easy to use at home, at school, or in an office. When using hand-held peak flowmeters, care must be taken to avoid partial occlusion of the flow exit orifice during exhalation. Partial occlusion decreases the amount of flow required to raise the flow indicator, resulting in overestimation of PEFR. This measurement can also be erroneously high if the patient uses a "spitting" action during exhalation.[5,35]

Maximum Inspiratory Pressure. MIP, or NIF, is the maximum negative pressure, expressed in centimeters of water, generated during inspiration against an occlusion. Connect the patient's airway to an inspiratory pressure gauge with an adapter that allows occlusion of the airway during inspiration. Instruct the patient to exhale, and then occlude the airway while the patient inhales with maximal effort, which results in measuring the maximum negative pressure.

MIP is an important measure to help differentiate weakness from other causes of restrictive lung disease. It can be an important differentiating point for children and young adults with various neuromuscular diseases. These patients usually have a combination of scoliosis and muscle weakness, both of which might contribute to reduced lung volumes. Measuring MIP helps in determining how much reduction might be caused by weakness. Because many neuromuscular diseases are progressive, MIP helps to document this progression. MIP may also indicate the patient's physical ability to take a deep breath and is often measured when weaning a patient from mechanical ventilation is being considered.

Complex Bedside Measurements. Automated and computed monitors allow the measurement of more complex breathing variables at the bedside. Usually these measurements are useful for weaning a child from mechanical ventilation, but they may also be helpful when evaluating the pulmonary status of a neuromuscular patient.

An example of such a measurement is the $P_{0.1}$, pronounced "P one hundred." It is similar to MIP but measures the negative pressure generated in the first one hundredth of a second. $P_{0.1}$ appears to be more indicative of the ability to sustain respiratory drive and predict successful extubation or weaning from mechanical ventilation.

Another such measure is the *tension time index* (TTI), which may assist in predicting successful weaning from mechanical ventilation. The TTI is essentially a measurement of the energy demand on the inspiratory muscles to tolerate the workload of breathing.[48] The TTI is the product of the inspiratory time/cycle time ratio and the integrated area under the pressure curve throughout the respiratory cycle. Unlike the adult measurement and similar to the RSBI, these advanced weaning predictors have no pediatric range that correlates with successful weaning.[48]

REFERENCES

1. Lemen RJ: Pulmonary function testing in the office, clinic, and home. In Chernick V, editor: *Kendig's disorders of the respiratory tract in children.* Philadelphia, Saunders, 1990, pp 147-154.
2. Hilman BC, Allen JL: Clinical application of pulmonary function testing in children and adolescents. In Hilman BC, editor: *Pediatric respiratory disease: diagnosis and treatment.* Philadelphia, Saunders, 1993, pp 98-107.
3. Hibbert ME, Couriel JM, Landau LI: Changes in lung, airway and chest wall function in boys and girls between 8 and 12 years. *J Appl Physiol* 1984; 57:304-308.
4. Pagtakhan RD et al: Sex differences in growth patterns of the airways and lung parenchyma in children. *J Appl Physiol* 1984; 56:1204-1210.
5. American Association for Respiratory Care: Clinical practice guideline: Infant/toddler pulmonary function tests. *Respir Care* 1995; 40:761-768.
6. Bates JH et al: Tidal breath analysis for infant pulmonary function testing. ERS/ATS Task Force on Standards for Infant Respiratory Function Testing, European Respiratory Society/American Thoracic Society. *Eur Respir J* 2000; 16:1180-1192.
7. Hanrahan JP et al: Pulmonary function measures in healthy infants. *Am Rev Respir Dis* 1990; 141:1127-1135.
8. Rosenfeld M et al: Effect of choice of reference equation on analysis of pulmonary function in cystic fibrosis patients. *Pediatr Pulmonol* 2001; 31:227-237.
9. Chatburn RL: Evaluation of pediatric pulmonary function: theory and application. *Respir Care* 1989; 34:597-610.
10. Hyatt RE: Expiratory flow limitation. *J Appl Physiol* 1983; 55:1-8.
11. Gardner RM: Pulmonary function laboratory standards. *Respir Care* 1989; 34:651-660.
12. American Thoracic Society: Standardization of spirometry, 1994 update. *Am J Respir Crit Care Med* 1995; 152:1107-1136.
13. Taussig LM et al: Standardization of lung function testing in children. *J Pediatr* 1980; 97:668-676.
14. Blonshine SB: Pediatric pulmonary function testing. *Respir Care Clin North Am* 2000; 6:27-40.
15. Hershenson M et al: The effect of chloral hydrate on genioglossus and diaphragmatic activity. *Pediatr Res* 1984; 18:516-519.
16. Desmond KJ et al: Redefining end of test (EOT) criteria for pulmonary function testing in children. *Am J Respir Crit Care Med* 1997; 156:542-545.
17. Frey U et al: Specifications for equipment used for infant pulmonary function testing. ERS/ATS Task Force on Standards for Infant Respiratory Function Testing, European Respiratory Society/American Thoracic Society. *Eur Respir J* 2000; 16:731-740.
18. Bancalari E: Pulmonary function testing and other diagnostic laboratory procedures. In Thibeault DW, Gary GA, editors: *Neonatal pulmonary care,* ed 2. Norwalk, Conn, Appleton-Century-Crofts, 1986, pp 195-234.
19. Coates AL et al: Liquid-filled esophageal catheter for measuring pleural pressure in preterm neonates. *J Appl Physiol* 1989; 67:889-893.
20. Cunningham MD, Desai NS: Methods of assessment and findings regarding pulmonary function in infants less than 1000 grams. *Clin Perinatol* 1986; 13:299.
21. Guslits BG et al: Comparison of methods of measurement of compliance of the respiratory system in children. *Am Rev Respir Dis* 1987; 136:727-729.
22. LaSouef PN, England SJ, Bryan AC: Passive respiratory mechanics in newborns and children. *Am Rev Respir Dis* 1984; 129:552-556.
23. Hayden MJ et al: Using low-frequency oscillation to detect bronchodilator responsiveness in infants. *Am J Respir Crit Care Med* 1998; 157:574-579.
24. Peslin R, Duvivier C: Reliability of thoracic gas volume derived from mechanical impedance at different levels of the vital capacity. *Respiration* 1999; 66:323-331.
25. Delacourt C et al: Use of the forced oscillation technique to assess airway obstruction and reversibility in children. *Am J Respir Crit Care Med* 2000; 161:730-736.
26. Tepper RS, Asdell S: Comparison of helium dilution and nitrogen washout measurements of functional residual capacity in infants and very young children. *Pediatr Pulmonol* 1992; 13:250-254.
27. Gerhardt T, Hehre D, Bancalari E: A simple method of measuring functional residual capacity in the newborn by N_2 washout. *Pediatr Res* 1985; 19:1165.
28. Morgan WJ: Evaluation of forced expiratory flow in infants. In Bhutani VK, Shaffer TH, Vidyasagar D, editors: *Neonatal pulmonary function testing.* Ithaca, NY, Perinatology Press, 1988.
29. Morgan WJ et al: Partial expiratory flow-volume curves in infants and young children. *Pediatr Pulmonol* 1988; 5:232-243.
30. LeSouef PN, Hughes DM, Landau LI: Effect of compression pressure on forced expiratory flow in infants. *J Appl Physiol* 1986; 61:1639-1646.
31. Tepper RS et al: Use of maximal expiratory flows to evaluate central airways obstruction in infants. *Pediatr Pulmonol* 1989; 6:272-274.
32. Maynard RC et al: Partial forced expiratory flow (PFEF) measurements in premature infants at discharge. *Pediatr Res* 1991; 29:324A.
33. Wahlig TM et al: Partial forced expiratory flow-volume measurement, radiographic severity score, and bronchodilator response in infants with chronic lung disease. *Respir Care* 1992; 37:1325.
34. Executive Summary: *Guidelines for the diagnosis and management of asthma.* Washington, DC, US Department of Health and Human Services, Pub No 91-3042A, 1991.
35. Lebowitz MD: The use of peak expiratory flow rate measurements in respiratory disease. *Pediatr Pulmonol* 1991; 11:166-174.
36. Gardner RM, Crapo RO, Nelson SB: Spirometry and flow volume curves. *Clin Chest Med* 1989; 10:145-154.
37. Buist AS: Tests of small airways function. *Respir Care* 1989; 34:446-454.
38. Green M, Mead J, Turner JM: Variability of maximum expiratory flow volume curves. *J Appl Physiol* 1974; 37:67-74.
39. Pennock BE, Rogers RM, McCaffree DR: Changes in spirometric indices: what is significant? *Chest* 1981; 80:97-99.

40. Reis AL: Measurement of lung volumes. *Clin Chest Med* 1989; 10:177-186.

41. Snow MG: Determination of functional residual capacity. *Respir Care* 1989; 34:586-596.

42. DuBois AB et al: A rapid plethysmographic method for measuring thoracic gas volume: a comparison with nitrogen washout method for measuring functional residual capacity in normal subjects. *J Clin Invest* 1956; 35:322-326.

43. Irvin CG: Airways challenge. *Respir Care* 1989; 34:455-469.

44. American Association for Respiratory Care: Clinical practice guideline for bronchial provocation. *Respir Care* 1992; 37:902-906.

45. American Thoracic Society: Guidelines for methacholine and exercise challenge testing, 1999. *Am J Respir Crit Care Med* 2000; 161:309-329.

46. Bhutani VK et al: Evaluation of neonatal pulmonary mechanics and energetics: a two factor least mean square analysis. *Pediatr Pulmonol* 1988; 4:150-158.

47. Mammel MC et al: Effect of spontaneous and mechanical breathing on dynamic lung mechanics in hyaline membrane disease. *Pediatr Pulmonol* 1990; 8:222-225.

48. Vassilakopoulos T, Spyros Z, Roussos C: The tension-time index and the frequency/tidal volume ratio are the major pathophysiologic determinants of weaning failure and success. *Am J Respir Crit Care Med* 1998; 158:378-385.

49. Chatila W et al: The unassisted respiratory rate–tidal volume ratio accurately predicts weaning outcome. *Am J Med* 1996; 101:61-67.

50. Venkataraman ST, Khan N, Brown A: Validation of predictors of extubation success and failure in mechanically ventilated infants and children. *Crit Care Med* 2000; 28:2991-2996.

51. Farias JA, et al: Weaning from mechanical ventilation in pediatric intensive care patients. *Intensive Care Med* 1998; 24(10):1070-1075.

52. Thiagarajan RR et al: Predictors of successful extubation in children. *Am J Respir Crit Care Med* 1999; 160:1562–1566.

53. Boros SJ et al: Using conventional infant ventilators at unconventional rates. *Pediatrics* 1984; 74:487.

54. Bhutani VK: Pulmonary function profile: computer analysis and pulmonary graphics. In Bhutani VK, Shaffer TH, Vidyasagar D, editors: *Neonatal pulmonary function testing*. Ithaca, NY, Perinatology Press, 1988.

55. Abramson AL et al: The use of tidal breathing flow volume loop in laryngotracheal disease of neonates and infants. *Laryngoscope* 1982; 92:922-926.

56. Fisher JB et al: Identifying lung overdistention during mechanical ventilation by using volume-pressure loops. *Pediatr Pulmonol* 1988; 5:10-14.

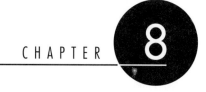

CHAPTER 8

Radiographic Assessment

J. David Ingram

Radiographic assessment of the chest and airway is often critical in patient evaluation by the respiratory care practitioner. The position of lines and tubes can be accurately determined. Visualized lung fields on the radiographs can be correlated with the physical examination. Airways can be assessed for patency and abnormalities.

RADIOGRAPHIC TECHNIQUE

Radiographs are obtained using a portable x-ray machine at the patient's bedside or by using equipment in the radiology department. Because the quality of the examination is better using the techniques and equipment available in the radiology department, portable radiographs should only be used whenever it is not safe or feasible to transport the patient. The radiographs may be viewed as hard-copy films or digitally on a monitor.

The standard radiographic evaluation of the chest comprises both a frontal view and a lateral view. The *frontal view* shows the position of a structure in relation to right and left as well as to center. With the addition of the *lateral view,* the structure can also be positioned in an anterior to posterior plane, and a more three-dimensional representation can be surmised. *Posteroanterior* (PA) frontal views are obtained upright with the chest against the radiographic plate and the x-ray beam going through the patient in a posterior to anterior path. When the radiograph is performed portably, the plate is placed between the patient's back and the bed with the x-ray tube in front of the patient's chest. The *anteroposterior* (AP) technique, with the beam passing from anterior to posterior, causes magnification of structures such as the heart, located in the anterior half of the chest. Therefore knowledge of how the frontal film was obtained (AP versus PA) is useful when deciding whether the heart size is different because of magnification or clinical change.

Although most chest radiographs are performed using frontal and lateral projections, other views may contribute additional information. The *lateral decubitus view* is a frontal projection performed with the patient lying on either the right side, *right-side down* lateral decubitus, or on the left side, *left-side down* lateral decubitus. The down side can be evaluated for presence of a mobile pleural effusion, whereas the up side may demonstrate a pneumothorax. These views may also be used if a foreign body lodged in a bronchus causes air trapping. The down-side lung normally loses volume but may remain expanded when a foreign body is obstructing airflow out through the bronchus.

Forced expiratory films may also be used to evaluate for foreign body aspiration. The technologist gently adds pressure to the abdomen during expiration. The obstructed lung will not decrease in size but remains normal to hyperexpanded (Fig. 8-1). In older and cooperative children the technologist can have the patient inspire and expire without assistance while obtaining the radiographs. *Oblique* views are typically used for rib fracture or pulmonary metastatic evaluations in the pediatric population.

Although the thoracic trachea and mainstem bronchi are demonstrated on chest radiographs, soft tissue frontal and lateral projections of the neck allow evaluation of the upper airway. These views may show mass effect on the airway from a retropharyngeal abscess or can show distortion of the tracheal caliber from croup and subglottic stenosis. Real-time imaging of the airway using fluoroscopy will show the dynamic collapse of tracheomalacia. If a barium swallow is performed as well, the presence of a vascular ring or tracheoesophageal fistula can be excluded.

NORMAL CHEST ANATOMY

The normal structures that are visualized on a chest radiograph are distinguishable because of differences in the absorption of the x-ray beam. Bone and metallic orthopedic hardware appear very white because of greater x-ray absorption and less exposure of the film. In contrast, air has little beam absorption, so well-expanded lungs appear relatively black. Soft tissue organs and fluid usually appear as shades of gray in between the white bones and black lungs. However, incorrect exposure of the film may alter the normal gray scale such that soft tissue organs can appear very white in an underexposed film. Therefore the technical quality of the film must be considered when viewing.

A chest film is a two-dimensional representation of a three-dimensional object. When an x-ray beam passes through the chest, the densities of all the structures that it encounters are added together. Thus a flat object such as a plate of atelectasis may add little to the opacity of the chest seen en face in one projection but may appear very opaque when viewed on edge in another projection. Pulmonary vessels appear as white dots when viewed in cross section but are fainter when viewed as tubes.

Differences in tissue density allow the viewer to discriminate between different structures. The heart, which is of soft tissue or waterlike density, is clearly demarcated by a distinct edge from the adjacent air-filled lung. However, if the lung becomes more waterlike in density from loss of air, as in atelectasis, or if the alveoli become filled with pus, as in pneumonia, the sharp edge between the heart and the lung is no longer apparent. The sign

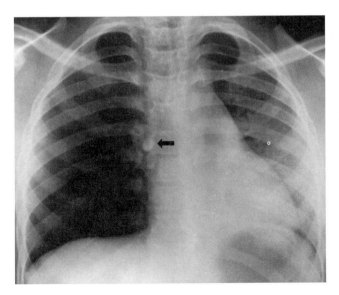

Fig. 8-1

Expiratory frontal chest radiograph shows normal decrease in left lung volume. Tooth *(arrow)* obstructs the right mainstem bronchus and causes air trapping in the right lung.

caused when two normal structures lose their distinct edge and blend imperceptibly is widely known as the *silhouette sign* (Fig. 8-2).

The normal structures that the respiratory care practitioner must evaluate on all chest films are the heart, lungs, and airway. Other structures that may be important in a specific patient include the diaphragm, bones, and organs in the upper abdomen. Although the heart is central in the chest, it normally projects more into the left hemithorax. Heart size may be accentuated by AP projection as well as decreased lung expansion. Pulmonary arteries and veins form confluent areas on either side of the heart called the right and left pulmonary *hila.* Enlargement of the hila may be caused by increased caliber of the pulmonary vessels or enlarged lymph nodes. The side of the aortic arch should also be noted. Normally the arch is on the left and causes a left lateral bulge of the superior mediastinum and a mild indentation on the trachea.

Fig. 8-2

A, The left lower lobe pneumonia abuts the diaphragm, leading to nonvisualization of the normal edge of the diaphram. The cardiac border is demarcated because the lingula is normally aerated. **B,** Only the right hemidiaphragm is visualized because the left is obscured by the left lower lobe pneumonia. Major fissure appears as an edge *(arrow).*

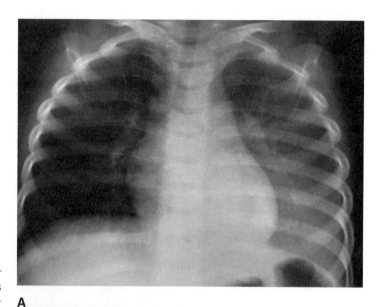

A

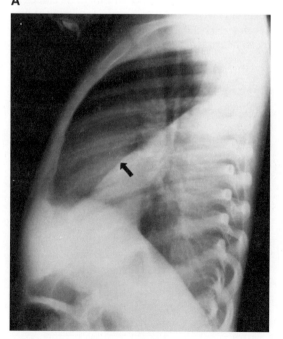

B

The mediastinum is composed of the heart, aorta, main pulmonary artery and proximal branches, origins of the great vessels from the aorta, superior vena cava, and thymus. Thymic tissue is usually prominent in the neonate and becomes less apparent with age due to regression of the thymus and growth of surrounding structures. Because it is an anterior mediastinal structure, the thymus in the small child fills the anterior clear space normally seen on the lateral view of a teenager or adult. On the frontal view it may only cause widening of the superior mediastinum. When it projects away from the mediastinum, typically into the right upper lung, it appears as a "sail" with a sharp inferior margin. The lateral margins often have a characteristic wavy contour (Fig. 8-3).

The right lung is divided into three lobes and the left lung into two lobes. Both lungs have upper and lower lobes, but the right lung also has a middle lobe. The lingula of the left upper lobe may be thought of as corresponding to the right middle lobe, at least in location. Separating the upper and lower lobes, the major fissures extend diagonally on the lateral view in an anteroinferior to posterosuperior plane. Fluid in the fissures increases their visibility. The minor fissure separates the middle lobe from the right upper lobe. It is horizontal in orientation on both frontal and lateral projections and terminates into the major fissure on lateral projection.

Lung density is greatly affected by the degree of inspiration. Poor inspiration will cause crowding of pulmonary vessels and airways leading to overall increase in lung density. When comparing the pres-ent chest radiograph to a prior film, the depth of inspiration should be taken into account and excluded as a cause for the change in the appearance of both the lungs and size of the heart. When viewing infant and pediatric radiographs, body rotation may be difficult to avoid. Evaluating thoracic symmetry helps when interpreting the loss of lung volume or increased density in this situation.

Evaluation of the trachea and mainstem bronchi should include the size as well as evidence of abnormal displacement or distortion by an adjacent mass. Truncation of a mainstem bronchus is often a sign of a mucus plug when the lung is collapsed. Although the right hemidiaphragm is usually slightly higher than the left because of the underlying liver, position of the diaphragms may indicate hemidiaphragm paralysis or abdominal pathology. Congenital fusion anomalies may be seen in the neonatal rib cage, and rib fractures may contribute to difficult ventilation in a trauma patient.

POSITIONING OF LINES AND TUBES

The frontal chest radiograph can readily assess the distance of the endotracheal tube (ETT) to the carina. The tube should be located between the thoracic inlet and the carina. If the tube is at the carina or in one of the mainstem bronchi, overaeration of one lung and atelectasis of the opposite lung may result. The position of the head, especially in a neonate, may result in a significant change in position of the ETT tip. The tip will advance toward the carina when the head is flexed. If a chest

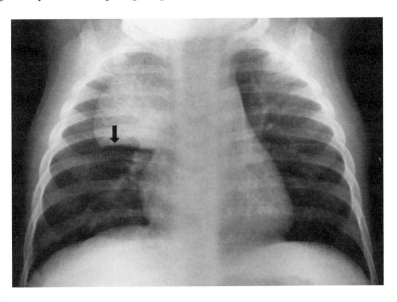

Fig. 8-3

Normal thymus abuts the minor fissure *(arrow)* and has curved lateral margin.

radiograph is obtained for suspected esophageal intubation, the stomach and possibly esophagus will be distended with air while the lungs will be underinflated. A lateral view would show the ETT in the esophagus. The positions of vascular catheters should also be evaluated and repositioned if necessary. If the tip of the catheter is in the right atrium, arrhythmia may result.

AIRWAY OBSTRUCTION

The adenoids are posterior to the nasopharynx on the lateral neck radiograph. The palatine tonsils are best seen between the oropharynx and nasopharynx. Enlargement of these normal lymphoid structures is a major cause of sleep-related apnea. Acutely, infection can also cause adenoidal and tonsillar enlargement leading to obstruction (Fig. 8-4).

Croup is the most common cause of upper airway obstruction in children, with a peak incidence of 6 months to 3 years. Most cases are viral induced

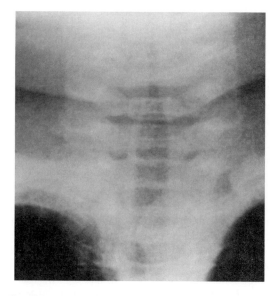

Fig. 8-5

"Steepling" of the subglottic airway is caused by croup.

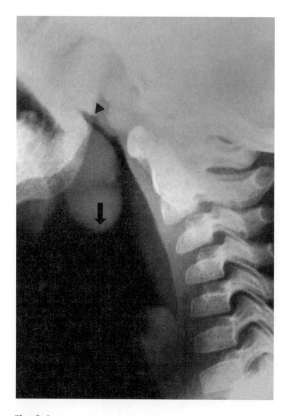

Fig. 8-4

Enlarged tonsils *(arrow)* appear to hang down into hypopharynx. Nasopharynx *(arrowhead)* is narrowed from enlarged adenoids located posterior and superior.

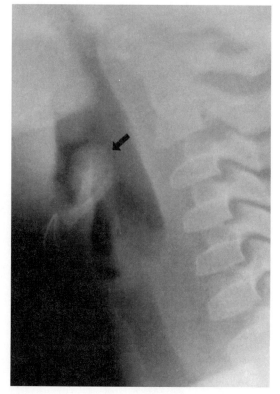

Fig. 8-6

Enlarged epiglottis *(arrow)* appears as a "thumb" projecting into the airway.

(parainfluenza) and cause inspiratory stridor with a barking cough. Frontal and lateral neck radiographs may show the characteristic subglottic narrowing below the vocal cords with loss of the normal "shouldering" of the airway and resultant "church steeple" appearance. The hypopharynx usually appears overdistended (Fig. 8-5).

Whereas croup usually improves within a few days using supportive therapy, *epiglottitis* is a life-threatening disease causing acute inspiratory stridor, fever, and dysphasia. The usual pathogen is *Haemophilus influenzae,* with the risk of infection now reduced by immunization programs. The diagnosis should be made by physical examination or by direct visualization through a scope. If a lateral radiograph of the neck is obtained, the epiglottis is enlarged, and the aryepiglottic folds are thickened with overdistention of the hypopharynx. The radiograph is performed upright in the position most comfortable for the patient to breathe. Because safety of the child is of primary concern, the radiograph should be performed portably in the emer-gency department (ED), where intubation can be performed quickly if necessary (Fig. 8-6).

Retropharyngeal cellulitis and *abscess* are usually preceded by an upper respiratory infection, often with cervical adenopathy. Spread of infection along lymph channels leads to enlargement of the retropharyngeal (prevertebal) soft tissues on the lateral neck radiograph with forward displacement and bowing of the airway (Fig. 8-7). Computed tomography (CT) is the modality of choice for distinguishing cellulitis from an abscess, which will appear as a walled-off fluid collection needing surgical drainage.

Occasionally the child being evaluated for stridor has aspirated a foreign body such as a peanut into the bronchus and the airway is blocked, or has ingested an object such as a coin into the esophagus, causing compression of the trachea. If the child is suspected of ingesting a coin or other object, a lateral radiograph of the neck and frontal views of the chest and abdomen are usually obtained to locate the object (Fig. 8-8). Nonradiopaque objects that are aspirated may be difficult to see unless outlined by air in the trachea or bronchi. Forced expiratory chest views, decubitus films, or fluoroscopy may be useful in showing the air trapping that may result when a foreign body is aspirated.

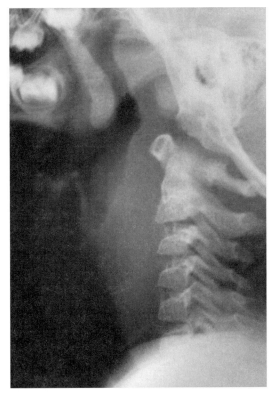

Fig. 8-7

Hypopharynx and trachea are displaced away from the cervical spine by the retropharyngeal abscess.

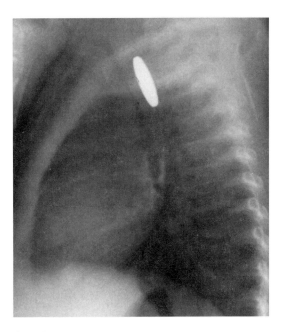

Fig. 8-8

Edema from the coin in the upper esophagus causes marked narrowing of the adjacent trachea. The child presented with stridor and difficulty with swallowing.

Tracheomalacia is diagnosed when the thoracic trachea abnormally collapses during expiration, leading to an expiratory wheeze. Although this may be seen in premature infants, other associations include tracheoesophageal fistula and vascular rings. The abnormal collapse may be easily demonstrated with airway fluoroscopy, which may be combined with a barium swallow to exclude a fistula or ring.[1,2]

RESPIRATORY DISTRESS IN THE NEWBORN

The various entities resulting in respiratory distress in the newborn may be combined under the mnemonic "CHAMPS" (Box 8-1).

One of the most common causes of respiratory distress in the newborn is *transient tachypnea of the newborn,* or *wet lung disease.* Conditions that decrease the thoracic squeeze to clear the lungs of fluid at delivery include cesarean section, mild or-moderate prematurity, maternal diabetes, and pre-cipitous delivery. The radiographic findings usually show mild vascular congestion with pulmonary edema and small pleural effusions. The chest film clears rapidly by 24 hours and is usually normal by 48 to 72 hours of age with conservative treatment.

Respiratory distress syndrome (RDS), or *hyaline membrane disease,* occurs in premature infants and is caused by a deficiency in pulmonary surfactant. By lowering the surface tension in the alveoli, surfactant prevents atelectasis. When surfactant is deficient, the chest radiograph shows the characteristic pattern of low lung volumes with a ground glass or granular pattern of alveolar collapse surrounding air bronchograms (Fig. 8-9).

The appearance of pleural effusions with increased heart size and edema several days after birth suggests patent ductus arteriosus. Whiteout of a lung or lobe may result from conditions such as pulmonary hemorrhage. Artificial surfactant given through the endotracheal tube may lead to rapid radiographic improvement, but it may also lead to asymmetric patterns of aeration if distributed unevenly. Gradual improvement over 1 week occurs with mild or moderate cases of RDS, but severe disease usually results in the chronic lung changes of *bronchopulmonary dysplasia* (BPD). This chronic disease is characterized by coarse, linear areas of scarring or atelectasis interspersed with areas of air trapping as well as shifting atelectasis. Both RDS and BPD may develop a variety of air leaks related to mechanical ventilation, including pneumothorax,

---

BOX 8-1

RESPIRATORY DISTRESS IN THE NEWBORN

C: Cardiac, congenital anomalies
H: Hyaline membrane disease
A: Airway
M: Meconium aspiration
P: Pneumonia
S: Surgical lesions

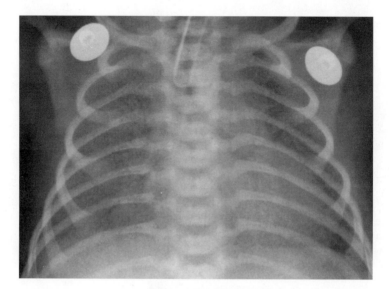

Fig. 8-9

Even after intubation, the lungs are hypoinflated and have a granular pattern with faint air bronchograms in this infant with respiratory distress syndrome.

pneumomediastinum, and pulmonary interstitial emphysema.

Pneumothoraces are the most common air leaks and are caused when air dissects in the pleural space surrounding the lung. On the frontal film of a supine patient, air is usually seen lateral to the lung but may be subpulmonic between the lung and diaphragm or medial next to the heart, where it mimics a pneumomediastinum (Fig. 8-10). If the hemithorax appears hyperlucent or the lateral costophrenic margin is too clearly visualized, a decubitus or cross-table lateral view may be helpful to exclude a pneumothorax. The upright chest film is preferred in older children in whom the pneumothorax accumulates above the lung apex.

When air dissects in the mediastinal tissues, it is called a *pneumomediastinum*. This air elevates the thymus, producing a "spinnaker sail" appearance, and may dissect under the heart, leading to a continuous diaphragm appearance (Fig. 8-11). A lateral decubitus film may cause a medial pneumothorax to shift to the elevated lateral pleural space, which distinguishes it from a pneumomediastinum. Air in a *pneumopericardium* surrounds only the heart and does not extend around other mediastinal structures such as the aorta. Neither a medial pneumothorax nor a pneumopericardium will elevate the thymus.

Pulmonary interstitial emphysema results from air dissecting in the interstitium of the lung. This

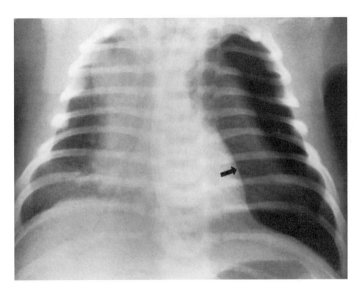

Fig. 8-10

Large left pneumothorax appears black and outlines the partially collapsed left lung and left cardiac border *(arrow)*.

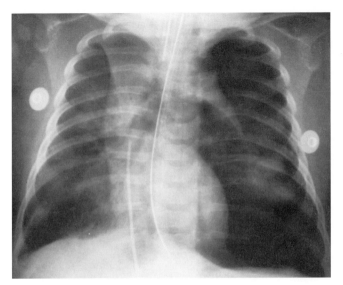

Fig. 8-11

Pneumomediastinum elevates the left lobe of the thymus to produce a "spinnaker sail" in this child who also has a large left pneumothorax.

appears as a diffuse pattern of random, small radiolucent bubbles combined with an irregular network of branching radiolucencies. Distribution is variable from entire lung to lobar to segmental. Interestingly, the pattern of involvement may shift from one lobe of one lung to another lobe in the other lung (Fig. 8-12).

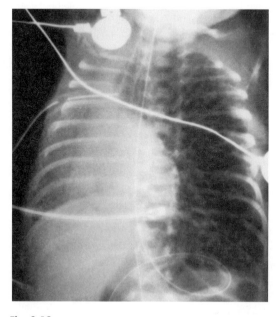

Fig. 8-12

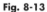

Massive pulmonary interstitial emphysema throughout the left lung causes shift of the mediastinum to the right and downward displacement of the left hemidiaphragm.

Although meconium staining of amniotic fluid occurs in 12% of deliveries, only 2% of these newborns develop *meconium aspiration syndrome* (MAS). Predisposing factors are postmaturity, intrauterine stress, and small size for gestational age. The aspirated meconium plugs bronchi and produces a chemical pneumonitis. The chest radiograph is characterized by coarse, patchy opacities secondary to atelectasis from bronchial obstruction alternating with areas of hyperinflation (Fig. 8-13). The severity of the radiographic abnormalities does not always correlate with the clinical severity of the disease. Likewise, an infant with relatively mild radiographic findings may be worse clinically due to persistent pulmonary hypertension. Pneumothoraces and pneumomediastinum develop in about 25% of infants with MAS. Resolution of the radiographic findings may take several weeks.

Although a variety of organisms may cause neonatal pneumonia, the most common is group B streptococcus, which is usually acquired transnatally. Premature rupture of the membranes and maternal infection are predisposing factors. The radiographic findings are variable and may mimic other disease entities. For example, pneumonia may have a pattern resembling RDS, but the presence of pleural effusions is rare in RDS but common in neonatal pneumonia (Fig. 8-14). Treatment is usually begun based on the clinical assumption of pneumonia, with the radiographs used to follow the progress of the disease.[3]

Two surgical entities that may cause a cystic appearance in the lung are congenital diaphragmatic hernia and cystic adenomatoid malformation. In *congenital diaphragmatic hernia,* bowel herniates

Fig. 8-13

Meconium aspiration appears as a coarse asymmetric pattern. Enlargement of the heart may be secondary to fluid overload in this infant.

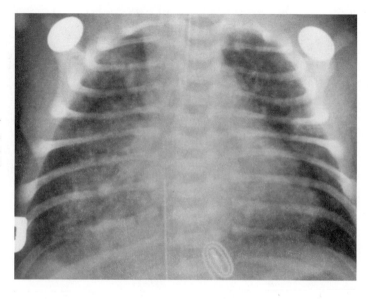

through the defect in the diaphragm, leading to a "cystic" appearance as the loops become air filled. If the stomach herniates as well, placement of a naso-gastric tube may confirm the diagnosis. Because the bowel is in the chest, the abdomen will appear scaphoid. Most of the hernias occur on the left. Patient outcome depends on the degree of pulmonary hypoplasia caused by compression of the developing lung tissue (Fig. 8-15).

Cystic adenomatoid malformation is a derange-ment in the normal pulmonary tissue development leading to cysts ranging from millimeters to sev-eral centimeters in size. Initially the cysts are fluid filled but become air filled over the first day or two of life. A large dominant cyst could mimic congenital lobar emphysema, whereas cysts appearing to fill one lung could mimic congenital diaphragmatic hernia. The presence of a normal amount of bowel in the abdomen would make a hernia unlikely.[4]

ATELECTASIS

Atelectasis is caused by an absence of air in the lung parenchyma from a myriad of causes, includ-ing bronchial obstruction or extrinsic compression. Most atelectasis is subsegmental in extent and appears as discoid or plate-like opacities, often radiating from the hila or located just above the diaphragm. Segments, lobes, and entire lungs may be collapsed, or atelectatic. This loss of volume may shift fissures toward the area of atelectasis, cause mediastinal shift toward the affected side, and elevate the ipsilateral diaphragm. Crowding of the pulmonary vascular and interstitial markings in the affected region will occur. The other lung or adjacent lobes may become more lucent secondary to hyperexpansion.

When atelectasis occurs in the right upper lobe, the minor fissure and posterior half of the major fissure shift upward. The collapsed right upper lobe appears as a triangular wedge of opac-ity adjacent to the superior mediastinum in the frontal radiograph and as a triangular wedge at the apex in the lateral radiograph. Because no minor fissure is present on the left, collapse of the left upper lobe appears different from the right, with the major fissure shifting in an ante-rior direction. The collapsed left upper lobe on frontal projection appears as an opacity in the up-per two thirds of the lung that obscures superior mediastinal and left cardiac borders and lacks a sharply defined border with the aerated lower lobe (Fig. 8-16). In lateral projection the left up-per lobe collapses adjacent to the anterior chest wall, with the major fissure defining the edge against the lower lobe. Isolated lingular atelecta-sis obscures the left cardiac border.

Right middle lobe collapse is commonly seen in asthmatic children and causes the major and minor fissures to approximate. The resultant triangular wedge or plate-like opacity is most diagnostic in

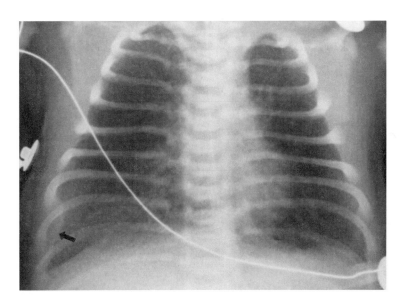

Fig. 8-14

Group B streptococcal pneumonia presents in this infant with hyperinflation, small right pleural effusion *(arrow),* and hazy infiltrative pattern.

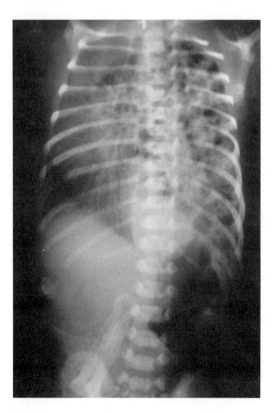

Fig. 8-15

Multiple "cysts" in the left hemithorax are air-filled loops of bowel that herniated through the defect in the left hemidiaphragm. The abdomen is scaphoid from decreased bowel content.

lateral projection and extends from the hilum to the anterior chest wall (Fig. 8-17). It is less defined in frontal projection and may appear as a vague loss of the right cardiac border. A special view called the *apical lordotic view* rotates the right middle lobe collapse on the frontal projection so that it is better seen as a triangular opacity contiguous with the right cardiac border.

Both right and left lower lobe atelectasis cause downward shift of the upper half of the major fissure and posterior shift of the lower half of the fissure. The lobe collapses posteromedially toward the posterior costophrenic sulcus and medial costovertebral angle. The sharp border of the adjacent diaphragm becomes obscured in both projections. In the lateral radiograph the normally more lucent appearing lower thoracic vertebral bodies appear denser than normal due to the x-ray beam having to penetrate through the adjacent collapsed lower lobe.

The previously described silhouette sign is useful in localizing suspected atelectasis. The right cardiac border loses its sharp definition with right middle lobe atelectasis, whereas the left border is associated with lingular pathology. The diaphragmatic border is lost when atelectasis or other pathology occurs in the adjacent lower lobe.[5]

PNEUMONIA

Viruses are the most common cause of *pneumonia* in children, especially in the outpatient population. Many bacterial pneumonias are superimposed over viral infections but may also be seen in hospitalized patients. Fungal and less common infections

Fig. 8-16

Left upper lobe collapse causes elevation of the left hemidiaphragm and crowding of the left ribs from volume loss. The cardiac and superior mediastinal borders are indistinct due to the "silhouette sign" while the diaphragm remains demarcated by the aerated left lower lobe.

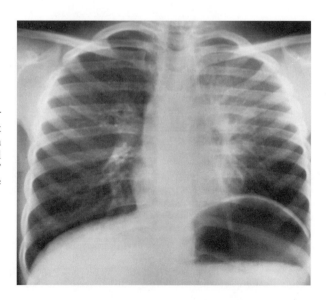

should be suspected in the immunocompromised patient.

Infections may involve primarily the airways, mainly the peripheral air spaces, or a combination of both. *Bronchiolitis* in the younger child and *bronchitis* in the older child are viral infections of the airways leading to a radio-

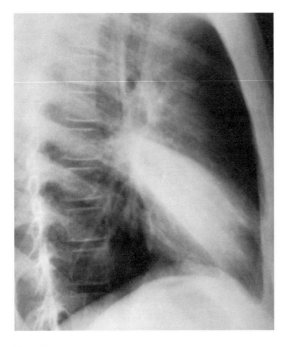

Fig. 8-17

Collapsed right middle lobe appears as a triangular wedge of increased density extending anteriorly and inferiorly toward the anterior chest wall and diaphragm.

graphic appearance of bronchial wall thickening. Hyperinflation of the lungs as well as linear areas of atelectasis secondary to airway plugging by mucus are often associated with airway inflammation.

Patchy areas of poorly defined parenchymal opacification characterize *bronchopneumonia*. The inflammation in the airways extends outward to involve the adjacent air spaces. The opacities may be caused by the air space inflammation as well as by atelectasis from associated mucus plugging of the peripheral airways. Air bronchograms occur when the open airways are surrounded by consolidated or collapsed air spaces. Both viral and bacterial pneumonias can cause a bronchopneumonia pattern. Although it may mimic other pulmonary diseases, *Mycoplasma* presents typically as a bronchopneumonia.

Filling of the peripheral air spaces with an infectious exudate causes a dense, consolidated appearance. The involvement may be limited to a segment of lung or spread to involve the entire lobe. Bacterial infections are usually the cause of consolidated, or *lobar,* pneumonia.

Pneumonia may be associated with hilar adenopathy and pleural effusions. When the pleura becomes infected, the resulting empyema may need to be surgically drained. Although decubitus films may be able to differentiate an uncomplicated mobile effusion from loculated fluid or thickening, both ultrasound and CT can be used to better characterize the pleural fluid or empyema. Pulmonary abscesses are rare complications, but pneumatoceles may occur after staphylococcal pneumonia. Round pneumonias are usually of pneumococcal origin (Fig. 8-18).[6-9]

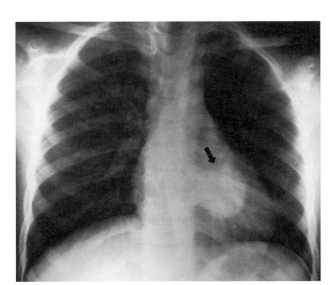

Fig. 8-18

Round pneumonia *(arrow)* in the left lower lobe simulates a mass.

ASTHMA

Asthma is caused by recurrent bronchospasm of the large intrathoracic airways leading to wheezing and labored breathing. Chest radiographs are usually obtained to exclude the presence of pneumonia causing the acute episode. Typical findings are hyperinflation and bronchial wall thickening. Mucus plugging of the airways may lead to atelectasis and obstructive emphysema. Atelectasis is the usual cause of a focal opacity in the lung, but persistence of the opacity for several days should raise suspicion of pneumonia. Pneumomediastinum occurs in a small percentage of children evaluated for an acute asthma attack.[7,9]

CYSTIC FIBROSIS

Cystic fibrosis is a genetic disorder found in Caucasians that causes increased viscosity of the respiratory mucus. This mucus is difficult to clear from the airways, leading to obstruction and promotion of bacterial infection. Early childhood radiographs may show nonspecific findings of airways disease with peribronchial thickening, atelectasis, and air trapping. As the disease progresses, finger-like mucoid impaction of the airways may be demonstrated along with abnormal dilation of the airways called *bronchiectasis*. Recurrent infections are common. Striking hyperinflation is seen in older patients, often with enlarged hila from pulmonary hypertension. Spontaneous pneumothoraces may occur from rupture of bullae or blebs (Fig. 8-19).[8]

ADULT RESPIRATORY DISTRESS SYNDROME

Although described in adults, *adult respiratory distress syndrome* (ARDS) may occur in children as well. An insult causes increased capillary permeability, pulmonary edema, and hemorrhage leading to acute respiratory failure. A partial list of causes includes trauma, infection, inhalation injury, aspiration, near drowning, and drugs. The disease passes through stages, starting with hyperinflation and eventually leading to extensive lung consolidation. Pneumothoraces and pneumomediastinum are common complications (Fig. 8-20).[8]

CHEST TRAUMA

When the injured child is evaluated in the ED, initial radiographs to screen for trauma usually include a frontal view of the chest. Lines and tubes inserted at the accident site or on arrival in the ED

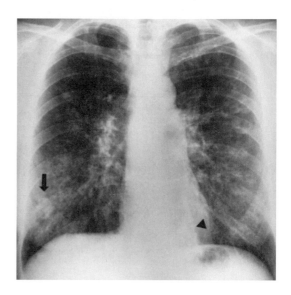

Fig. 8-19

Coarse interstitial markings, hyperinflation, bronchiectasis, mucus plugging *(arrow)*, atelectasis *(arrowhead)*, and enlarged pulmonary hila are all demonstrated in this child with cystic fibrosis.

should be assessed for position and effectiveness. A right mainstem intubation may lead to collapse of the left lung. The position of a chest tube may not be optimal for evacuating a pneumothorax, and the nasogastric tube may need to be advanced for placement in the stomach.

Consolidation in the patient with blunt trauma may result from pulmonary contusion with hemorrhage into the air spaces. Laceration of the lung may lead to a pneumothorax. The rib cage should be evaluated for fractures, especially adjacent to an area of lung injury. Multiple contiguous rib fractures may result in a flail chest with associated ventilation difficulties (Fig. 8-21).

Widening of the superior mediastinum suggests hemorrhage, and aortic injury should be considered. Children have prominent thymic tissue, so this should be excluded as the cause of mediastinal widening. Tracheal and bronchial fractures are rare but cause massive air leaks. Enlargement of the cardiac silhouette from a traumatic pericardial effusion is rare.

If the patient is undergoing CT for abdominal injury, a scan of the chest can easily be performed at the same time. CT of the chest is supplanting aortography for exclusion of aortic injury at many hospitals. The extent of pulmonary injury can also be better defined, with more injury often demonstrated on the CT than suspected on the chest radiograph. Positioning of the chest tubes can be more

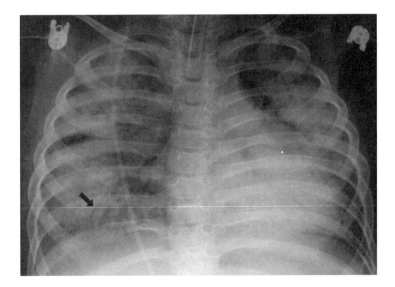

Fig. 8-20

Pneumonia was the precipitating precursor to ARDS, with densely consolidated lungs and air bronchograms (*arrow*).

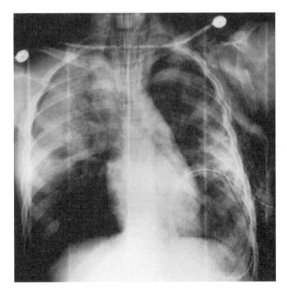

Fig. 8-21

Trauma to the chest resulted in extensive bilateral air leaks and densely consolidated pulmonary contusions. Multiple rib fractures are present.

precisely evaluated. However, the need for CT is usually made after assessment of the previously obtained chest radiographs.[7,8]

REFERENCES

1. Strife JL: Upper airway and tracheal obstruction in infants and children. *Radiol Clin North Am* 1988; 26(2):309-322.
2. Griscom NT: Diseases of the trachea, bronchi and smaller airways. *Radiol Clin North Am* 1993; 31(3):605-615.
3. Newman B, Bowen AD, Sang OK: A practical approach to the newborn chest. *Curr Probl Diagn Radiol* 1990; 19(2):41-84.
4. Newman B, Sang OK: Abnormal pulmonary aeration in infants and children. *Radiol Clin North Am* 1988; 26(2): 323-339.
5. Paré JA, Fraser R: *Synopsis of diseases of the chest.* Saunders, Philadelphia, 1983.
6. Eggli KD, Newman B: Nodules, masses, and pseudomasses in the pediatric lung. *Radiol Clin North Am* 1993; 31(3):651-666.
7. Hedlund GL, Kirks DR: Emergency radiology of the pediatric chest. *Curr Probl Diagn Radiol* 1990; 19(4):133-164.
8. Kirks DR: Practical pediatric imaging. In *Diagnostic radiology of infants and children,* ed 3. Philadelphia, Lippincott-Raven, 1998.
9. Hilton SV, Edwards DK: *Practical pediatric radiology.* Philadelphia, Saunders, 1994.

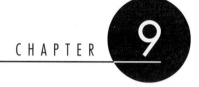

CHAPTER 9

Pediatric Flexible Bronchoscopy

Karl Kalavantavanich
Craig M. Schramm

Flexible fiberoptic bronchoscopy was first introduced for clinical practice in 1968, with the invention of flexible scopes containing fiberoptic bundles to illuminate and visualize the airways. The procedure was initially performed in adults due to the relatively large size of the fiberscopes, and most often by surgeons in operating suites. Since then the technique has proven to be easy to use, with high efficacy and portability. The development of smaller bronchoscopes in the late 1970s led to the widespread extension of this procedure to the pediatric population.[1] Pediatric flexible bronchoscopy is now performed by many medical specialists, including pediatric pulmonologists, otolaryngologists, surgeons, anesthesiologists, and pediatric intensivists. It is done in a variety of settings, including bronchoscopy suites, operating suites, intensive care units, and procedure rooms.[2-5]

INDICATIONS

Flexible bronchoscopy is indicated when (1) information valuable to the management of a patient cannot be obtained by less invasive techniques and (2) therapeutic interventions need to be directly administered to the airway (Box 9-1). As with any invasive procedure, the potential benefits to be gained in any given patient must be weighed against the risks of the procedure, even the most minor risk.

DIAGNOSTIC BRONCHOSCOPY

For diagnostic purposes, persistent or recurrent respiratory symptoms are the most common indication for flexible bronchoscopy, including stridor and abnormal voice, wheeze, and cough.

Stridor. Stridor is a common diagnostic indication for flexible bronchoscopy in infants. The possible

INDICATIONS FOR FLEXIBLE BRONCHOSCOPY

DIAGNOSTIC
AIRWAY ANATOMY EVALUATION
　Fistulas
　Hemangioma or tumors
　Stenosis or stricture
　Tracheal bronchus
　Tracheostomy evaluation
　Vascular rings

BRONCHOALVEOLAR LAVAGE AND BIOPSY
　Cytopathology
　• Lipid-laden macrophage
　• Heme-stained macrophage
　• Malignant cells
　Microbiology
　• Bacteria
　• Fungi
　• *Pneumocystis*
　• *Mycobacterium tuberculosis*
　• Viruses

FOREIGN BODY ASPIRATION

FUNCTIONAL AIRWAY EVALUATION
　Laryngo/tracheo/bronchomalacia
　Vocal cord dysfunction

HEMOPTYSIS

INHALATION INJURY

THERAPEUTIC
　Atelectasis
　Endotracheal intubation
　Foreign body aspiration
　Laser therapy

causes of recurrent or persistent stridor include vocal cord dysfunction, laryngeal pathology, subglottic stenosis, mass or tumor, and extrinsic compression of the tracheobronchial tree.

The *timing* of the stridor may give an important clue to its site of origin. The lumen of the extrathoracic airway is reduced during inspiration, when negative intraluminal pressures accompanying air movement into the lungs are less than extramural atmospheric pressure. Accordingly, lesions of the extrathoracic airway are accentuated during inspiration, and stridor is heard during the inspiratory phase. In contrast, the lumina of the intrathoracic central airways are narrowed during exhalation, when intraparenchymal pressure is greater than intraluminal pressure. Intrathoracic airway lesions will be functionally greater during exhalation and will elicit expiratory stridor. Such phase timing

is not always helpful, however, because large obstructions in the intrathoracic or extrathoracic airway may produce stridor during both phases of the respiratory cycle.

Stridor may also vary in *intensity* depending on the extent of a child's activity or agitation, which increases the child's minute ventilation. This increase in airflow will result in louder stridor.

Stridor is therefore a very dynamic process in children, and flexible bronchoscopy is ideally suited for its evaluation. Because flexible bronchoscopy is usually performed on a sedated but spontaneously breathing patient, the dynamics of the airways are preserved, without disruption by general anesthesia, positive-pressure ventilation, or the oral approach of rigid bronchoscopy. Of all indications of diagnostic pediatric flexible bronchoscopy, stridor receives the highest diagnostic yield of the procedure, identifying specific lesions in more than 80% of patients.[6,7]

The most common cause of inspiratory stridor is *laryngomalacia,* which is a prolapse of the epiglottis or aryepiglottic folds into the supraglottic space during inspiration. Laryngomalacia is caused by a congenital weakness in cartilage stiffness and redundant aryepiglottic tissue. The condition occurs in three patterns: (1) the prolapse of one or both arytenoids into the supraglottic space during inspiration, (2) the lateral enfolding across the airway of a soft epiglottis that is more omega than crescent shaped in a young infant, and (3) the anteroposterior bending of a soft epiglottis across the supraglottic space.

Other laryngeal lesions that can produce stridor include unilateral or bilateral abductor vocal cord paralysis from congenital lesions, birth trauma or recurrent laryngeal nerve injury after thoracic surgery, laryngeal papillomatosis, and laryngeal webs. Inspiratory or biphasic stridor may also arise from subglottic lesions, such as congenital or acquired subglottic stenosis, subglottic edema resulting from infection or chronic acid aspiration, or subglottic hemangiomas.

Tracheomalacia, caused by a congenital or acquired weakness in tracheal cartilaginous support, may cause inspiratory stridor but is more often associated with biphasic or expiratory stridor. Tracheomalacia may be seen in up to one third of patients with laryngomalacia. It is also present when the cartilage is deformed by a tracheoesophageal fistula or a vascular ring, and it may develop with longstanding tracheal inflammation, as seen in infants with bronchopulmonary dysplasia. If the weakness in support extends into the mainstem bronchi, the condition is termed *bronchomalacia.*

Additional causes of expiratory stridor include extrinsic tracheal or bronchial obstruction from vascular rings or slings, anomalous arteries, congenital heart disease, hilar adenopathy, or mediastinal mass lesions.

Wheeze. Recurrent wheezing is another common respiratory symptom in the pediatric population. Wheezing usually results from a more distal site of airway obstruction than stridor. The most frequent cause of recurrent wheezing in children is asthma, and most asthmatic patients do not require bronchoscopy as part of their evaluation. Exceptions to this rule include asthmatics with recurrent or persistent atelectasis (frequently of the right middle lobe) or asthmatics with gastroesophageal reflux (GER) who may have chronic aspiration. A flexible bronchoscopic evaluation is often indicated to investigate other causes of wheezing, particularly when the wheezing is unilateral, is present at birth or a very young age, or is refractory to asthma medications. Nonasthmatic causes of wheezing include anatomic abnormalities of the airway (e.g., bronchomalacia, stenosis, extrinsic compression of the left mainstem bronchus from a dilated heart), anomalies of great vessels (vascular ring), recurrent aspiration, or foreign body aspiration.

Cough. Some disorders may produce chronic cough in addition to wheezing, and bronchoscopy is often indicated because of chronic refractory cough. This indication is particularly strong when there is radiographic indication of bronchiectasis in an area of lung. There is little role for bronchoscopy in evaluating the cough that accompanies common childhood conditions such as upper and uncomplicated lower respiratory tract infections, sinusitis, postnasal drip syndrome, asthma, and exposure to environmental irritants. On the other hand, bronchoscopy should be considered to evaluate the possibilities of GER or aspiration, anatomic abnormalities of airways or large vessels, and any occult endobronchial lesions or foreign bodies, as well as to obtain culture specimens from children not responding to therapy.

Bronchoalveolar Lavage and Biopsy. Specimens are most often obtained through a pediatric bronchoscope by the instillation and return of lavage fluid into the airway. Such bronchoalveolar lavage (BAL) has emerged as a frequent indication for bronchoscopy, particularly for diagnosing a variety of microbiologic agents in complicated or refractory pneumonias, including bacterial, fungal, viral, mycobacterial, and *Pneumocystis* organisms. In addition, BAL can be used to evaluate for GER or aspiration for lipid-laden macrophages, pulmonary hemorrhage by hemosiderin-stained macrophages,

or malignancy by cytopathologic studies. Children with lobar atelectasis or consolidation may be treated conservatively with inhaled β-adrenergic agonists, corticosteroids, antimicrobial agents, and chest physiotherapy as the first line of treatment. If these measures fail to restore a collapsed area, bronchoscopy is justified for both diagnostic and therapeutic purposes.

The yield of BAL in the pediatric population is excellent. Biopsies may also be obtained through the larger flexible bronchoscopes. These may include mucosal biopsies for the evaluation of ciliary motion and ultrastructure, as well as transbronchial biopsies for the diagnosis of certain pulmonary conditions, especially rejection or infection in lung transplant patients.

Foreign Body Aspiration. The flexible bronchoscope may be used to rule out the presence of a foreign body in the lower airways of children in whom the diagnosis is not strongly suspected. However, when the presence of a foreign body is confirmed or highly suspected either by radiographic evaluation or by history, the preferred approach is to identify and remove the foreign body by rigid bronchoscopy. Although some authors believe that the flexible bronchoscope can be used for the therapeutic purpose of foreign body removal, rigid bronchoscopy is a better and safer approach in children. It allows better ventilation of the patient under general anesthesia and facilitates safer delivery of large foreign bodies through the subglottic area and the larynx compared with the flexible bronchoscope.

Hemoptysis. Flexible bronchoscopy is sometimes indicated in selected pediatric patients with hemoptysis who need visual inspection of the airways for localization of their bleeding sites. It can be useful for therapeutic purposes as well, by removal of blood clots and placement of single-lumen or double-lumen endotracheal tubes and balloon catheters to tamponade the bleeding portion of the lung. In massive hemoptysis, however, the flexible bronchoscope is usually inadequate because of its limited visualization and suction capabilities compared with rigid bronchoscopy.

Inhalation Injury. In patients with acute inhalation of a toxic or heated gas, flexible bronchoscopic evaluation of the upper and lower airways can be helpful in judging the extent of injury and determining the therapy and level of respiratory support needed. The decision for elective intubation with the assistance of bronchoscopy may be made if significant laryngeal edema is visualized.

THERAPEUTIC BRONCHOSCOPY

The flexible bronchoscope is an excellent therapeutic tool. It is very useful in placing an endotracheal tube in difficult intubation cases and is frequently used for removal of retained secretions or mucus plugs. Flexible bronchoscopy is especially beneficial in patients with atelectasis who do not respond to conventional therapy. If indicated, the bronchoscopist can selectively instill medications, such as acetylcysteine (Mucomyst), dilute sodium bicarbonate, recombinant human deoxyribonuclease I, or DNase (Pulmozyme), to help loosen secretions before bronchoscopic suctioning.

An emerging therapeutic area for flexible bronchoscopy is bronchoscopic laser surgery. A surgical team performs this procedure in an operating suite. The flexible bronchoscope can be passed through either a rigid bronchoscope or an endotracheal tube to treat the lesions located in the glottic to distal bronchi area. Lesions that have been successfully treated by this method include primary bronchial stenosis, tracheal stenosis, distal subglottic stenosis, tracheal papillomatosis, strictures in lung transplantation, and granulation tissue or tumors of the distal bronchi. Bronchoscopic laser surgery is done more frequently in adults, but the procedure can be performed safely and effectively in pediatric patients.[8]

CONTRAINDICATIONS

Flexible bronchoscopy has been shown to be a safe procedure, even when performed on very ill pediatric patients. However, certain conditions can place a patient at risk for complications (Box 9-2). Most are relative contraindications. If after careful evaluation the possible benefit of bronchoscopy outweighs the risks, the procedure should be performed by an experienced bronchoscopist.

Flexible bronchoscopy frequently causes *hypoxemia,* most often due to occlusion of the airway by the bronchoscope during the procedure and hypoventilation or apnea from sedation. Pulse oximeter and cardiac and respiratory tracings should be continuously monitored during and after the procedure. Supplemental oxygen should be provided to maintain oxygen saturation, optimally above 95%. If the patient is already hypoxemic, flexible bronchoscopy can further worsen the hypoxemia and place the patient at serious risk. Patients with impending respiratory failure may be electively intubated before the bronchoscopy, in anticipation of worsening ventilation and oxygenation during and after the procedure. Some patients may benefit from the administration of low-flow oxygen through the suction channel of the bronchoscope. This can be done by attaching a 1-ml syringe to oxygen tubing, inserting the syringe into the suction port, and administering 1 to 2 liters per minute of oxygen. The application of oxygen in this manner must be done with caution in young children, whose airways are substantially occluded by the bronchoscope. Similarly, such administration precludes wedging the scope in older patients because of the risks of barotrauma and pneumothorax.

Elective flexible bronchoscopy should not be performed in the patient who has cardiovascular instability, uncontrolled asthma, coagulopathy, pulmonary hypertension, severe upper airway obstruction, and superior vena cava obstruction, until these conditions are stabilized. It should be performed very selectively and with great caution in patients with acute laryngotracheitis because of the risks of sudden laryngospasm during the procedure and additional postprocedural airway edema that may severely compromise an already swollen airway. The bronchoscope should never be forcefully inserted past any area of airway narrowing to avoid further injury and compromise to that site. As noted earlier, the strong suspicion of foreign body aspiration is a relative contraindication to flexible and an indication for rigid bronchoscopy.

EQUIPMENT

FLEXIBLE BRONCHOSCOPE

The flexible bronchoscope may be divided into three sections: (1) insertion tube, (2) control head and eyepiece, and (3) light source connector.

Insertion Tube. The insertion tube is the flexible portion of the bronchoscope that is inserted into

---

BOX 9-2

CONTRAINDICATIONS TO FLEXIBLE BRONCHOSCOPY

ABSOLUTE CONTRAINDICATIONS
Inability to oxygenate the patient adequately
Cardiovascular instability
- Hypotension
- Malignant arrhythmias
- Myocardial infarction

RELATIVE CONTRAINDICATIONS
Coagulopathy
Hypercapnia with acidosis
Hypoxemia
Severe pulmonary hypertension
Severe upper airway obstruction
Superior vena cava obstruction
Uncooperative patient
Uncontrolled asthma
Uremia

the patient's airways. These tubes have the same working length of 55 cm, but they vary in outer diameter from less than 2.0 mm to 6.3 mm. The instruments most often used in pediatric patients are 2.2-mm-diameter scopes for neonates, 3.5- to 3.7-mm scopes for older children, and 4.5-mm scopes for adolescents (Fig. 9-1). The composition of the tubes varies somewhat according to the diameter. All scopes contain one or two fiberoptic bundles for light transmission from the light source to the airway, as well as one fiberoptic cable for transmission of the airway image from the tip of the scope to the eyepiece. These fiberoptic bundles consist of thousands of tiny (8-μm) glass fibers that are coated with a highly reflective glass material. These fibers transmit light and images by internal reflections at the core-coating interface. This arrangement of highly reflective, minute glass fibers accounts for the bronchoscope's flexibility and high image quality; however, it also imparts substantial fragility to the instrument.

The insertion tubes of the thinnest bronchoscopes, those less than 2.0 mm in diameter, only contain light and image bundles. They are nondirectable because they lack the cables necessary to direct the distal section of the scope. Appropriately, they have been nicknamed "spaghetti scopes," and their use is limited to visualization of an airway via insertion down an endotracheal tube.

Larger, flexible bronchoscopes have two control cables aligned 180 degrees from each other that connect a hinged bending section at the distal tip of the tube to a control lever at the head of the scope. These cables allow the operator to flex and extend the distal tip of the bronchoscope, in order to direct the passage of the scope through the airways. The 2.2-mm scopes have this directable capability, but they lack the third major component of the insertion tube, a suction channel. The larger scopes contain suction channels, varying in diameter from 1.2 mm in the 3.5- to 3.7-mm scopes to 3.2 mm in the 4.5-mm scopes. These suction channels allow for the suction of airway secretions, the instillation of lavage fluids or medications into the airway, and the passage of brushes and biopsy instruments for obtaining airway cytology and pathology specimens. The channel, direction cables, and fiberoptic bundles are enmeshed in a woven metal sheath and then enclosed in a nonlatex flexible plastic membrane.

Control Head and Eyepiece. The control head directs the insertion tube and use of the bronchoscope and transmits its images to the operator. Transmission is accomplished with an eyepiece and focusing ring. The operator may look through the eyepiece directly at the distal image. Alternately, the image can be split with a teaching head to allow for co-visualization by the operator and an observer. More often, the image is recorded by a camera attached to the eyepiece and displayed on a video monitor during the procedure. On directable bronchoscopes the control head contains the angulation lever, which regulates the cables attached to the bending tip of the scope. On the larger scopes there is also a channel port attached or in addition to a button that activates suction through the suction channel. Syringes attach to the port for airway lavage, and instruments may be passed through the port for the collection of airway specimens. A suction adapter extends at a right angle

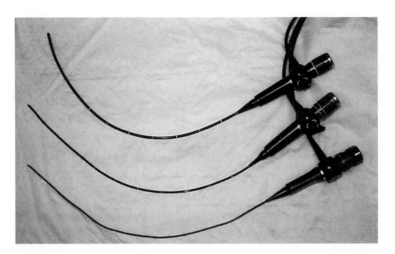

Fig. 9-1

Three different sizes of pediatric flexible bronchoscopes. *Top to bottom,* 4.5, 3.6, and 2.2 mm outer diameter. Note that all scopes have similar working tube lengths.

from the head of the bronchoscope and attaches to tubing connected to the suction source.

Light Source Connector. The control head is also attached to a cable. The other end of the cable contains the light source connector, for the transmission of light from a source to the fiberoptic cables in the insertion tube. The light source houses a bright halogen or xenon lamp, which provides adequate illumination via the fiberoptic cables.

VIDEO RECORDING EQUIPMENT

Video recording has proven to be valuable in flexible bronchoscopy procedures. Video allows the bronchoscopist to review the findings after the procedure, identifying or clarifying lesions missed during the actual procedure and at other times allowing for consultation with medical or surgical colleagues. Video of the taped procedure may also be shown to the patient and family when discussing the pathology and treatment plan. The video also provides a record of the findings, which may be used for comparison with past or future bronchoscopies.

PREPARATION

To perform an efficient and safe procedure with minimal complications, the practitioner needs to fully prepare the bronchoscopy area and equipment, medications, the patient, and the bronchoscopist and assistants.

EQUIPMENT AND SUPPLIES

The proper selection and preparation of equipment are important to ensure a safe and effective procedure. The preparation of this equipment and certain medications is usually the responsibility of the respiratory therapist who will assist in the procedure. Pediatric bronchoscopes come in many diameters, with the smaller ones used in patients who have small airways, such as neonatal patients or patients with airway obstruction. Smaller scopes do not have suction channels and are more difficult to handle because they are more rigid and lack directability. The larger bronchoscope has a suction channel and usually provides better visualization.

The light source, video recorder, and monitor are usually maintained on a portable bronchoscope cart. Equipment, such as 1% to 2% lidocaine spray, 2% lidocaine jelly for lubricant, syringes containing aliquots of 1% to 2% lidocaine, a Leuken's trap, 10-ml normal saline aliquots for lavage, and clean gauzes may be placed on top of the cart for easy access (Fig. 9-2). A cardiac monitor, pulse oximeter, and emergency resuscitation cart should also be placed at the bedside. The cart must contain an appropriately sized resuscitation

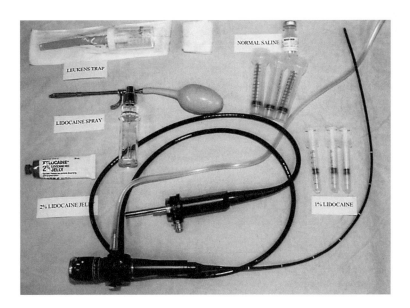

Fig. 9-2

Necessary equipment for basic pediatric flexible bronchoscopy includes bronchoscope, attached suction tube, 2% lidocaine jelly, lidocaine spray, 3 aliquots of 1-ml 1% lidocaine solution, Leuken's trap, gauze pads, and 3 to 5 aliquots of 10-ml normal saline for bronchoalveolar lavage. These items are placed on a clean drape on top of a portable bronchoscopy cart.

bag and mask, laryngoscopes and endotracheal tubes, and resuscitation medications. Wall suction and oxygen should be connected and turned on for prompt access if needed. Two sources of wall suction are ideal; one connected to the bronchoscope to clear the field of vision and to obtain specimens, and the other connected to a suction catheter for use if the patient has excessive oropharyngeal secretions or vomits during the procedure. On certain occasions, special equipment or medications may be needed, such as a swivel adapter for an endotracheal tube, positive end-expiratory pressure (PEEP) valves, tracheostomy tubes, wire brushes for cytology, transbronchial needle catheters, sodium bicarbonate, acetylcysteine, and DNase (Box 9-3).

During the procedure, nearly all pediatric patients require some type of sedation. The most common

---

BOX 9-3

EQUIPMENT AND SUPPLIES FOR PEDIATRIC FLEXIBLE BRONCHOSCOPY

BRONCHOSCOPE WITH LIGHT SOURCE
Endotracheal tube swivel adapter
Water-soluble lubricant

MONITORING EQUIPMENT
Cardiac monitor with electrode
   patches
Pulse oximeter with probes
Respiratory monitor
Sphygmomanometer
Stethoscope

OXYGEN AND AEROSOL EQUIPMENT
Aerosol mask
Cannula with naris prong clipped
Flowmeter
Nebulizer
Oxygen mask with nose cut out
Oxygen source
Oxygen tubing with connectors

SPECIMEN COLLECTION EQUIPMENT
Biopsy forceps
Channel brush
Fixative
Glass slides
Leuken's trap
Retrieval baskets and cages
Syringes with nonbacteriostatic saline for
   bronchoalveolar lavage
Transport media

SUCTION EQUIPMENT
Sterile gloves
Suction canisters
Suction catheters
Suction tubing
Tonsil-tip or Yankauer-type suction
   catheter
Vacuum suction source

INTRAVENOUS EQUIPMENT
Isotonic saline
IV sets
Syringes with flush solution

MEDICATIONS
TOPICAL ANESTHETICS
Lidocaine solution (1% to 2%)
Lidocaine viscous (2%)

SEDATIVES
Diazepam
Fentanyl
Meperidine
Midazolam
Morphine

AEROSOLS
Albuterol
Racemic epinephrine

EMERGENCY DRUGS
Atropine
Bicarbonate
Epinephrine (1:1000)
Flumazenil
Furosemide
IV corticosteroids
Naloxone
Phenobarbital
Succinylcholine

RESUSCITATION EQUIPMENT
Bite block
Endotracheal tubes
Extra batteries for laryngoscope
Extra light bulbs
Face masks
Laryngoscope with blades
Oral airways
Resuscitation bag with oxygen tubing attached
Stylets

VIDEO CAMERA WITH RECORDING EQUIPMENT

BRONCHOSCOPIST AND ASSISTANT EQUIPMENT
Eye protectors
Gloves
Gown
Mask
Scissors

approach is a conscious sedation. Intravenous (IV) drugs are preferable to intramuscular (IM) medications because of their quicker onset, shorter duration, and titratable dosage for optimal effects. Although a variety of sedative agents are available, the combination of a *benzodiazepine* (e.g., midazolam) and a *narcotic* (e.g., fentanyl or morphine) is widely accepted. In addition to sedative effects, the narcotic provides analgesic and antitussive effects, and the benzodiazepine offers anxiolytic effects and antegrade amnesia. The most common side effect of this combination is respiratory depression. Occasionally, benzodiazepines can induce cardiovascular depression, and narcotics can elicit muscular rigidity and impaired liver and kidney functions. Fortunately, if these complications occur, specific reversal agents, naloxone (0.01 mg/kg/dose) and flumazenil (0.2 mg/kg/dose), can be given to restore the patient's respiratory status. These antagonists, along with atropine and epinephrine for adverse cardiac events, should be immediately available.

Additional medications that should be available include aerosolized albuterol to treat any bronchospasm that may develop, aerosolized epinephrine for airway edema, and diphenhydramine and a corticosteroid to treat a potential anaphylactic reaction to the sedating medications.

PATIENT

Patient preparation includes a thorough history and physical examination before the procedure. Any radiographic studies are reviewed. Information regarding the child's current health status and drug allergies must be obtained. Elective bronchoscopic procedures should be postponed if the patient has a reversible condition or acute illness that may increase the risk for complications from the sedation or the procedure itself. An informed consent must be obtained with a thorough explanation of the procedure to the parents and, if able to understand, the patient. All patients must not take anything by mouth (NPO) 4 to 6 hours before the procedure to ensure an empty stomach and minimize the risk of aspiration.

The need for IV access to the patient is somewhat controversial. Flexible laryngoscopy may be performed in infants and cooperative older children with only topical anesthesia because it causes no more trauma than nasopharyngeal suctioning and can be equally brief when done by an experienced operator. Many bronchoscopists require IV access in all young children in whom the scope will be passed below the glottis. Although sufficient conscious sedation can be achieved with oral, intranasal, and IM agents in the absence of IV access, an IV line may prove lifesaving if rare complications arise.

For psychological support and patient comfort, parents should be allowed to stay with the patient as long as possible before starting the procedure. However, they should not overstimulate the patient, especially when conscious sedation is used. The importance of a calm, nonstimulating atmosphere in the bronchoscopy area cannot be overstated. This may be achieved by low-level lighting, calm and quiet actions by the bronchoscopist and support personnel, and a smooth prebronchoscopy routine. Premedication with a benzodiazepine 30 to 60 minutes before the procedure can help the patient relax prior to starting the procedure.

PERSONNEL

In general, the flexible bronchoscopy team includes a bronchoscopist, a nurse, and a respiratory therapist. All team members should be informed of the patient's diagnosis, indication for bronchoscopy, allergies, and biologic risks to the patient and team members. In addition, the team should be fully informed of the planned procedures and any difficulties that may arise. Everyone should wear a clean protective gown, gloves, mask, and eye protection. All body fluids, including BAL specimens, should be handled carefully using universal precautions.

Personnel safety is increased by identifying patients with potentially transmissible pathogens, such as hepatitis viruses, human immunodeficiency virus (HIV), and *Mycobacterium tuberculosis*. Approved HEPA filter masks should be worn for all procedures involving patients with suspected *M. tuberculosis* infection, and the procedure should be performed in a room that meets ventilation requirements for tuberculosis. The suspected patient should be kept in a respiratory isolation room before and after the procedure.

PROCEDURE

Most pediatric flexible bronchoscopies are performed with the patient in a supine position on a bed. The height of the bed should be adjusted to the bronchoscopist's comfort level. When the patient and bronchoscopy team are ready and all preparations are completed, the selected sedation is initiated. Appropriate sedation will decrease the patient's anxiety, discomfort, and unwanted physiologic effects. Nevertheless, many younger patients may need a gentle restraining system even when sedated.

CONSCIOUS SEDATION

Several different conscious sedation regimens have been used safely and successfully for pediatric flexible bronchoscopy. As noted earlier, one of the most widely accepted is a combination of a benzodiazepine (e.g., midazolam) and a narcotic (e.g., fentanyl or meperidine) given intravenously. The usual pediatric dose of IV midazolam ranges from 0.05 to 0.3 mg/kg to a maximal total dose of 0.4 to 0.6 mg/kg (or 6 to 10 mg). Typically, sedation is begun with a small dose (0.05 to 0.1 mg/kg) and is then titrated upward every 5 minutes to achieve the optimal sedative effect. The same approach is also used for IV fentanyl, 1 to 3 µg/kg to a maximal total dose of 5 to 10 µg/kg, starting with 1-µg/kg/dose and titrating upward every 5 minutes. Some bronchoscopists prefer a stronger sedative, such as IV ketamine (1 mg/kg/dose) or IV propofol (1 to 2 mg/kg/dose).[9]

Other combinations of drugs are given intramuscularly and include meperidine, promethazine, and chlorpromazine and the combination of droperidol, promethazine, and thorazine. The disadvantages of IM sedation include the inability to titrate the optimal dose of the medications and the lack of IV access in case of an emergency. However, the IM approach is sometimes justified for short procedures in stable children with difficult IV access.

Intranasal midazolam has also been shown to induce adequate sedation for pediatric patients undergoing endoscopic procedures or imaging studies.[10] The usual dosage of intranasal midazolam ranges from 0.2 to 0.5 mg/kg/dose.

Regardless of the method, optimal sedation is achieved when the child is sleepy and has minimal reaction to noxious stimuli, while still maintaining adequate ventilation and protective airway reflexes.

TOPICAL ANESTHESIA

Conscious sedation is augmented by the application of the local anesthetic agent, 1% to 2% lidocaine, to the nasal cavity, posterior pharynx, vocal cords, and tracheobronchial tree. Another technique is to pretreat the subject with an aerosol of 4 to 8 mg/kg of lidocaine given by a nebulizer.[11] Lidocaine 2% jelly may also be applied to the nares with a cotton-tipped applicator or small syringe. Care should be taken in small infants that the total lidocaine dosage does not exceed the maximal therapeutic range of 3 to 4 mg/kg. Toxic lidocaine levels have been reported with topical airway administration.

PATIENT MONITORING

Continuous cardiac, respiratory, and oximetry monitoring must be performed during and after the procedure. During the procedure the patient should be closely monitored for heart rate, respiratory rate, cardiac and respiratory tracings, oxygen saturation, clinical airway obstruction, chest wall movement, peripheral perfusion, and cyanosis. Ideally, oxygen saturation should be maintained above 95% at all times, with supplemental oxygen delivered to the patient by mask or blow-by if necessary. Occasionally a bronchoscopy may be required in a critically ill child whose oxygen saturation cannot be maintained above 95%. In this setting, if the potential benefits of the procedure outweigh its increased risks, the bronchoscopy may be performed with added caution. If a patient's cardiorespiratory status becomes unstable during any procedure, the bronchoscope must be withdrawn and the procedure stopped immediately. Appropriate emergency procedures should be performed.

TECHNIQUE

The bronchoscope may be balanced on the left hand (Fig. 9-3). The left thumb controls the angulation lever on the control head, and the right

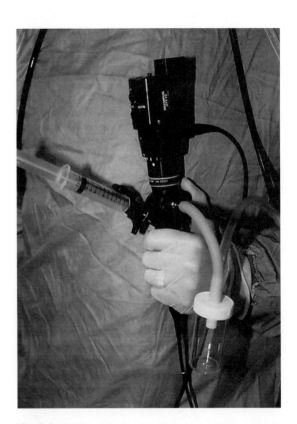

Fig. 9-3

Demonstration of holding the flexible bronchoscope in the operator's left hand. A video camera has been attached to the eyepiece of the control head of the bronchoscope. A 10-ml syringe has been inserted into the suction channel port, and a Leuken's trap has been placed in line with the suction tubing for specimen collection. The operator's thumb is positioned on the angulation lever, and the suction valve is situated just above the operator's index finger for easy activation.

thumb and index finger direct the insertion tube at the naris. Other bronchoscopists may prefer to hold the scope in their right hand and direct the tube with their left hand. Routes for bronchoscopic approaches include nasal, oral, and through endotracheal or tracheostomy tubes.

The most common route for pediatric patients is the *transnasal* approach. The flexible bronchoscope is lubricated with lidocaine jelly, or another sterile water-based lubricant, and then inserted through a nostril into the nasopharyngeal area. A topical decongestant (e.g., phenylephrine) may be administered to the nasal mucosa first to facilitate passage of the scope past edematous tissue and to reduce the risk of epistaxis. The nasopharyngeal and laryngeal anatomy is visualized. The vocal cords are assessed for movement and then anesthetized with lidocaine sprayed through a suction channel of the bronchoscope. Adequate laryngeal anesthesia is critical to avoid sudden laryngospasm. The bronchoscope is then passed through the vocal cords into the tracheobronchial tree. Another dose of 1% to 2% lidocaine is usually applied to the carina to minimize a cough reflex. The tracheobronchial anatomy is then examined.

If BAL is performed, the bronchoscopist wedges the bronchoscope in the selected segmental or subsegmental bronchi, and normal saline is instilled in 3 to 5 aliquots of up to 1 ml/kg per aliquot. The saline is then suctioned back through the suction channel. Typically, one-third to one-half the instilled volume is recovered with suctioning. A specimen is usually collected in a Leuken's trap and sent for microbiology or pathology studies. If a specimen is collected for microbiologic evaluation, suction should not be applied until the bronchoscope is inside the trachea, in order to minimize contamination of the channel with nasopharyngeal secretions. To avoid tipping over the trap and losing the specimen to the wall suction, special care should be taken to handle the specimen trap in an upright position. In special cases, consultation with the microbiologist or pathologist beforehand will ensure that the specimen is large enough for the requested study and is handled and sent appropriately. The bronchoscopist is usually responsible for ordering the tests and specimen handling. The whole procedure may be useless if the specimen is not handled and processed properly.

During the bronchoscopy the respiratory therapist is often responsible for connecting and disconnecting suction, attaching normal saline syringes and traps for lavage, and giving certain transbronchoscopic medications. The therapist and assisting nurse may divide responsibility for monitoring the patient's oxygenation and respiratory status, stabilizing the patient's head and upper airway, and comforting the patient. Because the bronchoscopist is focused on the procedure, the therapist and nurse are responsible for detecting and promptly notifying the bronchoscopist of any untoward patient occurrence. The respiratory therapist is also responsible for assisting in emergency respiratory management, such as maintaining patency of the patient's airway, suctioning oropharyngeal secretions, handling emergency equipment, and giving certain respiratory medications.

When performing flexible bronchoscopy in a patient who is being mechanically ventilated, the risk of further compromise to the patient's respiratory condition is higher with a partially occluded endotracheal tube. Special considerations should be made for maximizing the patient's ventilation and oxygenation and compensating for air leaks that may occur. In this situation the respiratory therapist is responsible for ventilator adjustment and stabilization of the endotracheal tube.

POSTPROCEDURAL MONITORING

Monitoring of the patient must continue after the procedure until the patient has fully awakened or has returned to preprocedural baseline status. Children, particularly anxious toddlers, often require large doses of medications, with the level of sedation increasing after the procedure, when the agents are still active and the child is no longer stimulated by the procedure. It is essential to continue to monitor the adequacy of the patient's oxygenation, ventilation, and airway patency until the sedation has completely resolved. Breath sounds should be followed for the development of any stridor or wheezing after the procedure. To prevent aspiration, oral fluids are withheld until the patient is fully awake and the topical laryngeal anesthesia has worn off, usually about 1 hour after administering the topical anesthetic.

COMPLICATIONS

In general, flexible bronchoscopy is a safe and well-tolerated procedure in pediatric patients, especially when it is performed by an experienced bronchoscopy team that employs careful monitoring and takes appropriate precautions. The most common complications include transient cough, respiratory depression, hypoxemia, and bronchospasm during the procedure. Cough is almost universally seen during and after the procedure, but it is usually self-limited and resolves within 24 hours. Minor epistaxis is common and does not require therapy. Respiratory depression is usually associated with oversedation and sometimes requires reversal agents (e.g., naloxone, flumazenil). Any bronchospasm is relieved promptly in most patients by bronchodilator aerosol treatments (e.g., albuterol).

A less common but potentially more serious complication is *laryngospasm*. This problem can be avoided by application of topical lidocaine to the vocal cords and minimal manipulation of the scope around the glottic area. If laryngospasm occurs, the bronchoscope must be withdrawn immediately and airway resuscitation initiated. These measures include jaw thrust, suction of secretions, and mask ventilation. Rarely, laryngospasm may become life threatening and require paralysis and endotracheal intubation.

Complications from BAL include fever and less frequently pneumonia. Other, more serious complications, including arrhythmias, pulmonary hemorrhage, and pneumothorax, are seldom encountered during pediatric flexible bronchoscopy. Deaths are extremely rare, with no bronchoscopy-related mortality reported in more than 2500 pediatric flexible bronchoscopy procedures.[12]

EQUIPMENT MAINTENANCE

Because the bronchoscope and its accessories are extremely fragile and expensive, special attention must be taken during care and cleaning and maintenance procedures. Proper care can increase the life span of the equipment, decrease repair and replacement costs, and reduce the potential risk of cross-contamination. Handling requires the avoidance of any excessive angulation or twisting of the scope, actions that can damage the quartz fiber bundles. Inadequate disinfection of a bronchoscope can result in serious outcome to a patient. The organisms most often responsible for cross-contamination between bronchoscopies are *Mycobacterium* and *Pseudomonas*.[3]

The flexible bronchoscope should be cleaned immediately after each procedure. Dried secretions or blood will prevent penetration of the disinfecting agent. Therefore the exterior surface should be wiped or gently scrubbed with a soft cloth or brush. The suction channel and port should be irrigated and flushed with water and then scrubbed with a special brush. If the suction valve is not disposable, it should be flushed thoroughly with a cleaning solution. The entire instrument is then rinsed copiously with tap water and immersed in a high-level disinfectant solution for 45 minutes.

Because flexible bronchoscopy is not a sterile procedure, cleaning a bronchoscope has not required routine sterilization, and high-level disinfection has been considered satisfactory. High-level disinfection is a cleaning method that inactivates all viruses, fungi, and vegetative microorganisms, but not necessarily all bacterial spores. The most common agent used is 2% glutaraldehyde. Immersion of a bronchoscope in glutaraldehyde for 10 minutes can destroy all bacteria, viruses, and 99.8% of mycobacteria, which increases to 100% if immersed for 45 minutes at 25° C.[3]

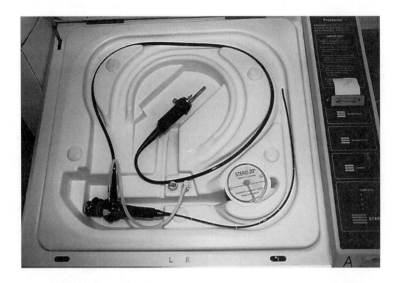

Fig. 9-4

Correct placement of flexible bronchoscope in STERIS cleaning apparatus, used for chemical sterilization of the instrument.

With increasing concern for more virulent and resistant microorganisms, many centers are adopting routine sterilization of their bronchoscopes. Two highly effective methods against all types of microorganisms are ethylene oxide gas sterilization and peracetic acid submersion. Ethylene oxide is noncorrosive and able to penetrate all portions of the bronchoscope without requiring high pressures. However, a venting cap must be placed to equalize the pressure between the interior and the exterior of the bronchoscope. The major disadvantage of ethylene oxide sterilization is that it is time-consuming, taking at least 12 to 16 hours to complete the process. An alternative method is the STERIS system (Fig. 9-4), an automated, microprocessor-controlled device using a sterilant concentrate, peracetic acid, as the active biocidal agent. This chemical sterilization process requires only 25 minutes. Once the disinfection or sterilization process is completed, the bronchoscope is rinsed with tap water and may be wiped with alcohol before storage in a dry, clean cabinet.

COMPARISON TO RIGID BRONCHOSCOPY

Rigid bronchoscopy is most often performed in the operating room by surgeons or otolaryngologists, with general anesthesia administered to the patient by an anesthesiologist. This procedure has some advantages over flexible bronchoscopy, including better control of the airway and ventilation and the ability to perform certain therapeutic maneuvers (e.g., foreign body removal, laser therapy). Relative disadvantages of rigid bronchoscopy are inability to allow inspection of distal airways, inability to assess the dynamic and natural state of the airways, and the complications associated with general anes-thesia. Thus the risks and benefits of each procedure must be carefully considered for each patient before choosing the bronchoscopic method. Occasionally the two procedures are coordinated and performed sequentially in the operating room for different diagnostic and therapeutic purposes in select patients.

REFERENCES

1. Wood RE: Spelunking in the pediatric airways: explorations with the flexible fiberoptic bronchoscope. *Pediatr Clin North Am* 1984; 31:785-799.
2. Johnson NT, Pierson DJ: Pulmonary diagnostic procedures. In Pierson DJ, Kacmarek RM, editors: *Foundations of respiratory care.* New York, Churchill-Livingstone, 1992, pp 621-640.
3. Wang KP, Mehta AC, editors: *Flexible bronchoscopy.* Cambridge, Mass, Blackwell Science, 1995.
4. Brutinel WM, Cortese DA: Fiberoptic bronchoscopy. In Burton GG, Hodgkin JE, Ward JJ, editors: *Respiratory care: a guide to clinical practice,* ed 4. Philadelphia, Lippincott, 1997, pp 281-294.
5. Hollinger LD, Lusk RP, Green CG, editors: *Pediatric laryngology and bronchoesophagology.* Philadelphia, Lippincott-Raven, 1997.
6. Barbato A et al: Use of the pediatric bronchoscope, flexible and rigid, in 51 European centers. *Eur Respir J* 1997; 10:1761-1766.
7. Godfrey S et al: Yield from flexible bronchoscopy in children. *Pediatr Pulmonol* 1997; 23:261-269.
8. Rimell FR: Pediatric laser bronchoscopy. *Int Anesthesiol Clin* 1997; 35:107-113.
9. Hertzog JH et al: Propofol anesthesia for invasive procedures in ambulatory and hospitalized children: experience in the pediatric intensive care unit. *Pediatrics* 1999; 103:e30.
10. Fishbein M et al: Evaluation of intranasal midazolam in children undergoing esophagogastroduodenoscopy. *J Pediatr Gastroenterol Nutr* 1997; 25:261-266.
11. Gjonaj ST, Lowenthal DB, Dozor AJ: Nebulized lidocaine administered to infants and children undergoing flexible bronchoscopy. *Chest* 1997; 112:1665-1669.
12. Nussbaum E: Pediatric fiberoptic bronchoscopy. *Clin Pediatr* 1995; 34:430-435.

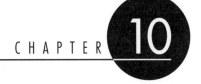

CHAPTER 10

Invasive Blood Gas Analysis and Cardiovascular Monitoring

Michael P. Czervinske

Evaluating an infant or child with respiratory impairment requires analyzing blood gases obtained through umbilical, arterial, capillary, or mixed-venous blood samples. To interpret these blood gas values correctly, the clinician must understand acid-base balance and gas exchange and be able to recognize normal and abnormal blood gas values. The techniques of blood gas sampling affect the results. This chapter reviews the procedures, indications, complications, and contraindications for each technique.

BLOOD GAS SAMPLING

Arterial blood gas (ABG) analysis is indicated when an accurate measurement of acid-base balance or pulmonary gas exchange is required.[1] This analysis may be needed in the diagnosis, evaluation of response to therapy, and therapy for patients with acute deterioration in status (Box 10-1).[2] Fig. 10-1 shows the various anatomic sites that provide access for percutaneous arterial puncture and catheterization.

PAIN CONTROL

Blood gas sampling can be a painful procedure, but the resulting information is frequently a vital part of patient management. After weighing the benefits of the procedure against potential pain, use one of the recommended techniques for controlling newborn and pediatric pain. Because painful procedures do not evoke vigorous responses to painful stimuli in critically ill newborns, many believe that the neonates are not being affected by pain.[3] However, infants probably have a higher sensitivity to painful procedures than older age groups.[4,5] Various methods, such as using an anesthetic cream, lidocaine injection, or a sucrose pacifier, are effective in helping to ameliorate the effects of pain. Depending on the type and duration of procedure, more potent short-acting analgesic or anesthetic agents may be appropriate.[6]

ARTERIAL SAMPLING SITES

Fig. 10-1 illustrates potential sites for arterial puncture or catheterization in infants or children. Avoid using the brachial and femoral sites; both feed large distal networks, and neither has collateral circulation. Also, the brachial pulse is difficult to palpate in infants and small children due to the naturally large fat pad located in that area of the arm. Injury to the brachial nerve can also result in serious complications. Only a highly skilled clinician should perform a brachial artery puncture if necessary.

BOX 10-1

INDICATIONS FOR BLOOD GAS ANALYSIS

1. Evaluation of ventilation (Pa_{CO_2})
2. Evaluation of acid-base balance (pH, Pa_{CO_2})
3. Evaluation of oxygenation (Pa_{O_2}, oxyhemoglobin)
4. Evaluation of oxygen-carrying capacity (Pa_{O_2}, oxyhemoglobin, hemoglobin, dyshemoglobin)
5. Evaluation of intrapulmonary shunt ($\dot{Q}_{SP}/\dot{Q}_T$)
6. Quantitation of response to therapy
   a. Supplemental oxygen
   b. Mechanical ventilation
7. Diagnostic evaluation
8. Monitoring of severity or progress of disease

Pa_{CO_2}, Partial pressure of carbon dioxide in arterial blood; *Pa_{O_2},* partial pressure of oxygen in arterial blood.

In a child, reserve the femoral artery for an emergency, and then only as last resort. In the neonate or infant, femoral artery puncture is not indicated. The femoral artery lies close to the femoral vein, nerve, and hip joint. Because of the proximity of these structures, likely damage to one may cause severe complications.[7]

The preferred site in both neonatal and pediatric populations is the *radial artery.* The radial artery provides good access as well as collateral circulation to the hand by the ulnar artery. No nerves or veins are directly adjacent to the radial artery, and the patient's wrist is easier to manipulate than other body parts. The bone and firm ligaments of the wrist make it easy to palpate, stabilize, and compress the radial artery.[1,7] Perform a modified Allen's test to ensure collateral circulation around the radial artery and to avoid complications. Avoid using the ulnar artery because it runs adjacent to the ulnar nerve.

Consider using the dorsalis pedis or posterior tibial artery if the radial artery is not acceptable. The temporal artery provides an alternate site for the premature or newborn infant. Access is generally good because two branches are close to the scalp. In most premature and neonatal patients, the temporal branches are larger than the radial artery.

MODIFIED ALLEN'S TEST

Use the modified Allen's test to verify the presence of collateral circulation to an extremity before puncturing the radial, posterior tibial, or dorsalis pedis artery. To assess blood flow to the hand, ask the child to make a tight fist. Occlude the radial and ulnar arteries by pressing them with the child's

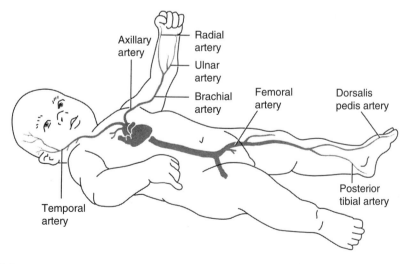

Fig. 10-1

Arterial sites that may be used for peripheral artery puncture in infants and children.

wrist between the index fingers and thumb using both hands, one on each artery. Keeping both arteries occluded, unclench the fist and note if the palm is blanched, which indicates impaired blood flow. Then remove the pressure from the ulnar artery. The palm will become pink within 5 seconds if the ulnar artery is patent and able to provide collateral circulation.[7]

Use the passive method for performing the modified Allen's test on an infant or child who cannot follow commands by gently squeezing or elevating the hand while occluding both arteries. Once the ulnar artery is released, interpret the results as previously described.[1] Allen's test can also be used to verify collateral circulation when using one of the arteries of the foot as a puncture site. Elevate the foot, and compress the dorsalis pedis and posterior tibial arteries. Release pressure from the artery that will not be punctured, and assess the nailbeds and sole of the foot for return of blood flow, which would confirm collateral circulation.[1,7]

ARTERIAL PUNCTURE

When infrequent sampling is required, obtain ABG samples by percutaneously puncturing one of the peripheral artery sites just discussed. Obtaining a blood gas sample from an infant or child generally is more difficult than in an adult and requires more patience, skill, and time. However, an experienced clinician using proper technique can quickly obtain a sample that yields accurate results. Two individuals are required to perform an arterial puncture on a child who is too young to understand the need for the test but strong enough to react to the procedure. On a small infant or neonate, a transilluminating light placed behind the wrist may help visualize the location of the radial artery.[1,7,8]

PROCEDURE

Performing a successful arterial puncture requires knowledge of the anatomy involved and proficient technical skills. Collect the equipment required for the arterial puncture (Box 10-2). Use the following sequence of technical steps as a guideline for performing the puncture.[1,7]

1. Wash hands and adhere to universal precautions for bloodborne pathogens using proper-fitting examination gloves, along with eye and splash protection.[9,10]
2. Palpate the pulse at the various sites (see Fig. 10-1) to determine the best site for testing.
3. Perform the modified Allen's test if appropriate for the artery being sampled.
4. Use an assistant to help restrain the child and immobilize the limb if required.

BOX 10-2

EQUIPMENT FOR ARTERIAL PUNCTURE AND BLOOD GAS COLLECTION

- 1-ml preheparinized* tuberculin syringe
- 25-gauge needle *or* preheparinized* 25-gauge butterfly needle infusion kit
- Correctly fitting examination gloves
- Povidone-iodine and alcohol wipe
- Sterile gauze
- Needle capping and protection device
- Eye and splash shield
- Patient label

*Use dry heparin or expel liquid heparin from the syringe and needle hub or butterfly set before starting the procedure.

5. Scrub the puncture site with an approved antiseptic swab and allow to air-dry, or use a sterile gauze pad. Do not blow on the site to dry it.
6. Palpate the artery again, and position the index and middle finger of the nondominant hand to stabilize the artery.
7. Maintain a clean field around the syringe and syringe kit while opening it. Prepare the kit for use, and heparinize the syringe if required. Remember to expel the heparin completely from the barrel of the syringe and hub of the needle.
8. Insert the needle of the syringe or butterfly catheter into the artery at a 35- to 45-degree angle with the bevel up, and advance it gently. Enter the artery from the direction opposite, or against, the blood flow. A flash in the hub of the syringe or butterfly catheter verifies that the needle penetrated the artery and is located in the lumen. In the small pediatric patient it is quite easy to pass through the artery with the needle. If a good pulse is palpated and no blood return occurs after the needle is inserted, pull the needle back incrementally and continue to watch for a flash of blood. If resistance is met when inserting the needle, slowly withdraw it immediately and change direction because it has most likely touched the bone.
9. Obtain the required amount of blood. Because the arterial pressure is usually high enough, manual aspiration is not required. If manual aspiration is required, however, the barrel of the syringe is withdrawn slowly. When using a butterfly catheter, attach the syringe to the catheter and slowly aspirate the correct amount of blood into the syringe. Maintain the sample amount as close to the

technically feasible minimum volume as possible.[2,7]

10. After obtaining the sample, withdraw the needle and immediately apply firm pressure to the puncture site with a sterile gauze pad for at least 5 minutes. Apply pressure for a longer period if the patient has a coagulopathy or is receiving anticoagulation therapy (e.g., heparin, warfarin, streptokinase). Avoid using pressure dressings. Patients should not apply the pressure because they may not press hard or long enough.

11. While holding the site, gently remove air bubbles from the sample. If using a butterfly catheter, remove it from the syringe.

12. Continue compressing the site, and seal the syringe using a one-handed safety cover device to seal the sample from the air. Gently roll the syringe between the hands or fingers to mix the specimen.[3]

13. Immediately apply the proper patient label to the specimen according to institutional policy.

14. For accurate results, analyze the sample immediately, or analyze room temperature samples within 10 to 15 minutes after they are drawn. Samples placed on ice should be analyzed within 1 hour.[11]

CONTRAINDICATIONS

The major contraindication to an arterial puncture is *lack of collateral circulation.* Punctures should not be performed at sites where the extremity has previously blanched, which may result from arterial obstruction or spasm. Do not puncture a site distal to or through a surgical shunt, as in a dialysis patient. Select an alternative site if a limb is infected or shows evidence of peripheral vascular disease.[11]

COMPLICATIONS

Hematoma formation is the most common complication during arterial puncture and is seen more often in brachial than in radial artery punctures. Minimize the risk of complication by immediately applying adequate pressure to the puncture site after the needle is withdrawn. As with any invasive procedure, infection is a possible complication but is relatively low with aseptic technique. Scarring, laceration of the artery, and hematoma formation are more likely to occur with repeated puncture of an artery.[8] Alternating puncture sites decreases this risk. Other complications associated with arterial punctures in infants and children include nerve damage, bleeding, obstruction of the artery by clots or spasms, trauma to the artery, and pain.

Because the median nerve is close to the brachial artery, the nerve may be punctured as well during the procedure, which will cause intense pain down the arm. Because the posterior tibial artery and nerve are also close to one another, special care should also be taken to avoid nerve damage during puncture of this artery. Although the femoral artery is much easier to puncture, complications in infants tend to occur more frequently, including thrombosis, nerve damage, and necrosis of the head of the femoral bone.[7]

Although gloves are worn and universal precautions applied during all arterial punctures, needle sticks remain a risk to the clinician and are the most frequent source of transmission of bloodborne pathogens to health care workers.[2,8-10] Most of these complications are avoided by having only thoroughly trained and highly skilled clinicians perform a puncture.

CAPILLARY BLOOD GAS SAMPLES

Capillary blood gas (CBG) sampling provides a frequent alternative to ABG analysis in the infant or child. Punctures for capillary samples are less invasive than arterial punctures, are easier and quicker to perform, and can be used when there is no arterial catheter for drawing ABG samples.[11-13] Drawing a CBG sample is usually less painful, but local anesthetic application helps alleviate pain associated with the procedure.[6,14]

Generally, a CBG sample correlates best with pH and arterial carbon dioxide tension ($Paco_2$) values. Correlation of capillary samples with arterial samples varies depending on the parameters measured.[11,15-17] When a capillary sample site is adequately "arterialized" and puncture and sampling procedures are performed correctly, the pH and carbon dioxide partial pressure (Pco_2) of capillary samples can accurately reflect those of arterial samples. Capillary oxygen partial pressure (Po_2) may correlate with arterial pressure (Pao_2) in isolated cases and must be assessed on an individual basis before using the capillary Po_2 monitor oxygenation. Frequently, capillary Po_2 will trend with arterial values given a clinically acceptable difference between capillary Po_2 and Pao_2.[11,16]

Accuracy of capillary samples is severely attenuated by the presence of hypotension, hypothermia, hypovolemia, and lack of perfusion.[11] Accuracy is especially compromised when trying to correlate capillary Po_2 with Pao_2. Conversely, correlation improves with hypoxemia as venous and arterial Po_2 converge. Certain situations may result in poorer capillary sampling correlation compared with normal conditions. Special consideration should be given to patients with circulatory defects. Decreased venous return, secondary to cor pulmonale or decreased cardiac output, leads to venous congestion and peripheral pooling, which may result in an increase in P_{CO_2}. Conversely, increased blood flow may result in a decreased capillary P_{CO_2}.[14]

Although capillary punctures are less invasive, obtain an arterial sample at some point to ensure correlation and accuracy. Use noninvasive monitors such as pulse oximeters or transcutaneous oxygen monitors to monitor oxygenation when arterial samples are not obtained.[13] However, many factors that lead to inaccurate CBG sampling may also affect accuracy of monitoring (see Chapter 11).[1]

PUNCTURE SITES

The least hazardous puncture site for infants is the *posterolateral foot*, just anterior to the heel (Fig. 10-2).[1,12] Avoid the posterior heel curvature and back of the heel because the lancet could puncture the bone and result in calcaneous osteomyelitis. Do not perform a capillary puncture on the medial aspect of the heel, which is the location of the posterior tibial artery. For children and some infants, use the palmar

or fleshy surface of the distal aspects of the fingers (middle or ring) and toes (Fig. 10-3).[11,12,14] The earlobes are a secondary site for puncture in children. In general, avoid punctures on the fingers and toes of neonates because of the higher risk of nerve damage in this area.[12] Do not use previous puncture sites or inflamed areas with an apparent or possible infection. As previously discussed, avoid extremities with localized swelling or edema because of the effect of extracellular or interstitial fluid on sample accuracy. Also, avoid cyanotic areas.[11]

PROCEDURE

Successful capillary puncture is not complicated, but it does requires proficient technical skill. Collect the equipment required (Box 10-3), and use the following sequence of steps as guide to collect a CBG sample.[1,7,12]

1. Select a puncture site and warm the area for 5 to 10 minutes. Use a warm (less than 42° to 45° C) wet cloth or disposable warming pack, and apply with caution.[1,7]
2. Give a 12% to 24% sucrose solution pacifier 2 minutes before the procedure, or apply an anesthetic cream or subcutaneous injection for pain control.[3,5-7]
3. Wash hands and adhere to universal precautions for bloodborne pathogens using proper-fitting examination gloves, along with splash protection.[8,9]

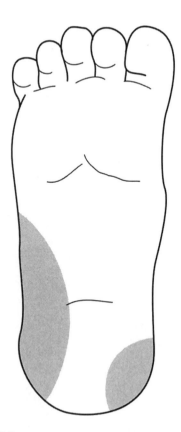

Fig. 10-2

Recommended puncture sites *(shaded areas)* in infant's heel to obtain capillary blood for analysis.

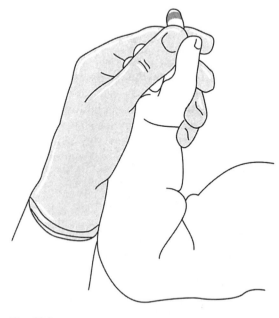

Fig. 10-3

Technique for grasping the finger for a capillary puncture, with recommended site for puncture *(shaded area)*.

4. Remove the warming device. Clean the site with an antiseptic, and dry with a sterile gauze pad; alcohol will hemolyze the blood.
5. Immobilize the area by properly grasping the puncture area and anchoring the hand on a hard surface (Figs. 10-3 and 10-4). Use an assistant to help restrain a child and immobilize the limb if required. Restrain infants by swaddling them in a blanket.[7]
6. *Finger or toe stick.* Hold the digit (patient's finger or toe) with the thumb, and support the digit behind or close to the nail using the forefinger (see Fig. 10-3). Keep fingertips well away from the puncture site.
7. *Heel stick.* Consider using venipuncture or a digit first because either may be less painful and require less resampling.[3-7] Hold the heel gently but firm. Wrap the forefinger around the infant's upper heel and ankle while holding the arch of the foot with the thumb (Fig. 10-4).
8. Position the lancet.
   a. For finger or toe stick, hold the lancet at a 10- to 20-degree angle to the longitudinal axis of the phalangeal bone. Do not direct it into the bone.
   b. For heel stick, hold the lancet between the thumb and index finger of the opposite hand perpendicular to the puncture site.
9. Poke the point of the lancet into the skin with one continuous, deliberate motion. Correct depth depends on the infant, but 1 to 2 mm is generally sufficient to produce a free-flowing drop of blood.[7,17] Use a mechanical puncture when available because most produce consistent results with less need for resampling.[7,18] Avoid superficial punctures and the need to repeat the puncture. Do not slice, dig, or make multiple punctures.[1,6,7,17]

10. Ease thumb pressure after the lancet is removed.
11. Wipe the first drop of blood, which may be contaminated with intracellular, interstitial, or lymphatic fluids, with a dry sterile gauze pad.
12. Apply moderate pressure to the heel or digit without massaging or squeezing until a free-flowing drop of blood appears. Squeezing or "milking" the sample may cause red blood cell hemolysis, especially in newborns, because their hematocrit levels are higher and their red blood cells more fragile. Squeezing also results in bruising and contamination of the specimen with lymphatic and venous drainage.
13. Collect the blood by placing the tip of the capillary tube into the blood droplet without touching the puncture wound. Hold the capillary tube angled horizontally, or slightly downward, with the colored ring away from the infant. Keep the tube in contact with the blood droplet until the required amount of blood fills the tube, usually 40 to 125 μl.[7] Maintaining contact with the droplet limits unnecessary exposure to air and reduces the incidence of air bubbles in the sample. Do

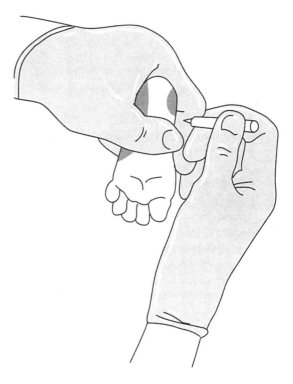

Fig. 10-4

Technique of stabilizing the heel for a capillary puncture.

BOX 10-3

EQUIPMENT FOR CAPILLARY PUNCTURE AND BLOOD GAS COLLECTION

- Warming device or warm damp cloth
- Lancet and mechanical puncture device
- Lancet disposal system
- Correctly fitting examination gloves
- Alcohol wipe
- Sterile gauze
- Adhesive bandage
- Eye and splash shield
- Preheparinized capillary tube
- Metal "flea," magnet, capillary tube caps (if required)
- Patient label

not scrape blood that has smeared onto the skin surface into the capillary tube. Scraping from the skin surface increases exposure to air and alters the partial pressure of the gases being measured.[1,7,12]

14. Apply pressure to the puncture site with a sterile gauze pad until the bleeding stops. Use an adhesive bandage only on a child old enough not to place it in their mouth and possibly aspirate it.

15. Label the tube with the proper patient information.

16. If the sample cannot be analyzed immediately after collection, insert a metal mixing "flea" into the capillary tube and seal it. Mix the sample by running a magnet gently back and forth along the tube, and place the sample on ice; this decreases the incidence of sample clotting. Remove the metal flea before analyzing the blood.

CONTRAINDICATIONS

Do not perform CBG sampling when accurate assessment of oxygenation or ABG values is necessary. Do not perform CBGs for routine blood gas monitoring when less painful or noninvasive measurements provide results that are more accurate.

Capillary puncture is contraindicated in neonates less than 24 hours old. A newborn has a low systemic output, and vasoconstriction tends to be maximal during this stage secondary to a decrease in environmental temperature and an increase in circulating catecholamines.[12,17,19,20] CBG sampling is not recommended in a patient with decreased peripheral blood flow, especially in the case of hypotension.[12,17,19] CBG sampling may be difficult to perform on a patient with polycythemia (hematocrit greater than 70%) because of the short clotting time. Do not use areas that are edematous, inflamed, or infected, or other areas previously mentioned. Avoid heel samples from ambulatory children who have formed calluses on the soles of their feet.[7,21]

COMPLICATIONS

Serious complications may result in medical management if capillary results do not accurately reflect the patient's condition. Consider potential errors in correlation with arterial values before deciding on a clinical course of action based on CBG values.[12,14,19]

Although capillary puncture is a relatively safe procedure, complications have been observed. Burns have been reported secondary to heel warming, but using a prepackaged warming kit that does not require an external heat source minimizes this problem. Other complications include infection, scarring, calcaneous osteomyelitis, calcifications, nerve damage, arterial laceration, bruising, cellulitis, hematoma, and bleeding.[1,11,12] Some of these complications may seem benign at first but lead to developmental delays in such milestones as grasping and walking.

ARTERIAL CATHETERS

For frequent blood gas sampling, use an umbilical artery catheter (UAC) in the newborn and a peripheral artery catheter or arterial line in the older infant or child. Arterial catheters provide access for arterial blood pressure analysis and ABG sampling. UAC and arterial catheters also allow blood pressure monitoring in patients who are hemodynamically unstable.

UMBILICAL ARTERY CATHETERIZATION

In the infant the umbilicus provides ready access to two arteries. Facing the child, the two umbilical arteries are located at about the 5 and 7 o'clock positions. Prompt catheterization is essential in neonates because these vessels will undergo arterial spasm in the presence of increased arterial oxygen, making cannulation difficult if not impossible.[7]

Two positions are typically used to place the tip of the UAC. In the *high position* the catheter overlies the sixth through eighth thoracic vertebrae (T6 to T8); this position avoids major tributaries of the aorta because it is below the ductus arteriosus and above the celiac access. The *low position* is usually at the third to fourth lumbar (L3 to L4) space, between the renal artery and aortic intersection and above the takeoff of the inferior mesenteric artery. Place the UAC to avoid the large tributaries supplied by these vessels to minimize trauma and hemodynamic disturbances of vital organs.[22]

The choice of high or low catheter placement is empiric. Hospitals tend to favor one site or the other; both are associated with their own set of complications related to hypoglycemia, hypotension, vasospasm, and embolic disturbances of organs distal to the catheter tip. A recent meta-analysis and literature reviews demonstrate a small advantage when using the high position over the low position.[23]

Determine the catheter length by measuring from the umbilicus to the shoulder, or use another institutionally established measurement. Using a nomogram, compare this measurement to the correct catheter insertion distance.[24-27]

Using sterile technique, insert the catheter into one of the arteries. The artery that is less tortuous will be easier to cannulate. Direct the tip toward

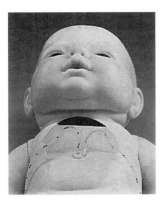

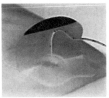

Fig. 10-5

NeoBridge is a one-piece umbilical catheter holder patterned after the umbilical catheter "bridge." It uses a hydrocolloid adhesive to minimize skin breakdown. (Courtesy Neotech Products, Chatsworth, Calif.)

the ipsilateral groin. Advance the catheter with a gentle downward pressure, using a rotating motion to allow the catheter to seek the arterial lumen. Advance it to a length of one-third the infant's body length plus 1 cm for the high position. Confirm patency and ease of blood flow, and connect the UAC to a prepared fluid-pressure-transducing system.[7,22]

Secure the catheter by suturing it into the umbilical artery, and tape it to the abdomen using the "goalpost" method (Fig. 10-5). Confirm catheter placement by chest and abdominal radiographs. A UAC may remain in place for several days to weeks as indicated by patient need.[1,22,27]

PERIPHERAL ARTERY CATHETERIZATION

The clinician must rely on peripheral arterial catheterization in the pediatric patient. An arterial line is also used for blood gas monitoring in an infant or a newborn without umbilical artery access.

Perform arterial line placement using either a percutaneous or a cutdown method. As noted, the most common site is the radial artery, with the posterior tibial and dorsalis pedis arteries occasionally used. Other monitoring sites, such as the brachial artery, superficial temporal artery, and femoral artery, are rarely used because of the increased risk of complications. Arterial catheter sizes range from

22 to 24 gauge for a neonate and 20 to 22 gauge for a pediatric patient.[28]

Before placing the arterial catheter, perform the modified Allen's test previously described to observe collateral blood flow to the hand or foot being punctured.[1,7] For small children and infants, use a transilluminating light to locate the radial artery when performing a radial artery puncture.[29]

PROCEDURE FOR SAMPLING

Use the following procedure as a guideline for drawing a blood for sample from an arterial or umbilical artery catheter.[1,28] Both catheters are connected to a heparinized infusion source and blood pressure–monitoring transducer.

1. Wash hands and adhere to universal precautions for bloodborne pathogens using proper-fitting examination gloves, along with eye and splash protection.[8,9]
2. Uncap the locking port of the three-way stopcock. Apply appropriate antibacterial solution to the stopcock port or rubber infusion port, depending on institutional procedures, and allow to dry.[1] Because multiple syringes are required, maintain a clean field around the site and a place to set the syringes that are not in use.
3. Attach a 3-ml syringe to the stopcock, or attach a syringe with a 25-gauge needle to the infusion port.
4. Turn stopcock off to infusion, aspirate 1.25 to 2.0 ml of blood diluted with the infusion fluid, and remove syringe. Do not discard this sample, and keep the tip sterile because it must be reinfused after the blood sample is acquired.
5. Close the stopcock by making a one-quarter turn between the syringe and the line to the flush solution.
6. Attach a sterile preheparinized syringe to the port. Switch the stopcock back one-quarter turn toward the infusion line to the off position and toward the sampling syringe to the on position.
7. Aspirate 0.25 to 1.0 ml of blood into the sampling syringe according to volume required by blood gas analyzer.
8. Close the stopcock by making a one-quarter turn between the syringe and the line to the flush solution, and remove the sample.
9. Reattach the syringe with the aspirated infusion volume, and switch the stopcock back one-quarter turn toward the infusion line in the off position and toward the sampling syringe in the on position. Slowly reinfuse the solution from the syringe.

10. Repeat the procedure for turning the stop-cock off the infusion line, remove the syringe, and attach a syringe prefilled with flush solution.
11. Open the stopcock back to the flush syringe, and infuse 0.5 to 1.5 ml of solution to flush blood from the line. Turn the stopcock off to the sampling port, and remove the flush syringe. Return the stopcock cap to its position.
12. Record the amount of blood sampled and flush solution infused to keep accurate input and output records.
13. Immediately apply the proper patient label to the specimen according to institutional policy.
14. For accurate results, analyze the sample immediately, or analyze room-temperature samples within 10 to 15 minutes after they are drawn. Samples placed on ice should be analyzed within 1 hour.[11]

When infusing or reinfusing solution into the umbilical or arterial line, tap any bubbles to the surface and expel them from the syringe before attaching it to the stopcock. When infusing, keep the syringe in a perpendicular position to allow air bubbles to rise toward the plunger. If bubbles form, tap them so they rise toward the plunger. Continue infusing the solution, but do not infuse air bubbles into the arterial line.

COMPLICATIONS

As with any invasive method of monitoring, peripheral artery catheterization carries an increased risk of infection.[27,30] The risk is greater when a catheter has been in place for longer than 72 hours. Some complications associated with the use of arterial catheters are related to thrombotic phenomena, either at the site of the catheter tip or distal to catheter placement.

The risk of *thrombosis* tends to depend on the size of the catheter and the duration of placement. Children younger than 5 years are at greater risk. Once significant perfusion or thrombotic problems are identified, remove the catheter as soon as possible, and manage the affected extremity to improve perfusion.

Hemorrhage may occur during insertion and if the catheter tubing is inadvertently disconnected. Pallor, decreased pulses, and poor capillary refill are all signs of ischemia. Although ischemia rarely occurs, continuously monitor the arterial pressure waveform. Injection of even a small amount of air into the arterial system can result in rapid and devastating air embolism to the brain.

UAC complications may also include intraventricular hemorrhage, altered mesenteric blood flow, and necrotizing enterocolitis.[27,31] These and other complications, such as misplacement into the iliac artery or infarction of various organ systems, including the kidney, liver, and spinal cord,[32,33] may result in life-threatening or prolonged severe disability.

MEASUREMENTS

The placement of arterial catheters allows the direct measurement of arterial blood pressure values, the systolic and diastolic pressures. Monitoring arterial pressure waveforms helps to determine the patency of the arterial line and the quality of the pulse pressure and to calculate the *mean arterial pressure* (MAP). The arterial line monitor calculates MAP internally. However, use the following formula to obtain an indirect measurement of MAP with a sphygmomanometer:

$$MAP = \frac{[(2 \times Diastolic) + Systolic]}{3}$$

MAP is often used as an indication of left ventricular afterload, thus representing the resistance against which the left ventricle must pump. The *pulse pressure* is the difference between the systolic and the diastolic blood pressure. A decreasing pulse pressure may indicate hypovolemia, and an increasing pulse pressure may indicate a restoration of normal volume status.

CENTRAL VENOUS CATHETERS

Indications for a central venous catheter are (1) cardiovascular instability; (2) intravascular volume disturbances (e.g., extreme dehydration, hemorrhage, increased intracranial pressure, renal failure, diabetic ketoacidosis); (3) administration of drugs, fluids, or nutritional support to the central circulation; and (4) the need for central venous pressure (CVP) monitoring.[34] Central venous catheterization is also indicated when other peripheral access sites have been exhausted. Placing a CVP line allows measurement of right atrial pressure (RAP) to assist in (1) managing fluid volume, (2) infusing fluid volumes larger than a peripheral intravenous (IV) catheter can accommodate, (3) administering total parenteral nutrition, and (4) providing a secure long-term venous site in the chronically ill child.[34-36]

MONITORING SITES

Techniques for central line placement in infants and children vary according to the patient's age and condition. Monitoring sites for central venous catheterization are locations where a peripheral vein can be cannulated by either the percutaneous or the cutdown method and the catheter can be advanced to a central location in the vena cava. The percutaneous technique is relatively safe and easy, with many potential sites.

The cutdown method, or surgical cannulation, reduces the risk of trauma to the vein and adjacent tissue. Cutdown also provides additional sites for patients with poor peripheral perfusion or lack of percutaneous sites. Cutdown locations include the internal and external jugular veins, common facial vein, brachial vessels, saphenous vein, and femoral veins. The cutdown technique requires experience to avoid surgical complications such as bleeding, inadvertent interruption of arterial flow, and dissection through vital structures such as muscles and nerves.

Common vessels used for percutaneous approaches are the external and internal jugular veins (the right is preferred over the left vein), subclavian vein, brachial veins, and saphenous vessels.[37-39] The umbilicus offers a unique site in the newborn because the umbilical vein is available for placement of a central catheter.[37]

PROCEDURE

Placement of the catheter is performed under sterile conditions with the child sedated and following the recommendations for pain control.[6] The site is usually anesthetized using lidocaine before the catheter is placed in the vein. Advance the catheter until an RAP waveform appears on the monitor. Connect a flush line and pressure transducer as with any indwelling catheter used for pressure monitoring. Confirm catheter placement with a chest radiograph.

COMPLICATIONS

The major complication of venous catheter use in general is catheter-related *sepsis*, especially when the catheter is in place longer than 72 hours.[34] Fungal sepsis is especially significant in the neonatal population.[40,41] In older children the additional complication of *pulmonary embolism* is significant.[42] Embolism appears to be an unrecognized clinical entity in the neonate.

The percutaneous approach may be difficult in patients with poor peripheral perfusion and in those with chronic disease who require many venous catheters. The cutdown method requires a higher degree of skill and training than the percutaneous approach to avoid complications. Dysrhythmias may occur if the catheter tip slips into the right ventricle. Inadvertent placement of the catheter tip in the left atrium is possible if the patient has a patent foramen ovale or atrial septal defect. Perforation of the trachea is rare but has occurred with insertion into the jugular vein. Saphenous and femoral vein sites tend to be at higher risk for thrombosis. Air embolus may occur during insertion and when tubing is disconnected.[42]

Catheterization should be discontinued at the first sign of inflammation or when the patient's condition no longer requires its use. Percutaneous sites should be rotated on a regular basis. Any vein may be safely reused after 4 to 7 days.

MEASUREMENTS

The placement of a central venous catheter allows measurement of the RAP, which represents the filling pressure of the right atrium. Systemic venous return, intravascular volume, tricuspid valve performance, myocardial function, and right ventricular pressure all affect the RAP. Normal values for RAP range from 2 to 7 cm H_2O but must be interpreted cautiously, because filling pressures vary with changes in thoracic and intrapleural pressure, such as during mechanical ventilation. The value of the RAP measurement is in monitoring trends and following changes in therapy.

Blood samples taken from the right atrium may represent mixed-venous samples. This approach demands caution, however, because catheter tip placement may be influenced by venous return from one portion of the body rather than the whole body. Analyzing mixed-venous oxygen saturation ($S\bar{v}O_2$) and P_{O_2} in mixed-venous blood provides information about overall tissue oxygenation and can be compared to arterial samples to monitor changes in oxygen consumption. The use of a catheter with light-transmitting fiberoptics allows continuous measurement of oxygen saturation.

Decreased CVP values usually indicate hypovolemia. Reduced CVP values occur during fluid imbalance, hemorrhage, extreme vasodilation, and shock. Increased CVP values may result from (1) hypervolemia, as with sudden fluid shifts or volume overload; (2) interference with the right ventricle's ability to pump blood, such as tricuspid valve regurgitation or stenosis, right ventricular failure or infarction, increased pulmonary vascular resistance, or cardiac tamponade; (3) increased systemic vasoconstriction; or (4) left ventricular failure.[39]

PULMONARY ARTERY CATHETERIZATION

The pulmonary artery catheter provides cardiovascular information unavailable in other noninvasive approaches about ventricular performance, volume status, and the effects of various pharmacologic therapies.[43] The pulmonary artery catheter is often referred to as a "Swan-Ganz" catheter and is indicated for critically ill patients with respiratory failure or profound shock requiring vasoactive drugs. It is used to assess left ventricular

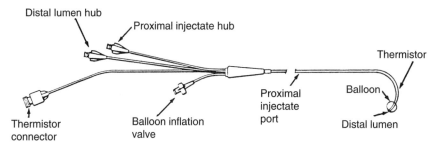

Fig. 10-6

Pulmonary artery (Swan-Ganz) thermodilution catheter. (From *Understanding hemodynamic measurements made with the Swan-Ganz catheter*. Irvine, Calif, Baxter Edwards Laboratories, 1989.)

function and shock, guide fluid management, and aid in diagnosing and managing pulmonary disease and cardiac dysfunction. Direct intracardiac and pulmonary pressure monitoring, along with cardiac output measurement and $P\bar{v}O_2$ monitoring, can be accomplished with a pulmonary artery catheter.[44,45]

Pulmonary artery catheters contain quadruple lumens and come in 5 French (for patients less than 18 kg) and 7 French. They are marked in 10-cm increments along the outside, and a balloon is fastened 1 to 2 mm from the tip. A four-lumen catheter has the following ports (Fig. 10-6):

- Proximal port for placement in the right atrium; this port terminates in an opening at the tip of the catheter and is used to measure RAP.
- Distal port for placement in the pulmonary artery; this lumen terminates in an opening at the tip of the catheter and lies in the pulmonary artery. It is used to measure pulmonary artery pressure (PAP) and pulmonary capillary wedge pressure (PCWP) and to sample mixed-venous blood.
- Port for the inflation of the balloon at the catheter tip; when inflated, the balloon should surround but not cover the tip of the catheter.
- Port for the temperature-measuring thermistor; this port connects to the cardiac output monitor. The thermistor wires transmit the temperature of the blood flowing over them to the cardiac output monitor.[46]

PROCEDURE

Place the patient in Trendelenburg's position if tolerable to prevent air embolism and enhance neck vein filling. Prime the catheter with IV flush solution, and test the integrity of the balloon by injecting air into it. Evacuate all the air in the tubing and pressure transducer. Place the catheter in a large vessel using a cutdown or percutaneous approach, and advance it until an RAP tracing appears on the monitor. Then slowly inflate the balloon with air, and float the catheter through the tricuspid valve into the right ventricle. Advance it farther into the pulmonary artery, then into a wedged position, where the catheter occludes the artery. As the catheter is advanced, observe the characteristic waveforms of each heart and vessel location to assist with placement (Figs. 10-7 and 10-8). Once the catheter is wedged, deflate the balloon, and confirm the pulmonary artery waveform on the monitor.

Demonstrate the ability to acquire a PCWP and a PAP by inflating and deflating the balloon. Then suture the catheter in place, and record the length of the catheter at the insertion site. The catheter should never be inserted to a length greater than that measured before placement. This avoids complications, such as knotting or unintentional wedging of the catheter without the balloon inflated. Obtain a chest radiograph immediately to rule out a pneumothorax and to verify the catheter's position.

Continuously monitor the catheter waveforms and pressures. On the monitor, maintain the catheter in position to produce a PAP waveform, except for those brief intervals when PCWP readings are obtained. To obtain a PCWP reading, attach a syringe to the balloon port and aspirate to ensure complete emptying of the balloon, which avoids overinflation and rupture. Normally, when inflating the balloon, you will feel some initial resistance. If there is no resistance, check the integrity of the balloon and discontinue inflation.[39,47] Observe as the waveform flattens out, using the mean of the peaks and troughs to determine the pressure to record.

COMPLICATIONS

At insertion, complications include bleeding, pneumothorax, tricuspid or pulmonic valve damage,

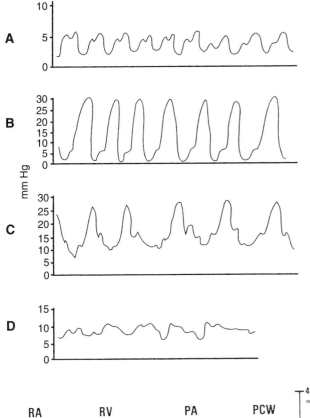

Fig. 10-7

Examples of pressure waveform patterns at various locations surrounding the heart. **A,** Central venous pressure. **B,** Right ventricular pressure. **C,** Pulmonary artery pressure. **D,** Pulmonary capillary wedge pressure.

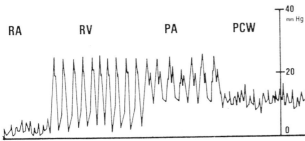

Fig. 10-8

Pressure waveforms as the catheter travels through the right atrium *(RA),* right ventricle *(RV),* and pulmonary artery *(PA),* becoming wedged (pulmonary capillary wedge pressure *[PCW]).* (From *Understanding hemodynamic measurements made with the Swan-Ganz catheter.* Irvine, Calif, Baxter Edwards Laboratories, 1989.)

right atrium or right ventricle perforation, and arrhythmias resulting from the catheter traversing the right ventricle. The most frequently observed arrhythmias are premature ventricular contractions and ventricular tachycardia. Overinflation of the balloon may result in rupture of the pulmonary artery, pulmonic valve obstruction, and air embolization. Pulmonary infarction may occur if the catheter is left in the wedge position for extended periods. The major complications remain catheter-induced thrombosis and sepsis.[47-51]

Positive-pressure ventilation affects PCWP measurements. Measurement error may result from changes in baseline during the inflation and exhalation. Other sources of measurement error are failure to zero-set or calibrate the transducer properly, misalignment of the transducer with the tip of the catheter in the pulmonary artery, and dampening of the waveform secondary to thrombus formation.[51]

MEASUREMENTS

The proximal port measures the RAP and the distal port the PAP (Box 10-4). A decrease in PAP usually indicates hypovolemia. An increase in PAP may indicate an increase in pulmonary vascular resistance, mitral stenosis, left ventricular failure, or hypervolemia. Increased PAP also may result from pulmonary edema or an increase in pulmonary blood flow, as with left-to-right shunts in congenital heart defects.

The PCWP reflects downstream pressures in the left side of the heart under conditions of absent flow in the pulmonary capillary bed. Variations in airway pressures, such as during mechanical ventilation

TABLE 10-1	**NORMAL RANGES OF DERIVED HEMODYNAMIC PARAMETERS**	
Parameter	Formula	Range
Cardiac index	CO/BSA	2.8-4.2 L/min/m²
Stoke volume	CO/HR	50-80 ml/beat
Stroke volume (SV) index	SV/BSA	30-65 ml/beat/m²
Systemic vascular resistance	MAP – LAP/CO	11-18 mm Hg/L/min
Pulmonary vascular resistance	PAP – PCWP/CO	1.5-3.0 mm Hg/L/min
Shunt fraction	$(Cc_{O_2} - Ca_{O_2})/(Cc_{O_2} - C\bar{v}_{O_2})$	Less than 5%

CO, Cardiac output; *BSA,* body surface area; *HR,* heart rate; *MAP,* mean arterial pressure; *LAP,* left atrial pressure; *PAP,* pulmonary artery pressure; *PCWP,* pulmonary capillary wedge pressure; *Cc$_{O_2}$,* pulmonary end-capillary oxygen content; *Ca$_{O_2}$,* arterial oxygen content; *C$\bar{v}_{O_2}$,* mixed-venous oxygen content.

with positive end-expiratory pressure (PEEP), can influence PCWP. The degree to which ventilation affects the relationship between PCWP and left atrial pressure depends on lung compliance. Therefore, PCWP should be measured at end expiration and without PEEP if tolerated by the patient. Measure the PCWP with PEEP to establish trends in changes in clinical conditions. If not caused by PEEP, increased PCWP usually indicates left ventricular failure, hypervolemia, or intravascular fluid overload. A catheter with a fiberoptic lumen provides continuous measurement of S$\bar{v}_{O_2}$ from the pulmonary artery.[46,52]

CARDIAC OUTPUT

Most cardiac output measurements use the *thermodilution technique.* Derive measurements from injecting a known volume of liquid at a set temperature, 22° to 24° C, or iced, 0° to 4° C, into the right atrium through the right atrial port of the catheter. Inject the solution with a rapid and constant motion. Enter the exact temperature and amount of liquid into the cardiac output computer. As the liquid mixes with the blood and passes through the right ventricle into the pulmonary artery, the thermistor measures the rate of change in blood temperature from the value entered into the computer. The computer calculates the rate at which the blood warms the liquid, which is proportional to blood flow, and yields cardiac output.

Perform three measurements. Discard the result of the first measurement, because this cools down the catheter, then average the remaining measurements. Complete all measurements during the same phase of the respiratory cycle because pulmonary artery blood flow is profoundly influenced by respiration, especially mechanical ventilation. By using the cardiac output and pressure measurements from the pulmonary and peripheral artery catheters, construct a complete hemodynamic profile of the patient (Table 10-1).[52-54]

PATIENT INFORMATION

Monitor and record several parameters when taking a blood gas sample. Document the specific puncture or sample site and whether it is arterial, venous, mixed venous, or capillary. Record the date and time of the sample, along with the patient's respiratory variables. Important respiratory variables are respiratory frequency, temperature, fraction of inspired oxygen (F$_{IO_2}$), and specific oxygen device. If the patient is mechanically ventilated, include the type of ventilator, mode of ventilation, tidal volume, peak inflation pressure, PEEP, and other relevant settings. Note the patient's position (e.g., upright in an infant seat), activity level (e.g., whether crying or breath holding), clinical appearance, and other signs of respiratory distress. Be sure to document any adverse reactions, along with the corrective action taken.

FREQUENCY

The clinical status of the patient, rather than an arbitrarily set time or frequency, should dictate the need for arterial and capillary punctures.[2,10,12] It is also important to understand that the infant, especially a very premature neonate, has a much smaller quantity of blood. Frequent blood sampling results in hypovolemia and anemia in these patients. During mechanical ventilation, wait 10 minutes after changing the F$_{IO_2}$ in a patient without chronic pulmonary disease to perform an ABG sample.[55] Samples should not be drawn until 20 to 30 minutes

TABLE 10-2	APPROXIMATE NORMAL RANGE OF ARTERIAL BLOOD GAS VALUES		
Parameter	**Newborn (Birth to 24 Hours)**	**Infant to Toddler (Up to 2 Years)**	**Child to Adult (Over 2 years)**
pH	7.3-7.4	7.3-7.4	7.35-7.45
Arterial carbon dioxide tension ($Paco_2$, mm Hg)	30-40	30-40	35-45
Arterial oxygen tension (Pao_2, mm Hg)	60-90	80-100	80-100
Bicarbonate (HCO_3^-) (mEq/L)	20-22	20-22	22-24

Modified from Pagtakhan RD, Pasterkamp H: Intensive care for respiratory disorders. In Chernick V, editor: *Kendig's disorders of the respiratory tract in children*, ed 5, Philadelphia, WB Saunders, 1990, pp 205-224.

TABLE 10-3	LABORATORY VALUES FOR ACID-BASE DISTURBANCES		
Disease	**pH**	**$Paco_2$**	**HCO_3^-**
METABOLIC ACIDOSIS			
Uncompensated	↓	N	↓
Partially compensated	↓	↓	↓
Compensated	N	↓	↓
METABOLIC ALKALOSIS			
Uncompensated	↑	N	↑
Partially compensated	↑	↑	↑
Compensated	N	↑	↑
RESPIRATORY ACIDOSIS			
Uncompensated	↓	↑	N
Partially compensated	↓	↑	↑
Compensated	N	↑	↑
RESPIRATORY ALKALOSIS			
Uncompensated	↑	↓	N
Partially compensated	↑	↓	↓
Uncompensated	N	↓	↓
MIXED ACIDOSIS	↓	↑	↓
MIXED ALKALOSIS	↑	↓	↑

$Paco_2$, Arterial carbon dioxide tension; *HCO_3^-,* bicarbonate.

after changing the Fio_2 of a spontaneously breathing patient without chronic pulmonary disease. Patients with chronic pulmonary disease should not have samples drawn for at least 30 minutes after an Fio_2 change.[2]

BLOOD GAS INTERPRETATION

Although a thorough discussion of blood gas interpretation is beyond the scope of this text, using the blood gas result requires some explanation of acid-base balance and gas exchange. *Gas exchange* refers to the exchange of oxygen and carbon dioxide between air and blood and then between blood

and tissue. Proper gas exchange depends on many factors, such as blood flow, cardiac output, metabolic rate, diffusion, shunting, and gas concentration of the inspired air. An abnormality in any of these factors will result in a change in blood gas values and possibly an increase in the work of the cardiopulmonary system. Usually, only three values are measured during blood gas analysis: pH, Pco_2, and Po_2. Bicarbonate (HCO_3^-) and oxygen saturation are also usually calculated. Occasionally, other non–blood gas values may be measured simultaneously, depending on the analyzer in use at the time.

Typically, interpretation of the blood gas involves (1) acid-base interpretation, to evaluate the pH and Pco_2 values, and (2) evaluation of oxygenation, or Po_2, separately. Normal Pao_2 and $Paco_2$ values reflect normal gas exchange, whereas an abnormality in gas exchange results in abnormal values. Recognizing normal and abnormal values helps in more completely understanding and interpreting blood gas values (Table 10-2).

ACID-BASE BALANCE

Assess acid-base balance by evaluating the pH, $Paco_2$, and HCO_3^- values for *acidosis* or *alkalosis* and the degree of compensation present (Table 10-3). $Paco_2$ is directly proportional to the adequacy of alveolar ventilation. Thus acid-base abnormalities are classified as primarily *respiratory* or *metabolic*. The amount to which the pH is balanced by the metabolic or respiratory processes determines the degree of compensation. Boxes 10-5 to 10-8 list common causes of metabolic acidosis/alkalosis and respiratory acidosis/alkalosis.

OXYGENATION

The *arterial partial pressure of oxygen* (Pao_2) reflects exchange of oxygen, or oxygenation. Oxygen moves into the airway and the alveolus, at which point a pressure gradient causes it to diffuse across the alveolocapillary membrane into the pulmonary capillary blood. It is then carried in the

---

BOX 10-5

CAUSES OF METABOLIC ACIDOSIS

Diarrhea
Small bowel, biliary, or pancreatic tube or
    fistula drainage
Hyperalimentation
Ingestion of chloride-containing compounds
• Calcium chloride
• Magnesium chloride
• Ammonium chloride
• Hydrochloric acid
Renal tubular acidosis
Renal failure
Carbonic anhydrase deficiency
Lactic acidosis
• Tissue hypoxia
• Sepsis
• Neonatal cold stress
Ketoacidosis
• Diabetes mellitus
• Starvation
Ingestion of toxins
• Salicylate poisoning
• Methanol poisoning
• Ethylene glycol poisoning
• Prolonged use of paraldehyde
Inborn errors of metabolism

Modified from Brewer ED: Disorders of acid-base balance. *Pediatr
Clin North Am* 1990; 37:429-447.

BOX 10-6

CAUSES OF METABOLIC ALKALOSIS

Vomiting
Nasogastric suctioning
Congenital chloride-wasting diarrhea
Dehydration
Drugs
• Diuretics
• Steroids
• Sodium bicarbonate
Cushing's syndrome
Bartter's syndrome
Hypokalemia
Hypochloremia
Chewing tobacco
Massive blood transfusion
Cystic fibrosis infants fed regular formula or
    breast milk (low in sodium)

Modified from Brewer ED: Disorders of acid-base balance. *Pediatr
Clin North Am* 1990; 37:429-447.

BOX 10-7

CAUSES OF RESPIRATORY ACIDOSIS

LUNG DISEASE
  Upper airway obstruction
  • Laryngotracheobronchitis (croup)
  • Epiglottitis
  • Foreign body
  Small airway obstruction
  • Asthma
  • Bronchiolitis
  Chronic obstructive pulmonary disease
  • Cystic fibrosis
  • Bronchopulmonary dysplasia
  • Bronchiectasis
  Pneumonia
  Pulmonary edema
  Respiratory distress syndrome
  Aspiration
  • Meconium
  • Foreign body
  Pulmonary hypoplasia

IMPAIRED LUNG MOTION
  Pleural effusion
  Pneumothorax
  Thoracic cage abnormalities
  • Flail chest
  • Scoliosis
  • Osteogenesis imperfecta
  • Thoracic dystrophy

APNEA

NEUROMUSCULAR DISORDERS
  Brainstem/spinal cord injury or tumor
  Paralysis of diaphragm
  Drug overdose/oversedation
  Muscular dystrophy
  Guillain-Barré syndrome
  Myasthenia gravis
  Poliomyelitis

OTHER
  Botulism
  Extreme obesity

Modified from Brewer ED: Disorders of acid-base balance. *Pediatr
Clin North Am* 1990; 37:429-447.

---

blood to the tissues in two forms: (1) dissolved in plasma and (2) in combination with hemoglobin. Although the amount of oxygen dissolved in plasma is small, it is critical because it determines the pressure gradients among the inspired air, the blood, and the tissues. Hemoglobin carries the majority of the oxygen as oxyhemoglobin.

The amount of oxygen in combination with hemoglobin is expressed as *arterial oxygen saturation* (SaO_2). The oxyhemoglobin dissociation curve illustrates the relationship between PaO_2 and SaO_2 (Fig. 10-9). The sigmoid shape of the curve shows that the hemoglobin loads and unloads oxygen at

BOX 10-8
CAUSES OF RESPIRATORY ALKALOSIS

Anxiety
Fever
Sepsis
Hypoxemia
• Pneumonia
• Atelectasis
• Pulmonary emboli
• Congestive heart failure
• Asthma
Central nervous system disorders
• Head injury
• Brain tumor
• Infection
• Cerebrovascular accident
• High altitude
Liver failure
Reye's syndrome
Hyperthyroidism
Salicylate poisoning
Mechanical ventilation

Modified from Brewer ED: Disorders of acid-base balance. *Pediatr Clin North Am* 1990; 37:429-447.

TABLE 10-4	**FACTORS THAT MAY SHIFT OXYHEMOGLOBIN DISSOCIATION CURVE**	
Increased Affinity (Shift to Left)		**Decreased Affinity (Shift to Right)**
Increased pH		Decreased pH
Decreased PCO_2		Increased PCO_2
Decreased temperature		Increased temperature
Decreased 2,3-DPG		Increased 2,3-DPG
Fetal hemoglobin		
Carboxyhemoglobin		
Methemoglobin		

PCO_2, Partial pressure of carbon dioxide (tension); *2,3-DPG*, 2,3-diphos-phoglycerate.

various pressures. The oxyhemoglobin dissociation curve is affected by several factors and may shift left or right (Table 10-4). A shift to the *right* results in a decrease in oxygen affinity and decrease in oxyhemoglobin. A shift to the *left* increases oxygen affinity and increases oxyhemoglobin.

The oxygen content of the blood, expressed as a percentage, is the sum of the oxygen dissolved in the plasma and the oxygen in combination with hemoglobin (Hb, g/dl). Oxygen content accurately reflects the amount of oxygen being transported to the tissues, as follows:

$$O_2 \text{ content} = [(Hb \times 1.34) \times Sao_2] + (Pao_2 \times 0.003)$$

ABNORMAL HEMOGLOBIN

Abnormal hemoglobins also have an effect on the hemoglobin's capacity to combine with oxygen. The following hemoglobins are sometimes encountered in the infant and pediatric population. *Fetal hemoglobin* accounts for approximately 85% of the hemoglobin in the full-term infant. It causes a shift to the left of the oxyhemoglobin dissociation curve and consequently an increased affinity of hemoglobin for oxygen. In utero this compensates for the low fetal Pao_2 and causes more oxygen to be picked up in the placenta. At about 6 months of age, all fetal hemoglobin should be converted to normal.

Methemoglobin forms when hemoglobin is oxidized to the ferric state. It causes the oxyhemoglobin dissociation curve to shift to the left, resulting in a decrease in hemoglobin's ability to combine with oxygen. Nitrate-containing molecules in medications and therapeutic gases may cause methemoglobinemia.

Carboxyhemoglobin forms when carbon monoxide combines with hemoglobin, which reduces the

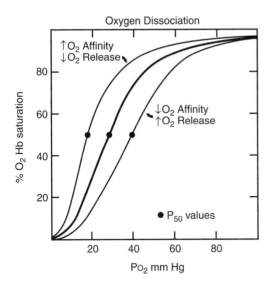

Fig. 10-9

Oxyhemoglobin dissociation curve illustrating the P_{50} value with the effects of right and left shifts of the curve. As the curve shifts to the right, the oxygen affinity of hemoglobin decreases, more oxygen is released at a given Po_2, and the P_{50} value increases. When the curve shifts to the left, there is increased oxygen affinity, less oxygen is released at a given Po_2, and the P_{50} value decreases. (From Oski FA: Fetal hemoglobin, the neonatal red cell, and 2,3-diphosphoglycerate. *Pediatr Clin North Am* 1972; 19:907-917.)

amount of oxygen that can attach to the hemoglobin. In carbon monoxide poisoning the patient has reduced oxygen content even though the PaO_2 may be normal (see Chapter 39). A left-shifted oxyhemoglobin dissociation curve compounds the tissue hypoxia further.

REFERENCES

1. Czervinske MP: Arterial blood gas analysis and other cardiopulmonary monitoring. In Koff PB, Eitzman DV, Neu J, editors: *Neonatal and pediatric respiratory care.* St Louis, Mosby, 1988.
2. American Association for Respiratory Care: Clinical practice guideline: blood gas analysis and hemoximetry, 2001 revision and update. *Respir Care* 2001; 46:498-505.
3. Johnston CC et al: Factors explaining lack of response to heel stick in preterm newborns. *J Obstet Gynecol Neonat Nurs* 1999; 28:587-594.
4. Anand KJS: Clinical importance of pain and stress in preterm newborn infants. *Biol Neonate* 1998; 73:1-9.
5. Johnston CC et al: Differential response to pain by very premature neonates. *Pain* 1995; 61:471-479.
6. Anand KJS, International Evidence-Based Group for Neonatal Pain: Consensus statement for the prevention and management of pain in the newborn. *Arch Pediatr Adolesc Med* 2001; 155:173-180.
7. NCCLS: *Procedures for the collection of arterial blood specimens,* ed 3, H11-A3, NCCLS, 1999.
8. American Association for Respiratory Care: Clinical practice guideline: sampling for arterial blood gas analysis. *Respir Care* 1992; 37:913-917.
9. Centers for Disease Control: Update: universal precautions for prevention of transmission of human immunodeficiency virus, hepatitis B virus, and other blood borne pathogens in health care settings. *MMWR* 1988; 37:377-388.
10. U.S. Occupational Safety and Health Administration: Occupational exposure to bloodborne pathogens, 29 CFR 1910.1030. *Federal Register,* December 1991.
11. Escalante-Kanashiro R, Tantalean Da Fieno J: Capillary blood gases in a pediatric intensive care unit. *Crit Care Med* 2000; 28:224-226.
12. American Association for Respiratory Care: Clinical practice guideline: capillary blood gas sampling for neonatal and pediatric patients. *Respir Care* 1994; 39:1180-1183.
13. McLain BI, Evans J, Dear PFR: Comparison of capillary and arterial blood gas measurements in neonates. *Arch Dis Child* 1988; 63:743-747.
14. Hess D: Detection and monitoring of hypoxemia and oxygen therapy. *Respir Care* 2000; 45:65-80.
15. Courtney SE et al: Capillary blood gases in the neonate: a reassessment and review of the literature. *Am J Dis Child* 1990; 144:168-172.
16. Harrison AM et al: Comparison of simultaneously obtained arterial and capillary blood gases in pediatric intensive care unit patients. *Crit Care Med* 1997; 25:1904-1908.
17. Kisling JA, Schreiner RL: Techniques of obtaining arterial blood from newborn infants. *Respir Care* 1977; 22:513-518.
18. Johnson KJ et al: Neonatal laboratory blood sampling: comparison of results from arterial catheters with those from an automated capillary device. *Neonat Network* 2000; 19(1):27-34.
19. Wayman T: Factors affecting capillary blood-gas values. *Respir Ther* 1980; 1:21-23.
20. Koch G, Wendel H: Comparison of pH, carbon dioxide tension, standard bicarbonate, and oxygen tension in capillary blood and in arterial blood during neonatal period. *Acta Paediatr Scand* 1967; 56:14.
21. Sell EJ, Hansen RC, Struck-Pierce S: Calcified nodules on the heel: a complication of neonatal intensive care. *J Pediatr* 1980; 96:473-475.
22. Symansky MR, Fox HA: Umbilical vessel catheterization: indications, management and evaluation of the technique. *J Pediatr* 1972; 80:820-826.
23. Barrington KJ: Umbilical artery catheters in the newborn: effects of position of the catheter tip. *Cochrane Library (Oxford)* 2000; 4.
24. MacDonald MG: Umbilical artery catheterization. In Avery GB, Fletcher MA, MacDonald MG, editors: *Neonatology: pathophysiology and management of the newborn.* Philadelphia, Lippincott/Williams & Wilkins, 1999, p 1338.
25. Dunn PM: Localization of the umbilical artery catheter by post-mortem measurement. *Arch Dis Child* 1966; 41:69-74.
26. Rosenfeld W et al: Evaluation of graphs for insertion of umbilical artery catheters below the diaphragm. *J Pediatr* 1981; 98:627-628.
27. Green C, Yohannan MD: Umbilical arterial and venous catheters: placement, use, and complications. *Neonat Network* 1998; 17(6):23-28.
28. Cole FS, Todres ID, Shannon DC: Technique for percutaneous cannulation of the radial artery in the newborn infant. *J Pediatr* 1978; 92:105-107.
29. Pearse RG: Percutaneous catheterization of the radial artery in newborn babies using transillumination. *Arch Dis Child* 1978; 53:549-554.
30. Eshali H et al: Septicaemia with coagulase negative staphylococci in a neonatal intensive care unit: risk factors for infection, and antimicrobial susceptibility of the bacterial strains. *Acta Paediatr Scand Suppl* 1989; 360:127-134.
31. Lott JW, Conner GK, Phillips JB: Umbilical artery catheter blood sampling alters cerebral blood flow velocity in preterm infants. *J Perinatol* 1996; 16:341-345.
32. Cumming WA, Burchfield DJ: Accidental catheterization of internal iliac artery branches: a serious complication of umbilical artery catheterization. *J Perinatol* 1994; 14:304-309.
33. Brown MS, Phibbs RH: Spinal cord injury in newborns from use of umbilical artery catheters: report of two cases and a review of the literature. *J Perinatol* 1988; 8:105-110.
34. Duck S: Neonatal intravenous therapy. *Neonat Intensive Care* 1998; 11(2):36-41.
35. Chiang VW, Baskin MN: Uses and complications of central venous catheters inserted in a pediatric emergency department. *Pediatr Emerg Care* 2000; 16:230-232.
36. Hamilton H, Fermo K: Clinical assessment of patients requiring IV therapy via a central venous route. *Br J Nurs* 1998; 7:451-460.
37. MacDonald MG: Umbilical vein catheterization. In Avery GB, Fletcher MA, MacDonald MG, editors: *Neonatology: pathophysiology and management of the newborn.* Philadelphia, Lippincott/Williams & Wilkins, 1999, p 148.
38. Kelly RE et al: Choosing venous access in the extremely low birth weight (ELBW) infant: percutaneous central venous lines and peripherally inserted catheters. *Neonat Intensive Care* 1997; 10(5):15-18.
39. Jordan W: Arterial catheters. In Blumer JL, editor: *A practical guide to pediatric intensive care.* St Louis, Mosby, 1990, p 825.
40. Green C, Yohannan MD: Umbilical arterial and venous catheters: placement, use, and complications. *Neonat Network* 1998; 17(6):23-28.

41. Trotter CW: Percutaneous central venous catheter-related sepsis in the neonate: an analysis of the literature from 1990 to 1994. *Neonat Network* 1996; 15(3):15-28.

42. Wynsma LA: Negative outcomes of intravascular therapy in infants and children. *AACN Clin Issues Adv Pract Acute Crit Care* 1998; 9:49-63.

43. Osgood CF, Watson MH, Slaughter MS: Hemodynamic monitoring in respiratory care. *Respir Care* 1984; 29:25.

44. Abou-Khalil B: Hemodynamic responses to shock in young trauma patients: need for invasive monitoring. *Crit Care Med* 1994; 22:633-639.

45. Katz RW, Pollack MM, Weibley RE: Pulmonary artery catheterization in pediatric intensive care. *Adv Pediatr* 1983; 30:169.

46. Marini JJ: Obtaining meaningful data from the Swan-Ganz catheter. *Respir Care* 1985; 30:572.

47. Pollack MM et al: Bedside pulmonary artery catheterization in pediatrics. *J Pediatr* 1980; 96:274.

48. Merl KE, Pauly-O'Neill SJ: Nursing care of the child with a pulmonary artery catheter. *Pediatr Nurs* 1987; 13(2):114-119.

49. Mermel LA et al: Guidelines for the management of intravascular catheter-related infections. *Infect Control Hosp Epidemiol* 2001; 22:222-242.

50. Randolph AG et al: Benefit of heparin in central venous and pulmonary artery catheters: a meta-analysis of randomized controlled trials. *Chest* 1998; 113:165-171.

51. Elliott CG, Zimmerman GA, Clemmer TP: Complications of pulmonary artery catheterization in the care of critically ill patients: a prospective study. *Chest* 1979; 76:647.

52. White KM: Completing the hemodynamic picture: SV_{O_2}. *Heart Lung* 1985; 14:272.

53. Moodie DS et al: Measurement of cardiac output by thermodilution: development of accurate measurements at flows applicable to the pediatric patient. *J Surg Res* 1978; 25:305.

54. Wyse SD et al: Measurement of cardiac output by thermal dilution in infants and children. *Thorax* 1975; 30:262.

55. Hess D et al: The validity of assessing arterial blood gases 10 minutes after an F_{IO_2} change in mechanically ventilated patients without chronic pulmonary disease. *Respir Care* 1985; 30:1037-1041.

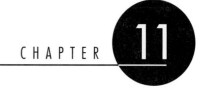

CHAPTER 11

Noninvasive Monitoring in Neonatal and Pediatric Care

Garry Sitler

Cardiorespiratory alterations are the most frequent problems encountered in sick pediatric or neonatal patients. Poor gas exchange and acid-base disturbances are characteristic of pediatric patients with cardiopulmonary failure. Noninvasive monitoring has provided the bedside clinician with the ability to monitor the patient's cardiopulmonary status continuously. These machines can detect subtle changes in patient condition before the appearance of clinical symptoms. Monitors can acquire data and display this information as a trend over several hours, which may lead to improved patient outcomes. In the managed care atmosphere, continuous noninvasive monitoring not only improves patient outcomes, but also is generally more cost-effective than serial laboratory testing.

PULSE OXIMETRY

The monitoring of oxygenation in the pediatric patient is critical to patient outcomes. *Hypoxemia* is one of the major causes of morbidity and mortality. *Hyperoxemia* can lead to lung damage and retinopathy of the premature. Pulse oximetry is useful for monitoring trends in oxygenation.

PRINCIPLES OF OPERATION

Oxygen is carried in the blood in two forms, bound and dissolved. Approximately 98% of the oxygen is *bound* to hemoglobin, and the other 2% is *dissolved* in the plasma.[1] The hemoglobin binds with oxygen in the pulmonary circulation and then releases oxygen at the tissue level. This affinity is displayed as the oxyhemoglobin dissociation curve. Arterial oxygen saturation (SaO_2) is the amount of hemoglobin that has bound with oxygen.

A pulse oximeter sensor measures oxygenation. The sensor has two light-emitting diodes (LEDs) that function as light sources and one photodiode as a light receiver (Fig. 11-1). One LED emits red light, and the other diode emits infrared light. As the light from the diodes passes through the blood

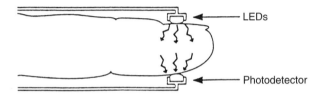

Fig. 11-1

Proper alignment of light-emitting diodes (LEDs) opposite the photodetector in sensor applied to finger. (From *Pulse oximetry,* note 7. Hayward, Calif, Nellcor, 1991.)

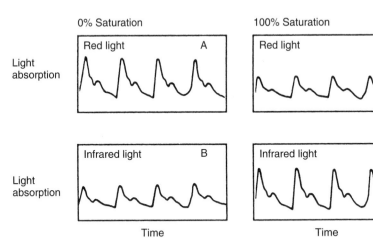

A = Desaturated blood viewed in red light, pulse signal larger because more light is absorbed.

B = Desaturated blood viewed in infrared light, pulse signal smaller because less light is absorbed.

C = Saturated blood viewed in red light, pulse signal smaller because less light is absorbed.

D = Saturated blood viewed in infrared light, pulse signal larger because more light is absorbed.

Fig. 11-2

Differences in light absorption between deoxygenated hemoglobin (0% saturation) and oxygenated hemoglobin (100% saturation) during pulsatile signals. (From *Clinical reference card,* no 1. Hayward, Calif, Nellcor, 1988.)

and tissue, some of the light from both the red and the infrared diodes is absorbed. The photodiode then measures the amount of light that passes through the body without being absorbed. By knowing the amount of light that is entering the body and the amount of light leaving the body, the amount of light absorbed is easily determined. This absorption of both the red and infrared light is used to determine the percentage of functional hemoglobin that is saturated with oxygen (Fig. 11-2). To measure arterial blood, the sensor detects pulsatile blood as it enters the tissue. SaO_2 is measured in both nonpulsatile and pulsatile states, and the ratio is corrected to determine functional saturation.

APPLICATION

Pulse oximeters are precalibrated. The calibration is built into the instrument's algorithm. Each sensor is calibrated during manufacture. The wavelength of the sensor diodes is checked and then coded into a calibration resistor. The instrument decodes the resistor each time it is turned on, at periodic intervals during use, or when a new sensor is used.

A variety of sensors are available for different clinical settings. The disposable bandage type for

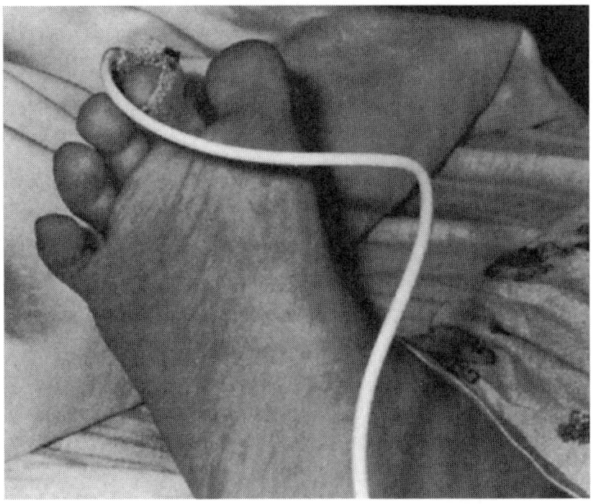

Fig. 11-3

Pulse oximeter probe attached to a child's toe.

wrapping around a finger or toe is used most often (Fig. 11-3). Application of the sensor is crucial to the quality of readings from the pulse oximeter. The sensor should be placed over a vascular area with the diodes and the photodiode directly opposite each other and in good contact with the skin. The palm of the hand, ball of the foot, and wrist are good sites in the neonate.[2] The fingers and toes of larger children are also good sites.[3] The sensors should be placed firmly to avoid falling off or motion artifact, but care should be taken to avoid overtightening and compromising the circulation.[4] The sensor sites should be changed routinely and the monitoring sites assessed for tissue injury. Finger and ear clips are also available for the larger patients. Care must be taken with the clip type of sensors because the clinician has no control over the spring tension and the pressure created on the extremity.

Most pulse oximeters have an indicator of pulse signal strength. A minimum level of pulse signal is needed to obtain an accurate SaO$_2$ reading. For best results, always make sure that the signal is as strong as possible and that the pulse oximeter's pulse rate reading corresponds to the patient's true heart rate.[5]

DISADVANTAGES

Pulse oximetry was originally developed by anesthesiologists for use in the operating room. In this well-controlled environment the patient is warm, still, and well perfused. As use of the pulse oximeter expanded to other areas of the hospital, the well-controlled environment was lost, and the problems of artifacts causing oximetry alarms arose. False alarms occurred more often because patients could be awake and moving and may poorly perfuse. Artifact can occur in two ways. First, if misinterpreted by the machine as a pulse wave, the artifact can corrupt the measurement and set off an alarm limit. Second, if the artifact obscures the pulse, the "loss of pulse" alarm could be triggered. Patient movement, electrical noise, and rapidly changing ambient light (e.g., fluorescent) can produce artifacts that affect pulse oximeters.[4]

Some studies are questioning the correlation of pulse oximeters and arterial blood gases in the neonate.[1] Neonatal patients with hyperbilirubinemia or anemia and those receiving hyperalimentation, intralipids, or inotropic infusions may not yield comparable data between pulse oximeters and arterial blood gases. Even when properly functioning, the pulse oximeter does not provide good information regarding hyperoxia in the neonatal patient. If the oximeter is reading a SaO$_2$ of 100%, the oxygen tension (PO$_2$) could be between 90 and 250 mm Hg. Proper site selection, understanding the principles of operation, and routinely assessing the patient to correlate the SaO$_2$ with other vital signs will help to minimize these problems and make the pulse oximeter a valuable clinical tool.[6-8]

TRANSCUTANEOUS MONITORING

In the hands of an experienced and trained clinician, a well-maintained and properly calibrated transcutaneous monitor will provide very accurate information regarding the pediatric patient's oxygenation status.[9] Transcutaneous measurement of PO$_2$ and carbon dioxide tension (PCO$_2$) provides immediate, continuous information on the body's ability to deliver oxygen to the tissues and to remove carbon dioxide by way of the cardiopulmonary system. It is, however, important to realize that the electrode is measuring the gas tension of the underlying tissue, *not* the arterial gas tension. When hemodynamic conditions are stable, transcutaneous measurements correlate well with arterial values, but this does not necessarily mean that the measured values will be identical.

PRINCIPLES OF OPERATION

Transcutaneous measurements of PO$_2$ and PCO$_2$ are based on the principle that a heating element in the sensor elevates the temperature in the underlying tissue. This increases the capillary blood flow to the tissue as well as the partial pressure of oxygen and carbon dioxide, and it makes the skin permeable to gas diffusion. Because metabolism in the tissue consumes oxygen and produces carbon dioxide, transcutaneous values differ from arterial values.[10] Usually the PO$_2$ is slightly lower than in the arteries, and the PCO$_2$ is slightly higher when measured transcutaneously.

APPLICATION

The most critical aspect to transcutaneous monitoring is the application and site selection of the sensor (Fig. 11-4). The site should be a highly vascular area such as the upper chest, abdomen, and thighs,

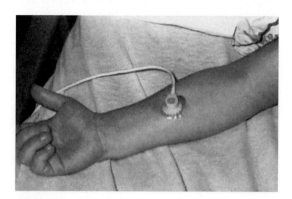

Fig. 11-4

Transcutaneous oxygen monitor electrode placed on a child's arm.

or the lower back if the patient is supine. Bony areas over the spine should be avoided. Another consideration when selecting a site is that the right side of the upper chest will give preductal oxygenation values, whereas the left side of the chest and the lower parts of the body will give postductal values.

Selecting a sensor temperature is important to proper operation.[11] The temperature range is usually 43° to 44° C, with the thicker skin requiring the higher temperature. The heating of the sensor requires that the site be changed on a routine basis to prevent thermal injuries. The frequency of the site changes ranges from 3 to 4 hours and can be increased to 2 or 3 hours if the skin at the site has a reaction or if the sensor is operated at higher temperatures.

Meticulously following the manufacturer's membrane changing procedure and calibration instructions will result in the most accurate readings. Once the machine has been prepared and the site selected, the skin must be cleaned to wipe away dead skin, oils, and medications. The accuracy of the sensor is improved by using 1 or 2 drops of contact gel. This liquid-to-liquid medium makes the diffusion of gases more efficient. The sensor is then attached to the skin with a fixation ring. This ring must seal the environment from the sensor and the skin.

DISADVANTAGES

The use of the transcutaneous monitor is labor intensive because it requires frequent site changes, membrane changes, and calibration. Properly trained clinicians are needed to care for the machine, select the sites, and apply the sensor.

The main physiologic factor relating to good correlation is good peripheral blood perfusion. The skin reacts to cold, shock, and certain drugs by contracting the superficial blood vessels and by opening the larger, deeper-lying arterioles to achieve a shunting effect. In case of exposure to cold, capillary blood flow is stopped to reduce the loss of body heat. Shock and certain cardiopulmonary medications will dilate the blood vessels, causing the blood pressure in the body to drop. In response to this drop in blood pressure, the body will shunt blood away from the skin and toward major organs. If the blood flow in the capillary bed is reduced, the capillary blood rapidly becomes more or less venous, with a considerably lower Po_2 and higher Pco_2. Therefore, in patients with impaired peripheral blood perfusion, large deviations may occur between central Po_2/ Pco_2 and the transcutaneous values.[12]

CAPNOMETRY

The measurement of oxygenation saturation with the pulse oximeter has revolutionized the assessment of oxygenation in patients with respiratory failure. The recent availability of noninvasive techniques for measuring end-tidal carbon dioxide ($ETco_2$) has shown great promise as a reliable alternative to blood gas analysis for assessing ventilatory status. Capnometry is one such technique.

PRINCIPLES OF OPERATION

The CO_2 concentration in a pediatric patient's expired breath can be measured continuously by infrared spectroscopy.[13,14] The displayed waveform produced by variations in CO_2 throughout the respiratory cycle is known as a *capnogram*. Variations in this waveform are associated with specific abnormalities. The infrared CO_2 analyzer consists of a source of infrared radiation, a chamber containing the gas sample, and a detector. The wavelength of the infrared rays is longer than visible light. Specific wavelengths are absorbed by specific gases; absorption bands from which the identity of the gas can be read are produced on the infrared spectrum. Gas concentration is measured by the reduction in intensity of the radiation within the same band and is compared with the effect of a reference gas mixture. *Mainstream* CO_2 analyzers have the infrared source and detectors on opposite sides of the primary stream, across which the rays must pass.

Analysis occurs in the sensor head, which is placed at the proximal end of the endotracheal tube (Fig. 11-5). *Sidestream* infrared CO_2 analyzers continuously aspirate a small sample of gas from the main respiratory flow. Analysis occurs within the machine. This method can cause inaccuracies if mucus or water from the humidity of the patient circuit is aspirated and the sampling line becomes occluded, or if the sample is contaminated with fresh gases, as in infants with small tidal volumes. Most analyzers have a mechanism to clear accumulated liquids and solids from the sample line.

INTERPRETATION OF CAPNOGRAM

Trending $ETco_2$ will give the bedside clinician a good sense of the adequacy of ventilation for the patient. An increase in $ETco_2$ from previous levels might indicate hypoventilation. The possibility of decreased tidal volume or respiratory rate should be investigated. A decrease in $ETco_2$ from previous levels might indicate hyperventilation. The interpretation of the capnogram (waveform display of the exhaled CO_2) can also help the clinician detect other ventilatory abnormalities.

The normal capnogram can be divided into four phases. *Phase A-B* is the inspiratory phase, during which the sensor detects no carbon dioxide. *Phase B-C* is the initial expiratory phase, during which

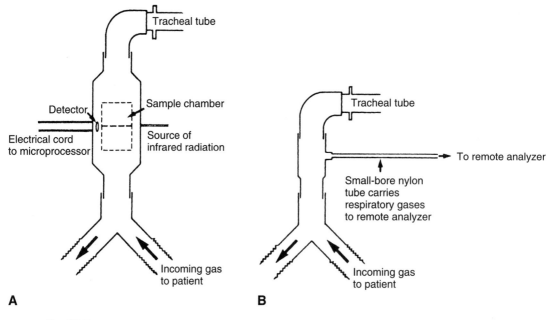

Fig. 11-5

Location of mainstream airway adapter (**A**) and sidestream adapter (**B**) in patient's airway. (From Stock MC: Non-invasive carbon dioxide monitoring. *Crit Care Clin* 1988; 4:511.)

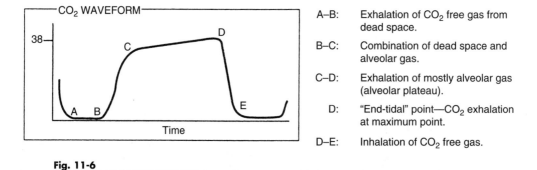

A–B:	Exhalation of CO_2 free gas from dead space.
B–C:	Combination of dead space and alveolar gas.
C–D:	Exhalation of mostly alveolar gas (alveolar plateau).
D:	"End-tidal" point—CO_2 exhalation at maximum point.
D–E:	Inhalation of CO_2 free gas.

Fig. 11-6

Normal capnogram. (From *Advanced concepts in capnography.* Hayward, Calif, Nellcor, 1988.)

carbon dioxide rapidly increases as the alveoli begin to empty. *Phase C-D* is the completion of expiration as the alveoli empty *(alveolar plateau)* and shows a slight increase in carbon dioxide. *Phase D-E* is the beginning of inspiration as the waveform returns to zero (Fig. 11-6).

DETECTION OF VENTILATION PROBLEMS

The clinician can use the capnogram to detect important ventilation problems in neonatal and pediatric patients.

Endotracheal Tube in Esophagus. A normal capnogram is the best evidence that the endotracheal

tube is in proper position and that ventilation is occurring. When the endotracheal tube is placed incorrectly in the esophagus, no CO_2 will be detected, or only small transient capnograms will be present.

Rebreathing. Rebreathing is characterized by an elevation in the A-B phase of the capnogram with a corresponding increase in ETCO_2. It indicates the rebreathing of the previously exhaled CO_2. Rebreathing can be caused by using an insufficient expiratory time or an inadequate inspiratory flow (Fig. 11-7).

Obstructed Airway. Obstruction to the expiratory flow of gas will be noted as a change in the

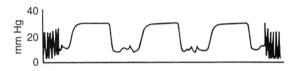

Fig. 11-7

Effect of rebreathing carbon dioxide on the capnogram. Note that the inspiratory level does not return to zero. (From Stock MC: Non-invasive carbon dioxide monitoring. *Crit Care Clin* 1988; 4:511.)

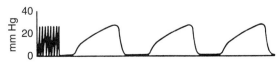

Fig. 11-8

Capnogram with sloping alveolar plateau representative of airway obstruction. (From Stock MC: Non-invasive carbon dioxide monitoring. *Crit Care Clin* 1988; 4:511.)

slope of the B-C phase of the capnogram. The B-C phase may diminish without a plateau. Obstruction can be caused by a foreign body in the upper airway, increased secretions in the airways, the patient having bronchospasms, or partial obstruction of the ventilator circuit (Fig. 11-8).

Paralyzed Patients. Patients who are paralyzed and receiving mechanical ventilation may develop a cleft in the C-D phase of the capnogram. The cleft may indicate a return in diaphragmatic activity and the need for additional paralytic agents (Fig. 11-9).

Pneumothorax. A stair stepping of the D-E phase of the capnogram, caused by unequal and incomplete emptying of the lungs, and a failure to return to baseline may suggest a pneumothorax (Fig. 11-10).

Cardiogenic Oscillations. Cardiogenic oscillations may be seen in patients with long expiratory times and slow respiratory rates. The oscillations will be seen in the D-E phase of the capnogram and are caused as the heart contracts and moves the lungs, causing gas flow (Fig. 11-11).

IMPEDANCE PNEUMOGRAPHY

Measuring the respiratory rate and assessing the breathing patterns are critical to the care of neonatal and pediatric patients, especially those susceptible to apnea. The incidence and number of apneic events or fluctuations in respiratory condition may suggest

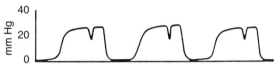

Fig. 11-9

Curare cleft in the alveolar plateau. (From Stock MC: Non-invasive carbon dioxide monitoring. *Crit Care Clin* 1988; 4:511.)

a changing respiratory status or alterations in central nervous system function. Rate counts—by observation, by placing a hand on the patient, or by auscultation—may be grossly inaccurate because of the time required for the measurement as well as the result of tactile stimulation, which may alter breathing patterns.

Impedance pneumography provides continuous, noninvasive monitoring of respiration. This method is easy to perform and is generally used in home care. One set of electrodes for both electrocardiographic and respiratory monitoring makes the application very simple. It must be understood that the monitor functions only as a *warning device* that sounds when breathing or heart rate (or both) is outside the set alarm limits. The monitor will not prevent any abnormal episodes from occurring.

PRINCIPLES OF OPERATION

The principle of impedance pneumography is based on the measurement of the difference in resistance (impedance) to electric current. The resistance to electric current in blood, muscle, fat, and air is different. Gas volume in the chest varies with each respiration, and blood volume varies with each cardiac cycle. Although the resistance of muscle and fat tissue is relatively stable during respiratory and cardiac cycles, the variation caused by respiration is greater than the variations created by changes in thoracic blood volume with each cardiac cycle. Therefore the electrical resistance of the chest increases as the lungs fill with air and decreases as the lungs empty.

The monitor passes an electric current between two electrodes placed on the patient's chest in the midaxillary line. *Impedance* is a function of the distance between the electrodes, which increases and decreases during the respiratory cycle with inspiration and expiration. The electric current changes as the chest expands and contracts, and the monitor interprets these changes as inhalation and exhalation and counts them as respiratory cycles. The smaller electrical resistance changes are also detected with each cardiac cycle and counted as heartbeats.

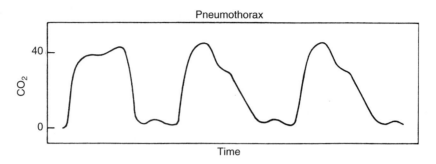

Fig. 11-10

Stair effect on the descending limb of the capnogram. (From Curley MA, Thompson JE: End tidal CO_2 monitoring in critically ill infants and children. *Pediatr Nurs* 1990; 16:397.)

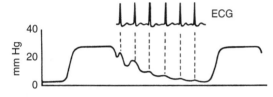

Fig. 11-11

Cardiogenic oscillations in synchrony with the ECG signal. (From Stock MC: Non-invasive carbon dioxide monitoring. *Crit Care Clin* 1988; 4:511.)

APPLICATION

The patient's chest should be washed to remove all soap, oil, powder, and lotion before the electrode pads are applied. The electrode pads are held in place by a foam belt that is placed under the patient's back and wrapped around the patient's chest, with the top of the belt usually at the patient's nipple line and held tight with adhesive strips (Fig. 11-12). The electrode pads are placed under each armpit, with the wires directed down toward the lower ribs. Correctly sized and placed electrodes are critical to obtaining a reliable signal. The belt should be snug, but with enough room to allow one finger to slide under it after it is closed. The electrode pads are connected to the monitor via lead wires. These wires carry the electric signals back to the monitor through a patient cable. The monitors have an alarm system that warns of problems with both the patient and the equipment.

Monitors can detect slow, fast, or absent respiratory rate and heart rate in the neonatal or pediatric patient. Most monitors can detect equipment problems involving the battery functions, lead wire, electrode pad, patient cable, and monitor.

The *event log* should be kept by the monitor if used in a home care situation. Events logged may

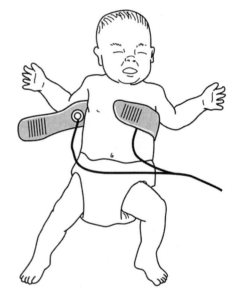

Fig. 11-12

Neonatal impedance pneumography. With the infant on a flat surface, the belt is positioned in line with the nipples. After the electrodes are placed, the belt is wrapped snugly around the infant's chest.

include alarms sounded, changes in the monitor controls and alarm settings, and times when the monitor is turned on and off.

DISADVANTAGES

Impedance pneumography is sensitive to body movement and postural changes that may alter the impedance of the patient interface. The sensitivity of the monitor may detect cardiogenic oscillations and count them as respirations. Impedance pneumography measures changes in chest wall configuration but cannot measure the effectiveness of ventilation.

Therefore, in obstructive apnea associated with absent effective gas flow, the monitor will display this activity as respirations, and no alarms may sound. The signal from the electrodes is only *qualitative,* and assumptions about tidal volume changes based on signal size can be erroneous. False apnea alarms often sound in conditions such as abdominal breathing, poor electrode placement, and restricted chest movement. Artifact may cause a monitor to fail to detect an actual apnea event, or the patient may move during an apneic event, with the monitor recognizing it as a breath. When interpreting the data from impedance pneumography, careful attention must be paid to the activity of the patient to ensure that the signal is free from artifact.

ELECTROCARDIOGRAPHY

The electrocardiogram (ECG) is a recording of body surface electric potentials generated by the heart. It is easy to perform and noninvasive and has been used for many years to provide important information about cardiac anatomy and pathology. More specifically, ECGs are indicated in the evaluation of arrhythmias, atrial or ventricular hypertrophy, electrolyte changes, myocardial or pericardial infections/inflammation, myocardial ischemia/infarction, and congenital heart disease.

In the intensive care unit the primary reasons for continuous monitoring of the ECG are to ensure an adequate heart rate and to sound an alarm if the heart rate drops below a set limit. To detect and record the electric potential created by the heart's activity, electrodes are attached to the patient on the left arm, right arm, and the left leg for typical six-lead intensive care monitoring. Careful attention should be paid to electrode placement on infants and small children; pediatric-sized electrodes should be used to guarantee recording from the proper area without overlapping the electrodes.

The quality of ECG recordings can be influenced by a number of technical problems that lead to artifact. Common sources are patient movement, shaking due to tremulousness, and interference from another electric source causing a fuzzy baseline.

CALORIMETRY

Although the resting metabolic rate (RMR) can be determined by a direct calorimeter, which directly measures heat production (changes in temperature), it is usually measured by indirect calorimetry. The preference for indirect over direct calorimetry is attributed to the cost and unavailability of direct calorimeters (only a few exist in the

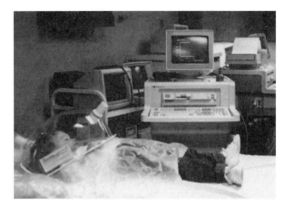

Fig. 11-13

Pediatric indirect calorimetry using metabolic cart with dilution canopy.

United States). In addition, direct calorimetry requires extensive time for equilibration and measurement. *Indirect calorimetry* measures oxygen consumption and carbon dioxide production.[15] From the rate of oxygen consumed and carbon dioxide produced, the clinician can calculate the corresponding energy expenditure.

The *Benedict-Roth respirometer apparatus,* which is a closed-circuit system, has been used for more than 100 years. In this method a known volume of pure oxygen is supplied to the subject, and carbon dioxide is constantly removed as it passes through soda lime without being measured. The decrease in the gas volume in this closed system is related to the rate of oxygen consumption, from which the RMR is then calculated.

The indirect calorimeters most often used are *open-circuit systems.* The patient inspires room air, and the expired air is then collected and analyzed for oxygen and carbon dioxide content. Normally, room air contains 20.93% oxygen and 0.003% carbon dioxide. The difference in content between the control (inspired air) and the sample (expired air) is assumed to be consumed or produced by the patient. Newer systems are computer driven and can make the calculations very quickly, allowing the measurement of RMR in a short time.

The most difficult task in obtaining reliable RMRs is proper preparation of the patient in a relaxed, postabsorptive state. All indirect calorimetry methods necessitate the collection and analysis of expired air. The use of a mouthpiece to collect the expired air requires less equilibration time but may cause patient discomfort. Such discomfort has been reported to result in higher RMRs than with a hood system (Fig. 11-13) or a respiration chamber.[16]

REFERENCES

1. Gibson LY: Pulse oximeter in the neonatal ICU: a correlational analysis. *Pediatr Nurs* 1996; 22:511-514.
2. Whyte RK, Jangaard KA, Dooley KC: From oxygen content to pulse oximetry: completing the picture in the newborn. *Acta Anaesthesiol Scand* 1995; 39:95-100.
3. Hanna D: Guidelines for pulse oximetry use in pediatrics. *J Pediatr Nurs* 1995; 10:124-126.
4. Barker SJ, Shah NK: The effects of motion on the performance of pulse oximeters in volunteers. *Anesthesiology* 1997; 86:101-107.
5. Dassel ACM et al: Effects of location of the sensor on reflectance pulse oximetry. *Br J Obstet Gynaecol* 1997; 104:910-916.
6. Wipperman CF et al: Continuous measurement of cardiac output by the Fick principle in infants and children: comparison with the thermodilution method. *Intensive Care Med* 1996; 22:467-471.
7. Tallon RW: Oximetry: state of the art. *Nurs Manage* 1996; 27:43-44.
8. Trivedi NS et al: Pulse oximeter performance during desaturation and resaturation: a comparison of seven models. *J Clin Anesth* 1997; 9:184-188.
9. Lewer BMF et al: Accuracy of transcutaneous carbon dioxide measurement. *Can J Anaesth* 1998; 45:186.
10. Carter B et al: A comparison of two transcutaneous monitors for the measurement of arterial Po_2 and Pco_2 in neonates. *Anaesth Intensive Care* 1995; 23:708-714.
11. Talbot A et al: Dynamic model of oxygen transport for transcutaneous Po_2 analysis. *Ann Biomed Eng* 1996; 24:294-304.
12. Tobias JD, Meyer DJ: Noninvasive monitoring of carbon dioxide during respiratory failure in toddlers and infants: end-tidal versus transcutaneous carbon dioxide. *Anesth Analg* 1997; 85:55-58.
13. Tobias JD, Lynch A, Garrett J: Alterations of end-tidal carbon dioxide during the intrahospital transport of children. *Pediatr Emerg Care* 1997; 12:249-251.
14. Abramo TJ et al: Noninvasive capnometry in a pediatric population with respiratory emergencies. *Pediatr Emerg Care* 1996; 12:252-254.
15. Coss-Bu JA et al: Resting energy expenditure in children in a pediatric intensive care unit: comparison of Harris-Benedict and Talbot predictions with indirect calorimetry values. *Am J Clin Nutr* 1998; 67:74-80.
16. Segal KR: Comparison of indirect calorimetric measurement of resting energy expenditure with a ventilated hood, face mask, and mouthpiece. *Am J Clin Nutr* 1987; 45:1420-1423.

Therapeutic Procedures for Treatment of Neonatal and Pediatric Disorders

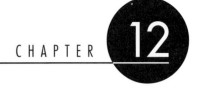

CHAPTER 12

Oxygen Administration

Sherry L. Barnhart

When Priestly discovered oxygen in 1774, it was viewed as a scientific curiosity. Today, oxygen plays an essential role in the survival of premature infants and critically ill children. We accept oxygen as effective therapy to prevent or relieve hypoxemia.[1]

The goal of oxygen therapy is to achieve adequate tissue oxygenation with the lowest fractional concentration of inspired oxygen (FIO_2) possible. Unfortunately, adverse reactions from the therapeutic use of oxygen are well documented in neonatal and pediatric patients. Just as the delivery system used to administer supplemental oxygen must suit the patient's size, physiologic needs, and therapeutic goals, it must also provide accurate and safe levels of oxygen in a variety of clinical conditions.[2]

INDICATIONS

DOCUMENTED OR SUSPECTED HYPOXEMIA

The correction of *hypoxemia* (low oxygen content in the blood) is the most common indication for oxygen therapy.[3] Left untreated, hypoxemia progresses to *hypoxia* (low tissue oxygen) and possibly *anoxia* (absent tissue oxygen), which if severe enough, leads to metabolic abnormalities and the development of acidosis.

Hypoxemia occurs as a result of decreased alveolar ventilation, decreased inspired oxygen, poor ventilation-perfusion relationships, intrapulmonary or cardiac shunting, diffusion defects, or short red blood cell transit times. In conditions such as anemia or carbon monoxide poisoning, the oxygen-carrying capacity of the blood is reduced despite the presence of normal arterial oxygen tension (PaO_2). Bradycardia, cardiac failure, hypotension, and hypothermia leave the circulatory system unable to provide adequate tissue oxygen. In rare cases, such as cyanide poisoning, the tissue is unable to accept and use oxygen, despite adequate oxygen delivery.[4] The documentation of hypoxemia through arterial blood gas sampling or pulse oximetry provides the most definitive evidence of

141

actual or impending tissue hypoxia (see Chapters 7 and 11).

Administration of oxygen is also appropriate if hypoxia is strongly suspected on clinical grounds. However, substantiation of the PaO_2 is required within an appropriate period after administration.[3,4] In emergency situations, such as severe respiratory distress, shock, or cardiopulmonary arrest, oxygen therapy is never withheld even if laboratory test results are unavailable.

EVIDENCE OF HYPOXEMIA

Measurement of Oxygen Tension and Saturation. In the child, PaO_2 less than 80 mm Hg and percentage of oxygen saturation (SpO_2) less than 95% usually indicate hypoxemia. Because fetal hemoglobin has a much greater affinity for oxygen, the oxygen dissociation curve is shifted to the left, allowing a higher saturation for any given PaO_2. The normal immediate postnatal PaO_2 of 60 mm Hg corresponds closely with an SpO_2 of 90%. For this reason, it is generally agreed that PaO_2 less than 60 mm Hg and SpO_2 less than 90% in the newborn indicate hypoxemia and necessitate administration of oxygen.

Clinical Signs and Symptoms. In the infant and child the earliest clinical manifestations of hypoxia are *tachycardia* and *tachypnea*. Worsening hypoxia results in decreased ventilation, apnea, and bradycardia. This is especially true in both the neonate and the term infant. Other physical signs of hypoxia include grunting, nasal flaring, retractions, paradoxical breathing, cyanosis, irritability, and increased restlessness.[5] Often the neonate or infant becomes lethargic and flaccid, with arms and legs extended in a "frog leg" position.

The presence of cyanosis has often been used to determine inadequate oxygenation. Although this clinical sign is somewhat useful in the pediatric and adult patient, its presence in infants is often a late sign of severe hypoxia. *Peripheral cyanosis* (acrocyanosis) is the bluish discoloration of the skin or extremities. It occurs when a decrease in body temperature results in poor peripheral circulation or vasoconstriction. *Central cyanosis* involves the warm and well-perfused areas of the tongue and mucous membranes. It does not occur until 4 to 6 g/dl of reduced hemoglobin is present in arterial blood. In the child and adult the reduced hemoglobin concentration at which cyanosis occurs corresponds to PaO_2 of approximately 50 to 60 mm Hg and SpO_2 of 85% to 90%. In the infant, fetal hemoglobin's stronger affinity for oxygen results in the PaO_2 falling to a significantly lower level before 5 g/dl of reduced hemoglobin is present in arterial blood. In

fact, by the time central cyanosis is present in the infant, oxygen delivery to the tissues is grossly insufficient. For this reason, the clinical impression of cyanosis in the infant must be confirmed by arterial blood gas analysis or pulse oximetry.

COMPLICATIONS

Complications of therapeutic oxygen administration are separated into two categories, the adverse physiologic effects and the equipment-related complications. Adverse reactions that result directly from using an oxygen delivery device are discussed later with the specific device. Although potential risks are present whenever oxygen is administered, the consequences of hypoxia are more severe.

In certain disorders, including cystic fibrosis and bronchopulmonary dysplasia (BPD), the normal response to ventilation is blunted because of chronic carbon dioxide retention. Abrupt and excessive increases in supplemental oxygen decrease the respiratory drive and result in *hypoventilation* or respiratory arrest.[6]

Oxygen's role in the development of *retinopathy of prematurity* (ROP) is controversial. It is believed to cause constriction of retinal and cerebral vessels in neonates and infants, leading to ischemia, varying degrees of retinal scarring, and permanent visual impairment, including blindness. Formerly referred to as "retrolental fibroplasia," ROP may resolve spontaneously or remain permanent. In addition to oxygen, many other factors appear to correlate with the development of ROP, including gestational age, intraventricular hemorrhage, sepsis, and low birth weight.[7] For this reason, oxygen administration to infants less than 37 weeks' gestation should not result in PaO_2 greater than 80 mm Hg.[8]

Absorption *atelectasis* may occur after high concentrations of oxygen increase the alveolar oxygen tension (PAO_2) and decrease the alveolar nitrogen. As the nitrogen is replaced by oxygen, the oxygen is rapidly absorbed into the blood and the gas volume decreases, resulting in atelectasis. *Pulmonary vasodilation* results from high FIO_2. As the pulmonary vasculature dilates and alveolar volumes decrease, areas of ventilation/perfusion mismatch occur with increased intrapulmonary shunting and worsening of arterial oxygen delivery. In patients with a hypoplastic left ventricle or a single ventricle, the increased PaO_2 that occurs with oxygen therapy has been reported to compromise the balance between pulmonary and systemic blood flow.[9] *Pulmonary fibrosis* has been reported to occur after oxygen administration to patients with paraquat poisoning and to those receiving the chemotherapeutic agent bleomycin.[10,11]

OXYGEN ADMINISTRATION

Many of the devices used to deliver supplemental oxygen to neonatal and pediatric patients are simply smaller versions of the adult devices. They are similarly classified in the same manner as either variable-performance oxygen delivery systems (low-flow and reservoir systems) or fixed-performance oxygen delivery systems (high-flow systems).

Variable-performance oxygen delivery systems include devices that are not capable of meeting the patient's inspiratory demand and therefore provide a *fractional concentration of delivered oxygen* (FDO_2) that varies with the patient's rate and depth of ventilation and the flow rate of the gas. These devices include nasal cannulas, nasopharyngeal catheters, tracheostomy oxygen adapters, simple oxygen masks, partial-rebreathing masks, and non-rebreathing masks.

Fixed-performance oxygen delivery systems include devices that can meet or exceed the patient's inspiratory demand and thereby provide an accurate FDO_2. These devices include air-entrainment masks, air-entrainment nebulizer systems, and oxygen blender systems. The last category of oxygen delivery devices includes enclosure systems that provide some means of controlling oxygen concentration, temperature, and humidity. These devices include oxygen hoods, oxygen tents, and closed incubators.[2]

VARIABLE-PERFORMANCE OXYGEN DELIVERY SYSTEMS

Nasopharyngeal Catheter. The nasopharyngeal catheter is a soft plastic tube with several holes at its distal tip. Oxygen flows from the catheter into the patient's oropharynx, which acts as an anatomic reservoir. The nasopharyngeal catheter comes in a variety of sizes, with the smallest size being 8 French (outer diameter). The catheter is best suited for providing a low FIO_2 of 0.24 to 0.3 in infants with chronic pulmonary disease and oxygen dependency. The FIO_2 varies with the patient's inspiratory flow. Flow rates from 0.25 to 1 L/min on 100% oxygen provide a variable FIO_2 of approximately 0.24 to 0.35.[12,13]

Indications and contraindications. Because the catheter can be firmly secured in position, it does not impose a barrier between the infant and caregivers. Feeding, bathing, and other activities are accomplished without interrupting oxygen delivery. Infants can be placed in a sitting position and can roll over, reach for objects, and even crawl while oxygen delivery is maintained. Catheters are not used in patients with maxillofacial trauma,

nasal obstruction such as choanal atresia and nasal polyps, and existing or suspected basilar skull fracture.[14,15] Catheter use may be limited by excessive mucus drainage, mucosal edema, or a deviated septum.[16]

Application. After the tip is lubricated with a sterile, water-soluble material, insert the catheter through the patient's nose into the oropharynx. Determine the proper distance to insert the catheter by gently advancing the catheter until the tip rests slightly above the uvula or by inserting the catheter to a depth equal to the distance from the ala nasi (tip of the nose) to the tragus (earlobe).[13,16] Take care during insertion so that nasal turbinates are not damaged or excessive nasal bleeding does not occur. After verifying the correct position of the catheter, tape the catheter to the patient's face, and connect it to a low-flow flowmeter (less than 3 L/min) and bubble humidifier with small-bore oxygen supply tubing. Catheters smaller than 8 French are less effective in oxygen delivery.[13] However, this may be too large for the premature or very small infant. In this case, insert a 5-French feeding tube in the same manner, and connect it to small-bore tubing.

Hazards and complications. Major problems associated with nasopharyngeal catheters involve the insertion and removal process, correct positioning, and obstruction of the catheter end. Nasal trauma and bleeding may occur if the catheter is forced into small or obstructed nasal passages. If the catheter is not secured properly and slips down past the oropharynx, gagging may occur and lead to vomiting and aspiration.[16] Excessive flow can produce pain in the frontal sinuses as well as gastric distention and impaired diaphragm movement.[13,14] Pneumocephalus is also a rare but possible complication.[17] The catheter can become blocked with mucus or blood, obstructing the flow of oxygen to the patient. For this reason, frequently clear the catheter to prevent occlusion of the distal holes. Observe the patient for evidence of catheter occlusion, and alternate the catheter between nares every 8 to 12 hours, changing it every 24 hours.[12,18] If an infant receiving oxygen by nasopharyngeal catheter becomes cyanotic and agitated or shows a decrease in food intake, or if there is a profound change in the ventilatory pattern, remove the nasopharyngeal catheter and initiate an alternative method of oxygen delivery.

Nasal Cannula. Infants and children with chronic pulmonary diseases, such as cystic fibrosis and BPD, as well as premature infants who survive neonatal respiratory disorders, often require prolonged supplemental oxygen administration. The most

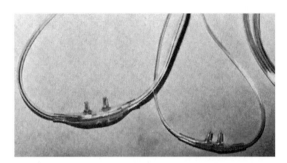

Fig. 12-1

Pediatric nasal cannula *(left)* and neonatal nasal cannula *(right)*. The major differences are the length and width of the prongs and the distance between the two prongs.

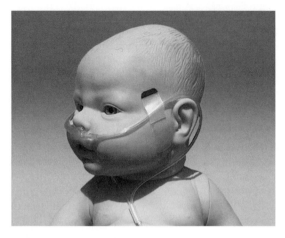

Fig. 12-2

NeoHold cannula/tubing holder. The 4-cm-long strip attaches to patients with hydrocolloid and has a clear flap that allows visualization of the tubing.

commonly used device for oxygen delivery to these patients is the nasal cannula (Fig. 12-1).

Application. Two soft prongs from oxygen supply tubing are inserted into the patient's nares. Oxygen flows from the cannula into the patient's nasopharynx, which acts as an anatomic reservoir. In the very small infant in whom the prongs appear to be too large, remove the prongs and position the cannula on the infant's face with the openings placed below the nose. Wrap the lightweight tubing around the ears, and hold it under the chin with an adjustable plastic notch. In the very small or very active infant, secure the cannula to the face with tape to prevent dislodgment, and position the tubing past the ears, securing it behind the head, instead of under the chin, to prevent airway obstruction. Skin irritation can result from material used to secure the cannula or from a local allergic reaction to polyvinyl chloride.[2] One alternative to using adhesive tape or stoma adhesive to secure the cannula to a neonatal patient's face is the NeoHold cannula/tubing holder (Fig. 12-2). This device is especially useful in holding cannula tubing to the fragile skin of the neonatal patient.

As with the nasopharyngeal catheter, the cannula is designed to provide low oxygen concentrations from approximately 24% to 45%, with the F_{IO_2} varying with the patient's inspiratory flow.[19,20] In the child, oxygen concentrations are controlled primarily by varying the flow rate of the gas. At low flow rates, oxygen concentrations decrease as a result of room-air entrainment that occurs during the patient's inspiration. In the small or premature infant, inspiratory flow rates are quite small and result in less room-air entrainment during inspiration. The F_{IO_2} is higher in infants receiving oxygen via nasal cannula than in adults and can exceed potentially toxic levels.[21] Several studies have documented high F_{IO_2} when supplemental oxygen is supplied to neonates via nasal cannula, ranging from 22% to 95% on various flows of 100% oxygen.[22-24]

Blenders and low-flow flowmeters. Two methods of providing oxygen through a nasal cannula are common in neonatal and pediatric units. The first method entails connecting the cannula to a flowmeter attached to an air-oxygen blender. The second method consists of simply connecting the cannula to a low-flow flowmeter.

Oxygen blenders set at specific oxygen concentrations can be used to regulate the F_{IO_2} to infants with nasal cannulas. With this method, adjust both the oxygen concentration and the flow rate of the gas to achieve the appropriate F_{DO_2}. With a cannula connected to the flowmeter on the blender, set the oxygen concentration at F_{IO_2} of 1.00 and the flow rate at 0.25. Some protocols begin the flow rate at 1 L/min. Adjust the flow rate, decreasing it until reaching the level necessary to maintain adequate oxygen saturation (S_{PO_2}) levels. Continue weaning by decreasing the flow rate until reaching the minimum flow setting of the flowmeter. Proceed with weaning by decreasing the oxygen concentration setting on the blender to maintain adequate S_{PO_2} levels, or until oxygen is no longer required. Although some centers lower the oxygen concentration first, a lower flow rate results in less variations in hypopharyngeal oxygen concentration.[24,25] Tables

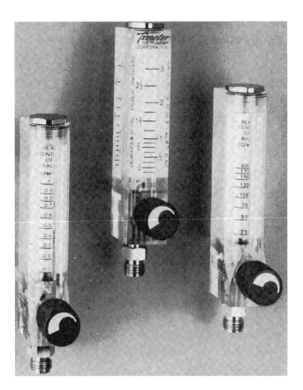

Fig. 12-3

Low-flow flowmeters. Flow rate capabilities range from 25 ml/min to 3 L/min. (Courtesy Timeter Instrument, St Louis.)

have been constructed to estimate hypopharyngeal oxygen concentrations at various settings, but reproducibility is affected by the range of infant sizes and variable breathing patterns.[23,25,26]

Because hypopharyngeal oxygen concentrations tend to be more stable when using lower flows, the use of a *low-flow flowmeter* helps to optimize continuous oxygen administration in the infant population (Fig. 12-3). Depending on the flowmeter, the flow rates range from 0.1 to 3.0 L/min, with some adjustable in increments of less than 0.125 L/min.[2] Using this method, connect the cannula to a low-flow flowmeter receiving 100% oxygen. Set an appropriate flow rate, as determined by Sp_{O_2}, and wean the oxygen by decreasing the flow rate in small increments of 0.1 to 0.2 L/min. Continue weaning in small increments until the minimum desired Sp_{O_2} is reached, or until oxygen is no longer required.

Inspired oxygen determination. Oxygen delivered by nasal cannula is measured in liters per minute (L/min) rather than F_{IO_2}. Tables and equations are available to translate a flow rate into an approximate F_{IO_2}. Two reasons exist for this need: to gauge the relative degree of respiratory compromise

BOX 12-1

REGRESSION EQUATION FOR ESTIMATING NASAL CANNULA F_{IO_2} AT LOW FLOW RATES*

Approximate F_{IO_2} = $(O_2 \text{ flow} \times 0.79)$
$+ [(0.21 \times V_E)/(V_E \times 100)]$

This equation is most predictive with an assumed tidal volume of 5.5 ml/kg for infants less than 1500 g.

F_{IO_2}, Fractional concentration of inspired oxygen; O_2 flow = ml/min; V_E, minute ventilation = (tidal volume × respiratory rate).

and to compare oxygen conditions in clinical studies. Tables and equations were distributed for this purpose in the multicenter STOP-ROP study on the safety of oxygen use and the progression of ROP.[25,27]

Because the concentration of oxygen inhaled into the lungs varies according to respiratory rate, tidal volume, inspiratory flow, and other factors such as mouth breathing, it is difficult to determine the F_{IO_2} with certainty.[25] An approximation of F_{IO_2} at low flows can be determined using the regression equation (Box 12-1).[24] This equation incorporates minute ventilation, but it does not account for changes in respiratory pattern and is more accurate for infants weighing less than 1500 g. Use such an equation only as a comparative estimate, and do not rely on it as an accurate determination of breath-to-breath F_{IO_2}.

Determine the measure of improvement during weaning from a nasal cannula by monitoring the amount of the incremental decreases in oxygen flow rate. During most routine clinical situations, approximating the F_{IO_2} from cannula flow is unnecessary. However the clinician should develop an awareness of the degree of oxygen requirement while assessing an infant.

Hazards and complications. Depending on the type of cannula, the flow rate, and the infant's anatomy, an increase in exhaled resistance can result in substantial inadvertent continuous positive airway pressure (CPAP) being delivered to an infant using a nasal cannula.[2,28] This occurs when using either the blender or the low-flow flowmeter to deliver supplemental oxygen. Substantial CPAP tends to occur more often when the cannula has large-diameter prong tips and when flow rates are set above 2 L/min.[22,28] This could be detrimental to an infant with obstructive pulmonary disease.[21] While the amount and certainty of CPAP may not be determined, keep in mind the possibility of such complications when improvement in response to nasal oxygen is less than expected.

Although the nasal cannula is relatively comfortable, lightweight, and easy to apply, the prongs are difficult to keep in the nares of active infants, often becoming displaced and resulting in loss of oxygen delivery.[29] Irritation to the nares can result from improperly sized cannulas or excessive oxygen flows. It is recommended that maximum flow be limited to 2 L/min in infants and newborns.[2]

Simple Oxygen Mask.   The simple oxygen mask is a lightweight plastic reservoir designed to fit over the patient's nose and mouth and is secured by an elastic strap around the patient's head (Fig. 12-4). Holes are located on both sides of the mask to allow exhalation, although the patient can draw in room air during inspiration. FIO_2 varies with the patient's inspiratory flow.[30] Flow rates from 6 to 10 L/min provide a variable FIO_2 of 0.35 to 0.5.[31]

Indications and contraindications.   Administration of oxygen with a simple mask is reserved for infants and children who need moderate concentrations of supplemental oxygen for short periods. Such situations include medical transport, emergency stabilization, postanesthesia recovery, and during medical procedures. The oxygen concentrations may be higher in patients with small tidal volumes, and therefore simple masks are not suitable for infants and small children who require low or precise concentrations of oxygen.[2-4]

Application.   The mask is secured around the patient's head by a strap, and oxygen is delivered to the mask from a flowmeter and bubble humidifier through small-bore tubing. The cone shape of the simple mask may act as a reservoir for accumulated

exhaled carbon dioxide if a minimal flow of gas is not maintained. In older children and adults, 6 L/min is the recommended minimum flow rate to flush accumulated carbon dioxide. However, modern masks are equipped with air-dilution ports that are more efficient at flushing carbon dioxide.

Hazards and complications.   Because these masks are strapped to the face, they often prove confining and are not well tolerated by infants and small children. In addition, the confinement of the mask interferes with eating and feeding, and aspiration of vomitus may be more likely. The elastic strap is often uncomfortable and can cause skin irritation with prolonged use.

Reservoir Masks.   A reservoir mask consists of a soft vinyl mask with a plastic bag attached to its front (Fig. 12-5). Oxygen source gas flows directly into the neck of the mask and is directed into the reservoir bag during exhalation. When the patient inhales, high concentrations of oxygen can be delivered from the bag through the mask. Currently, there are two types of reservoir masks: partial-rebreathing and nonrebreathing masks.

If functioning properly, reservoir masks have the advantage of providing high concentrations of oxygen. However, the tight fit necessary to achieve optimal performance makes the masks impractical for long-term therapy. As with the simple oxygen mask, elastic straps may be uncomfortable, confining, and not well tolerated by children. The use of reservoir masks is limited to short-term situations requiring high FIO_2 administration or specific gas mixture therapy.[2]

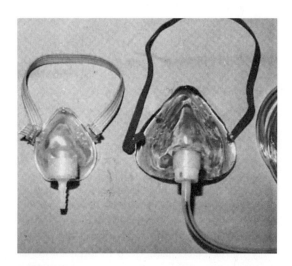

Fig. 12-4

Neonatal *(left)* and pediatric *(right)* simple oxygen masks.

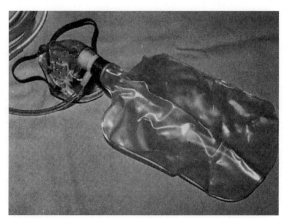

Fig. 12-5

Pediatric partial-rebreathing mask, a type of reservoir mask.

Partial-rebreathing mask. The partial-rebreathing mask is similar to a simple oxygen mask but contains a reservoir at the base of the mask. It is designed to conserve oxygen by receiving 100% oxygen along with a small portion of the patient's exhaled volume (approximately equal to the volume of the patient's "anatomic dead space"). The oxygen concentration of the exhaled gases combined with the supply of fresh oxygen permits the use of oxygen flows lower than those necessary for other devices, potentially conserving oxygen use. The remaining portion of the patient's exhaled volume is vented through open exhalation ports located on the sides of the mask.

The mask must fit the patient's face securely to minimize the amount of room air entrained during inspiration. Adjust the oxygen flow rate to a level sufficient to keep the bag partially inflated during inspiration, usually 6 to 15 L/min. If the reservoir bag becomes totally deflated when the patient inspires, increase the flow rate. When there is an adequate seal around the mask and an appropriate flow rate is maintained, an FIO_2 of up to 0.6 is delivered to the patient.[2,30] However, this FIO_2, as in other variable performance devices, is also influenced by the patient's ventilatory pattern.

Nonrebreathing mask. The nonrebreathing mask is similar in design to the partial-rebreathing mask but also has one-way valves that function to keep the patient from rebreathing any exhaled gas.[8] A one-way valve located between the face mask and the reservoir bag allows 100% source gas to enter the mask during inspiration, but unlike the partial-rebreathing mask, it prevents any of the patient's exhaled gas from entering the bag. Instead, the exhaled gas is directed through one-way leaflet valves located over the exhalation ports on the sides of the mask. The leaflet valves ensure minimal dilution from the entrainment of room air.

The nonrebreathing mask is designed to provide a higher FIO_2 than the simple and partial-rebreathing masks and the nasal devices.[19] If there is an adequate seal around the mask and the flow rate is sufficient to keep the bag partially inflated during inspiration, oxygen concentrations can conceivably reach greater than 90%. Because it is designed to provide almost 100% source gas, the nonrebreathing mask is the recommended device to deliver specific gas mixtures, as in helium-oxygen therapy, or specific concentrations from a blender.[3,4,31]

FIXED-PERFORMANCE OXYGEN DELIVERY SYSTEMS

Air-entrainment Mask. Air-entrainment masks, or *Venturi masks,* are examples of high-flow systems that provide the patient's entire inspiratory require-

ments while delivering predetermined, precise oxygen concentrations (Fig. 12-6). This is accomplished by providing a total flow of gas that exceeds the patient's ventilatory demands, thus eliminating dilution of the oxygen concentration with room air, as occurs in low-flow devices.

The performance of the mask is based on principles described by Bernoulli.[32] As 100% oxygen under pressure flows through a small jet orifice entering the mask, the velocity increases, creating viscous shearing forces. As a result, room air is entrained through open ports located at the base of a reservoir tube attached to the front of the mask. By varying the diameter of the jet orifice or the size of the entrainment ports, the amount of room air entrained can be proportionately changed, resulting in higher total flows and specific concentrations delivered to the patient's proximal airway.

Indications and contraindications. The air-entrainment mask is indicated for pediatric patients who require a controlled FIO_2 at either low or moderate levels. The common oxygen concentrations

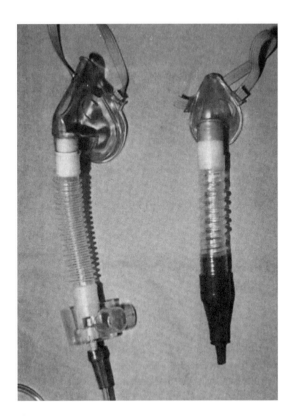

Fig. 12-6

Pediatric *(left)* and neonatal *(right)* air-entrainment masks. The pediatric size has the attachment used for aerosol delivery.

available range from 24% to 50%. In hypoxemic patients in whom increased breathing frequency and tidal volume may dilute F_{IO_2} concentrations from other variable-performance devices, the air-entrainment mask is the best choice because it maintains total flows in excess of the patient's inspiratory demand. For pediatric patients who tend to hypoventilate with increased oxygen concentrations, the air-entrainment mask is ideal because it maintains a constant F_{IO_2} even at low concentrations.

Application. An air-entrainment mask is designed to fit over the patient's nose and mouth and contains a short corrugated hose with a jet orifice that is connected to oxygen supply tubing. Because the high total flows produced by this system can be quite drying, humidification is provided using a bubble-diffusion humidifier. At the lower concentrations of 24% and 28%, oxygen flow through the small, restricted orifice creates excessive back pressure in the humidifier. For these levels of oxygen concentration, an alternative method is used in which a bland aerosol is applied through a 22-mm collar attached to the base of the corrugated hose at the air-entrainment ports. The device can be adapted to a tracheostomy collar and can be used without the application of aerosol, simply to prevent accidental occlusion of the air-entrainment ports, as might occur with bed linens.

Hazards and complications. Correct performance of the air-entrainment mask can be altered by resistance to the flow of gas that may occur distal to the restricted orifice. The resistance to flow at this particular point creates back pressure, resulting in less air entrainment. As a result, higher oxygen concentrations and lower total flows are delivered to the patient. If total flow decreases significantly, room air may be inhaled around and through the mask parts. This same phenomenon will also occur if the entrainment ports are partially or completely obstructed. Also, at the 50% setting, total gas flow from the device may not meet the patient's inspiratory flow requirements, resulting in the patient receiving a less than 50% oxygen concentration.

Air-entrainment Nebulizer. The gas-powered, large-volume or all-purpose nebulizer is another fixed-performance system that provides particulate water and contains an adjustable air-entrainment port that controls oxygen concentrations.[14,30] The addition of heat gives this type of system the advantage of providing 100% body humidity when clinically indicated. The nebulizer provides oxygen at fixed concentrations by adjusting the size of the air-entrainment port located at the top of the nebulizer lid. The small size of the nebulizer jet restricts

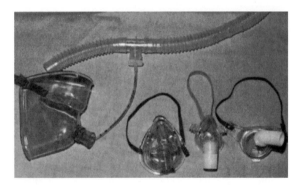

Fig. 12-7

Various aerosol attachments. *Left to right,* Face tent, T-piece attached to an endotracheal tube, pediatric aerosol mask, infant aerosol mask, and tracheostomy mask (collar).

maximum flow to 15 L/min from any 50-psi gas source.

Indications and contraindications. Air-entrainment nebulizers are used when high levels of humidity or aerosol are desired, as with a bypassed upper airway. Patient application devices used with the nebulizers include a tracheostomy collar, face tent, aerosol mask, or blow-by arrangement (Fig. 12-7).[2]

Application. Nebulizers may be used with many different devices. Each of these devices is attached to the nebulizer unit with 4 to 6 feet of large-bore corrugated tubing that allows high gas flows and maximal aerosol delivery to the patient. Both the aerosol mask and the face tent apparatus are primarily indicated for short-term administration of oxygen with high humidity, as in postextubation or postanesthesia hypoxemia. In the immediate postoperative recovery period, a blow-by method of oxygen administration set close to the patient's face may be more easily tolerated and thus more effective (Fig. 12-8).[33]

The tracheostomy mask and T-piece appliances are indicated for the delivery of high humidity and oxygen to pediatric patients with artificial airways. If a precise F_{IO_2} is required for the patient with a tracheostomy, the tracheostomy mask may be less desirable than the T-piece device, which can ensure delivery of a more exact F_{IO_2} because of its close fit on the endotracheal or tracheostomy adapter. This eliminates room-air entrainment, provided that the gas flow to the patient exceeds his or her inspiratory demand. The disadvantage of this system is that the weight of the T-piece and tubing assembly often creates torque on the endotracheal or tracheostomy tube, causing tracheal irritation and possible displacement.

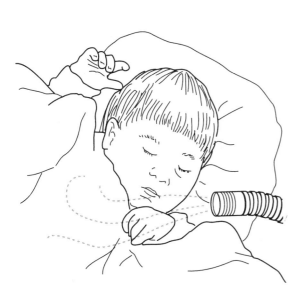

Fig. 12-8

Blow-by method of oxygen administration used in postanesthesia recovery rooms.

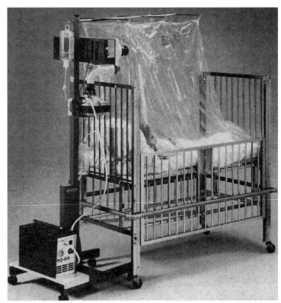

Fig. 12-9

Oxygen mist tent. (Courtesy Timeter Instrument, St. Louis.)

Hazards and complications. As with all masks used to deliver oxygen therapy to the pediatric patient, the aerosol mask and face tent frequently provoke unnecessary agitation and anxiety, especially in the treatment of postanesthesia hypoxemia. The weight of the tubing attached to a tracheostomy mask or T-piece device may cause irritation or displacement. The nebulizers are susceptible to contamination and are changed every 24 hours when applied to a patient with an artificial airway.[34] Condensate in the tubing may result in inadvertent lavage when attached to a tracheostomy or endotracheal tube.[2]

A cool mist is not recommended for newborns because of the potential to induce cold stress.[35] If the gas flow from the oxygen source is cool and is directed toward the infant's face, stimulation of the trigeminal nerves may cause alterations in the respiratory pattern and lead to apnea.[36] If heated, the gas-aerosol mixture at the patient is monitored and maintained at a temperature approximately equal to the desired environmental temperature.

ENCLOSURES

Oxygen Tent. In the past, oxygen tents were one of the primary methods of oxygen administration for both adults and children. At present, however, their use is very limited. Tents are designed to provide a cool, oxygen-enriched environment with high humidity. A high-output aerosol generator or large-volume nebulizer powered by oxygen or compressed air (with oxygen titrated into the system) produces a dense mist. The mist is cooled and circulated by a refrigerator unit and connected to a transparent canopy placed over the patient and secured under the mattress of the crib or bed (Fig. 12-9).[14]

Oxygen concentrations are quite variable and seldom reach greater than 50%, even with flow rates greater than 10 L/min and 100% oxygen source gas. This is primarily caused by leaks that occur when the tent is opened or inadequately sealed around the patient's bed. Because of variation in F_{IO_2}, the oxygen concentration should be monitored using an oxygen analyzer, placing the analyzer sensor near the patient's face.

Indications and contraindications. Tents are used most often to deliver supplemental oxygen and cool, high-humidity gas mixtures to pediatric patients with laryngotracheobronchitis,[37] those with artificial airways in whom direct attachment of a device to the airway is contraindicated, or to patients who are too large for hoods.[2] Only low- to moderate oxygen concentrations less than 40% can be achieved in a tent.

Hazards and complications. Electric shock or fire can result from sparks generated by nurse call devices, electric and battery-operated toys, vibrators, percussors, and static electricity. These devices should not be allowed under the tent canopy when in use. A dense fog or excessive condensation can develop inside the tent, which is frightening to the child and makes it difficult for the child to be observed. Loss of air in the circulation system may result in failure to cool the tent.[2] Check the tent frequently to ensure proper cooling and circulation and to empty the condensate collection bottle. Opening the tent decreases the oxygen concentration, and therefore nasal oxygen devices (e.g., nasal cannula) may be indicated during feeding and nursing care. Close monitoring of the patient is necessary because of the potential for asphyxiation if the patient becomes lodged between the mattress and the tent.[2]

Oxygen Hood. The most common method of administering short-term oxygen therapy to the neonate or infant is the oxygen hood (Fig. 12-10). The oxygen hood is a transparent enclosure constructed of clear plastic material in a cylinder or boxlike design. Oxygen is administered through large-bore corrugated tubing attached to the back of the hood. The hood surrounds the infant's head, leaving the body accessible for nursing care. This design also allows the infant to be placed in a neutral thermal environment, such as an incubator, and still receive controlled oxygen concentrations. Variations in hood design allow access to the infant's head by removing the top lid or by opening large ports on the sides or top of the hood.

Indications and contraindications. Hoods are indicated most often in neonates, infants, and small children who require supplemental oxygen with heated humidity. Hoods are used to provide a controlled FiO_2 and increased heated humidity to patients who are unable to tolerate other oxygen or humidification devices. An oxygen hood can also be used to perform an oxygen challenge (hyperoxia) test in a spontaneously breathing neonate.[2] Oxygen concentration in a hood can be varied from 21% to 100% and is more stable than that provided by a tent.[2]

Application. Oxygen is delivered to the hood through a heated air-entrainment nebulizer or with heated humidification using an oxygen blender or dual air and oxygen flowmeters. When using the heated air-entrainment nebulizer, power the nebulizer with compressed air, set the oxygen concentration dial at 100%, and bleed oxygen into the corrugated tubing through a T-piece adapter. In this way, oxygen concentrations are more easily regulated and noise levels are reduced.[38]

The oxygen blender system premixes oxygen concentrations and passes the blended gas through a heated humidifier before entering the hood. This allows more precise control over both oxygen concentrations and temperature and virtually eliminates noise inside the hood. With dual air and oxygen

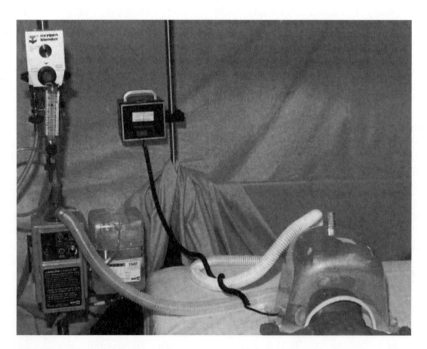

Fig. 12-10

Infant oxygen hood with gas delivered through an oxygen blender system with heated humidification. The oxygen analyzer sensor is placed inside the hood close to the infant's head.

flowmeters, both air and oxygen are titrated through the heated humidifier and tubing into the hood and analyzed until accurate prescribed oxygen concentrations are obtained. Regardless of which system is used, oxygen is analyzed on a continuous basis to ensure accurate concentrations.

When high oxygen concentrations are used, a layering effect occurs inside the hood, with the highest oxygen concentrations settling toward the bottom. For this reason, place the oxygen analyzer sensor as close to the infant's head as possible. It is also important that an adequate flow of gas be delivered to wash out any carbon dioxide that may accumulate inside the hood. Generally, flow rates greater than 7 L/min are adequate for most hoods.

It is important that adequate heat and humidity be maintained inside the hood. Administration of cool, dry gas induces cold stress in infants, resulting in increased oxygen consumption. Likewise, delivery of overheated gases induces apnea.[36] Temperature is maintained at or near body temperature with a thermometer placed inside the hood for continuous monitoring.

Oxygen hoods come in a variety of sizes to fit the very small neonate and very large infant. For patients too large for neonatal-size hoods, there are transparent enclosures in larger sizes called *tent houses* or *huts* (Fig. 12-11). For optimal temperature, flow, and oxygen control, choosing the proper-sized hood is imperative.

Hazards and complications. Opening the hood decreases the oxygen concentration and can result in hypoxia. If the hood is opened for an extended period, such as during feeding and nursing

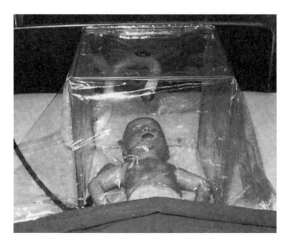

Fig. 12-11

Tent house for oxygen administration to larger infants. (Courtesy Nova Health Systems, Blackwood, NJ.)

procedures, it is appropriate to provide nasal oxygen with a cannula while the patient is eating or until the procedure is completed. Just as a loss of gas flow to the hood can result in hypoxia, hypercapnia, and even death, excessive oxygen concentrations can lead to irreversible complications. For these reasons, use an oxygen analyzer to monitor continuously the oxygen concentration in the hood and maintain high and low alarms on the analyzer at all times. Although the oxygen hood is usually well tolerated, irritation to the infant's skin, especially around the neck, may occur due to pressure from an improperly sized hood or to active movement of the patient. Cutaneous fungal infections have been associated with prolonged exposure to humidified oxygen in hoods.[39] High gas flow into the hood may produce noise levels that induce hearing impairment.[38]

Incubators. In 1893, Rotch presented a wooden box with hot water bottles known as a "brooder" that was to provide technology's answer to the uterus in the case of the premature infant.[40] Since that time, incubators have enjoyed both favorable and unfavorable status in the care of infants. The incubator is a clear Plexiglas enclosure that controls temperature and humidity and has the capability of delivering supplemental oxygen.

Indications and contraindications. In the past, incubators were used frequently as a primary mode of oxygen delivery in the premature infant.[1] At present, however, the primary purpose of an incubator is to provide a temperature-controlled environment to small infants with temperature instability.[2,14] Precise oxygen delivery is more effectively administered with the oxygen hood, which can be set up directly on the infant within the incubator.

Application. The temperature of the incubator is servo-controlled and maintained with a skin probe attached to the infant. Humidity is provided either by using a baffled blow-over water reservoir within the unit itself or by attaching an alternative humidification system.[14] Oxygen is provided by attaching small-bore tubing to a flowmeter and an inlet nipple connection to the incubator. Some units have two oxygen connections, one for low to moderate oxygen concentrations (approximately 40%) and one for high oxygen concentrations (near 100%). In some models, oxygen analyzers are incorporated with flow-controlling solenoids. When oxygen levels decrease to less than preset values, solenoids open and increase the oxygen flow rate until the analyzed value of oxygen equals the preset value on the controller.

Hazards and complications. The greatest disadvantage of the incubator is the inability to stabilize and maintain FIO_2 regardless of whether the unit has flow-controlling solenoids or conventional methods of oxygenation. This drawback results from the large open space within the incubator and the inherent leaks that occur.

MANUAL RESUSCITATION SYSTEMS

Neonatal and pediatric manual resuscitators are most often used to support ventilation in emergency situations. They are also used to hyperoxygenate patients intermittently before or during invasive procedures and during periods of apnea or bradycardia. Effective use of these devices depends not only on their physical structure and performance characteristics, but also on the knowledge and skill of the clinician. Two types of manual resuscitation systems are available for use in the neonatal and pediatric patient: the self-inflating system and the non–self-inflating system.

Self-inflating Resuscitation System.

The self-inflating systems for neonatal and pediatric use are similar in design and function to those used in adult resuscitation bags (Fig. 12-12). They consist of a self-inflating compressible bag that has a tidal volume range of 200 to 300 ml for neonates and 400 to 500 ml for pediatric patients.[41] One-way valves prevent the rebreathing of exhaled gas and allow source gas to be directed into the bag during inflation. Self-inflating systems are also equipped with pressure-relief valves that prevent the administration of excessive pressures. Most models have reservoirs that help to achieve high oxygen concentrations.

Although the self-inflating systems are the most frequently used devices for resuscitation efforts, several have failed to meet one or more of the American Society for Testing and Materials standards for safety.[42,43] First, pressure-relief valves within the systems are often activated over a wide range of pressures rather than the manufacturer's stated limits of 30 to 40 cm H_2O. In addition, activation of the pressure-relief valve causes a significant reduction in the delivered oxygen concentration from the units, even when a reservoir system is in place. Second, although the addition of a reservoir system increases the delivered oxygen concentrations, 100% oxygen is not readily achievable in any of these self-inflating manual resuscitators. Finally, some of the patient valve assemblies crack or break when dropped on hard surfaces, rendering them useless.

Non–self-inflating Resuscitation System.

The non–self-inflating, or *flow-inflating,* manual resuscitation bags consist of an anesthesia reservoir bag connected to a T-piece adapter and corrugated reservoir tube or a patient adapter with a pressure-relief valve (Fig. 12-13). The gas source is connected to an oxygen nipple adapter in front of the bag, and a pressure manometer is connected in-line between the patient adapter and gas source inlet.

A flow rate of gas at least two to three times the patient's minute ventilation (or ranging from 3 to 15 L/min) is sufficient to fill the bag and flush the reservoir tube, allowing exhaled gas to be continuously flushed out of the system.[41] During inspiration, fresh gas is delivered to the patient by compressing the bag. Excess gas exits simultaneously through the pressure-relief valve and prevents excessive ventilating pressures and volumes. The in-line pressure manometer is a critical component of the non–self-inflating bag and is used to monitor the peak inspiratory pressures and the positive end-expiratory

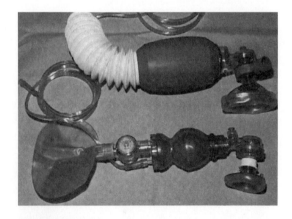

Fig. 12-12

Pediatric *(top)* and neonatal *(bottom)* self-inflating manual resuscitation bags.

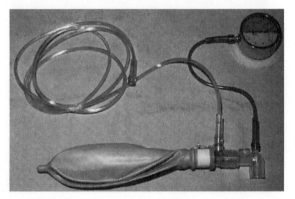

Fig. 12-13

Neonatal non-self-inflating manual resuscitation bag with in-line pressure manometer.

pressure (PEEP) maintained during ventilation. In intensive care settings, it is helpful to have manometers permanently mounted on the patient bed columns.

The non–self-inflating systems have the advantage of allowing more control over delivery pressures, inspiratory time, the addition of PEEP, and the assurance of delivering 100% oxygen or exact oxygen concentrations from an air-oxygen blender. Unfortunately, many clinicians are not adequately skilled in the operation of non–self-inflating bags. Technical problems, such as maintaining an adequate seal with the face mask or selection of the proper flow rate, often result in collapse of the anesthesia bag and reduced levels of ventilation.[44] For these reasons, the use of non–self-inflating resuscitation bags should be reserved for clinicians who are adequately trained and proficient in using such systems.

REFERENCES

1. The early history of oxygen use for premature infants: oxygen therapy and RLF. *Pediatrics* 1976; 57(suppl 2): 591-642.
2. American Association for Respiratory Care: Clinical practice guideline: selection of an oxygen delivery device for neonatal and pediatric patients. *Respir Care* 1996; 41(7): 637-646.
3. American Association for Respiratory Care: Clinical practice guideline: Oxygen therapy in the acute care hospital. *Respir Care* 1991; 36(12):1410-1413.
4. Fulmer JD, Snider GL, American College of Chest Physicians–National Heart, Lung, and Blood Institute: National Conference on Oxygen Therapy. *Chest* 1984; 86:234-247. Concurrent publication in *Respir Care* 1984; 29(9):922-935.
5. Guthrie RD, Hodson WA: Clinical diagnosis of pulmonary insufficiency: history and physical. In Thibault DW, Gregory GA, editors: *Neonatal pulmonary care*. Norwalk, Conn. Appleton-Century-Crofts, 1986.
6. Fisher AB: Oxygen therapy: side effects and toxicity. *Am Rev Respir Dis* 1980; 122(5, part 2):61-69.
7. George DS et al: The latest on retinopathy of prematurity. *Maternal Child Nurs* 1988; 13:254-258.
8. American Academy of Pediatrics, American College of Obstetricians and Gynecologists: *Guidelines for perinatal care*, ed 2. Chicago,1988; pp 246-247.
9. El-Lessy HN: Pulmonary vascular control in hypoplastic left-heart syndrome: hypoxic- and hypercarbic-gas therapy. *Respir Care* 1995; 40(7):737-742.
10. Fairshter RD et al: Paraquat poisoning: new aspects of therapy. *Q J Med* 1976; 45(180):551-565.
11. Ingrassia TS et al: Oxygen-exacerbated bleomycin pulmonary toxicity. *Mayo Clin Proc* 1991; 66:173-178.
12. Coffman JA, McManus KP: Oxygen therapy via nasal catheter for infants with bronchopulmonary dysplasia. *Crit Care Nurs* 1984; 4:22-23.
13. Shann F, Gatchalian S, Hutchinson R: Nasopharyngeal oxygen in children. *Lancet* 1988; 2(8622):1238-1240.
14. Thalken FR: Medical gas therapy. In Scanlan CL, Spearman CB, Sheldon RL, editors: *Egan's fundamentals of respiratory care*. St Louis. Mosby, 1990; pp 606-632.
15. Fremstad JD, Martin SH: Lethal complication from insertion of nasogastric tube after severe basilar skull fracture. *J Trauma* 1978; 18(12):820-822.
16. Guilfoile T, Dabe K: Nasal catheter oxygen therapy for infants. *Respir Care* 1981; 26(1):35-40.
17. Frenckner B et al: Pneumocephalus caused by a nasopharyngeal oxygen catheter. *Crit Care Med* 1990; 18(11): 1287-1288.
18. Givan DC, Wylie P: Home oxygen therapy for infants and children. *Indiana Med* 1986; 45:849-853.
19. Leigh JM: Variation in performance of oxygen therapy devices. *Anaesthesia* 1970; 25(2):210-222.
20. Ooi R, Joshi P, Soni N: An evaluation of oxygen delivery using nasal prongs. *Anaesthesia* 1992; 47(7):591-593.
21. Kuluz JW et al: The fraction of inspired oxygen in infants receiving oxygen via nasal cannula often exceeds safe levels. *Respir Care* 2001; 46(9):897-901.
22. Fan LL, Voyles JB: Determination of inspired oxygen delivered by nasal cannula in infants with chronic lung disease. *J Pediatr* 1983; 103(6):923-925.
23. Vain NE et al: Regulation of oxygen concentration delivered to infants via nasal cannulas. *Am J Dis Child* 1989; 143(12):1458-1460.
24. Finer NN, Bates R, Tomat P: Low flow oxygen delivery via nasal cannula to neonates. *Pediatr Pulmonol* 1996; 21(1):48-51.
25. Benaron DA, Benitz WE: Maximizing the stability of oxygen delivered via nasal cannula. *Arch Pediatr Adolesc Med* 1994; 148:294-300.
26. Stevens DP et al: Hypopharyngeal O_2 concentration in infants breathing O_2 by nasal cannula. *Respir Care* 1986; 31:988 (abstract).
27. STOP-ROP Multicenter Study Group: Supplemental therapeutic oxygen for prethreshold retinopathy of prematurity: a randomized, controlled trial. I. Primary outcomes. *Pediatrics* 2000; 105:295-310.
28. Locke RG et al: Inadvertent administration of positive end-distending pressure during nasal cannula flow. *Pediatrics* 1993; 91(1):135-138.
29. Thilo EH, Comito J, McCulliss D: Home oxygen therapy in the newborn: costs and parental acceptance. *Am J Dis Child* 1987; 141:766-768.
30. McPherson SP: Gas regulation, administration, and controlling devices. In *Respiratory care equipment*, ed 5. St Louis. Mosby, 1995; pp 66-73.
31. Redding JS, McAfee DD, Parham AM: Oxygen concentrations received from commonly used delivery systems. *South Med J* 1978; 71(2):169-172.
32. Scacci R: Air entrainment masks: jet mixing is how they work; the Bernoulli and Venturi principles are how they don't. *Respir Care* 1979; 24:928-931.
33. Amar D et al: An alternative oxygen delivery system for infants and children in the post-anesthesia care unit. *Can J Anaesth* 1991; 38:49-53.
34. Centers for Disease Control and Prevention: Guideline for the prevention of nosocomial pneumonia. *Respir Care* 1994; 39(12):1191-1236.
35. Scopes JW, Ahmed I: Ranges of critical temperatures in sick and premature newborn babies. *Arch Dis Child* 1966; 41:417-419.
36. Daily WJR, Klaus M, Meyer HBP: Apnea in premature infants: monitoring, incidence, heart rate changes, and an effect of environmental temperature. *Pediatrics* 1969; 43(4):510-518.
37. Skolnik NS: Treatment of croup. *Am J Dis Child* 1989; 143:1045-1049.
38. Beckham RW, Mishoe SC: Sound levels inside incubators and oxygen hoods used with nebulizers and humidifiers. *Respir Care* 1982; 27:33-40.
39. Lanska MJ, Silverman R, Lanska DJ: Cutaneous fungal infections associated with prolonged treatment in humidified oxygen hoods. *Pediatr Dermatol* 1987; 4(4):346 (letter).

40. Baker JP: The incubator controversy: pediatricians and the origins of premature infant technology in the United States, 1890 to 1910. *Pediatrics* 1991; 87:654-662.

41. Thompson JE, Farrell E, McManus M: Neonatal and pediatric airway emergencies. *Respir Care* 1992; 37: 582-597.

42. Barnes TA, McGarry WP: Evaluation of ten disposable manual resuscitators. *Respir Care* 1990; 35:960-968.

43. Finer NN et al: Limitations of self-inflating resuscitators. *Pediatrics* 1986; 77:417-420.

44. Kanter RK: Evaluation of mask-bag ventilation in resuscitation of infants. *Am J Dis Child* 1987; 141:761-763.

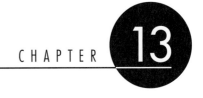

CHAPTER 13

Aerosols and Medication Administration

James B. Fink
Bruce K. Rubin

Decades of research have established the scientific principles underlying the use of therapeutic aerosols. In general, the advantages of aerosol therapy include a smaller but targeted dose, less cost, fewer side effects, efficacy comparable to or better than that observed with systemic administration of the drug, and usually a more rapid onset of action.[1] When inhaled drugs are delivered directly to the conducting airways, their systemic absorption is limited and systemic side effects are minimized, providing a high therapeutic index.[2] On the other hand, peptides and other macromolecules can be targeted to the terminal airways and alveoli for systemic administration across the pulmonary vascular bed. This is an exciting and evolving use for therapeutic aerosols.

The uses for aerosol devices vary widely, ranging from bronchodilators to insulin. New uses for aerosol devices continue to increase. Nebulizers, pressurized metered-dose inhalers (pMDIs), and dry powder inhalers (DPIs) are often used as aerosol generators because they produce respirable particles with a *mass median aerodynamic diameter* (MMAD) of 0.5 to 5.0 μm.[3] Although pMDIs and DPIs are chiefly used now to deliver bronchodilators and steroids, nebulizers can be used to administer antibiotics, mucoactive agents, and other drugs.[4] Given the appropriate formulation, even complex molecules can potentially be delivered by pMDI or DPI. The operating characteristics and limitations of aerosol-generating devices are major determinants of aerosol therapy efficacy. This chapter reviews the key principles of how aerosols are generated, deposited, and administered in the neonatal and pediatric patient.

AEROSOL CHARACTERISTICS

DEPOSITION OF PARTICLES

An *aerosol* is a group of particles that remain suspended in air for a relatively long time because of low terminal settling velocity. The *terminal settling velocity* of a particle is the velocity that the particle will fall in air due to gravity, which is related to the size and density of the particle. For a spherical particle, MMAD = $\delta\sqrt{\rho}$, where δ is the particle diameter and ρ the particle density.[5] Aerosols are also described by their *geometric standard deviation* (GSD), a measure of the particle size distribution. A *monodisperse* aerosol has a GSD less than 1.22, and a *heterodisperse* aerosol has a GSD greater than 1.22. Monodisperse aerosols are used for diagnostic and research purposes. Most therapeutic aerosols are heterodisperse, which means they contain a wider range of particle sizes. The greater the MMAD, the larger the median particle size, the greater the GSD, and the more heterodisperse is the aerosol. The particle size and size distribution of an aerosol are the major factors in determining deposition efficiency and distribution in the lung.

Gravitational sedimentation occurs when the aerosol particles lose inertia and settle because of suspension due to gravity. The greater the mass of the particle, the faster it settles, affecting particles down to 0.5 μm in diameter or less. Breath holding for 4 to 10 seconds after inhaling an aerosol increases the residence time for the particles in the lung, extending the time to allow deposition through gravitational sedimentation, especially in the last six generations of the airway.[6] This breath hold can increase deposition of the aerosol by up to 10%. For example, if normal deposition is 10%, the breath hold can increase total deposition to 11%. This marginal increase in deposition may explain why breath hold has not been demonstrated to significantly improve the clinical response to aerosolized medications. Breath holding after inhalation does not appear to influence the response to administration of a bronchodilator given by a DPI to children with asthma.[7]

Inertial impaction is the primary mechanism for deposition of particles 5 μm or greater and an important mechanism for particles as small as 2 μm. When a particle is traveling in a stream of gas that is diverted by a turn in the airway, the particle tends to continue traveling on its initial path and not travel with the flow of gas. Thus the particle impacts with the surface and deposits on the airway. This tendency increases with the velocity and mass of the particle. The higher the inspiratory flow of gas, such as during crying, the greater is the velocity and inertia of the particles, which increases the tendency for even smaller particles to impact and deposit in large airways. Common factors that increase the rate of inertial impaction of particles larger than 2 μm are turbulent flow, complex passageways, bifurcations, and inspiratory flows greater than 30 L/min.

Diffusion, also known as *brownian movement,* is the primary mechanism for deposition of particles less than 3 μm in diameter in the airway. As gas reaches the more distal regions of the lung, gas flow ceases. Aerosol particles bounce against air molecules and each other and deposit on contact with the airway surfaces. Particle deposition in the particle size range of 0.5 to 3.0 μm is reported to be divided between central and peripheral airways.[8]

Aerosol droplets in the respirable range (0.5 to 5.0 μm MMAD) have a better chance to deposit in the lower respiratory tract than larger or smaller particles.[7] For particles greater than 0.5 μm, the depth of penetration into the lung is inversely proportional to the particle's size, whereas particles less than 0.5 μm are so small, light, and stable that a significant proportion entering the lung do not deposit and are exhaled. Very large particles may go into suspension as an aerosol or may "rain out" before reaching the airway.

TRANSLOCATION OF AEROSOLS

To be effective as a therapeutic agent, an aerosol medication first must efficiently deposit in the airway and then must translocate across the mucous barrier, retaining bioactivity in this process. The optimal site of action depends on the agent administered. Bronchodilators and steroids need to reach the epithelium to be effective. Aerosolized antibiotics and mucolytics are most effective when dispersed in infected airway secretions at sites of maximal airway obstruction. Gene transfer therapy must not only access the epithelium through the mucous barrier but must then gain access to the submucous glands or basal progenitor cells of the epithelium.

Particle size, charge, solubility, and the biophysical properties of secretions all affect the ability of an aerosol to penetrate the mucous barrier. A consistent inverse relationship exists between molecular weight and particle diffusion through mucus, especially at molecular weights greater than 30 kD.[9] Turbulent flow and airway obstruction can affect the airway deposition pattern. Other factors limiting efficacy, especially of macromolecules, include binding to constituents of mucus, including mucin and deoxyribonucleic acid (DNA), and the breakdown of bioactive molecules by proteases and other enzymes. Translocation of macromolecules can be further compromised by the hypersecretion that accompanies inflammation and chronic pulmonary disease. These secretions can be a barrier to the penetration of any aerosol.[10,11]

The antibiotic diffusion barrier represented by mucin may be significant in vitro, particularly for nebulized antibiotics.[12] Some antibiotics bind to whole cystic fibrosis sputum, with the degree of binding dependent on the DNA concentration and the presence of acidic mucins.[13] Mucolytic agents might be able increase diffusion and increase antibiotic levels in sputum.[14] Similarly, treatment of the sputum-covered cells with recombinant human deoxyribonuclease (rhDNase) at 50 µg/ml significantly improved gene transfer.[15]

Factors promoting translocation include an effective surfactant layer and increased particle retention time. Mucus discontinuity in the airway may assist deposition and translocation. The translocation of particles through the mucus layer is likely to depend partly on the presence of bronchial surfactant. In vitro experiments have shown that pulmonary surfactant promotes the displacement of some particles from air to the aqueous phase and that the extent of particle immersion depends on the surface tension of the surface active film.[16,17]

DRUG DOSE DISTRIBUTION

In infants and small children the degree of aerosol penetration and the amount of particle deposition are reduced (Box 13-1). This reduction is an important consideration when determining dosing strategies for aerosolized medication delivery to small children. A correlation between tidal volume and aerosol effectiveness is not well established. Theoretically, larger breaths capture more aerosol with each individual breath. This relationship has not been shown clinically, however, possibly because partitioning of the tidal volume is regulated by both the delivered volume and the airway dimensions.

Dosing of aerosolized medication is an imprecise science. It is unclear how much, if any, drug is delivered to targeted areas of the lung with progressive disease states or during acute exacerbations. All the factors previously discussed decrease the rate and depth of aerosol deposition to the respiratory tract to as little as 1% of the medication

dose placed in a nebulizer, regardless of whether the patient is breathing spontaneously or intubated. High flow increases aerosol impaction in larger airways, whereas lower inspiratory flow can affect the integrity of high-resistance DPIs, reducing the amount of medication available for inhalation.

Humidity also influences medication delivery, especially for DPIs and in ventilator circuits. Droplets of solution may evaporate or grow, depending on the water content and temperature of the gas, and powder can clump or aggregate in high humidity. High ambient humidity can also result from a child *exhaling* into a DPI or from a DPI being brought into a warm indoor environment from the cold outdoors (or from inside a car on a very cold day), with condensation forming inside the device.[18]

Drug formulations dictate in part which aerosol options are available for medication delivery. Most solutions can be nebulized if the medication is *soluble* (corticosteroids are a notable exception), but the physical characteristics of the solution (or suspension) can affect particle size and nebulizer output. Furthermore, some macromolecules may not enter suspension well and can shatter into nonbioactive forms with the force of air required to generate an aerosol. Because of development costs, many aerosol medications are initially developed as nebulizer solutions and later reformulated for DPI or pMDI delivery.

Theoretically, if a particle can be milled to a respirable size while retaining bioactivity, it can be delivered by DPI or pMDI. However, development costs are greater for these devices than for nebulizer solutions. At present, DPI formulations are limited to only a few preparations. With more effective DPI devices being developed and the need to eliminate chlorofluorocarbon (CFC)–based propellants in accordance with the Montreal protocol, it is anticipated that a greater variety of DPI medications and devices will soon be commercially available. A greater variety of formulations are available for pMDIs, and more are being developed for the new hydrofluoroalkene (HFA)–based pMDIs.

AEROSOL DELIVERY

The most common methods of generating therapeutic aerosols are with a jet pneumatic nebulizer, ultrasonic nebulizer (USN), pMDI, and DPI. Older methods such as the spray "atomizer" or adding medications to room humidifiers are ineffective, and their use should be discouraged.

PNEUMATIC NEBULIZERS

Pneumatic nebulizers use the Bernoulli principle to drive a high-pressure gas through a restricted

---

BOX 13-1

FACTORS THAT REDUCE RATE AND DEPTH OF AEROSOL PARTICLE DEPOSITION IN NEONATAL AND PEDIATRIC PATIENTS

Large tongue in proportion to oral airway
Nose breathing
Narrow airway diameter
Fewer and larger alveoli
Fewer generations of airway
More rapid respiratory rate
Small tidal volume
Inability to hold breath and coordinate inspiration
High inspiratory flow rate during respiratory distress and crying

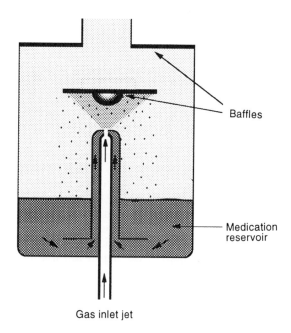

Baffles

Medication reservoir

Gas inlet jet

Fig. 13-1

Operating principle of a small-volume nebulizer. Baffles break the spray into aerosol particles, which are entrained in the gas flow and travel to the patient or fall back into the solution. (From Fink J, Cohen N: Humidity and aerosols. In Eubanks DH, Bone RC, editors: *Principles and applications of cardiorespiratory care equipment.* St. Louis. Mosby, 1994.)

orifice and draw the fluid into the gas stream from a capillary tube immersed in the solution. Shearing of the fluid stream in the jet forms the aerosol (Fig. 13-1). Impaction against a baffle removes larger particles and allows them to return to the reservoir.

An effective pneumatic nebulizer should deliver more than 50% of its total dose as aerosol in the respirable range in 10 minutes or less of nebulization time. Performance varies with diluent volume, operating flow, pressures, gas density, and manufacturer.[19] The amount of drug that is nebulized increases as the volume of diluent is increased. The residual volume of medicine that remains in commercial small-volume nebulizers (SVNs) varies from 0.5 to 2.0 ml depending on the specific device; thus increasing the fill volume allows a greater proportion of the active medication to be nebulized. For example, with a residual volume of 1 ml, a fill of 2 ml would only leave 50% of the nebulizer charge available for nebulization, whereas a fill of 4 ml would make 3 ml, or 75%, of the medication available for nebulization. No significant difference in clinical response has been shown with varying diluent volumes and flow rates.[20]

Droplet size and nebulization times are both inversely proportional to gas flow through the jet. The higher the flow to the nebulizer, the smaller the particle size generated and the shorter is the time required to nebulize the full dose.[21,22] Nebulizers that produce smaller particle sizes by use of baffles such as one way valves may have a lower total drug output per minute than the same nebulizer without baffling, requiring more time to deliver a standard dose of medication.

Gas density affects both aerosol generation and delivery of aerosol to the lungs, especially with low-density helium-oxygen mixtures. The lower the density of a carrier gas, the less turbulent the flow, which theoretically decreases aerosol impaction.[23] When using heliox to drive a jet nebulizer, the aerosol output is much less than with air or oxygen, requiring double the flow to produce a comparable output of respirable aerosol per minute. Thus, although helium increases the amount of aerosol reaching the lungs, it impairs the production of the aerosol suspension from the nebulizer.[24]

Humidity and temperature affect the particle size and the concentration of drug remaining in the nebulizer. Evaporation of water and adiabatic expansion of gas can reduce the temperature of the aerosol to as much as 5° C below ambient temperature. Aerosol particles entrained into a warm and fully saturated gas stream increase in size. These particles can also stick together, further increasing the MMAD, and with a DPI, this can severely compromise the output of respirable particles.

With three different fill volumes, albuterol delivery from the nebulizer was found to cease after the onset of inconsistent nebulization (sputtering).[25] Aerosol output declined by one half within 20 seconds of the onset of sputtering. The concentration of albuterol in the nebulizer cup increased significantly once the aerosol output declined, and further weight loss in the nebulizer was primarily caused by evaporation. The conclusion was that aerosolization past the point of initial jet nebulizer sputter is ineffective.

Nebulizer selection affects aerosol delivery. Only nebulizers that have been shown to work reliably under specific conditions, with specific medications, and with specific compressors should be used.[26] When used to treat small children or during mechanical ventilation, nebulizers producing aerosols with MMAD of 0.5 to −3.0 μm are more likely to achieve greater deposition in the lower respiratory tract.[5]

Continuous nebulization wastes medication because the aerosol is produced throughout the respiratory cycle and is largely lost to the atmosphere (Fig. 13-2, *A*). Patients with an inspiratory/expiratory

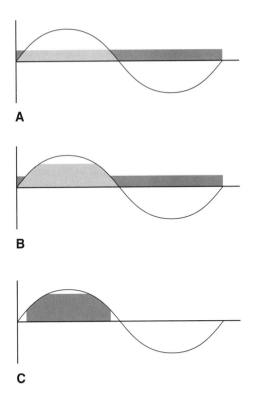

A

B

C

Fig. 13-2

Aerosol generated and inhaled during nebulization therapy. **A,** Continuous nebulization. **B,** Breath-enhanced nebulization. **C,** Breath-actuated nebulization.

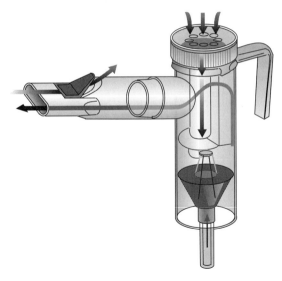

Fig. 13-3

Vented breath-enhanced nebulizer. (Modified from photo courtesy Pari, Midlothian, Va.)

(I:E) ratio of 1:3 lose a minimum of 75% of the aerosol generated to the atmosphere. If only 50% of the dose is available from the nebulizer as aerosol in the respiratory range and only 25% of that is inhaled by the patient, it is clear that less than 10% deposition is typically measured with nebulizer therapy.

A reservoir on the expiratory limb of the nebulizer conserves drug aerosol.[26] A simple approach is to place 6 inches of aerosol tubing on the expiratory side of the nebulizer T-tube device. Alternatively, select a commercial device such as the Piper or Circulaire system. These simple bag reservoirs hold the aerosol generated during exhalation, allowing the small particles to remain in suspension for inhalation with the next breath while larger particles rain out.

As another alternative to continuous nebulization, the thumb control port allows the patient to direct gas to the nebulizer only on inspiration. This improves efficiency only if there is good hand-breath coordination. Rather than having the patient control when nebulization occurs, a one-way valve system can be used to reduce aerosol waste.[27] In

this type of device, such as the Pari LC Jet Plus (Fig. 13-3), an inspiratory vent allows the patient to inhale air with the aerosolized drug and on exhalation, the inlet vent closes, and aerosol exits via a one-way valve near the mouthpiece, reducing aerosol waste. This breath-enhanced nebulizer increases inhaled dose by as much as 50% and decreases the amount of aerosol lost to the atmosphere (Fig. 13-2, *B*).

Breath-actuated nebulization occurs by actuating the device in coordination with inspiration. Nebulizing only during inspiration is more efficient than continuous or vented systems (Fig. 13-2, *C*). Breath-actuated nebulizers deliver the same or greater dose in the same amount of time as the continuous nebulizer. To nebulize the entire dose placed in the nebulizer, however, the demand system may take four times longer (delivering four times more drug) than the continuous nebulizer. One such nebulizer, the HaloLite (Profile Therapeutics,), uses a microprocessor and pressure transducer to regulate nebulization during the first half of inspiration. The AeroEclipse (Monaghan Medical Corporation) is a purely pneumatic device that nebulizes only during inspiration (Fig. 13-4).

A typical dose of albuterol sulfate solution is 2.5 mg (2500 μg). If only 34% (850 μg) leaves the nebulizer and is inhaled by the patient, and some of that drug deposits in the upper airways (50 μg) and is exhaled (500 μg), it should not be surprising that 12%

deposition of the nominal dose, typical of ambulatory adult patients, would be 300 µg (Fig. 13-5). In small children and infants, deposition can be less than 1%, representing less than 25 µg delivered to the lung.

Gas pressure and flow affect particle size distribution and output. A nebulizer that produces a MMAD of 2.5 µm when driven by a gas source of

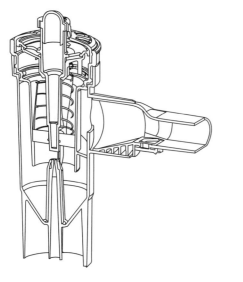

Fig. 13-4

Pneumatic breath-actuated nebulizer. (Courtesy Monaghan Medical, Plattsburgh, NY.)

50 psi at 6 to 10 L/min may produce a MMAD greater than 8 µm when operated on a home compressor (or ventilator) developing 10 psi. Insufficient flow can result in negligible respirable nebulizer output. Consequently, nebulizers used for home care should be matched to the compressor based on data supplied by the manufacturer so that the specific combination of equipment will efficiently nebulize the desired medications prescribed. European standards require equipment manufacturers to demonstrate that their nebulizer and compressor combination can nebulize the appropriate fill volume of drug within 10 minutes, deliver more than 50% of the drug in the nebulizer as respirable particles, and identify all medications with which the nebulizer and compressor might reliably meet these two criteria.[28] Until such time that standards are required in the United States, clinicians should ascertain that patients are only prescribed systems that have been demonstrated to meet these criteria.

Repeated use of a nebulizer will not alter MMAD, or output, as long as it is properly cleaned. Failure to clean the nebulizer properly results in degradation of performance from clogging the jet (Venturi) and buildup of electrostatic charge in the device.[29] The Centers for Disease Control and Prevention (CDC) recommends cleaning and disinfecting nebulizers or rinsing with sterile water between uses, then air drying.[30] Storing of multidose solutions at room temperature and reusing syringes to measure the solution

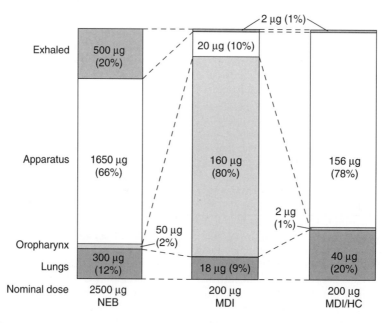

Fig. 13-5

Distribution of albuterol delivered via nebulizer, pressurized metered-dose inhaler (pMDI), and pMDI with holding chamber.

are the main sources of nebulizer microbial contamination.[31] The contamination appears to have been caused by storing multiple-dose solutions at room temperature instead of in a refrigerator and by reusing syringes to measure the solution. Refrigerating the solution and disposing of syringes every 24 hours help to eliminate bacterial contamination.

NEONATAL AND PEDIATRIC MEDICATION DELIVERY

Compared with adults, infants and children have a smaller airway diameter, their breathing rate is faster and irregular, nose breathing filters out large particles and deposits more medication in the upper airway, and mouthpiece administration often cannot be used. Cooperation and ability to perform the procedure effectively vary with the child's age and developmental ability.

For children who can tolerate a mask, the medication nebulizer can be fitted to an appropriate aerosol mask. There is no difference in clinical response between mouthpiece and close-fitting mask treatment, so compliance and preference should guide selection of the device[32] If the child cannot tolerate mask treatment, is not wearing the mask closely to the face, or becomes upset to the point of compromising oxygenation, a common strategy is use of a "blow-by" technique. With this method the practitioner directs the aerosol from the nebulizer toward the child's nose and mouth. No published data support the use of the blow-by technique, and aerosol deposition studies suggest that virtually no drug enters the airway with this technique.[33] Because blow-by wastes considerable resources with no evidence of effectiveness, it is more efficient to deliver medication by close-fitting mask when the patient is sound asleep.

Normal tidal breathing is the most effective method to administer aerosols to an infant. Mouth breathing enhances medication delivery to the airways in adults, but there are few data in infants who are preferential nose breathers. Crying is a long exhalation preceded by a very short and rapid inhalation that completely prevents lower airway deposition of an aerosol medication.[34] Thus, avoid administering aerosols to a crying child.

LARGE-VOLUME NEBULIZER

The large-volume pneumatic nebulizer (LVN) has a reservoir volume greater than 100 ml and can be used to administer an aerosol solution over a prolonged time. Indications for using LVN with a bland solution include humidifying medical gases when the upper airway is bypassed, controlling stridor with a cold aerosol, and inducing sputum. Because nebulizers provide a route of transmission

for pathogens, pass-over humidifiers and heater wire humidifiers are preferable.

LVNs work on the same principles as SVNs, except that the residual volume is greater and the effects of evaporation over time are more profound. When using the LVN to administer a solution containing medications such as bronchodilators, the medication becomes increasingly concentrated over time because of preferential evaporation of the diluent.

LVNs tend to be rather noisy. Caution should be exercised when using LVNs with incubators or hoods. The American Academy of Pediatrics recommends a sound level less than 58 dB to avoid hearing loss in patients in incubators and hoods. Many LVNs are designed to deliver controlled concentrations of oxygen and use a Venturi system to entrain air into the stream of gas administered to the patient. Standard entrainment nebulizers may deliver a fractional concentration of delivered oxygen (F_{DO_2}) approaching 1.00 but cannot provide a fractional concentration of inspired oxygen (F_{IO_2}) greater than 0.40. High-flow nebulizers are designed to deliver high flow rates of oxygen, bringing the F_{IO_2} up to 0.60 to 0.80. Closed dilution and gas injection nebulizers provide high-flow access to the nebulizer from two gas sources, allowing gas to mix without compromising F_{IO_2}.

SMALL-PARTICLE AEROSOL GENERATOR

The small-particle aerosol generator (SPAG) (ICN Pharmaceuticals) is a jet-type aerosol generator used to administer the antiviral agent ribavirin (Fig. 13-6). The SPAG incorporates a secondary drying chamber that reduces the MMAD to 1.2 μm, with a GSD of 1.4 and relatively high output. The SPAG reduces the 50 psi of line pressure medical gas to 26 psi, which is connected to two flowmeters controlling flow to the nebulizer and the drying chamber. As the aerosol leaves the medication reservoir, it enters the long cylindrical drying chamber, where additional flow of dry gas reduces the size of the aerosol particles through evaporation. The nebulizer flow is adjusted to maximum, approximately 7 L/min, with a total flow from both flowmeters equal to at least 15 L/min.

Ribavirin is an expensive antiviral agent that has been used to treat high-risk infants and children with severe respiratory syncytial virus (RSV) infections.[35] Ribavirin's effectiveness is poor, with few data to support its use for such a broad population. Additionally, concerns about the second-hand exposure of health care workers to ribavirin have resulted in recommendations to avoid open-air administration, use specific room filtration techniques, and use personal protective equipment (PPE) for staff and visitors.[36,37] Risks of using ribavirin during mechanical

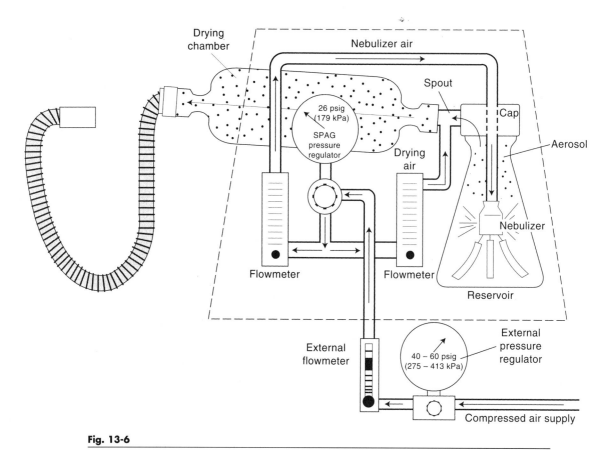

Fig. 13-6

Diagram of small-particle aerosol generator (SPAG), which may be used with a hood, tent, mask, or ventilator. (Courtesy ICN Pharmaceuticals, Costa Mesa, Calif.)

ventilation include delivering excessive volume and pressure.[38]

ULTRASONIC NEBULIZERS

The USN uses a piezoelectric crystal vibrating at a high frequency to create an aerosol. The crystal transducer converts electricity to sound waves, which creates motion or waves in the liquid immediately above the transducer. This motion disrupts the liquid surface and forms a geyser of droplets (Fig. 13-7). A large-volume USN generally does not lend itself to rigorous sterilization procedures, so these devices are usually designed to use disposable medication cups with a flexible diaphragm on the bottom.

USNs are capable of a broader range of aerosol output (0.5 to 7.0 ml/min) and higher aerosol densities than most conventional jet nebulizers. Particle size is affected by frequency, whereas output is affected by the amplitude of the signal. Particle size is inversely proportional to the frequency of vibrations. Frequency is usually device specific and is not user adjustable. For example, the DeVilbiss Portasonic operates at a frequency of 2.25 MHz and

produces a MMAD of 2.5 µm, and the DeVilbiss Pulmosonic operates at 1.25 MHz and produces particles in the 4- to 6-µm range. Large-volume USNs, used mainly for bland aerosol therapy or sputum induction, incorporate air blowers to carry the mist to the patient. Low flow rates of gas through the nebulizer are associated with higher mist density. Unlike jet nebulizers, the temperature of the solution placed in an USN increases during use. As the temperature increases, the drug concentration can also rise, increasing the likelihood of undesired side effects. In addition, some medications may be denatured by the increased operating temperature.[39]

A number of small-volume USNs are available for aerosol drug delivery.[40] Unlike the large USN, these systems do not always use a couplant compartment; instead, medication is placed directly into the manifold on top of the transducer connected to a battery-power source. The patient's inspiratory flow draws the aerosol from the nebulizer into the lung. As the USN operates, the aerosol remains in the medication cup/chamber until a flow of gas draws the aerosol from the nebulizer. Thus during exhalation, aerosol

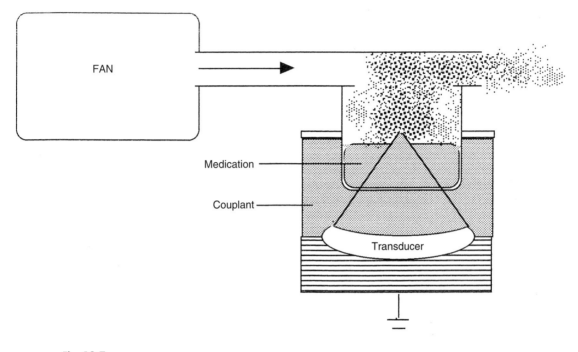

Fig. 13-7

Aerosol is produced in an ultrasonic nebulizer by focusing sound waves, which disrupt the surface of the fluid, creating a standing wave that produces droplets. Flow from a fan pushes the aerosol out of the chamber. (From Fink J, Cohen N: Humidity and aerosols. In Eubanks DH, Bone RC, editors: *Principles and applications of cardiorespiratory care equipment.* St. Louis. Mosby, 1994.)

generated by the USN remains in the chamber, awaiting the next breath.

Small-volume USNs have less dead space than SVNs, reducing the need for a large quantity of diluent to ensure delivery of drugs. The contained portable power source provides convenience and mobility. Both these theoretic advantages of USNs may be outweighed by their high cost, however, which can be as much as a hundred times greater than pMDI therapy. USNs have been promoted for administration of a wide variety of formulations, ranging from bronchodilators to antiinflammatory agents and antibiotics.[41] In general, however, USNs have been shown to be less effective than other delivery devices.[42]

In addition to the contamination risks of any aerosol device, several other hazards are associated with using an USN. Overhydration may occur when using an USN for prolonged treatment of a neonate, small child, or patients with renal insufficiency. The high-density aerosol from USNs has been associated with bronchospasm, increased airway resistance, and irritability in a substantial portion of the population.[43] Also, the structure of the medication may be disrupted by an acoustic power output rated greater than 50 watts/cm-cm.[44,45] Several ventilator manufacturers (Siemens, Nellcor-Puritan Bennett) are promoting the use of USNs for administration of aerosols during mechanical ventilation. The advantage of the USN during ventilation is that no driving gas flow is added to the circuit, changing ventilator parameters and alarm settings.[46] Disadvantages may be the weight of the USN in the ventilator circuit, tendency to heat up over time, and potential for reduced therapeutic efficacy of medications.

PRESSURIZED METERED-DOSE INHALERS

The pMDI is the most frequently prescribed method of aerosol delivery. Pressurized MDIs are used to administer bronchodilators, anticholinergics, antiinflammatory agents, and steroids. More formulations of these drugs are currently available for use by

Metered-dose inhaler

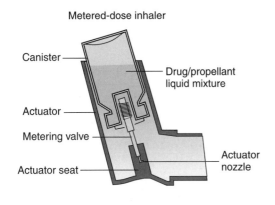

Metered-valve function

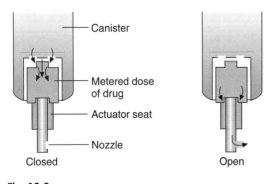

Fig. 13-8

Cross-sectional diagrams of pressurized metered-dose inhaler. (Modified from Rau JL Jr: *Respiratory care pharmacology,* ed 5. St. Louis. Mosby, 1998.)

pMDI than for use with other nebulization systems. Properly used, pMDIs are at least as effective as other nebulizers for drug delivery.[47] Therefore pMDIs are often the preferred method for delivering bronchodilators to spontaneously breathing, as well as intubated, ventilated patients.[48]

A pMDI is a pressurized canister containing a drug in the form of a micronized powder or solution that is suspended with a mixture of propellants along with a surfactant or a dispersal agent.[5] Dispersing agents are present in concentrations equal to or greater than that of the medication. In some patients these agents may be associated with coughing and wheezing.[49] The bulk of the spray, up to 80% by weight, is composed of a propellant, typically a CFC such as Freon. Adverse reactions to CFCs are extremely rare.[50-52] Due to international agreements to ban CFCs (Montreal protocol), new pMDIs are in development using environmentally safe propellants. The best new propellants are the HFAs, such as HFA133a.

The output volume of the pMDI varies from 30 to 100 μl and contains 20 μg to 5 mg of drug. Lung deposition is estimated at between 10% and 25% in adults, with high intersubject variability largely dependent on user technique. When proper technique and an accessory device are used, the pMDI delivers substantially more of the dose of medication to the lung than an SVN.

The pMDI canister contains a pressurized mixture containing propellants, surfactants, preservatives, and sometimes flavoring agents, with approximately 1% of the total contents being active drug. This mixture is released from the canister through a metering valve and stem that fits into an actuator boot, designed and tested by the manufacturer to work with the specific formulation (Fig. 13-8). Small changes in actuator design can change the characteristics and output of the aerosol from a pMDI.

Pressurized MDI actuation into a valved holding chamber decreases impaction losses by reducing the velocity of the aerosol jet,[5] allowing time for evaporation of the propellants and the particles to "age" before impacting on a surface. The nominal dose of medication with the pMDI is much smaller than with the nebulizer. The quantity of albuterol from a pMDI exiting the actuator nozzle is 100 μg with each actuation or 90 μg from the opening of the actuator boot; this is how pMDI aerosol actuations are characterized in the United States. Thus a dose of 2 to 4 actuations (200 to 400 μg nominal dose) is typically used. In ambulatory patients, 10% deposition may deliver a dose of 20 to 40 μg for an effective bronchodilator response.

Technique. Effective use of a pMDI is technique dependent. Up to two thirds of patients who use pMDIs *and* health professionals who teach pMDI use do not perform the procedure properly.[53,54] Box 13-2 outlines recommended steps for self-administering a bronchodilator using a pMDI.[55] Good patient instruction can take 10 to 30 minutes and should include demonstration, practice, and confirmation of patient performance (demonstration placebo units are available for this purpose). Repeated instruction improves performance.[56]

Infants, young children, and patients in acute distress may not be able to use a pMDI effectively. A "cold Freon effect" can occur when the aerosol plume reaches the back of the mouth and the patient stops inhaling. These problems can be corrected by using the proper pMDI accessory device (see next section).

Problems with home use of pMDI devices include not only poor technique but also poor storage. The pMDI should always be stored with cap on, both to prevent foreign objects from entering

OPTIMAL SELF-ADMINISTRATION TECHNIQUE FOR USING PRESSURIZED METERED-DOSE INHALER (pMDI)

1. Warm pMDI canister to hand or body temperature.
2. Shake the canister vigorously.
3. Assemble the apparatus, and uncap the mouthpiece.
4. Ensure that no loose objects are in the device that could be aspirated or could obstruct outflow.
5. Open the mouth wide.
6. Keep the tongue from obstructing the mouthpiece.
7. Hold the pMDI vertically with the outlet aimed at the mouth.
8. Place canister outlet between lips, or position pMDI 4 cm (two fingers) away from the mouth.*
9. Breathe out normally.
10. Begin to breathe in slowly (less than 0.5 L/sec).
11. Squeeze and actuate ("fire") the pMDI.
12. Continue to inhale to total lung capacity.
13. Hold breath for 4 to 10 seconds.
14. Wait 30 seconds between inhalations (actuations).
15. Disassemble the apparatus, and recap the mouthpiece.

*Open mouth technique is not recommended with ipratropium bromide.

the boot and to reduce humidity and microbial contamination. Pressurized MDIs should always be discarded when empty to avoid administering propellant without medication. Although it has been suggested that pMDIs can be tested for drug remaining by floating the canister in water, this technique can be difficult to perform and interpret and runs the risk of contaminating the device. It is easier and more accurate for the patient or parent to note when the medication was started, the number of doses to be taken each day, and the number of doses in the canister, and from this information to calculate a discard date. For example, if 200 actuations are in a canister (information always indicated on the canister label) and 4 "puffs" are taken per day, the canister should be discarded 50 days, or 7 weeks, after the start date. This discard date should be written on the canister label on the day the new canister is started.

Accessory Devices. A variety of pMDI accessory devices have been developed to overcome the two primary limitations of pMDI administration: hand-breath coordination problems and high oropharyngeal deposition. Accessory devices include flow-triggered pMDIs, spacers, and valved holding chambers.

Flow-triggered device. The Autohaler (3M) is a flow-triggered pMDI designed to reduce the need for hand-breath coordination by firing in response to the patient's inspiratory effort.[57] To use the Autohaler, the patient cocks a lever on the top of the unit that spring-loads the canister against a vane mechanism. When the patient's inspiratory flow exceeds 30 L/min, the vane moves, allowing the canister to be pressed into the actuator, firing the pMDI. This device is only available with the β-agonist pirbuterol in the United States, but other formulations are in development. The flow required to actuate the device may be too great for some children to generate, especially during acute exacerbations of disease.

Spacers and holding chambers. When properly designed, spacers and valved holding chambers (1) reduce oropharyngeal deposition of drug, (2) relieve the bad taste of some medications by reducing oral deposition, (3) eliminate the cold Freon effect, (4) decrease aerosol MMAD, (5) increase respirable particle mass, (6) improve lower respiratory tract deposition, and (7) significantly improve therapeutic effects.[40,56,58]

Spacers should be differentiated from valved holding chambers. A *spacer* device is a simple open-ended tube or bag that has sufficiently large volume to provide space for the pMDI plume to expand by allowing the propellant to evaporate. To perform this function, a spacer device must have an internal volume greater than 100 ml and must provide a distance of 10 to 13 cm between the pMDI nozzle and the first wall or baffle. Smaller, inefficient spacers can reduce respiratory dose by 60% and offer no protection against poor coordination between actuation and breathing pattern. Spacers with internal volumes greater than 100 ml generally provide some protection against early firing of the pMDI, although exhaling immediately after the actuation clears most of the aerosol from the device, wasting the dose.

The *valved holding chamber*, usually 140 to 750 ml in volume, allows the plume from the pMDI to expand. It incorporates a one-way valve that permits the aerosol to be drawn from the chamber during inhalation only, diverting the exhaled gas to the atmosphere and not disturbing remaining aerosol suspended in the chamber (Fig. 13-9). Patients with small tidal volumes may empty the aerosol from the chamber with five to six breaths, except when there is a large dead space. A valved holding chamber can also incorporate a mask for

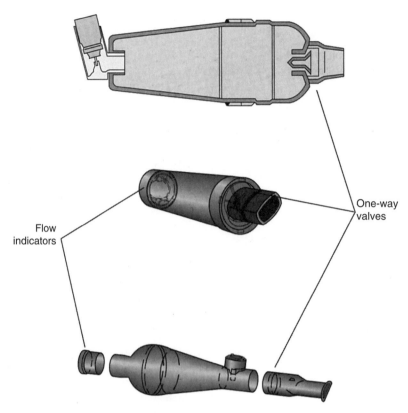

Fig. 13-9

MDI holding chambers are spacers with one-way valves that allow the chamber to be emptied only when the patient inhales by preventing the exhaled gas from entering the chamber. (From Fink J, Cohen N: Humidity and aerosols. In Eubanks DH, Bone RC, editors: *Principles and applications of cardiorespiratory care equipment.* St. Louis. Mosby, 1994.)

use in an infant or child (Fig. 13-10). These devices allow effective pMDI administration in a patient who is unable to use a mouthpiece because of size, age, coordination, or mental status.[59] With infants these masks should have minimal dead space, should be comfortable on the child's face, and should have a valved chamber that will open and close with the low inspiratory flow generated by the patient. Box 13-3 describes the correct technique for using a pMDI with a holding chamber.

Encouraging the use of a valved holding chamber, especially for infants, small children, and any child using steroids, reduces the need to coordinate the breath with actuation. Additionally, chambers reduce the pharyngeal dose of aerosol from the pMDI 10- to 15-fold over administration without a holding chamber. This decreases total body dose from swallowed medications, which is an important consideration with steroid administration.[58,60,61] The high percentage of oropharyngeal drug deposition with steroid pMDIs can increase the risk of

oral yeast infections (thrush). Rinsing the mouth after steroid can reduce this problem, but most pMDI steroid aerosol impaction occurs deeper in the pharynx, which is not easily rinsed. For this reason, steroid MDIs should always be used in combination with a valved holding chamber.

Wheezing Infants. Valved holding chambers make pMDIs more reliable than SVNs for aerosol administration. In one study, 34 infants between 1 and 24 months with acute asthma received two doses of terbutaline, 20 minutes apart, as either 2 mg/dose in 2.8 ml of 0.9% saline by nebulizer or 0.5 mg/dose (5 puffs) by pMDI with a valved holding chamber.[62] No difference was found in the rate of improvement or clinical score, and both devices were reported equally effective. Similarly, 60 children 6 years of age or less who had an acute asthma exacerbation were randomized to receive albuterol through nebulizer or pMDI with valved holding chamber for three treatments more than 1 hour.[63]

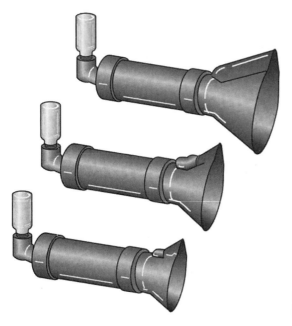

Fig.13-10

MDI holding chambers with masks for infants and children who are unable to use a mouthpiece design. (Redrawn from Fink J, Cohen N: Humidity and aerosols. In Eubanks DH, Bone RC, editors: *Principles and applications of cardiorespiratory care equipment.* St. Louis. Mosby, 1994.)

All patients showed improvement over baseline, with no difference between treatment groups.

In another study, 84 children were enrolled in the emergency department (ED) to receive inhaled medication with or without a valved holding chamber to determine whether a single brief demonstration of the proper use of a valved holding chamber would result in improved outcomes.[64] The valved holding chamber group reported significantly faster resolution of wheezing, fewer days of cough, and fewer missed days of school.

Evidence-based research does not support the belief that an SVN is better than a pMDI if the patient is not able to inhale with optimal technique. In fact, if unable to perform an optimal maneuver using a pMDI, the patient cannot perform an optimal maneuver using an SVN. Although optimal technique is always preferred, it is often difficult to attain with an infant, small child, or severely dyspneic patient. In such patients, an alternative may be to increase the pMDI or nebulizer dosage (see later discussion).

Care and Cleaning. Particles containing drug settle and deposit within these devices, causing a whitish buildup on the inner chamber walls. This residual drug poses no risk to the patient but should

---

OPTIMAL TECHNIQUE FOR USING pMDI WITH VALVED HOLDING CHAMBER

1. Warm pMDI to hand or body temperature.
2. Shake the canister vigorously, holding it vertically.
3. Assemble the apparatus.
4. Ensure that no loose objects are in device that could be aspirated or could obstruct outflow.
5. Place holding chamber in the mouth (or place mask completely over the nose and mouth), encouraging patient to breathe through the mouth.
6. Have patient breathe normally, and actuate at the beginning of inspiration.
7. For small children and infants, have them continue to breathe through the device for five or six breaths.
8. For patients who can cooperate, encourage larger breaths with breath holding.
9. Allow 30 seconds between actuations.

---

be rinsed out periodically. After washing a chamber or spacer with tap water, it is less effective for the next 10 to 15 puffs, until the static charge in the chamber (which attracts small particles) is once again reduced. Use of regular dish soap to wash the chamber reduces or eliminates this static charge.

Accessory devices either use the manufacturer-designed boot that comes with the pMDI or incorporate a "universal canister adapter" to fire the pMDI canister. Different formulations of pMDI drugs operate at different pressures, and devices have different orifice sizes in the boot specifically designed for use exclusively with the specific pMDI. Output characteristics of pMDIs will change when using an adapter with a different-size orifice; therefore spacers or holding chambers with universal canister adapters should be avoided. Devices that use the manufacturer's boot with the pMDI should be used, when available.

DRY POWDER INHALERS

DPIs create aerosols by drawing air through a dose of dry powder medication. The powder contains micronized drug particles (less than 5 μm MMAD) with larger lactose or glucose particles (greater than 30 μm in diameter), or it contains micronized drug particles bound into loose aggregates.[65] Micronized particles adhere strongly to each other and to most surfaces. Addition of the larger particles of the carrier decreases cohesive forces in the micronized drug powder so that separation into individual respirable particles (deaggregation) occurs more readily. Thus the carrier particles aid the flow of the drug

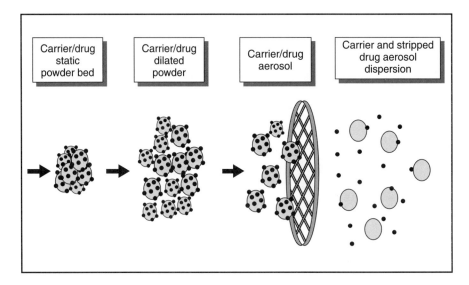

Fig. 13-11

As patient inhales through the dry powder inhaler, inspiratory flow is drawn from the powder bed, dilated, and drawn through a screen that strips drug from carrier, creating an aerosol dispersion. (Modified from Dhand R, Fink J: Dry powder inhalers. *Respir Care* 1999; 44:940-951.)

powder from the device. These carriers also act as "fillers" by adding bulk to the powder when the unit dose of a drug is very small. Usually the drug particles are loosely bound to the carrier,[66] and they are stripped from the carrier by the energy provided by the patient's inhalation (Fig. 13-11). The release of respirable particles of the drug requires inspiration at relatively high flow (30 to 120 L/min).[67,68] A high inspiratory flow results in pharyngeal impaction of the larger carrier particles that comprise the bulk of the aerosol. The oropharyngeal impaction of carrier particles gives the patient the sensation of having inhaled a dose.

The internal geometry of the DPI device influences the resistance offered to inspiration and the inspiratory flow required to deaggregate and aerosolize the medication. Devices with higher resistance require a higher inspiratory flow to produce a dose. Inhalation through high-resistance DPIs may improve drug delivery to the lower respiratory tract compared with pMDIs as long as the patient can reliably generate the required flow rate.[50,69] High-resistance devices have not been shown to improve either deposition or bronchodilation compared with low-resistance DPIs. DPIs with multiple components require correct assembly of the apparatus and priming of the device to ensure aerosolization of the dry powder. Periodic brushing is needed to remove any residual powder accumulated within some DPIs.

DPIs produce aerosols in which most of the drug particles are in the respirable range, with distribution of particle sizes (GSD) differing significantly among various DPIs.[51] High ambient humidity produces clumping of the dry powder, creating larger particles that are not as effectively aerosolized.[52] Air with a high moisture content is less efficient at deaggregating particles of dry powder than dry air, such that high ambient humidity increases the size of drug particles in the aerosol and may reduce drug delivery to the lung. Newer DPI devices contain individual doses more protected from humidity. Humidity can accumulate once opened or if the DPI is stored with the cap off or by condensation when the device is brought from a very cold environment into a warmer area.

Because the energy from the patient's inspiratory flow disperses the drug powder, the magnitude and duration of the patient's inspiratory effort influence aerosol generation from a DPI.[70] Failure to perform inhalation at a sufficiently fast inspiratory flow reduces the dose of the drug emitted from DPIs and increases the distribution of particle sizes within the aerosol with a variety of devices.[71,72] For example, the Diskus (Glaxo Wellcome) delivers approximately 90% of the labeled dose at inspiratory flow ranging from 30 to 90 L/min, whereas the dose delivered by the high-resistance Turbuhaler (Astra) is significantly lower at an inspiratory flow of 30 L/min compared to the dose delivered at

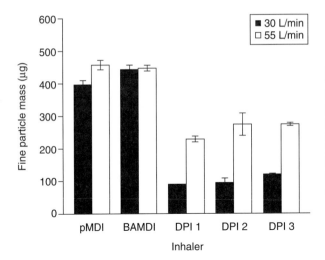

Fig. 13-12

Fine particle mass delivered from 1000-μg target dose (±SD) as a function of flow rate. *PMDI*, Pressurized metered-dose inhaler; *BAMDI*, breath-actuated MDI, Autohaler; *DPI 1*, Rotahaler; *DPI 2*, Turbuhaler; *DPI 3*, Diskhaler. (From Smith KJ, Chan H-K, Brown KF: Influence of flow rate on particle size distributions from pressurized and breath actuated inhalers. *J Aerosol Med* 1998; 11:231-245.)

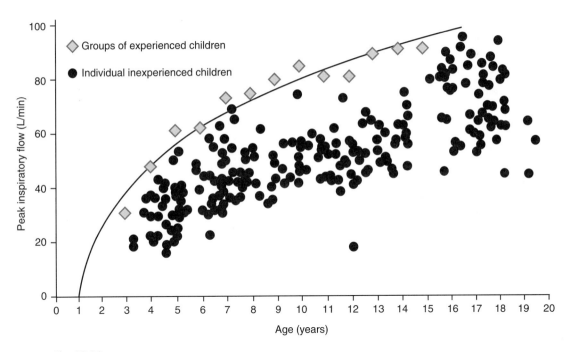

Fig. 13-13

Peak inspiratory flows in individual inexperienced children (Pederson et al, 1990) and groups of experienced children (Agertoft et al, 1995). (From Pederson S: Delivery options for the inhaled therapy in children over the age of 6 years. *J Aerosol Med* 1997; 10:41-44.)

90 L/min. The variability between doses at different inspiratory flows is higher with the Turbuhaler.[73,74] Fig. 13-12 shows the effect of two inspiratory flows (30 and 55 L/min) when using a pMDI, breath-actuated MDI (Autohaler), Rotahaler (DPI 1), Turbuhaler (DPI 2), and Diskhaler (DPI 3).[75] The peak inspiratory flow rate of children is limited and associated with age, making it

unlikely that a child less than 6 years old could reliably empty a DPI requiring greater than 50 L/min (Fig. 13-13).[75]

Active DPI delivery devices use a small motor and impeller or compressed gas propulsion to disperse the powder and are under investigation. Aerosol production and airway deposition when using these devices are influenced by the patient's

TABLE 13-1	DIFFERENCES IN INHALATION TECHNIQUE BETWEEN PRESSURIZED METERED-DOSE INHALER WITH HOLDING CHAMBER (pMDI/HC) AND DRY POWDER INHALER (DPI)	
Step	**pMDI/HC**	**DPI**
Shaking the inhaler	Yes	No
Actuation with inspiration	Optional	Essential
Inspiration	Slow, deep Improves deposition	Fast, prolonged Required for deposition
Interval between doses	30-60 sec	20-30 sec
Exhalation into device	Small decrease in dose	Large decrease in dose

TABLE 13-2	COMPARISON OF PRESSURIZED METERED-DOSE INHALER WITH HOLDING CHAMBER (pMDI/HC), DRY POWDER INHALER (DPI), AND NEBULIZER AS AEROSOL DELIVERY DEVICE		
Factor	**pMDI/HC**	**DPI**	**Nebulizer**
PERFORMANCE			
Most aerosol particles <5 μm in size	+	+	±
High pulmonary deposition	+	±	±
Low mouth deposition	+	±	−
Reliability of dose	+	±	±
Influenced by humidity	−	+	−
Physical and chemical stability	+	+	+
Breath actuated	−	+	−
Risk of contamination	−	−	+
CONVENIENCE			
Lightweight, compact	+	+	−
Multiple doses	+	+	−
Dose indicator	−	+	−
Dose counter	−	+	−
Inexpensive	+	+	−
Easy and quick operation	±	±	−
Suitable for all ages	+	−	+
Suitable for multiple clinical situations	+	±	+

inspiratory flow to a lesser extent than DPIs that rely solely on patient effort for aerosol production.

Breath coordination is also important when using DPIs. Exhalation into a DPI blows out the powder from the device and reduces drug delivery. Moreover, the humidity in the exhaled air reduces subsequent aerosol generation from the DPI. Therefore patients must be instructed not to exhale into a DPI.

DPIs are breath actuated and reduce the problem of coordinating inspiration with actuation. The technique of using DPIs differs in important respects from the technique employed to inhale drugs from a pMDI (Table 13-1). Although DPIs are easier to use than pMDIs, up to 25% of patients may use DPIs improperly.[75] DPIs are critically dependent on inspiratory airflow to generate the aerosol. Thus they should be used with caution, if at all, in the very young or ill child, weak patients, elderly persons, and those with altered mental status. Patients may need repeated instruction before they can master the technique of using DPIs, and periodic assessment is necessary to ensure that patients continue to use an optimal technique.[75] Clinicians must also learn the correct technique of using DPIs to train their patients in proper use of these devices.

DEVICE SELECTION AND COMPLIANCE

Whenever possible, patients should use only one type of aerosol-generating device for inhalation therapy. The technique of using each device is different, and repeated instruction is necessary to ensure that the patient uses the device appropri-

ately. The use of different devices for inhalation can be confusing for patients and may decrease their compliance with therapy.

At present, DPIs can be considered as alternatives to pMDIs for patients who can generate inspiratory flow rates greater than 30 to 60 L/min but are unable to use pMDIs effectively. DPIs are recommended for therapy for patients with stable asthma and chronic obstructive pulmonary disease (COPD), but not for patients with acute bronchoconstriction or children less than 6 years of age. Therefore one drawback of DPIs is that they do not substitute for pMDIs in all clinical situations. Moreover, dose adjustment may be needed when the same drug is administered by a DPI instead of a pMDI. Table 13-2 compares DPIs, pMDIs, and nebulizers. Deciding on the appropriate dose of inhaled corticosteroids may be a particularly vexing problem because it is difficult to determine bioequivalence with these agents. Further research is needed to determine equivalent dosages when both the drug and the device used for inhalation therapy are altered.[76,77]

To improve compliance, aerosol therapy should be administered along with some easily remembered activity of daily living. For twice-daily administration, medications can be kept with the toothbrush and inhaled just before brushing teeth. This approach also reduces aerosol corticosteroid deposition in the oral pharynx. It is always best to avoid the regular use of medication at school because the inconvenience can significantly reduce compliance and may embarrass some children. However, the availability of rescue medication at school (or day care or other caregiver's home) must be ensured. It helps to prepare written guidelines for medication use. Distribute these guidelines to all the places where the child stays, such as home, school, or at the residence of each parent if divorced or separated.[78]

It is helpful, at least initially, to keep a diary of medication use. Lack of response to inhaled asthma medication can be related to a number of factors, including incorrect technique of inhalation, inhaling empty canisters of medications thinking that they contain active drug, not taking preventive medications as prescribed, change in the child's environment, or misdiagnosis. For example, children with aspirated foreign body, gastroesophageal reflux disease, or psychogenic wheeze will have a poor response to asthma therapy. Infants with tracheomalacia or bronchopulmonary dysplasia may even become much worse after inhaling a bronchodilator aerosol because of increased dynamic airway collapse.[79]

EMERGENCY BRONCHODILATOR RESUSCITATION

When a patient comes to the ED with an acute exacerbation of asthma, the onset of the exacerbation is often 12 to 36 hours earlier. These children have often taken rescue medications without obtaining sufficient relief. They are anxious, uncomfortable, and exhausted. The goal of bronchodilator resuscitation is to provide relief of dyspnea as quickly as possible with minimal side effects.

Administration of selective β_2-agonists and anticholinergics such as ipratropium (Atrovent) by aerosol is usually the first therapy given. Albuterol (salbutamol outside the United States) reaches 85% of bronchodilator effect in the first 5 minutes after administration. The goal is to provide relief as soon as possible and to decrease the work of breathing until antiinflammatory medications take effect.

Although many ED physicians still use the SVN for treatment of acute asthma, a large number of studies clearly support that pMDI with a valved holding chamber is more effective and safer than nebulizer therapy. The national asthma guidelines recommend albuterol administration with either 2.5 or 5.0 mg by jet nebulizer, or 4 to 8 puffs of albuterol by pMDI with valved holding chamber at 20-minute intervals for the first hour.[80,81]

INTERMITTENT VERSUS CONTINUOUS THERAPY

When treating an acute exacerbation of asthma with a bronchodilator, if the patient does not experience relief of symptoms with standard dosing, other dosing strategies may be used. The frequency of administration is often increased to hourly, or even every 15 to 20 minutes, in the ED. Treatments can be continued at this frequency until symptoms are relieved. The standard SVN treatment takes 10 to 15 minutes and requires that a clinician be at the bedside constantly. An alternative is to provide continuous nebulization by having a nebulizer with an adequate volume of solution operate continuously at a controlled rate of medication delivery. Doses of albuterol between 7.5 and 15 mg/hr have been shown to be effective in treating acute exacerbation of asthma in adults and children.[82-85]

One strategy is to use an intravenous infusion pump to drip a premixed bronchodilator solution into a standard SVN. Another solution is to use an LVN that produces a MMAD in the respirable range and that is known to deliver a consistent output of medication at a specific flow. Albuterol solution and normal saline are mixed in the reservoir, and the LVN is operated at a specific flow, identified by the manufacturer, to deliver the desired dose. Several LVNs are now commercially available for continuous administration of bronchodilators. The HEART nebulizer (Westmed) has an output of approximately 30 ml/hr at a flow of 10 L/min for up to 6 or 8 hours. The HOPE nebulizer (B&B Medical) is a closed dilution nebulizer that allows drug output and oxygen administration (Fig. 13-14). The medication can be delivered through an aerosol mouthpiece or mask or in-line with a ventilator circuit. For patients with moderately severe asthma, continuous therapy and intermittent therapy have similar effect with either low-dose or high-dose β-agonists. For patients with a severe asthma exacerbation, or forced expiratory volume (FEV) less than 40% of predicted values, continuous therapy may work more rapidly.[85]

Although β_2-agonists are the first-line agents for acute exacerbation of asthma, data in both adults and children suggest that ipratropium bromide is synergistic with β-agonists for the therapy of acute asthma.[86-91] Combination bronchodilator therapy using albuterol and ipratropium in patients with severe asthma significantly reduced the percentage of patients hospitalized (Fig. 13-15).[92] It is important to remember that poor relief of acute asthma with bronchodilators may signify a nonasthmatic cause of wheezing, such as foreign body aspiration or tracheitis. Infants with bronchiolitis respond poorly to bronchodilator medications, which are therefore not recommended for this condition.

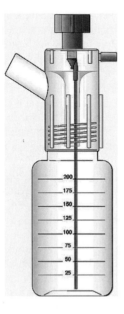

Fig. 13-14

Large-volume closed dilution nebulizer (HOPE) used for bronchodilator aerosol therapy in the emergency department. (Courtesy B & B Medical Technologies, Orangevale, Calif.)

UNDILUTED BRONCHODILATOR

A faster method of administering albuterol is by pouring undiluted medication into the nebulizer. We typically add diluent to the medication in the nebulizer to reduce the fraction of the dose that is trapped as residual volume. With undiluted administration, enough medication must be added to the nebulizer to exceed the residual volume of the nebulizer and to allow 1.0 to 2.0 ml of albuterol solution (5 to 10 mg) to be nebulized. Patients should be monitored closely during administration, and the treatment should be terminated when the patient has significant reduction of symptoms and begins to develop tremor or other side effect. Undiluted albuterol administered with specialty nebulizers achieves similar improvements in clinical status in less time. The osmolarity of undiluted medication may be a problem for some patients, especially children under 2 years.[93]

MECHANICAL VENTILATION

Deposition of aerosol in the endotracheal tube (ETT) and ventilator circuit was thought to reduce significantly the fraction of aerosol delivered to the lower respiratory tract. Until recently the consensus was that the efficiency of aerosol delivery to the lower respiratory tract in mechanically ventilated patients was much lower that that in ambulatory patients.[93] Data suggest that this might be overly pessimistic, however, because a variety of variables affect aerosol delivery during mechanical ventilation (Box 13-4).

FACTORS AFFECTING AEROSOL DELIVERY

Ventilator-Patient Interface. The ventilator circuit is typically a closed system that is pressurized

Fig. 13-15

Rates of hospitalization of asthmatic patients from the emergency department after treatment with control (albuterol) and ipratropium (with albuterol). In patients with moderate asthma, no difference was seen in hospitalization rate. In patients with severe asthma, benefits of combined therapy are significant. (From Qureshi F et al: Effect of nebulized ipratropium on the hospitalization rates of children with asthma. *N Engl J Med* 1998; 339:1030-1035. Copyright 1998 Massachusetts Medical Society. All rights reserved.)

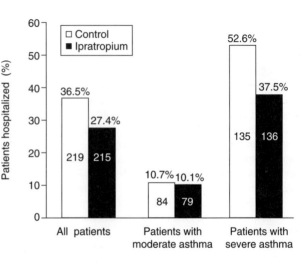

during operation, requiring the nebulizer or pMDI to be attached with connectors that maintain the integrity of the circuit during operation. The pMDI cannot be used with the actuator designed by the manufacturer, and use of a third-party actuator is required (Fig. 13-16). The size, shape, and design of these actuators greatly affect respirable drug available to the patient and may vary with different pMDI formulations.[94]

Breath Configuration. During *controlled mechanical ventilation* (CMV) the pattern and rate of inspiratory gas flow, as well as rate and pattern of breathing, differ from spontaneous respiration. Ambulatory

patients under normal stable conditions tend to have sinusoidal inspiratory flow patterns of about 30 L/min, whereas ventilators may use square or decelerating waves with considerably higher flow. Also, the airways are pressurized on inhalation when using CMV, whereas spontaneous inspiration is generated by negative airway pressure drawing gas deep into the lungs. All these factors can influence aerosol delivery to the lower respiratory tract.

Airway. Although the ETT is usually considered the first and major point of impaction of aerosol during mechanical ventilation, other factors are also important. In the mechanically ventilated patient, the conduit between the aerosol device and lower respiratory tract is narrower than the oropharynx. Abrupt angles, such as the 90-degree connector often used to connect the ventilator circuit Y-device to the ETT, result in points of impaction and turbulence not found in the normal

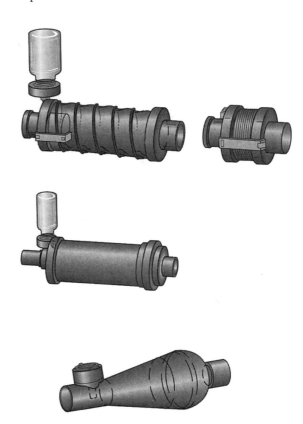

Fig. 13-16

MDI holding chambers to use in-line with mechanical ventilator circuits or in intubated patients or those with tracheostomies. (Redrawn from Fink J, Cohen N: Humidity and aerosols. In Eubanks DH, Bone RC, editors: *Principles and applications of cardiorespiratory care equipment.* St. Louis. Mosby, 1994.)

BOX 13-4

VARIABLES THAT AFFECT AEROSOL DELIVERY AND DEPOSITION DURING MECHANICAL VENTILATION

VENTILATOR RELATED
Mode
Tidal volume
Respiratory frequency
Duty cycle
Inspiratory flow waveform
Trigger mechanism

DEVICE RELATED
METERED-DOSE INHALER
Type of spacer or adapter
Position of spacer in circuit
Timing of actuation

NEBULIZER
Type of nebulizer
Fill volume
Gas flow
Cycling: inspiration versus continuous
Duration of nebulization
Position in circuit

CIRCUIT RELATED
Endotracheal tube
Inhaled gas humidity
Inhaled gas density

DRUG RELATED
Dose
Formulation
Aerosol particle size
Targeted site for delivery
Duration of action

PATIENT RELATED
Severity of airway obstruction
Mechanism of airway obstruction
Presence of dynamic hyperinflation
Patient-ventilator synchrony

airway. Although the ETT is narrower than the trachea, its smooth interior surface may create a more laminar flow path than the structures of the glottis and larynx and may be less of a barrier to aerosol delivery than the ventilator circuit. We recently reported that twice as much aerosol from the pMDI deposits in the ventilator circuit than in the ETT under both dry and humidified conditions during CMV, raising some doubt that the ETT is the primary barrier to aerosol.[95]

Environment. Ventilator circuits are typically designed to provide heat and humidity for inspired gas to compensate for bypassing the normal airway. Humidity can increase particle size and reduce deposition during CMV, but no data suggest that this reduction is unique to the ventilated patient. The ambulatory patient taking an aerosol in a hot, high-humidity climate may experience a similar reduction in delivered dose.

Response Assessment. The most common method to assess patient response to bronchodilator administration is through changes in expiratory flow. During mechanical ventilation forced expiratory maneuvers are impractical, poorly reproducible, and rarely performed, requiring other, less sensitive methods such as monitoring pressure changes (peak and plateau) during ventilator-generated breaths (e.g., passive inspiration). Other changes in mechanics consistent with bronchodilator therapy include decreasing pressures needed to deliver a set tidal volume during volume ventilation, decreased mean airway pressure (now continuously monitored electronically by most mechanical ventilators), and decreased requirement for supplemental oxygen. Chest auscultation for changes in wheezing is notoriously inaccurate and should *never* be used as the sole criterion for evaluating the effect of inhaled bronchodilators.

Nebulizer. Placement of a continuous nebulizer 30 cm from the ETT is more efficient than placement between the patient Y-device and the ETT because the inspiratory ventilator tubing acts as a spacer for the aerosol to accumulate between inspirations.[96] Addition of a spacer device between the nebulizer and ETT modestly increases aerosol delivery.[97] Operating the nebulizer only during inspiration is more efficient for aerosol delivery compared with continuous aerosol generation.[96]

Inhaler Adapters. Several types of commercial adapters are available to connect the pMDI canister to the ventilator circuit. Pressurized MDIs can be used with adapters that attach directly to the ETT, with in-line chamber or nonchamber adapters

placed in the inspiratory limb of the ventilator circuit. In vitro and in vivo studies have shown that the combination of a pMDI and an accessory device with a chamber results in a fourfold to sixfold greater delivery of aerosol than pMDI actuation into a connector attached directly to the ETT or into an in-line device that lacks a chamber.[59,97-100] When using the elbow adapter connected to the ETT, actuation of the pMDI out of synchrony with inspiratory airflow delivers very little aerosol to the lower respiratory tract. This observation may explain the lack of therapeutic effect with this type of adapter after administration of very high doses (100 puffs, 1.0 mg of albuterol) of aerosol from a pMDI in some studies.[101]

Aerosol Particle Size. In ambulatory patients, aerosols with a higher proportion of respirable particles (0.5 to 5.0 µm MMAD) are more efficient for aerosol delivery to the lower respiratory tract. In mechanically ventilated patients the ventilator circuit and ETT act as baffles that trap particles with larger diameter en route to the bronchi, and hygroscopic particles might increase further in size in the ventilator circuit. Wide variability exists in the MMAD of aerosols produced by different brands of nebulizers. Nebulizers producing aerosols smaller than 2 µm MMAD are likely to produce greater deposition in the lower respiratory tract of ventilator-supported patients.[92]

Endotracheal Tube. Aerosol impaction in the ETT can reduce the efficiency of aerosol delivery in mechanically ventilated patients. The efficacy of aerosol delivery decreases when narrow ETTs are used in pediatric ventilator circuits.[102,103] The efficiency with which various nebulizers deliver aerosols beyond the ETT did not vary among tube sizes ranging in internal diameter from 7 to 9 mm.[99]

Heating and Humidification. Humidification of inhaled gas decreases aerosol deposition with pMDIs and nebulizers by approximately 40%, probably because of increased particle loss in the ventilator circuit.[59,102-104] Therefore some investigators have proposed bypassing the humidifier during aerosol administration. Absence of humidification may not pose problems during the brief period required to administer a bronchodilator with a pMDI. Some nebulizers require up to 35 minutes to complete aerosolization, however, and inhalation of dry gas during this time can damage the airway.[59] In addition, the disconnection of the ventilator circuit required to bypass the humidifier interrupts ventilation and may increase the risk of ventilator-associated pneumonia. For routine bronchodilator treatment, we recommend using either a pMDI or a nebulizer with a humidified ventilator circuit.

Density of Inhaled Gas. The *Reynolds number* is calculated from the flow and density of a gas and the resistance of the tube through which the gas flows. Laminar flow becomes turbulent at Reynolds numbers greater than 1000. High inspiratory flow produces turbulence, whereas inhalation of a less dense gas such as helium-oxygen reduces the Reynolds number. Therefore breathing helium-oxygen may improve aerosol deposition. Studies in ambulatory patients with airway obstruction reveal higher aerosol retention when breathing helium-oxygen compared with air.[105,106] The effects of helium-oxygen mixtures on aerosol deposition during in vitro modeling of mechanical ventilation have been investigated, with preliminary reports of up to 50% increase in deposition of albuterol from a pMDI during CMV of a simulated adult patient.[107]

Ventilator Mode and Settings. The ventilator mode and settings of tidal volume, flow, and respiratory rate influence the characteristics of the airflow used to deliver aerosol in mechanically ventilated patients. For optimal aerosol delivery, actuation of a pMDI into a spacer needs to be synchronized with the onset of inspiratory airflow. Actuation of a pMDI into a cylindrical spacer synchronized with inspiration results in approximately 30% greater efficiency of aerosol delivery compared with actuation during exhalation.[59] When using an elbow adapter, actuation of a pMDI that was not synchronized with inspiratory airflow achieved negligible aerosol delivery to the lower respiratory tract. Aerosol can be delivered during assisted modes of ventilation, provided that the patient is breathing in synchrony with the ventilator. Albuterol deposition may be up to 23% higher during simulated spontaneous breaths than with controlled breaths of equivalent tidal volume.[104] For efficient aerosol delivery to the lower respiratory tract, the tidal volume of the ventilator-delivered breath must be larger than the volume of the ventilator tubing and ETT. Tidal volumes of 500 ml or greater in adults are associated with adequate aerosol delivery, but the higher pressures required to deliver larger tidal volumes can be detrimental to the lungs.

Aerosol delivery directly correlates with longer inflation times.[102,104] A longer inspiratory time allows a higher proportion of the aerosol generated by the nebulizer to be inhaled with each breath. Because nebulizers generate aerosol over several minutes, longer inspiratory times have a cumulative effect in improving aerosol delivery. However, pMDIs produce aerosol only over a portion of a single inspira-

tion, and the mechanism by which longer inspiratory times increase aerosol delivery is unclear. Aerosol particles that deposit in the ventilator tubing may be swept off the walls and entrained by longer periods of inspiratory flow.

In addition, the diluent volume and the duration of treatment influence nebulizer efficiency.[102] Approximately 5% of the nominal dose of albuterol administered by a pMDI is exhaled in mechanically ventilated patients, whereas less than 1% is exhaled with use of pMDIs in ambulatory patients.[104,108] The mean exhaled fraction (7%) with use of nebulizers in mechanically ventilated patients is similar to that with MDIs, but considerable variability exists between patients (coefficient of variation, 74%).[109]

TECHNIQUE OF AEROSOL ADMINISTRATION

In vitro studies have helped in understanding the technique of aerosol administration to achieve the greatest amount of aerosol deposition in the lower respiratory tract. In mechanically ventilated patients the technique of aerosol administration often requires a compromise between the optimal operating characteristics of the aerosol generator and the patient's pulmonary mechanics. For example, a longer inflation time increases aerosol deposition in the lung, but it may worsen dynamic hyperinflation for patients with airflow limitation.

In vitro the best delivery with a nebulizer during CMV (15%) is accomplished using a nebulizer (e.g., Aerotech II) that produces an MMAD less than 2 μm, but this can take 35 minutes to administer a test dose of medication. This dose was nebulized into a dry ventilator circuit, with a duty cycle of 0.5 at inverse-ratio ventilation.[109] Admittedly, this approach would be difficult to tolerate for a patient requiring mechanical ventilation. A common nebulizer that generates particles with MMAD of 3.5 μm takes half the time but may reduce the dose to the lung by up to 50%, reducing total deposition to 7.5%. Keeping the humidifier on during administration reduces delivery by another 40% (decreasing total deposition to 4%), and reducing duty cycle to a normal 0.25 reduces deposition to 2%.[102] This 2% of the nominal dose of 2500 μg would equate to 50 μg of albuterol delivered to the lung. This dose would be similar to the 60 μg of albuterol delivered from 4 puffs of a pMDI with chamber adapter in a humidified circuit, at 15% deposition.

Box 13-5 outlines a modification of the technique of aerosol administration with nebulizers to mechanically ventilated patients. Box 13-6 provides another strategy for bronchodilator therapy using a pMDI.[5]

BOX 13-5

TECHNIQUE FOR USING NEBULIZERS IN MECHANICALLY VENTILATED PATIENTS

1. Place drug solution in nebulizer to optimal fill volume (2 to 6 ml).*
2. Place nebulizer in inspiratory line about 30 cm from patient Y-piece.
3. Ensure airflow of 6 to 8 L/min through the nebulizer.†
4. Ensure adequate tidal volume (about 500 ml in adults). Attempt to use duty cycle greater than 0.3, if possible.
5. Adjust minute volume, sensitivity trigger, and alarms to compensate for additional airflow through the nebulizer, if required.
6. Turn off flow-by or continuous-flow mode on ventilator and remove heat moisture exchanger (if present) from between nebulizer and patient.
7. Observe nebulizer for adequate aerosol generation throughout use.
8. Disconnect nebulizer when no more aerosol is being produced.
9. Rinse with sterile water or air-dry between uses. Store nebulizer under aseptic conditions.
10. Reconnect ventilator circuit, and return to original ventilator and alarm settings. Confirm proper operation with no leaks in circuit.

*The volume of solution associated with maximal efficiency varies with different nebulizers and should be determined before using any nebulizer.
†The nebulizer may be operated continuously or only during inspiration; the latter method is more efficient for aerosol delivery. Some ventilators provide inspiratory gas flow to the nebulizer. Continuous gas flow from an external source can also be used to power the nebulizer.

BOX 13-6

TECHNIQUE FOR USING pMDIs IN MECHANICALLY VENTILATED PATIENTS

1. Minimize inspiratory flow rate during administration.
2. Aim for an inspiratory time (excluding the inspiratory pause) greater than 0.3 of total breath duration.
3. Ensure that the ventilator breath is synchronized with the patient's inspiration.
4. Shake the pMDI vigorously.
5. Place the canister in the actuator of a cylindrical spacer situated in the inspiratory limb of the ventilator circuit.*
6. Actuate the pMDI to synchronize with precise onset of inspiration by the ventilator.†
7. Allow passive exhalation.
8. Repeat actuations after 20 to 30 seconds until total dose is delivered.‡

*With pMDIs, it is preferable to use a spacer that remains in the ventilator circuit so that disconnection of the ventilator circuit can be avoided at the time of each bronchodilator treatment. Although bypassing the humidifier can increase aerosol delivery, it prolongs the time for each treatment and requires disconnection of the ventilator circuit.
†In ambulatory patients with pMDI placed inside the mouth, actuation is recommended briefly after initiation of inspiratory airflow. In mechanically ventilated patients in whom a pMDI and spacer combination is used, actuation should be synchronized with onset of inspiration.
‡The manufacturer recommends repeating the dose after 1 minute. However, pMDI actuation within 20 to 30 seconds after the prior dose does not compromise drug delivery.

CARE OF ACCESSORY DEVICES AND NEBULIZERS

Nebulizers placed in-line in the ventilator circuit can become contaminated with bacteria, which are then carried as microaerosols directly to the lower respiratory tract. This contamination may result from condensate within the ventilator circuit, which is subject to retrograde contamination from the patient. Such contamination has been documented even after single use of a nebulizer.[110,111] The CDC recommends that nebulizers should be sterile at the start of nebulization between patients, and should be removed from the ventilator circuit after each use, disassembled, and rinsed with sterile water or air-dried.[30] Care should be taken to store the nebulizer aseptically between uses. Failure to observe these guidelines has been associated with nosocomial pneumonia.[112]

Single-dose ampules of drug are preferred to multidose containers or bottles, which are more easily contaminated. Similarly, when the chamber spacer remains in the ventilator circuit between treatments, condensate collects inside. Using a heated wire circuit can reduce formation of condensate within the spacer. Care must be taken to prevent the condensate in the spacer from being washed into the patient's respiratory tract when the spacer is pulled open during use. When a noncollapsible spacer chamber is used to actuate a pMDI, it should be removed from the ventilator circuit between treatments. No studies demonstrate contamination problems with administration of aerosol from a pMDI during CMV.

The administration of medication by pMDI to the mechanically ventilated neonate may not be well tolerated. Leaving a chamber device in-line is not practical because of the increased compressible volume to the ventilator circuit. Depending on the FIO_2 and the propellant gas volume, an in-line pMDI actuation theoretically may result in a hypoxic gas mixture to an infant receiving a tidal volume less than 100 ml. It is possible to deliver a pMDI aerosol medication to the intubated neonate, especially for medications available only in pMDI preparations. However, it may be preferable to hand-ventilate the pMDI delivery of medication to the patient. If a chamber adapter is used, the infant must be removed from the circuit, the chamber placed in-line, and the infant reattached to the circuit before the pMDI is administered. The large dead space volume caused by placing a spacer or chamber at the end of the ETT must also be considered when administering pMDI medications to an infant.

BRONCHODILATOR ADMINISTRATION

A primary goal of aerosol therapy is to achieve the greatest amount of drug deposition in the lower respiratory tract. However, increased drug deposition in the lower respiratory tract does not necessarily correlate with greater therapeutic efficacy. The response to bronchodilator administration depends on the patient's airway geometry, severity of disease, presence of mucus, the effects of inflammation and other drugs, and the degree of airway responsiveness. Once a threshold response has been achieved, there is little demonstrated increase in bronchodilation with greater amounts of medication administered.

Studies on the dose-response to bronchodilators in mechanically ventilated patients found effects with administration of 2.5 mg of albuterol using a standard nebulizer even under less than optimal conditions or with 4 actuations (400 µg) with a pMDI.[113] The pMDI was administered to stable COPD patients through a humidified ventilator circuit, with a chamber-style adapter placed in the inspiratory limb at the Y-piece. Actuations were synchronized to inspiration, with a pause of 20 to 30 seconds between actuations. Minimal therapeutic advantage was gained by administering higher doses, but the potential for side effects was increased.[112,113] In the routine clinical setting, higher doses of bronchodilators may be needed for patients with severe airway obstruction or if the technique of administration is not optimal. Because these results were observed with humidified ventilator circuits, we do not recommend bypassing the humidifier for routine bronchodilator therapy. In summary, when the technique of administration is carefully executed, most stable mechanically ventilated patients with COPD achieve near maximal bronchodilation after administration of 4 puffs of albuterol with a pMDI or 2.5 mg with a nebulizer. Dosing requirements for infants and small children during mechanical ventilation have not been established.

INHALER VERSUS NEBULIZER

Many investigators have demonstrated that nebulizers and pMDIs are equally effective in the treatment of airway obstruction in ambulatory children.[18] Similarly, nebulizers and pMDIs produce similar therapeutic effects in mechanically ventilated patients.[106]

The use of pMDIs for routine bronchodilator therapy in ventilator-supported patients is preferred because of several problems associated with the use of nebulizers. The rate of aerosol production by nebulizers is highly variable, not only in nebulizers from different manufacturers, but also in different batches of the same brand.[18] Furthermore, the nature of the aerosol produced, especially the particle size, is also highly variable among different nebulizers. The issue is further complicated because the operating efficiency of a nebulizer changes with the pressure of the driving gas and with different fill volumes. Because the pressure of the gas supplied by a ventilator to drive the nebulizer during inspiration is lower than that supplied by a tank/air compressor unit, the efficiency of some nebulizers can be drastically decreased in a ventilator circuit. The gas flow driving the nebulizer produces additional airflow in the ventilator circuit, necessitating adjustment of tidal volume and inspiratory flow when the nebulizer is in use. When patients are unable to trigger the ventilator during assisted modes of mechanical ventilation because of the additional nebulizer gas flow, hypoventilation can result.[114] Therefore, before using a nebulizer in a ventilator-supported patient, it is imperative to characterize its efficiency in a ventilator circuit under the typical clinical conditions for which it will be used.

Another problem associated with the use of nebulizers is bacterial contamination. Unless the nebulizers are scrupulously cleaned and disinfected, they could be a source for aerosolization of bacteria and pneumonia.[111] In contrast, pMDI aerosols are easy to administer, involve less personnel time, provide a reliable dose of the drug, and are free from the risk of bacterial contamination. When pMDIs are used with a collapsible cylindrical spacer, the ventilator circuit need not be disconnected with each treatment, thus reducing the risk of ventilator-associated pneumonia.

For infants or children with increased work of breathing or poor I:E ratios and for those in whom intubation is imminent, a nebulizer adapted to a resuscitation bag can be used. The same F_{IO_2} is used in the nebulizer and the resuscitation bag. Flow to the nebulizer should be optimal for the nebulizer used, and flow to the bag should be reduced to compensate for the flow from the nebulizer. When using a bag and mask to deliver medication, care must be taken to avoid gastric insufflation, pulmonary hyperinflation, and hyperventilation or hypoventilation. The mask is used to create a good seal, and attempts must be made to time the inflation with the inspiratory effort. Care must be taken to stabilize the ETT to prevent accidental extubation with the added weight of the equipment. The patient is ventilated using the same pressures and rate as with the mechanical ventilator. It is theoretically helpful to deliver an occasional sigh by providing a slight inspiratory hold at the peak inspiratory pressure, thereby enhancing the volume and depth of medication delivered while providing additional time for deposition to occur in the airways.

HOME CARE AND MONITORING COMPLIANCE

With most therapeutic aerosols being administered in the home, patient education and adherence with written medicine and action plans are critical. Standard nebulizers and pMDIs have no intrinsic mechanism for tracking use or compliance. The pMDI also has no mechanism to track how many doses remain in the canister. If accurately completed, medication diaries can help to track medication use and the use of rescue medications while monitoring prescription refill records.

Several aerosol delivery devices entering the market can directly track use and monitor compliance. These devices range from electronic models integrated with the nebulizer that track number of breaths taken, size of breaths, and duration and frequency of treatment, to simple counting devices attached to the pMDI actuator boot. More sophisticated devices allow monitoring of both pMDI use and expiratory maneuvers for later transmission to the care provider's office. Some newer DPI devices contain a built-in counter that advances each time a dose is loaded. These devices also give a visual signal when few doses remain in the device.

OTHER MEDICATIONS FOR AEROSOL DELIVERY

ANTIBIOTICS

Aerosol antibiotics can deliver high concentrations of antibiotics to the airway with low systemic bioavailability, thus reducing toxicity. This approach is of particular importance in patients with cystic fibrosis (CF), who frequently require courses of antibiotic therapy.[115] In a recent study, 468 patients with CF were enrolled in a 6-month masked, placebo-controlled trial of preservative-free, nonpyrogenic tobramycin aerosol, alternating between 4-week courses of tobramycin and placebo. During treatment the patients received 300 mg of tobramycin in 5 ml of 2.25-mg/L saline. The forced expiratory volume in 1 second (FEV_1) increased by more than 11% by the end of 6 months, with a 36% reduction in the mean number of hospital days and a 10-fold reduction in sputum bacterial density.[116] This medication is now commercially available as TOBI (Chiron). Other antibiotics are being prepared for aerosol delivery including colistin for nebulization and gentamicin in a DPI. The emergence of bacterial resistance to these antibiotics is a real risk and must be closely monitored.

MUCOACTIVE AGENTS

Sputum is expectorated mucus mixed with inflammatory cells, cellular debris, polymers of DNA and F-actin, as well as bacteria. Mucus is usually cleared by airflow and ciliary movement, and sputum is cleared by cough. RhDNase I (dornase alfa, Genentech) was the first approved mucoactive agent for the treatment of CF.[9] Dornase alfa is safe and effective, even in patients with more severe pulmonary disease defined as an FVC less than 40% of predicted value.[117] Efficacy has not yet been demonstrated for therapy of acute exacerbations of CF lung disease or for the treatment of other chronic airway diseases.[118]

Other mucoactive agents under development include mucolytics such as nacystelin (acetylcysteine lysinate), thymosin β_4, and low-molecular-weight dextran; mucokinetic agents such as surfactant; and mucoregulatory agents such as indomethacin and macrolides.

SURFACTANT

Randomized, masked, placebo-controlled studies demonstrate that surfactant aerosol improves pulmonary function and sputum transportability in patients with chronic bronchitis and CF and that this effect is dose dependent with no significant side effects.[119] As a wetting and spreading agent, the surfactant also has the ability to increase the lower airway deposition of other aerosol medications, such as dornase alfa or gene therapy vectors, and may increase small particle translocation through the mucus layer.[16]

HYPEROSMOLAR AEROSOLS

Sputum induction using hypertonic saline inhalation has been used to obtain specimens for the diagnosis of pneumonia. In one study, 58 CF patients were randomly assigned to receive 10 ml of either 0.9% normal saline or 6% hypertonic saline twice daily by USN.[120] Spirometry was measured for 2 weeks during therapy and 2 weeks after therapy. At 2 weeks there was a significant increase in the FEV_1 in the hypertonic saline group, with a return to baseline by 28 days. Despite pretreatment with 600 μg of inhaled albuterol, several patients had an acute decrease in the FEV_1 after inhaling the hypertonic saline. Although ready availability and low cost make hypertonic saline attractive, high salt concentration inactivating tracheal antibacterial peptides (defensins) and increasing the risk of airway infection is a concern.[72,121]

GENE TRANSFER THERAPY

Gene transfer therapy represents a novel use for aerosols. Efforts in this arena have largely centered on complementary (copy) DNA transfer of the normal CF transmembrane regulator (CFTR) gene in CF patients. Gene transfer was first attempted by inserting the normal CFTR gene into a replication-defective *Adenovirus* vector with bolus bronchoscopic delivery of the vector. An unanticipated host immune response to the vector led to reevaluation of this strategy.[121]

For gene transfer to be effective, the vector and its package must be nonimmunogenic, stable to shear forces during aerosolization, and safe to transfected cells. The vector should not increase cell turnover. It should either stably integrate into the progenitor (basal) cell genome or be safe and effective with repeated administration and should be able to reach the cellular target of relevance. Part of the difficulty with CF is that this cellular target has not been clearly identified as epithelial cell, goblet cell, submucous gland, or all of these. The amount of gene and vector and persistence in the airway must also be determined for each vector and delivery system.

Virus vectors that have been studied include adenoviruses, adeno-associated virus, and lentivirus. *Adenoviruses* naturally target the airway epithelium. *Adeno-associated viruses* are very small organisms that require a "helper" virus to replicate. These viruses are capable of site-directed insertion into DNA, reducing the risk of insertional mutagenesis (initiating cancer by activation of an oncogene or inactivation of an oncogene suppressor). *Lentiviruses* are retroviruses such as human immunodeficiency virus (HIV). They are able to transfect cells that are not terminally differentiated, such as the basal or airway progenitor cell, but insertional mutagenesis is a substantial risk.

The primary nonvirus vectors studied to date have been cationic *liposomes.* These lipid capsules are able to form complexes with DNA and then enter cells. With the first generation of liposome vectors, the efficiency of gene transfer was poor; however, this has improved dramatically with newer systems. The development of this technology will result in revolutionary aerosol generators.[122,123]

AEROSOLS FOR SYSTEMIC ADMINISTRATION

Aerosols can be targeted to different sites in the airway. Depending on the intrapulmonary behavior of each molecule, the aerosol mode of administration allows airway secretion, cellular delivery, or systemic delivery. Most medications are targeted to the airway epithelium, including the neuromuscular plexus (bronchodilators) and inflammatory cells (corticosteroids). Agents such as the P2Y ion channel activators are targeted directly to the ciliated epithelium. Mucolytics, proteases, and antibiotics are targeted to secretions in the airway rather than to the epithelial cells.

Very small particles targeted to the alveolus can be effective for systemic delivery of macromolecules through the extensive pulmonary vascular bed. Insulin is likely to be the first such medication introduced for systemic administration through aerosol administration, but other peptides and macromolecules are under development. Considerations for systemic administration include cost, convenience, efficacy, and safety. The pulmonary behavior of an inhaled molecule is not predictable and must be studied individually.

INSULIN

Insulin was one of the first medications to be administered by aerosol.[122] Because of the nebulizer and insulin formulation available at that time, absorption and efficacy were highly unpredictable. This has changed dramatically with the development of ultrafine particles and aerosol devices that can efficiently and reliably target the alveolar space.

With a rapid and smooth onset of action and elimination of the necessity for injections with their attendant risks and discomfort, inhaled insulin has great potential for clinical use. Intrapulmonary insulin administration to healthy subjects can induce significant hypoglycemia and a clinically relevant increase in serum insulin concentrations.[123] Once plasma glucose levels are normalized, postprandial glucose levels can be maintained below diabetic levels by delivering insulin into the lungs 5 minutes before ingestion of a meal.[124,125]

SUMMARY

The use of therapeutic aerosol medications is evolving from a basis of optimizing the delivery of asthma medications to the airway, to understanding how the extensive pulmonary vascular bed can be used for the systemic administration of a variety of macromolecules. Evolving and novel uses of therapeutic aerosols will require understanding aerosol generation, deposition, and translocation, as well as target organ physiology and pharmacology.

REFERENCES

 1. Newhouse MT, Dolovich MB: Control of asthma by aerosols. *N Engl J Med* 1986; 315:870-874.

2. Janson C: Plasma levels and effects of salbutamol after inhaled or i.v. administration in stable asthma. *Eur Respir J* 1991; 4:544-550.

3. Brain JD, Valberg PA: Deposition of aerosol in the respiratory tract. *Am Rev Respir Dis* 1979; 120:1325-1373.

4. Gross NJ, Jenne JW, Hess D: Bronchodilator therapy. In Tobin MJ, editor: *Principles and practice of mechanical ventilation*. New York. McGraw-Hill, 1994; pp 1077-1123.

5. Fink JB, Dhand R: Aerosol therapy. In Fink JB, Hunt G, editors: *Clinical practice in respiratory care*. Philadelphia. Lippincott-Raven, 1998.

6. Dolovich M: Physical principles underlying aerosol therapy. *J Aerosol Med* 1989; 2(2):171.

7. Pedersen S: Delivery systems in children. In Barnes PJ et al, editors: *Asthma*. Philadelphia. Lippincott-Raven, 1997; pp 1915-1929.

8. Yu CP, Nicolaides P, Soong TT: Effect of random airway sizes on aerosol deposition. *Am Ind Hyg Assoc J* 1979; 40:999-1005.

9. Desai MA, Mutlu M, Vadgama P: A study of macromolecular diffusion through native porcine mucus. *Experientia* 1992; 48:22-26.

10. Bolister N et al: The diffusion of beta-lactam antibiotics through mixed gels of cystic fibrosis–derived mucin and *Pseudomonas aeruginosa* alginate. *J Antimicrob Chemother* 1991; 27:285-293.

11. King M, Kelly S, Cosio M: Alteration of airway reactivity by mucus. *Respir Physiol* 1985; 62:47-59.

12. De Sanctis GT et al: Hyporesponsiveness to aerosolized but not to infused methacholine in cigarette-smoking dogs. *Am Rev Respir Dis* 1987; 135:338-344.

13. Bataillon V et al: The binding of amikacin to macromolecules from the sputum of patients suffering from respiratory diseases. *J Antimicrob Chemother* 1992; 29:499-508.

14. Taskar VS et al: Effect of bromhexeine on sputum amoxycillin levels in lower respiratory infections. *Respir Med* 1992; 86:157-160.

15. Stern M et al: The effect of mucolytic agents on gene transfer across a CF sputum barrier in vitro. *Gene Ther* 1998; 5:91-98.

16. Schürch S et al: Surfactant displaces particles toward the epithelium in airways and alveoli. *Respir Physiol* 1990; 80:17-32.

17. Kharasch VS et al: Pulmonary surfactant as a vehicle for intratracheal delivery of technetium sulfur colloid and pentamidine in hamster lungs. *Am Rev Respir Dis* 1991; 144:909-913.

18. Newhouse MT, Kennedy A: Rapid temperature change from +25° C to −15° C impairs powder deaggregation in Bricanyl Turbuhaler. *J Aerosol Med* 1999; 12:113.

19. Hess D et al: Medication nebulizer performance: effects of diluent volume, nebulizer flow, and nebulizer brand. *Chest* 1996; 110(2):498-505.

20. Johnson MA et al: Delivery of albuterol and ipratropium bromide from two nebulizer systems in chronic stable asthma: efficacy and pulmonary deposition. *Chest* 1989; 96:1-10.

21. Hadfield JW, Windebank WJ, Bateman JRM: Is driving gas flow clinically important for nebulizer therapy? *Br J Dis* 1986; 80:550-554.

22. Douglas JG et al: A comparative study of two doses of salbutamol nebulized at 4 and 8 L/min in patients with chronic asthma. *Br J Dis* 1986; 80:55-58.

23. Hess DR et al: The effect of heliox on nebulizer function using a beta-agonist bronchodilator. *Chest* 1999; 115:184-189.

24. Goode ML et al: Improvement in aerosol delivery with helium-oxygen mixtures during mechanical ventilation. *Am J Respir Crit Care Med* 2001; 163(1):109-114.

25. Malone RA et al: Optimal duration of nebulized albuterol therapy. *Chest* 1993; 104:1114-1118.

26. Thomas SH et al: Improving the efficiency of drug administration with jet nebulisers. *Lancet* 1988; 1:126.

27. Newnham DM, Lipworth BJ: Nebulizer performance, pharmacokinetics, airways and systemic effects of salbutamol given via a novel nebulizer system (Ventstream). *Thorax* 1994; 49:762-770.

28. Nebuliser Project Group of the British Thoracic Society Standards of Care Committee: Current best practice for nebuliser treatment. *Thorax* 1997; 52:S4-S16.

29. Standaert TA et al: Effects of repetitive use and cleaning techniques of disposable jet nebulizers on aerosol generation. *Chest* 1998; 114:577-586.

30. Centers for Disease Control and Prevention: Guideline for prevention of nosocomial pneumonia. *Respir Care* 1994; 39(12):1191-1236.

31. Oie S, Kamiya A: Bacterial contamination of aerosol solutions containing antibiotics. *Microbios* 1995; 82:109-113.

32. Lowenthal D, Kattan M: Facemasks versus mouthpieces for aerosol treatment of asthmatic children. *Pediatr Pulmonol* 1992; 14:192-196.

33. Dolovich MB et al: Pulmonary aerosol deposition in chronic bronchitis: intermittent positive pressure breathing vs quiet breathing. *Am Rev Respir Dis* 1967; 115:397-402.

34. Ilesa R, Listera P, Edmunds AT: Crying significantly reduces absorption of aerosolised drug in infant. *Arch Dis Child* 1999; 81:163-165.

35. American Academy of Pediatrics Committee on Infectious Diseases: Use of ribavirin in the treatment of respiratory syncytial virus infection. *Pediatrics* 1993; 92(3):501-504.

36. Harrison R: Reproductive risk assessment with occupational exposure to ribavirin aerosol. *Pediatr Infect Dis J* 1990; 9:S102-S105.

37. Kacmarek RM, Kratohvil J: Evaluation of a double-enclosure double-vacuum unit scavenging system for ribavirin administration. *Respir Care* 1992; 37:37-45.

38. Adderly RJ: Safety of ribavirin with mechanical ventilation. *Pediatr Infect Dis J* 1990; 9:S112-S114.

39. Phillips GD, Millard FJL: The therapeutic use of ultrasonic nebulizers in acute asthma. *Respir Med* 1994; 88(5):387-389.

40. Summer W et al: Aerosol bronchodilator delivery methods' relative impact on pulmonary function and cost of respiratory care. *Arch Intern Med* 1989; 149:618-622.

41. Yuksel B, Greenough A: Comparison of the effects on lung function of two methods of bronchodilator administration. *Respir Med* 1994; 88:229-233.

42. Nakanishi AK et al: Ultrasonic nebulization of albuterol is no more effective than jet nebulization for the treatment of acute asthma in children. *Chest* 1997; 97(6):1505-1508.

43. Lewis RA et al: Ultrasonic and jet nebulizers: differences in the physical properties and fractional deposition on the airway responses to nebulized water and saline aerosols. *Thorax* 1984; 39:712 (abstract).

44. Doershuk CF et al: Evaluation of jet type and ultrasonic nebulizers in mist tent therapy for cystic fibrosis. *Pediatrics* 1968; 41:723-732.

45. Boucher RGM, Kreuter J: Fundamentals of the ultrasonic atomization of medicated solutions. *Ann Allergy* 1968; 26:59.

46. Thomas SH et al: Delivery of ultrasonic nebulized aerosols to a lung model during mechanical ventilation. *Am Rev Respir Dis* 1993; 148(4, part 1):872-877.

47. Lin YZ, Hsieh KH: Metered dose inhaler and nebulizer in acute asthma. *Arch Dis Child* 1995; 72:214-218.

48. American Association for Respiratory Care: Clinical practice guideline: Selection of aerosol delivery device. *Respir Care* 1992; 37(8):891-897.

49. Newhouse MT, Dolovich M: *Aerosol therapy in children: basic mechanisms of pediatric respiratory disease, cellular and integrative.* New York. Dekker, 1991.

50. Svartengren K et al: Added external resistance reduces oropharyngeal deposition and increases lung deposition of aerosol particles in asthmatics. *Am J Respir Crit Care Med* 1995; 152:32-37.

51. Hill LS, Slater AL: A comparison of the performance of two modern multidose dry powder asthma inhalers. *Respir Med* 1998; 92:105-110.

52. Rajkumari NJ, Byron PR, Dalby RN: Testing of dry powder aerosol formulations in different environmental conditions. *Int J Pharmacol* 1995; 113:123-130.

53. Larsen JS et al: Evaluation of conventional press-and-breathe metered-dose inhaler technique in 501 patients. *J Asthma* 1994; 31(3):193-199.

54. Guidry GG et al: Incorrect use of metered dose inhalers by medical personnel. *Chest* 1992; 101(1):31-33.

55. Newman SP, Pavia D, Clarke SW: Simple instructions for using pressurized aerosol bronchodilators. *J R Soc Med* 1980; 73:776-779.

56. De Blaquiere P et al: Use and misuse of metered-dose inhalers by patients with chronic lung disease: a controlled randomized trial of two instruction methods. *Am Rev Respir Dis* 1989; 140:910-916.

57. Hampson NB, Mueller MP: Reduction in patient timing errors using a breath-activated metered dose inhaler. *Chest* 1994; 106(2):462-465.

58. Toogood JH et al: Use of spacer to facilitate inhaled corticosteroid treatment of asthma. *Am Rev Respir Dis* 1984; 129:723-729.

59. Diot P, Morra L, Smaldone GC: Albuterol delivery in a model of mechanical ventilation: comparison of metered-dose inhaler and nebulizer efficiency. *Am J Respir Crit Care Med* 1995; 152:1391-1394.

60. Salzman GA, Pyszczynski DR: Oropharyngeal candidiasis in patients treated with beclomethasone dipropionate delivered by metered-dose inhaler alone and with Aerochamber. *J Allergy Clin Immunol* 1988; 81:424-428.

61. Rubin BK: Pressurized metered-dose inhalers and holding chambers for inhaled glucocorticoid therapy in childhood asthma. *J Allergy Clin Immunol* 1999; 103:1224.

62. Closa RM et al: Efficacy of bronchodilators administered by nebulizers versus spacer deivces in infants with acute wheezing. *Pediatr Pulmonol* 1998; 26:344-348.

63. Williams JR, Bothner JP, Swanton RD: Delivery of albuterol in a pediatric emergency department. *Pediatr Emerg Care* 1996; 12:263-267.

64. Cunningham SJ, Crain EF: Reduction of morbidity in asthmatic children given a spacer device. *Chest* 1994; 106:753-757.

65. Ganderton D: The generation of respirable clouds from coarse powder aggregates. *J Biopharm Sci* 1992; 3: 101-105.

66. Dolovich M et al: Measurement of the particle size and dosing characteristics of a radiolabelled albuterol-sulphate lactose blend used in the SPIROS dry powder inhaler. In Dalby RN, Byron P, Farr SY, editors: *Respiratory drug delivery.* Buffalo Grove, NY. Interpharm Press, 1996; pp 332-335.

67. Engel T et al: Peak inspiratory flow rate and inspiratory vital capacity of patients with asthma measured with and without a new dry powder inhaler device (Turbuhaler). *Eur Respir J* 1990; 3:1037-1041.

68. Pederson S, Hansen OR, Fuglsang G: Influence of inspiratory flow rate on the effect of a Turbuhaler. *Arch Dis Child* 1990; 65:308-310.

69. Thorsson L, Edsbacke S, Conradson TB: Lung deposition from Turbuhaler is twice that from a pressurized metered-dose inhaler (pMDI). *Eur Respir J* 1994; 7:1839-1844.

70. Timsina MP et al: The effect of inhalation flow on the performance of a dry powder inhalation system. *Int J Pharm* 1992; 81:199-203.

71. Hindle M, Byron PR: Dose emissions from marketed dry powder inhalers. *Int J Pharm* 1995; 116:169-177.

72. Gansslen M: Uber inhalation von insulin. *Klin Wochenschr* 1925; 4:71

73. Bisgaard H et al: Inspiratory flow rate through the Diskus/Accuhaler inhaler and Turbuhaler inhaler in children with asthma. *J Aerosol Med* 1995; 8:100.

74. Smith KJ, Chan H-K, Brown KF: Influence of flow rate on particle size distributions from pressurised and breath actuated inhalers. *J Aerosol Med* 1998; 11:231-245.

75. Pederson S: Delivery options for the inhaled therapy in children over the age of 6 years. *J Aerosol Med* 1997; 10:41-44.

76. Fok TF et al: Aerosol delivery to non-ventilated infants by metered dose inhaler: should a valved spacer be used? *Pediatr Pulmonol* 1997; 24(3):204-212.

77. Kesten S et al: Patient handling of a multidose dry powder inhalation device for albuterol. *Chest* 1994; 105:1077-1081.

78. Rubin BK, Newhouse MH, Barnes PJ: *Conquering childhood asthma.* Decker, Hamilton, Canada,1998.

79. Rubin BK: Tracheomalacia as a cause of respiratory compromise in infants. *Clin Pulm Med* 1999; 6:195-197.

80. National Asthma Education and Prevention Program Expert Panel Report II: *Guidelines for the diagnosis and management of asthma.* National Institutes of Health, 1997.

81. Schuh S et al: High-versus low-dose, frequently administered nebulized albuterol in children with severe acute asthma. *Pediatrics* 1989; 83:513-518.

82. Colacone A et al: Continuous nebulization of albuterol (salbutamol) in acute asthma. *Chest* 1990; 97:693-697.

83. Portnoy J, Aggarwal J: Continuous terbutaline nebulization for the treatment of severe exacerbations of asthma in children. *Ann Allergy* 1988; 60:368-371.

84. Rebuck AS et al: Nebulized anticholinergic and sympathomimetic treatment of asthma and chronic obstructive airways disease in the emergency room. *Am J Med* 1987; 82:59-64.

85. Amado M, Portnoy J: A comparison of low and high doses of continuously nebulized terbutaline for treatment of severe exacerbations of asthma. *Ann Allergy* 1988; 60:165 (abstract).

86. Rubin BK, Albers GM: Use of anticholinergic bronchodilation in children. *Am J Med* 1996; 100:49S-53S.

87. Zorc JJ et al: Ipratropium added to asthma treatment in the pediatric emergency department. *Pediatrics* 1999; 103:748-752.

88. Lanes SF et al: The effect of adding ipratropium to salbutamol in the treatment of acute asthma: a pooled analysis of three trials. *Chest* 1998; 114:365-372.

89. Lin RY et L: Superiority of ipratropium plus albuterol over albuterol alone in the emergency department management of adults asthma: a randomized clinical trial. *Ann Emerg Med* 1998; 31:208-213.

90. Qureshi F et al: Effect of nebulized ipratropium on the hospitalization rates of children with asthma. *N Engl J Med* 1998; 339:1030-1035.

91. Schuh S et al: Efficacy of frequent nebulized ipratropium bromide added to frequent high-dose albuterol therapy in severe childhood asthma. *J Pediatr* 1995; 127:842.

92. Qureshi F et al: Effect of nebulized ipratropium on the hospitalization rates of children with asthma. *N Engl J Med* 1998; 339(15):1030-1035.

93. American Association for Respiratory Care: Aerosol consensus statement. *Chest* 1991; 100:1106-1109.

94. Fink JB, Dhand R: Bronchodilator therapy in mechanically ventilated patients. *Respir Care* 1999; 44:53-69.

95. Fink JB et al: Reconciling in vitro and in vivo measurements of aerosol delivery from a metered-dose inhaler during mechanical ventilation and defining efficiency-enhancing factors. *Am J Respir Crit Care Med* 1999; 159:63-68.

96. Hughes JM, Saez J: Effects of nebulizer mode and position in a mechanical ventilator circuit on dose efficiency. *Respir Care* 1987; 32:1131-1135.

97. Harvey CJ et al: Effect of a spacer on pulmonary aerosol deposition from a jet nebulizer during mechanical ventilation. *Thorax* 1995; 50:50-53.

98. Rau JL, Harwood RJ, Groff JL: Evaluation of a reservoir device for metered-dose bronchodilator delivery to intubated adults: an in vitro study. *Chest* 1992; 102:924-930.

99. Bishop MJ, Larson RP, Buschman DL: Metered dose inhaler aerosol characteristics are affected by the endotracheal tube actuator/adapter used. *Anesthesiology* 1990; 73:1263-1265.

100. Fuller HD et al: Efficiency of bronchodilator aerosol delivery to the lungs from the metered dose inhaler in mechanically ventilated patients: a study comparing four different actuator devices. *Chest* 1994; 105:214-218.

101. Manthous CA et al: Metered-dose inhaler versus nebulized albuterol in mechanically ventilated patients. *Am Rev Respir Dis* 1993; 148:1567-1570.

102. O'Riordan TG et al: Nebulizer function during mechanical ventilation. *Am Rev Respir Dis* 1992; 145:1117-1122.

103. Garner SS, Wiest DB, Bradley JW: Albuterol delivery by metered-dose inhaler with a pediatric mechanical ventilatory circuit model. *Pharmacotherapy* 1994; 14:210-214.

104. Fink JB et al: Deposition of aerosol from metered-dose inhaler during mechanical ventilation: an in vitro model. *Am J Respir Crit Care Med* 1996; 154:382-387.

105. Svartengren M et al: Human lung deposition of particles suspended in air or in helium/oxygen mixture. *Exp Lung Res* 1989; 15:575-585.

106. Anderson M et al: Deposition in asthmatics of particles inhaled in air or in helium-oxygen. *Am J Respir Crit Care Med* 1993; 147:524-528.

107. Fink J et al: Heliox increased delivery of albuterol from a MDI during mechanical ventilation: in in vitro model. *Am J Respir Crit Care Med* 1997; 155:A268.

108. Moren F, Andersson J: Fraction of dose exhaled after administration of pressurized inhalation aerosols. *Int J Pharm* 1980; 6:295-300.

109. O'Riordan TG, Palmer LB, Smaldone GC: Aerosol deposition in mechanically ventilated patients: optimizing nebulizer delivery. *Am J Respir Crit Care Med* 1994; 149:214-219.

110. Craven DE et al: Contaminated medication nebulizers in mechanical ventilator circuits: a source of bacterial aerosols. *Am J Med* 1984; 77:834-838.

111. Hamill RJ et al: An outbreak of *Burkholderia* (formerly *Pseudomonas*) *cepacia* respiratory tract colonization and infection associated with nebulized albuterol therapy. *Ann Intern Med* 1995; 122:762-766.

112. Thomas SHL et al: Pulmonary deposition of a nebulized aerosol during mechanical ventilation. *Thorax* 1993; 48: 154-159.

113. Dhand R et al: Dose response to bronchodilator delivered by metered-dose inhaler in ventilator-supported patients. *Am J Respir Crit Care Med* 1996; 154:388-393.

114. Beaty CD, Ritz RH, Benson MS: Continuous in-line nebulizers complicate pressure support ventilation. *Chest* 1989; 96:1360-1363.

115. Rubin BK: Emerging therapies for cystic fibrosis lung disease. *Chest* 1999; 115:1120-1126.

116. Ramsey BW et al: Efficacy of aerosolized tobramycin in patients with cystic fibrosis. *N Engl J Med* 1993; 328: 1740-1746.

117. Mccoy K, Hamilton S, Johnson C: Effects of 12-week administration of dornase alfa in patients with advanced cystic fibrosis lung disease. *Chest* 1996; 110:889-895.

118. Wilmott RW et al: Aerosolized recombinant human DNase in hospitalized cystic fibrosis patients with acute pulmonary exacerbations. *Am J Respir Crit Care Med* 1996; 153:1914-1917.

119. Anzueto A et al: Effects of aerosolized surfactant in patient with stable chronic bronchitis: a prospective randomized controlled trial. *JAMA* 1997; 278:1426-1431.

120. Eng PA et al: Short-term efficacy of ultrasonically nebulized hypertonic saline in cystic fibrosis. *Pediatr Pulmonol* 1996; 21:77-83.

121. Knowles MR et al: A controlled study of adenovirus-vector-mediated gene transfer in the nasal epithelium of patients with cystic fibrosis. *N Engl J Med* 1995; 333: 823-831.

122. Flotte TR, Carter BJ: In vivo gene therapy with adeno-associated virus vectors for cystic fibrosis. *Adv Pharmacol* 1997; 4:199-209.

123. Mallet JP, Diot P, Lemarie E: Inhalation route for administration of systemic drugs. *Rev Malad Respir* 1997; 14:257-267.

124. Heinemann L, Traut T, Heise T: Time-action profile of inhaled insulin. *Diabet Med* 1997; 14:63-67.

125. Jedle JH, Karlberg BE: Intrapulmonary administration of insulin to healthy volunteers. *J Int Med* 1996; 240:93-98.

126. Laube BL, Benedict GW, Dobs AS: The lung as an alternative route for delivery for insulin in controlling postprandial glucose levels in patients with diabetes. *Chest* 1998; 114:1734-1739.

Airway Clearance Techniques and Lung Volume Expansion

Brian K. Walsh
Kathy Davidson

Classic airway clearance techniques are designed to remove secretions from the lungs and include postural drainage, percussion, chest wall vibration, and coughing. Newer techniques considered part of chest physical therapy (CPT) are maneuvers to improve the efficacy of cough, such as the forced expiration technique (FET); positive expiratory pressure (PEP) therapy; high-frequency chest compression (HFCC); and specialized breathing techniques, such as autogenic drainage (AD). Because all of these techniques share the same goal—removal of bronchial secretions—the term *bronchial drainage* is often employed to describe them collectively. This term may be preferable to CPT because it highlights the aims, rather than the means, of treatment. This chapter is devoted to describing and analyzing bronchial drainage techniques and how they should be applied to the infant or pediatric patient with lung disease or respiratory impairment.

HISTORY AND CURRENT STATUS OF AIRWAY CLEARANCE TECHNIQUES

Postural drainage was used as early as 1901 in the treatment of bronchiectasis.[1] In the 1960s and 1970s we saw an increase in the use of CPT.[2] It was introduced in many U.S. hospitals concurrent with a wave of mounting criticism of intermittent positive-pressure breathing (IPPB) therapy. Many institutions found that the routine use of IPPB was replaced with routine use of CPT. Beginning in the late 1970s, experts in the field began to point to the lack of evidence to support the routine use of CPT in pulmonary disorders such as pneumonia and chronic bronchitis.[3] However, despite a steady stream of criticism, the use of CPT appears to have increased dramatically in the past decade.[4-12]

CHEST PHYSICAL THERAPY TECHNIQUES

Classic CPT has four components: (1) postural drainage, (2) percussion, (3) vibration of the chest wall, and (4) coughing.

POSTURAL DRAINAGE

Postural drainage attempts to use gravity to move secretions from peripheral airways to the larger bronchi, from which they are more easily expectorated. The patient is placed in various positions, each designed to drain specific segments of the lung, and may be supported by rolled towels, blankets, or pillows. Figs. 14-1 and 14-2 illustrate postural drainage positions used in infants and children.[13] Other versions incorporating minor variations have also been published.[2,14,15] Postural drainage can be performed with or without percussion or vibration. When accompanied by percussion or vibration, each position is maintained for 1 to 5 minutes, depending on the severity of the patient's condition. When percussion or vibration is omitted, longer periods of simple postural drainage can be performed.

PERCUSSION

Percussion is believed to loosen secretions from the bronchial walls. While the patient is in the various postural drainage positions, the clinician percusses the chest wall using a cupped hand (Fig. 14-3). The areas to be percussed are illustrated in Figs. 14-1 and 14-2. Clinicians should not percuss over bony prominences; over the spine, sternum, abdomen, last few ribs, sutured areas, drainage tubes, kidneys, or liver; or below the rib cage. The ideal frequency of percussion is unknown; however, some reports recommend a frequency of 5 to 6 Hz (300 to 360 blows/min), whereas others recommend slow, rhythmic clapping.[14,16] Several devices can be used for percussion, including soft face masks as well as those commercially designed, such as "palm cups" and mechanical percussors (Fig. 14-4). Infants and children may have CPT performed in the lap of the clinician. However, if the patient is mechanically ventilated or has multiple tubes and intravenous lines in place, it may be preferable to perform therapy with the patient in the bed. Catheters, tubes, and indwelling lines are easily dislodged in infants and young children, and appropriate care must be taken.

POSTURAL DRAINAGE AND PERCUSSION

Many investigations have been conducted to determine the relative importance of percussion, vibration, and postural drainage. In a study designed to determine the contribution of these maneuvers to clearance of mucus, there was no demonstration of improvement in clearance of mucus from the lung when percussion, vibration, or breathing exercises were added to postural drainage.[17] These investigators also showed that FET was superior to simple coughing and when combined with postural drainage was the most effective form of treatment.[18] Other studies have reported that (1) percussion without postural drainage or cough produced minimal change in clearance of mucus; (2) when compared with simple postural drainage, chest percussion actually reduced the amount of sputum mobilized; and (3) manual self-percussion did not increase the amount of sputum expectorated compared with simple postural drainage in a group of patients with cystic fibrosis (CF).[19-21]

VIBRATION OF THE CHEST WALL

Vibrations are an additional method of transmitting energy through the chest wall to loosen or move bronchial secretions. Unlike in percussion, the clinician's hand does not lose contact with the chest wall during the procedure. Vibrations are performed by placing both hands (one over the other) over the area to be vibrated and tensing and contracting the shoulder and arm muscles while the patient exhales. To prolong exhalation, the patient may be asked to breathe through pursed lips or make a "hissing" sound. As with percussion, the ideal frequency is unknown, although some recommend 10 to 15 Hz.[22] It is unclear how well clinicians are able to perform vibrations at this frequency. Several mechanical vibrators are commercially available. An electric toothbrush with foam padding covering the bristle or a padded syringe barrel attached to the handle of the toothbrush can be used with an infant. Some models of mechanical percussors or vibrators are appropriate only for the newborn or premature infant, whereas other models are appropriate for the larger child. When evaluating such devices, the clinician should consider if the appearance and sound of the device will be frightening and if the amount of force is appropriate for the size of the patient. All percussion and vibration devices should be cleaned after each use.

CHEST PHYSICAL THERAPY IN THE NEWBORN

Collapse of the right upper lobe after extubation is a common complication in the premature infant, and routine treatment of premature infants after extubation is common.[23,24] Treatment may be given to the right upper lobe only and need not be prolonged, nor does it require the routine use of percussion. A treatment length of 5 minutes is sufficient, and vibration

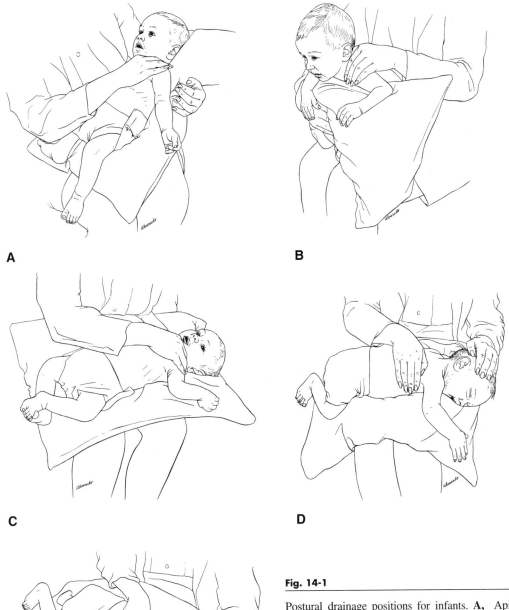

Fig. 14-1

Postural drainage positions for infants. **A,** Apical segment of the right upper lobe and apical subsegment of the apical-posterior segment of the left upper lobe. **B,** Posterior segment of the right upper lobe and posterior subsegment of the apical-posterior segment of the left upper lobe. **C,** Anterior segments of right and left upper lobes. **D,** Superior segments of both lower lobes. **E,** Posterior basal segments of both lower lobes.

Continued

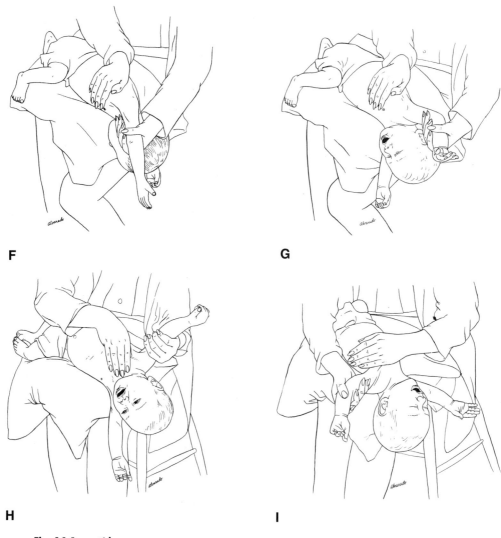

Fig. 14-1, cont'd

Postural drainage positions for infants. **F,** Lateral basal segment of the right lower lobe. Lateral basal segment of the left lower lobe is drained in a similar fashion but with the right side down. **G,** Anterior basal segment of the right lower lobe. The segments on the left side are drained in a similar fashion but with the right side down. **H,** Right middle lobe. **I,** Left lingular segment of lower lobe. (From Waring WW: Diagnostic and therapeutic procedures. In Chernick V, editor: *Kendig's disorders of the respiratory tract in children,* ed 5. Philadelphia. WB Saunders, 1990; pp 86-87.)

is applied to the right upper lobe in one of the three standard drainage positions every 1 to 3 hours for 24 to 48 hours.[24]

Patients with esophageal atresia and tracheoesophageal fistula often require assistance in mobilization of thick secretions. Aspiration of oropharyngeal secretions, leading to atelectasis or pneumonia, is common. If surgical repair has been performed, deep endotracheal suctioning (beyond the tip of the endotracheal tube) is contraindicated because the suction catheter may reopen the closed fistula. Likewise, nonintubated patients should rarely have the catheter advanced more than 7 cm because this makes removal of secretions more difficult. Occasionally, tracheal suction under direct vision using a laryngoscope is necessary. If the fistula has been closed, Trendelenburg positioning may be used. This is especially helpful if the patient has difficulty clear-

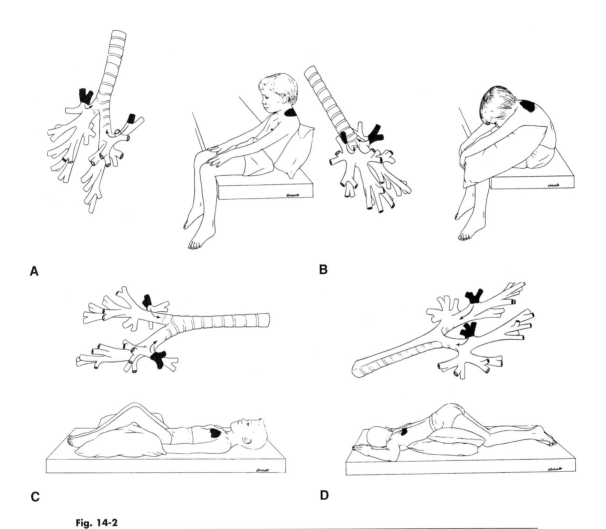

Fig. 14-2

Postural drainage positions for the child or adult. The model of the tracheobronchial tree above the child illustrates the segmental bronchi being drained. The stippled area over the child's chest illustrates the area to be percussed or vibrated. The area is described in the parentheses. **A,** Apical segment of right upper lobe and apical subsegment of apical-posterior segment of left upper lobe (area between the clavicle and top of the scapula). **B,** Posterior segment of right upper lobe and posterior subsegment of apical-posterior segment of left upper lobe (area over the upper back). **C,** Anterior segments of right and left upper lobes (area between clavicle and nipple). **D,** Superior segments of both lower lobes (area over middle of back at tip of scapula, beside spine). *Continued*

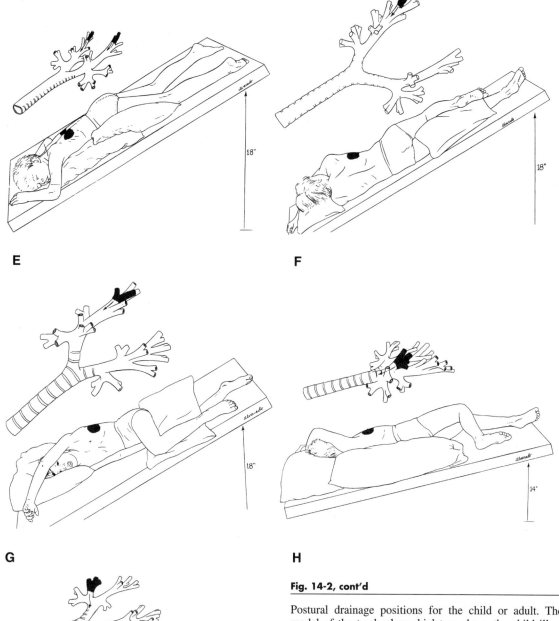

E

F

G

H

I

Fig. 14-2, cont'd

Postural drainage positions for the child or adult. The model of the tracheobronchial tree above the child illustrates the segmental bronchi being drained. The stippled area over the child's chest illustrates the area to be percussed or vibrated. The area is described in the parentheses. **E,** Posterior basal segments of both lower lobes (area over lower rib cage, beside spine). **F,** Lateral basal segment of right lower lobe. Segment on left is drained in a similar fashion but with the right side down (area over middle portion of rib cage). **G,** Anterior basal segment of left lower lobe. Segment on right is drained in a similar fashion but with the left side down (area over lower ribs, below the armpit). **H,** Right middle lobe (area over right nipple; below breast in developing females). **I,** Left lingular segment of lower lobe (area over left nipple; below breast in developing females). (From Waring WW: Diagnostic and therapeutic procedures. In Chernick V, editor: *Kendig's disorders of the respiratory tract in children,* ed 5. Philadelphia. WB Saunders, 1990; pp 84-85.)

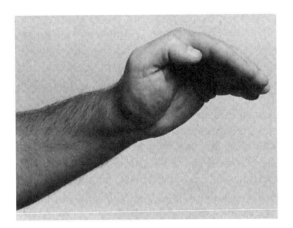

Fig. 14-3

Proper cupping of hand for percussion.

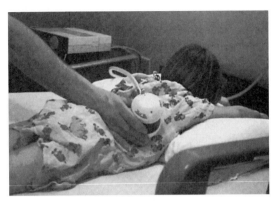

Fig. 14-4

Percussion being performed on a child using a manual percussor.

ing oral secretions by swallowing. These patients should not be routinely placed flat on their backs because this promotes aspiration of oral secretions. Given that a thoracotomy has been performed to repair the defect, use of a small mechanical vibrator may be preferable to chest percussion.

The clinician must be careful to avoid excessive movement (extension or extreme turning) while treating the infant. Esophageal atresia is repaired by performing an anastomosis of the distal and proximal esophagus. Excessive head movement may result in its disruption. Many other patients often require CPT in the neonatal intensive care unit. Usually, such patients have been intubated for some time and have responded to prolonged intubation with excessive production of secretions.

CHEST PHYSICAL THERAPY IN YOUNG CHILDREN

When performing CPT on young children, the clinician must make a special effort to secure the patient's confidence and cooperation. Some children may have seen CPT performed on other patients and may conclude that it is a painful procedure. Spending a few moments to gain the child's confidence is well worth the effort. Assigning the same clinician to treat the child as often as is practical may be useful in establishing a rapport. Likewise, allowing the child as much control over the situation as possible, such as deciding which lobes will be treated first, may increase the child's sense of control and reduce hospitalization-related anxiety. Having a parent available during therapy, especially when the child is unfamiliar with CPT, is useful as well.

CPT may be extremely uncomfortable for the postoperative patient, and routine use of CPT in these patients may actually promote atelectasis. Some patients, however, suffer from excessive secretions or mucus plugging and atelectasis. Performing CPT in these patients can be difficult. Adequate analgesia is essential, and attempts should be made to schedule CPT shortly after pain medication is administered. Coughing is also a considerable source of discomfort in pediatric patients postoperatively. Cough efficacy can be improved if the patient is taught to splint the wounds when coughing. Holding a pillow over the incision may also be useful in minimizing movement of the incision when coughing.

Adverse Consequences

Several conditions common to the full-term or preterm newborn suggest that these infants may be at risk for increased complications from CPT; therefore modification of routine CPT procedures is advisable. Because the newborn has high chest wall compliance, the loss of lung volume due to chest wall compression (e.g., from percussion) may be greater in the infant than in the adult.[25] For this reason, some institutions routinely omit chest wall percussion in neonatal CPT treatments, opting instead for the use of small vibrators. Because an infant's chest wall is not as thick as an adult's, and the infant's ribs are more cartilaginous, a gentler touch is required during therapy.[26] Hypoxemia has been reported after CPT in the newborn.[27-30] Handling infants, for whatever reason, frequently results in hypoxemia. It is therefore essential that oxygenation be monitored during CPT in infants.

Routine application of CPT in the preterm infant has been associated with an increased risk of intraventricular hemorrhage (IVH).[31] The preterm infant is unable to adequately regulate cerebral blood flow, and changes in blood pressure often lead to increased intracranial pressure and volume, with rupture of immature blood vessels. Trendelenburg positioning and chest wall percussion would seem likely to increase cerebral blood flow and to reduce venous return, further increasing the risk of IVH. Therefore these procedures should be used sparingly, if at all, in infants at risk. If possible, CPT should be withheld from infants at high risk for IVH (i.e., very premature infants in the first few days of life).

Critically ill newborns are unable to adequately maintain body temperature and are therefore routinely placed in isolettes (incubators) or under radiant warmers. Caregiver interventions of any kind, including CPT, interfere with maintaining temperature stability, especially for infants in closed isolettes. Treatment time with these patients should be kept to a minimum, usually between 5 and 10 minutes. If a patient is in a temperature-regulated environment, special attention must be given to preventing heat loss during therapy.

The trachea and bronchi of the newborn appear especially vulnerable to damaging effects from endotracheal tubes and suction catheters. Consequences of deep endotracheal suctioning include the development of bronchial stenosis and granulomas. Avoiding deep endotracheal suctioning minimizes these risks.[32] Therefore, when suctioning intubated infants after CPT, the suction catheter should not be routinely advanced beyond the end of the endotracheal tube. If there is evidence of persistent secretion retention despite adequate suction of the endotracheal tube, the suction catheter can be carefully and slowly advanced 1 or 2 cm beyond the tip of the endotracheal tube.

Many infants in the neonatal intensive care unit are sensitive to handling. This is especially true of the preterm infant as well as the full-term infant with pulmonary hypertension, who may develop hypoxemia or bradycardia in response to excessive stimulation. Many clinicians believe that the adverse consequences of handling can be minimized by clustering as many caregiver interventions as possible, thereby leaving the infant undisturbed for longer periods. Minimizing excessive light and sound associated with therapy is also desirable.

COUGH

All CPT sessions should end with a period of coughing. Patients with minimal lung disease should be able to clear the lungs after one or two attempts. Those with severe lung disease may need more prolonged coughing periods. Prolonged periods of unproductive coughing should be avoided because they may tire the patient. The clinician should emphasize effective, productive coughing. Infants may require nasopharyngeal suction to stimulate a cough, whereas patients with artificial airways may require endotracheal suctioning.

The following procedures are sometimes incorporated into CPT treatments, or used independently, with the aim of promoting bronchial drainage: (1) FET, (2) PEP therapy, (3) AD, and (4) automatic HFCC.

FORCED EXPIRATION TECHNIQUE

FET is also known as "huff" coughing. This maneuver requires the patient to forcibly exhale, from a middle to low lung volume, with an open glottis. This is repeated several times, following which the patient coughs to remove any loosened mucus.[33] FET can be used alone or in conjunction with other forms of therapy. It is designed to prevent dynamic airway collapse by preventing the explosive pressure changes associated with coughing.[8,33] Studies have documented that patients with long-standing lung disorders that are characterized by destruction or weakening of the bronchial wall, such as CF and bronchiectasis, have ineffective coughing secondary to dynamic airway compression while coughing.[34] The developers of this technique now use the term *active cycle of breathing* to refer to FET. They emphasize the importance of interspersing "huff" coughs with periods of deep, relaxed breathing. This helps prevent bronchospasm and ensures sufficient lung volume to promote an effective cough.

COUGHING AND FORCED EXPIRATION TECHNIQUE

Over the years, a number of investigators have demonstrated that the single most important component of CPT is vigorous coughing.[35-39] Simple postural drainage has been reported to improve secretion clearance, whereas the addition of percussion did not.[36] Several other studies in patients with CF and other chronic lung diseases likewise support the notion that vigorous coughing, especially when used in conjunction with FET, may be as effective as postural drainage and percussion.[37,38,40]

Many clinicians, however, are reluctant to abandon postural drainage, percussion, or vibration in favor of simple FET, especially in patients needing life-long assistance with secretion removal, such as those with CF. A 3-year prospective study in children with CF demonstrated that conventional CPT, performed twice a day, was more effective than FET used at the same frequency.[41] Patients performing

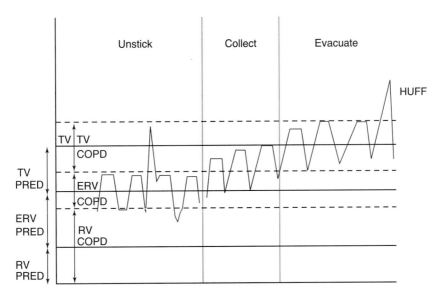

Fig. 14-5

Graphic illustration of the depth of successive breaths by lung volumes using the autogenic drainage technique. *TV,* Tidal volume; *ERV,* expiratory reserve volume; *RV,* residual volume; *HUFF,* Huff maneuver; *PRED,* predicted; *COPD,* chronic obstructive pulmonary disease.

FET in this study had an average age of slightly younger than 12 years. In contrast, patients in studies that showed FET to be successful were older.[38,40] This suggests that forms of self-care may be more effective in adolescents than in younger children, who perhaps require more supervision. Likewise, comparison of studies on the efficacy of exercise as pulmonary therapy in CF suggests that self-therapy is more effective in older patients.[42,43]

POSITIVE EXPIRATORY PRESSURE THERAPY

PEP therapy uses an expiratory resistor, coupled with the patient's active expiration, to generate positive airway pressure throughout expiration. This prevents dynamic airway collapse and improves clearance of mucus.[44] It is widely used in Europe, and increasingly in the United States, as an adjunct or substitute for conventional CPT in the treatment of CF or bronchiectasis, and to a lesser extent in postoperative patients. A variety of devices are available to serve as expiratory resistors. PEP therapy is essentially the same as the "blow-bottles" that have been used to prevent postoperative atelectasis.[45] Both PEP therapy and FET are advocated as forms of simple, self-treatment for patients with CF.

AUTOGENIC DRAINAGE

AD is a series of breathing exercises designed to mobilize secretions in patients with bronchiectasis or CF.[46-48] To loosen secretions from the smallest airways, the patient begins breathing in a slow, controlled manner, first at the expiratory reserve volume (ERV) level. The volume of ventilation is then increased, with the patient breathing in the normal tidal volume range but exhaling approximately halfway into the ERV. This moves secretions from the peripheral to the middle airways. Finally, the depth of inspiration is increased, with the patient inhaling maximally to total lung capacity and exhaling as before about halfway into the ERV. Fig. 14-5 graphically illustrates the autogenic drainage technique. Advocates of AD claim that its simplicity (no devices or clinicians are needed) and efficacy make it an ideal form of self-treatment for patients with CF.

POSITIVE EXPIRATORY PRESSURE THERAPY AND AUTOGENIC DRAINAGE

PEP therapy, AD, and HFCC have been shown to be highly effective. PEP therapy, especially, has been shown by a number of researchers to be beneficial in mobilizing secretions and preserving pulmonary function in CF patients, and with FET it was marginally superior to simple FET and postural drainage.[49-56] Less information is available on AD, although a few reports indicate it is highly effective and that compliance is improved.[46-48,57]

HIGH-FREQUENCY CHEST COMPRESSION

A commercially available device (ThAIRpy Bronchial Drainage System, American Biosystems) has been developed that compresses the entire chest wall at high frequencies by means of a snug-fitting inflatable vest connected to a high-performance air compressor (Fig. 14-6). Intermittent chest wall compression produces brief periods of high expiratory air flow, which loosens and mobilizes mucus from bronchial walls.[58] The device is widely used in patients with CF (see Chapter 35).

HFCC has also been evaluated in a long-term study. After a 22-month period of using HFCC as the sole form of CPT, patients experienced a small but significant improvement in pulmonary function. In contrast, after a similar period on conventional manual CPT, pulmonary function declined somewhat.[58] HFCC does not require the patient to perform postural drainage (known to be effective for sputum mobilization) and incorporates rapid percussion (generally demonstrated to be ineffective). What accounts for this seeming paradox? HFCC compresses the chest at frequencies up to 22 Hz, which is much higher than can be generated by manual percussion (5 to 8 Hz). Furthermore, compression is usually applied only on exhalation.

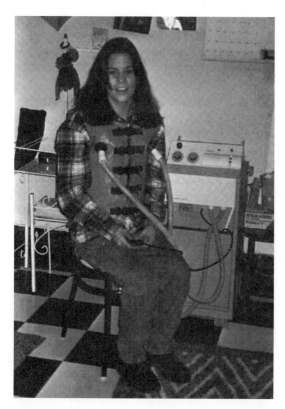

Fig. 14-6

Patient wearing an inflatable vest during high-frequency chest compression therapy in the home.

In the initial studies with HFCC, the developers of this device measured expiratory volumes and flows and selected the frequencies that resulted in the highest values for these variables. High expiratory air flow is maintained with HFCC, even at low lung volumes. The result is multiple, brief periods of high expiratory air flow (or more precisely air velocity), similar to "huff" coughing or FET.[59]

High expiratory air velocity at low lung volumes produces the greatest air-mucus interaction and hence mucus mobilization. HFCC does not directly dislodge mucus from the bronchial wall, as conventional percussion is thought to do, but instead simulates multiple coughs or FETs by generating high expiratory air velocities. Because the compressive phase of HFCC is brief (as short as 0.02 second at a frequency of 22 Hz) and the glottis remains open during therapy, it is unlikely that dynamic airway collapse occurs, as happens with natural coughing in patients with bronchiectasis or CF.

Manual percussion bears little resemblance to HFCC. In contrast to HFCC, manual percussion is rarely, if ever, adjusted to produce optimal expiratory air flow to simulate cough or FET. In addition, it is given during inspiration as well as expiration, which may limit the deep breathing that is essential for producing high expiratory air velocities. Finally, manual percussion is applied only to a small portion of the chest wall at once, which may be insufficient to generate adequate expiratory flows.

EFFECTIVENESS OF TECHNIQUES

Proponents of conventional CPT techniques often describe the problem that CPT aims to treat as abnormal (excessive, thick, tenacious) secretions. Although this is partially correct, therapies that would seem to attack this problem directly have proved disappointing. Manual, low-frequency chest percussion does not seem to jar mucus loose from the airways, nor does chest wall vibration. Of the therapies that do work—postural drainage, PEP, AD, FET, and the HFCC system—all attempt to prevent or compensate for dynamic airway collapse. Postural drainage attempts to move mucus passively, by force of gravity, past the damaged, collapsible portions of the airways and toward less-diseased, more rigid central airways. The remaining therapies attempt to prevent dynamic airway collapse while at the same time produce high expiratory air velocity at low lung volumes. This develops the shearing forces required to mobilize sputum.[4] A novel explanation for the efficacy of simple postural drainage is suggested by Lannefors and Wollmer, who demonstrated improved mucus clearance in the dependent lung of patients undergoing postural drainage.[60] For most patients, lung volumes and airway diameter are reduced in the dependent lung but ventilation is increased. These factors result in increased air movement at high velocity, which increases turbulence and shearing in small airways and results in greater mobilization of mucus.

Deep breathing associated with vigorous exercise has also been shown to be an effective technique for mobilization of secretions in patients with CF.[61,62] To accommodate the increased ventilatory demands of exercise, rate and depth of breathing are increased and active exhalation may occur. Hence, vigorous exercise produces a ventilatory pattern that, like AD or FET, increases air velocity at low lung volumes and promotes sputum mobilization.

"Take a deep breath and you'll feel better." This is a sound piece of advice that was given long before the advent of incentive spirometry or IPPB. Taking a deep breath to total lung capacity, either by sighing or yawning, is a normal, unconscious maneuver performed periodically to keep the lungs inflated and to avoid ventilation-perfusion mismatch.[63] When the breathing pattern becomes one of tidal ventilation without periodic maximal inflation, atelectasis ensues within a few hours.[64] Variations in the normal pattern of breathing may result in respiratory complications and an increase in postoperative morbidity and mortality. Changes in the breathing patterns of pediatric patients are most often caused by increased sedation, narcotics, pain, fluid overload, parenchymal lung damage, fear and anxiety, and abdominal or thoracic surgery. It has been estimated that 10% to 40% and even as many as 70% of patients undergoing abdominal or thoracic surgery experience postoperative pulmonary complications,[65,66] consisting of atelectasis, pneumonia, pulmonary embolism, and hypoxemia. These conditions are believed to be caused by reduced diaphragmatic movement (especially after upper abdominal surgery), changes in chest wall muscle tone, and secretion retention, all of which result in decreased lung volumes.[67]

The modalities and methods used to increase a child's lung volume can be classified as (1) voluntary—using the patient's own effort and initiative to sustain a deep breath (incentive spirometry) and (2) applied—providing the patient with a positive-pressure–generated breath to achieve an increase in lung volume (IPPB). In this chapter these methods of lung volume expansion therapy are discussed as they relate to the pediatric patient.

INCENTIVE SPIROMETRY

Incentive spirometry, also referred to as sustained maximal inspiration, was introduced in the early 1970s in an effort to prevent postoperative pulmonary complications.[68,69] It was designed to encourage patients to improve their inspiratory volumes while visualizing their inspiratory effort. Forced expiratory maneuvers using devices such as blow bottles, blow gloves, and balloons have been prescribed in the past to prevent postoperative complications; however, they have been associated with the development of atelectasis and do not result in the same physiologic effects as incentive spirometry.[70-72] Although it is still debated which methods are most effective for the prevention and management of postoperative pulmonary complications, it is estimated that incentive spirometry is prescribed in 95% of all U.S. hospitals for prophylaxis and treatment of postoperative atelectasis.[73-77] The objectives of incentive spirometry are to prevent or reverse atelectasis, improve lung volumes, and improve inspiratory muscle performance (including use of the diaphragm).[70]

INDICATIONS, CONTRAINDICATIONS, AND COMPLICATIONS

Clinical conditions that may benefit from incentive spirometry are listed in Box 14-1.[70] Clinical symptoms often include fever, increased work of breathing, tachypnea, hypoxia, and evidence of atelectasis on the chest radiograph. For incentive spirometry to be effective in the pediatric patient, he or she must be able to cooperate and understand the procedure and to be able to breathe volumes exceeding his or her normal tidal volume.

Incentive spirometry is contraindicated in patients who cannot cooperate or follow instructions concerning the proper use of the device. The child may be uncooperative, physically disabled, or simply too young to effectively perform the maneuvers. Alternative methods to improve lung volumes should then be considered.[78,79]

The majority of problems that patients experience with incentive spirometry are the result of inadequate supervision or instruction, or both. These two factors account for a large number of ineffective treatments.[80] Hyperventilation may occur in the patient who performs the maneuvers too rapidly, and he or she may complain of lightheadedness or

---

BOX 14-1

INDICATIONS FOR INCENTIVE SPIROMETRY

Abdominal surgery
Thoracic surgery
Surgery in patients with pulmonary disease
Atelectasis
Restrictive lung defects associated
  with quadriplegia
Restrictive lung defects associated
  with a dysfunctional diaphragm

tingling in the fingers. The patient may also complain of fatigue during the procedure. These complaints can be alleviated by coaching the patient to slow down and rest between each maneuver. Pain from surgical incisions is frequently encountered postoperatively and can be decreased by splinting the surgical area with a pillow during deep breathing and coughing. Airway closure and bronchospasm may occur if the patient exhales forcefully to less than functional residual capacity before taking a deep inspiration. Again, this can be avoided with proper coaching by the clinician. Hypoxia may develop if the patient's oxygen therapy is interrupted, especially when a mask is used. This can be prevented by using a nasal cannula during therapy.

DEVICES

The original Bartlett-Edwards incentive spirometer operated on a piston-bellows principle and was designed to fall open by gravity at a preset volume. A battery-operated light was activated when the patient inhaled from the spirometer and the preset volume was reached. To keep the light on, the patient had to continue to inhale. The light went off when the patient's glottis closed or total lung capacity was reached.[81] There are many different types and brands of incentive spirometers, including disposable and nondisposable devices. They are classified according to how inhalation is activated: (1) volume-oriented or (2) flow-oriented.

Most of the current volume-oriented incentive spirometers are based on the original Bartlett-Edwards spirometer. A volume is preset as a goal, and the patient is instructed to inhale until the preset goal is reached. The spirometer volume is measured according to the amount of volume displaced during the inhalation. Flow-oriented spirometers operate by using a floating ball or bar that is raised by the negative flow generated with inspiration. The more rapid and forceful the inspiratory flow, the higher the ball rises. Although differences in the inspiratory work of breathing among the various incentive spirometers have been reported, in terms of clinical outcome the differences among the devices appear to be negligible.[82,83] The device used will vary from one institution to another and may even vary among patients within the institution. Regardless of the type, the operator's instructions should be read and universal precautions followed.[84]

PROCEDURE

Because the effectiveness of incentive spirometry relies mainly on the patient's effort and cooperation, it is essential that the procedure is understood. Even though incentive spirometry is routine to the clinician, it is not routine to the patient, and its impor-

tance, as well as its technique, should be thoroughly explained. The teaching session should be conducted preoperatively, before the child experiences the pain and trauma of surgery. The parents should be involved in the teaching process whenever possible because they eventually assume the role of coach. The explanation should include the reason for therapy, how to use the incentive spirometry device, the goals of therapy, what is expected postoperatively, the importance of an effective cough, and how the patient may feel after surgery. The use of charts and pictures is especially effective with young patients. Explaining to the older patient that he or she normally sighs every 6 to 10 minutes and that the spirometer helps to make up for this is a simple way to emphasize the reason for the therapy. The specific incentive spirometer used should be shown to the child and family. A demonstration unit can be used to show the child exactly how to breathe and how the spirometer functions. The patient should then demonstrate its use. It may take several attempts before the patient can effectively use the device. If the patient cannot be instructed preoperatively, the postoperative teaching should be carried out only after the patient is awake and alert enough to follow instructions. If preoperative instruction has taken place, the postoperative teaching should briefly review the procedure and specifically convey to the patient the frequency and duration prescribed by the physician (Fig. 14-7).

APPLICATION

The patient should be positioned in an upright sitting position or a semi-Fowler position so that there is minimal restriction to chest expansion. This may not be possible depending on the type of surgery or injuries that the patient might have received. The chest should be auscultated and the volume goal on the incentive spirometer preset. In the postoperative patient, the goal should begin with 75% of the preoperative volume and be increased or decreased according to the patient's ability. The patient should be instructed to exhale normally and then to place the mouth tightly around the mouthpiece and to inhale as slowly and deeply as possible through the mouth. Inspiring slowly will assist in even distribution of air to the alveoli. The breath should be held at end inspiration for 3 to 5 seconds and followed by a normal exhalation.[70] The patient should then remove the mouthpiece and exhale slowly. The patient should be allowed a short time to rest between maneuvers to help prevent fatigue and dizziness. A nose clip can be used for the patient who continues to inhale through the nose. The maximum volume of air the patient inhales is noted. (When teaching the use of this device preoperatively, the volume obtained should be

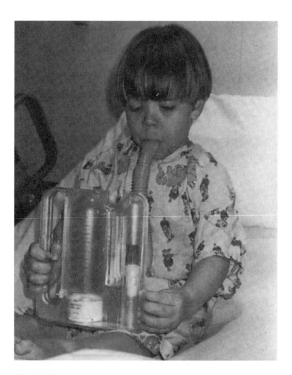

Fig. 14-7

Child using incentive spirometry device.

recorded and used postoperatively as a baseline.) The number of maneuvers to be performed per session should be either prescribed by the physician or set by departmental policy. Several sources have suggested 5 to 10 *effective* breaths per treatment as an adequate frequency.[70] The patient should cough during the session whenever it is felt necessary and then again when the maneuvers have been completed. The postoperative patient may need assistance with splinting of the incision during coughing as well as during deep breathing. A pillow or folded blanket can be placed over the incision area. The inspiratory volume goal may be increased when the patient reaches the preset goal repeatedly. Breath sounds should be assessed after coughing, and the incentive spirometer should be left within the patient's reach before the clinician leaves the room. The patient should be encouraged to perform the maneuvers independently between scheduled sessions. The frequency of sessions varies with the patient and may be prescribed as often and specifically as once per hour or as variably as three times per day.[16,17]

ASSESSMENT OF THERAPY

Documentation of the patient's response during therapy should include the following: (1) heart rate, (2) respiratory rate, (3) breath sounds, (4) inspiratory volume or flow achieved, (5) number of goals achieved, (6) description of cough and sputum production, (7) patient effort and tolerance, (8) how many maneuvers the family has tried/agreed to get the patient to do per hour, and (9) any patient complaints or adverse reactions, or both, and the corrective action taken. Therapy is considered effective if atelectasis is prevented or resolved and inspiratory muscle performance is improved.[70] Clinical signs of this would include a decreased respiratory rate, normal temperature, normal pulse rate, normal or improved breath sounds that were previously absent or diminished, a normal chest radiograph, improved oxygenation, and increased vital capacity and peak expiratory flows.[70]

Although there have been numerous studies evaluating the therapeutic value of incentive spirometry, it is difficult to compare them because of the variation in patients and study design.[85] However, a number of studies have indicated that incentive spirometry, along with other deep breathing maneuvers, is effective in reducing pulmonary complications when used correctly.[75,77,86-89] A study comparing the efficacy of postoperative incentive spirometry between children and adults concluded that incentive spirometry is as effective in reducing the incidence of atelectasis in children who have undergone cardiac surgery.[90]

INTERMITTENT POSITIVE-PRESSURE BREATHING

IPPB is the intermittent, short-term delivery of positive pressure to a patient for the purpose of improving lung expansion, delivering aerosolized medications, and assisting ventilation.[91] Since its inception in 1947 and its introduction into the medical arena in 1948, IPPB has been one of the most controversial topics in respiratory care.[92] It was one of the most popular therapeutic modalities prescribed in the 1960s and 1970s and was regarded as the panacea to all pulmonary ailments. Not until the American College of Chest Physicians' conference on oxygen therapy in September 1983, when both its overuse and its doubtful efficacy were discussed, did IPPB decline as a treatment modality.[93] Today newly practiced modalities, such as bilevel positive airway pressure (BiPAP) and incentive spirometry, have rendered the prescription of IPPB more selective than in the past.[94,95]

INDICATIONS, CONTRAINDICATIONS, AND COMPLICATIONS

Clinically, IPPB is given to provide a significantly larger inhaled volume at a physiologically advantageous inspiratory to expiratory pattern than the patient can produce with spontaneous ventilation. If this goal is met, there should be improvement in the cough mechanism, distribution of ventilation, and delivery of medication.[96] In the pediatric population, however, the hazards and potential complications that can result from its use render it unpopular and ineffective among infants and children.[97] It is indicated most often in the older patient who needs increased lung expansion but has failed to respond to other modes of treatment, such as incentive spirometry, chest physiotherapy, deep-breathing exercises, and BiPAP. This includes patients with neuromuscular disease or chest wall deformity that inhibits maximum inspiratory efforts. Medication can also be delivered via IPPB to these patients. However, studies have continued to report that the delivery of medications via IPPB depends on the technique and that the first mode of choice for aerosolized medication therapy should be a small-volume nebulizer or metered-dose inhaler.[98-100]

The absolute contraindication to IPPB is a tension pneumothorax; however, there are other factors that should be considered carefully before IPPB therapy is recommended. Because the effectiveness of applying IPPB therapy hinges on the cooperation of the patient, any infant or child who most likely would not cooperate and who has difficulty coordinating deep breathing should not be considered for this therapy. (Asynchronous breathing as well as breathing against the high positive pressure could result in increased work of breathing.) According to the American Association for Respiratory Care's clinical practice guideline for IPPB, other clinical contraindications include increased intracranial pressures (greater than 15 mm Hg); recent facial, oral, or skull surgery; tracheoesophageal fistula; recent esophageal surgery; active hemoptysis; active, untreated tuberculosis; radiographic evidence of blebs; hemodynamic instability; nausea; and swallowing of air.[91] Because IPPB is so rarely used in pediatrics, it is possible that the clinician may be inexperienced in administering the therapy and unable to provide optimal respiratory care. When this situation arises, the objective of providing a safe, effective treatment may be unattainable, and it is in the patient's best interest not to have the treatment administered.

Complications associated with IPPB therapy are listed in Box 14-2.[91,101,102] This list demonstrates the need for an experienced clinician to administer the therapy and to monitor the patient and the equipment closely. Should adverse reactions occur, the treatment should be discontinued and the physician notified of the situation.

EQUIPMENT

The equipment used during an IPPB treatment includes the IPPB device, the circuit, the patient application device, and the volume measuring device. Although the addition of a humidifier is not essential, it is recommended in patients with mucus

---

> **BOX 14-2**
>
> **COMPLICATIONS ASSOCIATED WITH INTERMITTENT POSITIVE-PRESSURE BREATHING**
>
> Bronchospasm
> Gastric distention and ileus
> Nosocomial infection
> Decreased venous return
> Hyperventilation
> Hypoventilation
> Impaction of secretions
> Fatigue
> Air trapping
> Volutrauma, pneumothorax
> Hemoptysis
> Reduction of respiratory drive in patients with chronic hypercarbia

---

retention. The most popular IPPB devices used in pediatric patients are the Bird series (Bird Products), the Puritan-Bennett series (Puritan-Bennett), and the Monaghan 515 (Monaghan Medical). The devices vary in design and in flow, volume, and pressure capabilities.[103] The patient application devices are dependent on the patient's needs and include a mouthpiece, lip-mouth seal, mask, or endotracheal tube/tracheostomy adapter. A nose clip should be available for the patient who uses either a mouthpiece or lip seal. The volume measuring device can be either a volume spirometer (such as that used with the Puritan-Bennett MA-1 ventilator) or a hand-held spirometer. Suctioning equipment should be available, as should containers for collecting or disposing of sputum.[91]

PROCEDURE

An explanation of the equipment and the procedure should be given to the patient. The equipment may be frightening, and the clinician should soothe and encourage the patient by explaining exactly what the patient will feel and how the IPPB machine will perform. Manually cycling the machine on and listening to the gas flow may be helpful in alleviating some of the patient's fears. Allowing the patient to examine the mouthpiece (lip seal, mask, or adapter) and circuit before therapy begins may also help. A thorough explanation of the proper breathing pattern is essential *before* therapy begins. The patient should be encouraged to inhale slowly with the machine and to exhale passively, not forcefully.

Application. The patient should be placed in a sitting position if possible and therapy initiated at low pressures (10 cm H_2O). The pressure can be gradually increased until one of the following conditions

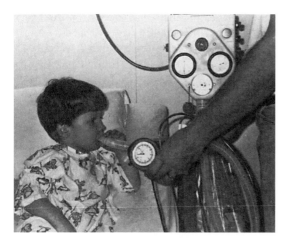

Fig. 14-8

Intermittent positive-pressure breathing (IPPB) therapy administered to child with respirometer attached to exhalation valve for exhaled volume monitoring.

is met: (1) the pressure provides the set volume goal, (2) further increase in pressure provides a minimal increase in volume, or (3) the patient becomes intolerant of the pressure increase. The gas flow rate should be set by the clinician and will vary depending on the individual patient (Fig. 14-8).

Monitoring. The patient and equipment should be monitored closely during therapy. The heart rate and respiratory rate should be obtained before, during, and after each treatment. Breath sounds should be assessed before and after each treatment and any time the patient complains of respiratory difficulty or chest pains. With the goal of therapy being to generate a tidal volume during IPPB that is at least 15 ml/kg or to exceed one third of inspiratory capacity, it is essential that tidal volume be monitored.[104] To determine if lung volume is being augmented, the patient's tidal volume should be monitored before (spontaneous breathing) and several times during therapy. The exhaled gas is measured during therapy at the exhalation valve with either a respirometer or spirometer. If the tidal volume delivered during IPPB therapy is not greater than that during spontaneous breathing, the therapy is of little, if any, value to the patient. The patient's peak flow should also be monitored before and after treatment.

ASSESSMENT OF THERAPY

Document the following with each IPPB treatment: (1) heart rate, (2) respiratory rate, (3) breath sounds, (4) pressure used (beginning and end of therapy), (5) tidal volume obtained (before and during therapy), (6) machine controls used (i.e., sensitivity, flow), (7) Fio_2 values, (8) medication aerosolized, (9) peak flow, (10) description of cough and sputum production, (11) patient cooperation and tolerance, (12) duration of therapy, and (13) any patient complaints or adverse reactions and the corrective action taken.

IPPB therapy is believed to be effective if the therapeutic goals are met, including (1) an augmented tidal volume during IPPB (15 ml/kg or more than one third inspiratory capacity), (2) an increase in peak flow or forced expiratory volume in 1 second (FEV_1), (3) a more effective cough, (4) secretion clearance, (5) improved breath sounds, and (6) an improved chest radiograph.[91]

When compared with other aerosol delivery devices, IPPB in the pediatric patient is both equipment and labor intensive.[91] With this in mind, perhaps thought should be given *not* to whether IPPB is effective in delivering aerosols but rather to whether IPPB is the most effective method of delivery.[105] However, although there are other less expensive and less invasive lung expansion maneuvers, there remain patients who fail to respond to these maneuvers but who do benefit from IPPB. If there are no observable benefits from the therapy, however, its use cannot be justified.

COMPLICATIONS OF CHEST PHYSICAL THERAPY

Numerous studies have demonstrated that CPT can be detrimental, especially when applied in patients with little or no sputum production. Reported complications of CPT range from rare reports of complete airway obstruction and respiratory arrest to bronchospasm and hypoxemia.

HYPOXEMIA

The most commonly cited adverse effect of CPT is hypoxemia. Several studies have reported hypoxemia in infants receiving CPT.[27-30] Hypoxemia has also been documented in studies of adolescent and adult patients receiving CPT and was reported to occur more often in patients with preexisting cardiovascular complications, with minimal sputum production, and when mucoid rather than mucopurulent secretions were present. It occurred in patients with good pulmonary function and also when supplemental oxygen was being used.[106-111] Tachypnea and tachycardia may occur in patients who experience hypoxemia during CPT.

There may be a variety of reasons why CPT often causes hypoxemia. Among the proposed mechanisms are ventilation-perfusion ($\dot{V}/\dot{Q}$) abnormalities caused by postural changes, atelectasis, bronchospasm, alterations in cardiac output and oxygen consumption, and incomplete expectoration of mobilized secretions. In addition, each of the CPT techniques may contribute to hypoxemia to differing degrees.

Position. Most studies of the effects of posture on oxygenation in adults would suggest that putting the diseased portion of the lung uppermost, as in postural drainage therapy, improves oxygenation.[112-114] This is a consequence of improved perfusion of the healthy, dependent lung tissue at the expense of the diseased, elevated lung segments. Thus, at least for patients with localized, unilateral lung disease, $\dot{V}/\dot{Q}$ abnormalities secondary to postural changes are an unlikely explanation for CPT-associated hypoxemia in patients outside of infancy. Infants, however, have better oxygenation when the affected side is dependent (i.e., the good lung is up).[115] This may in part be the result of higher baseline pulmonary artery pressures, which would mitigate the effects of gravity on pulmonary blood flow. Hence, alterations in $\dot{V}/\dot{Q}$ relationships as a direct result of postural changes are a possible explanation for CPT-associated hypoxemia in infants. Patients with generalized lung disease may respond differently to postural changes, however, and careful monitoring of oxygenation with position changes may be warranted. Position changes during CPT may also result in hypotension or hypertension.

Percussion. Several studies report that chest percussion, rather than postural changes, is responsible for CPT-associated hypoxemia.[29,106-108] These studies suggest that chest percussion causes significant $\dot{V}/\dot{Q}$ abnormalities, and unless counterbalanced by removal of a substantial quantity of mucus and improvement in $\dot{V}/\dot{Q}$ ratios, the net change will be a deterioration in $\dot{V}/\dot{Q}$ relationships and hypoxemia.

Atelectasis. Both human and animal studies have shown an increase in atelectasis when CPT was given.[67,68] Vigorous chest percussion has been noted to produce pressure swings in the chest of up to 30 cm H_2O. Such pressures generated by intermittent compression or percussion of the chest wall would seem sufficient to expel appreciable quantities of air from the lung, especially if chest wall compliance is high. Chest wall vibration, in contrast to percussion, has been associated with hypoxemia in some studies.[28-30,116,117] This reflects the fact that vibration may or may not be associated with chest wall compression, depending on the techniques or equipment used, whereas chest percussion invariably causes chest wall compression.

Bronchospasm. An additional explanation for the association of chest percussion with hypoxemia is the observation that chest percussion can cause bronchospasm in susceptible patients, especially when sputum production is minimal. Administering bronchodilators before therapy may be desirable, especially when CPT is applied in patients with reactive airway disease.

Increased Oxygen Consumption. Oxygen consumption is increased during CPT.[118,119] If significant shunting is present, or if an increase in cardiac output is not produced, increased oxygen consumption can be manifested by decreased Pa_{O_2}.

Gastroesophageal Reflux. Gastroesophageal reflux (GER) is a common cause of respiratory problems in infants and children, and CPT is often ordered for patients who have GER. One study found that in patients with GER, CPT resulted in a fivefold increase in reflux episodes, compared with periods when CPT was not given.[120] This increase in GER was seen even though treatments were withheld up to 3.5 hours after the infant's last feeding. The study did not link the increase in reflux episodes to any particular aspect of CPT, such as head-down positioning. GER may cause severe esophagitis, bronchospasm, or pneumonia and has been linked to apnea and sudden infant death syndrome.[121] Therefore CPT should be given only when the benefits of treatment clearly outweigh the risks of aggravated GER. Although withholding treatment as long as possible after an infant's feeding is advisable, it clearly will not eliminate the risks involved.

AIRWAY OBSTRUCTION AND RESPIRATORY ARREST

Although CPT can be an effective means of removing bronchial foreign bodies in children, it may also result in acute upper airway obstruction and death.[122] This is especially true when the foreign body consists of organic material, such as seeds or nuts, that may increase in size (secondary to water absorption) after a period in the lung. Vomiting and aspiration may also occur during CPT, especially if therapy is given soon after the patient has eaten. Therefore at least 1 hour should be allowed after the last meal or feeding before beginning CPT. Patients receiving continuous feedings through gastric tubes should have the feedings turned off at least 30 minutes before therapy. More time may be needed in patients with a history of vomiting or reflux. For patients in whom feedings cannot be interrupted, Trendelenburg (head-down) positioning should not be used.

INTRACRANIAL COMPLICATIONS

Studies in preterm infants have reported that certain positions of the infant's head may increase intracranial pressure and that routine application of CPT, especially in the first few days of life, can significantly increase the risk of IVH.[31,123] CPT procedures in the child or adult with a recent head injury can also increase intracranial pressure.[124] Because of these concerns, many institutions do not place premature infants or patients with head injuries in the Trendelenburg position during CPT.

RIB FRACTURES AND BRUISING

Rib fractures have been reported as a complication of chest percussion in preterm infants with bronchopulmonary dysplasia.[125] The infants in this study suffered from rickets secondary to long-term parenteral nutrition. Improvement in nutritional therapy for preterm infants, however, should make rickets a rare finding in the infant with bronchopulmonary dysplasia. Infants with the rare condition of osteogenesis imperfecta are also at high risk of rib fractures. Bruising may occur in some patients, especially in the very small premature infant and the child with vitamin K deficiency. Most patients are more comfortable if percussion or vibration is performed with the skin covered by a pajama top or T-shirt. If the patient is not wearing pajamas or clothing, a lightweight blanket or towel should be placed on the chest and back. Excessive padding, however, should be avoided.

AIRWAY TRAUMA

In all patients, extreme care must be taken to maintain a proper airway. Infants and children with artificial airways in place can be accidentally extubated during CPT, especially if they are being mechanically ventilated. The ventilator tubing or endotracheal tube, or both, are easily pulled during position changes, and extubation may result. When turning the patient, condensation in the ventilator tubing can be inadvertently drained into the patient's airway, which may result in bronchospasm and respiratory distress. Special attention should also be given to patients who receive CPT during the first 24 hours after a tracheostomy because hemorrhage may occur if therapy is given too vigorously.[26] Therefore, for patients in intensive care units or those with artificial airways in place, suction equipment as well as a manual resuscitator and mask should be readily available, preferably at the patient's bedside.

SELECTION OF PATIENTS FOR CHEST PHYSICAL THERAPY

CPT is ordered for a multiplicity of conditions, including acute respiratory infections, postoperative complications, CF, and asthma, to name a few. Evidence is increasing, however, that CPT is required in only a limited number of conditions, all of which are characterized by chronic, excessive sputum production.

CONDITIONS IN WHICH CHEST PHYSICAL THERAPY MAY NOT BE BENEFICIAL

A variety of studies in children and adults have demonstrated that CPT may not be beneficial in certain conditions.

In studies of the effects of CPT in children hospitalized with severe exacerbation of asthma, no difference was found in the rate of improvement of pulmonary function, even in the most severe cases.[126] Other studies in adults with reactive airway disease have shown that chest percussion can cause bronchospasm and hypoxemia.[108,127,128] Selected patients with asthma may benefit from CPT, especially when copious secretions or obstructive atelectasis are present. However, bronchospasm and hypoxemia should be well controlled before treatment. CPT is no substitute for adequate treatment with bronchodilating agents. It is also essential that a patient with asthma be well hydrated before CPT is begun.

Although bronchiolitis is characterized by increased secretions, studies have reported CPT to be of minimal value. CPT made no difference in the length of hospital stay or the severity or duration of symptoms in patients with bronchiolitis, even when associated pneumonia or atelectasis was present.[129] It also produced no beneficial changes in lung mechanics or work of breathing in patients with bronchiolitis.[130] The failure of CPT to produce an effect in bronchiolitis most likely results from the fact that the disease affects the smaller, peripheral airways, where CPT techniques are generally not effective.[8]

Several studies have evaluated the role of CPT in pneumonia and have reported that CPT either had no effect or actually delayed resolution, especially in young adults.[129,131,132]

In a study of a group of closely matched pediatric cardiac surgery patients, Reines and colleagues reported that those treated with CPT had twice the incidence of atelectasis as did the control group (68% versus 32%), who received deep-breathing instruction, coughing, or suction as appropriate.[133] Moreover, atelectasis was more severe and the duration of hospitalization prolonged in the CPT group.

CPT to the right upper lobe every 1 to 2 hours for 24 hours after extubation is a common practice in many neonatal intensive care units. This practice is based on a report by Finer and associates that claimed a dramatic reduction in the risk of right upper lobe atelectasis after extubation when CPT was given.[134] However, it is unclear from the study if suctioning alone or CPT was responsible for the results.

CONDITIONS IN WHICH CHEST PHYSICAL THERAPY MAY BE BENEFICIAL

In contrast to the reports criticizing its effectiveness, CPT has been shown to be beneficial in patients with acute and chronic conditions characterized by excessive secretion production or mucus plugging of large airways that does not clear with coughing or suction. "Excessive secretions" usually means 30 ml of sputum per day in adults. Obviously, lesser amounts would qualify as excessive secretions in children. CPT is also useful in the treatment of obstructive atelectasis. Fig. 14-9 illustrates the process of evaluation of the pediatric patient for CPT.

Acute Lobar Atelectasis. The majority of patients with acute atelectasis secondary to mucus plugs respond with one CPT treatment.[23,135,136] If patients fail to respond to several CPT treatments, the atelectasis most likely is caused by conditions not amenable to CPT, and therapy should be discontinued. The presence of an air bronchogram, suggesting no mucus obstruction of the airways, has been shown to predict a poor response to CPT.[23,136] Although a period of CPT after resolution of the atelectasis may be warranted, prolonged CPT should not be necessary. As discussed earlier, CPT is not useful in the prevention of the return of atelectasis, except in patients with large amounts of secretions.

Cystic Fibrosis. CPT has been widely employed as a mainstay of treatment for the pulmonary complications of CF. In fact, much of our knowledge of CPT comes from studies conducted in patients with CF.[41,136] Current issues in the application of CPT in these patients include the following questions: (1) Which techniques are most effective? (2) How can self-care be promoted? and (3) How can compliance with therapy be improved?

Effective techniques are those that foster high expiratory air velocity at low lung volume, such as FET, PEP therapy, HFCC, vigorous exercise, and AD. Postural drainage is also a useful adjunct to PEP therapy or FET. Although little evidence is available to support the routine use of manual chest percussion in the treatment of CF, and although some CF centers (especially in Europe) have abandoned the routine use of manual chest percussion, most CF treatment centers in the United States still consider it an integral component of CPT. Many patients will expect percussion to be a part of their CPT treatments, especially when hospitalized. Therefore elimination of chest percussion from routine CPT treatments should not be carried out arbitrarily. Radical changes in CPT practice for patients facing a lifelong battle with excessive pulmonary secretions should be made only after careful deliberation and consultation with the pulmonary physicians responsible for their care.

Fig. 14-9

Algorithm for evaluating patients for chest physical therapy.

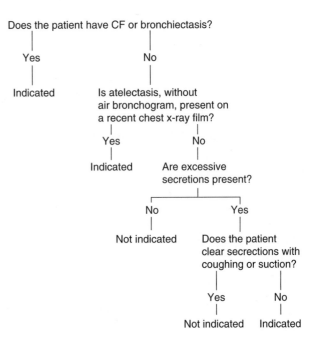

The issue of promoting self-care is especially important when dealing with patients with CF and their families. Patients with CF differ from most patients receiving CPT in that they need to employ some technique or techniques for removal of bronchial secretions on a daily basis for the rest of their lives. Current practices, especially those that require the routine application of chest percussion by a second person, often give the message that CPT is a passive technique, that it is something that is done "to" rather than "by" the patient. This may promote passivity and dependence on parents or other caregivers. As a result, compliance is often poor, and treatments become a frequent source of arguments in families of patients with CF, with difficulties increasing as the patient grows older.[40,137] Also, because CPT must be administered by a parent two or more times a day, it may interfere with normal adolescent developmental processes, such as increasing autonomy and separation from parents. Therefore increasing the patient's ability to perform self-care is essential. All patients with CF, especially as they approach adolescence, should be well instructed in one of the forms of self-care, such as PEP, AD, FET with or without postural drainage, or HFCC. Vigorous exercise, such as running or swimming, is also an effective form of self-therapy in well-motivated patients. The techniques selected will depend on patient preference and learning ability, the preferences of the attending physician and, in the case of HFCC, the ability to arrange financing. Patients and their families often report improved compliance with self-care over parent-administered CPT, and treatment-related conflicts are minimized.[40]

Follow-up and consistency are essential when teaching bronchial drainage techniques. Reteaching may be necessary at intervals, and most patients with CF and their families are often interested in learning new developments in CPT. Families often need assistance in adapting CPT practices to changing life circumstances, such as the patient entering school, traveling, entering college, and leaving home.

CF patients with advanced disease often have hemoptysis. CPT is usually withheld until the bleeding is controlled because vigorous coughing may aggravate the bleeding or dislodge clots. Likewise, CPT may need to be withheld in patients with pneumothorax, another common complication of advanced CF. Patients with end-stage disease may be especially reluctant to cooperate with CPT, especially the Trendelenburg positioning that is required. Supplemental oxygen may allow some patients with advanced disease to tolerate postural drainage. Withholding percussion may also improve the patient's ability to maintain the Trendelenburg position. Some investigators have reported that PEP therapy is better tolerated than postural drainage and percussion in patients with end-stage disease.[44]

Neuromuscular Disease or Injury. CPT is often used in many patients with neuromuscular injury or disease, and survival is often improved when CPT, coughing, turning, and deep breathing are incorporated into routine care (see Chapter 44).[10,138-140] Prolonged postural drainage is often especially helpful. However, patients with acute head injury should have well-controlled intracranial pressures before CPT is initiated.

Lung Abscess. There are some patients with lung abscesses who may be successfully treated with CPT, especially older children.[141] Fearing that discharge of large amounts of infected material may spread the infection and lead to acute respiratory distress, some clinicians are reluctant to use CPT in the treatment of lung abscess.[22] Likewise, hemoptysis is a common complication in patients with lung abscess, and CPT may increase this risk. These concerns must be balanced against the knowledge that alternative treatments for lung abscess, such as lung resections, are also risky.

CONTRAINDICATIONS

Frank hemoptysis, empyema, foreign body aspiration, and untreated pneumothorax are often considered contraindications to all components of CPT. Withholding CPT, especially percussion, is sometimes recommended when the platelet count is low (less than 50,000 cells/mm^3). CPT is also usually withheld in the immediate postoperative period after tracheostomy, tracheobronchial reconstruction, and selected other conditions in which postoperative movement is extremely dangerous. Chest percussion should not be performed directly over fractured ribs, areas of subcutaneous emphysema, or recently burned or grafted skin. Some conditions may require modification of therapy or omission of certain components of CPT.

LENGTH AND FREQUENCY OF THERAPY

Treatments for patients with CF or bronchiectasis should be performed for at least 30 minutes, with many patients benefiting from therapy lasting 45 minutes or longer. Patients with severe dyspnea may require rest periods, which will further prolong therapy. Most pediatric respiratory care departments limit routine CPT treatments to 15 to 20 minutes.[142] CPT is rarely needed more than every 4 hours, although selected patients may benefit from more frequent suctioning or coughing. CPT orders should be evaluated at least every 48 hours in patients in intensive care units, at least every 72 hours in acute care patients, or whenever there is a change in the patient's status.[143]

THERAPY MODIFICATION

Many patients require modification of therapy because of medical or surgical procedures. Percussion may be extremely painful for patients postoperatively, and the use of manual vibration or mechanical vibrators is sometimes better tolerated. Also, clinicians should be careful to avoid percussion over implanted devices, such as ventricular-peritoneal shunts or implantable venous access devices (often used in patients with CF). Percussion is also omitted in patients with brittle bones, for example, in those with rickets or osteogenesis imperfecta.

Many patients may not tolerate Trendelenburg positioning. Included in this group are those with severe GER, recent intracranial trauma or surgery, increased intracranial pressure, abdominal distention or ascites, compromised diaphragm movement, uncontrolled hypertension, and severe cardiopulmonary failure.[143] With careful monitoring, simple side-to-side positioning may be attempted in these patients. The patient with a gastrostomy tube or chest tube, or both, may also require modifications in drainage positions.

Patients receiving CPT often have a disorder affecting only one lobe. These patients do not need CPT in all 11 positions but rather an abbreviated CPT treatment that uses postural drainage positions for the affected lobe only.

Infants and small children are unable to perform maneuvers such as FET or AD. Some clinicians have attempted to mimic these techniques with gentle chest wall compression during the expiratory phase, allowing the child to exhale to less than functional residual capacity. Like AD or FET performed in cooperative older patients, this technique results in increased expiratory air velocity at low lung volumes, improving mucus mobilization.

MONITORING DURING THERAPY

Patients in an intensive care unit who require CPT should have continuous monitoring of Sao_2, heart rate, and respiratory rate. Breathing pattern, skin color, and breath sounds should also be noted.[143] Patients not in an intensive care unit who require high oxygen concentrations or who have a condition presenting a high risk of respiratory or cardiac failure should also have these variables monitored. Other patients with mild respiratory distress should have pulse and respiratory rate as well as breathing pattern, skin color, and breath sounds measured before and after therapy. This is especially true for younger patients who cannot verbalize complaints of distress. Routine monitoring of heart rate and respiratory rate for patients with chronic respiratory disorders, such as CF, is probably not warranted and may inadvertently give the message that CPT is harmful. When performing percussion or vibration on patients who are connected to cardiopulmonary monitors, the alarm on the monitor may become activated because of interference from the percussion or vibration. It is best to refrain from turning the monitor alarms completely off.

EVALUATION OF THERAPY

Because the goal of CPT is to promote the removal of excessive bronchial secretions, the single most important variable in evaluating the effectiveness of CPT is the amount of secretions expectorated with therapy. Changes in sputum production, breath sounds, vital signs, chest radiographic findings, blood gas values, and lung mechanics may indicate a positive response to the therapy.[143] However, removal of excessive bronchial secretions is not always associated with an immediate change in blood gases, breath sounds, or lung mechanics. Patients with advanced CF, for example, almost always have audible rales before and after therapy, whereas pulmonary function and blood gas determinations change little.

Patients undergoing mechanical ventilation may have measurements of lung mechanics as well as noninvasive blood gas monitoring data readily available. If so, the clinician should note any changes associated with therapy. A deterioration in these variables, especially if unaccompanied by removal of secretions, suggests that therapy should be modified or discontinued.

DOCUMENTATION OF THERAPY

When charting CPT treatments, the clinician should describe the techniques used (e.g., postural drainage, percussion, AD), which lobes were treated, and what positions the patient was placed in. If certain segments or positions are omitted, this should be documented as well as the reason why this was done. The clinician should also note if suctioning was performed. To document the response to therapy, pretreatment and posttreatment breath sounds, vital signs, and the amount and quality of sputum expectorated should be noted.

REFERENCES

1. Ewart W: The treatment of bronchiectasis and of chronic bronchial affections by posture and respiratory exercises. *Lancet* 1901; 2:70-72.
2. Gaskell DV, Webber BA: *The Brompton Hospital guide to chest physiotherapy.* Oxford. Blackwell Scientific Publications, 1973.
3. Murray JF: The ketchup-bottle method. *N Engl J Med* 1979; 300:1155-1157.
4. Sutton PP et al: Chest physiotherapy: a review. *Eur J Respir Dis* 1982; 63:188-201.
5. Kirilloff LH et al: Does chest physical therapy work? *Chest* 1985; 88:436-444.
6. Sutton P: Chest physiotherapy: time for a reappraisal. *Br J Dis Chest* 1988; 82:127-137.
7. Selsby D: Chest physiotherapy may be harmful in some patients. *BMJ* 1989; 298:541-542.
8. Selsby D, Jones JG: Chest physiotherapy: physiological and clinical aspects. *Br J Anaesth* 1990; 64:621-631.
9. Pavia D: The role of chest physiotherapy in mucus hypersecretion. *Lung* 1990; 168(Suppl):614-621.
10. Stiller KR: Chest physiotherapy for the medical patient: are current practices effective? *Aust N Z J Med* 1990; 20:183-187.
11. Eid N et al: Chest physiotherapy in review. *Respir Care* 1991; 36:270-282.
12. Lewis RM: Chest physical therapy: time for a redefinition and a renaming. *Respir Care* 1992; 37:419-421.
13. Waring WW: Diagnostic and therapeutic procedures. In Chernick V, editor: *Kendig's disorders of the respiratory tract in children,* ed 5. Philadelphia. WB Saunders, 1990; pp 77-95.
14. Hough A: *Physiotherapy in respiratory care: a problem solving approach.* London. Chapman & Hall, 1991.
15. Cystic Fibrosis Foundation: *Consumer fact sheet: an introduction to chest physical therapy.* Bethesda, MD. Cystic Fibrosis Foundation, 1992.
16. Mellins RB: Pulmonary physiotherapy in the pediatric age group. *Am Rev Respir Dis* 1974; 110 (2, Suppl): 137-142.
17. Sutton PP et al: Assessment of percussion, vibratory shaking, and breathing exercises in chest physiotherapy. *Eur J Respir Dis* 1985; 66:147-152.
18. Sutton PP, Parker RA, Webber BA: Assessment of the forced expiration technique, postural drainage and directed coughing in chest physiotherapy. *Eur J Respir Dis* 1983; 64:62-68.
19. van der Schans CP, Piers DA, Postma DS: Effect of manual percussion on tracheobronchial clearance in patients with chronic airflow obstruction and excessive tracheobronchial secretion. *Thorax* 1986; 41:448-452.
20. Murphy MB, Concannon D, FitzGerald M: Chest percussion: help or hindrance to postural drainage. *Ir Med J* 1983; 76:189-190.
21. Webber B et al: Evaluation of self-percussion during postural drainage using the forced expiration technique. *Physiother Pract* 1985; 1:42-45.
22. Faling LJ: Chest physical therapy. In Burton GG, Gee GN, Hodgkin JE, editors: *Respiratory care: A guide to clinical practice,* ed 3. Philadelphia. JB Lippincott, 1991; pp 625-654.
23. Marini JJ, Pierson DJ, Hudson LD:. Acute lobar atelectasis: a prospective comparison of fiberoptic bronchoscopy and respiratory therapy. *Am Rev Respir Dis* 1979; 19: 971-978.
24. Finer NN, Boyd J: Chest physiotherapy in the neonate: a controlled study. *Pediatrics* 1978; 61:282-285.
25. O'Bradovich HM, Chernick V: The functional basis of respiratory pathology. In Chernick V, editor: *Kendig's disorders of the respiratory tract in children,* ed 5. Philadelphia. WB Saunders, 1990; pp 3-47.
26. Walters P: Chest physiotherapy. In Levin DL, Morris FC, Moore GC, editors: *A practical guide to pediatric intensive care.* St Louis. Mosby, 1979; pp 395-403.
27. Holloway R et al: Effect of chest physiotherapy on blood gases of neonates treated by intermittent positive pressure respiration. *Thorax* 1969; 24:421-426.
28. Fox WW, Schwartz JG, Schaffer TH: Pulmonary physiotherapy in neonates: physiologic changes and respiratory management. *J Pediatr* 1978; 92:977-981.
29. Curran CL, Kachoyeanos MK: The effects on neonates of two methods of chest physical therapy. *MCN* 1979; 4: 309-313.
30. Walsh CM et al: Controlled supplemental oxygenation during tracheobronchial hygiene. *Nurs Res* 1987; 36: 211-215.
31. Raval D et al: Chest physiotherapy in preterm infants with RDS in the first 24 hours of life. *J Perinatol* 1987; 7:301-304.
32. Green CG: Assessment of the pediatric airway by flexible bronchoscopy. *Respir Care* 1991; 36:555-568.
33. Pryor JA: The forced expiration technique. In Pryor JA, editor: *International perspectives in physical therapy, 7: Respiratory care.* Edinburgh. Churchill Livingstone, 1991; pp 79-100.
34. Zapletal A et al: Chest physiotherapy and airway obstruction in patients with cystic fibrosis: a negative report. *Eur J Respir Dis* 1983; 64:426-433.
35. Oldenburg FA et al: Effects of postural drainage, exercise, and cough on mucus clearance in chronic bronchitis. *Am Rev Respir Dis* 1979; 120:739-745.
36. Rossman C et al: Effect of chest physiotherapy on the removal of mucus in patients with cystic fibrosis. *Am Rev Respir Dis* 1982; 126:131-135.
37. DeBoeck C, Zinman R: Cough versus chest physiotherapy. *Am Rev Respir Dis* 1984; 129:132-134.
38. Bain J, Bishop J, Olinsky A: Evaluation of directed coughing in cystic fibrosis. *Br J Dis Chest* 1988; 82: 138-148.
39. van Hengstum M et al: Conventional physiotherapy and forced expiratory manoeuvres have similar effects on tracheobronchial clearance. *Eur Respir J* 1988; 1: 758-761.
40. Klig S et al: A biopsychosocial examination of two methods of pulmonary therapy. *Pediatr Pulmonol* 1989; 4(Suppl):145.
41. Reisman J et al: Role of conventional physiotherapy in cystic fibrosis. *J Pediatr* 1988; 113:632-636.
42. Holzer FJ, Schnall R, Landau LI: The effect of a home exercise programme in children with cystic fibrosis. *Aust Paediatr J* 1984; 20:297-302.
43. Blomquist M et al: Physical activity and self treatment in cystic fibrosis. *Arch Dis Child* 1986; 61:362-367.
44. Mahlmeister MJ et al: Positive-expiratory-pressure mask therapy: Theoretical and practical considerations and a review of the literature. *Respir Care* 1991; 36:1218-1230.
45. Iverson LIG et al: Comparative study of IPPB, the incentive spirometer and blow bottles: The prevention of atelectasis following cardiac surgery. *Ann Thorac Surg* 1978; 25:197-200.
46. Schoni MH: Autogenic drainage: a modern approach to physiotherapy in cystic fibrosis. *J R Soc Med* 1989; 82(16, Suppl):32-37.

47. David A: Autogenic drainage—The German approach. In Pryor JA, editor: *International perspectives in physical therapy, 7: Respiratory care.* Edinburgh. Churchill Livingstone, 1991; pp 65-78.

48. Davidson AGF et al: Long-term comparison of conventional percussion and drainage physiotherapy versus autogenic drainage in cystic fibrosis. *Pediatr Pulmonol* 1992 (abstract); 8(Suppl):298.

49. Falk M et al: Improving the ketchup bottle method with positive expiratory pressure, PEP, in cystic fibrosis. *Eur J Respir Dis* 1984; 65:423-432.

50. Tonnesen P, Stovring S: Positive expiratory pressure (PEP) as lung physiotherapy in cystic fibrosis: a pilot study. *Eur J Respir Dis* 1984; 65:419-422.

51. Tyrell JC, Hiller EJ, Martin J: Face mask physiotherapy in cystic fibrosis. *Arch Dis Child* 1986; 61:598-600.

52. Oberwaldner B, Evans JC, Zach MS: Forced expirations against a variable resistance: a new chest physiotherapy method in cystic fibrosis. *Pediatr Pulmonol* 1986; 2: 358-367.

53. Van Asperen PP et al: Comparison of a positive expiratory pressure (PEP) mask with postural drainage in patients with cystic fibrosis. *Aust Paediatr J* 1987; 23: 283-284.

54. Falk M, Andersen JB: Positive expiratory pressure (PEP) mask. In Pryor JA, editor: *International perspectives in physical therapy, 7: Respiratory care.* Edinburgh. Churchill Livingstone, 1991; pp 51-63.

55. Oberwaldner B et al: Chest physiotherapy in hospitalized patients with cystic fibrosis: A study of lung function effects and sputum production. *Eur Respir J* 1991; 4:152-158.

56. Mortensen J et al: The effects of postural drainage and positive expiratory pressure physiotherapy on tracheobronchial clearance in cystic fibrosis. *Chest* 1991; 100: 1350-1357.

57. Lindemann H et al: Autogenic drainage: efficacy of a simplified method. *Acta Univ Carol* 1990; 36:210-212.

58. Warwick WJ, Hansen LG: The long-term efficacy of high-frequency chest compression on pulmonary complications of cystic fibrosis. *Pediatr Pulmonol* 1991; 11: 265-271.

59. Warwick WJ: High frequency chest compression moves mucus by means of sustained staccato coughs. *Pediatr Pulmonol* 1991 (abstract); 6(Suppl):283.

60. Lannefors L, Wollmer P: Mucus clearance with three chest physiotherapy regimes in cystic fibrosis: a comparison between postural drainage, PEP, and physical exercise. *Eur Respir J* 1992; 5:748-753.

61. Zach M et al: Cystic fibrosis: physical exercise versus chest physiotherapy. *Arch Dis Child* 1982; 57:587-589.

62. Andreasson B et al: Long-term effects of physical exercise on working capacity and pulmonary function in cystic fibrosis. *Acta Paediatr Scand* 1987; 76:70-75.

63. Bartlett RH et al: Physiology of yawning and its application to postoperative care. *Surg Forum* 1970; 21:223-224.

64. Bartlett RH: Incentive spirometry. In Kacmarek R, Stoller J, editors: *Current respiratory care: techniques and therapy.* St Louis. Mosby, 1988.

65. Bartlett RH: Post-traumatic pulmonary insufficiency. In Cooper P, Nyhus L, editors: *Surgery annual.* New York. Appleton-Century-Crofts, 1971.

66. Ali J et al: Consequences of postoperative alterations in respiratory mechanics. *Am J Surg* 1974; 128:376-382.

67. Meyers JR et al: Changes in residual capacity of the lung after operation. *Arch Surg* 1975; 110:567-583.

68. Bartlett RH, Gazzaniga AB, Geraghty TR: Respiratory maneuvers to prevent postoperative pulmonary complications: a critical review. *JAMA* 1973; 224:1017-1021.

69. Bakow ED: Sustained maximal inspiration: a rationale for its use. *Respir Care* 1977; 22:379-382.

70. American Association for Respiratory Care: Clinical practice guideline: incentive spirometry. *Respir Care* 1991; 36:1402-1405.

71. Harken DE: A review of the activities of the thoracic center for the III and IV hospital groups, 160th general hospital European theater of operations, June 10, 1944 to Jan 1, 1945. *J Thoracic Cardiovasc Surg* 1946; 15:31-43.

72. Iverson LIG et al: A comparative study of IPPB, the incentive spirometer and blow bottles: the prevention of atelectasis following cardiac surgery. *Ann Thoracic Surg* 1978; 35:197-200.

73. O'Donohue WJ: National survey of the usage of lung expansion modalities for the prevention and treatment of postoperative atelectasis following abdominal and thoracic surgery. *Chest* 1985; 87:76-80.

74. Oikkonen M et al: Comparison of incentive spirometry and intermittent positive pressure breathing after coronary artery bypass graft. *Chest* 1991; 99:60-65.

75. Stock MC et al: Prevention of postoperative pulmonary complications with CPAP, incentive spirometry, and conservative therapy. *Chest* 1985; 87:151-157.

76. Stock MC et al: Comparison of continuous positive airway pressure, incentive spirometry, and conservative therapy after cardiac operations. *Crit Care Med* 1984; 12:969-972.

77. Celli BR, Rodriguez KS, Snider GL: A controlled trial of intermittent positive pressure breathing, incentive spirometry, and deep breathing exercises in preventing pulmonary complications after abdominal surgery. *Am Rev Respir Dis* 1984; 130:12-15.

78. Craven JL et al: The evaluation of incentive spirometry in the management of postoperative pulmonary complications. *Br J Surg* 1974; 61:793-797.

79. Bartlett RH: Respiratory therapy to prevent pulmonary complications of surgery. *Respir Care* 1984; 29:667-679.

80. Scuderi J, Olsen GN: Respiratory therapy in the management of postoperative complications. *Respir Care* 1989; 34:281-291.

81. Bartlett RH et al: Studies on the pathogenesis and prevention of postoperative pulmonary complications. *Surg Gynecol Obstet* 1973; 137:925-933.

82. Mang H, Obermayer A: Imposed work of breathing during sustained maximal inspiration: comparison of six incentive spirometers. *Respir Care* 1989; 34:1122-1128.

83. Lederer DH, Van de Water JM, Indech RB: Which deep breathing device should the postoperative patient use? *Chest* 1980; 77:610-613.

84. Centers for Disease Control: Update: universal precautions for prevention of transmission of human immunodeficiency virus, hepatitis B virus, and other bloodborne pathogens in health care settings. *Morb Mortal Wkly Rep* 1988; 37:377-388.

85. Schwieger I et al: Absence of benefit of incentive spirometry in low-risk patients undergoing elective cholecystectomy. *Chest* 1986; 89:652-656.

86. Davies BL, Macleod JP, Ogilvie HM: The efficacy of incentive spirometers in postoperative protocols for low-risk patients. *Can J Nurs Res* 1990; 22:19-36.

87. Gale GD, Sanders DE: Incentive spirometry: its value after cardiac surgery. *Can Anaesth Soc J* 1980; 27:475-480.

88. Jung R et al: Comparison of three methods of respiratory care following upper abdominal surgery. *Chest* 1980; 78:31-35.

89. Gooding JM et al: Is incentive spirometry valuable as an addition to traditional respiratory maneuvers? *Respir Care* 1977 (abstract); 22:414.

90. Krastins I et al: An evaluation of incentive spirometry in the management of pulmonary complications after cardiac surgery in the pediatric population. *Crit Care Med* 1982; 10:525-528.

91. American Association for Respiratory Care: Clinical practice guideline: intermittent positive pressure breathing. *Respir Care* 1993; 38:1189-1195.

92. Motley HL et al: Use of intermittent positive pressure breathing combined with nebulization in pulmonary disease. *Am J Med* 1948; 5:853-856.

93. Eubank DH, Bone RC: Intermittent positive pressure breathing. In Eubank DH, Bone RC, editors: *Comprehensive respiratory care: a learning system module.* St Louis. Mosby, 1985; pp 430-450.

94. Chang N, Levison H: The effect of nebulized bronchodilator administration with or without IPPB on ventilatory function in children with cystic fibrosis and asthma. *Am Rev Respir Dis* 1972; 106:867.

95. Baker JP: Magnitude of usage of intermittent positive pressure breathing. *Am Rev Respir Dis* 1974; 110S:170-177.

96. Agency for Health Care Policy and Research: Health technology reports: intermittent positive pressure breathing (IPPB) therapy. 1991, Number 1.

97. Burgess WR, Chernick V: Humidity and aerosol therapy. In Burger WR, Chernick V, editors: *Respiratory therapy in newborn infants and children.* New York. Thieme-Stratton, 1982; pp 74-84.

98. Jasper AC et al: Cost-benefit comparison of aerosol bronchodilator delivery methods in hospitalized patients. *Chest* 1987; 91:614-618.

99. Summer W et al: Aerosol bronchodilator delivery methods: Relative impact on pulmonary function and cost of respiratory care. *Arch Intern Med* 1989; 149:618-623.

100. American Association for Respiratory Care: Clinical practice guideline: selection of aerosol delivery device. *Respir Care* 1992; 37:891-897.

101. Bierman CW: Pneumomediastinum and pneumothorax complicating asthma in children. *Am J Dis Child* 1967; 114:43.

102. Moore RB, Cotton EK, Dinnery MA: The effect of IPPB on airway resistance in normal and asthmatic children. *J Allergy Clin Immunol* 1972; 49:137.

103. McPherson SP: *Respiratory therapy equipment.* St Louis. Mosby, 1985.

104. Oldenburg FA et al: Effects of postural drainage, exercise, and cough on mucus clearance in chronic bronchitis. *Am Rev Respir Dis* 1979; 120:739-745.

105. Imle CP: Adjuncts to chest physiotherapy. In Mackenzie CF, editor: *Chest physiotherapy in the intensive care unit.* Baltimore. Williams & Wilkins, 1981; pp 187-198.

106. Connors AF et al: Chest physical therapy: The immediate effect on oxygenation in acutely ill patients. *Chest* 1980; 79:559-564.

107. McDonnell T, McNicholas WT, Fitzgerald MX: Hypoxaemia during chest physiotherapy in patients with cystic fibrosis. *Ir J Med Sci* 1986; 155:345-348.

108. Gormezano J, Branthwaite MA: Pulmonary physiotherapy with assisted ventilation. *Anaesthesia* 1972; 27:249-257.

109. Gormezano J, Branthwaite MA: Effects of physiotherapy during intermittent positive pressure ventilation. *Anaesthesia* 1972; 27:258-264.

110. Huseby J et al: Oxygenation during chest physiotherapy. *Chest* 1976 (abstract); 70:430.

111. Tyler ML et al: Prediction of oxygenation during chest physiotherapy in critically ill patients. *Am Rev Respir Dis* 1980 (abstract); 121:218.

112. Dhainaut JF, Bons J, Bricard C: Improved oxygenation in patients with extensive unilateral pneumonia using the lateral decubitus position. *Thorax* 1980; 35:792-793.

113. Emolina C et al: Positional hypoxemia in unilateral lung disease. *N Engl J Med* 1981; 304:523-525.

114. Rivara D: Positional hypoxemia during artificial ventilation. *Crit Care Med* 1984; 12:436-438.

115. Heaf DP et al: Postural effects on gas exchange in infants. *N Engl J Med* 1983; 308:1505-1508.

116. Holody B, Goldberg HS: The effect of mechanical vibration physiotherapy on arterial oxygenation in acutely ill patients with atelectasis or pneumonia. *Am Rev Respir Dis* 1981; 124:372-375.

117. Mohsenifar Z et al: Mechanical vibration and conventional chest physiotherapy in outpatients with stable chronic obstructive lung disease. *Chest* 1985; 87:463-485.

118. Weissman C et al: Effect of routine intensive care interactions on metabolic rate. *Chest* 1984; 86:815-818.

119. Weissman C, Kemper M: The oxygen uptake-oxygen delivery relationship during ICU interventions. *Chest* 1991; 99:430-435.

120. Vandenplas Y et al: Esophageal pH monitoring data during chest physiotherapy. *J Pediatr Gastroenterol Nutr* 1991; 13:23-26.

121. Orenstein SR, Orenstein DM: Gastroesophageal reflux and respiratory disease in children. *J Pediatr* 1988; 112:847-858.

122. Kosloske A: Tracheobronchial foreign bodies in children: back to the bronchoscope and a balloon. *Pediatrics* 1980; 66:321.

123. Emery JR, Peabody JL: Head position affects intracranial pressure in newborn infants. *J Pediatr* 1983; 103:950-954.

124. Ersson U et al: Observations on intracranial dynamics during respiratory physiotherapy in unconscious neurosurgical patients. *Acta Anaesth Scand* 1990; 343:99-103.

125. Purohit DM, Caldwell C, Levkoff AH: Multiple rib fractures due to physiotherapy in a neonate with hyaline membrane disease. *Am J Dis Child* 1975; 129:1103-1104.

126. Asher MI et al: Effects of chest physical therapy on lung function in children recovering from acute severe asthma. *Pediatr Pulmonol* 1990; 9:146-151.

127. Campbell AH, O'Connell JM, Wilson F: The effects of chest physiotherapy upon the FEV1 in chronic bronchitis. *Med J Aust* 1975; 1:33-35.

128. Wollmer P et al: Inefficiency of chest percussion in the physical therapy of chronic bronchitis. *Eur J Respir Dis* 1985; 66:233-239.

129. Webb MSC et al: Chest physiotherapy in acute bronchiolitis. *Arch Dis Child* 1985; 60:1078-1079.

130. Quittell LM et al: The effectiveness of chest physical therapy (CPT) in infants with bronchiolitis. *Am Rev Respir Dis* 1988 (abstract); 137:406.

131. Graham WGB, Bradley DA: Efficacy of chest physiotherapy and intermittent positive-pressure breathing in the resolution of pneumonia. *N Engl J Med* 1978; 299:624-627.

132. Britton S, Bejstedt M, Vedin L: Chest physiotherapy in primary pneumonia. *BMJ* 1985; 290:1703-1704.

133. Reines HD: Chest physiotherapy fails to prevent postoperative atelectasis in children after cardiac surgery. *Am Surg* 1982; 48(2):59-62.

134. Finer NN et al: Postextubation atelectasis: a retrospective review and a prospective controlled study. *J Pediatr* 1979; 94:110-113.

135. Stiller K et al: Acute lobar atelectasis: a comparison of two chest physiotherapy regimens. *Chest* 1990; 98:1336-1340.

136. Desmond J et al: Immediate and long-term effects of chest physiotherapy in patients with cystic fibrosis. *J Pediatr* 1983; 103:538-542.

137. Currie DC et al: Practice, problems and compliance with postural drainage: a survey of chronic sputum producers. *Br J Dis Chest* 1986; 80:249-253.

138. Hammon W, Martin RJ: Chest physiotherapy for acute atelectasis. *Phys Ther* 1981; 61:217-220.

139. MacKenzie CF, Shing B, McAslun TC: Chest physiotherapy: the effect on arterial oxygenation. *Anesth Analg* 1978; 57:28-30.

140. McMichan JC, Michel L, Westbrook PR: Pulmonary dysfunction following traumatic quadriplegia. *JAMA* 1980; 243:528-531.

141. Kosloske A et al: Drainage of pediatric lung abscess by cough, catheter, or complete resection. *J Pediatr Surg* 1986; 21:596-600.

142. Lewis R: Chest physical therapy in pediatrics: a national survey. *Respir Care* 1991 (abstract); 36:1307-1309.

143. American Association for Respiratory Care: Clinical practice guideline: postural drainage therapy. *Respir Care* 1991; 36:1418-1426.

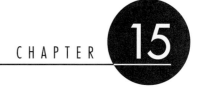

CHAPTER 15

Airway Management

Ian N. Jacobs
Mary M. Pettignano
Robert Pettignano

Recognizing the child who is in respiratory distress or failure is an integral step in caring for the critically ill child. Ensuring adequate oxygenation and ventilation is a major goal in managing any ill child. In the acute setting this is best accomplished by using a bag and mask in patients of all ages. Establishing and maintaining the airway is a crucial part of this effort, and it is one of the unique and challenging aspects of pediatric acute and critical care.

INTUBATION

Rapid and unencumbered intubation of the trachea depends on knowledge of the upper airway anatomy, the indications for intubation, the appropriate use of airway equipment, and the medications available to facilitate translaryngeal intubation. The ability to perform safe and rapid laryngoscopy and endotracheal (ET) tube placement enables the clinician to immediately manage and secure the airway in any emergency.

INDICATIONS

The indications for translaryngeal intubation are numerous; however, all can be placed in one of four broad categories, which can be defined by the four "Ps":
- *P*ulmonary function
- *P*rovide an airway
- *P*rotect the airway
- *P*ulmonary hygiene

When considering intubation because of a lack of pulmonary function, deficits in oxygenation as well as ventilation must be considered. Acute ventilatory dysfunction can be defined as a $PaCO_2$ of greater than 50 to 60 mm Hg with a pH of less than 7.3. A patient with hypoxemia can be defined as one with a PaO_2 of less than 60 mm Hg or an FIO_2 of greater than or equal to 0.60. This assumes cardiac disease is not contributing to an intracardiac shunt. These guidelines have been established as indicators of severe oxygenation or ventilation failure based on the fact that acidosis with a pH less than 7.2 may result in myocardial irritability and calcium and potassium disturbances.

It is difficult to reliably administer an FIO_2 of greater than 0.6 without an ET tube. Therefore a patient with a decreasing oxygen saturation that is unresponsive to increases in oxygen concentration is a candidate for intubation. Other disease processes that fall in the pulmonary function category include apnea requiring mechanical ventilation, central nervous system disease requiring respiratory support, and other forms of respiratory distress or failure.

Upper airway obstruction may also require an artificial airway. Processes classified in this category are diseases such as laryngotracheobronchitis, epiglottitis, adenoidal hypertrophy, tonsillar hypertrophy, and laryngomalacia. Head and neck trauma is also a possible reason to intubate, but it requires a specialized approach depending on the nature of the injury.

Intubation to protect the airway is most commonly performed when there is loss of protective airway reflexes such as gag, cough, and swallowing. Intubation in this scenario is necessary to minimize aspiration of oropharyngeal or gastric secretions that may lead to aspiration pneumonia. Patients at risk include those with neuromuscular disturbances, such as Guillain-Barré syndrome, and, more commonly, those who are comatose secondary to drug ingestion.

Finally, under the category of pulmonary hygiene, there are patients with persistent or recurring lobar or whole-lung atelectasis with an inability to clear secretions. These patients usually have inadequate ventilatory reserve, as evidenced by a vital capacity of less than 20 mg/kg and a negative inspiratory force of less than –20 cm H_2O.

EQUIPMENT

Anticipating and preparing for intubation by collecting the proper equipment is essential. The equipment necessary for intubation is listed in Box 15-1. Using the mnemonic MSMAID facilitates preparation so that essential equipment is not inadvertently omitted (Table 15-1).

Endotracheal Tubes. Once a decision has been made to undertake translaryngeal intubation, the appropriate size and type of ET tube must be identified. The ET tubes most commonly used are sterile, disposable, and made of clear nontoxic plastic or polyvinyl chloride. The tubes have markings placed longitudinally 1 cm apart and can be used as reference points for proper placement once endotracheal intubation is accomplished (Fig. 15-1). The distal end of the ET tube should contain a side port, termed *the Murphy eye,* to prevent complete

TABLE 15-1	EQUIPMENT PREPARATION
Monitors	ECG, pulse oximeter, BP, stethoscope
Suction	Apparatus, Yankauer tube, catheter without relief valve, sterile catheter
Machine	Bag and mask, ventilator
Airway	Masks, oronasal airways, endotracheal tubes, laryngoscopes (handles, blades, bulbs, batteries), forceps
Intravenous	Two patent intravenous lines
Drugs	Anesthetic and resuscitative agents

ECG, Electrocardiogram; *BP,* blood pressure.

BOX 15-1

ESSENTIAL AIRWAY EQUIPMENT FOR INTUBATION

Laryngoscope handles (2)
Curved and straight laryngoscope blades
Endotracheal tubes (3 sizes)
Stylet
Bag and mask
Suction set-ups (2)
Suction catheter to fit endotracheal tube
Tonsil suction (Yankauer tube)
Foam donut head rest
Oropharyngeal airway
Magill forceps or Kolodny hemostats
1-inch tape
Benzoin

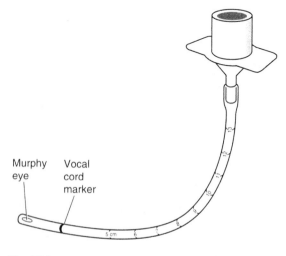

Murphy eye   Vocal cord marker

Fig. 15-1

Endotracheal tube with distance markings.

obstruction of the ET tube if mucoid secretions occlude the end hole. The appropriate ET tube size is determined by the patient's age and size. Suggested ET tube diameters based on age and size are listed in Table 15-2. The appropriate ET tube for any child 1 year of age or older may be determined by the following formula[1]:

$$\text{Internal diameter (mm)} = \text{age in years} \div 4 + 4$$

Accurate selection of an ET tube takes into consideration the child's size and length.[2-4] To be prepared for any emergency, ET tubes one-half size smaller and one-half size larger than the estimated or calculated size should always be available. The trachea becomes adult in size at 12 to 14 years of age. The appropriate ET tube size for adult females is between 7 and 8.5 mm; for adult males, it is between 8 and 10 mm.[5]

Cuffed and Uncuffed Tubes. Because the cricoid cartilage is the narrowest portion of the pediatric airway until about 8 years of age, use of an uncuffed ET tube is recommended until that time. As the child grows, the airway becomes more adult-like and tubular, with the vocal cords, not the subglottic space, becoming the smallest cross-sectional area of the airway.[6] At this age, a cuffed ET tube helps create a seal to occlude unwanted air leaks during positive-pressure ventilation. The cuff also helps to reduce the likelihood of pulmonary aspiration, although this is not guaranteed. The deflated cuff on the distal cuff end of the ET tube increases the outer diameter of the tube by approximately 0.5 mm when compared with uncuffed tubes. To compensate for the increased diameter of the cuffed

tube, a smaller sized tube, 0.5 to 1 mm, is inserted when no cuff is present.

Laryngoscope Blades and Handles. The laryngoscope is the instrument used to expose the glottic opening during intubation. It consists of two parts: a handle and a blade. The handle is available in two sizes: large and small. The handle also contains batteries that power a light source incorporated into the blade. The large handle is recommended for an adult, but it is also suitable for an infant, child, or adolescent. Because of its size and ease of manipulation, the small handle should be used for a premature infant or newborn.

Although many types of laryngoscope blades are available, the curved (MacIntosh) and straight (Miller) blades are most common. The straight blade is preferred for an infant or small child, and the curved blade is most commonly used when intubating an adult. Each blade requires a different technique for exposing the glottis. When a straight blade is used, the epiglottis is actually lifted with the tip of the blade and pressed against the base of the tongue (Fig. 15-2). The advantage of this technique is inherent in the fluffy U-shaped epiglottis of

TABLE 15-2	GUIDELINES FOR PEDIATRIC TRACHEAL TUBE SIZE	
Child's Age	**Internal Diameter (mm)**
Premature	
1000 g	2.5
1000-1500 g	3.0
1500-2500 g	3.5
Normal newborns	3.5-4.0
6-12 months	4.0-4.5
1-2 years	4.5
4 years	5.0
6 years	5.5
8 years	6.0
10 years	6.5
Greater than 12 years	
Female	7.0-8.5
Male	8.0-10.0

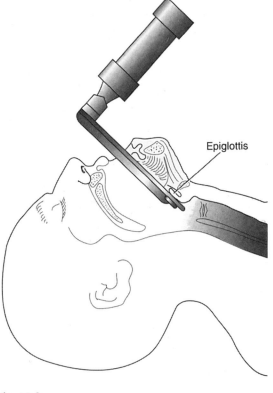

Fig. 15-2

Direct laryngoscopy using a straight (Miller) blade.

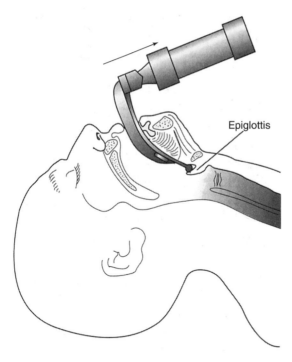

Epiglottis

Fig. 15-3

Direct laryngoscopy using a curved (MacIntosh) blade and demonstrating proper lifting technique. Note the upward and forward lift while the wrist is held straight.

an infant or small child. In contrast, the tip of the curved blade is placed in the vallecula, the space between the epiglottis and the base of the tongue, and as the laryngoscope is pulled forward, it elevates the epiglottis and exposes the glottis (Fig. 15-3).[7] This method may also be helpful to visualize the cords when using a straight blade during intubation of a small newborn.[1] Although different blades and handles are recommended for intubation, ease of use, comfort with a particular instrument, and personal preference are the important guides to determining which technique to use. The MacIntosh curved blade, for example, has a wider flange, which provides better control of the tongue. This may be helpful in intubation of a small infant or child, whose anatomy is such that the tongue can be a major obstacle to success.

Suction Equipment. Suctioning both the upper and lower airway will contribute to both successful intubation and maintaining a patent airway. Suctioning equipment should be immediately accessible in anticipation of airway problems in any intensive care unit or operating room suite. Portable suction devices are available for use during the transportation of intubated patients or in those who may require air-

way intervention. In addition to the vacuum device, a regulator, a connecting tube, a tonsillar tip suction handle, such as a Yankauer, and several standard sterile suction catheters, with and without a control port, are required.

The suction device is located at the head of the bed, and the regulator is set at a medium setting, between 80 and 120 mm Hg suction.[8] The tonsillar tip handle is used to quickly clear the upper airway of large amounts of liquid or particulate matter. Using the suction catheter without a control port during intubation allows the clinician to continuously visualize the glottic opening without stopping to occlude the control port. Finally, once the intubation is successful, the sterile suction catheter with a control port can be placed through the ET tube to suction pulmonary secretions. Suctioning is indicated for pulmonary hygiene and to obtain secretions for possible diagnostic purposes, such as a Gram's stain or culture.

INTUBATION PROCEDURE

The indication for translaryngeal intubation will determine the most appropriate technique to use during the process. The options available to the clinician are orotracheal intubation, nasal or blind nasal intubation, awake intubation, or anesthetized intubation using neuromuscular blockers, amnesic agents, and sedatives. Universal precautions, wearing gloves and eye protection, should be observed with all intubation procedures to reduce the risk of transmitting infectious diseases.

OROTRACHEAL INTUBATION

In the majority of cases, translaryngeal intubation takes place with the patient supine. The height of the bed or stretcher should be such that the patient's head is level with the clinician's xiphoid process. This allows direct visualization of the airway without putting undue stress or strain on the clinician. Because the larynx in the pediatric patient is anterior and cephalad, placing a small towel or roll underneath the patient's occiput optimally aligns the axes of the mouth, pharynx, and larynx. Flexing the neck forward and the head backward maintains the "sniffing" position.[9] Because an infant's or small child's occiput is more prominent than the older child's, the sniffing position may be obtained without the use of head elevation. Head elevation in these patients may push the airway farther anterior, making translaryngeal intubation more difficult.

If the patient is breathing spontaneously, the application of 100% oxygen for 2 to 5 minutes with a bag and mask with or without applying positive pressure is sufficient to fully oxygenate and denitrogenate the lungs. In the event that there are no spontaneous respirations, four maximal breaths of 100% oxygen over 30 seconds accomplishes the same goal. Adjuvant agents, such as sedatives, amnesic agents, or neuromuscular blockers, are administered at this point to facilitate airway exposure. If the patient is at risk for regurgitation and aspiration, cricoid pressure is applied to compress the esophagus against the cervical vertebrae (Sellick's maneuver).[10] The cricoid pressure is not withdrawn until a secure airway is assured. Cricoid pressure may help prevent the gastric distention associated with bag and mask ventilation of the pediatric airway.[11]

Once the patient is fully oxygenated, the mouth is opened wide using the forefinger and thumb in a scissoring motion. This is accomplished by depressing the mandible with the thumb of the right hand and applying pressure on the upper teeth with the index finger of the same hand. Once the mouth has been opened, the upper airway is suctioned as necessary.

To use the laryngoscope, the handle is grasped midshaft with the left hand and the blade is inserted on the right side of the patient's mouth, sweeping the tongue toward the left. The laryngoscope is advanced forward in the midline while a forward and upward motion is exerted, as shown in Fig. 15-3. Individual blade preference determines whether the epiglottis is lifted with the tip of a straight blade or exposed by placing the tip of the curved blade in the vallecula. It is important to remember that throughout this portion of the technique the wrist cannot be flexed or rotated. Such motion causes undue pressure on the upper teeth and can chip or dislodge them. Pressure on the maxillary ridge in the small infant or child can cause hematoma and damage to unerupted teeth.

Fig. 15-4 illustrates the glottic structures as viewed through the laryngoscope. After visualizing of the glottic opening, the appropriate-sized ET tube is held in the right hand and is introduced into the right side of the patient's mouth to avoid obstructing the view of the glottic opening. The tip of the ET tube is advanced through the glottic opening so that the single black ring, the cord guide, lies just distal to the opening of the glottis. If the ET tube is marked with three rings, it should be inserted until the double black ring is distal to the glottic opening. In the event that the child is old enough to have a cuffed ET tube, the tube is advanced until the cuff is distal to the vocal cords.

The proper ET tube position is in the mid trachea or about 2 cm above the carina. In an adult, this is at the 21- to 23-cm mark. For the child, correct ET tube placement for oral intubation is estimated by using the following formula[12]:

$$12 + (age \div 2)$$

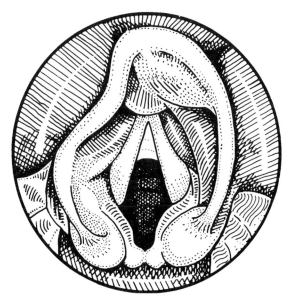

Fig. 15-4

Glottic structures viewed through the laryngoscope. (From Grundfast KM, Harley E: Vocal cord paralysis. *Otolaryngol Clin North Am* 1989; 22:582.)

Any attempt at intubation should not exceed 30 seconds. In the event that the glottic opening cannot be visualized or the ET tube cannot be placed in that time period, the attempt should be aborted. The patient's airway should be reestablished by bag and mask ventilation to ensure adequate oxygenation before another attempt at intubation is made.

The chest is auscultated after intubation to assess correct tube position. Breath sounds should be heard bilaterally over the lateral chest wall. Auscultating over the anterior chest wall of an infant or neonate can cause gastric sounds from an esophageal intubation to be mistaken for adequate breath sounds. Proper tube position must be assessed by one or several other methods, such as observing chest wall movement, observing condensation in the ET tube during exhalation, palpating the ET tube in the suprasternal notch, calorimetry, or capnometry. The last procedure is helpful because esophageal intubation may cause an initial observation of carbon dioxide, but within one to two breaths a negligible amount of carbon dioxide is observed.[13,14] A chest radiograph is the most common method of assessing tube position, although the results are not immediately available. Each of the methods suggested for assessing proper ET tube placement has the potential for false-positive re-

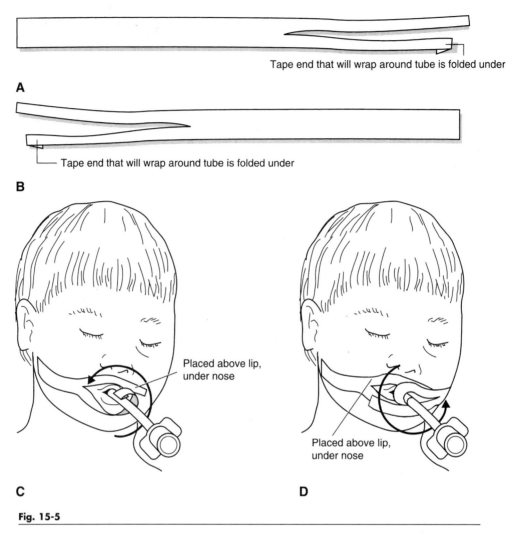

Fig. 15-5

Steps used to secure the ET tube with tape. **A** and **B,** Slit two pieces of tape, making a Y on one end of each piece (as shown). Turn under the end of the tape that will be wrapped around the ET tube. This will make tape removal easier. **C,** Apply benzoin to the area below the nose and across the cheeks (where tape will be placed). Attach one piece of tape to the cheek and below the nose, wrapping the bottom of the Y around the ET tube. The tape should be placed under the tube (chin side) first, then wrapped around the top of the tube. **D,** Repeat step **C** on the other side of the face.

sults. The best method of ensuring proper ET tube placement is direct visualization.

The ET tube is secured by preparing the skin with tincture of benzoin. Two strips of tape are cut long enough to go from the lateral aspect of the right eye to the lateral aspect of the left eye. Each piece is split into a Y shape with the arms of the Y two-thirds the length of the tape. The tape should have a width that will easily fit on the upper lip and around the ET tube. One end of the tape is secured to the cheek and wrapped around the tube in a "barber pole" fashion (Fig. 15-5). The necessary equipment (Box 15-2) for securing the ET tube is assembled before attempting the intubation. Other taping methods may be used to secure the tube, as long as the method can be performed by all clinicians involved in airway care and is fast and secure. The centimeter mark at which the ET tube is secured must be marked.

There are various devices available to secure the ET tube as an alternative to using tape. Fig. 15-6 illustrates an example of one of these devices. When selecting a device to secure the tube it is important that it does not occlude access to the mouth, provides minimal tube movement when the head moves, and secures without creating decubitus ulcers at pressure points. Additionally, the same rules apply as with taping methods: fast, easy, and can be applied by all clinicians. The evidence that these devices help reduce the incidence of accidental extubations is inconclusive. However, it does suggest that these devices may be more effective on a small infant than a larger infant or child.[15,16]

NASOTRACHEAL INTUBATION

Once a patent and stable airway has been established using the orotracheal route, switching to a nasal tube can follow. The patient's nares are prepared by spraying a vasoconstrictive agent, such as phenylephrine, into the opening. This decreases mucosal swelling and inflammation. An ET tube of a size that will pass easily through the nares is used. Depending on the patient's anatomy, this may be the same size as the tube selected for orotracheal intubation or, as is usually the case, approximately one size smaller.

The tube is lubricated with either petroleum jelly or 2% lidocaine jelly. Then the tube is inserted into the nares until approximately one half of it is passed through the nose. While an assistant holds the existing oral ET tube in the left corner of the mouth, the glottis is exposed in the same manner as for orotracheal intubation. Once the nasal tube is visualized in the hypopharynx, the tip of the tube is grabbed with a Magill or Kolodny forceps held in the right hand and the nasal tube is lifted up and in front of the opening to the larynx. When direct visualization of the glottic opening is ensured, the assistant is asked to remove the orotracheal tube. Then the nasotracheal tube is advanced immediately into the trachea. Difficulty in passing the tube through the cords may be encountered because of the upward curve of the ET tube and the limited mobility of the forceps in the small pharyngeal opening. Gentle rotation of the tube to the right or left may allow easier passage. Additionally, the assistant may gently advance the tube from above while the clinician guides the ET tube through the glottic opening.

Proper tube position is assessed using the methods described previously. For depth of nasal intubations, the following formula is used:

$$15 + (age \div 3)$$

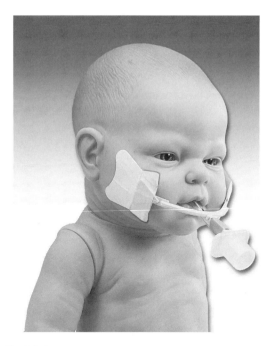

Fig. 15-6

The Neobar. A commercial adaptation of the Logan Bow for stabilizing an infant endotracheal tube. (Courtesy of Neotech Products, Inc., Chatsworth, Calif.)

The centimeter mark at the nares is noted and the ET tube is taped securely in place. The major contraindications to nasotracheal intubation are a bleeding diathesis, such as thrombocytopenia, abnormal clotting times, facial trauma, and suspected basilar skull fracture.

BLIND NASAL INTUBATION

The larynx of an infant or small child is anterior and cephalad, making intubation more difficult. This anatomic difference between adults and children makes attempts at blind nasal intubation almost uniformly unsuccessful. Wisdom recommends that attempts at a blind nasal intubation be vigorously discouraged, owing to the potential for damaging the airway and making further intervention and intubation more difficult and dangerous.

ORAL VERSUS NASAL INTUBATION

One of the most frequently used arguments for nasal over oral intubation is patient comfort. Although it is believed that a nasal tube is more comfortable than an oral tube, recent evidence may dispute this and, in fact, there may be no difference between the two.[17] In the small infant and pediatric population, there is less effort in securing and maintaining a nasotracheal tube in the proper position. Salivation, which interferes with the adhesiveness of the tape, is not stimulated, so the ET tube does not slip out of position as readily. Usually it is not a problem in the nasally intubated patient with teeth biting down on the ET tube, which can cause an occlusion or hole. Although oral hygiene is facilitated, ET tube suctioning may be more difficult.

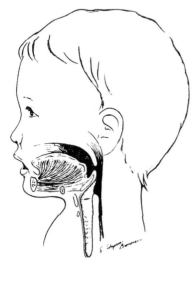

A

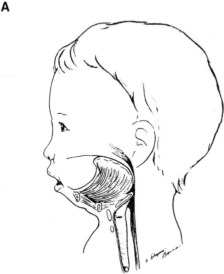

B

Fig. 15-7

Anatomic features of the normal larynx (**A**), and of the larynx in the presence of mandibular hypoplasia (**B**). In the presence of mandibular hypoplasia, the posterior displacement of the tongue makes the larynx appear more anteriorly situated than normal. (From Handler SD: Craniofacial surgery: otolaryngological concerns. *Int Anesthesiol Clin North Am* 1988; 26:62.)

Disadvantages to nasal intubation include a predisposition to sinusitis, pressure necrosis of the nares, and bleeding complications associated with passing the ET tube through the nares and upper airway. A higher incidence of postextubation atelectasis among very low-birth-weight infants has also been reported.[17]

APPROACHES TO THE DIFFICULT AIRWAY

Some children may present challenging problems that may make intubation difficult or impossible. These include patients with craniofacial syndromes, orofacial trauma or infections, and complete laryngeal obstruction. The clinician should have additional options available to secure the airway in the event that orotracheal intubation is not successful. Other methods of securing an airway include anterior commissure intubation, flexible fiberoptic intubation, or emergency tracheotomy.

Anterior Commissure Intubation. Children with craniofacial malformations may present a significant challenge to a straightforward intubation. In addition, many of these children require intubation for plastic reconstructive surgery. The child with the hypoplastic mandible is a very challenging problem. This would include children with Pierre Robin sequence (retrognathia, glossoptosis, and cleft palate), Treacher Collins syndrome, and hemifacial microsomia. The young patient with the Pierre Robin sequence has a larynx that is exceedingly difficult to expose. In such cases, the larynx is high,

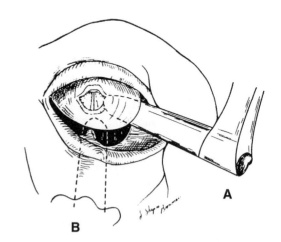

A

B

Fig. 15-8

Laryngoscope placed laterally in the right oral commissure (**A**), permitting more complete visualization of the larynx when the instrument is passed in the standard midline position (**B**). (From Handler SD: Craniofacial surgery: otolaryngological concerns. *Int Anesthesiol Clin North Am* 1988; 26:62.)

anterior, and concealed by the tongue base (Fig. 15-7). During intubation the clinician may be only able to visualize the tips of the arytenoid cartilages. Handler described a technique known as *anterior commissure intubation* using the Holinger anterior commissure laryngoscope. This rigid and tubular style laryngoscope offers excellent exposure of the endolarynx (Fig. 15-8). The narrow end of the laryngoscope is placed into the laryngeal inlet, and the ET tube can be passed directly into the scope with a long alligator forceps and advanced as the laryngoscope is withdrawn (Fig. 15-9). This technique may be useful to intubate the child who cannot be intubated with a standard laryngoscope and thus avoid an emergency tracheotomy without an airway.[18]

Flexible Fiberoptic Intubation. When the larynx cannot be visualized with a rigid endoscope, the flexible fiberoptic bronchoscope offers several advantages for intubation. First, the flexible scope

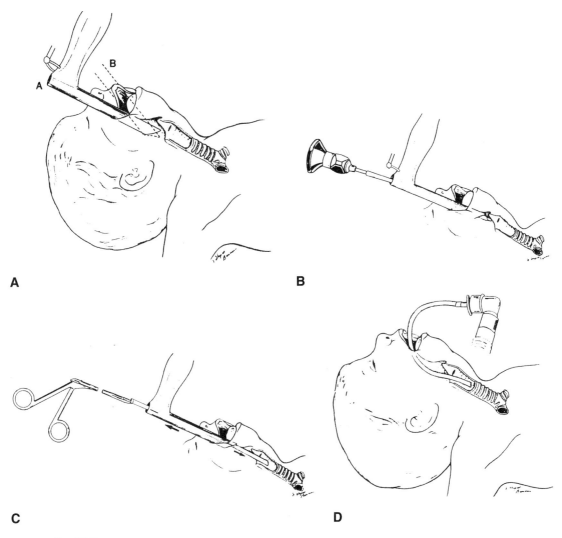

Fig. 15-9

Laryngoscopy and intubation. **A,** With laryngoscope in lateral position (A), approximately 30 degrees of anterior angulation is gained over the standard midline position (B), thus permitting more complete visualization of the larynx. **B,** Endotracheal tube (without 15-mm anesthetic adapter) is inserted into the barrel of the laryngoscope under direct vision. In this example, an optical stylet is used. **C,** Endotracheal tube is grasped with alligator forceps and advanced slightly *(small arrow)* as the laryngoscope is withdrawn *(large arrow)*. **D,** Anesthetic adapter (15 mm) is replaced, and ventilation is begun. (From Handler SD: Craniofacial surgery: otolaryngological concerns. *Int Anesthesiol Clin North Am* 1988; 26:63.)

can navigate into an endolarynx that is impossible or difficult to expose with the rigid scope. This enables the clinician to pass an ET tube over the flexible scope once the flexible scope is inside the trachea. Second, the flexible scope facilitates nasotracheal intubation, which may be a more secure airway in certain clinical situations, such as hypopharyngeal masses, craniofacial anomalies, and muscular dystrophy. The older child or young adult with certain muscular dystrophies may have such severe contractures that they are impossible to expose with the anterior commissure laryngoscope. In such cases the best option for a controlled intubation is with the flexible fiberoptic scope.

Although their discussion is beyond the scope of this chapter, there are several other methods of orotracheal intubation worth mentioning. These include finger intubation of the trachea, retrograde tracheal intubation, intubation with the laryngeal mask airway, and several new fiberoptic laryngoscopes such the Bullard and Neustein laryngoscopes.[19-24]

Emergency Tracheotomy. In the infant and small child it is preferred to perform a tracheotomy after the airway has been secured. In most cases endotracheal intubation is preferred yet not always possible. Circumstances under which endotracheal intubation may be difficult or impossible include severe trauma or hemorrhage, craniofacial problems, and the newborn with complete laryngeal obstruction. The alternative approaches to securing the airway are dictated by the urgency of the clinical situation and the age of the patient. These include tracheotomy under local anesthesia, mask ventilation, or cricothyroidotomy.

In an older patient with airway obstruction who can cooperate, a tracheotomy under local anesthesia is preferred. The infant with near-total laryngeal obstruction may require face mask or laryngeal mask airway ventilation during tracheotomy. In the emergency setting, an option in older children and adolescents is a cricothyroidotomy in which the tracheotomy is inserted into the cricothyroid membrane. This is a relatively expeditious way of placing an emergency tracheostomy tube in older patients.[25] In infants and small children, an emergency cricothyroidotomy may be difficult to perform and other options are less difficult and safer.

Epiglottitis. In recent years the frequency of epiglottitis has decreased dramatically as the vaccine for *Haemophilus influenzae* type b has all but eliminated most of the typeable strains of *H. influenzae*. Today epiglottitis is a rare disorder and experience with its emergency management is declining. Epiglottitis is a true pediatric emergency. It is

important to follow the same basic airway management principles and to be fully prepared if adherence to basic principles cannot be maintained.

The child with clinical manifestations of epiglottitis should not undergo a visual examination in the emergency department (see Chapter 33). The child should not be stimulated and should be kept as calm as possible. The patient should be accompanied by medical personnel with the appropriate airway skills to accomplish emergency intubation to an area where diagnosis can be confirmed by a soft tissue, lateral neck radiograph (Fig. 15-10). Radiologic findings include thickening of the epiglottis and aryepiglottic folds and the classic "thumbprint" sign. Once the diagnosis has been established, arrangements should be made for immediate transport to the operating room for intubation by an anesthesiologist, with back up by an otorhinolaryngologist in the event an emergency tracheostomy is required. An emergency tracheotomy set and bronchoscope should be available and ready for use. Intubation is done by the anesthesiologist after a slow mask induction with continuous spontaneous ventilation. Then a valleculae laryngoscope is used to expose the epiglottis and endolarynx. This confirms the diagnosis and exposes the airway for intubation. The larynx is orally intubated, and then a nasotracheal tube is placed. Check the leak pressure daily and attempt extubation when there is a leak of 10 to 20 cm H_2O around an age-appropriate ET tube. Generally, 48 to 56 hours of intubation and intravenous antibiotics is needed before extubation is successful.

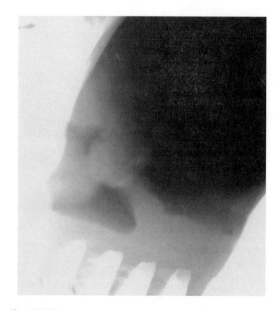

Fig. 15-10

Lateral soft tissue neck radiograph revealing epiglottitis.

ARTIFICIAL AIRWAY CUFF MANAGEMENT

The cuff is inflated once proper placement of the ET or tracheostomy tube is ensured. If the patient has a large leak with the cuff deflated, then the cuff is inflated. To inflate the cuff, a 5- or 10-ml syringe is attached to the pilot balloon and gradually air is added to the cuff. Positive pressure applied through the ET tube should produce an audible escape of air, or leak, at less than or equal to 20 cm H_2O. The leak should be auscultated for over the larynx. Intracuff pressures are maintained at less than 20 to 25 cm H_2O because higher pressures are associated with ischemia and necrosis of the tracheal mucosa and can lead to tracheal stenosis.

Cuff pressures should be checked approximately every 8 hours to guarantee that the pressure does not exceed the recommended levels. If a cuff pressure-measuring device is not available, the minimal leak test can be performed. To inflate the cuff to minimal leak, the cuff is inflated until no air leak is noted during the application of positive pressure. Then a small amount of air is withdrawn from the cuff until a slight leak is auscultated. During certain positive-pressure applications, the minimal occlusion technique may be necessary. The procedure is the same as that just described, with the exception that enough air is left in the cuff to prevent a leak.

If large amounts of air are required in the cuff and a leak persists, one of two possibilities exists: (1) the cuff is damaged or (2) it has not been advanced totally through the cords. The latter problem can be identified by direct laryngoscopy. According to present recommendations, a cuffed ET tube should not be used in a patient younger than 8 years of age. In patients younger than 8 years, the cricoid cartilage, the narrowest portion of the airway, serves as a functional cuff. In the neonate, the leak pressure should be kept at less than or equal to 10 cm H_2O if possible to prevent tracheal damage.

PATIENT MONITORING

Continuously evaluating the patient undergoing intubation is essential to ensure a safe and effective outcome. Before the airway is manipulated, the heart rate, capillary refill, blood pressure, and oxygen saturation should be monitored and recorded. Under ideal circumstances, a precordial stethoscope is used to continuously monitor heart tones and breath sounds. At a minimum, the patient's heart rate, blood pressure, and oxygen saturation should be monitored continuously. A continuous electrocardiogram monitors the heart for dysrhythmias. Noninvasive means of monitoring blood pressure include palpation, auscultation, and automated

devices. Pulse oximetry and patient color best indicate oxygen saturation during intubation. A single individual should be made responsible for the task of monitoring the patient continuously during the procedure. If, at any time, acceptable values or rhythms are breached, the clinician should be warned and attempts at intubation stopped. The airway should be reestablished without delay using a bag and mask.

COMPLICATIONS

Serious complications from endotracheal intubation may occur at any time during or after the intubation procedure. The immediate complications encountered during intubation include both mechanical processes and reflex reactions. Immediate mechanical complications include tissue trauma, perforation or laceration of the pharynx or larynx, esophageal intubation, and pneumothorax. Risks involving autonomic reflexes include laryngospasm and bronchospasm, resulting in hypoxia, cardiac dysrhythmias, and hypotension. Stimulation of the vagal reflex leads to severe bradycardia and arterial hypotension.

After intubation takes place, the spectrum of complications changes. ET tube obstruction secondary to kinking, biting, blood, and secretions becomes more prominent. Cuff ruptures are also prominent on cuffed tubes. The incidence of accidental extubation has been reported to be between 3% and 13% and appears to be more common in infants younger than 1 year of age. Aspiration, endobronchial intubation, and atelectasis are not uncommon. Laryngeal edema is a common complication associated with intubation. The edema may be glottic, supraglottic, or subglottic. Subglottic edema is more common because of the infant's small airway; it can cause narrowing of the trachea and may require urgent reintubation. The incidence of clinically significant subglottic stenosis has been reported to be 2% to 6% of the pediatric population. Maxillary sinusitis and nosocomial pneumonia are long-term infectious complications associated with significant mortality and morbidity.

EXTUBATION

The most important question to consider when evaluating a patient for extubation is whether there has been improvement or reversal of the disease process that initially mandated the intubation. Before extubation, the patient must be hemodynamically stable, must be able to breathe spontaneously with an adequate tidal volume and respiratory pattern, and must have adequate muscle strength to protect the airway.

Hemodynamic stability is manifested by normal cardiac output, capillary refill, urine output, and blood pressure. The patient should be alert and awake with evidence of adequate muscle strength. In older children, muscle strength is evaluated by measuring maximum inspiratory pressure during airway occlusion and vital capacity. A maximum inspiratory pressure greater than 20 cm H_2O and a vital capacity greater than 20 ml/kg in an adult correlate with successful extubation. It is important to point out that these tests, although used in the pediatric population, have not been validated by prospective trials. Additionally, adequate airway reflexes include being able to gag, swallow, and cough. The gag reflex can be stimulated by placing a tongue blade in the posterior pharynx, and a cough reflex can be evaluated as the trachea is stimulated during suctioning.

ACCIDENTAL EXTUBATION

The reported incidence of accidental extubation in the pediatric and neonatal intensive care population is between 3% and 13%. Other methodologies of reporting the number of accidental extubations have focused on accidental extubation per 100 intubated days. This rate varies from 0.72 per 100 intubated days in the neonatal intensive care unit to 1.1 per 100 intubated days in the pediatric intensive care unit.[26] Risk factors associated with accidental extubation include failure to secure the ET tube properly, lack of adequate sedation, failure to provide adequate restraint, and performing a procedure, such as chest radiography, on a patient. In the adult population, deliberate self-extubation despite sedation and restraints also contributes to unplanned extubations. Although death can result from self-extubation in any population, it is an infrequent complication. Despite its potential for adverse outcome, self-extubation is usually well tolerated by most patient populations.

EQUIPMENT

As in the intubation procedure, anticipation and preparation are essential in accomplishing a smooth extubation. The equipment necessary for extubation includes a bag and mask set-up, suction equipment, adhesive remover, and all the equipment previously listed for intubation (see Box 15-1). This ensures a proactive approach to patient care in the event that the patient does not tolerate extubation.

PROCEDURE

Pulmonary function is optimized by administering aerosolized β-agonists as needed and suctioning the oropharynx and trachea before extubation. If the patient has been receiving enteral feedings, the feedings are discontinued for approximately 6 hours before the planned extubation. Although this allows gastric emptying, it does not guarantee that the aspiration of gastric contents will not occur.

To reduce the risk of hypoxemia, the patient is placed on 100% oxygen and manually ventilated, occasionally with hyperinflation. If a cuffed tube is in place, the cuff should be deflated. While the ET tube is held in place, the tape is removed from the face and tube with an adhesive remover. One large breath is administered and the ET tube is withdrawn from the trachea near peak inflation. The majority of patients will then cough and begin to breathe spontaneously. It is not unusual, especially in small children, for a short interval of breathholding to occur. However, this must be distinguished from the more severe complication of laryngospasm. Oxygen is administered by the most appropriate means available, such as a face tent, face mask, or oxyhood. The oxygen concentration is titrated to maintain an oxygen saturation level that is clinically indicated.

The tube should not be removed during a cough or at end-expiration. During a cough, the tissues of the trachea are collapsed into the air column and tighten around the ET tube. If the patient is extubated at this point, he or she will not have sufficient lung inflation for an effective cough and may aspirate oral secretions.

EXPLANATION TO PATIENT AND PARENT

Before extubation of any patient, the extubation procedure and possible complications should be explained. Guidelines regarding the need for reintubation should be discussed in depth with either the patient or the patient's family. The first two topics are delineated in detail in other sections of this chapter. It is essential that any explanation be clear, using a vocabulary easily understood by the patient and parents. The patient and parents must be aware that every effort has been made to adequately evaluate the patient's readiness for extubation but that there is a possibility that reintubation may be required. A review of possible scenarios requiring reintubation may help alleviate the parental disappointment associated with this apparent setback. Common scenarios include, but are not limited to, laryngospasm that will not respond to conservative therapy, the development of postextubation stridor that is not amenable to therapy, and hypoxemia or hypercarbia associated with a patient's inability to maintain adequate oxygenation and ventilation. It is important to relieve as much of patient or parental anxiety as possible. Reassurances that the procedure will be as painless, effortless, and smooth as possible aid in a successful and atraumatic extubation.

COMPLICATIONS

Sore throat and hoarseness are common complaints after extubation. The presence of an ET tube may cause edema of the laryngeal structures. Once extubation is successfully accomplished, postextubation stridor can develop within minutes and usually peaks within 8 hours. This condition has been well described and occurs frequently in the pediatric population. Corticosteroids, aerosolized racemic epinephrine, and helium/oxygen mixtures have all been used to treat this complication.[27] Laryngospasm, another known complication postextubation, is caused by stimulating the larynx when removing the ET tube or from pooled secretions that may drain into the airway.

Difficulty with extubation can be associated with poor pulmonary function or can occur secondary to mechanical complications. Patients who have not been adequately assessed with regard to their pulmonary status may not tolerate extubation. An ineffective cough and gag reflex will predispose the patient to aspiration of secretions or gastric contents, possibly leading to alveolar collapse and pneumonitis. A mechanical problem related to extubation is the failure to deflate the ET tube cuff, resulting in direct trauma and the potential for laryngeal edema.

EXTUBATION FAILURE

A child may fail one or more controlled attempts at extubation for a number of reasons. These include pathologic processes of both the upper and lower airway as well as the general medical and neurologic condition of the patient. In the premature infant the lungs may not be developed enough for the child to breathe without ventilatory support or positive pressure. In these cases the infant may need time for further pulmonary development. In addition, the child who is neurologically compromised or oversedated may not be able to breathe spontaneously and protect the airway. One must wait for the child's neurologic status to improve.

Some children may have congenital or acquired causes for obstruction of the upper airway that will prevent a successful extubation. These include choanal atresia, severe laryngomalacia, vocal cord paralysis, laryngeal edema, stenosis (congenital or acquired), subglottic cysts, hemangiomas, and tracheomalacia. In these situations the child does well with minimal or no ventilator support but develops a problem as soon as the ET tube is removed.

Treatment Strategies. First, the reason for extubation failure and/or the site of obstruction must be determined. It is important to know the degree of ventilatory support that is required before extubation. Children who cannot be weaned from mechanical ventilation may have underlying pulmonary or central neurologic pathology. In such cases, long-term ventilation may need to be considered. In contrast, the child who easily weans from mechanical ventilation but cannot be extubated may have significant upper airway obstruction. In such a case, endoscopy may be useful in determining the site and cause of the problem. The child should undergo a direct laryngoscopy and bronchoscopy in the operating room to localize the site of obstruction. Treatment then depends on the specific pathology. The child with subglottic stenosis may need surgical intervention and may be considered for an anterior cricoid split to achieve extubation. The patient with a subglottic cyst or hemangioma may require laser ablation of the lesion. The infant with bilateral choanal atresia requires immediate surgical repair with stenting. The child with distal tracheomalacia may have a vascular compression and will require additional tests such as magnetic resonance angiography to define the vascular pathology. When there are vascular anomalies, cardiovascular intervention may be necessary.

Nasal Mask Ventilation, Heliox. To ease the transition to spontaneous ventilation or when there is residual upper airway obstruction, noninvasive positive-pressure mask ventilation may be helpful. A nasal face mask that fits over the nose and mouth is used to deliver both inspiratory and expiratory pressure. The so-called BiPAP (bilevel positive airway pressure) system may be a useful method to transition the patient to spontaneous respiration after extubation. In the event that a fixed narrow opening such as in subglottic stenosis or laryngeal edema is the cause of difficulty, a helium-oxygen mixture (Heliox) may be beneficial. Its lower density may reduce the viscosity of air flow and decrease airway resistance. Mixtures of helium to oxygen are available in 80% helium/20% oxygen and 70% helium/30% oxygen. Additional oxygen can be titrated into these mixtures; however, as the concentration of oxygen increases, the density of the gas decreases, as does efficacy. When the upper airway obstruction has resolved, one can then gradually reduce and stop the Heliox.

Anterior Cricoid Split. The child with evolving subglottic stenosis and a normal lower airway may be a good candidate for an anterior cricoid split (ACS). The criteria are listed in Box 15-3.[28] The best candidate for ACS has an isolated subglottic laryngeal pathologic process and no pulmonary or other airway problems. Before one embarks on a cricoid split procedure other causes of airway obstruction should be ruled out. The main purpose of the ACS is to decompress the subglottic airway by splitting the cricoid ring and stenting the laryngeal framework for 7 to 14 days. Because the postoperative care is a critical component of the success of this procedure, it should only be undertaken in an institution in which there is a pediatric intensive care unit.

Once candidacy is confirmed, the child is intubated and positioned with the neck hyperextended

---

BOX 15-3

CRITERIA FOR THE ANTERIOR CRICOID SPLIT

1. Extubation failure on at least two occasions secondary to subglottic laryngeal pathology.
2. Weight greater than 1500 g.
3. No ventilator support for at least 10 days before repair.
4. Supplemental O_2 requirement less than 30%.
5. No congestive heart failure for 1 month before repair.
6. No acute respiratory tract infection.
7. No antihypertensive medication for 10 days before repair.

Modified with permission from Myer CM III, Cotton RT, Shott SR, editors: *The pediatric airway: an interdisciplinary approach.* Philadelphia. Lippincott-Raven, 1995; p 122.

---

in the same position used to do a tracheotomy. A horizontal neck incision affords exposure to the upper two tracheal rings and the thyroid cartilage. Two nylon stay sutures are placed in the paramedian position on the cricoid cartilage. A midline vertical incision is made through the cricoid cartilage, the first two tracheal rings, and the lower portion of the thyroid cartilage (Fig. 15-11). The child is kept nasally intubated for 7 to 14 days with an age-appropriate-sized ET tube. Ventilator support with continuous neuromuscular blockade may be necessary. If the child is accidentally extubated, then reintubation may be quite hazardous. Dexamethasone is started 24 hours before extubation, and the child is extubated when extubation criteria are met.

TRACHEOTOMY

The child who is not a candidate for extubation or the ACS may require a tracheotomy. The decision to perform tracheotomy is based on the future airway prognosis, as well as on the family's ability to care for an artificial airway at home. Before proceeding with a tracheotomy the risks as well as the significant burden for the family must be considered.

TRACHEOTOMY INDICATIONS

The three main indications for tracheotomy in infants and children are airway obstruction, long-term ventilation, and pulmonary hygiene. Children with congenital or acquired upper airway obstruction may

Fig. 15-11

Anterior cricoid split procedure. A midline laryngofissure extends from the inferior half of the thyroid cartilage to the second tracheal ring. (From Walner DL, Cotton RT: Acquired anomalies of the larynx and trachea. In Cotton RT, Myer CM, editors: *Practical pediatric otolaryngology*. Philadelphia. Lippincott-Raven, 1999; p 525.)

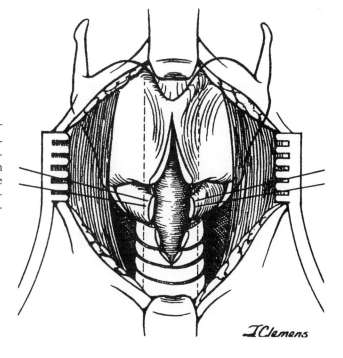

require a tracheotomy at an early age if extubation cannot be accomplished. Congenital laryngeal stenosis, which varies in severity, may require a tracheotomy at a very early age or even in the delivery room. Bilateral vocal cord paralysis, which is usually secondary to central neurologic causes, such as Arnold-Chiari malformation, results in severe airway obstruction. Tracheotomy may be required in about 66% of these cases.[29] In many cases the vocal cord paralysis resolves within several years. Acquired laryngeal stenosis is related to prematurity, prolonged intubation, traumatic intubation sepsis, and so on. Premature children with bronchopulmonary dysplasia require a tracheotomy for long-term ventilation. In addition, children with neurologic problems, especially if they have impairment of brain stem function, may develop difficulties with pulmonary hygiene requiring a tracheotomy.

TRACHEOTOMY TUBES

Tracheotomy tubes come in various dimensions and materials, and selecting a tracheotomy tube is an important issue. The age, size, and medical condition of the patient determine the type of tracheotomy tube selected. Tracheotomy tubes come in various sizes, which are usually chosen based on age (Table 15-3). Tracheotomy tubes have three dimensions: inner diameter (ID), outer diameter (OD), and length. The depth of the tube from the flange is usually related to the length of the tube. The dimensions of three common brands of tracheotomy tubes are compared in Table 15-4.

When selecting a tube, the shape and composition must be considered in addition to the size. Some tubes are made of polyvinyl chloride, which is rigid, whereas other brands are made of silicone and require wire reinforcement. Softer does not always equal better. Whereas softer tube composition may be used to overcome pressure ulcerations, it does not aid in healing ulcerations caused by friction forces. Most of the time, patient comfort will dictate which material to use in a clinical situation.

An arched tube is curved in the shape of one fourth of a circle and is short. An angled tube is curved into a 90-degree bend and slightly longer than the arched tube. Each tube must be positioned correctly in the airway to optimize performance. Malpositioning of these tubes may result in kinking, mainstem intubation, or occluding on the anterior or posterior wall of the trachea (Fig. 15-12).[30] However, once the tube warms to body temperature, it usually conforms to the shape of the airway. Sometimes changing the tube to a different shape may overcome a stoma track that is difficult to cannulate.

A cuffed tracheotomy tube may be needed for a child requiring higher ventilatory pressures for chronic lung disease. There are three basic types of cuffs, high volume low-pressure, foam cuff, and tight-to-shaft (TTS). The first two are inflated with air, whereas the last requires saline. Customized tracheotomy tubes may be needed in certain situations. The type of cuff is decided by the team and ordered specifically for each patient. It is important to avoid overinflation of the cuff. This may lead to problems with tracheal erosion and stenosis. It is essential to visualize the tracheotomy endoscopically with the cuff inflated with the usual amount of saline or air. The cuff should not be causing pressure necrosis on the distal tracheal mucosa. If the cuff appears tight, then less air or saline is used. The technique for determining minimal leak or minimal occlusion pressures for tracheotomy tube cuffs is the same as described for ET tube cuffs.

There are several types of tracheotomy ties that caretakers may use. These include tracheotomy string or twill tape, felt with a Velcro fastener (Fig. 15-13), and metal chain. Each has its advantages and disadvantages and depends on the individual preference of the caretakers. The latter two facilitate cleaning and are easier to remove in an emergency.

PROCEDURE AND TECHNIQUE

There are special concerns with respect to tracheotomy in the infant and small child. First the anatomic characteristics make it more difficult to localize the trachea than in adults. The major landmarks including the cricoid and thyroid cartilage are not prominent. The trachea is smaller and not as superficial, and it is more mobile and easy to push over to one side. Furthermore, the rapid placement of the tracheotomy in the cricothyroid membrane (cricothyroidotomy) is contraindicated in an infant or small child but may be performed in an emergent situation in an older child or adolescent.

Routine tracheotomy for infants and small children requires careful dissection with an established airway such as an orotracheal tube. If the airway is not already established, then the child may undergo bronchoscopy or intubation before tracheotomy. Occasionally, a tracheotomy is performed in older children or adolescents with the use of local anesthesia, but this should be avoided if possible in small children. The airway is usually managed by mask ventilation or using a laryngeal mask airway when performing the procedure on difficult airways, such as with the Pierre Robin sequence.

Once the airway is established, the child is positioned for tracheotomy (Fig. 15-14). All indwelling feeding tubes are removed from the esophagus. A shoulder roll is used for hyperextension. The anesthesiologist is at the patient's head and has access to the airway at all times. A transverse incision is made

TABLE 15-3	AGE AND TRACHEOTOMY TUBE SIZE*					
Age	Size	French	Inside Diameter (mm)	Outside Diameter (mm)	Length (mm)	
SHILEY†						
Premature	00	14	3.1	4.5	30, 39	
Newborn-3 mo	0	15	3.4	5.0	32, 40	
3-10 mo	1	17	3.7	5.5	34, 41	
10-12 mo	2	18	4.1	6.0	42	
13-24 mo	3	21	4.8	7.0	44	
2-9 yr	4	24	5.5	8.0	46	
9 yr +	4 adult	26	5.0	8.5	67	
9 yr +	6 adult	30	7.0	10.0	78	
	8 adult	36	8.5	12.0	84	
	10 adult	39	9.0	13.0	84	
HOLINGER‡						
Premature	000	13	2.1	4.1	26, 30, 33, 36, 40, 46	
Premature	00	13	2.4	4.5	26, 30, 33, 36, 40, 46	
Newborn	0	15	2.9	5.0	26, 30, 33, 36, 40, 46	
Newborn-3 mo	1	17	3.0	5.5	30, 33, 36, 40, 46	
3-10 mo	2	18	3.3	6.0	30, 33, 40, 46	
10-24 mo	3	21	4.4	7.0	33, 40, 50, 55, 60	
2-7 yr	4	24-25	5.3	8.0	50, 55, 60	
8-9 yr	5	27	6.1	9.0	63, 68	
10 yr +	6	30	7.1	10.0	63, 68, 73	

From Myer CM, Cotton RT, Shott SR, editors: *Pediatric airway: an interdisciplinary approach*. Philadelphia. Lippincott-Raven, 1995; p 165.
*Ages adapted from Bluestone CD, Stool SE, editors: *Pediatric otolaryngology*, vol 2. Philadelphia. WB Saunders, 1983. This information is a guide. Individual adaptation may be necessary.
†From Mallinckrodt Medical TPI Inc., Irvine, California.
‡From Pilling-Weck Co., Research Triangle Park, North Carolina, 1986. Sizes may vary with Holinger tubes manufactured by other companies.

through skin and subcutaneous tissue. The strap muscles are separated to identify the midline, and careful midline dissection is performed to avoid pneumothorax. The upper tracheal cartilages are identified. Occasionally, the isthmus of the thyroid gland must be divided to expose the upper tracheal rings. The tracheotomy tube is usually placed between the second and third tracheal rings. One surgeon holds the tracheotomy tube while an assistant secures the tube. Two stay sutures, which are removed after the first tracheotomy tube change, are placed on either side of the midline (Fig. 15-15). A vertical midline incision is made, and the tracheotomy tube is inserted. If a cuff tracheotomy is used, then the cuff is inflated with saline or air.

COMPLICATIONS

In the 1970s, the mortality rate from tracheotomy was reported as high as 24%.[27] More recent reports indicate mortality rates ranging from 0.5% to 3%.[28-30] This may be attributed to improvements in monitoring techniques such as pulse oximetry as well as frequency of medical follow-up visits and heightened vigilance. Avoidable deaths can be prevented by a thorough education program for all persons caring for the child in the hospital and the home. The ability to recannulate in case of accidental decannulation, proper airway assessment, good hygiene, and adequate systemic hydration are important factors for a successful long-term outcome for a tracheotomized infant or child. Teaching the parents or caregivers to teach others caring for the child how to care for the tracheotomy site is a critical component of this training.[30]

The most common reasons for death of a tracheotomy-dependent child are plugging of the tube with mucus and accidental decannulation. Plugging with mucus occurs when thick, viscous mucus obstructs the lumen of the tracheotomy tube. Several factors that lead to this problem include dehydration, infection, and lack of humidity. Many children with bronchopulmonary dys-

			Inside Diameter	Outside Diameter	
Age	Size	French	(mm)	(mm)	Length (mm)
PORTEX§					
Newborn	0	15	3.0	5.0	36
Newborn-3 mo	1	16	3.5	5.5	40
3-10 mo	2	18	4.0	6.0	44
10-12 mo	—	19	4.5	6.5	48
2-7 yr	3	21	5.0	7.0	48.5
8-11 yr	4 adult	24	6.0	8.1	55
12 yr +	6 adult	30	7.0	9.7	75
	7 adult	33	8.0	11.0	82
	8 adult	36	9.0	12.1	87
	9 adult	40	10.0	13.5	98
ARGYLE‖					
Premature	000		2.5	4.0	34.4
Premature	00		3.0	4.7	35.9
—	—	—	—	—	—
Newborn-3 mo	0		3.5	5.4	38.5
3-10 mo	1		4.0	6.0	41
10-12 mo	2		4.5	6.6	45.5
2.7 yr	3 adult	22	5.0	7.3	52.1
2-9 yr	4		5.5	7.8	56.5
9 yr +	5 adult	26	6.0	8.5	61.6
9 yr +	Adult	30	7.0	10.0	
	Adult	33	8.0	11.0	
	Adult	37	9.0	12.3	
	Adult	40	9.5	13.3	

TABLE 15-3 AGE AND TRACHEOTOMY TUBE SIZE—CONT'D

§From Concord Portex, Keene, New Hampshire.
‖From Sherwood Medical, St. Louis, Missouri. Formerly Dover brand.

plasia develop frequent exacerbations of mucus plugging with increased bronchorrhea. Tracheitis, either viral or bacterial, may also lead to an increase in thick secretions. These problems can be avoided with appropriate hydration, antibiotics, chest physiotherapy, and frequent suctioning. Sometimes the use of a humidifier or passive humidification device may help alleviate thick secretions. Acute mucus plugging requires emergency suctioning. The tube is changed immediately if the suctioning does not relieve the obstruction. Then the previously mentioned treatments are performed to help prevent a recurrence of the problem.

Another serious complication is accidental dislodgment of the tracheotomy tube. This accounts for most of the tracheotomy-related deaths. Accidental dislodgment may occur during play activity or tracheotomy care or when the child is alone. Immediate reinsertion is required. Occasionally this may be difficult during an emergency situa-

tion. If the same size of tracheotomy tube cannot be inserted, then an attempt is made to insert a tube that is one size smaller. If this is unsuccessful, the patient is ventilated with a bag and mask until additional medical help arrives. Parents are usually sent home with a mask and bag for use in case of an emergency. When there is a critical airway and there is no reserve airway around the tracheotomy tube, such as total laryngeal stenosis, then insertion of an ET tube into the tracheotomy site is an acceptable alternative approach to securing the airway.

Other complications associated with tracheostomy use include bleeding, stomal and suprastomal granulation tissue, tracheal erosion, and suprastomal tracheomalacia. External granulations may be removed or cauterized. Suprastomal granulation is not routinely removed during endoscopy unless there is bleeding or obstruction beyond the distal end of the tracheotomy tube. Suprastomal granulation is also removed just before decannulation. Tracheal granulation usually recurs if the tracheotomy tube is left in place. In contrast, obstructive granulation tissue in the distal airway should be removed early. Suprastomal tracheomalacia may also be repaired at the time of decannulation.

TABLE 15-4	DIMENSIONS OF THREE COMMONLY USED TRACHEOTOMY TUBES		
Cannula	Inner Diameter (mm)	Outer Diameter (mm)	Overall Length (mm)
SHILEY			
3.0 Neonatal (00NT)	3.0	4.5	30
3.5 Neonatal (0NT)	3.5	5.2	32
4.0 Neonatal (1NT)	4.0	5.9	34
3.0 Pediatric (00PT)	3.0	4.5	39
3.5 Pediatric (0PT)	3.5	5.2	40
4.0 Pediatric (1PT)	4.0	5.9	41
4.5 Pediatric (2PT)	4.5	6.0	42
5.0 Pediatric (3PT)	5.0	7.1	44
5.5 Pediatric (4PT)	5.5	7.7	46
PORTEX			
3.0	3.0	5.0	36
3.5	3.5	5.8	40
4.0	4.0	6.5	44
4.5	4.5	7.1	48
5.0	5.0	7.7	50
5.5	5.5	8.3	52
BIVONA NEONATAL			
2.5	2.5	4.0	30
3.0	3.0	4.7	32
3.5	3.5	5.3	34
4.0	4.0	6.0	36
BIVONA PEDIATRIC			
2.5	2.5	4.0	38
3.0	3.0	4.7	39
3.5	3.5	5.3	40
4.0	4.0	6.0	41
4.5	4.5	6.7	42
5.0	5.0	7.3	44
5.5	5.5	8.0	46

Bleeding from the tracheotomy tube is usually related to tracheitis, but occasionally it may be caused by granulation polyps or even erosion into a major vessel such the innominate artery. Innominate artery bleeding may require thoracic surgery surgical intervention. In addition, suction trauma causes bleeding that is usually self-limited. Suctioning beyond the end of the tracheotomy tube should not be done so as to avoid direct tracheal trauma and bleeding. Routine care of a tracheotomy includes interval bronchoscopies every 6 months to ensure there are no major problems developing with the tracheotomy.

Other problems with a chronic tracheotomy include speech delay and problems with phonation. The underlying airway lesion may limit phonation such as in the child with total laryngeal stenosis. In addition, the ventilator or the tracheotomy tube itself may block the flow of air. Unless there is a critical airway, the child with a tracheotomy may be fitted for a Passy-Muir speech valve. This valve allows one-way flow of air up through the glottis to allow phonation (Fig. 15-16).[31]

Moreover, many tracheotomized children have significant swallowing difficulties and problems with certain food textures. These problems may be related to the tracheotomy tethering the airway and preventing elevation of the larynx during deglutition or to actual food aversion by the child, who may be protecting the airway. In addition, the sense of smell and taste may be altered in a child who is bypassing the nasal airway. Close work with a speech and swallowing therapist is essential for the young child or infant with a tracheotomy. [31]

TRACHEOTOMY TUBE CHANGES

Safe tracheotomy tube changes are a very important part of routine tracheotomy care. It is essential that the child's parents or caretakers learn proper tracheotomy tube care before the child is discharged.[32] Preparation is the key to safety. It is always imperative to have proper equipment around for the tracheotomy change, as listed in Box 15-4. It is also important to perform routine tracheotomy tube changes during daytime hours when everyone is alert and a "partner" is available. Proper lighting

Fig. 15-12

Midsagittal section of a trachea with tracheotomy tube in position. This reveals two common problems: suprastomal granulation tissue *(white arrow)* and suprastomal collapse *(black arrow)*. (From Gray RF, Todd NW, Jacobs IN: Tracheostomy decannulation in children: approaches and techniques. *Laryngoscope* 1998; 108:10.)

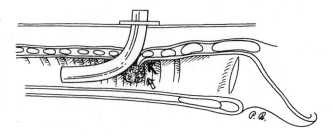

and position are essential. It is best to perform a routine tracheotomy tube change with two people. One must always communicate with the helper, be prepared for the worst, and remain calm.

At least 2 hours should have passed after the last feeding before the tracheotomy tube is changed. All supplies and emergency equipment are assembled. The role of the partner is determined and then the child is positioned on a shoulder roll with the neck hyperextended to make tube insertion easier. It is important to be prepared for any emergency

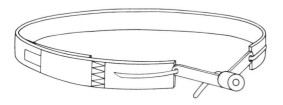

Fig. 15-13

Diagram of a Velcro tracheostomy securing system using Velcro ties.

such as a difficult cannulation or significant bradycardia or desaturation.

First, the child is adequately hyperoxygenated. During the routine tube change, the person inserting the tracheotomy tube takes charge. On this person's count, the "partner" removes the old tracheotomy tube and the person changing the tracheotomy tube places it at a right angle into the stoma and quickly advances it into the airway. The partner listens for breath sounds and then reattaches the ventilator if required. After the change, the stoma is cleaned and dressed with gauze to protect the skin. The tracheotomy ties are threaded and secured, and then the correct tension is checked for. The ties should be tight enough to hold the tube in place without movement yet not bind or pinch the neck.[32]

TRACHEOTOMY HOME CARE

Many of the complications of tracheotomy take place in the home. Therefore, an optimal home-care environment is essential. Parents and caregivers should be able to smoothly and quickly perform tracheotomy tube changes even in an urgent situation and should be trained in cardiopulmonary

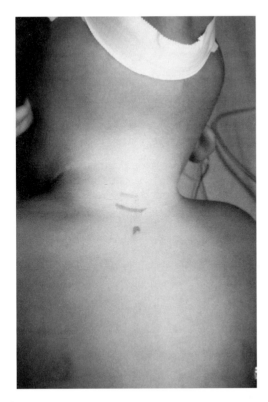

Fig. 15-14

An infant in a hyperextended position for tracheotomy.

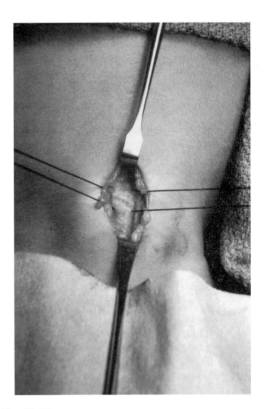

Fig. 15-15

Tracheotomy procedure with twostay sutures placed on either side of the tracheotomy incision.

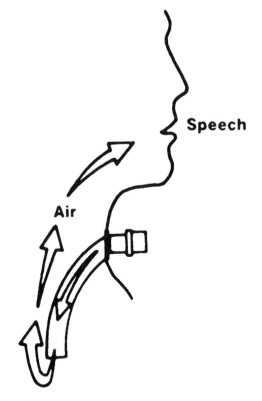

Fig. 15-16

Passy-Muir tracheostomy speaking valve enabled by redirecting exhaled air around the tracheostomy tube and through the larynx and upper airway.

resuscitation. They must be able to perform routine functions such as suctioning and cleaning. In addition, adequate tracheotomy equipment should be available. This includes such items as spare tracheotomies, smaller size tracheotomy, tracheotomy ties, dressing, suction catheters, suction machine, humidity devices, and monitors (Box 15-5). For monitoring, a pulse oximeter is preferred over an apnea monitor, since the apnea monitor will not detect an obstructed tracheotomy tube. Home nursing care is also required and depends on the clinical and family situation. Generally for a child who is tracheotomy and ventilator dependent, a parent can be expected to manage at least 8 hours of care alone and have up to 16 hours of nursing care per day.[33] However, each family has unique needs, resources, and capabilities. In addition, different insurance companies allow varying amounts of home nursing support.

DECANNULATION

Using a standard approach to routine decannulation in children promotes safe and expeditious removal of the tracheotomy tube once it is no longer required. Three conditions must be met before decannulation. First, the original condition requiring the tracheotomy must be resolved or improved, and all comorbid conditions should be stable. For instance, has the child's cardiac or pulmonary status improved? In addition, one might postpone decannulation if there is upcoming surgery that affects the airway.[34] Second, the airway must be adequate to handle the respiratory requirements of the patient. The entire airway should be evaluated endoscopically before decannulation to determine patency. Lastly, the child must be able to protect the airway.

The airway is evaluated with both flexible and rigid laryngoscopy and bronchoscopy in the operating room with the patient under general anesthesia. A pediatric flexible fiberoptic scope is passed through the nose to rule out choanal atresia, septal deformities, adenotonsillar obstruction, or laryngeal stenosis. Esophageal reflux may be inferred in the presence of supraglottic edema or laryngotracheal cobblestoning. The dynamic characteristics of the larynx, such as supraglottic collapse and vocal fold

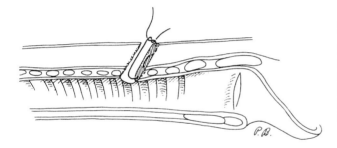

Fig. 15-17

Repair of suprastomal collapse using absorbable sutures placed on the collapsing suprastomal cartilage and tied to the stomal skin. (From Gray RF, Todd WN, Jacobs IN: Tracheostomy decannulation in children: approaches and techniques. *Laryngoscope* 1998; 108:10.)

mobility, are evaluated. Normal laryngeal reflexes and mobility are important to demonstrate. Then airway patency is assessed using rigid laryngoscopy and bronchoscopy. Immobile vocal cords are palpated to rule out glottic fixation. Suprastomal and other obstructing granulation polyps are excised with a forceps or laser, and bleeding is controlled with cautery or vasoconstrictive solutions, such as oxymetazoline. Suprastomal collapse is repaired surgically by hooking the collapsing segment and passing a suture from the cartilage to the tracheostoma skin (Fig. 15-17). In some cases, tracheal collapse may be severe enough to require an open tracheoplasty. After the procedure, the same size tracheotomy tube is inserted and decannulation is deferred until later that day, or the following day, when the patient has recovered from anesthesia.

There are several reasons why a child may not be ready for decannulation. First, the original condition may not have resolved. If the child had a tracheotomy tube in place for upper airway obstruction, then there may still be some degree of dynamic collapse while asleep, leading to sleep apnea. A monitored sleep study in a laboratory may help determine if the obstruction has resolved.[35] Other examples are diminished vocal cord abduction from posterior glottic stenosis or vocal cord paralysis and may require reconstructive surgery.

Decannulation Methods. There are three methods of decannulation: immediately remove the tube, downsize and cap the tube, or extubate after single-stage laryngotracheal reconstruction. All three methods are performed in a carefully monitored environment. The clinical situation as well as the preference of the clinician determines which method to use.

Once the airway is deemed adequate, the first method is removing the tracheotomy tube in a monitored environment, such as the postanesthesia care unit. This is scheduled for a time when the child is fully awake and alert. The child is monitored with pulse oximetry and kept calm in a parent's arms. Then the tube is gently removed. The stoma may be covered with gauze. The child is discharged to the floor once the criteria are met for discharge from the unit. Occasionally an insecure child may develop decannulation panic and may need the tracheotomy tube replaced.

The other common method involves downsizing the tracheotomy with a significantly smaller tube. Then, while monitoring the patient, the tube is capped or plugged and the child is allowed to breathe around it. If the child has normal gas exchange without tachypnea or respiratory distress for at least 24 hours, then the tracheotomy tube can be removed. The child is observed for at least another 24 hours. The disadvantage to this technique is with the borderline airway; the small tracheotomy tube may lead to airway obstruction, whereas complete removal would not.

Airway Reconstruction. When there is acquired or congenital laryngeal or tracheal stenosis, the child may require laryngotracheal reconstruction (LTR) before decannulation. Acquired subglottic stenosis is usually related to ET tube intubation. The treatment depends on the patient's age and the severity and location of stenosis. The infant with subglottic stenosis may present with failure of extubation, or an older child may present with a tracheotomy tube in place and mature stenosis. The challenge becomes repairing the stenosis so the child may safely undergo decannulation.

The first step in evaluating a tracheotomy-dependent child with subglottic stenosis is a comprehensive history to determine if the child is ready for decannulation (Box 15-6). The airway is fully evaluated endoscopically as previously described. Oral intubation is performed with various-sized ET tubes and the leak test is performed on each tube. One can infer the caliber of the airway and degree of stenosis from age if the tube size leaks at 10 to 15 mm H_2O (Fig. 15-18).[36] There are a number of approaches depending on the age, medical condition, and degree of stenosis. In some cases of mild stenosis the airway may grow as the child gets older.[37] Laser treatment may be useful for thin webs or mild stenosis; however, most cases of severe subglottic stenosis require open reconstructive surgery.

There are many surgical approaches of LTR, again depending on the situation.[38] For circumferential stenosis with good cartilaginous support, an anterior costal (rib) cartilage graft without stenting will be adequate (Fig. 15-19). When there is posterior glottic stenosis or severe loss of cartilaginous support, then a posterior split with costal cartilage grafting and a short stenting period may be required (Fig. 15-20). For severe or total stenosis of the high trachea or subglottis, then a partial cricotracheal resection (PCTR) rather than a traditional LTR would be indicated (Fig. 15-21).[38]

Stenting and postoperative care depend on the situation. If the patient requires a short period of stenting, the procedure may be accomplished in a single-stage manner and the tracheotomy tube removed at the time of surgery. With PCTR the child may be left intubated nasally after the resection if the child has excellent pulmonary status. For longer periods of stenting, staged LTR may be used with synthetic stents secured into the airway for varying periods of time.

Providing a safe and adequate airway while preserving or improving normal laryngeal functions, such as voice and protection during swallowing, is the goal of LTR or PCTR. However, voice and swallowing functions may be impaired by the surgery. An absolute contraindication to LTR or PCTR is gross impairment in the swallow mechanism because the stenosis is actually protecting against chronic aspiration. As our understanding of wound healing, swallowing, and laryngeal biomechanics improves, so will the outcome for LTR and PCTR.

SUCTIONING

Suctioning secretions from the airway or ET tube maintains patency, prevents aspiration, assists an ineffective cough, and can be used to obtain specimens for diagnostic purposes. Because suctioning is not a benign procedure, recognizing when it is or is not indicated is important. Some specific indications include auscultating decreased breath sounds implicating a possible mucus plug, difficulty during mechanical ventilation possibly resulting from ET tube occlusion or airway secretions, decreasing oxygen saturation, and the visible presence of

---

BOX 15-6

EVALUATION FOR DECANNULATION

Prematurity and gestational age
Birth weight
Number of intubations and duration
Traumatic intubations
Voice
What happens when the tracheotomy tube is removed during tube changes?
Mechanical ventilation and how long?
Continuous positive airway pressure or oxygen?
Cyanotic events or blue spells with the tracheotomy tube in position?
Recent hospitalizations for respiratory events?
Oral feedings? Aspiration?
Weight gain or failure to thrive?
Overall medical status?
Upcoming surgeries?

Classification of Stenosis with Actual Endotracheal Tube Size:									
Patient age		ID 2.0	ID 2.5	ID 3.0	ID 3.5	ID 4.0	ID 4.5	ID 5.0	ID 5.5	ID 6.0
Premature	No detectable lumen	NO								
		40	NO							
		58	30	NO						
0-3/12		68	48	26	NO					
3/12-9/12		75	59	41	22	NO				
9/12-2		80	67	53	38	20	NO			
2		84	74	62	50	35	19	NO		
4		86	78	68	57	45	32	17	NO	
6		89	81	73	64	54	43	30	16	NO
	Grade IV	Grade III			Grade II			Grade I		

Fig. 15-18

Proposed grading system for subglottic stenosis based on endotracheal tube sizes. *NO,* No obstruction; *ID,* inner diameter. (From Myer CM, O'Connor DM, Cotton RT: Proposed grading system for subglottic stenosis based upon endotracheal tube sizes. *Ann Otol Rhinol Laryngol* 1994; 103:319.)

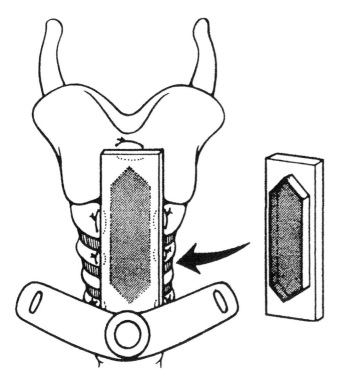

Fig. 15-19

Laryngotracheoplasty using an anteriorly placed costal cartilage graft. (From Walner DL, Cotton RT: Acquired anomalies of the larynx and trachea. In Cotton RT, Myer CM, editors: *Practical pediatric otolaryngology*. Philadelphia. Lippincott-Raven, 1999; p 528.)

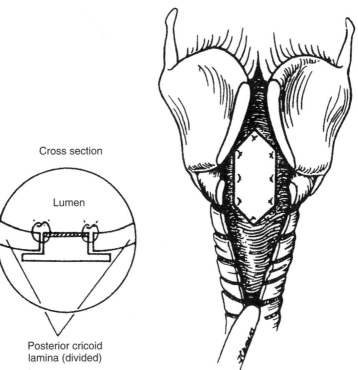

Cross section

Lumen

Posterior cricoid
lamina (divided)

Fig. 15-20

A posteriorly placed costal cartilage graft maintains excellent expansion of the cricoid and glottis. (From Walner DL, Cotton RT: Acquired anomalies of the larynx and trachea. In Cotton RT, Myer CM, editors: *Practical pediatric otolaryngology*. Philadelphia. Lippincott-Raven, 1999; p 528.)

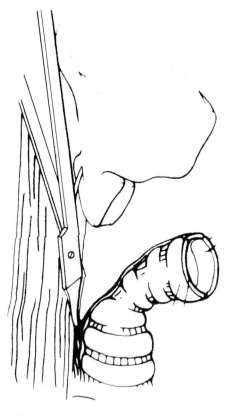

Fig. 15-21

Partial cricotracheal resection. Dissection of the stenotic trachea away from the esophagus. (From Walner DL, Cotton RT: Acquired anomalies of the larynx and trachea. In Cotton RT, Myer CM, editors: *Practical pediatric otolaryngology*. Philadelphia. Lippincott-Raven, 1999; p 532.)

secretions.[39] Although there are no absolute contraindications to suctioning, relative contraindications include patients with thrombocytopenia, epiglottitis, an unsecured airway, and labile cardiovascular or respiratory conditions. It is best to suction only when required and avoid potential complications by repeatedly suctioning without indication.

PROCEDURE

The necessary equipment for suctioning is gathered before initiating the procedure. This includes oxygen, a resuscitation bag and mask, suction catheters, sterile gloves, lavage fluid, a stethoscope, and a suction regulator to set the appropriate vacuum pressure. The vacuum pressure is set at 60 to 80 mm Hg in a neonate and 80 to 100 mm Hg in a pediatric patient. The appropriate catheter length is determined by measuring the length of the ET tube or tracheotomy tube against the suction catheter. The

proper length should pass the end of the tube but not touch the carina.[40] Optimally, the catheter should be less than one half the size of the internal diameter of the ET tube to avoid the total obstruction of the tube.

The patient's breath sounds, heart rate and pattern, respiratory rate and pattern, arterial oxygen saturation, and excessive ventilator pressures are monitored continuously. As with all procedures, an adequate explanation of the process must be provided to the patient and family before the procedure. The patient is ventilated with an FIO_2 of at least 0.1 to 0.2 greater than the oxygen being delivered at the time of the intervention, or an FIO_2 of 1.0 when necessary. The same peak inspiratory pressures and positive end-expiratory pressure as set on the ventilator are used.

To suction, the catheter is moistened with sterile water or saline and, without applying suction, inserted into the airway to the predetermined length, or until resistance is met. It is pulled back 0.5 to 1.5 cm, and intermittent suction is applied using the thumb port while withdrawing and rotating the catheter. Hypoxemia and atelectasis are avoided by keeping the duration of suctioning to less than 10 seconds a pass, and less than 5 seconds when applying the vacuum. The patient is oxygenated and ventilated between passes while observing the patient's vital signs on the monitors. Breath sounds are checked to evaluate the need for repeating the procedure. The need for further suctioning is reevaluated based on the patient's clinical status. Potentially, rotating the head to the right facilitates entry into the left mainstem bronchus, whereas turning the head to the left facilitates entering the right mainstem bronchus.

Although not always required, instilling a lavage solution may be necessary to remove mucus plugs or thick, tenacious secretions. Lavage or irrigating solutions include wetting agents such as normal saline, detergents such as sodium bicarbonate, and mucolytics such as *N*-acetylcysteine. For the neonatal patient, small incremental amounts are instilled to a volume of 0.5 to 1 ml. In the older child, 2 to 5 ml is instilled. Lavage is followed with manual ventilation and subsequent suctioning. Bagging the instilled solution into the ET tube allows it to disperse throughout the lung fields to help liquefy and loosen secretions. Before instilling any solution, it is important to know the patient's pertinent clinical history. Careful attention must be paid to the amount of solution instilled in the patient who is salt or fluid restricted. Certain types of wetting agents, such as sterile water or hypertonic saline solution, cause mucosal irritation, bronchospasm, and overhydration.

NASOTRACHEAL SUCTION

Blind nasotracheal suctioning requires that all of the previously mentioned equipment used for ET tube suctioning be readily available.[41] The procedure for blind nasotracheal suctioning differs in that an ET tube is not present. An infant is placed in the sniffing position, and the head and neck of an older child are slightly hyperextended. The suction catheter is lubricated with water or soluble jelly and placed in the nares. With the clinician facing the patient, the catheter is inserted slightly medial to the septum. The natural curve of the catheter is used as a guide to advance it over the top of the palate. When the catheter reaches the oropharynx, it is advanced into the tracheobronchial tree during inspiration. The catheter is pulled back 0.5 to 1.0 cm once resistance is felt, and suction is intermittently applied as previously described.

Hypoxemia, bradycardia with resultant hypotension, bronchospasm, laryngospasm, airway trauma, hemorrhage, infection, and aspiration are all potential complications of blind nasotracheal suctioning. The most frequent complication in the neonatal patient is hypoxemia and subsequent bradycardia. The incidence of this complication can be reduced by frequent bagging between suctioning, limiting suction time, and increasing the FiO_2. Before the procedure is begun in the premature infant and unstable neonate, careful monitoring of the blood pressure is performed because hypertension associated with the procedure predisposes the patient to intracranial hemorrhage.

BULB SUCTION

The bulb syringe is a manually operated device for use in the home or hospital. It is important to be gentle when using it because vigorous suctioning can lead to bleeding and airway damage. The bulb syringe is squeezed gently and held down. It is inserted in the area of mucus, and the pressure on the bulb is released to suction the mucus. Once the syringe is removed from the nasal passage, secretions are removed with a combination of squeezes, and the syringe is cleansed with water and wiped with gauze pads. The bulb syringe should be cleansed thoroughly after each use and allowed to air dry.

CLOSED TRACHEAL SUCTION SYSTEMS

As the frequency of suctioning increases, the need for a closed tracheal suction system or special suctioning adapter becomes imperative. These systems are necessary to prevent alveolar collapse associated with the loss of distention from positive end-expiratory pressure during suctioning and to reduce suction-related pulmonary infections.[39] Closed tracheal suction systems are designed to allow minimal disruption with mechanical ventilation, prevent the loss of positive end-expiratory pressure, and avoid hypoxia. This system is added to an adapter, as well as an irrigation port, protective sleeve, closed lock and control valve, and markings on the suction catheter to determine approximate depth of suctioning. This system can remain in-line with the circuit for 24 hours and is readily accessible for use. Additional advantages include less contamination of the sheathed catheter, a decrease in airborne particles being introduced into the ET tube, and a faster return to the preoxygenation baseline.

There are some disadvantages with these systems. Bacterial growth can occur if the catheter is not changed in a timely manner. Failure to pull the catheter back fully into the correct position can cause damage to or occlude the airway. Other disadvantages may be leaving the continuous suction in the "on" position, causing hypoxemia, and causing increased dead space if an inappropriate adapter size is used.

REFERENCES

1. International Guidelines for Neonatal Resuscitation: An Excerpt from the Guidelines 2000 for Cardiopulmonary Resuscitation and Emergency Cardiovascular Care: International Consensus on Science. *Pediatrics* 2000; 106(3):E29.
2. Keep PJ, Manford ML: Endotracheal tube sizes for children. *Anaesthesia* 1974; 29:181-185.
3. Hinkle AJ: A rapid and reliable method of selecting endotracheal tube size in children. *Anesth Analg* 1988; 67:S-592.
4. Luten RC et al: Length-based endotracheal tube and emergency equipment selection in pediatrics. *Ann Emerg Med* 1992; 21:900-904.
5. Brunel W et al: Assessment of routine chest roentgenograms and physical examination to confirm endotracheal tube position. *Chest* 1989; 96:1043-1045.
6. Berry FA, Yemen TA: Pediatric airway in health and disease. *Pediatr Clin North Am* 1994; 41:153-180.
7. Behar PM, Todd NW: Resuscitation of the newborn with airway compromise. *Clin Perinatol* 1999; 26:717-732.
8. Zander J, Hazinski MF: Pulmonary disorders: airway obstruction. In Hazinski MF, editor: *Nursing care of the critically ill child,* ed 2. St Louis. Mosby-Year Book, 1992.
9. Westhorpe RN: The position of the larynx in children and its relationship to the ease of intubation. *Anaesth Intensive Care* 1987; 15:384-388.
10. Selleck BA: Cricoid pressure to control regurgitation of stomach contents during induction of anesthesia. *Lancet* 1961; 2:404-406.
11. Moynihan RJ et al: The effect of cricoid pressure on preventing gastric insufflation in infants and children. *Anesthesiology* 1993; 78:652-656.
12. Tochen ML: Orotracheal intubation in the newborn infant: a method for determining depth of tube insertion. *J Pediatr* 1979; 95:1050-1051.
13. MacLeod BA et al: Verification of endotracheal tube placement with colorimetric end-tidal CO_2 detection. *Ann Emerg Med* 1991; 20:267-270.

14. Sum-Ping ST, Mehta PA, Anderton JM: A comparative study of methods of detection of esophageal intubation. *Anesth Analg* 1989; 69:627-632.

15. Brown MS: Prevention of accidental extubation in newborns. *Am J Dis Child* 1988; 142:1240-1243.

16. Volsko TA, Chatburn RL: Comparison of two methods for securing the endotracheal tube in neonates. *Respir Care* 1997; 42:288-291.

17. Spence K, Barr P: Nasal versus oral intubation for mechanical ventilation of newborn infants. *Cochrane Database Syst Rev* 2000; 2:CD000948.

18. Handler SD: Craniofacial surgery: otolaryngologic concerns. *Int Anesthesiol Clin* 1988; 26:61-63.

19. Hancock PJ, Peterson G: Finger intubation of the trachea in newborns. *Pediatrics* 1992; 89:325-326.

20. Fontarosa PB et al: Sitting oral-tracheal intubation. *Ann Emerg Med* 1988; 17:336-338.

21. Barriot P, Riou B: Retrograde technique for tracheal intubation in trauma patients. *Crit Care Med* 1988; 16:712-713.

22. Neustein SM: The Neustein laryngoscope: a new solution to difficult intubation. *Anesthesiol Rev* 1992; 54-59.

23. Verdile VP et al: Nasotracheal intubation using a flexible lighted stylet. *Ann Emerg Med* 1990; 19:506-510.

24. Pennant JH, White PF: The laryngeal mask airway. *Anesthesiology* 1993; 79:144-163.

25. Peak DA, Roy S: Needle cricothyroidotomy revisited. *Pediatr Emerg Care* 1999; 15:224-226.

26. Kallstrom TJ, Salyer JW: The incidence of accidental extubations in the neonatal intensive care unit. *Respir Care* 1989; 34:1006-1012.

27. Duncan PG: Efficacy of helium-oxygen mixtures in the management of severe viral and postintubation croup. *Can Anaesth Soc J* 1979; 26:206-208.

28. Cotton RT, Seid AB: Management of the extubation problem in the premature child: anterior cricoid split as an alternative to tracheotomy. *Ann Otol Rhinol Laryngol* 1980; 89:509-511.

29. Rosin DF et al: Vocal cord paralysis in children. *Laryngoscope* 1990; 100:1174-1179.

30. Czervinske MP: Pediatric tracheostomy: clinical perspectives part 2. *AARC Times* 1999; 23(9):33-36

31. Fearon B, Cotton RT: Surgical correction of subglottic stenosis of the larynx in infants and children: a progress report. *Ann Otol Rhinol Laryngol* 1974; 83:428-443.

32. Wetmore RF, Handler SD, Potsic WP: Pediatric tracheostomy: experience during the past decade. *Ann Otol Rhinol Laryngol* 1982; 91:628-632.

33. Kenna MA, Reilly JS, Stool SE: Tracheotomy in the preterm infant. *Ann Otol Rhinol Laryngol* 1987; 96:68-71.

34. Crysdale WS, Feldman RI, Natio K: Tracheotomies: a 10-year experience in 319 children. *Ann Otol Rhinol Laryngol* 1998; 97:439-443.

35. Orringer MK: The effects of tracheostomy tube placement on communication and swallowing. *Respir Care* 1999; 44:845-853.

36. Czervinske MP: Pediatric tracheostomy: clinical perspectives part I. *AARC Times* 1999; 23(9):31-33.

37. Panitch HB et al: Guidelines for home care of children with chronic respirator insufficiency. *Pediatric Pulmonol* 1996; 21:52-56.

38. Gray RF, Todd NW, Jacobs IN: Tracheostomy decannulation in children: approaches and techniques. *Laryngoscope* 1998; 108:8-12.

39. Tunkel DE et al: Polysomnography in the evaluation of readiness for decannulation in children. *Arch Otolaryngol Head Neck Surg* 1996; 122:721-724.

40. Myer CM, O'Conner DM, Cotton RT: A proposed laryngotracheal stenosis grading system based on endotracheal tube size. *Ann Otol Rhinol Laryngol* 1994; 103:319.

41. Holinger LD: Treatment of severe subglottic stenosis without tracheotomy. *Ann Otol Laryngol Rhinol* 1982; 91:407.

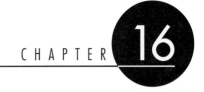
Surfactant Replacement

Douglas F. Willson

HISTORY

The successful introduction of surfactant therapy into clinical care is testimony to the value of basic science research. There are few better examples of how discoveries in the laboratory can be directly translated into improved patient care. The phenomenal success of surfactant replacement in respiratory distress syndrome (RDS) has prompted investigation into the possible role of surfactant therapy in other types of acute lung injury.[1-12] It is clear that qualitative and quantitative surfactant abnormalities are present in many non-RDS types of acute lung injury and that the expanding role of surfactant replacement must be explored.

The seeds were sown in the early nineteenth century with the observations of Pierre Simon de Laplace. In his theory of capillary action he described the relationship of trans-surface pressure and surface tension at a gas-fluid interface in a sphere:

$$P_{TS} = \frac{2\gamma}{r}$$

where P_{TS} is the trans-surface or distending pressure, γ is surface tension, and r is the radius of the sphere. More than a century later, von Neergaard applied the concept of a "tension" existing between gas-fluid interfaces to explain his observations on the pressure:volume relationship of the lung.[13,14] He observed that lower pressures were required to inflate the lung with a liquid than with air once the air-fluid interface was eliminated. He hypothesized this was because of the work required to overcome surface tension at the alveolar air-fluid interface predicted by Laplace's theory.

Twenty years later, Macklin postulated the existence of a "mucoprotein" lining in the lung that had the surface tension–lowering properties observed by von Neergaard.[15] In 1955, Pattle extracted a waxy substance from lung washings that had surface tension–lowering properties.[16] Clements subsequently confirmed this in 1957, but it was Avery and Mead, in 1959, who demonstrated that this substance was absent in the lungs of preterm infants.[17,18] Finally, in 1980, Fujiwara and colleagues reported success in producing and using surfactant replacement for preterm infants with RDS.[19] The release of surfactant for clinical use in the United States by the Food and Drug Administration in 1990 resulted in a measurable reduction in perinatal mortality and morbidity.[20] The use of exogenous surfactants for treatment of lung injury beyond the neonatal period is only now being studied but may offer similar promise.

SURFACTANT PHYSIOLOGY

Surfactant acts to lower surface tension. Surface tension is the consequence of the imbalance in opposing forces at the interface between two phases of matter. As an example, consider the interface between a liquid and a gas (Fig. 16-1): the forces between molecules in the liquid are stronger than those in the gas.[21] This results in molecules at the liquid surface being disproportionately pulled back into the fluid, creating a tension at the surface that resists disruption. In a spherical structure, such as an alveolus, these surface interactions increase as the alveolus gets smaller, according to Laplace's law, resulting in a tendency to collapse. These air-fluid interfaces exist in small airways as well and may result in resistance to air passing through any narrowing of these areas.[22]

Surfactant modifies surface tension at the interface by spontaneously forming a film at the surface, a process known as *adsorption.* Both the speed and degree of adsorption are inherent properties of a surfactant. Most surfactants, including pulmonary surfactants, are amphipathic molecules. Amphipathic means the molecules have both hydrophilic and hydrophobic groups, or moieties, in their structure.

The hydrophilic moiety orients toward the polar side of the interface, in this case the aqueous alveolar surface, and the hydrophobic moiety orients toward the nonpolar inspired gas side. This, in effect, creates a new interface with lower surface tension.

Although not entirely accurate, the lung can be thought of as a very large number of interconnected bubbles. These bubbles form the interface between the gaseous environment and the wet alveolar surface. If this interface were solely between air and water, that is, without surfactant, two consequences would ensue: (1) every breath would take a considerable amount of pressure to expand the lung, comparable to the 80 to 90 cm H_2O pressure required for a newborn's first breath, and (2) the lung would rapidly collapse during exhalation.

Pulmonary surfactant not only lowers surface tension at all lung volumes but, more importantly, also decreases surface tension as alveolar surface decreases (Fig. 16-2). If surface tension did not decrease with decreasing lung volume, alveoli of different size would require different distending pressures. Small alveoli would empty into large ones and there would be an overall tendency for the lung to coalesce into a smaller number of large alveoli as lung volume diminished. Surfactant not only decreases surface tension but also reduces it to a greater degree at low lung volume and counteracts the effect of decreasing alveolar size.

Functionally surfactant increases lung compliance, promotes homogeneous gas distribution during inhalation, and allows a residual volume of gas to be evenly distributed throughout the lung during exhalation; that is, it maintains functional residual capacity. In the absence of surfactant, distribution of ventilation becomes uneven, the lungs become

Fig. 16-1

A, Pressure/volume relationship of air-filled versus liquid-filled lung from von Neergaard's original data (1929). **B,** The difference in recoil attributed to a liquid-air interface (i.e., "bubble lining") that is eliminated by a liquid-only interface. (From Hills BA: *Biology of surfactant.* Cambridge, UK. Cambridge University Press, 1988.)

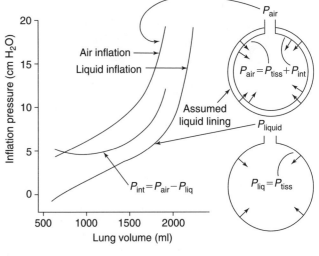

A
B

stiff, and atelectasis ensues during exhalation. The result is increased work of breathing, hypoxia, and respiratory failure, the clinical picture exemplified by preterm infants with RDS.

SURFACTANT COMPOSITION

Natural surfactant is a complex mixture of phospholipids, neutral lipids, and proteins.[23,24] See Table 16-1 for a list of the various components of surfactant. Phospholipids, mostly consisting of phosphatidylcholine, constitute the major component. The phospholipid components in surfactant are not unique, and are found in most biologic membranes. Neutral lipids, mostly cholesterol, make up about

10%, and proteins constitute the remaining 10%. It is likely that each of the components is important in adsorption, film formation, and the behavior of the film at the alveolar surface.

Four surfactant-associated proteins have been identified and usually are referred to as SP-A, B, C, and D.[25] SP-A is a large, collagen-like glycoprotein with a molecular weight of 26,000 to 36,000 daltons and is the most abundant of the surfactant-associated proteins.[26,27] It is thought to be important in the regulation of surfactant metabolism, as well as in tubular myelin formation.[28] SP-D is another collagen-like protein that forms large oligomers. It has only been recently identified, and its role is unclear.[29] SP-A and SP-D are hydrophilic proteins

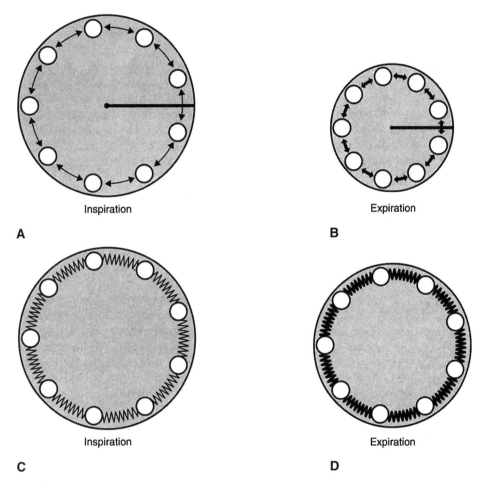

Inspiration

A

Expiration

B

Inspiration

C

Expiration

D

Fig. 16-2

A, Alveolar surface tension is a manifestation of the strong attraction between the molecules that are aligned on the surface of the alveoli. **B,** During expiration, when the alveolar radius is smaller, the attraction between the molecules is stronger and there is greater tendency for collapse. **C,** When surfactant is present, it spreads over the alveolus and dilutes the molecules. **D,** During expiration, the surfactant is compressed and the alveolar surface tension is lowered. This stabilizes the alveoli and prevents collapse of those with smaller radii.

TABLE 16-1	COMPONENTS OF PULMONARY SURFACTANT	
LIPIDS		90%-95%
Phospholipids		
Saturated phosphatidylcholine		45%
Unsaturated phosphatidylcholine		20%
Phosphatidylglycerol		8%
Other phospholipids		5%
Neutral lipids		10%
Other lipids		2%
PROTEINS		5%-10%
Loosely associated (mainly serum)		0%-5%
Surfactant apoproteins		
Hydrophilic proteins, SP-A, SP-D[25]		2%-4%
Hydrophobic proteins, SP-B, SP-C[25]		1%-2%

Modified from Rooney SA: The surfactant system and lung phospholipid biochemistry. *Am Rev Respir Dis* 1985; 131:439-460.

and are lost in the lipid extraction process used in most commercial preparations. Surfactant proteins B and C are hydrophobic molecules and extract with the phospholipids in commercial surfactants. SP-B and SP-C are relatively small proteins present in approximately equal amounts. These two are vital to spreading and surfactant film formation at the alveolar surface. The presence of SP-B and SP-C is probably the primary reason for the greater efficacy of natural relative to synthetic surfactants.

SURFACTANT METABOLISM

The metabolism of surfactant is complex and incompletely understood. Surfactant is synthesized in the type II alveolar pneumocyte (or pneumatocyte). The phospholipid components are synthesized in the endoplasmic reticulum and transported through the Golgi apparatus to the lamellar bodies (Fig. 16-3).[30,31] Lamellar bodies are subcellular organelles secreted from type II alveolar cells. They are composed of tightly packed membrane-like structures, the composition of which is identical to the surfactant isolated from the alveolar space. Lamellar bodies make their way to the cell surface and are extruded, seeming to unwind over the alveolar surface into a lattice-like construction called tubular myelin (Fig. 16-4).[32] During this process the tubular myelin becomes studded with regularly spaced particles that are thought to be SP-A, which is believed to play a primary role in regulating surfactant metabolism.[33,34]

The next step involving adsorption of phospholipid from this tubular myelin structure onto the alveolar surface film is not understood, but tubular myelin appears to be an alveolar storage form of

surfactant in dynamic equilibrium with the alveolar surface film. The alveolar surface film is composed of nearly pure dipalmitoyl phosphatidylcholine (DPPC).[35] The half-time for turnover of human surfactant is not known, but in animals such as rats and rabbits it is 5 to 10 hours.[36] Secretion and clearance are balanced, with 90% of the surfactant being recycled by the type II pneumocyte (or pneumatocyte). Studies using labeled surfactant introduced into the airways have shown the majority being taken up directly by the pneumocyte (or pneumatocyte) and being repackaged in lamellar bodies and eventually resecreted.[37] The remaining 10% are cleared by alveolar macrophages.

SURFACTANT DYSFUNCTION IN ACUTE LUNG INJURY

The role of surfactant deficiency in RDS is well established. Also, there is ample evidence of surfactant dysfunction in other causes of acute lung injury. The degree of dysfunction may actually correlate with the severity of respiratory failure.[38] How much surfactant dysfunction contributes to ultimate morbidity and mortality is less clear and is likely dependent on the particular type and degree of lung insult.

Pulmonary injury is not a static phenomenon. The role of surfactant dysfunction is dependent on the stage of the disease in question. Abnormalities in surfactant quantity or pool size, composition, metabolism, and inactivation of surfactant have been described in acute respiratory distress syndrome (ARDS) and other types of acute lung injury (Box 16-1).[39] These are important issues to consider when evaluating the potential efficacy of exogenous surfactant as a therapy.

ALTERED SURFACTANT POOL

The evidence related to altered surfactant pool size in acute lung injury is inconsistent. Decreases, increases, and no changes in pool size have all been reported.[38,40-42] This confusion reflects the difficulty in quantifying surfactant material obtained from bronchoalveolar lavage. Different clinical factors or types of lung injury may have completely different results. For example, prolonged exposure to 85% oxygen results in type II alveolar cell hyperplasia and increased surfactant secretion, whereas 100% exposure decreases alveolar cell numbers and surfactant secretion.[43,44] At present, no firm conclusions can be drawn regarding the effects of acute lung injury on the quantity of surfactant.

ALTERED SURFACTANT COMPOSITION

A consistent finding in studies of acute lung injury is that alterations in the composition of surfactant

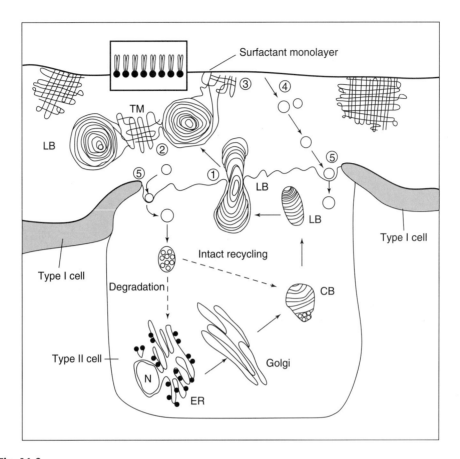

Fig. 16-3

Schematic diagram of surfactant metabolism. Generally accepted pathways are indicated by solid arrows. Probable pathways are indicated by broken arrows. *N,* Nucleus; *ER,* endoplasmic reticulum; *CB,* composite body; *LB,* lamellar body; *TM,* tubular myelin; *1,* secretion of LB; *2,* conversion of LB into TM; *3,* generation of monolayer from TM material; *4,* formation of small aggregate material from monolayer; *5,* reuptake of surfactant material. (Redrawn from Batenburg JJ: Biosynthesis, secretion, and recycling of surfactant components. In Robertson B, Taesch HW, editors: *Surfactant therapy for lung disease.* New York. Marcel Dekker, 1985.)

occur. These findings include a decrease in surfactant-associated proteins in patients with ARDS and decreases in the quantities of phosphatidylcholine and phosphatidylglycerol along with an increase in sphingomyelin and other phospholipids.[45,46] Furthermore, these abnormalities appear to reverse with recovery from acute lung injury.[47] The relationship of these abnormalities in surfactant composition to lung dysfunction is unknown, but surfactant isolated from animal models of lung injury has abnormal surface activity in vitro.[48,49]

ALTERED SURFACTANT METABOLISM

A body of evidence exists to support that surfactant metabolism may be altered in acute lung injury. Animals injured with hyperoxia have decreased incorporation of surfactant precursors into lung tissue that reverses with recovery.[50] Other animal models show more rapid conversion of large to small surfactant forms that have very poor surface tension–lowering properties.[51] Bronchoalveolar lavage specimens from patients with ARDS also support evidence of altered surfactant metabolism, showing increased levels of proteases and alterations in the density profiles of surfactant.[52]

SURFACTANT INACTIVATION

Inactivation by proteins is the most consistent surfactant abnormality seen in acute lung injury. Albumin, hemoglobin, fibrin, complement, and other proteins may gain access to the alveolar space secondary to alveolar-capillary membrane damage

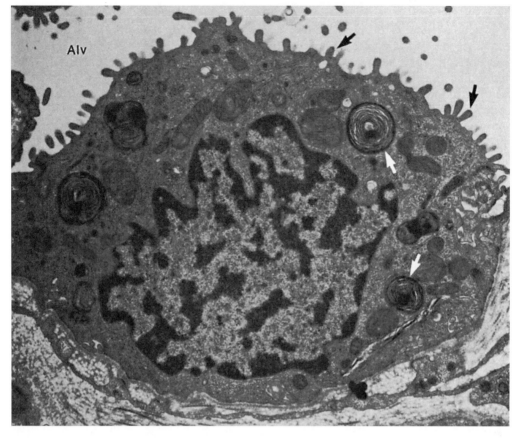

A

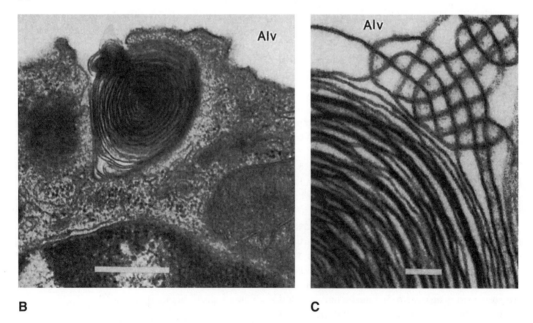

B   **C**

Fig. 16-4

A, Type II cell from a human lung, showing characteristic lamellar inclusion bodies *(white arrows)* within the cell, which are the storage sites of intracellular surfactant. Microvilli *(black arrows)* are projecting into the alveolus. **B,** Beginning exocytosis of a lamellar body into the alveolar space of a human lung. **C,** Secreted lamellar body and newly formed tubular myelin (lattice-look) in the alveolar liquid in a fetal rat lung. Membrane continuities between outer lamellar bodies and adjacent tubular myelin provide evidence of intraalveolar tubular myelin formation. (From Murray JF: *The normal lung,* ed 2. Philadelphia. WB Saunders, 1986. Courtesy of Dr. Mary C. Williams.)

and have shown in vitro to diminish surfactant's surface tension–reducing properties.[52-54] Proteins compete with surfactant for the air-fluid interface and interfere with monolayer formation.[55] Regardless of the event initiating capillary permeability, pulmonary edema results in surfactant inactivation, which leads to diminished lung compliance, increased intrapulmonary shunting, and atelectasis

BOX 16-1

FACTORS CONTRIBUTING TO SURFACTANT ABNORMALITIES IN ACUTE LUNG INJURY

Small alveolar surfactant pool size
Rapid turnover and dependence on recycling to maintain pool
Accelerated conversion to inactive forms of surfactant
Inhibition of biophysical properties by edema fluid
Inactivation of components by proteases and oxidants
Depletion of selected components with type of injury (SP-A, phosphatidylglycerol)

Modified from Jobe AH, Ikegami M: Surfactant and acute lung injury. *Proc Assoc Am Physicians* 1998; 110:489-495.

characteristic of ARDS (Fig. 16-5).[56] Interestingly, the surfactant appears to be unaltered and displays normal surface tension–reducing properties when separated from the protein using a centrifuge.[57]

VARIABLES IN SURFACTANT THERAPY

The effectiveness of surfactant therapy in surfactant-deficient preterm infants is indisputable. Evidence justifying the use of exogenous surfactant in other conditions is less substantial, however. Human studies are confounded by differences in type of surfactant, mode of delivery, timing of administration, and the underlying disease process. Animal data are similarly limited, and the relevance of the most common animal model, surfactant washout by warm saline lavage, to types of acute lung injury other than RDS is questionable. Each of these confounding variables must be addressed to analyze the literature regarding surfactant therapy for nonneonatal lung disease.

TYPES OF SURFACTANT

Surfactant composition is similar for all mammalian species. A number of different types of exogenous surfactants have been studied for use in ARDS.[58] The composition of pharmaceutical surfactants differs greatly and is determined largely by the extraction or

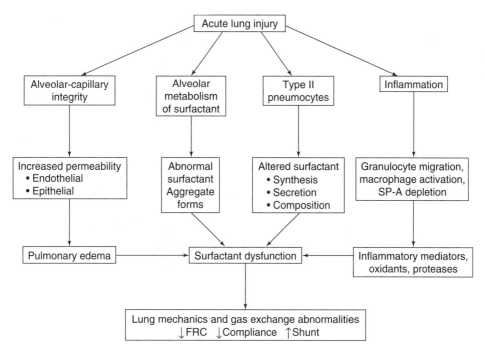

Fig. 16-5

Four pathways that contribute to surfactant dysfunction during acute lung injury. (From Jobe AH, Ikegami M: Surfactant and acute lung injury. *Proc Assoc Am Phys* 1998; 110:489-495.)

TABLE 16-2	COMMON COMMERCIAL SURFACTANTS		
Generic Name	**Trade Name**	**Preparation**	**Manufacturer**
Beractant	Survanta	Bovine lung mince extract with added DPPC, tripalmitin, and palmitic acid	Abbott Laboratories (USA)
Surfactant-TA	Surfacten	Bovine lung mince extract with added DPPC, tripalmitol-glycerol, and palmitic acid	Tokoyo Tanabe (Japan)
Porcine surfactant	Curosurf	Porcine lung mince, chloroform-methanol extract (liquid-gel chromatography)	Chiesi Pharmaceuticals (Italy)
Calf lung surfactant extract (CLSE)	Infasurf	Bovine lung wash, chloroform-methanol extract	Forrest Laboratories (USA)
SF-RI 1	Alveofact	Bovine lung wash, chloroform-methanol extract	Boehringer (Germany)
Artificial lung expanding compound (ALEC)	Pneumactant	DPPC and phosphatidyl-glycerol in 7:3 ratio	Britannia Pharmaceuticals (UK)
Colfosceril palmitate, hexadecanol tyloxapol (CPHT)	Exosurf	DPPC with 9% hexadecanol and 6% tyloxapol	Burroughs Wellcome (USA)

Modified from Kattwinkel J: Surfactant: evolving issues. *Clin Perinatol* 1998; 25:17-32.

synthetic process.[59] Table 16-2 lists some of the commercially available surfactants.

Natural surfactants are recovered from lung or amniotic fluid. They contain large surfactant aggregates and have excellent surface active properties. Unfortunately, they are difficult to manufacture and carry an infection risk. Currently no unmodified natural surfactants are available.

Modified natural surfactants are sterile lipid extracts of minced lung or alveolar lavage, some of which are modified by the addition or removal of compounds to improve surface activity. Whereas their lipid composition resembles that of endogenous surfactant, SP-A and SP-D are lost in the extraction process and SP-B and SP-C are present in variable amounts dependent on the specific surfactant. Minced lung surfactants (e.g., Survanta) may also be contaminated with nonsurfactant lipids and proteins. Modified natural surfactants generally have excellent surface activity both in vitro and in vivo.

Artificial surfactants are mixtures of synthetic compounds that approximate the lipid composition of natural surfactant but have no protein component. These compounds behave similarly to natural surfactants in vitro but tend to be less effective in vivo, probably because of differences in adsorption at the air-fluid interface. They are inexpensive and there is no risk of infection. Exosurf and ALEC are examples of artificial surfactants.

Synthetic natural surfactants are artificial surfactants with genetically engineered surfactant proteins added. These are likely to become available as the genes for the surfactant-associated proteins are identified and cloned.[60] A completely synthetic surfactant, known as KL_4-surfactant, has been undergoing clinical trials. It uses SP-B–mimicking peptides and behaves like a modified natural surfactant.[61]

Differences in the composition of commercially available surfactants may be important. The modified natural surfactants have been shown to be superior to artificial surfactants at improving oxygenation, decreasing mortality, and lowering the incidence of retinopathy and bronchopulmonary dysplasia in human neonates.[62-65] Studies in animals suggest that natural surfactants resist inactivation by protein and spread more rapidly at the alveolar surface.[66] This is likely caused by the presence of the surfactant proteins B and C. Differences in duration of improved oxygenation and lung compliance have been demonstrated when comparing two different modified natural surfactants in lambs: Survanta and Infasurf.[67,68] These results may reflect either the greater amount of SP-B in Infasurf or the greater amount of nonsurfactant lipid and protein contamination found in Survanta. Thus all surfactants are not equivalent and efficacy may depend on the formulation.

TIMING OF ADMINISTRATION

The timing of surfactant administration may also be important in determining efficacy. In preterm animal models, surfactant replacement before ventilation is

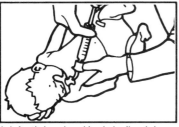
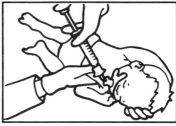

1. Infant's head and body inclined down, head turned to the right.

2. Head and body inclined down, head turned to the left.

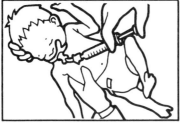
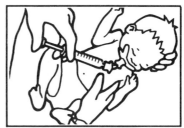

3. Head and body inclined up, head turned to the right.

4. Head and body inclined up, head turned to the left.

Fig. 16-6

Positioning of infant for instillation of Survanta exogenous surfactant. (Courtesy Ross Products Division, Abbott Laboratories. Columbus, OH, 1984.)

established prevents the development of bronchiolar epithelial injury and subsequent lung damage.[69] Studies in preterm human infants at high risk for development of RDS show that early, or prophylactic, treatment is superior to treatment given once RDS has developed.[70,71] This may be related to two factors: more uniform distribution when surfactant is administered before ventilator-induced lung injury can occur and avoiding ventilator-induced lung injury owing to improved lung compliance.

The pathophysiology of ARDS is more complex and the lung injury is more heterogeneous from its inception.[72] Timing of surfactant administration may be even more critical. Additionally, as in RDS, ventilator-induced lung injury can occur rapidly and is not responsive to surfactant. Because both factors may impede the distribution of administered surfactant, it is reasonable to assert that early treatment of acute lung injury is likely to be more effective than later treatment. As previously discussed, there is evidence that surfactant dysfunction occurs early in the course of many types of acute lung injury and contributes to the characteristic decreased lung compliance, atelectasis, and hypoxia seen. Early treatment should improve the distribution of administered surfactant and moderate the degree of ventilatory support needed.

One rabbit model demonstrates that rabbits given a modified natural surfactant at 6 hours as opposed to 3 hours after lung lavage had less sustained improvement in oxygenation and ventilation, a high incidence of barotrauma, and pathologic processes showing greater inflammation and hyaline membrane formation.[73] Unfortunately, timing of surfactant administration has not been routinely addressed in the studies of surfactant therapy for nonneonatal lung injury.

METHOD OF DELIVERY

Two approaches to surfactant administration have been taken: instilling a bolus down the endotracheal tube and aerosolizing it into the inspired gas. When instilling a bolus, the patient is positioned to allow gravity to aid in the distribution during administration (Fig. 16-6). This is the approach adopted for most clinical trials. Although this works well for neonates, in larger patients the volume of surfactant required makes it expensive. Additionally, it is more labor intensive and can lead to transient airway obstruction and hypoxia. In contrast, aerosolizing surfactant requires smaller volumes, is less labor intensive, and generally does not acutely change ventilation.

Results have been inconsistent when comparing bolus to aerosolized administration in animal models. In a uniform lung injury model with repeated saline lavage. aerosolized Survanta resulted in greater improvement in oxygenation and compliance than instilled Survanta, despite a much smaller total dose.[74] However, in other studies with nonuniform lung injury, aerosolization resulted in preferential distribution to already ventilated lung units with little to none of the surfactant reaching nonventilated areas and no improvement in oxygenation.[75,76] In another study with heterogeneous lung injury, instilled bovine lung extract surfactant (BLES) was significantly better than aerozolized BLES, but aerosolized Survanta was significantly better than instilled Survanta.[77] Thus the best method of delivery may depend on the type of surfactant and the model used. Additionally, the mode of ventilation and type of aerosol generator may also influence the efficacy of the aerosol delivery approach.[78]

No comparative human trial of instillation versus aerosolization has been published. The ideal dose and method of surfactant delivery are unclear but represent significant issues because of cost and relative untoward effects. It is reasonable to deduce that some combination of bolus administration followed by aerosolization would be the ideal approach.

MODELS OF ACUTE LUNG INJURY

The most commonly used animal lung injury model is lung lavage. Repeated lavage with warm saline results in surfactant washout and a subsequent inflammatory response comparable to RDS. Early surfactant replacement with this method effectively reverses the clinical signs and symptoms of respiratory distress, just as it does in preterm infants with RDS (Fig. 16-7). How relevant this model is to lung injuries other than RDS is unclear.

The hyperoxic lung injury model is mimicked by exposure to 100% oxygen until the alveoli become permeable to protein and decrease surfactant synthesis in type II cells.[44,50] Bronchoalveolar lavage samples from this type of model reveal markedly diminished phospholipid levels and surfactant with severely impaired dynamic surface activity. These changes are similar to those described in patients dying of ARDS and can be ameliorated by treatment with exogenous surfactant.[79]

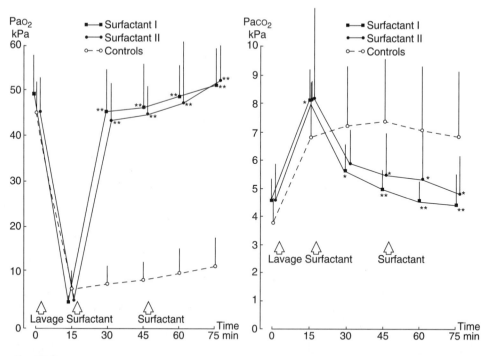

Fig. 16-7

Gas exchange after lung lavage in an experimental model of acute respiratory distress syndrome. After treatment with surfactant, blood gases are restored to prelavage levels. Note the effect on Pao_2 was more rapid than $Paco_2$. (From Berggren P et al: Gas exchange and lung morphology after surfactant replacement in experimental adult respiratory distress syndrome induced by repeated lung lavage. *Acta Anaesthesiol Scand* 1986; 30:321-328.)

Oleic acid injection produces an abrupt and severe hemorrhagic pulmonary edema that does not appear to respond to surfactant.[80,81] Nitroso-*N*-methyl-urethane (NNNMU) instillation produces a more subacute lung injury with worsening respiratory function over several days. With NNNMU, large doses of surfactant appear helpful but not curative.[82,83] In other models, treatment with exogenous surfactant is somewhat effective. These include hydrochloric acid, smoke inhalation, viral infection, and bilateral vagotomy. In these models the primary effect of exogenous surfactant is most likely the reversal of the endogenous surfactant inhibition by protein that has leaked into the alveolar space.[84-87] Although more complex and less standardized, these models are probably more comparable to human ARDS, as is their variable response to surfactant administration.

As straightforward as surfactant administration would seem, many factors appear to influence efficacy and make interpretation of both animal and human studies difficult. Further study is necessary, and it is likely that many questions concerning these confounding variables will remain unanswered until large-scale human trials are performed.

NEONATAL CLINICAL STUDIES

Most of the human clinical studies and the bulk of the clinical experience with surfactant are in preterm neonates. A decade after the initial failures of nebulized DPPC, the first successful clinical trial of surfactant therapy for neonates with RDS was reported in 1980.[19,88] Since then, numerous randomized and controlled clinical trials of RDS have been reported with remarkably positive results. These studies have demonstrated that surfactant delivered by instillation decreases mortality among infants with RDS.[20,89] Differences in morbidity are less impressive, with no significant difference in the incidence of bronchopulmonary dysplasia or intraventricular hemorrhage; however, there is a significant decrease in air leaks. A higher incidence of patent ductus arteriosus has been reported in surfactant-treated infants, although surfactant replacement does not appear to interfere with the action of indomethacin in closing the patent ductus arteriosus.[90-92] An increase in the incidence of apnea of prematurity has also been reported in surfactant-treated infants.[10,12,93]

More specific aspects of surfactant therapy in RDS have been addressed in recent studies. Comparative trials show natural surfactants to be more effective than synthetic surfactants.[62,63,94] Prophylactic treatment appears to be better than rescue treatment for those infants at highest risk—neonates from 29 to 30 weeks' gestation.[70,71] Beyond 30 to 32 weeks' gestation, the incidence of RDS decreases with gestational age, so rescue therapy is adequate and avoids treating many infants unnecessarily. The dose used is extrapolated to completely replace the normal surfactant pool: 100 mg/kg of phospholipid. Treatment regimens have varied somewhat, but most protocols have used multiple doses, usually scheduled 6 to 12 hours apart, beginning either in the delivery room or at the first clinical sign of respiratory distress. Multiple dosing strategies up to four doses have been shown to further reduce mortality and morbidity in infants with RDS.[11,95]

Surfactant has also been used in neonates with lung injury not related to prematurity. Surfactant deficiency and subsequent improvement after replacement have been reported in models and infants with congenital diaphragmatic hernia.[96,97] Similarly, meconium aspiration syndrome appears to respond favorably to exogenous surfactant. In a prospective trial infants with meconium aspiration syndrome treated with Survanta showed cumulative improvement in gas exchange and outcome relative to control infants.[98] Finally, in uncontrolled studies, the treatment of bacterial pneumonia in neonates with exogenous surfactant resulted in significant and sustained improvement in oxygenation.[99,100]

NONNEONATAL CLINICAL STUDIES

Small uncontrolled pilot studies and case reports support the use of exogenous surfactant in nonneonatal respiratory failure.[101-103] However, controlled studies have shown mixed results.

No improvement occurred after 5 days of continuously nebulized Exosurf in adults with sepsis-induced ARDS.[104] The negative results may have been related to the use of a synthetic instead of natural surfactant, the use of nebulization rather than instillation, and the fact that less than 5% of the total surfactant dose actually reached the lung with the aerosol delivery system.

Another controlled study evaluated the effectiveness of multiple doses of the modified natural surfactant Survanta in adults with ARDS.[105] Improvement in oxygenation was seen, but significant differences in mortality were only noted in the two groups receiving the larger dose of surfactant. There were no mortality differences when controls were compared with all treated patients.

A randomized controlled trial of porcine lung surfactant in 20 infants with respiratory syncytial virus infection showed immediate improvement in oxygenation and a significant reduction in time on mechanical ventilation and in the intensive care unit.[107] No

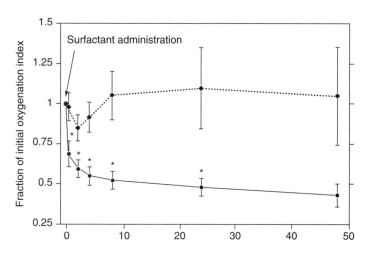

Fig. 16-8

Changes in oxygenation after surfactant. Circles, surfactant group; diamonds, placebo group. (From Willson DF et al: Instillation of calf's lung surfactant extract (Infasurf) is beneficial in pediatric acute hypoxemic respiratory failure. *Crit Care Med* 1999; 27:188-195.)

differences in mortality were seen, but they were not expected, owing to the small sample size.

Similar findings were demonstrated in a controlled trial of calf lung surfactant extract, Infasurf, in children with hypoxemic respiratory failure.[108] A striking and nearly immediate improvement in oxygenation relative to the control population was evidenced (Fig. 16-8). There was a 32% reduction in time on mechanical ventilation and a 30% reduction in stay in an intensive care unit (Table 16-3).

Although promising, the results of these studies are confounded by inconsistencies in dosing, timing of administration, surfactant formulation, randomization, and differences in patient populations. Surfactant administration in nonneonatal lung injury appears to be safe. Bolus instillation can be associated with transient hypoxemia, but allergic or other immune-mediated responses have not been reported. The only consistently reported complication has been an increased incidence of pulmonary hemorrhage, but this has only been reported in preterm neonates.[89]

FUTURE DIRECTIONS

Specific tasks related to surfactant administration need continued attention. The best mode of delivery needs to be determined because of its impact on efficacy, adverse effects, and costs. Which patients will benefit from surfactant administration and which will not need to be identified more carefully. Better and less expensive formulations of surfactant need to be developed. Synthetic surfactants, perhaps with genetically engineered surfactant-associated proteins that can be made in bulk, are likely to be less expensive and more effective, with less risk to the patient. These tasks are particularly pressing because of the phenomenal cost of this intervention. The natural surfac-

TABLE 16-3	LONG-TERM OUTCOME VARIABLES OF SURFACTANT VS. PLACEBO IN CHILDREN WITH RESPIRATORY FAILURE (MEAN ± SD)		
Variable	**Surfactant**	**Placebo**	**P value**
Days of mechanical ventilation	9.0 ± 10.4	13.2 ± 8.4	
Geometric mean	5.3	10.7	.03
Days in PICU*	11.7 ± 11.6	16.7 ± 9.2	
Geometric mean	8.1	14.4	.03
Days on oxygen*	13.5 ± 15	16.9 ± 11	
Geometric mean	7.6	13.9	.06
Days in hospital*	19.7 ± 15.9	23.1 ± 12.1	
Geometric mean	14.0	20.4	.12
Deaths	3	2	NS
ECMO	1	1	NS

Modified from Willson DF et al: Instillation of calf's lung surfactant extract (Infasurf) is beneficial in pediatric acute hypoxemic respiratory failure. *Crit Care Med* 1999; 27:188-195.

*In patients surviving without ECMO: excludes 5 who died and 2 placed on ECMO.

PICU, Pediatric intensive care unit; *ECMO,* extracorporeal membrane oxygenation.

tants are expensive to produce, and the cost of the drug will undoubtedly remain high.

In evaluating the studies that will be performed and reported over the next several years, we should remember that the initial trial of surfactant in human neonates, using aerosolized DPPC, was unsuccessful. It was not due to a flawed concept but to an ineffective surfactant and a poor delivery method. This delayed the introduction of this very effective therapy for over a decade. Proving or disproving the effectiveness of exogenous surfactant in other types of lung injury will be more difficult because of the many factors discussed in this chapter. It is vital that studies be continued to prevent adopting surfactant replacement prematurely into our therapeutic regimens and to prevent its premature dismissal as another failed therapy.

Surfactant replacement is unequivocally effective in treating surfactant-deficient preterm infants. Current evidence suggests that it may prove useful as an adjunctive therapy when surfactant dysfunction is a contributing, rather than a causative, factor of respiratory failure. Thus surfactant replacement offers promise to improve the disturbed lung physiology and allow moderation of ventilator support. It is not, however, a cure for the underlying lung injury. However, this approach may be adequate because the mortality from acute lung injury in children appears to be decreasing without surfactant replacement, perhaps owing to a better understanding of ventilator support.[103,108,109] The combination of better ventilator support and a better understanding of the role of surfactant administration may further improve the outcome for acute respiratory failure.

REFERENCES

1. Enhorning G et al: Prevention of neonatal respiratory distress syndrome by tracheal administration of surfactant: a randomized clinical trial. *Pediatrics* 1985; 76:145-153.
2. Shapiro DL et al: Double blind, randomized trial of a calf lung surfactant extract administered at birth to very premature infants for prevention of respiratory distress syndrome. *Pediatrics* 1986; 76:593-599.
3. Merritt TA et al: Prophylactic treatment of very premature infants with human surfactant. *N Engl J Med* 1996; 315:785-790.
4. Ten Centre Study Group: Ten Centre trial of artificial surfactant (artificial lung expanding compound) in very premature babies. *BMJ* 1987; 294:991-996.
5. Collaborative European Multicenter Study Group: Surfactant replacement therapy for severe neonatal respiratory distress syndrome: an international randomized clinical trial. *Pediatrics* 1988; 82:683-691.
6. Kendig JW et al: Surfactant replacement therapy at birth: final analysis of a clinical trial and comparisons with similar trials. *Pediatrics* 1988; 92:756-762.
7. Soll RF et al: Multicenter trial of single dose modified bovine surfactant extract (Survanta) for prevention of respiratory distress syndrome. *Pediatrics* 1990; 85:1092-1102.
8. Fujiwara T et al: Surfactant replacement therapy with a single postventilatory dose of a reconstituted bovine surfactant in preterm neonates with respiratory distress syndrome: final analysis of a multicenter, double-blind, randomized trial and comparison with similar trials. *Pediatrics* 1990; 90:753-764.
9. Corbet A et al: Decreased mortality rate among small premature infants treated at birth will a single dose of synthetic surfactant: a multicenter controlled trial. *J Pediatr* 1991; 118:277-284.
10. Long W et al: Effects of two rescue doses of synthetic surfactant on mortality rate and survival without bronchopulmonary dysplasia in 700- to 1350-gram infants with respiratory distress syndrome. *J Pediatr* 1991; 118:595-605.
11. Speer CP et al: Randomized European multicenter trial of surfactant replacement therapy for severe neonatal respiratory distress syndrome: single versus multiple doses of Curosurf. *Pediatrics* 1992; 89:13-20.
12. Horbar JD et al: Decreasing mortality associated with the introduction of surfactant therapy: an observational study of neonates weighing 60l to 1300 grams at birth. *Pediatrics* 1993; 92:19l-196.
13. Von Neergaard K: Neue Affasungen über einen grudnbegriff Atemmedranik: Die Retraktionskraft der Lunge, abhängig von der oberflachen Spannung en den Alveolen. *Z Die Gesamte Exp Med* 1929; 66:373-394.
14. Hills BA: *The biology of surfactant.* Cambridge, UK. Cambridge University Press, 1988; p 3.
15. Macklin CC: The pulmonary alveolar mucoid film and pneumocytes. *Lancet* 1954; 1:1099-1104.
16. Pattle RE: Properties, function, and origin of the alveolar lining layer. *Nature* 1955; 175:1125-1126.
17. Clements JA: Surface tension of lung extracts. *Proc Soc Exp Biol Med* 1957; 95:170-172.
18. Avery ME, Mead J: Surface properties in relation to atelectasis in hyaline membrane disease. *Am J Dis Child* 1959; 97:517-523.
19. Fujiwara T et al: Artificial surfactant therapy in hyaline membrane diseases. *Lancet* 1980; 1:55-59.
20. Wegman ME: Annual summary of vital statistics—1990. *Pediatrics* 1991; 88:1081-1092.
21. Hills BA: *The biology of surfactant.* Cambridge, UK. Cambridge University Press, 1988; p 10.
22. Enhorning G: From bubbles to babies: the evolution of surfactant replacement therapy. *Biol Neonate* 1997; 71(suppl 1):28-31.
23. Rooney SA: The surfactant system and lung phospholipid biochemistry. *Am Rev Respir Dis* 1985; 131:439-460.
24. Cockshutt A, Weitz J, Possmayer F: Pulmonary surfactant-associated protein A enhances the surface activity of lipid extract surfactant and reverses inhibition by blood proteins in vitro. *Biochemistry* 1990; 29:8424-8429.
25. Hawgood S: Surfactant: Composition, structure, and metabolism. In Crystal RG et al, editors: *The lung: scientific foundations,* ed 2. Philadelphia. Lippincott-Raven, 1997; p 560.
26. White RT et al: Isolation and characterization of the human pulmonary surfactant apoprotein gene. *Nature* 1985; 317:361-363.
27. Whitsett JA et al: Hydrophobic surfactant associated protein in whole lung surfactant and its importance for biophysical activity in lung surfactant extracts used for replacement therapy. *Pediatr Res* 1986; 20:460-467.
28. Chung J et al: Effect of surfactant associated protein A on the activity of lipid extract surfactant. *Biochem Biophys Acta* 1989; 1002:348-358.
29. Crouch E et al: Molecular structure of pulmonary surfactant protein D (SP-D). *J Biol Chem* 1994; 269:17311-17319.
30. Hawgood S, Clements JA: Pulmonary surfactant and its apoproteins. *J Clin Invest* 1990; 86:1-6.
31. Wright JR, Clements JA: Metabolism and turnover of lung surfactant. *Am Rev Respir Dis* 1987; 135:426-444.
32. Williams MC: Conversion of lamellar body membranes into tubular myelin in alveoli of fetal rate lungs. *J Cell Biol* 1977; 72:260-277.
33. Suzuki Y, Fujita Y, Kogishi K: Reconstitution of tubular myelin from synthetic lipids and proteins associated with pig pulmonary surfactant. *Am Rev Respir Dis* 1989; 140: 75-81.
34. Kuroki Y, Mason RJ, Voelker DR: Pulmonary surfactant apoprotein A structure and modulation of surfactant secretion by rat alveolar type II cells. *J Biol Chem* 1988; 263:3388-3394.

35. Clements JA: Composition and properties of pulmonary surfactant. In Villee CA, Villee DB, Zuckerman J, editors: *Respiratory distress syndrome.* New York. Academic Press, 1973; pp 77-95.

36. King RJ, MacBeth MC: Interaction of the lipid and protein components of pulmonary surfactant: role of phosphatidylglycerol and calcium. *Biochim Biophys Acta* 1981; 647:159-168.

37. Williams MC: Uptake of lectins by alveolar type II cells: subsequent deposition into lamellar bodies. *Proc Natl Acad Sci USA* 1984; 81:6383-6387.

38. Pison U et al: Surfactant abnormalities in patients with respiratory failure after multiple trauma. *Am Rev Respir Dis* 1989; 140:1033-1039.

39. Jobe AH, Ikegami M: Surfactant and acute lung injury. *Proc Assoc Am Physicians* 1998; 110:489-495.

40. Gregory T et al: Surfactant chemical composition and biophysical activity in acute respiratory distress syndrome. *J Clin Invest* 1991; 65:1976-1981.

41. Pison U et al: Altered pulmonary surfactant in uncomplicated and septicemia-complicated courses of acute respiratory failure. *J Trauma* 1990; 30:19-26.

42. Low RB et al: Bronchoalveolar lavage lipids during development of bleomycin-induced fibrosis in rats. *Am Rev Respir Dis* 1988; 138:709-713.

43. Young SL et al: Pulmonary surfactant lipid production in oxygen exposed rat lungs. *Lab Invest* 1982; 46:570-576.

44. Holm BA et al: Pulmonary physiological and surfactant changes during injury and recovery from hyperoxia. *J Appl Physiol* 1985; 59:1402-1409.

45. Gregory T et al: Surfactant chemical composition and biophysical activity in acute respiratory distress syndrome. *J Clin Invest* 1991; 65:1976-1981.

46. Pison U et al: Phospholipid lung profile in adult respiratory distress syndrome—evidence for surfactant abnormality. *Prog Clin Biol Res* 1987; 236A:517-523.

47. Lewis JF, Jobe AH: Surfactant and the adult respiratory distress syndrome. *Am Rev Respir Dis* 1993; 147:218-233.

48. Ueda T, Ikegami M, Jobe A: Surfactant subtypes: in vitro conversions, in vivo function, and effects of serum proteins. *Am J Respir Crit Care Med* 1994; 149:1254-1259

49. Veldhuizen RAW et al: Pulmonary surfactant subfractions in patients with the acute respiratory distress syndrome. *Am J Respir Crit Care Med* 1995; 152:1867-1871.

50. Holm BA et al: Type II pneumocyte changes during hyperoxic lung injury and recovery. *J Appl Physiol* 1988; 65:2672-2678.

51. Huguchi R, Lewis J, Ikegami M: In vitro conversion of surfactant subtypes is altered in alveolar surfactant isolated from injured lungs. *Am Rev Respir Dis* 1991; 145:1416-1420.

52. Seeger W et al: Alveolar surfactant and adult respiratory distress syndrome: pathogenetic role and therapeutic prospects. *Clin Invest* 1993; 71:177-190.

53. Kobayashi T et al: Inactivation of exogenous surfactant by pulmonary edema fluid. *Pediatr Res* 1991; 29:353-356.

54. Bruni R et al: Inactivation of surfactant in rat lungs. *Pediatr Res* 1996; 39:236-240.

55. Holm BA, Enhorning G, Notter RH: A biophysical mechanism by which plasma proteins inhibit lung surfactant activity. *Chem Phys Lipids* 1988; 49:4-55.

56. Holm BA, Matalon S: Role of pulmonary surfactant in the development and treatment of adult respiratory distress syndrome. *Anesth Analg* 1989; 805-818.

57. Ikegami M, Jacobs H, Jobe AH: Surfactant function in the respiratory distress syndrome. *J Pediatr* 1983; 102:443-447.

58. Merritt TA et al: Exogenous surfactant treatments for neonatal respiratory distress syndrome and their potential role in the adult respiratory distress syndrome. *Drugs* 1989; 38:591-611.

59. Kattwinkel J: Surfactant: evolving issues. *Clin Perinatol* 1998; 25:17-32.

60. Glaser SW et al: cDNA and deduced amino acid sequence of human pulmonary surfactant-associated proteolipid SPL (Phe). *Proc Natl Acad Sci U S A* 1987; 84:4007-4011.

61. Cochrane CG et al: Bronchoalveolar lavage with KL4-surfactant in models of meconium aspiration syndrome. *Pediatr Res* 1998; 44:705-715.

62. Horbar JD et al, for the National Institute of Child Health and Human Development Neonatal Research Network: A multicenter randomized trial comparing two surfactants for the treatment of neonatal respiratory distress syndrome. *J Pediatr* 1993; 123:757-766.

63. Sehgal SS et al: Modified bovine surfactant (Survanta) versus a protein-free surfactant (Exosurf) in the treatment of respiratory distress syndrome in preterm infants: a pilot study. *J Natl Med Assoc* 1994; 84:46-52.

64. Vermont Oxford Trials Network: A multicenter randomized trial comparing synthetic surfactant to modified bovine surfactant in the treatment of neonatal respiratory distress syndrome. *Pediatr Res* 1994 (abstract no. 1542); 35:259.

65. Hudak ML et al: Exosurf for the treatment of RDS: a 21 center randomized double-masked comparison trial. *Pediatr Res* 1994 (abstract no. 1370); 35:231.

66. Seeger W et al: Surfactant inhibition by plasma proteins: differential sensitivity of various surfactant preparations. *Eur Respir J* 1993; 6:971-977.

67. Cummings JJ et al: A controlled clinical comparison of four different surfactant preparations in surfactant deficient preterm lambs. *Am Rev Respir Dis* 1992; 145:999-1004.

68. Bloom BT et al: Randomized double-blind multicenter trial of Survanta and Infasurf. *Pediatr Res* 1994 (abstract no. 1942); 35:326.

69. Nilsson R et al: Surfactant treatment in experimental hyaline membrane disease. *Eur J Respir Dis* 1981; 62:441-449.

70. Kattwinkel J et al: Prophylactic administration of calf lung surfactant extract is more effective than early treatment of respiratory distress syndrome in neonates of 29 through 32 weeks gestation. *Pediatrics* 1993; 92:90-98.

71. Kendig JW et al: A comparison of surfactant as immediate prophylaxis and as rescue therapy in newborns of less than 30 weeks' gestation. *N Engl J Med* 1991; 324:865-871.

72. Gattinoni L et al: Relationships between lung computed tomographic density, gas exchange, and PEEP in acute respiratory failure. *Anesthesiology* 1988; 69:824-832.

73. Ito Y et al:. Timing of exogenous surfactant administration in a rabbit model of acute lung injury. *J Appl Physiol* 1996; 80:1357-1364.

74. Lewis JF et al: Physiologic responses and surfactant distribution in saline-lavaged sheep given instilled vs nebulized surfactant. *J Appl Physiol* 1993; 74:1256-1264.

75. Lewis JF et al: Physiologic responses and distribution of aerosolized surfactant (Survanta) in a non-uniform model of lung injury. *Am Rev Respir Dis* 1993; 147:1364-1370.

76. Lewis J et al: Aerosolized surfactant is preferentially deposited in normal versus injured regions of the lung in a heterogeneous lung injury model. *Am Rev Respir Dis* 1992; 145:A184.

77. Lewis JF et al: Evaluation of exogenous surfactant treatment strategies in an adult model of acute lung injury. *J Appl Physiol* 1996; 80:1156-1164.

78. Dijk PH, Heikamp A, Oetomo SB: Surfactant nebulization versus instillation during high frequency ventilation in surfactant–deficient rabbits. *Pediatr Res* 1998; 44:699-704.

79. Matalon S, Holm BA, Notter RH: Mitigation of pulmonary hyperoxic injury by administration of exogenous surfactant. *J Appl Physiol* 1987; 756-761.

80. Seeger W et al: Alterations of alveolar surfactant function after exposure to oxidative stress and to oxygenated and native arachidonic acid in vitro. *Biochim Biophys Acta* 1985; 835:58-67.

81. Zeller M et al: Effects of aerosolized artificial surfactant on repeated oleic acid injury in sheep. *Am Rev Respir Dis* 1990; 141:1014-1019.

82. Ryan SF et al: Correlation of lung compliance and quantities of surfactant phospholipids after acute alveolar injury from *N*-nitroso-*N*-methylurethane in the dog. *Am Rev Respir Dis* 1981; 123:200-204.

83. Harris JD et al: Effect of exogenous surfactant instillation on experimental acute lung injury. *J Appl Physiol* 1989; 66:1846-1851.

84. Eijking EP et al: Surfactant treatment of respiratory failure induced by hydrochloric acid aspiration in rats. *Anesthesiology* 1993; 78:1145-1151.

85. Nieman GF et al: Comparison of exogenous surfactants in the treatment of wood smoke inhalation. *Am J Respir Crit Care Med* 1995; 152:597-602.

86. VanDaal GJ et al: Surfactant replacement therapy improves pulmonary mechanics in end-stage influenza A pneumonia in mice. *Am Rev Respir Dis* 1992; 145: 859-863.

87. Berry D, Ikegami M, Jobe A: Respiratory distress and surfactant inhibition following vagotomy in rabbits. *J Appl Physiol* 1986; 61:1741-1748.

88. Chu J et al: Neonatal pulmonary ischemia: clinical and physiologic studies. *Pediatrics* 1967; 40:709-782.

89. Jobe AH: Pulmonary surfactant therapy. *N Engl J Med* 1993; 328:861-868.

90. Raju TNK et al: Double-blind controlled trial of single dose treatment with bovine surfactant in severe hyaline membrane disease. *Lancet* 1987; 1:651-665.

91. Ferrara TB et al: Survival and follow-up of infants born at 23-26 weeks of gestational age: effects of surfactant therapy. *J Pediatr* 1994; 124:119-124.

92. Kaapa P et al: Pulmonary hemodynamics after synthetic surfactant replacement in neonatal respiratory distress syndrome. *J Pediatr* 1993; 123:115-119.

93. Bose C et al: Improved outcome at 28 days of age for very low birth weight infants treated with a single dose of synthetic surfactant. *J Pediatr* 1990; 117:947-953.

94. Hudak ML et al: A multicenter randomized masked comparison trial of natural versus synthetic surfactant for the treatment of respiratory distress syndrome. *J Pediatr* 1996; 128:396-406.

95. Dunn MS, Shennan AT, Possmayer F: Single- versus multiple-dose surfactant replacement therapy in neonates of 30 to 36 weeks' gestation with respiratory distress syndrome. *Pediatrics* 1990; 86:564-571.

96. Suen HC et al: Biochemical immaturity of lungs in congenital diaphragmatic hernia. *J Pediatr Surg* 1993; 28:471.

97. Glick PL et al: Pathophysiology of congenital diaphragmatic hernia. III: Exogenous surfactant for the high-risk neonate with CDH. *J Pediatr Surg* 1992; 27:866.

98. Findlay RD, Taeusch HW, Walther FJ: Surfactant replacement therapy for meconium aspiration syndrome. *Pediatrics* 1996; 97:48.

99. Auten RL et al: Surfactant treatment of full-term newborns with respiratory failure. *Pediatrics* 1991; 87:101.

100. Fetter WPF et al: Surfactant replacement therapy in neonates with respiratory failure due to bacterial sepsis. *Acta Paediatr* 1995; 84:14.

101. Perez-Benavides F, Riff E, Franks C: Adult respiratory distress syndrome and artificial surfactant replacement in the pediatric patient. *Pediatr Emerg Care* 1995; 11:153-155.

102. Spragg RG et al: Acute effects of a single dose of porcine surfactant on patients with acute respiratory distress syndrome. *Chest* 1995; 105:195-202.

103. Willson DF et al: Calf's lung surfactant extract in acute hypoxemic respiratory failure in children. *Crit Care Med* 1996; 24:1316-1322.

104. Anzueto A et al: Aerosolized surfactant in adults with sepsis-induced ARDS. *N Engl J Med* 1996; 334:1417-1421.

105. Gregory TJ et al: Bovine surfactant therapy for patients with acute respiratory distress syndrome. *Am J Respir Crit Care Med* 1997; 155:1309-1315.

106. Vos GD, Rijtema MN, Blanco CE: Treatment of respiratory failure due to respiratory syncytial virus pneumonia with natural surfactant. *Pediatr Pulmonol* 1996; 22:412-415.

107. Luchetti M et al: Porcine-derived surfactant treatment of severe bronchiolitis. *Acta Anaesthesiol Scand* 1998; 42:805-810.

108. Willson DF et al: Instillation of calf's lung surfactant extract (Infasurf) is beneficial in pediatric acute hypoxemic respiratory failure. *Crit Care Med* 1999; 27:188-195.

109. Verbrugge SJ, Gommers D, Lachmann B: Conventional ventilation modes with small pressure amplitudes and high positive end-expiratory pressure levels optimize surfactant therapy. *Crit Care Med* 1999; 27:2724-2728.

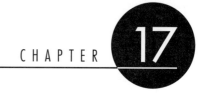

CHAPTER

Mechanical Ventilators

Barry Grenier

The mechanical ventilators originally used to ventilate infants and older pediatric patients were modifications of adult ventilators.[1] In the early 1970s, however, Kirby and associates[2] described a "new" pediatric ventilator, and the relatively simple continuous-flow time-cycled machine became the predominant design of infant ventilators produced after that time. Although Kirby and colleagues described their machine as a volume ventilator, the practice of pressure limiting became so popular that the terms *infant ventilator* and *pressure ventilator* were often used interchangeably. Older pediatric patients continued to be ventilated with modified adult, or volume, ventilators or with machines with the same design characteristics as adult ventilators.

More recent advances in ventilator technology, particularly the use of microprocessor control, have greatly increased the sophistication of mechanical ventilators and blurred traditional boundaries between ventilator types and ventilation techniques. It is now common for ventilators to offer a choice of pressure or volume (more accurately, flow) control as well as a variety of inspiratory flow waveforms. Microprocessors, and the electromechanical valves that they control, are capable of adjusting flow rates very rapidly and in a wide range, eliminating many of the limitations to flow and tidal volume delivery inherent in the design of earlier ventilators. As a result, it is often possible for a single ventilator to be used to ventilate a wider range of patients. Even the distinction between infant ventilator and adult ventilator is no longer always clear cut.

In this chapter, first a system is presented for classifying mechanical ventilators and for understanding ventilator function. Then, a number of machines currently used to ventilate infants and older pediatric patients are reviewed in this context.

VENTILATOR CLASSIFICATION

Citing the problems with traditional classification schemes, Chatburn proposed a new approach to the understanding and classification of mechanical ventilators.[3-5]

The remainder of this section summarizes Chatburn's classification system, which uses input power, power conversion and transmission, control, and output as a framework for describing mechanical ventilators.

INPUT POWER

Input power refers to the power source (or sources) required by the ventilator to perform the work of ventilation. Input power can be pneumatic or electric. Pneumatic power is usually provided by compressed gas pressurized to about 50 pounds per square inch gauge (psig). Electric power can be either alternating current (AC) or the direct current (DC) of a battery.

Ventilators can be designed to use either one or both input power sources.[6] The original Baby Bird (Bird Products) is an example of a pneumatically powered ventilator. Electrically powered ventilators such as the Puritan-Bennett MA-1 (Puritan-Bennett) and Emerson 3-MV (J.H. Emerson) may use a pneumatic source to increase the oxygen concentration of inspired gas, but interruption of the gas source does not disrupt basic ventilator function. Most ventilators currently in use require both pneumatic and electric power for operation. Typically, pneumatic power provides the ventilator's driving force whereas electricity powers the mechanism or mechanisms controlling the particular manner in which the gas is delivered.

POWER CONVERSION AND TRANSMISSION

Power conversion and transmission describes the mechanism or mechanisms that the ventilator uses to create and control gas flow to the patient. Together these devices can be referred to as the drive mechanism and include the ventilator's compressor and output control valves.

The force (or pressure) needed to effect a flow of gas may be generated by a device outside of the ventilator (an external compressor) or by a device that is part of the ventilator's design (an internal compressor). Pistons and cylinders, diaphragms, bellows, and rotating vanes have been used most often as internal compressors.

A ventilator's compressor is often described in conjunction with the motor used to drive it and the linkage between the motor and compressor. Motor and linkage types can be categorized as electric motor/rotating crank and piston, electric motor/rack and pinion, and direct-drive electric motor. In addition, compressed gas can be considered as the motor that drives a compressor. For example, compressed gas can be used to power a diaphragm or bellows, which, in turn, supplies flow to the patient. Compressed gas may also be used to inflate the lungs directly. The pressure of compressed gas is generally reduced to a "usable" level by a regulator.

The valves that are used to control the gas flow created by the compressor are called *output control valves*. These devices operate under the influence of the control circuit and include inspiratory flow control valves and exhalation valves. Common types of output control valves are pneumatic diaphragms (frequently used as exhalation valves), pneumatic poppet valves, electromagnetic poppet valves (solenoids), and electromagnetic proportional valves. The latter type of valve regulates flow by varying the size of the valve opening and is often used to "pattern" inspiratory flow.

CONTROL

Control Circuit. The control circuit is the subsystem that performs the logic and decision-making functions of the ventilator and regulates the drive mechanism or output control valves, or both, to produce the desired ventilator output. Ventilators may use one or more types of control circuit, which have been categorized as follows:

Mechanical control circuits (used in early ventilators) use levers, pulleys, and cams. Pneumatic control circuits rely on gas pressure to operate diaphragms, Venturi devices, and pistons. Fluidic control circuits use minute gas flows to operate pressure switches and timing mechanisms. Electric control circuits use only simple switches. Electronic control circuits use components such as resistors, capacitors, and transistors or combinations of components in integrated circuits. The most sophisticated form of electronic control is provided by a microprocessor.

A ventilator's control scheme can be open loop or closed loop. With both types of control, an input (pressure, volume, or flow setting) is added to a system to obtain a desired output. Control is closed loop when an output variable is measured and compared with a reference (the control settings), and the input is modified as needed to more closely approximate the desired output. Closed loop control is also known as feedback or servo control. If an input is selected and no information is fed back to modify the input (i.e., close the loop), the system is open loop.

Control Variables and Waveforms. The variables involved in the mechanics of ventilation are pressure, volume, and flow. The relationships among these variables are described by a mathematical model, the *equation of motion for the respiratory system*. A simplified form of this equation can be found in Fig. 17-1. The equation of motion demonstrates that if any single variable is specified, the specified variable is independent of anything

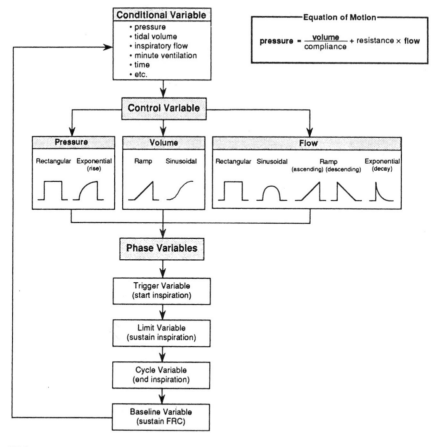

Fig. 17-1

A new paradigm for understanding mechanical ventilators based on a mathematical model known as the equation of motion for the respiratory system. The model illustrates that during inspiration the ventilator can control only one variable at a time. The diagram shows common waveforms for each control variable. Pressure, volume, flow, and time are also used as phase variables that determine the characteristics of each ventilatory cycle. The diagram is drawn as a flow chart to emphasize that each breath may have a different set of control and phase variables, depending on the mode of ventilation used. (From Chatburn RL: Classification of mechanical ventilations. *Respir Care* 1992; 37:1009-1025.)

else in the equation. Furthermore, the other two variables are dependent on the specified (independent) variable.

Because only one variable can serve as the independent variable at a given time, it follows that only one variable can be controlled by a ventilator at any one time. The variable that a ventilator controls to effect inspiration is the control variable. Pressure, volume, and flow generally serve as control variables, although a ventilator can theoretically control time (the implied variable) as well.

The pattern that a variable produces during inspiration is its inspiratory waveform. A waveform plots the magnitude of a variable (vertical axis) over inspiratory time (horizontal axis). Common inspiratory waveforms for each of the control variables are shown in Fig. 17-1. Although these waveforms are idealized, they are representative of waveform types produced by ventilators in current use.

The control variable is characterized by the ability to maintain a constant behavior despite the load, that is, changes in respiratory system resistance and compliance, imposed on the ventilator. Therefore the ability of a particular variable to retain its characteristic waveform in the face of changes in compliance and resistance distinguishes it as the control variable. The criteria for determining the control variable used by a ventilator are set forth in the algorithm in Fig. 17-2.

Pressure. If the pressure waveform does not change with changes in patient compliance and

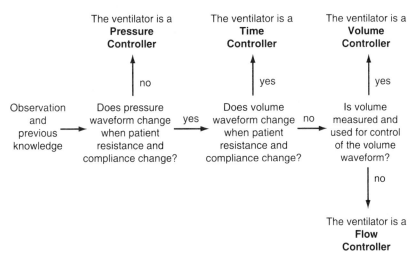

Fig. 17-2

Criteria for determining the control variable during a ventilator-assisted inspiration. (From Chatburn RL: Classification of mechanical ventilations. *Respir Care* 1992; 37:1009-1025.)

resistance, the control variable is pressure. If the ventilator causes airway pressure to rise to greater than body surface pressure to effect inspiratory gas flow, the ventilator is a positive-pressure controller. Infant ventilators are generally used as positive-pressure controllers. If the ventilator causes body surface pressure to drop to less than airway pressure to create the gradient for gas flow, the ventilator is a negative-pressure controller (e.g., the Emerson Iron Lung, J. H. Emerson Co.).

Volume. If the pressure waveform changes significantly with changes in resistance and compliance, the volume waveform is examined. If the volume waveform remains unchanged, the flow waveform also remains unchanged because volume and flow are functions of each other (i.e., flow is the change of volume over time and volume is flow divided by time).

The factor that distinguishes a volume controller from a flow controller is that a volume controller must measure volume and use the signal to control the volume waveform. Volume can be directly measured as the displacement of a piston or bellows (or similar device). With ventilators that use a piston or bellows compressor drive mechanism, controlling the excursion of the device controls the volume waveform. Examples of this type of volume controller are the Puritan-Bennett MA-1 and the Emerson 3-MV. Alternatively, a volume signal can be derived from the integration of a flow signal.

Flow. If the volume (and flow) waveform remains essentially unchanged with changes in

patient compliance and resistance, and delivered volume is not directly measured or used as a feedback signal, flow is the variable controlled by the ventilator. The Servo 900C (Siemens Medical Systems), Servo 300A (Siemens Medical Systems), Drager Evita 4 (Drager), Puritan-Bennett 840 (Puritan-Bennett), and V.I.P. Bird (Bird Products) are all flow controllers when delivering volume preset breaths, that is, they all measure flow and calculate volume. An infant ventilator that does not reach its preset pressure limit can be considered a flow controller rather than a pressure controller.

Time. If both pressure and volume outputs (and therefore pressure and volume waveforms) are significantly altered by changes in the imposed load, control must be defined in terms of the inspiratory and expiratory times. Thus time is the control variable. Some high-frequency ventilators can be best classified as time controllers.

Dual control of the inspiratory phase. Dual control is possible if a ventilator has the capability to switch from one control variable to another if a certain condition is met, or not met, during the inspiratory phase.[7] An example of dual control of inspiration is volume-assured pressure-support ventilation (VAPSV). With VAPSV, inspiration is initially pressure controlled with variable gas flow to meet the patient's inspiratory demand. If a target tidal volume is not delivered during the pressure-controlled portion of the breath, the ventilator switches to flow control with a constant inspiratory flow rate to meet the tidal volume target.

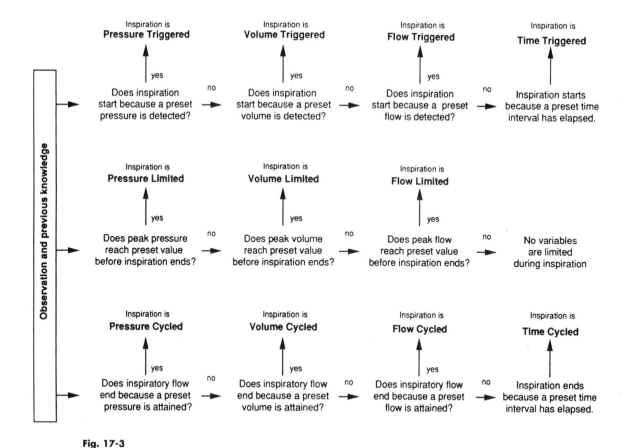

Fig. 17-3

Criteria for determining the phase variables during a ventilator-assisted breath. (From Chatburn RL: Classification of mechanical ventilations. *Respir Care* 1992; 37:1009-1025.)

Phase Variables.   Mushin and colleagues divided the ventilatory cycle into four phases: the change from expiration to inspiration, inspiration, the change from inspiration to expiration, and expiration.[8] Phase variables (Fig. 17-3) are the variables (pressure, volume, flow, and time) that are measured and used by the ventilator to initiate, sustain, or end a ventilatory phase.

Trigger.   The variable responsible for initiating inspiration (the changeover from expiration to inspiration) is referred to as the trigger variable. Time is the trigger variable if inspiration is initiated by the ventilator at the end of a period determined by the set ventilator rate, whether or not spontaneous breathing occurs. If the inspiratory phase is initiated by patient effort, one of the remaining variables—pressure, volume, or flow—is used as the trigger variable. Commonly, a ventilator senses patient effort as the drop in baseline pressure to a preset value. Volume and flow can also be used as trigger variables. Frequently, ventilators include a

control that permits mandatory breaths to be manually triggered by the operator.

Considerable interest has been generated in the potential benefits of patient synchronization in the infant population. The Drager Babylog 8000 Plus (Drager) permits volume triggering of mandatory breaths.

The V.I.P. Bird Infant-Pediatric Ventilator (Bird Products) incorporates a flow trigger. With the Star Sync option, the Infant Star 500 (Puritan-Bennett) can be triggered by the change in pressure caused by the movement of the abdomen preceding inspiration.

The degree of patient effort required to trigger inspiration is referred to as the ventilator's *sensitivity,* which is adjusted by changing the set value of the trigger variable.

Limit.   A variable that reaches a preset value before the end of inspiration is referred to as a limit variable. Pressure, volume, and flow can be limited. Time, however, cannot be a limit variable. If a preset time is reached during inspiration, the inspiration must be terminated.

Infant ventilators are generally pressure limited. During inspiration, circuit pressure rises and is maintained at the preset pressure level until inspiration is terminated at the end of the inspiratory time interval. Ventilators used to deliver volume preset breaths often limit flow to a preset peak value. Inspiration is volume limited if an inspiratory pause is added to the inspiratory time of a volume preset breath.

Cycle. The end of inspiration (i.e., the change-over from inspiration to expiration) occurs because a particular measured variable reaches a preset value. The variable responsible for terminating the inspiratory phase is the cycle variable. Pressure, volume, flow, and time can all act as cycle variables.

Many of the newer microprocessor-controlled ventilators require selection of a peak flow rate and tidal volume, suggesting that inspiration is cycled because a certain volume has been delivered. In fact, these ventilators do not measure volume. Rather, they control flow rates over an interval of time necessary to deliver the desired tidal volume at the selected flow rate to produce a predetermined flow waveform. Because the inspiratory phase is cycled at the end of this predetermined inspiratory time interval, the breath is actually time cycled. Pressure support breaths are typically cycled when inspiratory flow falls to a predetermined flow rate or percentage of the peak flow needed to reach the set pressure limit. Infant ventilators are generally time cycled. A ventilator may also have a back-up or safety-cycle variable. For example, inspiration may be pressure cycled if airway pressure reaches the value set on the high airway pressure alarm.

Baseline. With the changeover to expiration, flow, volume, and pressure return to their baseline values. Normally, expiratory flow ceases (and pressure and volume return to baseline) before the end of the expiratory phase. The variable controlled by the ventilator during the expiratory phase is the baseline variable. Although theoretically, pressure, volume, or flow can be controlled during the expiratory phase, the easiest variable to control from a practical standpoint is pressure. Positive end-expiratory pressure (PEEP) or continuous positive airway pressure (CPAP) is baseline pressure that is positive in relation to body surface pressure.

Modes of Ventilation. Fig. 17-2 emphasizes that each breath has a specific pattern of control and phase variables and that the pattern may change from one breath to the next. A ventilator may deliver only mandatory breaths, may allow spontaneous breaths between mandatory breaths, or may combine different types of mandatory and spontaneous breaths. The breath types, or combinations of breath types, permitted by a particular ventilator are dictated by the operational modes available on the ventilator. However, a mode name does not specifically describe the pattern or patterns of ventilation for that given mode. Thus a mode of ventilation can be more precisely described as a specific pattern of control and phase variables for both mandatory and spontaneous breaths.

Conditional Variables. Depending on the mode of ventilation, the ventilator must choose which pattern of control and phase variables to implement for each breath. The ventilator selects a particular pattern when a certain variable reaches a preset threshold value. A variable responsible for causing the ventilator to select a particular pattern of control and phase variables is the conditional variable. If the conditional variable reaches a certain preset value, one pattern is selected; if not, another pattern is selected.

For example, a ventilator may use pressure and time as conditional variables in the synchronized intermittent mandatory ventilation (SIMV) mode. In this example, breaths are either patient (pressure) triggered or machine (time) triggered, depending on whether the SIMV timing window is "open" or "closed" and if a patient effort is detected.

Spontaneous versus Mandatory Breaths. All breaths can be categorized as either spontaneous or mandatory, depending on the degree of control the patient can exert over the initiation and termination of the breath. A breath is spontaneous if it is initiated by the patient and can be terminated with sufficient activity of the ventilatory muscles or by the effects of respiratory system mechanics. A mandatory breath is a ventilator-assisted breath that is either initiated or terminated by the ventilator.

Spontaneous breaths can be ventilator assisted (e.g., pressure support) or unassisted. Spontaneous breaths from demand flow systems or from continuous flow through the patient circuit are unassisted breaths. To provide demand flow, however, the ventilator responds to patient effort throughout the spontaneous inspiratory phase, so it is appropriate to describe the breath in terms of its phase variables. Because the ventilator provides flow in an attempt to maintain a constant baseline pressure, inspiration is pressure limited. When continuous flow alone is used, the ventilator does not respond to patient effort, and these spontaneous breaths are not controlled.[9]

OUTPUT

As a breath is delivered, changes in volume, pressure, and flow occur simultaneously over the course of inspiratory time. The magnitude of the changes in volume, pressure, and flow and the patterns produced by these variables constitute the ventilator's output and are represented by output waveforms.

The ventilator determines the control waveform, which by definition should not be significantly altered by the load imposed on the ventilator. The shapes of the other waveforms are a function of the control waveform and the patient's compliance and resistance. However, waveforms used to represent ventilator output are idealized. Because no ventilator is an ideal controller, even the control waveform will only approximate the ideal. Also, waveforms recorded during ventilation may be deformed by artifact caused by vibration and turbulence in the patient circuit.

The location of the devices used to measure output variables affects the output values and the shape of output waveforms. Pressure, volume, and flow measurements made inside the ventilator are invariably different from measurements made at the patient airway because of the effects of the patient circuit. Pressure measured back inside the ventilator on the inspiratory side is higher than pressure measured at the airway because of both the resistance and compliance of the patient circuit. Circuit compliance also causes volume and flow at the patient airway to be less than that leaving the ventilator. The relative amount of volume "lost" in the patient circuit may be particularly significant with ventilation of infants and small children. Measurement of exhaled volume made inside the ventilator includes volume compressed in the patient circuit during inspiration and will not reflect the changes in compressed volume that may occur.

ALARM SYSTEMS

The purpose of ventilator alarms is to warn of inadvertent changes in ventilator performance and patient status. Thus ventilator alarm systems have been designed to monitor the mechanical and electronic functions of the ventilator and the variables involved in the mechanics of breathing—pressure, volume, flow, and time. Alarms can be categorized according to the same framework used to classify other ventilator functions.

Input Power Alarms. Alarms that signal loss of the power source or sources required for ventilator operation are the input power alarms. Alarms that indicate loss of electric power are activated with the interruption of that power, or they may signal a low battery state if the ventilator is operating on battery power. An alarm that indicates loss of pneumatic power is activated when there is a loss or critical reduction of compressed air or oxygen pressure.

Control Circuit Alarms. Activation of control circuit alarms may signal that a control is set improperly or warn of the incompatibility of a combination of control settings (e.g., an inverse inspiratory to expiratory [I:E] ratio). Control circuit alarms may also signal a fault in the control circuit itself, such as a failure of a microprocessor or related system. Alarms of this type may carry a generic warning such as "ventilator inoperative" or may include specific error codes to facilitate troubleshooting.

Output Alarms. Output alarms are activated when the value of a control variable or other ventilator output (e.g., inspired gas) falls outside an acceptable range. Alarm thresholds may be able to be adjusted by the operator, may automatically be set by the ventilator based on control settings, or may have fixed thresholds set at the factory. Output alarms may signal changes in patient status or changes in ventilator performance.

Pressure alarms include those for high and low peak airway pressure, high and low mean airway pressure, high and low baseline pressure, and failure of airway pressure to return to baseline within a specified period. Alarms for high and low exhaled tidal volume and high and low exhaled minute ventilation warn of unacceptable values for volume and flow output, respectively. Alarms associated with time include those for high and low respiratory rate, an inspiratory time that is too long or too short, and an expiratory time that is too short or too long. Apnea alarms (an expiratory time that is too long) fall into this category. Alarms for inspired gas include those for high and low gas temperature and high and low F_{IO_2}. Expired gas alarms include those for exhaled carbon dioxide tension and exhaled oxygen tension.

CRITICAL CARE VENTILATORS

BEAR CUB 750VS INFANT VENTILATOR

The Bear Cub 750vs (Viasys Healthcare, Bear Medical) (Fig. 17-4) is a pneumatically and electrically (AC or internal battery) powered infant ventilator. Power conversion and transmission are accomplished by pressure regulators, mechanical flow control valves, and a pneumatic exhalation valve. The Bear Cub is electronically (microprocessor) and pneumatically controlled and functions as a pressure or flow controller. Mandatory breaths are time or

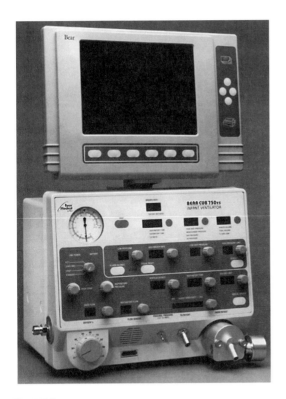

Fig. 17-4

Bear Cub 750vs Infant Ventilator. (Courtesy Bear Medical, Palm Springs, Calif.)

flow triggered, pressure or flow limited, and time cycled. A continuous gas flow is available for spontaneous breathing.[10] An enhanced Bear Cub, the Bear Cub 750PSV, is also available.

Power Conversion and Transmission. The Bear Cub 750vs utilizes compressed air and oxygen in a range of 30 to 80 psig. Air and oxygen pressures are reduced by separate pressure regulators, and the balanced gases are mixed at the air-oxygen blender, a mechanical proportioning valve. Gas flow is regulated by dual mechanical needle valves (flowmeters): the inspiratory flow control valve and the base flow control valve. The inspiratory solenoid switches the gas flows, providing the inspiratory flow rate during the inspiratory phase of mandatory breaths and base flow during the expiratory phase. Blended gas flows past a subambient/overpressure relief valve, dump valve, and pressure transducer before entering the inspiratory limb of the patient circuit.

Gas flow from the expiratory limb of the patient circuit is regulated by the pneumatic exhalation valve. The exhalation solenoid determines which of two control pressures—inspiratory (PIP) or base-line (PEEP)—is applied to a control diaphragm. When the inspiratory control pressure is transmitted, the control diaphragm moves a control pin and exhalation diaphragm against the exhalation valve opening. This action closes the exhalation valve and diverts gas flow to the patient. If circuit pressure reaches the inspiratory control pressure, the exhalation diaphragm opens slightly to vent excess gas flow. At the end of the inspiratory phase, the exhalation solenoid switches the control pressure to baseline. As a result, the control diaphragm and pin retract, the valve opens, allowing exhalation, and circuit pressure drops to set baseline pressure.

A jet Venturi is used to decrease flow resistance in the expiratory limb and eliminate inadvertent PEEP.

Control. The Bear Cub 750vs can be operated in the assist-control (A/C), SIMV/intermittent mandatory ventilation (IMV), and CPAP modes. When placed in the standby mode, the ventilator discontinues all electronic function except the charging system for the internal battery. Pressure support and a backup ventilation mode are available on the Bear Cub 750PSV.

Mandatory breaths are pressure or flow controlled. Inspiration is pressure limited if airway pressure reaches set inspiratory pressure (0 to 72 cm H_2O) and time cycled at the end of the set inspiratory time interval (0.1 to 3.0 seconds). The inspiratory flow setting (1 to 30 L/min) determines inspiratory flow rate. The ventilator effectively becomes a flow controller if the pressure limit is set higher than the actual pressure reached during the inspiratory time interval. In this case, mandatory breaths are flow limited. With the flow sensor in line and functional, mandatory breaths are volume cycled to expiration if measured inspiratory volume reaches the set volume limit (5 to 300 ml). Alternately, the inspiratory phase is pressure cycled if airway pressure reaches the high-pressure alarm limit.

In the A/C mode all breaths are mandatory and are either time triggered at the set ventilator rate (1 to 150 breaths per minute) or flow triggered if the patient's spontaneous inspiratory effort is sufficient to meet the set trigger sensitivity criteria. The Bear Cub 750vs uses a double hot wire anemometer type sensor to measure flow rate bidirectionally at the patient airway. Assist (trigger) sensitivity is set in a range of 0.2 to 5.0 L/min. In SIMV/IMV, mandatory breaths are time or flow triggered at the set ventilator rate. Depressing the manual breath button triggers a single mandatory breath. Mandatory breaths can be manually triggered in all modes.

The set base flow rate (1 to 30 L/min) determines the rate of continuous gas flow available for

TABLE 17-1	CONTROL AND PHASE VARIABLES FOR MANDATORY AND SPONTANEOUS BREATHS IN THE OPERATIONAL MODES AVAILABLE ON THE BEAR CUB 750VS INFANT VENTILATOR							
	Mandatory				Spontaneous			
Mode	Control	Trigger*	Limit	Cycle	Control	Trigger	Limit	Cycle
SIMV/IMV	Pressure, flow†	Time, flow	Pressure, flow†	Time, volume,‡ pressure‡	—	—	—	—
A/C	Pressure, flow†	Time, flow	Pressure, flow†	Time, volume,‡ pressure‡	N/A	N/A	N/A	N/A
CPAP	—	—	—	—	—	—	—	—

Modified from Chatburn RL, Lough MD, Primiano FP Jr: Mechanical ventilation. In Chatburn RL, Lough MD, editors: *Handbook of respiratory care,* ed 2. St Louis. Mosby, 1990; pp 159-223.
SIMV, Synchronized intermittent mandatory ventilation; *IMV,* intermittent mandatory ventilation; *A/C,* assist/control; *CPAP,* continuous positive airway pressure; *N/A,* not applicable; —, ventilator does not respond.
*Mandatory breaths can be manually triggered in all modes.
†Applies if airway pressure does not reach the set pressure limit.
‡Secondary or safety cycle variable.

spontaneous breathing in the CPAP mode or between mandatory breaths in the SIMV/IMV mode. Baseline pressure is set in a range of 0 to 30 cm H_2O with the PEEP/CPAP control. The oxygen percentage control regulates the blender proportioning valve to produce oxygen concentrations in a range of 21% to 100%. The mechanical over pressure relief valve is an additional safety mechanism set to relieve circuit pressure in a range of 15 to 75 cm H_2O.

With the Bear Cub 750PSV, base gas flow and inspiratory gas flow rates are set separately. Pressure support breaths are patient (flow) triggered, pressure limited at the set pressure support level, and cycled to expiration when inspiratory flow falls to 10% of the peak flow rate. Alternately, inspiration is terminated if either a set volume or time limit is reached before the flow-cycling threshold. Flow cycling can also be applied to non-pressure support breaths in the A/C and SIMV modes.

Table 17-1 summarizes the control and phase variables for mandatory and spontaneous breaths in the operational modes available on the Bear Cub 750vs ventilator.

Output

Waveforms. If mandatory breaths are pressure controlled, the inspiratory pressure waveform can be nearly rectangular or exponential, depending on specific control settings. The resulting flow and volume waveforms are exponential. When used as a flow controller, the ventilator produces an approximately rectangular inspiratory flow waveform. In this case, the pressure and volume waveforms are shaped like an ascending ramp.

Monitoring. Airway pressure is measured at the patient Y-connector and displayed throughout the ventilatory cycle on the ventilator's analog manometer. Peak inspiratory pressure and mean airway pressure are derived from measurements made by an electronic proximal pressure transducer and are displayed digitally.

Expiratory tidal volume, expiratory minute volume, breath rate, and a patient-trigger indicator are derived from the flow measurements made by the flow sensor at the patient airway. The flow sensor has a range of 0.2 to 40 L/min. Tube leak is calculated as the difference between the inspiratory and expiratory tidal volume expressed as a percentage of inspiratory volume. The inspiratory time for both mandatory and spontaneous breaths, as well as expiratory time and I:E ratio for mandatory breaths, is also displayed.

The Bear Cub 750vs is equipped with both analog and digital connections. A Bear Graphics Display is an option.

Alarms

Input power alarms. The low gas supply alarm activates if either the air or oxygen pressure falls below 24 ± 2 psig. With the loss of one gas supply, the ventilator continues to operate using the remaining available gas supply. In the event of complete pneumatic power loss, a fail-to-cycle alarm activates and spontaneous breathing can be accomplished through the subambient valve if the patient generates an inspiratory pressure of approximately 3 cm H_2O. The ventilator's line power indicator changes from green to red if AC power is lost and the ventilator switches to battery power. If all electric power is lost, the indicator is extinguished. The low battery alarm signals that the internal battery has approximately 5 minutes of power remaining. A fully charged battery will power the ventilator for approximately 30 minutes.

Control circuit alarms. The fail to cycle alarm activates if the ventilator detects an internal or external malfunction. An incompatible settings alarm indicates an inappropriately set inspiratory pressure (relative to set PEEP), inspiratory time, flow rate, or volume limit. If the ventilator detects a flow sensor malfunction or disconnect, the flow sensor alarm activates and volume monitoring and patient-triggering functions are lost.

Output alarms. The Bear Cub 750vs is equipped with operator-adjustable alarms for low inspiratory pressure, high inspiratory pressure, low PEEP/CPAP, and high breath rate. The apnea alarm interval can be set at 5, 10, 20, or 30 seconds. The patient circuit and prolonged pressure alarms activate for conditions resulting in sustained increased pressure in the ventilator or patient circuit.

The Bear Cub 750vs is equipped with a remote nurse call connection to signal alarm conditions.

DRAGER BABYLOG 8000 PLUS INFANT VENTILATOR

The Drager Babylog 8000 Plus (Drager) (Fig. 17-5) is a pneumatically and electrically powered infant ventilator. The Babylog employs an electronic (microprocessor) and pneumatic control circuit to regulate a drive mechanism composed of pressure regulators, a bank of electromagnetic flow-control valves, and a pneumatic diaphragm exhalation valve. The ventilator can be used as a pressure or flow controller. Mandatory breaths are volume or time triggered, pressure or flow limited, and time cycled. Continuous flow is available for spontaneous breathing. Alternately, spontaneous breaths can be volume triggered, pressure limited, and flow cycled.[11]

Power Conversion and Transmission. The Babylog uses compressed air and oxygen in the range of 45 to 90 psig. Air and oxygen regulators reduce and match the source gas pressures and establish the constant pressure necessary for gas blending and flow regulation. The digital blender-flow control system is composed of two sets of 10 solenoid valves, one set each for air and oxygen flows. The size of the valve openings is graduated so that the opening size of each valve in a set is twice as large as that of the preceding valve. The total number and size combination of open valves determines flow rate to the patient. The proportion of open valves for air and oxygen deter-

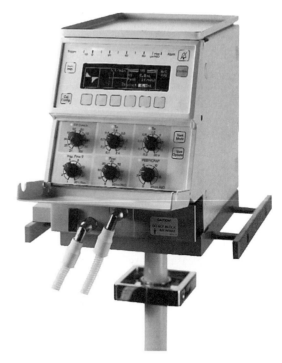

Fig. 17-5

Drager Babylog 8000 Plus Infant Ventilator. (Courtesy Drager, Telford, Penn.)

mines the oxygen concentration of inspired gas.[12] A continuous flow of gas passes a nonreturn valve, a pneumatic safety valve, an oxygen sensor, and the inspiratory pressure sensor before entering the inspiratory limb of the patient circuit.

Flow from the expiratory limb of the patient circuit is controlled by a pneumatic diaphragm exhalation valve. A solenoid-regulated PEEP-peak inspiratory pressure (PIP) control valve generates the inspiratory and expiratory control pressures applied to the exhalation valve to either direct gas flow to the patient or maintain baseline pressure. If the pressure in the patient circuit exceeds the pressure on the control side of the diaphragm, excess gas is vented out through the exhalation valve. An injector (Venturi) built into the exhalation valve block produces a negative pressure designed to prevent inadvertent PEEP in the patient circuit. Pressure is measured at the exhalation block by the expiratory pressure sensor.

Control. The Drager Babylog 8000 Plus can be operated in the following modes: IMV/continuous mandatory ventilation (CMV), SIMV, assist-control (A/C), and CPAP. A pressure support ventilation (PSV) mode and a volume guarantee (VG) option are also available.

Pressure-controlled mandatory breaths are pressure limited at the set inspiratory pressure limit (10 to 80 cm H_2O) and time cycled at the end of the set inspiratory time interval. The inspiratory flow rate is determined by the inspiratory flow setting (1 to 30 L/min). If airway pressure does not reach the set pressure limit, mandatory breaths are flow controlled and flow limited. Inspiration is pressure cycled before the end of set inspiratory time if the high inspiratory pressure alarm is activated.

In the IMV/CMV mode, mandatory breaths are time triggered at the set breath rate. The mandatory breath rate is determined as function of the inspiratory time (0.1 to 2 seconds) and expiratory time (0.2 to 30 seconds) settings and has a range of 2 to 150 breaths per minute. In the A/C and SIMV modes, a mandatory breath is volume triggered if the patient's measured inspiratory volume equals the set trigger volume (0.2 to 3 ml). Volume is derived from flow measured by a direction-sensitive hot-wire anemometer flow sensor integrated into the Y-connector of the patient circuit. The flow signal is leak compensated so as to decrease the potential for autotriggering. If a spontaneous breath is not detected in the A/C and SIMV modes, a mandatory breath is time triggered at the end of an interval determined by the set breath rate. Mandatory breaths can be triggered manually in all modes.

Spontaneous breathing between mandatory breaths and in the CPAP mode is passively supported by continuous flow. The rate of continuous flow available for spontaneous breathing may be set separately from the inspiratory flow rate for mandatory inspiration using the VIVE (variable inspiratory flow-variable expiratory flow) function. If this function is not used, the set inspiratory flow rate determines the continuous flow available for spontaneous breathing.

In the PSV mode, breaths are primarily patient triggered, pressure limited to the set inspiratory pressure level, and cycled to expiration when the inspiratory flow rate drops to 15% of the measured peak inspiratory flow rate. Alternately, inspiration is time cycled if inspiratory flow does not fall to the flow-cycling threshold before the end of the set inspiratory time interval. Patient triggering occurs if spontaneous inspiratory volume meets the set volume-triggering criteria. In the absence of spontaneous effort, pressure-limited breaths are time triggered at a "backup" rate dictated by the inspiratory and expiratory time settings; flow cycling remains in effect.

With the volume guarantee (VG) option, a target tidal volume (2 to 100 ml) is set. Based on the exhaled tidal volume measurements from previous breaths, the ventilator adjusts the inspiratory pressure limit breath to breath, as needed, to deliver the target tidal volume. Thus VG is volume targeted and pressure controlled. VG can be used in the A/C, SIMV, and PSV modes. VG does not affect the triggering and cycling criteria otherwise applicable in each mode.

Baseline pressure is set in a range of 0 to 25 cm H_2O with the PEEP-CPAP control. The inspired oxygen concentration is set between 21% and 100% with the oxygen concentration control. The optional nebulizer utilizes room air at a flow rate of 2 L/min, so actual FIO_2 will decrease for the duration of the nebulizer treatment.

Table 17-2 summarizes the control and phase variables for mandatory and spontaneous breaths in the operational modes available on the Babylog 8000 Plus.

Output

Waveforms. If mandatory breaths are pressure controlled, the inspiratory pressure waveform can be nearly rectangular or exponential, depending on specific control settings. The resultant volume and flow waveforms are exponential. Used as a flow controller, the ventilator produces an approximately rectangular inspiratory flow waveform. Pressure and volume waveforms are approximately ramp shaped.

Monitoring. The pressure or flow waveform is displayed in real time on the ventilator's monitoring screen. The sweep speed and scaling of waveforms are automatically adjusted.

Airway pressure is calculated from measurements made by the inspiratory and expiratory pressure sensors. The ventilator displays peak pressure, mean airway pressure, and baseline pressure (PEEP). Airway pressure is also continuously displayed on a bar graph.

Volume measurements include tidal volume, minute volume, and the fraction of minute volume contributed by spontaneous breathing. Endotracheal tube leakage is calculated from the difference between inspiratory and expiratory volumes. Displayed volumes are derived from flow measurements; and because of the position of the flow sensor just proximal to the endotracheal tube adapter, they are not affected by continuous flow or gas compressed in the patient circuit. The measurement range of the flow sensor is 0.2 to 30 L/min. Breathing frequency is also calculated from the flow signal.

The Babylog 8000 Plus calculates and displays the lung mechanics parameters of resistance, dynamic compliance, respiratory time constants, C20/C, and the rate-volume ratio (RVR). Inspired oxygen concentration is measured by the internal

TABLE 17-2	CONTROL AND PHASE VARIABLES FOR MANDATORY AND SPONTANEOUS BREATHS IN THE OPERATIONAL MODES AVAILABLE ON THE DRAGER BABYLOG 8000 PLUS INFANT VENTILATOR							
	Mandatory				**Spontaneous**			
Mode	**Control**	**Trigger***	**Limit**	**Cycle**	**Control**	**Trigger**	**Limit**	**Cycle**
IMV/CMV	Pressure, flow†	Time	Pressure, flow†	Time, pressure‡	—	—	—	—
A/C§	Pressure, flow†	Time, volume	Pressure, flow†	Time, pressure‡	N/A	N/A	N/A	N/A
SIMV§	Pressure, flow†	Time, volume	Pressure, flow†	Time, pressure‡	—	—	—	—
CPAP	—	—	—	—	—	—	—	—
PSV§	N/A	N/A	N/A	N/A	Pressure	Volume, time	Pressure	Flow, time,‡ pressure‡

Modified from Chatburn RL, Lough MD, Primiano FP Jr: Mechanical ventilation. In Chatburn RL, Lough MD, editors: *Handbook of respiratory care,* ed 2. St Louis. Mosby, 1990; pp 159-223.
IMV, Intermittent mandatory ventilation; *CMV,* continuous mandatory ventilation; *A/C,* assist/control; *SIMV,* synchronized intermittent mandatory ventilation; *CPAP,* continuous positive airway pressure; *PSV,* pressure support ventilation; *N/A,* not applicable; —, ventilator does not respond.
*Mandatory breaths can be manually triggered in all modes.
†Applies if airway pressure does not reach the set pressure limit.
‡Secondary or safety cycle variable.
§When the volume guarantee (VG) option is active, the ventilator varies the inspiratory pressure limit as needed to deliver a target tidal volume. Thus VG breaths are pressure controlled. VG does not alter the trigger and cycle variables otherwise in effect.

oxygen sensor near the ventilator's main flow outlet. A 24-hour trend of values for FIO_2, as well as minute volume, mean airway pressure, compliance, resistance, and RVR, is accessible.

The Babylog is equipped with analog and digital output connections.

Alarms. Ventilator alarms and alerts are grouped hierarchically as advisory, caution, and warning messages and are communicated in text on the ventilator's display screen. In addition, each grouping has a distinct audible signal intended to communicate an appropriate level of urgency. Alarm and alert messages are stored in the ventilator's "log," along with time of occurrence.

Input power alarms. A low air or low oxygen pressure alarm is activated if the respective gas pressure drops to less than 43.5 psig. The failure of one gas source causes the blender-flow control valves to be supplied with the remaining gas source. An electric power alarm occurs if operating voltages fall outside an acceptable range. If gas supply or electric power fails, ambient air can be drawn into the circuit via the nonreturn valve for spontaneous breathing.

Control circuit alarms. Failure of the microprocessor or associated components activates a ventilator malfunction alarm, which is accompanied by

a specific error code message. Advisory messages signal faults in the electronic circuitry for individual ventilator controls. Failure of the pressure or flow sensor is also identified. A failure of the flow sensor inactivates patient triggering, flow/volume monitoring and associated alarms, and the volume guarantee function.

Additionally, the ventilator alerts the operator to incompatible ventilator settings (i.e., mandatory breath rate exceeding 150 breaths per minute and inspiratory pressure set less than 5 cm H_2O above PEEP) or to settings that fall outside of "usual" ranges (i.e., inverse I:E ratio, inspiratory pressure greater than 40 cm H_2O, PEEP greater than 8 cm H_2O).

Output alarms. Alarm limits for high inspiratory pressure and for low and high baseline pressure are automatically set relative to the specific control settings. If excess pressure builds in the circuit, the ventilator responds by opening the exhalation valve. The safety valve vents pressure if other high-pressure safety mechanisms fail. Airway pressure measurements are also used to trigger alarms that signal circuit obstruction or a leak in the patient circuit. An alarm that indicates endotracheal tube obstruction is activated if the flow sensor does not detect gas movement during a complete mandatory breath cycle.

A high breath rate alarm limit and high and low thresholds for exhaled minute volume are operator selected. An apnea alarm condition occurs when no ventilation is detected (by the flow sensor) within the set apnea time interval. High and low oxygen concentration alarms are automatically set to $\pm 4\%$ of the selected oxygen concentration.

PURITAN-BENNETT INFANT STAR 500 VENTILATOR

The Infant Star 500 (Puritan-Bennett) (Fig. 17-6) is an electrically (AC or internal battery) and pneumatically powered, electronically (microprocessor) and pneumatically controlled infant-pediatric ventilator. Power conversion and transmission are accomplished by pressure regulators, an electromagnetic proportional manifold, and a pneumatic diaphragm exhalation valve. The Infant Star 500 can be used as a pressure or flow controller. Mandatory breaths are time triggered, pressure or flow limited, and time cycled. Mandatory breaths can also be patient triggered with the use of the Star Sync accessory. Continuous flow is available for spontaneous breathing. Additionally, spontaneous breaths can be pressure triggered, pressure limited, and pressure cycled.[13]

Power Conversion and Transmission. The Infant Star 500 utilizes compressed air and oxygen in a range or 35 to 90 psig. Pressure regulators reduce and match gas pressure to 38 psig for mixing in the oxygen blender. Blended gas is stored in a gas accumulator and is then further reduced in pressure to 18 psig by another pressure regulator before entering the flow-proportioning manifold.

The proportional manifold is a bank of six fixed-orifice solenoid valves that control gas flow to the patient circuit. Flow rate is a function of the 18 psig driving pressure and the opening sizes of the solenoid outlets. The flow output of each of the manifold solenoids ranges from 2 to 16 L/min. The control microprocessor opens individual valves or combinations of valves as needed to produce the required flow. Gas from the proportional manifold flows past a pressure transducer and pressure relief valve to the patient circuit.

Gas from the expiratory limb of the patient circuit is controlled by a pneumatic diaphragm exhalation valve. When the exhalation valve diaphragm is pressurized by gas from the IMV regulator, the valve closes and gas flow is directed to the patient. During the expiratory phase, the diaphragm is pressurized by gas from the PEEP regulator to maintain baseline pressure in the patient circuit. The microprocessor controls the selector valve that regulates which of the two pressures is applied to the diaphragm. A servo-regulated jet Venturi in the exhalation valve block creates a negative pressure designed to reduce

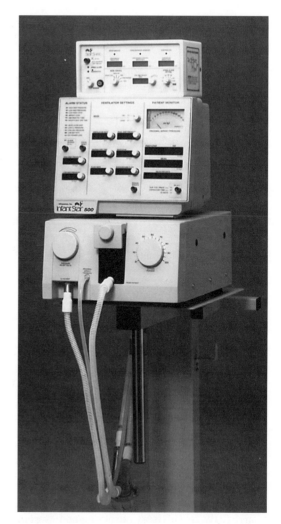

Fig. 17-6

Puritan-Bennett Infant Star 500 Ventilator. (Courtesy Puritan-Bennett, Pleasanton, Calif.)

resistance to expiratory gas flow and minimize inadvertent PEEP in the patient circuit.

Control. Two basic modes of operation are available on the Infant Star 500: CPAP and IMV. Additionally, A/C and SIMV are available if the Star Sync accessory is incorporated into the ventilator's control circuit.

In IMV, mandatory breaths are time triggered at an interval determined by the ventilator rate setting (0 to 150 breaths per minute). Initially, gas is delivered at the set flow rate (4 to 40 L/min); however, as proximal pressure approaches the set inspiratory pressure (5 to 90 cm H_2O), gas flow decreases as the microprocessor directs the proportional manifold to provide only the flow needed to maintain the set

TABLE 17-3	**CONTROL AND PHASE VARIABLES FOR MANDATORY AND SPONTANEOUS BREATHS IN THE OPERATIONAL MODES AVAILABLE ON THE PURITAN-BENNETT INFANT STAR 500 VENTILATOR**							
	Mandatory				**Spontaneous**			
Mode	**Control**	**Trigger***	**Limit**	**Cycle**	**Control**	**Trigger**	**Limit**	**Cycle**
IMV	Pressure, flow†	Time	Pressure, flow†	Time, pressure‡	Pressure§	Pressure§	Pressure§	Pressure§
CPAP	N/A	N/A	N/A	N/A	Pressure§	Pressure§	Pressure§	Pressure§
SIMV‖	Pressure, flow†	Time, pressure¶	Pressure, flow†	Time, pressure‡	Pressure§	Pressure§	Pressure§	Pressure§
A/C‖	Pressure, flow†	Time, pressure¶	Pressure, flow†	Time, pressure‡	N/A	N/A	N/A	N/A

Modified from Chatburn RL, Lough MD, Primiano FP Jr: Mechanical ventilation. In Chatburn RL, Lough MD, editors: *Handbook of respiratory care,* ed 2. St Louis, Mosby, 1990; pp 159-223.
IMV, Intermittent mandatory ventilation; *CPAP,* continuous positive airway pressure; *SIMV,* synchronized intermittent mandatory ventilation; *A/C,* assist/control; *N/A,* not applicable.
*Mandatory breaths can be manually triggered in all modes.
†Applies if airway pressure does not reach the set pressure limit.
‡Secondary or safety cycle variable.
§Applies only if demand flow is provided in addition to the available continuous flow.
¶Star Sync utilizes a small pressure-sensing balloon placed on the patient's abdomen to detect the movement accompanying a spontaneous breathing effort.
‖Available only if Star Sync accessory is in use.

pressure limit. The breath is time cycled at the end of the selected inspiratory time interval (0.1 to 3 seconds) or pressure cycled before inspiratory time elapses if the high inspiratory pressure alarm is activated. If the ventilator is set so that actual peak pressure does not reach the set pressure limit, the ventilator effectively becomes a flow controller and mandatory breaths are flow limited.

The background flow control setting (2 to 32 L/min) establishes the rate of continuous gas flow available for spontaneous breathing between mandatory breaths. Additionally, if proximal pressure drops 1 cm H_2O below set baseline, demand flow is provided as necessary to return pressure to baseline. Thus demand flow is pressure triggered, pressure limited, and pressure cycled.

Patient triggering of mandatory breaths (SIMV or A/C) can be accomplished by using the Star Sync accessory. Star Sync uses a small pressure-sensing balloon placed on the infant's abdomen to detect intraabdominal pressure changes caused by movement of the diaphragm. Star Sync interprets this pressure change as a spontaneous breathing effort and triggers the ventilator to inspiration. Trigger sensitivity is not adjustable. Star Sync also operates in a CPAP-backup mode.

Baseline pressure is set with the PEEP/CPAP control (0 to 24 cm H_2O). The oxygen percentage control determines the inspired oxygen concentration (21% to 100%) by adjusting the blender's proportioning valve for air and oxygen mixing.

A mechanical relief valve is set as a safety pressure limit in a range of 5 to 120 cm H_2O. The manual breath button permits the operator to manually trigger mandatory breaths in all modes.

Table 17-3 summarizes the control and phase variables for mandatory and spontaneous breaths in the Infant Star 500's operating modes.

Output

Waveforms. When the Infant Star 500 is used as a pressure controller, the inspiratory pressure waveform may approximate a rectangle or may be exponential, depending on the particular control settings. In either case, the volume waveform demonstrates an exponential rise and the flow waveform exhibits an exponential decay. Used as a flow controller, the Infant Star 500 produces an approximately rectangular inspiratory flow waveform. The resulting pressure and flow waveforms are ascending ramp shaped.

Monitoring. Airway pressure is measured by the proximal pressure transducer and digitally displayed as PEEP/CPAP, peak inspiratory pressure, and mean airway pressure. Airway pressure is also displayed on an analog meter. Duration of positive pressure is a measured value that approximates inspiratory time for mandatory breaths. Values for expiratory time and I:E ratio are calculated based on the inspiratory time and breath rate settings.

The Star Sync unit monitors and displays spontaneous breath rate, synchronous assisted (patient-triggered) breath rate, and controlled (time-triggered) breath rate.

The Infant Star 500 is equipped with analog and digital output connections.

Alarms

Input power alarms. Low air pressure and low oxygen pressure alarms are activated if air or oxygen supply pressures drop to less than 35 to 45 psig (depending on manufacturing date). If either air or oxygen gas pressure is lost, the ventilator maintains operation using the remaining available gas. In the event of a main electrical power loss, the external power loss alarm activates and the ventilator maintains operations using its rechargeable battery (for a minimum of 30 minutes at full charge). The low-battery alarm signals that 5 to 10 minutes of battery power remains before complete discharge.

Control circuit alarms. The ventilator inoperative alarm is activated in the event of microprocessor failure, exhalation valve failure, complete discharge of the internal battery, or other electronics failure. With this alarm condition, ventilator gas flow ceases and a vent valve opens to atmosphere to permit spontaneous breathing.

The insufficient expiratory time alarm indicates that the set inspiratory time and ventilator rate result in an insufficient expiratory time (0.2 to 0.3 second, depending on the set breath rate). In this case, the ventilator preserves the minimum expiratory time interval.

Additionally, the PIP display flashes if PIP is set less than 5 cm H_2O greater than the set PEEP/CPAP.

Output alarms. The ventilator is equipped with operator-adjustable alarms for high and low inspiratory pressure. The low PEEP/CPAP alarm is automatically set relative to the set baseline pressure. The purpose of the obstructed tube alarm is to detect excessive patient circuit pressure or conditions interfering with active exhalation. Specific alarm violations—labeled A01 through A05—are displayed in the ventilator's selected data window. The alarm signaling an airway leak is designed to detect leaks in the patient circuit that might otherwise be masked by high levels of gas flow triggered by the demand flow system. The Star Sync unit supplements ventilator alarms with an apnea alarm.

The Infant Star 500 is equipped with a remote alarm connection.

Sechrist IV-200 SAVI Infant Ventilator

The Sechrist IV-200 SAVI Ventilator (Sechrist Industries) (Fig. 17-7) is a pneumatically and electrically powered ventilator that employs pneumatic,

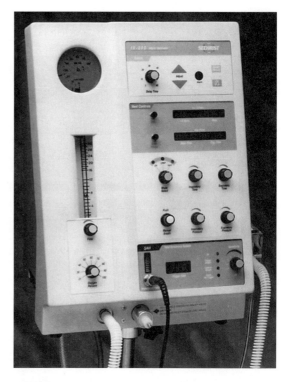

Fig. 17-7

Sechrist IV-200 SAVI Infant Ventilator. (Courtesy Sechrist Industries, Anaheim, Calif.)

electronic, and fluidic control of a pneumatic diaphragm exhalation valve. The IV-200 is a pressure or flow controller. Mandatory breaths are time triggered, pressure or flow limited, and time cycled. Inspiration may also be triggered and cycled by a thoracic impedance signal. Continuous flow is available for spontaneous breathing.[14]

Power Conversion and Transmission. Compressed air and oxygen at 50 psig supply an internal gas blender. The compressed air source also feeds the fluidic control circuit. The blender mixes air and oxygen to the desired concentration and a flow control needle valve regulates continuous gas flow to the patient circuit.

All gas flow from the expiratory limb of the patient circuit is controlled by a pneumatic diaphragm exhalation valve. A microprocessor-controlled solenoid valve regulates the backpressure that acts on the fluidic control circuit, determining which of two control pressures (inspiratory or baseline) is transmitted to the exhalation valve diaphragm. During the inspiratory phase, the inspiratory control pressure is applied to the diaphragm, closing the exhalation valve and directing gas flow to the patient. When pressure in the patient circuit reaches the control pressure, the exhalation valve vents excess gas flow to maintain the set pressure limit. With a switch from inspiratory to baseline control pressure, gas from the patient circuit flows out through the exhalation valve and pressure in the patient circuit is maintained at the baseline setting.

An injector jet in the exhalation block creates a slight negative pressure on the patient side of the exhalation valve, eliminating inadvertent PEEP caused by circuit resistance to continuous and expiratory gas flow.

Control. The Sechrist IV-200 can be operated in two modes: vent and CPAP. The vent mode can be used to provide either IMV or assist-control ventilation. Mandatory breaths are pressure or flow controlled.

When the ventilator is used to provide IMV, mandatory breaths are time triggered at a rate determined by the inspiratory time (0.10 to 2.9 seconds) and expiratory time (0.3 to 60 seconds) settings. Thus the ventilator has a breath rate range of 1 to 150 breaths per minute. The selected inspiratory and expiratory times, as well as the resulting breath rate and I:E ratio, are displayed digitally.

Mandatory breaths are pressure limited at the set inspiratory pressure (5 to 70 cm H_2O) and time cycled at the end of the selected inspiratory time interval. If set so that pressure in the patient circuit does not reach the set pressure limit, the ventilator functions as a flow controller and inspiration is flow limited. The proximal airway pressure waveform control is a needle valve that varies the response time of the exhalation valve. The waveform control can be set to produce a pressure waveform ranging from nearly rectangular to approximately sinusoidal.

The SAVI (Synchronized Assisted Ventilation of Infants) system uses the change in electrical impedance caused by chest movement during inspiration and expiration to patient trigger mandatory breaths. With SAVI, IMV becomes A/C ventilation. SAVI processes the impedance signal generated by a neonatal cardiorespiratory monitor. As the chest expands during inspiration, impedance increases. When the impedance value reaches the set sensitivity threshold, SAVI sends a trigger signal to the ventilator's microprocessor to initiate a machine-assisted inspiratory phase as described previously. Sensitivity is set using a nongraduated control with a range of minimum to maximum. Moving the sensitivity setting from minimum toward maximum increases the trigger sensitivity by decreasing the impedance value that SAVI must detect as the trigger value.

When SAVI is employed, the inspiratory phase is cycled to expiration by the impedance signal if the change in thoracic impedance indicates the onset of active expiration before the end of the set inspiratory time interval. If SAVI is switched off, or if the impedance signal is lost, the IV-200 reverts to IMV and breaths are time triggered, pressure limited, and time cycled according to the ventilator settings.

The continuous gas flow rate (0 to 32 L/min) is regulated using the blender flowmeter and determines the flow rate for mandatory inspiration as well as the continuous flow available for spontaneous breathing in both the vent and CPAP modes. Expiratory pressure (baseline pressure) can be set in an approximate range of –2 to 20 cm H_2O. A slightly negative baseline pressure is possible because of the action of the injector jet at the exhalation valve.

Mandatory breaths can be manually triggered in both operational modes. Inspiration is pressure limited and sustained for as long as the manual breath button is depressed. The manual breath control is independent of ventilator electronics; therefore manual breaths can be given as long as pneumatic power is available.

The oxygen concentration control on the Sechrist air-oxygen mixer is set between 21% and 100%. A spring-loaded safety pressure relief valve can be set in an approximate range of 15 to 85 cm H_2O.

Table 17-4 summarizes the control and phase variables for both mandatory and spontaneous breaths in the IV-200's operational modes.

Output

Waveforms. If the waveform control is set to produce a rectangular pressure waveform, the flow waveform exhibits an exponential decay and the volume waveform shows an exponential rise. A sinusoidal pressure waveform dictates that the volume and flow waveforms are also sinusoidal. If the ventilator functions as a flow controller, the inspiratory flow waveform is approximately rectangular and the pressure and volume waveforms are ascending ramp shaped.

Monitoring. An electronic pressure manometer on the ventilator provides a bar graph display of airway pressure that simulates the movement of a mechanical pressure gauge. Mean airway pressure is displayed digitally and is the average of the mean pressure of the last four machine-delivered breaths updated with each breath.

The SAVI unit displays information related to patient triggering. A bar graph provides a visual indicator of the changes in thoracic impedance over

TABLE 17-4	CONTROL AND PHASE VARIABLES FOR MANDATORY AND SPONTANEOUS BREATHS IN THE OPERATIONAL MODES AVAILABLE ON THE SECHRIST IV-200 SAVI VENTILATOR							
	Mandatory				Spontaneous			
Mode	Control	Trigger*	Limit	Cycle	Control	Trigger	Limit	Cycle
Vent-IMV	Pressure, flow†	Time	Pressure, flow†	Time	—	—	—	—
Vent-A/C‡	Pressure, flow†	Time, patient§	Pressure, flow†	Time, patient§	N/A	N/A	N/A	N/A
CPAP	—	—	—	—	—	—	—	—

Modified from Chatburn RL, Lough MD, Primiano FP Jr: Mechanical ventilation. In Chatburn RL, Lough MD, editors: *Handbook of respiratory care,* ed 2. St Louis. Mosby, 1990; pp 159-223.

IMV, Intermittent mandatory ventilation; *A/C,* assist/control; *CPAP,* continuous positive airway pressure; *N/A,* not applicable; —, ventilator does not respond.

*Mandatory breaths can be manually triggered in all modes. Inspiration extends for as long as the manual button is pressed.

†Applies if airway pressure does not reach the set limit.

‡Available only if the SAVI (synchronized assisted ventilation of infants) system is employed.

§With SAVI, mandatory breaths are patient triggered, and may be cycled to expiration, by the change in electrical impedance caused by chest movement during inspiration and expiration.

the inspiratory/expiratory cycle. A trigger breath indicator flashes with every patient-triggered breath and the patient trigger rate is digitally displayed.

Alarms

Input power alarms. No specific ventilator alarms signal the failure of either electric or pneumatic power. However, the Sechrist air-oxygen mixer is equipped with a low inlet pressure alarm. An inlet pressure differential of more than 23 psig triggers an audible pneumatic alarm. This condition also causes a proportioning system bypass so that the gas of the higher pressure supplies the patient circuit.

Control circuit alarms. If set inspiratory time exceeds expiratory time, the ventilator's inverse I:E light illuminates. With the SAVI system on, the control breath indicator flashes with every time-triggered (non–patient-triggered) breath. Persistent failure to detect a patient trigger (impedance signal) results in a progression from an alert to an alarm condition. If SAVI cannot detect an impedance signal, the ventilator reverts to IMV.

Output alarms. High and low airway pressure alarms are incorporated into the electronic pressure manometer. Limits for the pressure alarm are operator adjustable. The low pressure alarm is activated in response to a number of conditions, including circuit leaks (low airway pressure), circuit disconnection (loss of pressure), microprocessor failure (failure to trigger or cycle a breath), electric or pneumatic power loss, and prolonged inspiration.

The Sechrist Model 600 airway pressure monitor is an accessory that can be used with the IV-200

to enhance monitoring and alarm capabilities. The monitor can also be equipped with a vent to ambient pressure feature that vents patient circuit pressure to near ambient pressure if an overpressure condition is detected. Importantly, the reset button should not be pressed before the cause of an overpressure condition is resolved because resetting the system allows pressure to be generated in the patient circuit.

V.I.P. BIRD INFANT-PEDIATRIC VENTILATOR

The V.I.P. Bird (Viasys Healthcare, Bird Products) (Fig. 17-8) is electrically and pneumatically powered and electronically (microprocessor) controlled. Power conversion and transmission are accomplished with a pressure regulator, an electromagnetic proportional flow-control valve, and an electromagnetic exhalation valve. The V.I.P. functions as a pressure or flow controller. Mandatory breaths are time, pressure, or flow triggered; flow or pressure limited; and time cycled. Continuous flow is available for spontaneous breathing, or spontaneous breaths may be pressure triggered, pressure limited, and pressure or flow cycled.[15-17] An enhanced version of the V.I.P., the V.I.P. Bird Gold, has been introduced.

Power Conversion and Transmission. The V.I.P. Bird uses compressed air and oxygen in a range of 40 to 75 psig. At the oxygen blender, air and oxygen pressures are equalized and the gases mixed. Blended gas is directed past a 100 psig relief valve to the gas accumulator. This reservoir stores gas during the expiratory phase, increasing the ventilator's flow delivery capability to up to 120 L/min.

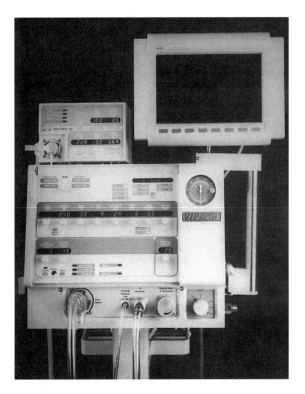

Fig. 17-8

V.I.P. Bird Infant-Pediatric Ventilator. (Courtesy Bird Products, Palm Springs, Calif.)

A pneumatic regulator establishes a consistent system pressure so that gas is supplied to the flow-control valve at 25 psig.

The flow-control valve is an electromechanical proportioning device that converts the rotary motion of an electric step motor driver to the linear motion of a plunger to regulate the size of the valve opening. Flow rates to the patient are a function of the system driving pressure and the size of the valve opening. With a system pressure of 25 psig, gas flow rates are essentially unaffected by downstream (patient circuit) pressures up to 5 psig (350 cm H_2O). From the flow-control valve, gas enters the patient circuit.

Gas flow from the expiratory limb of the patient circuit is regulated by an electromagnetic exhalation valve. The exhalation valve uses a linear motor and plunger to control the valve opening. The microprocessor regulates the exhalation valve plunger to direct inspiratory gas flow to the patient, to permit exhalation, and to maintain the set baseline pressure in the patient circuit during the expiratory phase. A jet Venturi in the exhalation manifold is used to help overcome inadvertent PEEP caused by continuous gas flow through the expiratory limb of the patient circuit.

Control The V.I.P. Bird can be operated in the following modes: volume-cycled (S)IMV/CPAP, volume-cycled A/C, time-cycled (S)IMV/CPAP, and time-cycled A/C. In addition, pressure support can be used to augment spontaneous breaths in the volume-cycled (S)IMV/CPAP mode. The V.I.P. Gold includes a pressure control mode and volume-assured pressure support (VAPS) in both A/C and SIMV/CPAP.

In the volume-cycled A/C and (S)IMV/CPAP modes, mandatory breaths are volume preset. To deliver a volume preset breath, the microprocessor moves the flow-control valve driver in the predetermined sequence necessary to deliver the selected tidal volume (20 to 995 ml) at the set flow rate (3 to 100 ml/min). Inspiration is terminated at the end of the time interval necessary to complete the predetermined flow-control valve sequence. Therefore mandatory breaths are, in essence, flow controlled, flow limited, and time cycled. Alternately, inspiration is pressure cycled if airway pressure reaches the value set on the high airway pressure alarm.

In the volume-cycled A/C and (S)IMV/CPAP modes, mandatory breaths are pressure triggered if patient effort drops airway pressure by an amount equal to the set assist sensitivity (off, 1 to 20 cm H_2O) or time triggered at the end of an interval dictated by the breath rate control setting (0 to 150 breaths per minute). In the A/C mode, all breaths are mandatory. In the (S)IMV/CPAP mode, the spontaneous breathing permitted between mandatory breaths is supported by demand flow if patient effort drops airway pressure by an amount equal to the assist sensitivity setting. CPAP with demand flow is implemented by turning the set breath rate to zero in the volume-cycled (S)IMV/CPAP mode.

Pressure support of 1 to 50 cm H_2O can be set in the volume-cycled (S)IMV/CPAP mode. A pressure support breath is pressure (i.e., patient) triggered as described earlier, pressure limited to the selected pressure support level set above PEEP, and cycled to expiration when gas flow from the inspiratory control valve drops to a predetermined percentage of the delivered peak inspiratory flow rate. The ventilator chooses the exact flow-cycling criteria (5% to 25% of peak flow) based on the delivered tidal volume. If inspiratory flow fails to fall to the predetermined flow-cycling threshold, inspiration is time cycled at the end of the set inspiratory time interval.

In the time-cycled (S)IMV/CPAP and A/C modes, the V.I.P. functions as a pressure controller and incorporates the flow sensor of the Partner volume monitor into the ventilator's control scheme. The Partner flow sensor is of the differential pressure type and is designed to be placed at the patient airway with size 4.5 or smaller endotracheal tubes. The inspiratory flow signal is used to trigger patient-initiated breaths and may be used to flow-cycle inspiration as described later.

In the time-cycled modes, mandatory breaths are either time triggered at an interval determined by the breath rate setting or flow triggered if the infant's spontaneous inspiratory flow rate is sufficient to meet the set triggering sensitivity (0.2 to 5 L/min). Inspiration is pressure limited at the set high-pressure limit (3 to 80 cm H_2O) and time cycled at the end of the set inspiratory time interval (0.1 to 3.0 seconds). Alternately, flow can be chosen as the cycling variable by setting the termination sensitivity percentage (5% to 25%, in 5% increments). In this case, breaths are pressure limited and cycled to expiration when the measured inspiratory flow rate falls to the percentage of peak flow set using the termination sensitivity. Inspiration is time cycled if the inspiratory flow rate does not fall to the set flow-cycling threshold before the end of set inspiratory time. When the time-cycled assist control mode is selected and ventilator controls are set so that inspiration is flow triggered and flow cycled, breath delivery becomes the functional equivalent of pressure support.

In the time-cycled (S)IMV/CPAP mode, the flow control setting (3 to 40 L/min) determines the inspiratory flow rate for mandatory breaths, as well as the rate of continuous flow available for spontaneous breathing (to a maximum of 15 L/min) between mandatory breaths. Additionally, demand flow is triggered if patient effort drops airway pressure 1 cm H_2O below set baseline and is provided as necessary to return pressure to baseline. Thus demand flow is pressure triggered, pressure limited, and pressure cycled. In the time cycled (S)IMV/CPAP mode, CPAP with continuous flow is implemented by turning the breath rate setting to zero.

Baseline pressure is set in a range of 0 to 24 cm H_2O with the PEEP/CPAP control. The oxygen percentage control regulates the proportioning valve in the gas blender to provide the desired oxygen concentration (21% to 100%). The overpressure relief control regulates a mechanical relief valve that acts as a safety limit for pressure in the patient circuit. The manual soft key permits mandatory breaths to be manually triggered in all modes. These breaths are pressure or flow controlled depending on the selected operational mode and specific control settings.

The VIP Gold offers flow triggering in all modes, a choice of square or decelerating inspiratory flow waveform in volume control modes, adjustable rise

time, and pressure support of spontaneous breaths in SIMV for all breath types. In the volume-assured pressure support (VAPS) modes, inspiration is initially pressure limited with variable decelerating gas flow. If necessary, the ventilator transitions to flow-limited inspiration at a constant flow rate to meet a target tidal volume. Thus VAPS is pressure or pressure and flow controlled and flow or volume cycled.

Table 17-5 provides a summary of the control and phase variables for mandatory and spontaneous breaths in the operational modes available on the V.I.P. Bird Ventilator.

Output

Waveforms. When the V.I.P. is used as a pressure controller, the inspiratory pressure waveform for mandatory breaths may approach a rectangular shape or may be exponential, depending on the specific control settings. The resulting volume and flow waveforms are exponential. Used as a flow controller, the ventilator produces an essentially rectangular inspiratory flow waveform; pressure and volume waveforms are ascending ramp shaped.

Monitoring. A monitoring window digitally displays values for PIP, mean airway pressure, breath rate, inspiratory time, and I:E ratio. A scan function allows each parameter to be displayed in sequence.

PIP and mean airway pressure values reflect pressure at the patient Y-connector measured by the proximal pressure transducer. PIP for all positive pressure breaths is displayed. Proximal airway pressure is also displayed on a mechanical pressure gauge. The displayed breath rate is the average number of breaths per minute and includes all mandatory breaths plus spontaneous breaths detected by the ventilator.

The microprocessor-based Partner volume monitor displays inspiratory tidal volume, expiratory tidal volume, minute volume, breath rate, and real-time inspiratory and expiratory flow rate. All values are derived from flow measured by the flow sensor placed at the patient airway.

With the V.I.P. Gold, both inspiratory and expiratory hold maneuvers can be performed in its volume-targeted modes.

Alarms

Input power alarms. The low inlet gas alarm activates when system pressure falls to less than 22.5 psig or rises to more than 27.5 psig. If pressure drops to less than 20 psig or rises to greater than 30 psig for more than 1 second, a ventilator-inoperative condition results. The air-oxygen blender has a separate pneumatic input alarm. If the

TABLE 17-5 **Control and Phase Variables for Mandatory and Spontaneous Breaths in the Operational Modes Available on the V.I.P. Bird Infant-Pediatric Ventilator**

Mode	Mandatory				Spontaneous			
	Control	Trigger*	Limit	Cycle	Control	Trigger	Limit	Cycle
Volume-cycled SIMV	Flow	Time, pressure	Flow	Time, pressure‡	Pressure	Pressure	Pressure	Pressure
Volume-cycled A/C	Flow	Time, pressure	Flow	Time, pressure‡	N/A	N/A	N/A	N/A
Time-cycled SIMV	Pressure, flow†	Time, flow	Pressure, flow†	Time, flow,¶ pressure‡	Pressure§	Pressure§	Pressure§	Pressure§
Time-cycled A/C	Pressure, flow†	Time, flow	Pressure, flow†	Time, flow,¶ pressure‡	N/A	N/A	N/A	N/A
Pressure support‖	N/A	N/A	N/A	N/A	Pressure	Pressure	Pressure	Flow, time,‡ pressure‡
CPAP (demand flow)	N/A	N/A	N/A	N/A	Pressure	Pressure	Pressure	Pressure
CPAP (continuous flow)	N/A	N/A	N/A	N/A	Pressure§	Pressure§	Pressure§	Pressure§

Modified from Chatburn RL, Lough MD, Primiano FP Jr: Mechanical ventilation. In Chatburn RL, Lough MD, editors: *Handbook of respiratory care*, ed 2. St Louis. Mosby, 1990; pp 159-223.
SIMV, Synchronized intermittent mandatory ventilation; *A/C,* assist-control; *CPAP,* continuous positive airway pressure; *N/A,* not applicable.
*Mandatory breaths can be manually triggered in all modes.
†Applies if airway pressure does not reach the set pressure limit within the set inspiratory time interval.
‡Secondary or safety cycle variable.
§Applies only if demand flow is provided in addition to the available continuous flow.
¶Applies if ventilator is set to flow cycle using termination sensitivity.
‖Considered here as separate mode, but can be used to support spontaneous breaths in the volume-cycled SIMV mode.

pressure differential between the two gas sources exceeds 20 psig, the gas with the higher pressure is used by the ventilator and the resulting oxygen concentration will be either 100% or 21%. Loss of electric power activates the ventilator-inoperative alarm.

Control circuit alarms. If a failure of the microprocessor or related components is detected by the ventilator's ongoing self-diagnostics, the ventilator-inoperative alarm is activated and a specific error code may be displayed.

Incompatible ventilator settings are signaled by the slow flashing of the digital displays of the parameters primarily involved in creating the incompatibility. These include tidal volume, breath rate, inspiratory time, and peak flow. In addition, the ventilator limits the values of incompatible settings in an attempt to preserve a "safe" or "acceptable" ventilatory pattern. If the set inspiratory time for a mandatory breath exceeds expiratory time (inverse I:E ratio), an alert is signaled visually.

Output alarms. In the volume-cycled A/C and (S)IMV/CPAP modes, the pressure-limit setting becomes the high airway pressure alarm setting. In the time-cycled A/C and (S)IMV/CPAP modes, the high prolonged pressure alarm is automatically set to activate if proximal pressure exceeds the high-pressure limit plus 10 cm H_2O. The high prolonged pressure alarm also acts as a high-PEEP alarm in all modes. The low peak pressure and low PEEP/

CPAP alarms have operator-selected alarm thresholds. The circuit fault alarm is activated if unacceptable pressure differentials occur among the ventilator's various pressure transducers and may signal a problem in the patient circuit or a pressure transducer fault.

The apnea alarm is activated if the interval between detected breaths exceeds the time interval of the alarm setting. The ventilator's apnea alarm is not active in modes utilizing continuous flow. The apnea interval select switch is an internal ventilator control that can be set to 20, 40, or 60 seconds. The Partner volume monitor is equipped with additional operator-adjustable alarms for apnea, low minute volume, and high breath rate.

DRAGER EVITA 4 VENTILATOR

The Drager Evita 4 (Drager) (Fig. 17-9) is a pneumatically and electrically powered, electronically (microprocessor) and pneumatically controlled ventilator designed for adult and pediatric use. An option for extending use to the neonatal range is also available. Power conversion and transmission are accomplished by pressure regulators, dual electromagnetic proportional flow control valves, and a pneumatic exhalation valve. The Evita 4 is a flow or pressure controller. Mandatory breaths are time or flow triggered; flow, volume, or pressure limited; and time cycled. Spontaneous breaths are flow or pressure triggered, pressure limited, and flow or pressure cycled.[18,19]

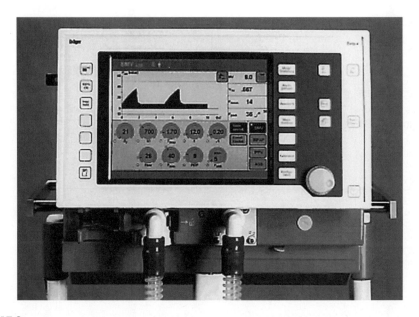

Fig. 17-9

Drager Evita 4 Ventilator. (Courtesy Drager, Telford, Penn.)

Power Conversion and Transmission. The Drager Evita 4 utilizes compressed air and oxygen in a range of 43.5 to 87 psig. The gases are regulated down to a pressure of about 29 psig before entering parallel air/oxygen electromagnetic proportional flow control valves. Each valve is composed of a linear motor and driver that regulates the size of the valve opening. A microprocessor controls the position of the motor and driver of both valves to proportion the gases to the set oxygen concentration and to provide the required inspiratory gas flow. The inspiratory gas flow rate is calculated by the microprocessor from the gas pressure and the size of the inspiratory valve opening as determined by the position of the valve driver. Blended gas flows past the oxygen sensor and the inspiratory pressure transducer before entering the patient circuit.

Gas from the expiratory limb of the patient circuit is controlled by a pneumatic exhalation valve. The PEEP/PIP solenoid valve generates a control pressure that is applied to the exhalation valve diaphragm. During the inspiratory phase of a mandatory breath, the inspiratory control pressure is applied, closing the exhalation valve. During pressure-controlled ventilation, this "floating" exhalation valve opens and closes as needed to maintain the target pressure limit and to accommodate the patient's spontaneous breathing activity. Excess gas flow is vented through the valve to atmosphere. With the onset of the expiratory phase, control pressure to the exhalation diaphragm switches to the PEEP setting. The exhalation valve diaphragm moves away from the valve opening, allowing exhalation to occur, and circuit pressure drops to baseline. The expiratory pressure sensor monitors pressure at the exhalation valve. The expiratory flow sensor measures expiratory gas flow.

Control. The Evita 4 can be operated in the following ventilation modes: CMV, SIMV, mandatory minute ventilation (MMV), pressure control ventilation (PCV+), airway pressure release ventilation (APRV), and CPAP. Pressure support can be used to augment spontaneous breaths in the SIMV, PCV+, MMV, and CPAP modes. The AutoFlow and pressure-limited ventilation (PLV) extensions can be used to modify mandatory breaths in the CMV, SIMV, and MMV modes. Additionally, an apnea ventilation mode is available. Selection of the adult or pediatric patient range determines the range of available tidal volume, set inspiratory flow rate, and maximum inspiratory flow availability (adult: 180 L/min; pediatric: 60 L/min). The ventilator can be configured to choose default ventilation control settings based on the entered ideal patient body weight.

NeoFlow is an available option that extends the patient range of the Evita 4 to infants and neonates as small as 0.5 kg. NeoFlow utilizes a hot wire anemometer-type flow sensor located at the patient Y-connector. The flow sensor provides the signal for patient triggering as well as flow and volume monitoring. These flow and volume measurements are compensated for gas leakage around the endotracheal tube. When NeoFlow is used in the CMV, SIMV, and MMV modes, AutoFlow is always active. With NeoFlow, the Evita 4 provides a base gas flow of 6 L/min through the patient circuit and an inspiratory gas flow rate of up to 30 L/min.

The "basic" mandatory breath in the CMV, SIMV, and MMV modes is flow controlled and requires setting tidal volume (adult: 100 to 2000 ml, pediatric: 20 to 300 ml, neonatal: 3 to 100 ml), breath rate of 0 to 100 breaths per minute (0 to 150 breaths per minute with NeoFlow), inspiratory flow rate (adult: 6 to 120 L/min, pediatric/neonatal: 6 to 30 L/min), and inspiratory time (0.1 to 10 seconds). During inspiration, gas is delivered at the set flow rate (flow limit) for the duration of time necessary to deliver the set tidal volume; the inspiratory phase is time cycled at the end of the set inspiratory time interval. If the tidal volume is delivered before the end of set inspiratory time, inspiratory flow ceases and an inspiratory pause occurs for the remainder of the inspiratory time interval. Depending on the duration of the inspiratory pause, inspiratory pressure may plateau.

If the PLV option is used, a maximum pressure (P_{max}) is set. The mandatory breath is initially delivered at the set flow rate, as described earlier. However, if peak inspiratory pressure reaches the set P_{max}, the ventilator effectively becomes a pressure controller, limiting inspiratory pressure to the set P_{max}. In this case, the inspiratory gas flow rate does not remain constant. If the measured inspiratory volume reaches the set tidal volume before the end of the set inspiratory time interval, inspiratory gas flow ceases and volume is held (limited) until the end of the inspiratory phase. If inspiratory gas flow does not reach zero before the end of set inspiratory time, the set tidal volume will not be delivered.

If the AutoFlow function is used, the ventilator acts as a pressure controller. Set tidal volume becomes a target tidal volume. Based on the measured tidal volume and inspiratory pressure of previously delivered mandatory breaths, the ventilator incrementally adjusts the pressure limit for subsequent breaths to maintain the target tidal volume. Thus inspiration is pressure limited at the pressure that the ventilator calculates is necessary to deliver the target tidal volume and time cycled at the end of set inspiratory time. Alternately, the inspiratory phase is volume cycled before the end of the set inspiratory time interval if measured volume reaches the set high inspired tidal volume alarm setting. With AutoFlow, the ventilator coordinates the action of the inspiratory flow control valves and exhalation valve to accommodate spontaneous breathing at any point during both the inspiratory and expiratory phases.

In the CMV mode, all breaths are mandatory. These breaths are either time triggered at an interval determined by the set breath rate or flow triggered if a patient's spontaneous inspiratory flow rate meets the set flow trigger sensitivity (1 to 15 L/min; 0.3 to 15 L/min with NeoFlow). In SIMV, mandatory breaths are time or flow triggered at the set SIMV breath rate. Spontaneous breaths between mandatory breaths are supported with demand flow. Demand flow is triggered when circuit pressure falls 0.2 cm H_2O below set PEEP and is provided, as needed, to maintain the PEEP setting. In the CPAP mode, all breaths are spontaneous and are supported by demand flow. Spontaneous breaths in the CPAP and SIMV modes may also be pressure-supported as described later.

The MMV mode provides mandatory breaths only to the extent that spontaneous minute volume does not meet the preselected minimum minute ventilation. Minimum minute volume is a product of the breath rate and tidal volume settings. If exhaled minute volume drops below minimum, mandatory breaths are time or flow triggered, as needed, to maintain the target minute volume. In MMV, spontaneous breaths may be pressure supported or simply supported with demand flow.

In the PCV+ mode, mandatory breaths are time or flow triggered at the set breath rate, pressure limited at the set inspiratory pressure level, and time cycled at the end of the set inspiratory time interval. As with AutoFlow, spontaneous breathing is permitted at any point during either the inspiratory or expiratory phase. Pressure support can be set to augment spontaneous breaths that occur between mandatory breaths.

Pressure support ventilation (PSV) must be patient triggered. With PSV, patient triggering occurs if the spontaneous inspiratory flow rate reaches the set flow-trigger sensitivity or if inspired volume exceeds 25 ml (12 ml in the pediatric mode; 1 ml with NeoFlow). PSV is pressure limited to the set pressure support level (0 to 80 cm H_2O) and cycled to expiration when inspiratory flow falls to a percentage of peak flow determined by the patient range selection. The flow cycling threshold is 25% of peak inspiratory flow in the adult mode, 6% of peak flow in the pediatric mode, and 15% of peak flow in the neonatal mode. Alternately, inspiration is time cycled if inspiratory flow does not fall to the flow-

cycling threshold within 4 seconds (1.5 seconds in the pediatric mode; at the end of the set inspiratory time interval with NeoFlow).

Airway pressure release ventilation (APRV) permits spontaneous breathing at two levels of positive airway pressure. The magnitude, as well as the duration, of the high and low levels of positive pressure is set separately. Typically, the patient breathes spontaneously at the higher pressure with only brief periods of release to the lower pressure level.

The pressure rise time setting determines the rate of increase in airway pressure from baseline (at the onset of inspiration) to the set pressure limit for all pressure-controlled breaths. Rise time is set in a range of 0 to 2 seconds and influences the ventilator's initial inspiratory gas flow rate. With rise time set to zero, the ventilator seeks to reach target pressure almost immediately, requiring a relatively high initial inspiratory flow rate. Increasing rise time causes peak pressure to be reached later in the inspiratory phase. For example, setting rise time to 0.5 second directs the ventilator to reach the target inspiratory pressure 0.5 second from the onset of inspiration. Increasing rise time effectively reduces the peak inspiratory flow rate delivered during inspiration. Rise time can be used to modify mandatory breaths in the PCV+ mode, AutoFlow mandatory breaths in all modes, and PSV breaths. Additionally, rise time determines how quickly the high pressure level is reached during APRV.

Baseline pressure is set in a range of 0 to 35 cm H_2O using the PEEP/CPAP control. Activation of the intermittent PEEP function provides increased end-expiratory pressure ("expiratory sighs") for two mandatory breaths every 3 minutes in the CMV mode. Oxygen concentration is set in a range of 21% to 100%. Oxygen concentration can be temporarily increased above what is set by pressing the suction O_2 key. Activation of the "neb" control key supplies gas flow to a micronebulizer for up to 30 minutes. Pressing and holding the inspiratory hold button creates an inspiratory pause for up to 15 seconds. Apnea ventilation provides mandatory ventilation at predetermined settings if the ventilator detects apnea.

Table 17-6 summarizes the control and phase variables for mandatory and spontaneous breaths in the operational modes available on the Drager Evita 4 Ventilator.

Output

Waveforms. To deliver volume-preset, flow-controlled breaths, the Evita 4 utilizes a constant inspiratory flow rate that produces an approximately rectangular inspiratory flow waveform. The resulting pressure and volume waveforms are an ascending

TABLE 17-6 CONTROL AND PHASE VARIABLES FOR MANDATORY AND SPONTANEOUS BREATHS IN THE OPERATIONAL MODES AVAILABLE ON THE DRÄGER EVITA 4 VENTILATOR

Mode	Mandatory				Spontaneous			
	Control‖	Trigger*	Limit	Cycle	Control‖	Trigger	Limit	Cycle
CMV	Flow, pressure†	Time, flow	Flow, volume, pressure†	Time, volume,‡ pressure‡	N/A	N/A	N/A	N/A
CMV-AutoFlow	Pressure	Time, flow	Pressure	Time, volume,‡ pressure‡	N/A	N/A	N/A	N/A
SIMV	Flow, pressure†	Time, flow	Flow, volume, pressure†	Time, volume,‡ pressure‡	Pressure	Pressure	Pressure	Pressure
SIMV-AutoFlow	Pressure	Time, flow	Pressure	Time, volume,‡ pressure‡	Pressure	Pressure	Pressure	Pressure
MMV	Flow, pressure†	Time, flow	Flow, volume, pressure†	Time, volume,‡ pressure‡	Pressure	Pressure	Pressure	Pressure
MMV-AutoFlow	Pressure	Time, flow	Pressure	Time, volume,‡ pressure‡	Pressure	Pressure	Pressure	Pressure
PCV+	Pressure	Time, flow	Pressure	Time, pressure‡	Pressure	Pressure	Pressure	Pressure
CPAP	N/A	N/A	N/A	N/A	Pressure	Pressure	Pressure	Pressure
PS§	N/A	N/A	N/A	N/A	Pressure	Flow	Pressure	Flow, time,‡ pressure‡
APRV	Pressure	Time	Pressure	Time	Pressure	Pressure	Pressure	Pressure

Modified from Chatburn RL, Lough MD, Primiano FP Jr: Mechanical ventilation. In Chatburn RL, Lough MD, editors: *Handbook of respiratory care*, ed 2. St Louis. Mosby, 1990; pp 159-223.

CMV, Continuous mandatory ventilation; *N/A*, not applicable; *SIMV*, synchronized intermittent mandatory ventilation; *MMV*, mandatory minute ventilation; *CPAP*, continuous positive airway pressure; *PS*, pressure support; *PCV+*, pressure-controlled ventilation; *APRV*, airway pressure release ventilation.

*Mandatory breaths can be manually triggered.

†Applies if the pressure-limited ventilation (PLV) function is used.

‡Secondary or safety cycle variable.

§Considered here as a separate mode, but can be used to support spontaneous breaths in the SIMV, MMV, PCV+, and CPAP modes.

‖The Rise Time setting can be used to modify the shape of the inspiratory pressure waveform for all mandatory pressure-controlled breaths and pressure-supported spontaneous breaths.

ramp shape. If set volume is delivered before the end of set inspiratory time, both the pressure and volume waveforms tend to form a plateau from the point that inspiratory gas flow stops. If circuit pressure reaches the set P_{max} (added using the PLV function), the flow waveform exhibits an exponential decay beginning at the point that the pressure limit is reached. The pressure waveform, which is initially ramp-shaped, forms a plateau.

The inspiratory pressure waveform for pressure-controlled mandatory breaths (PCV+ and Auto-Flow) is greatly influenced by the pressure rise time setting. If rise time is set to 0, the pressure waveform is essentially rectangular. The addition of rise time creates a ramp up to the pressure plateau. The ramp becomes less steep as rise time is increased. With pressure control, the resulting inspiratory flow waveform exhibits an exponential decay and the volume waveform shows an exponential rise. As rise time is added, the magnitude of the inspiratory flow waveform decreases (reflecting a decrease in peak flow rate).

Monitoring. The Evita 4 monitoring screen can be operator configured to display different combinations of numeric and graphic data. Values for peak pressure, mean airway pressure, plateau pressure, and PEEP are displayed numerically on the ventilator's monitoring screen. Exhaled tidal volume and minute ventilation are derived from measurements made by the ventilator's hot wire anemometer-type expiratory flow sensor. However, these measurements are corrected to eliminate the effects of gas compressed in the patient circuit and thus reflect effective volume delivery. When the NeoFlow option is utilized, monitored flow and volume values reflect measurements made at the patient airway (Y-connector). Breath rate includes both mandatory and spontaneous breaths.

The Evita 4 has the ability to calculate and display a number of pulmonary mechanics measures, including compliance, resistance, intrinsic (auto) PEEP, the volume of trapped gas, and occlusion pressure ($P = 0.1$ maneuver). The ventilator integrates data from its mainstream end-tidal carbon dioxide and flow sensors to yield volumetric CO_2-related values for CO_2 production (Vco_2), dead space, and dead space to tidal volume ratio. Graphics monitoring includes waveforms for pressure, flow, volume, and exhaled CO_2 as well as flow-volume and pressure-volume loops. O_2 concentration is measured by a sensor located near the inspiratory flow control valve. Values for most of the just-listed monitored values are stored and may be displayed as trends.

Analog and digital output connections are available.

Alarms. Alarms and alerts on the Evita 4 are prioritized and identified by differing audible and visual signals and text messages to indicate the specific level of urgency.

Input power alarms. A low air or oxygen supply pressure alarm is activated if the respective gas pressure falls below 43.5 psig. A high gas supply pressure alarm occurs if either gas pressure exceeds 87 psig. Loss of either supply gas will cause an automatic switchover to the remaining supply gas. A failure-to-cycle alarm activates if no gas flow is delivered by the ventilator.

Control circuit alarms. A number of alarm messages signify problems with the ventilator's control components. These include failure of the flow sensor, malfunction of the gas blender, loss of the expiratory pressure measurement, and malfunction of the exhalation valve.

Output alarms. Output alarms include an operator-adjustable high airway pressure alarm and a low airway pressure alarm that is automatically set 5 cm H_2O above the PEEP setting. A high PEEP alarm activates owing to a sustained increase in circuit pressure. Alarm limits for high tidal volume, high and low minute volume, apnea, and high spontaneous breath rate are operator adjustable. The low-volume alarm indicates that the delivered inspiratory tidal volume did not reach set tidal volume. Alarm limits for high and low oxygen concentration are automatically set relative to the selected oxygen concentration. High and low alarm limits for end-tidal CO_2 can also be set.

PURITAN-BENNETT 840 VENTILATOR

The Puritan-Bennett 840 (Puritan-Bennett) (Fig. 17-10) is a pneumatically and electrically (AC or internal battery) powered, electronically (microprocessor) controlled ventilator designed for use with infant, pediatric, and adult patients. Power conversion and transmission are accomplished with pressure regulators, dual proportional solenoid flow control valves, and an electromagnetic exhalation valve. The Puritan-Bennett 840 is a flow or pressure controller. Mandatory breaths are time, pressure, or flow triggered; flow, volume, or pressure limited; and time cycled. Spontaneous breaths are flow or pressure triggered, pressure limited, and flow cycled.[20,21]

Power Conversion and Transmission. The Puritan-Bennett 840 utilizes compressed air and oxygen in a range of 35 to 100 psig. Compressed air can be supplied by the optional 806 compressor unit. Air

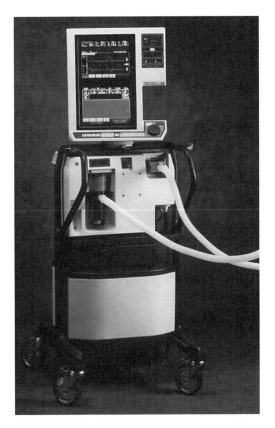

Fig. 17-10

Puritan-Bennett 840 Ventilator. (Courtesy Puritan-Bennett, Pleasanton, Calif.)

and oxygen gas pressures are reduced and matched to approximately 11 psig for use at separate proportional solenoid flow control valves. A microprocessor regulates the opening size of each solenoid to proportion gases to the set oxygen concentration and to provide the required inspiratory gas flow. The flow rate for each valve is calculated by the microprocessor as a function of the driving pressure of each gas and the size of the valve opening as determined by the position of the solenoid. Blended gas passes a safety valve and the inspiratory pressure transducer before entering the patient circuit.

Gas from the expiratory limb of the patient circuit is controlled by an electromagnetic exhalation valve. The exhalation valve adjusts rapidly and in small increments (in conjunction with the inspiratory flow control valves) to regulate breath phasing. During the inspiratory phase, the exhalation valve closes so that inspiratory gas flow is directed to the patient. During pressure-controlled ventilation, the exhalation valve opens and closes as needed to maintain the set inspiratory pressure limit. At the

end of the inspiratory phase for all breath types, the valve opens to permit exhalation and then adjusts as necessary to maintain the set baseline pressure. Circuit pressure is measured at the exhalation valve by the expiratory pressure transducer, and gas flow through the valve is measured by the expiratory flow sensor.

Control. The Puritan-Bennett 840 can be operated in the following modes: A/C, SIMV, and spontaneous. Mandatory breaths in the A/C and SIMV modes can be set as either pressure control or volume control. Pressure support can be used to augment spontaneous breaths in all modes that permit spontaneous breathing. An apnea ventilation mode and a safety ventilation mode are also available. The BiLevel mode is an available option.

When the volume-controlled mandatory breath type is chosen, tidal volume, peak flow rate, and flow pattern must be set. The ventilator's tidal volume range is 25 to 2500 ml. However, the ideal body weight (IBW; range 3.5 to 150 kg) entered during the patient set-up procedure determines the absolute limits for tidal volume and peak flow rate settings. The peak flow range is 3 to 150 L/min when the entered IBW is greater than 24 kg or 3 to 60 L/min if the IBW is less than or equal to 24 kg. The inspiratory flow pattern can be set to square (rectangular) or descending ramp shaped. Based on the patient circuit compliance calculated by the ventilator, tidal volume is compensated for compressible volume loss so that the volume actually delivered to the patient more closely approximates set tidal volume.

To deliver a volume-controlled mandatory breath, the ventilator determines the inspiratory time interval necessary to deliver the set tidal volume at the set peak flow rate to produce the selected flow pattern. The ventilator accomplishes compliance compensation by increasing the actual inspiratory flow rate above set so the compensated volume is delivered in the originally determined inspiratory time interval. Because the ventilator regulates inspiratory flow rate in a fixed pattern until the end of a predetermined inspiratory time interval, volume-controlled mandatory breaths are more specifically flow controlled, flow limited, and time cycled. Alternately, a volume-controlled breath is cycled to expiration if circuit pressure reaches a high pressure alarm threshold. Setting plateau time (0 to 2 seconds) creates an inspiratory pause and increases total inspiratory time.

Pressure-controlled mandatory breaths are pressure limited to the set inspiratory pressure level (5 to 90 cm H_2O above PEEP) and cycled to expiration at the end of the set inspiratory time interval. With changes in the set breath rate, inspiratory time is ultimately determined by the selection of one of the following three parameters as the primary timing parameter: inspiratory time (0.2 to 8 seconds), expiratory time (minimum 0.2 second), or I:E ratio (maximum 4:1). Pressure-controlled breaths are alternately cycled to expiration if circuit pressure reaches a ventilator-determined pressure above the set pressure limit.

When a pressure-controlled breath is triggered, the ventilator delivers gas at the flow rate necessary to reach and maintain the set pressure limit. Maximum inspiratory flow rate with pressure control is 200 L/min with IBW set at greater than 24 kg or at 80 L/min with an IBW of 24 kg or less. Inspiratory flow rate is also influenced by the flow acceleration percentage setting (1% to 100%). The flow acceleration percentage setting dictates how quickly inspiratory pressure rises to the set pressure limit after the initiation of a pressure-controlled breath. Increasing the flow acceleration percentage value directs the ventilator to reach the pressure limit more quickly, resulting in a higher peak inspiratory flow rate.

In A/C, all breaths are mandatory and are either time triggered at the end of a time interval dictated by the ventilator rate setting (1 to 100 breaths per minute) or patient triggered by spontaneous breathing effort. In SIMV, mandatory breaths are time or patient triggered at the set ventilator breath rate.

The patient trigger variable can be set as either pressure or flow. Pressure triggering requires patient spontaneous effort to drop circuit pressure below baseline by an amount equal to set trigger sensitivity (0.1 to 20 cm H_2O below PEEP). To accomplish flow triggering the ventilator delivers a base gas flow through the patient circuit during the expiratory phase of all breaths. This base flow is equal to the flow rate set as the trigger sensitivity plus 1.5 L/min. As the patient breathes from the base flow, the ventilator detects a difference in the inspiratory and expiratory flow measurements. Flow triggering occurs when this flow rate differential equals the value set as the trigger sensitivity (0.5 to 20 L/min). A backup pressure-triggering threshold of –2 cm H_2O is in effect when flow triggering is selected.

Spontaneous breaths in the SIMV, spontaneous, and BiLevel modes can be pressure-supported or supported with the ventilator's demand flow system. Pressure-supported breaths are patient (pressure or flow) triggered, pressure limited to the set pressure support level (0 to 70 cm H_2O set above PEEP), and flow cycled to expiration when the measured inspiratory flow rate falls to an operator-selected expiratory sensitivity setting. Expiratory sensitivity is set as a percentage (1% to 45%) of the peak inspiratory flow rate needed to reach the

set pressure limit. Peak inspiratory flow rate is also influenced by the set flow acceleration percentage. Increasing the flow acceleration percentage increases the initial inspiratory flow rate (and vice versa) as described earlier for pressure-controlled mandatory breaths. As a safety mechanism, pressure support is cycled to expiration if inspiratory flow does not fall to the set flow-cycling threshold at the end of a ventilator-determined time interval based on the entered ideal body weight. Pressure support is also pressure cycled if circuit pressure exceeds the set pressure limit by a ventilator-determined increment.

Demand flow, like pressure support, is patient (pressure or flow) triggered. When a patient effort is detected, the ventilator regulates the flow control valves to provide the gas flow necessary to reach and maintain set PEEP plus 1.5 cm H_2O (the pressure limit). Demand flow is terminated by the same cycling criteria described for pressure support.

The optional BiLevel mode establishes two levels of positive airway pressure: low PEEP (0 to 45 cm H_2O) and high PEEP (5 to 90 cm H_2O). Spontaneous breathing—with or without pressure support—is permitted on both levels of positive pressure. The change from one pressure level to the other is primarily determined by operator-selected time intervals. However, the ventilator attempts to synchronize the change in pressure level to the patient's spontaneous breathing activity and uses the set patient triggering criteria to switch from the low to the high pressure level. To synchronize the change from the high to the low pressure level, the ventilator uses the cycling criteria outlined for pressure support and demand flow. When the high and low PEEP time intervals are set to create only a brief drop to the low PEEP level, the mode resembles airway pressure release ventilation (APRV). The high PEEP time interval can be set to a maximum of 30 seconds.

Apnea ventilation provides a backup mode of ventilation if the ventilator detects an apnea condition. Apnea ventilation settings are operator selected and include the choice of pressure-controlled or volume-controlled mandatory breaths. A safety ventilation function institutes default ventilation settings intended to be safe for all patient types (infant to adult) if the ventilator senses circuit connection before the completion of the startup sequence.

The PEEP control sets baseline pressure in a range of 0 to 45 cm H_2O. The $O_2\%$ setting determines the oxygen concentration (21% to 100%). An inspiratory pause of up to 7 seconds or an expiratory pause of up to 20 seconds can be operator initiated. A mandatory breath can be manually triggered in all modes using the manual inspiration key. The characteristics of a manually triggered breath are determined by current ventilator settings. Pressing the manual inspiration key when the ventilator is set in the BiLevel mode causes a change from one pressure level to the other.

Table 17-7 summarizes the control and phase variables for both mandatory and spontaneous breaths in the Puritan-Bennett 840's operational modes.

Output

Waveforms. Flow-controlled (volume control) mandatory breaths can be delivered in either a rectangular or a descending ramp-shaped inspiratory flow pattern. If the rectangular inspiratory flow waveform is selected, the resulting pressure and volume waveforms are ascending ramp shaped. If the descending ramp flow waveform is chosen, the pressure and volume waveforms tend to rise exponentially.

The shape of the inspiratory pressure waveform produced during the delivery of a pressure-controlled mandatory breath is influenced by the flow acceleration percentage setting. A flow acceleration setting of 100% causes inspiratory pressure to rise very rapidly to the set pressure limit. In this case, the inspiratory pressure waveform is approximately rectangular. If the flow acceleration percentage is decreased, inspiratory pressure rises more slowly, causing the initial portion of the pressure waveform to be ramp shaped. The resulting inspiratory flow and volume waveforms exhibit an exponential rise. The magnitude of the inspiratory flow waveform (peak flow) decreases as the flow acceleration percentage setting is decreased.

Monitoring. The Puritan-Bennett 840 presents output data both numerically and graphically. Graphics options include pressure time, flow time, volume time, and pressure volume displays. The breath-type display indicates the type (control, assist, or spontaneous) and phase (inspiration or exhalation) of the currently delivered breath.

Airway pressure values are calculated from measurements made by the pressure sensors located in the ventilator's inspiratory and expiratory compartments. These include end-expiratory pressure, end-inspiratory (plateau) pressure, maximum circuit pressure, and mean circuit pressure. Measurements of intrinsic (auto-) PEEP and total PEEP are made during an operator-initiated expiratory pause. In addition, static compliance and resistance are calculated during an inspiratory pause maneuver.

Exhaled tidal volume, spontaneous minute volume, and (total) exhaled minute volume values are derived from the flow measurement made by a hot wire anemometer flow sensor located at the exhalation valve. These volume measurements are circuit compliance compensated. Total (spontaneous and mandatory) respiratory rate and I:E ratio are also displayed. Delivered $O_2\%$ reflects oxygen concentration measured by the internal oxygen sensor. The oxygen sensor can be enabled or disabled by the operator.

The Puritan-Bennett 840 is equipped with a digital output connection.

Alarms. The Puritan-Bennett 840 classifies alarms as low, medium, and high urgency and uses both visual and audible signals to indicate the appropriate level of urgency. Additionally, the ventilator suggests actions to remedy specific alarm conditions. Alarm events are chronologically entered into an alarm log. The log can store up to 50 alarm messages for subsequent review.

Input power alarms. If either gas pressure falls below the minimum required for ventilator operation, the no air supply or no O_2 supply alarm activates to indicate the specific gas loss and the ventilator continues operation using the remaining available gas. Failure of the optional air compressor activates the compressor inoperative alarm.

The low AC power alarm indicates that external electrical power has dropped below a level acceptable for ventilator operation. The AC power loss alarm indicates that AC power is not available and that the internal battery is supporting ventilator function. A fully charged battery generally sustains operation for at least 30 minutes. The inoperative battery alarm indicates that a battery is installed but not functional. The low battery alarm activates when less than 2 minutes of battery power remains. The loss of power alarm signals that both AC and battery power are insufficient for ventilator operation.

Control circuit alarms. A device alert is triggered if a system fault is detected during ongoing testing of the ventilator's electronic and pneumatic function. A high urgency device alert causes a ventilator inoperable condition and opening of a safety valve to allow the patient to breathe spontaneously from room air. A procedure error alarm activates if the patient is attached to the ventilator before completion of the startup procedure.

Output alarms. Most of the ventilator's adjustable output alarm limits are initially set based on the entered patient ideal body weight, but they may be subsequently operator adjusted. Operator-set alarms include those for apnea, high circuit

TABLE 17-7 CONTROL AND PHASE VARIABLES FOR MANDATORY AND SPONTANEOUS BREATHS IN THE OPERATIONAL MODES AVAILABLE ON THE PURITAN-BENNETT 840 VENTILATOR

Mode	Mandatory				Spontaneous			
	Control¶	Trigger*	Limit	Cycle	Control¶	Trigger	Limit	Cycle
A/C—volume control	Flow	Time, pressure, flow	Flow, volume	Time, pressure†	N/A	N/A	N/A	N/A
A/C—pressure control	Pressure	Time, pressure, flow	Pressure	Time, pressure†	N/A	N/A	N/A	N/A
SIMV—volume control	Flow	Time, pressure, flow	Flow, volume	Time, pressure†	Pressure	Pressure, flow	Pressure	Flow, time,† pressure†
SIMV—pressure control	Pressure	Time, pressure, flow	Pressure	Time, pressure†	Pressure	Pressure, flow	Pressure	Flow, time,† pressure†
Bilevel‡	Pressure	Time, pressure, flow	Pressure	Time, flow, pressure	Pressure	Time, flow, pressure	Pressure	Time, pressure, flow
Spontaneous	N/A	N/A	N/A	N/A	Pressure	Pressure, flow	Pressure	Flow, time,† pressure†
Pressure support§	N/A	N/A	N/A	N/A	Pressure, flow	Pressure	Pressure	Flow, time,† pressure†

Modified from Chatburn RL, Lough MD, Primiano FP Jr: Mechanical ventilation. In Chatburn RL, Lough MD, editors: *Handbook of respiratory care*, ed 2. St Louis. Mosby, 1990; pp 159-223.

A/C, Assist-control; *SIMV,* synchronized intermittent mandatory ventilation; *N/A,* not applicable.

*Mandatory breaths can be manually triggered in all modes.

†Secondary or safety cycle variable.

‡For the purpose of illustrating ventilator behavior in the Bilevel mode, the high PEEP level is here considered the mandatory breath and the low PEEP level the spontaneous breath. In fact, spontaneous breathing is permitted on both the high and low PEEP levels.

§Considered here as a separate mode, but can be used to support spontaneous breaths in the SIMV, Spontaneous, and Bilevel modes.

¶The Flow Acceleration % control can be used to modify the shape of the inspiratory pressure waveform for pressure-controlled mandatory breaths and pressure-supported spontaneous breaths.

pressure, high and low exhaled minute volume, low exhaled spontaneous tidal volume, low exhaled mandatory tidal volume, high exhaled tidal volume (spontaneous or mandatory), and high respiratory rate.

The inspiration too long alarm activates if, during the delivery of a spontaneous breath, inspiratory flow rate does not decrease to the flow cycling threshold (expiratory sensitivity setting) before the end of the ventilator-determined maximum inspiratory time. The ventilator is also equipped with a circuit disconnect alarm, a high internal pressure alarm, and a circuit occlusion alarm. If a severe circuit occlusion is detected, the ventilator discontinues normal operation, opens its safety valve, and periodically attempts to deliver a pressure-controlled breath (occlusion status cycling) while monitoring for the persistence of the occlusion.

The Puritan-Bennett 840 is equipped with a remote alarm connection.

NEWPORT WAVE VM200
INFANT-PEDIATRIC-ADULT VENTILATOR

The Newport Wave VM200 (Newport Medical Instruments) (Fig. 17-11) is the integration of the Newport Compass monitor with the Model E200 Wave Ventilator. The Wave VM200 is an electrically and pneumatically powered, electronically (microprocessor) and pneumatically controlled ventilator designed to support infant, pediatric, and adult patients. Power conversion and transmission are accomplished with a pressure regulator, an electromagnetic proportional flow-control valve, and a pneumatic diaphragm exhalation valve. The Wave is a flow or pressure controller. Mandatory breaths are time or pressure triggered; flow, volume, or pressure limited; and time cycled. Spontaneous breaths can be pressure triggered, pressure limited, and flow or pressure cycled. Continuous flow is also available for spontaneous breathing.[22,23]

Power Conversion and Transmission. The Newport Wave uses compressed air and oxygen in a range of 35 to 70 psig. The air-oxygen mixer proportions the gases to the desired oxygen concentration and regulates the system pressure to 29 psig. Blended gas is stored in a gas accumulator that supplies a proportional flow-control valve. The flow-control valve uses an electromagnetic coil and plunger to regulate gas flow through the valve opening. The amount of electric current applied to the coil determines the position of the plunger. Gas from the flow-control valve is monitored by a differential pressure flow sensor and a mechanical pressure manometer before entering the inspiratory limb of the patient circuit.

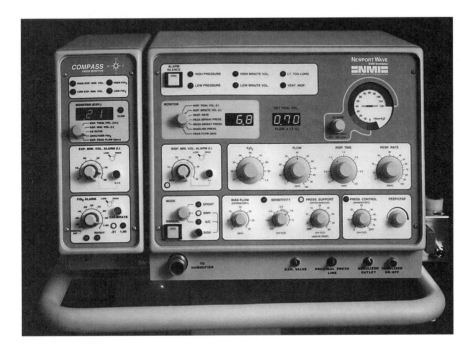

Fig. 17-11

Newport Wave VM200 Infant-Pediatric-Adult Ventilator. (Courtesy Newport Medical Instruments, Newport Beach, Calif.)

Gas from the expiratory limb of the patient circuit is controlled by a pneumatic exhalation valve that uses a balloon diaphragm to regulate the valve opening. Pressure inside the balloon is determined either by gas from the main flow outlet manifold (to direct inspiratory flow to the patient) or by a flow of gas that is regulated by the PEEP control needle valve (to maintain baseline pressure). A combination solenoid-pneumatic interface valve is switched on and off to control which of the two gas sources is transmitted to the balloon to control the breath phase. An electronic pressure transducer monitors pressure at the exhalation valve.

Control. The Newport Wave provides the option of either flow-controlled (volume preset) or pressure-controlled mandatory breaths in both the A/C and SIMV modes. A spontaneous mode is also available, and pressure support can be used to augment spontaneous breaths in the SIMV and spontaneous modes.

Volume preset mandatory breaths are flow limited at the set flow rate (1 to 100 L/min) and time cycled at the end of the set inspiratory time interval (0.1 to 3 seconds). Set tidal volume (30 to 2000 ml) is calculated as the product of the flow rate and inspiratory time settings and is displayed digitally. Using signals from the inspiratory flow sensor, the microprocessor adjusts the flow-control valve as necessary throughout the inspiratory phase to ensure that the set flow rate is maintained. Volume preset breaths can be volume limited with an inspiratory pause (10%, 20%, 30% of set inspiratory time).

Pressure-controlled mandatory breaths are pressure limited at the level determined by the pressure control setting (0 to 80 cm H_2O) and time cycled at the end of the set inspiratory time interval. Inspiratory flow rate is regulated by the microprocessor and will not exceed the set flow rate. Both pressure-controlled and flow-controlled mandatory breaths are pressure cycled before the end of the set inspiratory time interval if airway pressure reaches the high-pressure alarm setting.

Mandatory breaths (pressure or flow controlled) are pressure triggered when patient effort drops proximal pressure by an amount equal to the sensitivity setting (0 to –5 cm H_2O). In the A/C mode, breaths are pressure triggered with each spontaneous effort that meets the sensitivity criteria or are time triggered at a frequency determined by the respiratory rate setting (0 to 100 breaths per minute). In the SIMV mode, mandatory breaths are pressure or time triggered at the set respiratory rate. In SIMV, spontaneous breathing is allowed between mandatory breaths.

Spontaneous breaths in the spontaneous and SIMV modes can be supported with demand flow or continuous flow (set as bias flow: 0 to 30 L/min) or a combination of the two. Demand flow is pressure triggered if a spontaneous breath drops proximal airway pressure by an amount equal to the set sensitivity, pressure limited, and pressure cycled when airway pressure returns to within 0.5 cm H_2O of set baseline.

Pressure support is pressure triggered by patient effort and pressure limited at the level determined by the pressure support setting (0 to 60 cm H_2O) plus PEEP. Pressure support is flow cycled when inspiratory flow falls to a microprocessor-determined threshold based on the peak flow used to reach the pressure limit and elapsed inspiratory time. As a safety mechanism, pressure support is pressure cycled if airway pressure rises 2 cm H_2O above the set pressure support level or is time or volume cycled if inspiratory flow fails to drop to the required flow-cycling threshold.

Mandatory breaths can be manually triggered in all modes. Additionally, sigh breaths may be set in both the SIMV and A/C modes. Sighs are triggered every hundredth breath, are pressure or flow limited, and are time cycled at the end of a time interval equal to 1.5 times set inspiratory time.

Baseline pressure is controlled in a range of 0 to 45 cm H_2O using the PEEP/CPAP control knob. The inspired oxygen concentration is determined by the FIO_2 control setting (21% to 100%). Gas flow to a micronebulizer is controlled with the nebulizer on/off button. An adjustable pressure relief valve (0 to 120 cm H_2O) acts as a safety popoff valve.

Table 17-8 summarizes the control and phase variables for mandatory and spontaneous breaths in the operational modes available on the Wave VM200.

Output

Waveforms. Because volume preset (flow controlled) mandatory breaths are delivered at a constant flow rate, the inspiratory flow waveform is essentially rectangular. As a result, the volume and pressure waveforms are ascending ramp shaped.

When delivering pressure-controlled mandatory breaths, the Wave produces a pressure waveform that can vary from nearly rectangular to exponential, depending on the inspiratory flow rate setting. The resulting flow waveform exhibits an exponential decay and the volume waveform exhibits an exponential rise.

Monitoring. Output data are digitally displayed in the ventilator monitoring window and on the Compass monitor. Specific output parameters are chosen using multi-position selector dials.

Peak pressure and mean pressure reflect airway pressure measured by the proximal pressure

TABLE 17-8	CONTROL AND PHASE VARIABLES FOR MANDATORY AND SPONTANEOUS BREATHS IN THE OPERATIONAL MODES AVAILABLE ON THE NEWPORT WAVE VM200 VENTILATOR						
	Mandatory				**Spontaneous**		
Mode	**Control**	**Trigger***	**Limit**	**Cycle**	**Control**	**Trigger**	**Limit**	**Cycle**
A/C	Pressure	Time, pressure	Pressure	Time, pressure†	N/A	N/A	N/A	N/A
	Flow	Time, pressure	Flow, volume	Time, pressure†	N/A	N/A	N/A	N/A
SIMV	Pressure	Time, pressure	Pressure	Time, pressure†	Pressure‡	Pressure‡	Pressure‡	Pressure‡
	Flow	Time, pressure	Flow, volume	Time, pressure†	Pressure‡	Pressure‡	Pressure‡	Pressure‡
Spontaneous	N/A	N/A	N/A	N/A	Pressure‡	Pressure‡	Pressure‡	Pressure‡
Pressure support§	N/A	N/A	N/A	N/A	Pressure	Pressure	Pressure	Flow, pressure,† time,† volume†

Modified from Chatburn RL, Lough MD, Primiano FP Jr: Mechanical ventilation. In Chatburn RL, Lough MD, editors: *Handbook of respiratory care,* ed 2. St Louis. Mosby, 1990; pp 159-223.

A/C, Assist/control; *SIMV,* synchronized intermittent mandatory ventilation; *N/A,* not applicable.

*Mandatory breaths can be manually triggered in all modes.

†Secondary or safety cycle variable.

‡Applies to demand flow; ventilator may not respond if continuous flow is set.

§Considered here as a separate mode but can be used to support spontaneous breaths in the SIMV and spontaneous modes.

transducer. Baseline pressure is calculated by the microprocessor using measurements from the proximal and exhalation valve pressure transducers. An electronic manometer displays pressure measured at the main flow outlet.

Inspiratory tidal volume and minute volume are derived from inspiratory flow sensor measurements that are corrected for the delivered continuous flow. Because of the flow sensor location proximal to the main flow outlet, these measurements include volume lost because of leaks or gas compression in the patient circuit. Also, a tidal volume of 4 ml or less is regarded as zero, and the use of continuous flow will affect spontaneous inspiratory volume measurements because volume drawn from the continuous gas flow will not be detected. Respiratory rate includes all breaths that cause the inspiratory flow control valve to produce an inspiratory tidal volume of more than 4 ml. Peak flow is the maximum inspiratory flow rate for each breath as measured at the flow-control valve.

The Compass ventilation monitor provides measurements of expired tidal volume, expired minute volume, I:E, peak expiratory flow rate, and analyzed FIO_2. Displayed volumes are integrated from flow measurements made at the exhalation valve by a hot wire anemometer-type flow sensor (range: 1 to 400 L/min). Communication with the ventilator provides for continuous correction of expiratory volume measurements to offset the bias flow sup-

plied by the inspiratory flow-control valve. As with inspiratory volume measurements, expiratory volume measurements include gas volume compressed in the patient circuit.

The Wave VM200 is equipped with both analog and digital output connections.

Alarms

Input power alarms. The gas supply source failure alarm is activated if either source gas pressure falls to less than 35 psig. In the event of total input gas failure, a one-way valve opens to ambient air if spontaneous breathing generates an adequate negative pressure (less than 4 cm H_2O).

If the electric power supply is interrupted, a power failure alarm is activated and remains activated for at least 10 minutes. Both input power alarms are audible only.

Control circuit alarms. A failure of the electronics system or related components activates the ventilator-inoperative alarm, and the ventilator ceases to function. The alarm indicating that inspiratory time is too long is activated if the rate and inspiratory time control settings result in an I:E ratio greater than 1:1 (3:1 with the I:E override in effect).

Output alarms. The Wave's output alarms are high and low airway pressure and high and low (inspiratory) minute volume. The Compass monitor adds alarms for high and low exhaled minute volume and high and low F_{IO_2}. The alarm limits for these alarms are operator selected. The minute volume alarm has a dual scale: 0 to 5 L/min for neonates and pediatric patients and 0 to 50 L/min for adults.

Siemens Servo 900C Ventilator

The Siemens Servo 900C (Fig. 17-12) is an electrically and pneumatically powered, electronically controlled ventilator. The drive mechanism of the 900C incorporates a spring-loaded bellows and electromagnetic inspiratory and expiratory output control valves. The Servo 900C is a pressure or flow controller. Mandatory breaths are time or pressure triggered; pressure, flow, or volume limited; and time cycled. Spontaneous breaths are pressure triggered, pressure limited, and flow cycled.[24,25]

Power Conversion and Transmission. Gas from an external compressor feeds a spring-loaded bellows. The bellows stores gas and maintains a constant working pressure that determines the gradient for gas flow to the patient. Working pressure is adjusted upward and downward by means of a mechanical control "key" that increases or decreases the tension of the springs compressing the bellows. A safety valve just beyond the bellows outlet opens if the bellows overfills or if pressure exceeds approximately 120 cm H_2O, the maximum working pressure.

Gas from the bellows flows through a strain gauge-type inspiratory flow transducer, through the inspiratory valve, and past the inspiratory pressure transducer to the inspiratory limb of the patient circuit. The electromagnetic proportional inspiratory valve consists of a rubber tube, or flow channel, positioned between the fixed arm and movable arm of a scissors-like clamp. A step motor controls the position of the movable arm of the clamp, opening and closing the scissors valve in discrete "steps" to regulate gas flow from the bellows to the patient circuit.

Gas from the expiratory limb of the patient circuit passes through the expiratory flow transducer, the expiratory pressure transducer, and the expiratory valve before exiting the ventilator. The expiratory flow transducer is identical to the inspiratory flow transducer except that it is heated to about 60° C to prevent condensation. A linear motor controls the movable arm of the expiratory scissors valve used to regulate expiratory flow.

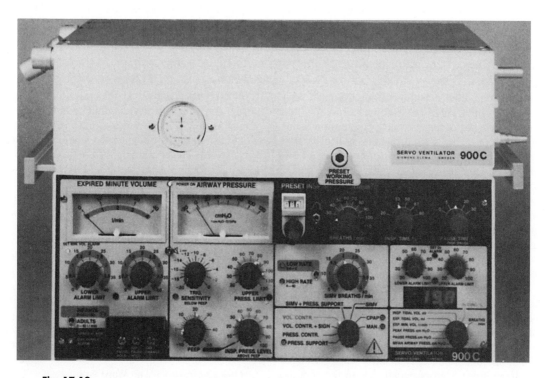

Fig. 17-12

Siemens Servo 900C Ventilator. (Courtesy Siemens Medical Systems, Danvers, Mass.)

Control. The Servo 900C can be operated in the following modes: volume control, volume control plus sigh, SIMV, pressure support, SIMV plus pressure support, pressure control, CPAP, and manual.

In the modes offering volume control and SIMV, mandatory breaths are volume preset and flow controlled. Inspiration is flow limited at the peak flow rate that the ventilator calculates is necessary to deliver the desired tidal volume in the set inspiratory time interval using the selected flow waveform. Actual flow is measured by the inspiratory flow transducer and is used to adjust the inspiratory scissors valve to more closely approximate the required flow. Inspiration is time cycled at the end of the inspiratory time interval or pressure cycled before the end of the set inspiratory time if inspiratory pressure reaches the value set on the high-pressure alarm.

Tidal volume is set indirectly as a function of the preset inspiratory minute volume (0.5 to 40 L/min) and the ventilator's breath rate (5 to 120 breaths per minute) settings. Either a rectangular or a modified sinusoidal (ascending-descending ramp) inspiratory flow waveform can be selected. Inspiratory time is set as a percentage (20%, 25%, 33%, 50%, 67%, or 80%) of the ventilatory cycle time dictated by the breath rate setting. The addition of an inspiratory pause (0%, 5%, 10%, 20%, or 30% of ventilatory cycle time) extends and volume-limits the inspiratory phase of a volume preset breath. If the combined inspiratory and pause times exceed 80% of the ventilatory cycle, the ventilator reduces pause time as necessary to preserve 20% of cycle time for expiration.

In the volume-control mode, mandatory breaths are pressure triggered whenever patient effort drops circuit pressure to the set trigger sensitivity level (0 to -20 cm H_2O) or time triggered at an interval determined by the breath rate setting. In the SIMV mode, mandatory breaths are pressure triggered by patient effort or time triggered at a rate determined by the SIMV breath rate control. This control is graduated in two scales: a low-rate range of 0.4 to 4 breaths per minute and a high-rate range of 4 to 40 breaths per minute.

Spontaneous breaths in the SIMV and CPAP modes are supported by demand flow, which is pressure triggered if patient effort is sufficient to drop airway pressure to the set sensitivity threshold, pressure limited to the set baseline pressure, and flow cycled when inspiratory flow drops to 25% of the peak flow rate necessary to return airway pressure to baseline.

In the pressure-control mode, pressure-controlled mandatory breaths are pressure triggered or time triggered as in the volume-control mode. Using feed-back from the inspiratory pressure transducer, the step motor adjusts the inspiratory valve opening to produce the flows necessary to reach and maintain the set inspiratory pressure limit (0 to 100 cm H_2O, set above baseline). Inspiration is time cycled at the end of the set inspiratory time interval (percentage inspiratory time plus percentage pause time) or pressure cycled if inspiratory pressure reaches the high-pressure alarm setting.

Pressure support is pressure controlled and pressure triggered if patient effort drops baseline pressure by an amount equal to the set trigger sensitivity, and it is pressure limited at the set inspiratory pressure level (above baseline). Pressure-supported breaths are flow cycled when the measured flow rate drops to 25% of the peak inspiratory flow rate needed to reach the pressure limit. Alternately, inspiration is pressure cycled if measured pressure reaches 3 cm H_2O above the set inspiratory pressure limit or time cycled at the end of a time interval equal to 80% of the ventilatory cycle time dictated by the breath rate setting.

Use of the manual mode requires the addition of a special bag-valve system. This mode is used primarily in the anesthesia setting and is mentioned here only for completeness.

A positive baseline pressure can be set in a range of 0 to 50 cm H_2O with the PEEP control. The expiratory scissors valve is servo-regulated to maintain baseline pressure based on the expiratory pressure transducer measurements. The PEEP control is also graduated to a range of 0 to -10 cm H_2O. The application of a negative baseline pressure requires the use of an optional gas-driven Venturi attachment placed on the expiratory outlet.

Because an external gas blender must be used with the Servo 900C, inspired oxygen concentration is determined by the control on the blender in use. The gas change button effects a rapid change of gas in the patient circuit. The inspiratory pause hold button sustains lung inflation for as long as the button is depressed. When the expiratory pause hold button is pushed, an expiratory pause is sustained until the push button is released.

Table 17-9 provides a summary of the control and phase variables for mandatory and spontaneous breaths in each of the operational modes available on the Servo 900C.

Output

Waveforms. If a rectangular inspiratory flow waveform is selected, waveforms for both pressure and volume are ascending ramp shaped. A modified sinusoidal inspiratory flow pattern results in pressure and volume waveforms that are also quasi-sinusoidal. The ability of the ventilator to

TABLE 17-9	CONTROL AND PHASE VARIABLES FOR MANDATORY AND SPONTANEOUS BREATHS IN THE OPERATIONAL MODES AVAILABLE ON THE SIEMENS SERVO 900C VENTILATOR							
	Mandatory				**Spontaneous**			
Mode	**Control**	**Trigger**	**Limit**	**Cycle**	**Control**	**Trigger**	**Limit**	**Cycle**
Volume control	Flow	Time, pressure	Flow, volume	Time, pressure*	N/A	N/A	N/A	N/A
Volume control + sigh	Flow	Time, pressure	Flow, volume	Time, pressure*	N/A	N/A	N/A	N/A
SIMV	Flow	Time, pressure	Flow, volume	Time, pressure*	Pressure	Pressure	Pressure	Flow, pressure
SIMV + pressure support	Flow	Time, pressure	Flow, volume	Time, pressure*	Pressure	Pressure	Pressure	Flow, time,* pressure*
Pressure control	Pressure	Time, pressure	Pressure	Time, pressure*	N/A	N/A	N/A	N/A
Pressure support	N/A	N/A	N/A	N/A	Pressure	Pressure	Pressure	Flow, time,* pressure*
CPAP	N/A	N/A	N/A	N/A	Pressure	Pressure	Pressure	Flow, pressure

Modified from Chatburn RL, Lough MD, Primiano FP Jr: Mechanical ventilation. In Chatburn RL, Lough MD, editors: *Handbook of respiratory care*, ed 2. St Louis. Mosby, 1990; pp 159-223.
SIMV, Synchronized intermittent mandatory ventilation; *CPAP*, continuous positive airway pressure; *N/A*, not applicable.
*Secondary or safety cycle variable.

produce the selected flow waveform is contingent on a working pressure high enough to maintain an adequate pressure gradient for gas delivery. If the peak inspiratory pressure necessary to deliver a breath approaches the set working pressure, the flow waveform exhibits an exponential decay. In this case, the pressure and volume waveforms are also exponential.

Pressure-controlled mandatory breaths produce an approximately rectangular inspiratory pressure waveform. In response, the volume waveform exhibits an exponential rise and the flow waveform shows an exponential decay.

Monitoring. Peak pressure, pause pressure, and mean airway pressure values are based on measurements made by the inspiratory pressure transducer. An analog pressure meter displays pressure measured at the expiratory pressure transducer. Inspired tidal volume and expired tidal volume values are derived from measurements made by the inspiratory and expiratory flow transducers, respectively. Expired minute volume is displayed digitally and on an analog meter. Breaths per minute is a running average of respiratory rate and includes all patient- and ventilator-triggered breaths. Oxygen concentration is measured by an oxygen analyzer at the ventilator gas inlet.

The Servo 900C is equipped with an analog output connection for recording pressure and flow waveforms.

Alarms

Input power alarms. In the event of electric power loss, ventilator functions cease, a slow audible signal sounds, and the "power on" indicator light is extinguished. The inspiratory and expiratory valves open, permitting the patient to breathe spontaneously from available gas. A loss of pneumatic power activates the gas supply alarm.

Output alarms. The high airway pressure alarm is activated if airway pressure reaches the alarm setting. Activation of the high-pressure alarm cycles an inspiratory phase in progress. This alarm must be set lower than the working pressure to be functional.

High and low minute volume alarm limits are set relative to the displayed exhaled volume derived from flow measured by the expiratory flow transducer. Each of these alarm controls has an infant and adult scale. The apnea alarm functions in modes that permit spontaneous breathing and becomes activated if the ventilator fails to detect a mandatory or spontaneous breath in a 15-second period.

A high and low oxygen concentration alarm is functional if the oxygen-measuring cell is engaged.

Failure to set the oxygen concentration or minute volume alarms is signaled by a persistent blinking of the alarm indicator light.

SIEMENS SERVO 300A VENTILATOR

The Siemens Servo 300A (Siemens Medical Systems) (Fig. 17-13) is a pneumatically and electrically (AC and internal battery) powered, electronically controlled ventilator designed for neonatal, pediatric, and adult use. Power conversion and transmission are accomplished with two electromagnetic proportional flow control valves and an electromagnetic exhalation valve. The 300A is a flow or pressure controller. Mandatory breaths are time, flow, or pressure triggered; flow, volume, or pressure limited; and time cycled. Spontaneous breaths are flow or pressure triggered, pressure limited, and flow cycled.[26]

Power Conversion and Transmission. Compressed air and oxygen in a range of 29 to 94 psig feed separate inspiratory flow control valve units. Gas flow through each unit is regulated by an

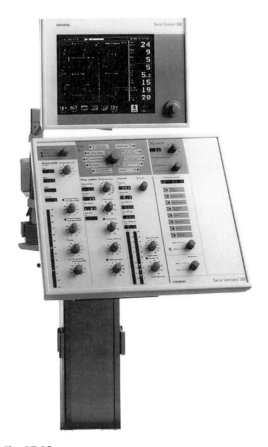

Fig. 17-13

Siemens Servo 300A Ventilator. (Courtesy Siemens Medical Systems, Danvers, Mass.)

electromagnetic proportional solenoid. The air and oxygen valves operate together to produce total inspiratory gas flow at the set oxygen concentration. Gas flow rate is a function of gas pressure and the valve opening size as determined by the solenoid position. Flow rate is measured in each unit by separate differential pressure-type flow sensors. Air and oxygen are mixed in the inspiratory flow channel before entering the patient circuit. The flow channel also includes the inspiratory pressure transducer and a spring-loaded safety valve that opens in the event of power failure or if pressure exceeds 120 cm H_2O.

Gas from the expiratory limb of the patient circuit is monitored by the expiratory flow sensor and the expiratory pressure transducer before passing through the exhalation valve. The exhalation valve consists of the expiratory solenoid valve and a flexible rubber tube. The solenoid squeezes the tube to close the exhalation valve and to regulate expiratory gas flow to maintain set baseline pressure.

Control. The Servo 300A can be operated in the following modes: volume control, SIMV (volume control) plus pressure support, pressure control, SIMV (pressure control) plus pressure support, pressure-regulated volume control, volume support, pressure support/CPAP, and Automode. Additionally, each mode functions in one of three patient ranges: adult, pediatric, and neonatal.

In the volume control and SIMV (volume control) plus pressure support modes, mandatory breaths are volume preset and flow controlled. Inspiration is flow limited to the peak flow rate that the ventilator's microprocessor calculates is necessary to deliver the set tidal volume in the set inspiratory time interval. The actual inspiratory flow rate is measured at the air/oxygen flow control valves and is used to adjust the position of the inspiratory solenoid valves as need throughout the inspiratory phase to maintain the required inspiratory flow rate. Inspiration is time cycled or is pressure cycled before the end of set inspiratory time if airway pressure reaches the set upper pressure alarm limit.

The available range of set (and measured) tidal volume and maximum inspiratory flow rate is dictated by the particular patient range selected by the clinician. Available tidal volume in the three patient ranges is adult, 50 to 3999 ml; pediatric, 10 to 399 ml; and neonatal, 2 to 39 ml. Maximum inspiratory flow rate for the adult, pediatric, and neonatal patient ranges is 200 L/min, 33 L/min, and 13 L/min, respectively.

Inspiratory time is set as a percentage (10% to 80%) of the total ventilatory cycle time determined by the CMV breath rate setting. An inspiratory pause time (0% to 30% of total cycle time) can also be added. Combined inspiratory and pause times cannot exceed 80% of the total ventilatory cycle time.

In the pressure-controlled and the SIMV (pressure control) plus pressure support modes, mandatory breaths are pressure limited at the set pressure control level (0 to 100 cm H_2O, set above baseline). The ventilator regulates inspiratory gas flow to maintain the set pressure limit for the duration of the inspiratory phase. Inspiration is time cycled at the end of the set inspiratory time interval.

Patient-triggered breaths are either pressure or flow triggered, depending on the selected trigger sensitivity setting. During the expiratory phase of all breaths, the ventilator applies a continuous (bias) gas flow. The initial portion of a spontaneous breath is drawn from this bias flow. The specific bias flow rate is dictated by the patient range selection and is delivered with both flow and pressure triggering. When flow is chosen as the patient trigger variable, a breath is triggered when the difference in the bias flow rate measured by the inspiratory and expiratory flow sensors equals the trigger sensitivity setting. The flow trigger sensitivity is set in a nongraduated range and is also influenced by the patient range selected. If pressure is chosen as the trigger variable, patient triggering occurs when inspiratory effort drops circuit pressure by an amount equal to the set trigger sensitivity (0 to –17 cm H_2O).

In the volume-controlled and pressure-controlled modes, all breaths are mandatory and are either patient triggered if inspiratory effort is sufficient to meet the triggering sensitivity criteria or time triggered at an interval determined by the CMV breath rate setting. In the SIMV plus pressure support modes (both volume control and pressure control), mandatory breaths are patient or time triggered at a rate dictated by the SIMV breath rate setting. Spontaneous breaths are permitted between mandatory breaths.

In the pressure support/CPAP mode, all breaths are spontaneous. These spontaneous breaths, as well as spontaneous breaths in the SIMV modes, can be either pressure supported or simply supported with demand flow from the inspiratory flow control valves. In either case, the ventilator provides gas flow if the spontaneous breathing effort is sufficient to meet the set trigger sensitivity criteria.

If pressure support is added, spontaneous breaths are pressure limited to the set pressure support level (0 to 100 cm H_2O, set above baseline). Pressure-supported breaths are flow cycled when the measured inspiratory flow rate drops to 5% of the peak inspiratory flow needed to reach the set pressure limit. Alternately, the inspiratory phase is pressure cycled if airway pressure exceeds the set pressure limit by 3 cm H_2O or time cycled at the end of a time interval equal to 80% of the set ventilatory cycle time or a time constant based on previously measured spontaneous inspiratory time. If pressure support is not added, the ventilator delivers the demand flow necessary to maintain the set baseline pressure (PEEP). Demand flow is terminated by the same cycling criteria described for pressure support.

In pressure-regulated volume control (PRVC) and volume support modes, the ventilator adjusts inspiratory pressure as needed breath to breath based on the pressure/volume relationship of previous breaths. Once triggered, the ventilator delivers the inspiratory gas flow needed to reach and maintain the pressure limit that the ventilator calculates is necessary to approximate a target (set) tidal volume. Thus PRVC and volume support breaths are pressure controlled. The ventilator adjusts the pressure limit in increments of up to 3 cm H_2O per breath but will not exceed an operator-selected absolute upper pressure limit.

In PRVC, breaths are patient or time triggered, pressure limited, and time cycled at the end of the set inspiratory time interval. In volume support, breaths must be patient triggered, are pressure limited, and are cycled to expiration when the inspiratory flow rate drops to 5% of the peak flow rate needed to reach the ventilator-determined pressure limit. The cycling criteria for volume support breaths (including secondary cycling criteria) are identical to that of pressure supported breaths; and, as with pressure support, inspiratory time is variable. If the apnea alarm is activated in volume support, the ventilator will automatically switch to PRVC.

The automode function, when activated, directs the ventilator to automatically switch back and forth between a "control" mode and a "support" mode depending on the patient's spontaneous breathing activity. AutoMode offers three combinations of control/support modes: pressure control/pressure support, volume control/volume support, and pressure-regulated volume control/volume support.

The inspiratory rise time % setting determines how quickly peak pressure (with pressure-controlled breaths) or peak flow (with volume-controlled breaths) is reached during the inspiratory phase. Rise time is set in a range of 0% to 10% of total ventilatory cycle time. Adding or increasing rise time effectively decreases initial inspiratory flow rate. Inspiratory rise time is functional in all modes and affects all ventilator-assisted breaths, both mandatory and spontaneous.

Baseline pressure in a range of 0 to 50 cm H_2O is set with the PEEP control knob. Oxygen concentration is set in a range of 21% to 100%. Turning the oxygen breaths control knob provides 100% oxygen for 20 breaths or 1 minute. Mandatory breaths can be manually triggered in all modes. Activation of the inspiratory pause hold causes the ventilator's inspiratory and expiratory valves to close at end-inspiration, creating an inspiratory hold to a maximum of 5 seconds. An expiratory pause hold creates an expiratory pause that can be sustained for up to 30 seconds.

Table 17-10 summarizes the control and phase variables for mandatory and spontaneous breaths in the operational modes available on the Servo 300A ventilator.

Output

Waveforms. Pressure-controlled mandatory breaths (in the pressure control, SIMV-pressure control, and PRVC modes) produce an approximately rectangular inspiratory pressure waveform if inspiratory rise time % is set to zero. However, the addition of rise time creates a ramp up to the pressure plateau. The ramp becomes more pronounced as rise time is increased. With pressure-controlled breaths, the resulting flow waveform exhibits an exponential decay and the volume waveform shows an exponential rise. As rise time is added, the magnitude of the flow waveform (peak flow) decreases.

Mandatory breaths in the volume control modes produce an essentially rectangular inspiratory flow waveform if inspiratory rise time is set to zero. The addition of rise time creates an ascending ramp to the flow plateau that becomes more pronounced as rise time is increased. The magnitude of the flow waveform (peak flow) increases as rise time is increased to deliver the set tidal volume in the set inspiratory time because, as rise time is increased, peak flow is reached later in the inspiratory phase. Pressure and volume waveforms are an ascending ramp shape.

Monitoring. A bar graph continuously displays airway pressure measured by the inspiratory and expiratory pressure transducers. Peak airway, mean airway, and pause pressure are digitally displayed breath to breath. End-expiratory pressure is also digitally displayed. Inspired tidal volume and expired tidal volume are derived from measurements made at the inspiratory flow control valves and expiratory flow sensor, respectively, and include both mandatory and spontaneous breaths. Expired minute volume is displayed digitally and on a bar graph. Because of the location of the flow sensors inside the ventilator, all volume measurements include compressible volume lost in the patient circuit. Measured breaths per minute is a running average of all patient-triggered and ventilator-triggered breaths. Oxygen concentration is measured at the inspiratory flow channel and is displayed digitally.

The Servo 300A is equipped with analog and digital output connections. The Servo Screen 390 is

TABLE 17-10 · Control and Phase Variables for Mandatory and Spontaneous Breaths in the Operational Modes Available on the Siemens Servo 300A Ventilator

Mode	Mandatory				Spontaneous			
	Control§	Trigger*	Limit	Cycle	Control§	Trigger	Limit	Cycle
Volume control‡	Flow	Time, flow, pressure	Flow, volume	Time, pressure†	N/A	N/A	N/A	N/A
Pressure control‡	Pressure	Time, flow, pressure	Pressure	Time, pressure†	N/A	N/A	N/A	N/A
PRVC‡	Pressure	Time, flow, pressure	Pressure	Time, pressure†	N/A	N/A	N/A	N/A
SIMV (volume control) + PS	Flow	Time, flow, pressure	Flow, volume	Time, pressure†	Pressure	Flow, pressure	Pressure	Flow, pressure,† time†
SIMV (pressure control) + PS	Pressure	Time, flow, pressure	Pressure	Time, pressure†	Pressure	Flow, pressure	Pressure	Flow, pressure,† time†
PS/CPAP	N/A	N/A	N/A	N/A	Pressure	Flow, pressure	Pressure	Flow, pressure,† time†
Volume support	N/A	N/A	N/A	N/A	Pressure	Flow, pressure	Pressure	Flow, pressure,† time†

Modified from Chatburn RL, Lough MD, Primiano FP Jr: Mechanical ventilation. In Chatburn RL, Lough MD, editors: *Handbook of respiratory care*, ed 2. St Louis. Mosby, 1990; pp 159-223.

PRVC, Pressure-regulated volume control; *SIMV,* synchronized intermittent mandatory ventilation; *PS,* pressure support; *CPAP,* continuous positive airway pressure; *N/A,* not applicable.

*Mandatory breaths can be manually triggered in all modes.

†Secondary or safety cycle variable.

‡If AutoMode is activated, ventilator automatically switches between "control" mode and "support" mode depending on spontaneous breathing activity.

§The inspiratory rise time setting can be used to modify the shape of the control waveform (pressure or flow) for mandatory and spontaneous breaths in all modes.

an optional ventilator graphics and mechanics monitoring package that provides the ability to monitor a variety of scalar waveforms, loops, and mechanics parameters.

Alarms. The Servo 300A prioritizes alarm conditions and communicates the specific level of urgency by a combination of audible, visual, and textual alerts. Most audible alarms can be temporarily silenced for a period of up to 2 minutes.

Input power alarms. The air or oxygen gas supply alarm activates if the respective gas pressure is lost or falls outside of the working range of 24 to 96 psig. In the event of main electrical power failure, the AC electrical power loss alarm activates and the ventilator automatically switches over to internal battery power. A fully charged battery maintains ventilator operation for about 30 minutes. Low battery power and loss of battery power are signaled by specific alarm messages.

Control circuit alarms. If ventilator controls are set so that the resulting inspiratory flow rate exceeds the maximum flow rate for the selected patient range setting, the technical alarm is activated and an "over-range" text message is displayed. A variety of other technical error messages are displayed in the event of electronic and control circuit problems.

Output alarms. The upper (high) pressure alarm is activated and inspiration cycled to expiration if airway pressure reaches the alarm setting. The high continuous pressure alarm is activated if measured airway pressure is equivalent to set PEEP plus 15 cm H_2O for more than 15 seconds.

High and low minute volume alarms are set relative to the measured expiratory minute volume. The alarm setting automatically rescales when the ventilator's neonatal patient range is selected. The apnea alarm is activated if the time interval between two triggered breaths exceeds 20 seconds in the adult patient range, 15 seconds in the pediatric range, and 10 seconds in the neonatal range.

High and low oxygen concentration alarms are automatically set to ±6% of the set oxygen concentration. Additionally, disconnection of the oxygen analyzer sensor elicits an O_2 sensor alarm.

HOME CARE VENTILATORS

PURITAN-BENNETT LP-10 AND LP-6 PLUS VENTILATORS

The Puritan-Bennett LP-10 (Fig. 17-14) and LP-6 Plus Ventilators (Puritan-Bennett) are electrically powered (AC, internal battery, or external 12 volt

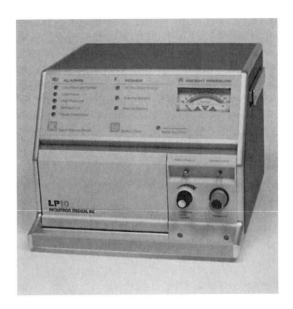

Fig. 17-14

Puritan-Bennett LP-10 Ventilator. (Courtesy Puritan-Bennett, Pleasanton, Calif.)

battery) and electronically (microprocessor) and pneumatically controlled. Power conversion and transmission are accomplished by a brushless motor and piston and an external pneumatic exhalation valve. The difference between the LP-10 and LP-6 Plus is that only the LP-10 has a pressure limit control. Mandatory breaths are time or pressure triggered, pressure limited (LP-10 only), and volume or pressure cycled. Spontaneous breathing is not actively supported by the ventilator.[27]

Power Conversion and Transmission. During the return (back) stroke of the motor-driven piston, gas is drawn into the ventilator through an inlet valve on the rear panel and accumulated in the piston cylinder. With the forward stroke of the piston, gas flows past a nonadjustable pressure-relief valve before entering the patient circuit. A separate gas line branches from the main gas flow channel to regulate the exhalation valve of the patient circuit. This gas flow pressurizes the exhalation valve diaphragm during the mandatory inspiratory phase so that the main gas flow through the circuit is directed to the patient.

Control. The LP-10 and LP-6 Plus can be operated in the A/C, SIMV, and pressure-cycle modes. In the stand-by mode, only the ventilators' battery recharging function is active. Both ventilators also provide backup ventilation.

Breath rate (1 to 38 breaths per minute), tidal volume (100 to 2200 ml), inspiratory time (0.5 to 5.5 seconds), and patient effort (–10 to +10 cm H_2O) are set in all modes. In the assist-control and pressure-cycle modes, all breaths are mandatory and are either time triggered at an interval determined by the breath rate setting or pressure triggered with each spontaneous breathing effort that drops circuit pressure to the set patient effort threshold. In SIMV, mandatory breaths are time or pressure triggered at the set breath rate. To accomplish spontaneous breathing between mandatory breaths in the SIMV mode, the patient must draw gas through the piston chamber or through the exhalation valve of the patient circuit.

When used as a volume controller in the A/C and SIMV modes, the microprocessor controls the stop point of the piston during its backstroke (refilling) so that the set tidal volume is delivered during the forward stroke. The microprocessor also regulates piston speed to deliver the tidal volume over the set inspiratory time interval. Inspiration cycles to expiration when the piston reaches its full forward position and the set tidal volume is delivered. Inspiration is cycled prematurely if circuit pressure reaches the set high pressure alarm limit. The range of inspiratory flow rate is 20 to 100 L/min.

In the pressure-cycle mode, the inspiratory phase is cycled to expiration when inspiratory pressure reaches the set high (pressure) alarm limit, although the alarm itself does not sound. In this mode, inspiratory time and tidal volume are variable. If inspiratory pressure does not reach the set cycling pressure, inspiration is volume cycled as described earlier.

The LP-10 can also function as a pressure controller if the pressure limit control (15 to 50 cm H_2O) is used. The pressure limit control is a mechanical spring-loaded valve that functions independently of the electronic control system. During the inspiratory phase, the ventilator piston delivers the set tidal volume (as earlier), but if inspiratory pressure reaches the set pressure limit, gas is vented to atmosphere, maintaining the set pressure limit until the tidal volume is completely displaced by the piston. Specific tidal volume and inspiratory time settings determine whether (and how fast) the pressure limit is reached.

If the set SIMV breath rate is less than 6 breaths per minute and the ventilator does not detect a patient breathing effort before the end of the apnea time interval (20 seconds in SIMV, 10 seconds in A/C and pressure cycle modes), the ventilator switches to backup ventilation. Backup ventilation delivers mandatory breaths at a rate of 10 per minute at the set tidal volume.

PEEP can be applied using an external PEEP valve that attaches to the exhalation valve of the patient circuit. Because patient effort can be set up to +10 cm H_2O, patient triggering can be PEEP compensated to that level. Supplemental oxygen can be titrated into the patient circuit at the ventilator's gas flow outlet or supplied by means of an optional oxygen accumulator attached to the gas inlet.

Table 17-11 summarizes the control and phase variables for mandatory and spontaneous breaths in the operational modes available on the Puritan-Bennett LP-10 and LP-6 Plus ventilators.

Output

Waveforms. The action of the motor and piston of the LP-10 and LP-6 Plus creates a sinusoidal inspiratory flow pattern during delivery of the set tidal volume. When the pressure limit control is

TABLE 17-11	**CONTROL AND PHASE VARIABLES FOR MANDATORY AND SPONTANEOUS BREATHS IN THE OPERATIONAL MODES AVAILABLE ON THE PURITAN-BENNETT LP-10 AND LP-6 PLUS VENTILATORS**							
	Mandatory				**Spontaneous**			
Mode	**Control**	**Trigger**	**Limit**	**Cycle**	**Control**	**Trigger**	**Limit**	**Cycle**
A/C	Volume, pressure*	Time, pressure	N/A, pressure*	Volume, pressure†	N/A	N/A	N/A	N/A
SIMV	Volume, pressure*	Time, pressure	N/A, pressure*	Volume, pressure†	—	—	—	—
Pressure cycled	Pressure, volume‡	Time, pressure	N/A	Pressure, volume‡	N/A	N/A	N/A	N/A

Modified from Chatburn RL, Lough MD, Primiano FP Jr: Mechanical ventilation. In Chatburn RL, Lough MD, editors: *Handbook of respiratory care,* ed 2. St Louis. Mosby, 1990; pp 159-223.

A/C, Assist/control; *SIMV,* synchronized intermittent mandatory ventilation; *N/A,* not applicable; —, ventilator does not respond.

*Applies only to the LP-10, when pressure limit is used.

†Secondary or safety cycle variable.

‡Applies if tidal volume is set so that inspiratory pressure does not reach the set cycling threshold.

used (LP-10 only), an approximately rectangular pressure waveform can be produced depending on specific control settings.

Monitoring. Airway pressure throughout the ventilatory cycle is displayed on an analog pressure gauge that reflects proximal pressure measured in the patient circuit. Patient triggering is indicated by the breathing effort display.

Alarms. The LP-10 and LP-6 Plus group alarm conditions into five alarm categories: power switchover, low power, setting error, low pressure/apnea, and high pressure. Alarm conditions are further detailed only if an optional printer is connected. The ventilators also have a remote alarm connection.

Input power alarms. With the loss of AC power, the ventilator automatically switches to battery power and activates the power switchover alarm. The low power alarm activates when approximately 5 minutes of internal battery power remains.

Control circuit alarms. A setting error alarm indicates that ventilator controls are set inappropriately or beyond the capability of the ventilator. An uninterrupted audible alarm tone signals the loss of microprocessor function.

Output alarms. The low pressure/apnea alarm is activated by a variety of conditions including the following: circuit pressure remains below the low pressure alarm setting for two consecutive breaths; the low pressure alarm is set lower than PEEP or higher than the pressure limit setting (LP-10 only); failure of the ventilator to detect a patient-triggered breath within the applicable apnea time interval; and failure of the leak portion of the ventilators' self test. The high pressure alarm activates if circuit pressure reaches the high pressure alarm control setting (the high pressure alarm setting plus 10 cm H_2O during operation in the pressure cycle mode) or if the pressure relief valve fails during a system self test.

Puritan-Bennett Companion 2801 Ventilator

The Puritan-Bennett Companion 2801 Ventilator (Puritan-Bennett) (Fig. 17-15) is electrically powered (AC, internal battery, or external 12-volt battery) and electronically (microprocessor) and pneumatically controlled. For power conversion and transmission, the ventilator utilizes an electric motor-driven piston and an external pneumatic exhalation valve. The Companion 2801 is primarily a volume controller that can also function as a pressure controller. Mandatory breaths are time or pressure triggered,

flow or pressure limited, and volume cycled. Spontaneous breaths are not actively supported.[28]

Power Conversion and Transmission. Gas flow is created by the movement of a rotating crank and piston driven by an electric gear motor. During the backstroke of the piston (expiratory phase), gas is drawn into the piston chamber through a one-way inlet valve and filter located on the right side-panel of the ventilator. The forward stroke of the piston displaces the cylinder volume, directing gas past two pressure-limiting valves and through the one-way outlet valve into the patient circuit.

The exhalation valve solenoid controls a separate gas flow to a mushroom valve in the exhalation manifold of the patient circuit. During the inspiratory phase, this gas flow pressurizes (closes) the valve, directing gas flow to the patient.

Control. The Companion 2801 can be operated in the control, A/C, and SIMV modes. A no-ventilation mode setting permits recharging of the internal battery without other ventilator functions.

All operational modes require setting tidal volume (50 to 2800 ml), flow (average inspiratory flow rate, 20 to 120 L/min), and breath rate (1 to 69 breaths per minute). To ensure the set tidal volume, the microprocessor determines the position to which the piston moves during its backstroke (refilling). When a mandatory breath is triggered, the microprocessor directs the electric motor to move the piston at the speed needed to deliver the cylinder volume at the set flow rate (i.e., flow limit). Inspiration cycles to expiration when the cylinder volume is

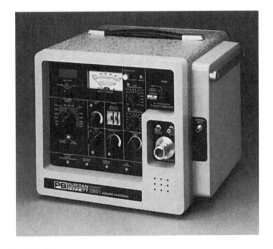

Fig. 17-15

Puritan-Bennett Companion 2801 Ventilator. (Courtesy Puritan-Bennett, Pleasanton, Calif.)

completely displaced by the movement of the piston to its full forward position. Inspiratory time is a function of set tidal volume and flow rate. Inspiration is prematurely cycled if circuit pressure reaches the high pressure alarm setting.

Mandatory breaths may be pressure controlled using the pressure limit control, a spring-loaded mechanical valve with a range of 10 to 100 cm H_2O. The pressure limit control is not graduated and must be set while observing circuit pressure on the ventilator's pressure gauge. If inspiratory pressure reaches the pressure limit setting, the pressure-limiting valve vents the remainder of the piston cylinder volume to atmosphere, maintaining the set pressure limit. The set flow rate and tidal volume influence how quickly pressure reaches the set limit.

In the control and A/C modes, all breaths are mandatory. In the control mode, mandatory breaths are time cycled at the set breath rate. In A/C mode, breaths are either time triggered or patient triggered if inspiratory effort drops circuit pressure to the pressure set using the sensitivity control (–10 to +10 cm H_2O).

In the SIMV mode, mandatory breaths are time or pressure (patient) triggered at the set breath rate. To accomplish spontaneous breathing between mandatory breaths, the patient must draw gas through the piston chamber or through the exhalation valve during the expiratory phase. If the breath rate is set to less than 8 breaths per minute in the SIMV mode and the ventilator fails to detect a patient inspiratory effort within 45 seconds, the ventilator switches to apnea ventilation. In apnea ventilation, mandatory breaths are delivered at a rate of 12 per minute; all other breath variables are determined by the control settings as described earlier.

Sigh breaths can be delivered in all operational modes. When activated, three successive sigh breaths are delivered every 10 minutes at the set sigh volume (50 to 2800 ml). Sigh breaths can also be manually triggered. PEEP can be created by adding a PEEP valve to the external exhalation manifold. Patient trigger sensitivity can be set to as high as approximately +10 cm H_2O to compensate for externally applied PEEP. Supplemental oxygen can be supplied using an optional oxygen accumulator that attaches to the ventilator's right side-panel.

Table 17-12 summarizes the control and phase variables for mandatory and spontaneous breaths in the operational modes available on the Puritan-Bennett Companion 2801 ventilator.

Output

Waveforms. The motion of the Companion 2801's piston creates a sinusoidal inspiratory flow (and volume) waveform. The resulting inspiratory pressure waveform is also sinusoidal. When the ventilator is set to pressure limit inspiration, the pressure waveform exhibits a plateau and may approximate a rectangular shape depending on the specific control settings.

Monitoring. Proximal airway pressure is displayed throughout the inspiratory and expiratory cycle on an analog pressure gauge. A digital monitoring window with a three-position switch displays electronically measured values for average inspiratory flow rate, I:E ratio, and the volume of gas displaced by the piston. A sensitivity indicator flashes with each patient breathing effort that drops proximal airway pressure to the set sensitivity threshold. The sigh indicator illuminates when the

TABLE 17-12	CONTROL AND PHASE VARIABLES FOR MANDATORY AND SPONTANEOUS BREATHS IN THE OPERATIONAL MODES AVAILABLE ON THE PURITAN-BENNETT COMPANION 2801 VENTILATOR							
	Mandatory				**Spontaneous**			
Mode	**Control**	**Trigger***	**Limit**	**Cycle**	**Control**	**Trigger**	**Limit**	**Cycle**
Control	Volume, pressure‡	Time	Flow, pressure‡	Volume, pressure†	—	—	—	—
A/C	Volume, pressure‡	Time, pressure	Flow, pressure‡	Volume, pressure†	N/A	N/A	N/A	N/A
SIMV	Volume, pressure‡	Time, pressure	Flow, pressure‡	Volume, pressure†	—	—	—	—

Modified from Chatburn RL, Lough MD, Primiano FP Jr: Mechanical ventilation. In Chatburn RL, Lough MD, editors: *Handbook of respiratory care,* ed 2. St Louis. Mosby, 1990; pp 159-223.

A/C, Assist/control; *SIMV,* synchronized intermittent mandatory ventilation; *N/A,* not applicable; —, ventilator does not respond.
*Sigh breaths can be manually triggered.
†Secondary or safety cycle variable.
‡Applies only if pressure limit control is used to limit inspiratory pressure.

next mandatory breath is scheduled to be a sigh breath.

Alarms

Input power alarms. With the loss of AC electric power, the Companion 2801 automatically switches to battery power and signals the changeover with an audible "chirping." The power indicator shows which of the three power sources is in use. A low battery alarm indicates that the voltage of the battery in use (internal or external) is below approximately 11.9 volts. Complete battery discharge is signaled by continuous long audible pulses.

Control circuit alarms. A continuous nonpulsating audio alarm and flashing front panel lamps indicate a microprocessor malfunction. The ventilator also alerts the operator when control settings result in an inverse I:E of 1:0.8 or less or in the inability of the ventilator to deliver breaths at the set rate.

Output alarms. The Companion 2801 is equipped with operator-adjustable high and low circuit pressure alarms. The apnea alarm activates if the ventilator fails to detect a patient inspiratory effort within a 15-second time interval (in SIMV) or if airway pressure remains above the low pressure alarm setting for 15 seconds or two breath cycles. The Companion 2801 is equipped with a remote alarm connection.

BEAR 33 VENTILATOR

The Bear 33 (Viasys Healthcare, Bear Medical) (Fig. 17-16) is an electrically (AC, external battery, or internal battery) powered, electronically (micro-processor) and pneumatically controlled ventilator. Power conversion and transmission are accomplished with a motor-driven piston and the external pneumatic exhalation valve of a patient circuit. The Bear 33 is a volume controller. Mandatory breaths are time or pressure triggered, flow limited, and volume cycled. Spontaneous breathing is permitted but not actively supported by the ventilator.[29]

Power Conversion and Transmission. The Bear 33 utilizes AC power, external battery power, or internal battery power in this order of priority, depending on availability. A rotary motor and piston create the gas flow for ventilation. During the piston's backstroke (expiratory phase), fresh gas is drawn into the piston cylinder through a filter and one-way inlet valve. The forward stroke of the piston (inspiratory phase) displaces the cylinder volume, causing gas to flow past the cylinder bypass check valve and an overpressure relief valve before entering the patient circuit. The overpressure relief valve opens if system pressure exceeds approximately 85 cm H_2O.

A separate gas flow branches from the main gas flow to supply the exhalation valve of the patient circuit. During the inspiratory phase, this gas source inflates the exhalation valve balloon, closing the valve and diverting the main gas flow to the patient. In the absence of gas flow to the exhalation valve during the expiratory phase, the balloon depressurizes to allow exhalation.

Control. The Bear 33 can be operated in one of the following three modes: control, A/C, and SIMV.

Ventilator controls include volume (100 to 2200 ml, set in 10-ml increments), breath rate (2 to

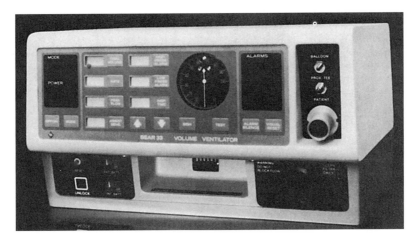

Fig. 17-16

Bear 33 Ventilator. (Courtesy Bear Medical, Palm Springs, Calif.)

40 breaths per minute), and peak flow (20 to 120 L/min). Based on the set tidal volume, the ventilator's microprocessor controls the stop position of the piston during its backstroke (refilling). During the inspiratory phase of a mandatory breath, the microprocessor regulates piston speed so that the gas volume is delivered at a rate determined by the peak flow setting (the flow limit). Thus inspiratory time is a function of the volume and flow rate settings. Inspiratory time is displayed on the front panel of the ventilator and must be in a range of 0.25 to 4.99 seconds. Inspiration is volume cycled when the piston reaches its full forward position, completely displacing cylinder volume. Inspiration is pressure cycled before the set volume is delivered if circuit pressure reaches the set high pressure alarm value.

In the control mode, mandatory breaths are time triggered at an interval determined by the set breath rate. In A/C, all breaths are mandatory and are either time triggered or patient triggered if inspiratory effort causes circuit pressure to fall to the set assist sensitivity setting (−9 to +19 cm H_2O). In SIMV, mandatory breaths are either time or pressure (patient) triggered at the set breath rate. Spontaneous breathing is permitted between mandatory breaths in both the SIMV and control modes. The patient must draw in the gas for spontaneous breathing either through the piston bypass check valve, which opens if inspiratory effort drops circuit pressure to approximately −0.2 cm H_2O, or through the relaxed exhalation valve during the backstroke of the ventilator piston. Because spontaneous breathing is also permitted between the time-triggered mandatory breaths in the control mode, this mode can be regarded as IMV.

An external PEEP valve must be attached to the exhalation manifold of the patient circuit to create positive baseline pressure. Assist sensitivity can be set up to +19 cm H_2O to compensate for externally applied PEEP. Supplemental oxygen can be delivered utilizing the oxygen accumulator accessory. If the sigh breath control is activated, sigh breaths 1.5 times the set tidal volume are delivered at a rate of 6 per hour. Sigh breaths can also be triggered manually.

Table 17-13 summarizes the control and phase variables for mandatory and spontaneous breaths in the operational modes available on the Bear 33 ventilator.

Output

Waveforms. The motion of the Bear 33 piston produces sinusoidal inspiratory flow and volume waveforms. The resulting inspiratory pressure waveform is also sinusoidal.

Monitoring. Airway pressure, measured in the patient circuit, is displayed throughout the ventilatory cycle on an analog pressure gauge. Tidal volume, peak flow rate, and inspiratory time are also displayed, but reflect set or calculated—versus measured—values. The letter "A" appears on the sensitivity display when a mandatory breath is patient triggered.

Alarms

Input power alarms. The power source change alarm activates when the ventilator switches from a higher to lower priority electric power source (e.g., from AC to external battery). A low internal battery alarm indicates that internal battery power is less than 25% of full capacity. Failure of the internal power supply or battery power insufficient to operate the ventilator results in a ventilator inoperative condition.

TABLE 17-13	**CONTROL AND PHASE VARIABLES FOR MANDATORY AND SPONTANEOUS BREATHS IN THE OPERATIONAL MODES AVAILABLE ON THE BEAR 33 VENTILATOR**							
	Mandatory				**Spontaneous**			
Mode	Control	Trigger*	Limit	Cycle	Control	Trigger	Limit	Cycle
Control	Volume	Time	Flow	Volume, pressure†	—	—	—	—
A/C	Volume	Time, pressure	Flow	Volume, pressure†	N/A	N/A	N/A	N/A
SIMV	Volume	Time, pressure	Flow	Volume, pressure†	—	—	—	—

Modified from Chatburn RL, Lough MD, Primiano FP Jr: Mechanical ventilation. In Chatburn RL, Lough MD, editors: *Handbook of respiratory care,* ed 2. St Louis. Mosby, 1990; pp 159-223.
A/C, Assist/control; *SIMV,* synchronized intermittent mandatory ventilation; *N/A,* not applicable; —, ventilator does not respond.
*Sigh breaths can be manually triggered.
†Secondary or safety cycle variable.

Control circuit alarms. The ventilator inoperative alarm also activates if the ventilator fails to cycle, with a timing circuit failure, or if ventilator control settings result in inspiratory time outside the acceptable range of 0.25 to 4.99 seconds.

Output alarms. High and low pressure alarms are operator adjustable. The apnea alarm is activated if the ventilator fails to detect a spontaneous or mandatory breath within a 20-second time period.

REFERENCES

1. Banner MJ, Blanch P, Desautels DA: Mechanical ventilators. In Kirby RR, Banner MJ, Downs JB, editors: *Clinical applications of ventilatory support.* New York. Churchill Livingstone, 1990; pp 401-503.
2. Kirby RR et al: A new pediatric volume ventilator. *Anesth Analg* 1970; 50:533-537.
3. Chatburn RL: A new system for understanding mechanical ventilators. *Respir Care* 1991; 36:1123-1155.
4. Chatburn RL: Classification of mechanical ventilators. *Respir Care* 1992; 37:1009-1025.
5. Chatburn RL, Lough MD, Primiano FP Jr: Mechanical ventilation. In Chatburn RL, Lough MD, editors: *Handbook of respiratory care,* ed 2. St Louis. Mosby, 1990; pp 159-223.
6. Spearman CB, Sanders HG Jr: Physical principles and functional designs of ventilators. In Kirby RR, Banner MJ, Downs JB, editors: *Clinical applications of ventilatory support.* New York. Churchill Livingstone, 1990; pp 63-104.
7. Branson RD, MacIntyre NR: Dual control modes of mechanical ventilation. *Respir Care* 1996; 41:294-302.
8. Mushin M, Rendell-Baker W, Thompson PW: *Automatic ventilation of the lungs,* ed 3. Oxford. Blackwell-Scientific, 1980; pp 62-166.
9. Branson RD, Chatburn RL: Technical description and classification of modes of ventilator operation. *Respir Care* 1992; 37:1026-1044.
10. *Instruction manual: Bear Cub 750vs Infant Ventilator.* Riverside, Calif. Bear Medical Systems, 1996.
11. *Operating instructions: Babylog 8000 plus Infant Care Ventilator,* Software 5.n, ed 1. Telford, Penn. Drager, Inc, 1997.
12. Frembgen S: Extending the power of conventional ventilation. *Neonatal Intensive Care* 1991; 4:30-36.
13. *Operating instructions: Infant Star® 500/950 Ventilators.* Pleasanton, Calif. Puritan-Bennett, Inc, 1996.
14. *User's manual: Model IV-200 SAVI System, Rev 7.* Anaheim, Calif. Sechrist Industries, Inc, 1997.
15. *Instruction manual: V.I.P. Bird Infant-Pediatric Ventilator.* Palm Springs, Calif. Bird Products Corp, 1991.
16. *Instruction manual: Bird Partner Volume Monitor.* Palm Springs, Calif. Bird Products Corp, 1991.
17. *Flow synchronization upgrade: addendum to the V.I.P. Bird Infant-Pediatric Ventilator and Partner Volume Monitor instruction manuals.* Palm Springs, Calif. Bird Products Corp, 1992.
18. *Operating instructions: Evita 4 Intensive Care Ventilator.* Chantilly, Vir. Drager, Inc, 1996.
19. *NeoFlow Neonatal Mode: addendum to operating instructions Evita 4* (as of software 2.n) *Evita 2 dura* (as of software 3.10). Telford, Penn. Drager, Inc, 1999.
20. *Operator's and technical reference manual: 840™ Ventilator System.* Carlsbad, Calif. Nellcor Puritan-Bennett Inc, 1998.
21. *BiLevel Option/800 Series Ventilators.* Carlsbad, Calif. Puritan-Bennett, Inc, 1998.
22. *Operating manual: Newport Wave Ventilator Model E200.* Newport Beach, Calif. Newport Medical Instruments Inc, 1998.
23. *Operating/service manual: Compass Ventilation Monitor Model VM200.* Newport Beach, Calif. Newport Medical Instruments, Inc, 1993.
24. *Operating manual: Siemens Servo Ventilator 900C,* English ed 3. Solna, Sweden. Siemens-Elema AB, 1984.
25. *Service manual: Siemens Servo Ventilator 900C/L,* English ed 3. Solna, Sweden. Siemens-Elema AB, 1984.
26. *Operating manual 8.0/9.0: Servo Ventilator 300/300A,* English ed 1. Solna, Sweden. Siemens-Elema AB, 1996.
27. *Users manual: LP-6 Plus Volume Ventilator and LP-10 Volume Ventilator with Pressure Limit.* Minneapolis, Minn. Aequitron Medical, 1994.
28. *Operating instruction manual—Issue B: Companion 2801 Volume Ventilator.* Lenexa, Kan. Puritan-Bennett Corp, 1990.
29. *Instruction Manual: Bear 33 Volume Ventilator: Clinical, #50000-10133.* Riverside, Calif. Bear Medical Systems, Inc, 1984.

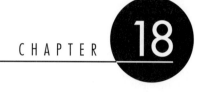

CHAPTER **18**

Continuous Positive Airway Pressure

Michael P. Czervinske

First introduced in the 1930s as continuous distending pressure, continuous positive airway pressure (CPAP) was reintroduced by Gregory and associates in 1971 as therapy for premature infants with respiratory distress syndrome (RDS), known at the time as idiopathic RDS. Despite the use of positive-pressure ventilation in these infants, atelectasis persisted. After observing expiratory grunting in these infants, Gregory and associates believed that the grunting played a role in decreasing or preventing the atelectasis. However, after intubation, the tube interrupted the grunting maneuver by preventing exhalation against a closed glottis. Gregory and associates believed that CPAP could replicate the physiologic effect of grunting. With CPAP, infants who were given a 25% chance of survival actually had an 80% survival rate.[1] After this pioneering research, CPAP became a standard therapy for early intervention of RDS, as well as therapy for other disorders, including apnea of prematurity, obstructive apnea, tracheobronchial malacia, and problems resulting in pulmonary volume loss.

PHYSIOLOGIC EFFECTS OF CONTINUOUS POSITIVE AIRWAY PRESSURE

There are several terms used to describe the application of positive pressure on expiration (Table 18-1). CPAP occurs when positive pressure is applied to the airways throughout the respiratory cycle of a spontaneously breathing patient.[2,3] CPAP applied to the neonate or pediatric patient has various physiologic effects on several organ systems, including the pulmonary, cardiovascular, central nervous, and renal systems.

PULMONARY SYSTEM

Applying CPAP maintains positive inspiratory and expiratory pressures and therefore increases mean airway pressure. Elevating mean airway pressure throughout both respiratory phases prevents early

TABLE 18-1	TERMS USED TO DESCRIBE POSITIVE PRESSURE
Term	**Definition**
CPAP	Application of positive airway pressure throughout the respiratory cycle to spontaneously breathing patients
EPAP	Application of positive airway pressure during exhalation to spontaneously breathing patients, with airway pressure becoming subatmospheric during inspiration
CDP	Application of either positive or negative pressure to maintain increased transpulmonary pressures throughout the respiratory cycle to spontaneously breathing patients
PEEP	Application of positive airway pressure during exhalation to a mechanically ventilated patient

CPAP, Continuous positive airway pressure; *EPAP,* expiratory positive airway pressure; *CDP,* continuous distending pressure; *PEEP,* positive end-expiratory pressure.

BOX 18-1

OVERALL EFFECTS OF CPAP

PHYSIOLOGIC
Increases mean airway pressure
    Increases functional residual capacity
    Improves static compliance
    Improves minute ventilation
    Improves oxygenation
    Prevents early terminal airway closure
    Decreases critical opening pressure of collapsed alveoli
    Minimizes distance of alveolar stretch
    Uniformly distributes transpulmonary pressure
    Redistributes lung fluid
    Maintains integrity of surfactant
    Alters control of breathing reflexes
    Decreases work of breathing

MECHANICAL
    Pneumatic stent of obstructed airway structures
    Continuous stimulation preventing apnea

---

terminal airway closure and improves ventilation to areas with a low ventilation-perfusion ratio.[3] The resulting reduction in airway resistance improves ventilation and oxygenation.[3,4] Uniform distribution of transpulmonary pressures maintains the patency of these terminal airways, whereas the upper and larger airways are kept patent by means of the direct distending effect of CPAP.[4,5]

Neonatal pulmonary compliance includes characteristics of the chest wall and rib cage. High chest wall compliance and insufficient elastic recoil to maintain an adequate functional residual capacity (FRC) result in low resting lung volumes. The neonate must begin each inspiration from a low resting lung volume and generate high opening pressures with each breath. Added to this is a surfactant deficiency in the premature neonate. All of this greatly increases the work of breathing (WOB) and may lead to respiratory distress, muscle fatigue, and apnea. The application of CPAP can stabilize the chest wall and provide an adequate FRC as well as reduce the WOB.[3,6-8]

The increase in FRC after CPAP is applied results in expansion of previously collapsed alveoli, accomplished in part by improving collateral ventilation.[9] An increase in respiratory rate may result when applying CPAP to an infant with RDS. This is believed to be caused by stimulation of the Hering-Breuer reflex when the FRC is increased.[10,11] CPAP increases alveolar and pulmonary vascular pressures independently of interstitial pressure. The increase in pressure across the capillary wall increases the

movement of water into the interstitium of the lung.[12] The redistribution of lung fluid also helps improve FRC.

PaO_2 usually increases after CPAP is applied.[13,14] The optimum level of CPAP produces maximum alveolar recruitment, FRC, and PaO_2, with the least amount of cardiac embarrassment, overdistention, or reduction in pulmonary blood flow. Surpassing optimum CPAP levels results in a fall in PaO_2 and a rising $PaCO_2$.[14,15] An optimum level of CPAP prevents alveolar collapse, reduces consumption of surfactant, and may even enhance surfactant production via cholinergic mechanisms.[7,16] Box 18-1 summarizes the overall effects of CPAP.[3,7,16,17]

CARDIOVASCULAR SYSTEM

CPAP increases intrathoracic pressure and may reduce venous return and compromise cardiac output. Any decrease in venous return reduces right ventricular preload, which decreases cardiac output and leads to a decrease in right ventricular end-diastolic volume and stroke volume. Cardiac function may also be compromised from changes in coronary perfusion caused by CPAP. Coronary perfusion depends on a pressure gradient to supply blood flow to the myocardium. Altering systemic and intrathoracic pressure may decrease myocardial perfusion and left ventricular function.[18] Lung compliance plays an important role in the transmission of pressure to the intrathoracic structures. The stiffer the lungs, the lesser the amount of pressure transmitted to the vascular system. CPAP may lead to a reduction in pulmonary vascular resistance (PVR) because of improved oxygenation. However, excessive levels of CPAP in a neonate with relatively normal lung compliance may compress the pulmonary vasculature, causing a rise in PVR and dead space ventilation. Additionally, an increase in PVR results in a shift of the intraventricular septum to the left and inhibits left ventricular filling, further decreasing cardiac output. When properly administered, CPAP produces a reduction in PVR and reduces the amount of right-to-left shunting via the patent ductus arteriosus and foramen ovale, thereby improving oxygenation.[19]

RENAL SYSTEM

CPAP causing reduced cardiac output may decrease renal perfusion and urine output. Changes in cardiac output may also stimulate the pituitary gland to secrete antidiuretic hormone, which further reduces urinary output.[20]

INTRACRANIAL PRESSURE

A reduced venous return can lead to an increase in intracranial pressure (ICP). A change in cerebral blood flow is a risk factor for intraventricular hemorrhage in the preterm infant. Increased incidences of intraventricular hemorrhage have not been associated with nasal or endotracheal tube (ETT) CPAP,[21] although such complications have been associated with older devices used to apply infant CPAP.[7]

INDICATIONS

The indications for CPAP in the neonatal and pediatric population fall into two categories: (1) clinical states that require an increased FRC and (2) clinical states that require positive pressure to maintain the patency of hypotonic airways (Box 18-2).[17,22] Because CPAP therapy is designed to assist spontaneously breathing patients, it is necessary that the patients for whom it is used have an intact respiratory drive.[2]

Early intervention with CPAP, especially when combined with surfactant administration, significantly alters the course of RDS in the newborn. Early intervention leads to a marked reduction in the severity of the disease, as well as prevents further alveolar collapse, thus enhancing surfactant stabilization and production.[7,16,23,24] These actions reduce the need for mechanical ventilation and high F_{IO_2} levels. Infants eventually requiring assisted ventilation tend to have reduced distending pressures and a less severe clinical course, with a marked reduction in barotrauma, and ventilator time.[16,23,25]

BOX 18-2

INDICATIONS FOR CONTINUOUS POSITIVE AIRWAY PRESSURE

DECREASED FUNCTIONAL RESIDUAL CAPACITY
Pneumonia
Pneumonitis
Atelectasis
Pulmonary edema
Smoke inhalation
Meconium aspiration
Postoperative thoracotomy
Respiratory distress syndrome
Transient tachypnea of the newborn
Congenital heart defects with left-to-right shunting

HYPOTONIC AIRWAYS
Mixed apnea
Apnea of prematurity
Obstructive sleep apnea
Tracheobronchial malacia

OTHER
Physiologic continuous positive airway pressure
Weaning from mechanical ventilation

When an infant is being weaned from mechanical ventilation, CPAP must be applied with caution. CPAP through an ETT, or tracheotomy tube, can assist in assessing the infant's ability to maintain adequate spontaneous ventilation before extubation. Once the ability to wean is established, the infant can be extubated from a low rate of 8 or 10 breaths per minute and placed on nasal CPAP to avoid complications associated with an elevated WOB through the ETT.[24,26] Early extubation to nasal CPAP in preterm infants avoids later complications of intubation and mechanical ventilation that lead to failure to extubate. It is not associated with an increase in complications related to nasal CPAP.[27]

One of the most common uses for nasally applied CPAP is to reduce apnea spells related to apnea of prematurity. As discussed earlier, CPAP stabilizes the compliant chest wall of the newborn as well as increasing FRC and stimulating respiration by altering stretch receptor reflexes.[28,29] Additionally, control of the respiratory center in newborns is influenced by sleep state, which may also be altered by applying CPAP.[29] The resulting stimulation increases respiratory rate and helps to prevent apnea.[10,11]

CPAP may reduce respiratory distress in patients with congenital heart defects, especially those associated with increased pulmonary blood flow, such as atrial septal defect, ventricular septal defect, patent ductus arteriosus, and endocardial cushion defect.

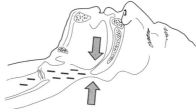

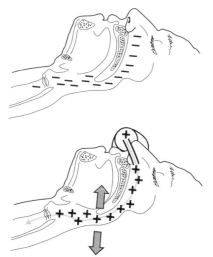

Fig. 18-1

Top left, Normal patent upper airway. *Top right*, Tongue obstructing upper airway. *Bottom*, CPAP distending structures of oropharynx, preventing obstruction by the tongue and soft palate.

Patients with these defects have decreased lung compliance, reduced FRC, and hypoxemia. Pulmonary edema may also be present. Increasing intrathoracic pressures can reduce pulmonary blood flow through the pulmonary artery and pulmonary capillaries.[7,18]

During the postoperative period, CPAP is useful in patients who have undergone thoracotomy. Atelectasis is common in these patients and often develops in the area of the lung closest to the surgical site. Applying CPAP reverses atelectasis, stabilizes the chest wall, improves overall ventilation, and maintains an adequate FRC. CPAP can also be helpful in treating patients who have undergone abdominal surgeries that result in compression of the lungs postoperatively, such as procedures for gastroschisis, omphalocele, and short-gut syndrome.

Disorders that require positive pressure to stent the airways open respond to CPAP. The positive pressure of CPAP exerts force to stabilize the airway walls, thereby reducing the tendency for collapse.[4,5,7] Disorders in this category include tracheobronchial malacia, obstructive sleep apnea, and mixed apnea. Abnormal tracheal cartilage characterizes congenital, or iatrogenic, tracheobronchial malacia. Respiratory distress, airway collapse, air trapping, and the inability to wean from assisted ventilation are frequent problems in these patients.[30-32] Supporting these obstructing structures with an artificial airway and CPAP helps preserve airway patency (Fig. 18-1).[4,5]

Questions continue to exist concerning physiologic positive end-expiratory pressure (PEEP) or CPAP. The initial study analyzed the PaO_2 and FRC in 16 intubated patients at varying levels of PEEP and after extubation. It was concluded that 2 cm H_2O of PEEP mirrored the effects of the glottis in the nonintubated infants.[33] Adult studies have not

been conclusive; however, for intubated infants, low levels of PEEP or CPAP are indicated to reduce the possible risk of decreased FRC and atelectasis.[34,35]

CPAP must be used cautiously in the infant with meconium aspiration. In the acute phase, meconium aspiration leads to a ball-valve type of obstruction and a chemical pneumonitis with unstable airways. The results are a combination of focal areas of atelectasis and alveolar overdistention. Ventilation-perfusion abnormalities lead to hypoxia, hypercarbia, and acidosis. CPAP levels of 4 to 6 cm H_2O may help stabilize the distal airways, thereby improving areas of atelectasis and avoiding even greater distention of already hyperinflated areas. The objective is to allow these areas to return to normal function. However, many patients with meconium aspiration also have pulmonary hypertension and increased PVR. Any further increase in the PVR caused by CPAP can worsen the degree of right-to-left shunting via the foramen ovale and patent ductus arteriosus.[7,22]

COMPLICATIONS AND CONTRAINDICATIONS

ADVERSE PHYSIOLOGIC RESPONSES

Overdistention caused by CPAP administration may lead to several pulmonary problems, including barotrauma, reduced static lung compliance, decreased pulmonary capillary blood flow, increased WOB, reduced minute ventilation, carbon dioxide retention, excessive expiratory work, and ventilation-perfusion mismatch. In clinical situations such as patchy or unilateral lung disease, the positive pressure maintained by CPAP may further distend the hyperinflated portions of the lung and cause excessive intraalveolar pressure. This increased pressure results in a decreased pulmonary capillary blood flow to hyperinflated lung units and shunts the blood to the low-pressure, poorly ventilated alveoli, thereby increasing venous admixture and hypoxemia.[36]

The reported incidence of pulmonary barotrauma ranges from 0.5% to 38%, with the average being approximately 10%.[37-40] Many factors interrelate to produce the syndrome of barotrauma, including (1) the nature and degree of lung disease; (2) the age of the patient, with infants and children having a higher incidence; (3) ventilator settings; and (4) level of CPAP used. Pneumothorax is the most dangerous manifestation of pulmonary barotrauma. Venous return can become compromised to the point of cardiovascular collapse and require resuscitation. Another barotrauma complication that occurs in infants is pulmonary interstitial emphysema.

Cardiovascular depression is the most often cited adverse physiologic response to CPAP. The addition of positive intrathoracic pressure in patients with compromised cardiac function or hypovolemia can decrease cardiac output to the point of life-threatening hypotension. In patients with chronic right ventricular dysfunction, the application of CPAP can significantly affect pulmonary blood flow and cause an increased PVR, resulting in extra work for the right ventricle. Many patients, however, can be successfully treated with volume expanders or inotropic agents, or both, to prevent these adverse cardiovascular effects.[17,41]

CPAP may increase the ICP and decrease cerebral perfusion pressure to the point that cerebral ischemia and neurologic damage occur. Patients with an increased ICP or those who are at risk of an increased ICP may be treated with CPAP; however, the ICP and neurologic function should be closely monitored.[22] If CPAP is applied, measures to lower the ICP should be instituted, such as cerebral diuresis and elevation of the head of the bed.[20,42]

The application of positive pressure has been documented to decrease urine output as well as creatinine clearance and urinary sodium secretion.[43] The decrease in venous return and cardiac output that may develop during CPAP can aggravate previously compromised renal function. If reduced urine output occurs, treatment with fluids or drugs that increase renal blood flow should be considered.

AIRWAY COMPLICATIONS

Complications associated with the airway are usually related to the device used to deliver the CPAP. The most frequent complications associated with CPAP are related to the artificial airway used to provide CPAP (ETT or tracheostomy tube) and include mucosal damage, pressure necrosis, malposition of the tube, tracheal erosion, tracheal steno-

sis, and accidental extubation. The most common complication is partial or complete obstruction of the airway.

Mask-delivered CPAP is associated with other complications, such as aerophagia, gastric distention, aspiration of gastric contents, damage to facial tissue, nasal bridge pain, and eye irritation.[7,22] Orogastric tubes may be used to decompress the stomach and relieve the distention. CPAP delivered through nasal prongs may cause nasal irritation, septal distortion, or mucosal damage. Nasal prongs may become plugged with mucus, kink, or become displaced with patient movement or when equipment is attached.

MECHANICAL FAILURE

As with any electric- or gas-powered system, the loss of the power source is an ongoing hazard. All CPAP systems should contain an alarm, either built in or added, as an auxiliary system to notify the caregiver of a mechanical failure. Oxygenation should be monitored continuously using a transcutaneous monitor or a pulse oximeter.

CONTRAINDICATIONS

Before CPAP is started, each patient is carefully evaluated and the benefits and risks involved are considered. Although there are no absolute contraindications to CPAP therapy, there are several clinical situations in which the benefits of therapy are minimal or in which extreme caution is required.[2,41] These situations include (1) untreated or tension pneumothorax, (2) increased frequency of apneic episodes, (3) respiratory failure with inability to maintain an effective tidal volume without mechanical ventilation, and (4) severe cardiovascular instability. One contraindication exists, however, for using infant nasal CPAP. CPAP should not be used if a congenital diaphragmatic hernia is suspected because nasal CPAP may increase intestinal gas distention within the thorax.[32]

DELIVERY SYSTEMS

Several devices are available to supply CPAP in infants and children.[8,44-49] For the purpose of this chapter, the term *system* is used to describe the gas source, pressure-producing unit, and various components of that unit, such as the circuit, heat and humidification source, reservoir bag, and alarms. The term *patient interface* refers to the device used to deliver CPAP from the system to the patient. A CPAP system may be a relatively small anesthesia bag system, a freestanding reservoir system, or a mechanical ventilator-supplied system (Fig. 18-2). Systems operate using either continuous flow or demand flow.

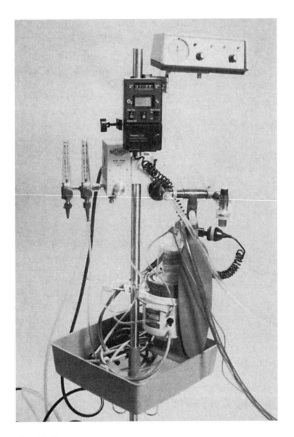

Fig. 18-2

Freestanding CPAP system with reservoir bag.

CONTINUOUS-FLOW SYSTEM

A continuous-flow system provides a noninterrupted supply of gas and does not require the infant to initiate a breath to begin gas flow (Fig. 18-3). Also, some infant ventilators offer continuous flow as an option for providing CPAP. Setting the flow two to three times the patient's estimated minute ventilation usually provides adequate flow. To verify adequate flow delivery, the clinician should observe the manometer and set the flow so that pressure fluctuates less than 2 cm H_2O during inspiration and does not drop below 2 cm H_2O.[2,22,41] To monitor pressure and possible disconnections, with this type of flow delivery, the pressure sensing line is placed as close to the patient interface as possible. Adding a reservoir bag to the circuit theoretically helps compensate for fluctuations in volume and system pressure. The flow and volume should be large enough to allow a vital capacity breath from the bag while maintaining it fully distended.[17]

Another type of continuous-flow system utilizes a fluidic nasal interface and a flow generator (Fig. 18-4).[44] The design of the nasal interface pro-

vides flow to the infant during inspiration and directs flow away from the infant during exhalation. Some have referred to this as a variable flow device, and others call it a fluid device.[50,51] The design helps stabilize airway pressure during the entire respiratory cycle and reduce the work associated with breathing against the continuous flow.[44] These devices require a flow driver unit that controls FIO_2, monitors pressure, and provides alarms. An increase in FRC, lower respiratory rate, and a lower oxygen requirement are reported when compared with conventional CPAP systems.[50,52]

Caution must be used when applying these systems because such increases in lung volume may result in higher than expected tidal volume and possible air leak complications, especially after surfactant administration. Careful monitoring and prudent application of initial pressure will alleviate such a problem. Additionally, some studies have not been able to determine a statistical difference between improvement with conventional CPAP and variable-flow CPAP.[53,54] However, despite similar improvement with either method of applying CPAP flow, WOB indices appear to be reduced during variable-flow style CPAP.[50]

DEMAND-FLOW SYSTEM

The demand-flow system is the one most often incorporated into mechanical ventilators. It requires the patient to initiate the release of gas flow by triggering, or opening, a valve. Common triggering mechanisms are flow, pressure, or possibly abdominal motion. Flow triggering during CPAP has been shown in adults to reduce the WOB when compared with pressure triggering.[55] Most modern infant ventilators incorporate flow triggering as the means of initiating CPAP flow. The gas flow to the patient is directly related to the patient's inspiratory effort: the greater the inspiratory effort, the more flow to the patient. As an additional measure to reduce work, most demand-flow systems now incorporate a low background, or bias, flow rather than triggering from a static state between breaths.[45] Using a demand-flow system allows for monitoring pulmonary mechanics along with alarm parameters and pressure levels.[2,22]

Care should be taken to ensure that a patient's WOB is not increased when a demand-flow system is used.[2] Rebreathing of exhaled gases may occur if a patient is unable to trigger the demand valve. The introduction of a background flow into ventilator demand systems has minimized this problem, with flow set high enough to prevent auto cycling. Adding a reservoir bag or additional continuous flow to demand CPAP devices should be avoided because it will prevent sufficient change in patient flow to trigger demand flow from the ventilator.

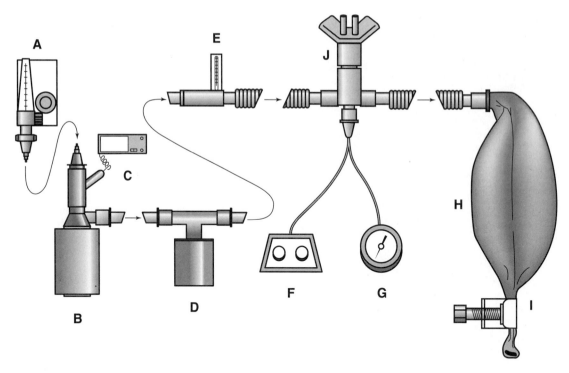

Fig. 18-3

Continuous flow CPAP system with nasal prongs. **A,** Blender or O_2-air gas flow. **B,** Heater-humidifier. **C,** O_2 analyzer. **D,** Water trap. **E,** Thermometer. **F,** High-low pressure alarm. **G,** Pressure manometer. **H,** Reservoir bag. **I,** Pigtail clamp (flow resistor). **J,** Nasal prongs.

Fig. 18-4

Illustration of the SensorMedics fluidic NCPAP generator, with a swivel and flex joint to reduce torque to the infant's nose. The middle line is the inspiratory flow line that produces the fluidic change in flow between inspiration and expiration. (Courtesy SensorMedics, Inc., Yorba Linda, Calif.)

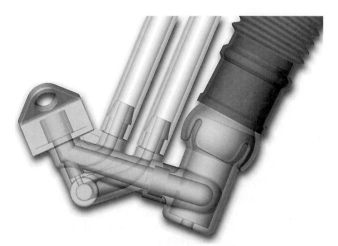

In a patient demonstrating respiratory muscle fatigue and impending respiratory failure, minimizing the WOB by applying CPAP may help prevent respiratory insufficiency. When comparing continuous- and demand-flow systems, it is important to consider the exact mechanism related to initiating flow and how each design impacts WOB. Early studies using pressure triggering favored continuous flow to reduce WOB.[56] Since then, flow triggering has demonstrated significant reduction in WOB studies with CPAP and may have advantages when compared with continuous-flow CPAP in some preterm infants.[45,54,57,58]

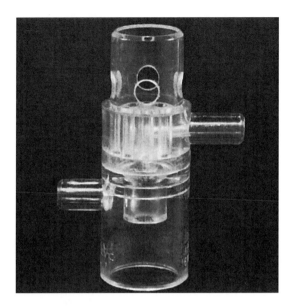

Fig. 18-5

Dupaco Carden device (Carden valve). (Courtesy MPI-Dupaco, Oceanside, Calif.)

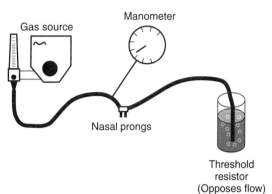

Fig. 18-6

Continuous flow CPAP system demonstrating a threshold resistor.

RESISTORS

Either a flow or threshold resistor controls the pressure level during CPAP.[22] The resistor opposes the flow and the resulting baseline pressure forms from the backpressure in the circuit. Resistors are an important element when evaluating devices because they affect the WOB. However, factors that affect WOB depend on the individual resistor's design and the entire CPAP system used, rather than on the type of resistor used.[58-60]

A flow resistor requires a continuous flow and uses a variable or fixed orifice that restricts gas flow as it exits the system (see Fig. 18-3). Some anesthesia bags use a variable orifice to adjust the CPAP level with an adjustable clamp or pigtail adaptor. When a fixed orifice is used, the CPAP level is adjusted by varying the flow rate. A flow resistor usually works best in a clinical situation requiring low flow and low pressure.[22]

The Dupaco Carden Device (MPI-Dupaco) is a type of flow resistor (Fig. 18-5). It is a small, lightweight, plastic device that attaches directly to the endotracheal or tracheostomy tube. By entraining gas from around a jet, it creates a resistance to expiratory flow, thereby resulting in CPAP. It has two ports, one to attach a proximal airway pressure manometer and the other for the source gas. Because of the flow dynamics through the device, the amount of flow is approximately equal to the amount of CPAP. For example, a flow rate of 5 L/min results in a CPAP of 5 cm H_2O,

and a flow rate of 8 L/min results in a CPAP of 8 cm H_2O. Additional small holes may be desired for ease of air entrainment at lower flow rates or as a safety mechanism in case of occlusion of gas outflow. Dead space volume of the valve alone is approximately 2 ml; however, other adapters may increase it. The device may be used continuously or while transporting a patient requiring CPAP. It is also designed to accept humidification systems, which attach to the open end opposite the airway. By using a simple flow driver, or other humidified oxygen source, such as an oxygen enricher, a simple CPAP system can be adapted for hospital or home use.

A threshold resistor produces CPAP by applying a force to oppose gas flow at the outlet and prevent the system pressure from dropping to less than the desired level. Pressure is placed against the one-way valve or diaphragm by any number of methods, including a spring-tension device, water column, or opposing gas flow (Fig. 18-6).

A threshold resistor usually works best in a clinical situation requiring higher flow and higher pressure.[22] At low flows, a threshold resistor will vibrate, or oscillate, as a result of the capacitance of the resistor. At very low flows, a critical volume builds up at the resistor before it discharges, creating a vibrating, honking, or oscillating effect. The lower the flow, the lower the frequency of oscillation. The formula of flow integrated over time determines the critical volume. Although such a volume may be small, or possibly insignificant, compared with tidal volume, in certain circumstances it may have beneficial physiologic effects.[61,62] Oscillation during CPAP possibly improves gas exchange, lowers WOB, and helps calm and comfort the infant. However, it does not appear to alter blood gas values, and any benefit may depend on the entire system versus this one component. The oscillation may also cause discomfort and irritation if the nasal prongs or artificial airway does not fit properly.[22]

ADDITIONAL SYSTEM COMPONENTS

In addition to the fresh gas source and a pressure-producing device, other components that must be incorporated into a CPAP system include a heater and humidifier, a disconnect and high pressure alarm, as well as a circuit, and a patient interface device. The circuit should be flexible and lightweight to prevent traction and torque on the patient interface device. A pressure relief or "pop-off" device prevents excessive pressure from developing in the circuit and is advisable for all systems. A guideline to setting the pop-off valve is 2 to 4 cm H_2O greater than the desired CPAP level. For example, for a CPAP of 6 cm H_2O, the pop-off valve should be set at 8 to 10 cm H_2O. A pressure manometer is necessary to monitor proximal airway pressures. When oxygen is being delivered, an oxygen analyzer with alarms is included in the circuit. As discussed previously, an anesthesia bag may be added to a continuous-flow system using a flow resistor.

PATIENT INTERFACE DEVICES

A wide range of patient interface products are available to apply CPAP from the system to the patient. Originally, CPAP was administered using an ETT and then a plastic head chamber.[1] Nasal devices were introduced shortly afterward, relying on an infant's preference for nasal breathing.[63] When a device is selected, its potential resistance to gas flow and effect on WOB should be considered first, along with the airway anatomy.[59,64] Then ease and comfort of securing the device are considered, and its stability once it is secured.[22,44,50,52]

HEAD AND FACE CHAMBERS

Although the head and face chamber appliances are not commonly used, they will be included for the sake of completeness (Fig. 18-7). These devices have been used infrequently because of the complications and impracticalities associated with their use.[31,52] The main advantage of the chamber is its ability to supply CPAP quickly and noninvasively. However, both are cumbersome and impede access to the patient's head and face.[22,65] To obtain consistent CPAP levels, the head chamber must have a tight seal at the neck. This has resulted in intracranial hemorrhage and hydrocephalus secondary to compression of the neck and associated vessels.[7,66] There have also been incidents of severe neck ulcerations and nerve palsies with the use of the head chamber.[67,68]

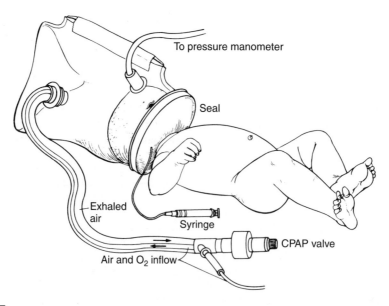

Fig. 18-7

Head chamber for CPAP application. (From Goldsmith JP, Karotkin EH, editors: *Assisted ventilation of the neonate,* ed 2. Philadelphia. WB Saunders, 1988.)

Because the entire head is within the closed chamber, excessive noise levels are a concern.[7,20,65] This problem has been reduced with effective noise suppression techniques.[20]

The face chamber is essentially a large mask that covers the entire face and is held in place by negative pressure.[7,69] During use, the patient is placed in a cradle, which may limit free patient movement. Because the chamber does not seal at the neck, many of the complications associated with head chambers are eliminated, although access to the patient remains limited. Attaching the face chamber has been infrequently associated with small cutaneous scars at the hairline.[7] Both head and face chambers are only used with infants and require placing a gastric tube to avoid abdominal distention.[22]

FACE MASKS

A face mask is effective in delivering CPAP to both infant and pediatric patients. A face mask is often used initially with a bag-valve-mask as a mechanism to quickly assess the patient's clinical response to the application of CPAP.[20,22] Usually it follows a short period of manual ventilation, but it may also be used as a method to rapidly improve oxygenation before beginning manual ventilation. If it is successful, mask CPAP is then replaced with another device designed for long-term use. Thus the potential for deleterious effects is reduced.

A lightweight mask with an inflatable face seal helps to avoid most of the complications associated with mask CPAP.[70] When the mask is manually secured to the patient's face, avoid occluding the nose and mouth and take special care to avoid pressure on the eyes and soft tissue under the chin. A tight seal is not mandatory for effective CPAP therapy. As long as the CPAP pressure is maintained, a minimal leak around the mask is permissible.[41]

Avoid using a mask to provide CPAP for a prolonged period of time. Although such an approach is helpful for obstructive sleep apnea or respiratory failure in an adult, it should be used cautiously with an infant. Disadvantages to using the facial mask for CPAP therapy are that it is difficult to provide mouth care and many infants will not tolerate having the mask secured to their face. Complications associated with use of the face mask include facial and ocular tissue trauma, gastric distention resulting in emesis and aspiration, and cerebral hemorrhage.[20,22,71] Facial trauma complications can be reduced by careful positioning and frequent repositioning of the mask. The incidents of brainstem and intracranial hemorrhage are most likely a result of the method used to affix the mask and are not related to mask use itself.[22,71,72] The

dead space volume of neonatal and pediatric masks can be significant; however, Goldman and colleagues reported no increase in carbon dioxide or rebreathing with the use of a mask.[64] A gastric tube may be placed to help decrease gastric distention and prevent emesis and aspiration. Patients with unstable facial fractures, extensive facial lacerations, laryngeal trauma, recent tracheal or esophageal anastomosis, or basilar skull fractures may require a patient interface device other than a face mask.[73]

ENDOTRACHEAL AND TRACHEOSTOMY TUBES

Rarely should an ETT be used to initiate CPAP on a newborn.[1,22] An ETT is used to supply CPAP only when weaning from mechanical ventilation, and then CPAP with an ETT is maintained for as short a time as possible. An extended weaning period causes an increase in WOB, owing to the small diameter tube, and risks fatigue, thus delaying extubation. The infant is extubated early from a low mechanical ventilator rate (6 to 10 breaths per minute) and placed on nasal CPAP.[26,74] This avoids many complications associated with mechanical ventilation, prevents reintubation, and maintains optimum lung function.[27]

Applying CPAP through a tracheostomy tube permits maintaining CPAP levels for an infant requiring prolonged ventilator assistance or who had a tracheostomy tube placed in the treatment of tracheobronchial malacia. Care of the patient receiving CPAP through a tracheostomy tube is similar to that of any other mechanically ventilated infant. The complications encountered are similar as well. Increased airway resistance can be a factor, although in most patients the increase is well tolerated, owing to the shorter length of the tracheostomy tube.[20,22,59,75] Leaks are common but are compensated for by using a slightly higher gas flow rate.

NASOPHARYNGEAL TUBES AND PRONGS

Nasopharyngeal tubes or prongs are essentially catheters placed into the nasal pharyngeal cavity that bypass the resistance of the nasal airway. Nasopharyngeal devices have several advantages over other devices. They allow delivery of CPAP directly to the airway, bypassing the nasal airway structures. Also, they are easily secured, are less likely to be displaced, and seem to be better tolerated by infants.[59,76] Securing nasopharyngeal CPAP devices is similar to securing a nasal ETT, so familiarity with such methods may be an advantage to their use. An alternative for securing nasopharyngeal prongs and tubes is a product such as the modern Logan bow device called the NeoBar (Neotech Products).

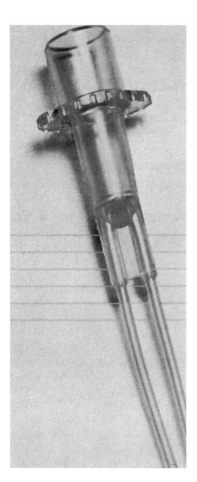

Fig. 18-8

V-SIL binasal pharyngeal prongs. (Courtesy Vesta, Inc., Franklin, Wisc.)

The Binasal Airway (Neotech Products) is a bilateral nasopharyngeal device consisting of two soft silicone pharyngeal catheters inserted through both nares (Fig. 18-8). The silicone prongs are inserted into the nasopharynx just to the point at which they can be secured. It is not necessary to insert the entire length of the prongs into the nares. The extra length allows the infant some movement without displacing the prongs.

An ETT can be used as a nasopharyngeal tube by inserting it unilaterally through a naris and into the nasopharynx. The depth of insertion is estimated by measuring the distance from the earlobe to the tip of the chin or nose. Enough length is left to secure the tube, and the excess length is trimmed to help reduce resistance (Fig. 18-9). The correct position of a nasopharyngeal device is confirmed by visualizing or feeling the tip of the catheters directly

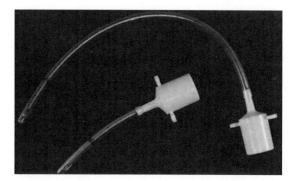

Fig. 18-9

Untrimmed *(top)* and trimmed *(bottom)* uncuffed endotracheal tubes. Trimming the length of an endotracheal tube reduces the resistance to exhaled gas flow during CPAP.

above the epiglottis. ETTs are radiopaque, and the position of the tube can be seen on a radiograph. The silicone prongs are not radiopaque.

Although reported as tolerated well by infants, nasopharyngeal CPAP has complications associated with its use. The tubes have a longer and smaller lumen than shorter devices, which may contribute significantly to airway resistance.[49,59,63,77-79] Other complications include nasal tissue trauma, obstruction of the tube and infant airway, kinking, gastric distention, emesis, and aspiration.[22,59,78] As with all nasal CPAP devices, there is also a tendency for the tube or prongs to become displaced in an active infant.

Proper positioning, as well as evaluating the prongs and nasal airway patency with gentle passes of a suction catheter, helps to prevent and identify obstruction or kinking. Properly heating and humidifying the gas assists in preventing dried secretions. Inserting a gastric tube minimizes gastric distention, but it may obstruct the open nares when using unilateral CPAP. Routine tube changes and careful attention to positioning help avoid nasal mucosal damage.

NASAL PRONGS

In 1973, Kattwinkel and co-workers devised a nasal prong that was a modification of Agostino's nasopharyngeal prong.[63,65] Today, nasal prongs are commonly used for nasal CPAP in infants (Fig. 18-10). Nasal prongs are short cannula-type devices that insert 0.5 to 1 cm into both nares.[31,50] They are wider and shorter than nasopharyngeal devices for the same size infant and therefore contribute less to airway resistance. The resistance of nasal prong devices to backflow varies significantly, depending on the size of the prong and patient.[59,72,76]

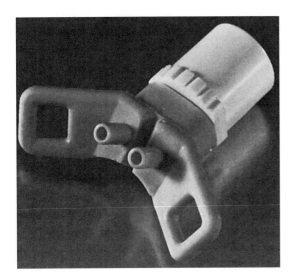

Fig. 18-10

Argyle nasal prongs for CPAP application. (Courtesy Sherwood Medical, St. Louis, Mo.)

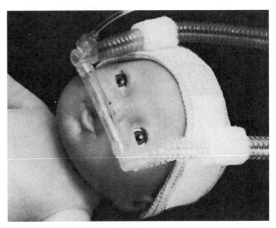

Fig. 18-11

Securing system and nasal prongs for CPAP therapy. This system includes a knit cap that fits over the infant's head and two sections of Velcro securing tape. The Velcro is placed on the hat and holds the CPAP circuit tubing in place. (Courtesy Hudson RCI, Temecula, Calif.)

Advantages of using nasal prongs include their low cost, ease of accessibility to the patient, single administration, and ability to maintain effective CPAP.[7,65,76] Recently, the use of early nasal prong CPAP therapy has been shown to yield significant decreases in the incidence of chronic lung disease.[25,26,76,80] Meta-analysis studies show that nasal prongs are slightly more effective than nasopharyngeal tubes in preventing reintubation and in reducing oxygen requirements.[24,74] However, none of these studies were controlled for CPAP level or the various other system components that may also contribute to successful weaning using nasal CPAP.

There are various methods for securing nasal prongs to the patient. Most manufacturers include bonnets or head straps for securing the prongs in the package. The type of securing method chosen depends primarily on patient tolerance and ability to maintain the prongs in the proper position (Fig. 18-11). The infant's mouth should not be taped shut, because the infant is a preferential nose breather and the mouth serves as a pop-off valve for excessive pressure.

There are several disadvantages to using nasal prongs to deliver CPAP. The most frequently reported problem is keeping the prongs in place, especially with an active infant. Secondly, prongs may not correctly fit a neonatal patient, despite several size selections from each manufacturer. Commonly reported complications resulting from incorrect sizing or overzealous securing mechanisms include nasal septal distortion, nasal irritation, and pressure necrosis. A common nickname for this appearance is the "pig nose" effect. There is no standard for prong sizes or securing mechanisms, so experimenting with different manufacturers' products helps minimize this problem. Products should be used that do not require pressing against the nasal septum to maintain a seal and that optimize the infant's comfort.

Other disadvantages are loss of pressure during mouth breathing or crying or obstruction of the prongs or nasal passages with secretions. Complications related to dysphagia secondary to CPAP have been reported to include gastric distention, emesis, and aspiration.[36]

NASAL MASKS

Nasal masks for infants initially required a custom-molded fit to be effective, which made them impractical for use in the intensive care nursery. Although limited sizes are commercially available for infants, applying nasal CPAP with a device designed for adult obstructive sleep apnea is not usually practical.

Infant masks are available to use with variable flow CPAP devices (Fig. 18-12). The size range is limited; however, they provide effective CPAP pressures and are generally tolerated by most infants. Advantages to using a nasal mask are twofold. The

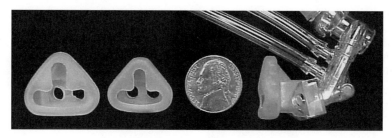

Fig. 18-12

Silicone nasal masks used for CPAP provided by a fluidic flow generator. (Courtesy SensorMedics, Inc., Yorba Linda, Calif.)

resistance to gas flow through the mask is less than anatomic upper airway resistance.[59,81] Tolerating a nasal device is largely dependent on comfort, and a mask does not rely on a prong entering the naris. Additionally, a mask may be beneficial when trying to secure the nasal device onto an infant with craniofacial abnormalities.

When a nasal mask is used, a slightly higher flow is usually necessary to clear the increased dead space of the mask and to compensate for leaks. Complications associated with the nasal mask include possible eye irritation caused by leaks around the mask and damage to facial tissue from improper fixation of the mask.

APPLICATION

When initiating CPAP, a pressure of 3 to 6 cm H_2O is a common starting point. The CPAP level is increased in increments of 2 cm H_2O. The FIO_2 that the patient was receiving before therapy is maintained. Generally, 12 cm H_2O is maximum pressure attainable when applying nasal CPAP because the mouth acts as a pop-off valve. The pressure and FIO_2 are increased to attain the desired PaO_2. However, it is best to change only one parameter at a time. Once an adequate level of CPAP is attained, oxygen requirements stabilize, respiratory frequency falls, and the signs of respiratory distress improve.

Box 18-3 lists the clinical signs indicating that CPAP has failed and that intubation and mechanical ventilation are indicated. Recognizing CPAP failure and the need to intubate and mechanically ventilate is paramount for the neonatal patient because fatigue progresses rapidly. Fatigue of the respiratory muscles and deteriorating pulmonary disease are the most frequent causes of failed CPAP. A rise in $PaCO_2$, or fall in PaO_2, after increasing the CPAP pressure may indicate that the optimal CPAP level has been exceeded.[82] If this occurs, the pressure can be reduced or the patient can be intubated, whichever is indicated.

BOX 18-3

RECOGNIZING FAILURE OF CPAP ADMINISTRATION

Decreasing pH ($<$7.25)
Increasing $PaCO_2$ ($>$50 to 60 mm Hg)*
Increasing FIO_2 ($>$0.6 to 0.7)
Decreasing PaO_2 ($<$60 to 80 mm Hg)†
Nasal CPAP $>$ 12 cm H_2O
Frequent apnea with bradycardia

*Higher ranges may apply with permissive hypercapnia.
†Range should be consistent with clinical state and the presence of congenital heart anomalies.

MONITORING

Pressure is monitored at the patient airway, and a low pressure, or disconnect, alarm is attached. This is the minimal monitoring of CPAP pressure required. However, besides loss of pressure to the patient, backpressure from the resistance across the prongs may prevent the low pressure or disconnect alarm from sounding. Other monitors with alarms, such as a pulse oximeter, transcutaneous monitor, or bradycardia alarm, should also be used with a low pressure, or disconnect, alarm. When CPAP is provided through a ventilator, whether nasal or by ETT, other alarm parameters are set to appropriate levels to monitor tidal volume or system flow.

The patient's pulmonary status and cardiovascular function are monitored frequently. Respiratory frequency should be observed closely, along with any pattern or changes that may indicate respiratory muscle fatigue and impending need for assisted ventilation. If possible, bedside pulmonary function testing should be performed, with compliance, resistance, volumes, and capacities assessed.[82,83] A chest radiograph is obtained as often as indicated, or if the patient's clinical status deteriorates.

Heart rate and blood pressure are monitored continuously in the acute phase of the therapy, with lessened emphasis as the patient's condition stabilizes. When CPAP levels are being increased, or when surfactant is used, capillary refill should be monitored. A slow refill, that is, longer than 2 seconds after blanching, indicates a potential drop in cardiac output. Urine output should be monitored carefully in critically ill patients because it is a direct indicator of renal blood flow.

Infants and children who are anxious, agitated, and inconsolable may be exhibiting early signs of compromised neurologic function. However, it cannot be overemphasized that before sedating the patient, or diagnosing neurologic compromise, airway obstruction and hypoxia should be ruled out. Also, changes in duration of apnea with bradycardia spells should be watched for.

WEANING

Weaning should be considered when the patient is stable, has no incidents of apnea, and exhibits acceptable vital signs, blood gas values, and chest radiographic findings. The patient is weaned from the FIO_2 first, in decreasing increments of 0.03 to 0.05, down to 0.40. Then the patient is weaned from CPAP pressure while the FIO_2 is continuing to be decreased to 0.21 to 0.3. If the patient has been on long-term, or chronic, positive pressure, then the pressure is reduced in increments of 1 cm H_2O. Otherwise, the CPAP is reduced in increments of 2 cm H_2O down to 2 to 3 cm H_2O, which approximates physiologic levels in the patient.[22,33]

SUMMARY

Infant nasal CPAP has a wide variety of applications, ranging from stabilizing the chest wall and improving FRC, to pneumatically stenting flaccid airway structures, to treating apnea of prematurity. CPAP is an important intervention in the treatment of pulmonary complications related to premature birth. It continues to grow in popularity as newer, more ergonometric, systems are deployed into clinical use. Various factors affect work of breathing. Whereas many studies evaluate one component or another, each aspect of the system should be considered to minimize the work of breathing and to optimize comfort and effectiveness.

REFERENCES

1. Gregory G et al: Treatment of the idiopathic respiratory distress syndrome with continuous positive pressure. *N Engl J Med* 1971; 248:1333-1340.
2. American Association for Respiratory Care: Clinical practice guideline: application of continuous positive airway pressure to neonates via nasal prongs or nasopharyngeal tube. *Respir Care* 1994; 39:817-823.
3. Saunders RA, Milner AD, Hopkins IE: The effects of continuous positive airway pressure on lung mechanics and lung volumes in the neonate. *Biol Neonate* 1976; 29:178-186.
4. Miller MJ et al: Effects of nasal CPAP on supraglottic and total pulmonary resistance in preterm infants. *J Appl Physiol* 1990; 68:141-146.
5. Miller RW et al: Effectiveness of CPAP in the treatment of bronchomalacia in infants: a bronchoscopic documentation. *Crit Care Med* 1986; 14:125-135.
6. Higgins RD, Richter SE, Davis JM: Nasal CPAP facilitates extubation of very low birth weight neonates. *Pediatrics* 1991; 88:999-1003.
7. Jonson B et al: CPAP: modes of action in relation to clinical application. *Pediatr Clin North Am* 1980; 27:687-697.
8. Field D, Vyas H, Milner A: CPAP via a single nasal catheter in preterm infants. *Early Hum Dev* 1985; 11:273-280.
9. Gregory GA et al: The time course changes in lung function after a change in CPAP. *Clin Res* 1977 (abstract); 25:193A.
10. Speidel BD, Dunn PM: Effect of continuous positive airway pressure on breathing pattern of infants with respiratory distress syndrome. *Lancet* 1975; 1:302-304.
11. Speidel BD, Dunn PM: Use of nasal CPAP to treat severe recurrent apnea in very preterm infants. *Lancet* 1976; 2:658-660.
12. Kumar A et al. Continuous positive-pressure ventilation in acute respiratory failure. *N Engl J Med* 1970; 283:1430-1436.
13. Fox WW et al: The PaO$_2$ response to changes in end expiratory pressure in the newborn respiratory distress syndrome. *Crit Care Med* 1977; 5:226-229.
14. Bonta BW et al: Determination of optimal CPAP for the treatment of IRDS by measurement of esophageal pressure. *J Pediatr* 1977; 91:449-454.
15. Suter PM, Fauley HB, Isenberg MD: Optimum end-expiratory airway pressure in patients with acute pulmonary failure. *N Engl J Med* 1975; 292:284-289.
16. Hegyi T, Hiatt IM: The effect of CPAP on the course of respiratory distress syndrome. *Crit Care Med* 1981; 9:38-41.
17. Engelke SC, Roloff DW, Kuhns LR: Postextubation nasal continuous positive airway pressure: a prospective controlled study. *Am J Dis Child* 1982; 136:359-361.
18. Gregory GA: Continuous positive airway pressure (CPAP). In Thibeault DW, Gregory GA, editors: *Neonatal pulmonary care*. Menlo Park, Calif. Addison-Wesley, 1979.
19. Roberton NRC: Prolonged continuous positive airways pressure for pulmonary oedema due to persistent ductus arteriosus in the newborn. *Arch Dis Child* 1974; 49:585-587.
20. Khambatta HF, Baratz RA: IPPB, plasma ADH and urine flow in conscious man. *J Appl Physiol* 1972; 33:362.
21. Aidinis SJ, Lafferty J, Schapiro HM: Intracranial responses to PEEP. *Anesthesiology* 1976; 45:275-296.
22. Czervinske MP: Continuous positive airway pressure. In Koff PB, Eitzman D, Neu J, editors: *Neonatal and pediatric respiratory care*. St Louis. Mosby, 1993; pp 263-284.
23. Verder H et al: Nasal continuous positive airway pressure and early surfactant therapy for respiratory distress syndrome in newborns of less than 30 weeks' gestation. *Pediatrics* 1999; 103:24-26.
24. Bachman TE: Evidenced based medicine: NCPAP in weaning preterm infants from ventilators. *Neonatal Intensive Care* 2000; 13(4):15-19.
25. De Klerk AM, De Klerk RK: Nasal continuous positive airway pressure and outcomes of preterm infants. *J Paediatr Child Health* 2001; 37(2):161-167
26. So BH et al: Application of nasal continuous positive airway pressure to early extubation in very low birthweight

infants. *Arch Dis Child Fetal Neonatal Ed* 1995; 72: F191-193.

27. Davis P et al: Randomised, controlled trial of nasal continuous positive airway pressure in the extubation of infants weighing 600 to 1250 g. *Arch Dis Child Fetal Neonatal Ed* 1998; 79:F54-57.

28. Martin RJ et al: The effect of a low continuous positive airway pressure on the reflex control of respiration in the preterm infant. *J Pediatr* 1977; 90:976-981.

29. Kattwinkel J: Neonatal apnea: pathogenesis and therapy. *J Pediatr* 1977; 90(3):342-347.

30. MacMahon HE, Ruggieri J: Congenital segmental bronchomalacia: report of a case. *Am J Dis Child* 1969; 188: 923-926.

31. Neijens HJ, Kerrebijn KF, Smalhout B: Successful treatment with CPAP of two infants with bronchomalacia. *Acta Paediatr Scand* 1978; 67:293-296.

32. Thompson JE, Farrell E, McManus M: Neonatal and pediatric airway emergencies. *Respir Care* 1992; 37:582-599.

33. Berman LS et al: Optimum levels of CPAP for tracheal extubation of newborn infants. *J Pediatr* 1976; 89:109-112.

34. Annest S, Gottbieb M, Paloski W: Detrimental effects of removing end-expiratory pressure prior to endotracheal extubation. *Ann Surg* 1983; 191:539-545.

35. Smith R: Physiologic PEEP. *Respir Care* 1988; 33:620-625.

36. Vender J: Complications and physiologic alternations of positive airway pressure therapy. *Anesth Clin North Am* 1987; 5:807-817.

37. Cullen DJ, Caldera DL: The incidence of ventilator-induced barotrauma in critically ill patients. *Anesthesia* 1979; 50:185-190.

38. De la Torre F, Tomasa A, Klamburg J: Incidence of pneumothorax and pneumomediastinum in patients with aspiration requiring ventilatory support. *Chest* 1977; 72:141-144.

39. Peterson GW, Horst B: Incidence of pulmonary barotrauma in a medical ICU. *Crit Care Med* 1983; 11:67-69.

40. Dimitriou G, Greenough A, Laubscher B: Lung volume measurements immediately after extubation by prediction of "extubation failure" in premature infants. *Pediatr Pulmonol* 1996; 21:250-254.

41. Branson RD, Hurst JM, DeHaven CB: Mask CPAP: state of the art. *Respir Care* 1985; 30:846-857.

42. Shapiro HM: Intracranial hypertension: therapeutic and anesthetic consideration. *Anesthesia* 1975; 43:445-471.

43. Hall SV, Johnson EE, Hedley-White J: Renal hemodynamics and function with continuous positive-pressure ventilation in dogs. *Anesthesia* 1974; 41:452-461.

44. Moa G, Nilsson K, Zetterstrom H: A new device for administration of nasal CPAP in the newborn: an experimental study. *Crit Care Med* 1988; 16:1238-1242.

45. Radermacher P, Breulmann M, Felber H: CPAP with a Siemens Servo 900C ventilator during weaning in infants. *Intensive Care Med* 1991; 17:189.

46. Cox J, Boehm J, Millare E: Individual nasal masks and intranasal tubes. *Anesthesia* 1974; 29:597-600.

47. Shehabi Y, Hillman KM, Nairn M: Tests of six continuous flow CPAP devices. *Anesth Intensive Care Med* 1991; 19: 237-243.

48. Hillman K et al: A new continuous positive airway pressure (CPAP) device. *Anesth Intensive Care Med* 1991; 19: 233-236.

49. Caliumi-Pellegrrini G: Twin nasal cannula for administration of continuous positive airway pressure to newborn infants. *Arch Dis Child* 1974; 49:228.

50. Courtney SE et al: Lung recruitment and breathing pattern during variable versus continuous flow nasal continuous positive airway pressure in premature infant: an evaluation of three devices. *Pediatrics* 2001; 107:304-308.

51. Bachman TE: Evidenced based medicine: NCPAP in weaning preterm infants from ventilators. *Neonatal Intensive Care* 2002; 15(1):16-19.

52. Mazzella M et al: A randomized control study comparing the infant flow driver with nasal continuous positive airway pressure in preterm infants. *Arch Dis Child Fetal Neonatal Ed* 2001; 85:F86-90.

53. Kavvadia V, Greenough A, Dimitriou G: Effect on lung function of continuous positive airway pressure administered either by infant flow driver or a single nasal prong. *Eur J Pediatr* 2000; 159:289-292.

54. Ahluwalia DK, White DK, Morley CJ: Infant flow driver or single prong nasal continuous positive airway pressure: short-term physiological effects. *Acta Paediatr* 1998; 87: 325-327.

55. Branson RD et al: Comparison of pressure and flow triggering systems during continuous positive airway pressure. *Chest* 1994; 106:540-544.

56. Bingham RM, Hatch D, Helms P: Assisted ventilation and the Servo ventilator in infants. *Anaesthesia* 1986; 41: 168-172.

57. Sanders RC et al: Work of breathing associated with pressure support ventilation in two different ventilators. *Pediatr Pulmonol* 2001; 32:62-70.

58. Heulitt MJ et al: Comparison of work of breathing between two neonatal ventilators utilizing a neonatal pig model. *Pediatr Crit Care Med* 2000; 2:170-175.

59. Czervinske MP, Durbin CG, Gal TJ: Resistance to gas flow across 14 CPAP devices for newborns. *Respir Care* 1986; 31:18-21.

60. Banner MJ et al: Flow resistance of expiratory positive pressure valve systems. *Chest* 1986; 90:212.

61. Lee KS et al: A comparison of underwater bubble continuous positive airway pressure with ventilator-derived continuous positive airway pressure in premature neonates ready for extubation. *Biol Neonate* 1998; 73(2):69-75.

62. Nekvasil R et al: High frequency "bubble" oscillation ventilation in the neonatal period. *Cesk Pediatr* 1992; 47(8): 465-470.

63. Agostino R et al: Continuous positive airway pressure (CPAP) by nasal cannulae in the respiratory distress syndrome (RDS) of the newborn. *Pediatr Res* 1973 (abstract); 7:50.

64. Goldman SL, Brady JP, Dumpit FM: Increased work of breathing associated with nasal prongs. *Pediatrics* 1979; 64:160-164.

65. Kattwinkel J, Fleming D, Cha C: A device for administration of CPAP by the nasal route. *Pediatrics* 1973; 52:170-178.

66. Vert P, Andre M, Sibout M: Continuous positive airway pressure and hydrocephalus. *Lancet* 1973; 2:319.

67. Krauss DR, Marshal R: Severe neck ulceration from CPAP head box. *J Pediatr* 1975; 86:286.

68. Turner T, Evans J, Brown JK: Monoaresis: complications of CPAP. *Arch Dis Child* 1975; 50:128.

69. Ahlström H, Jonson B, Svenningsen NW: Continuous positive airway pressure treatment by a face chamber in idiopathic respiratory distress syndrome. *Arch Dis Child* 1976; 51:31.

70. Covelli HD, Weled BJ, Beekman JF: Efficacy of continuous positive airway pressure administered by face mask. *Chest* 1982; 81:147-150.

71. Pape KE, Armstrong DL, Fitzhardinge PM: Central nervous system pathology associated with mask ventilation in the very low birth weight infant: a new etiology for intracerebellar hemorrhages. *Pediatrics* 1976; 58:473.

72. Tanswell AK: Continuous distending pressure in the respiratory distress syndrome of the newborn: who, when, and why? *Respir Care* 1982; 2:257-266.

73. Klopfenstein CE, Foster A, Suter PM: Pneumocephalus: a complication of CPAP after trauma. *Chest* 1980; 78: 656-657.

74. Davis PG, Henderson-Smart DJ: Extubation from low-rate intermittent positive airway pressure versus extubation after a trial of endotracheal continuous positive airway pressure in intubated preterm infants. In *The Cochrane Library*, Issue 1, 2002. Oxford: Update Software.

75. Katz JA, Kraemer RW, Gjerde GE: Inspiratory work and airway pressure with CPAP delivery systems. *Chest* 1985; 88:519.

76. Jones DB, Deveau D: Nasal prong CPAP: a proven method for reducing chronic lung disease. *Neonatal Network* 1991; 10:7-15.

77. Boros SJ: Prolonged apnea of prematurity therapy with continuous airway distending pressure delivered by nasopharyngeal tube. *Clin Pediatr* 1976; 15:123.

78. Levene M: Hazards of nasal CPAP. *Lancet* 1977; 1:1157.

79. Norogroder M, Mackvanying N, Eidelman A: Nasopharyngeal ventilation in respiratory distress syndrome. *J Pediatr* 1973; 82:1059.

80. Higgins RD, Richter SE, Davis JM: Nasal continuous positive airway pressure facilitates extubation of very low birth weight neonates. *Pediatrics* 1991; 88:999-1003.

81. Abbasi S, Bhutani V: Pulmonary mechanics and energetics of normal, non-ventilated low birthweight infants. *Pediatr Pulmonol* 1990; 8:89-95.

82. Andreasson B et al: Measurement of ventilation and respiratory mechanics during continuous positive airway pressure (CPAP) treatment in infants. *Acta Paediatr Scand* 1989; 78:194-204.

83. Teague WG, Darnall RA, Suratt PM: A noninvasive constant flow method for measuring respiratory compliance in newborn infants. *Crit Care Med* 1985; 13:965-969.

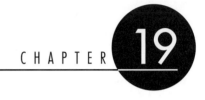

CHAPTER 19

Mechanical Ventilation of the Neonate and Pediatric Patient

Brian K. Walsh
Michael P. Czervinske

Neonatal and pediatric mechanical ventilation presents some of the most clinically challenging situations in respiratory care. The neonatal and pediatric population encompasses a wide range of weights, ages, and sizes. In this chapter, a *neonate* is defined as any newborn younger than 42 weeks' gestation and a *pediatric patient* represents any child older than 3 months of age. Children are not small adults, and infants are not small children.[1] Most of the concepts presented in this chapter are the same for both pediatric and neonatal applications; however, there are other situations that are quite unique to the neonatal or pediatric patient. To manage neonatal and pediatric mechanical ventilation effectively, the clinician must combine the principles described in this chapter with the knowledge of how airway anatomy and pulmonary physiology mature.

OBJECTIVES AND INDICATIONS FOR MECHANICAL VENTILATION

The physiologic objectives for mechanical ventilation in a neonate or pediatric patient are basically the same as for those in an adult patient. They are (1) to manipulate alveolar ventilation, (2) to improve oxygenation, (3) to improve lung volume, and (4) to reduce the work of breathing. Generally, mechanical ventilation is instituted to increase the Pao_2, correct respiratory acidosis, reduce respiratory distress, prevent or reverse atelectasis, reduce respiratory muscle fatigue, manage intracranial pressure, lower oxygen consumption, and stabilize the chest wall for adequate lung expansion. Box 19-1 lists clinical situations in which mechanical ventilation is indicated.[1-6]

BOX 19-1

CLINICAL INDICATIONS FOR (BUT NOT LIMITED TO) MECHANICAL VENTILATION

PULMONARY DISORDERS
RESTRICTIVE PROCESS
    Acute respiratory distress syndrome (ARDS)
    Pulmonary hemorrhage
    Pulmonary hypoplasia/agenesis
    Congenital pneumonia
    Pneumothorax/air leaks
    Pleural effusion/chylothorax
    Aspiration syndromes (blood, amniotic fluid)
    Flail chest
    Bronchopleural fistula
    Abdominal distention
    Diaphragmatic hernia
    Congenital lung cysts, tumors
    Rib cage anomalies
    Extrinsic masses

OBSTRUCTIVE PROCESS
    Meconium aspiration
    Asthma
    Bronchiolitis
    Cystic fibrosis
    Bronchopulmonary dysplasia

AIRWAY
    Laryngomalacia
    Tracheomalacia
    Choanal atresia
    Pierre Robin syndrome
    Micrognathia
    Nasopharyngeal tumor
    Subglottic stenosis

EXTRAPULMONARY DISORDERS
NEUROLOGIC/MUSCULAR
    Myasthenia gravis
    Muscular dystrophy

    Guillain-Barré syndrome
    Cerebral edema
    Cerebral hemorrhage
    Spinal cord injury/disease
    Phrenic nerve damage

HYPOVENTILATION
    Sleep apnea
    Overdose/poisoning
    Postoperative recovery

INCREASED INTRACRANIAL PRESSURE
    Infection
    Head trauma
    Near-drowning
    Reye's syndrome

CARDIOVASCULAR DYSFUNCTION
    Cardiac shunting
    Cyanotic heart disease
    Circulatory collapse
    Hypovolemia
    Anemia
    Polycythemia
    Congestive heart failure
    Postoperative cardiac surgery
    Persistent pulmonary hypertension

METABOLIC
    Acidosis
    Hypoglycemia
    Hypothermia
    Hyperthermia

TYPES OF MECHANICAL VENTILATION

Mechanical ventilation can be employed in a variety of ways, which are defined by the dominant feature of each type of ventilator.[7] Fig. 19-1 compares the differences between the flow and pressure waveforms of volume and pressure ventilation. Although ventilators of the past could deliver only one form of ventilation, the modern microprocessor ventilators are capable of delivering both volume and pressure ventilation and of producing a wide variety of flow and pressure waveforms.

PRESSURE VENTILATION

Pressure ventilation uses a pressure setting as the main feature to define inflation. Pressure ventilators are classified as positive pressure or negative pressure.[7] Positive-pressure ventilators use a high external pressure gradient to drive a gas mixture into the lungs and produce inflation. They are generally more suitable in the critical care environment because they allow a more detailed definition of the inflation waveform and entire respiratory cycle.

Negative-pressure ventilation forces gas flow into the lungs by using a vacuum to externally expand the thorax. The chest wall pressure drops to less than the airway opening pressure, and air flows into the lungs. The main advantage of a negative-pressure ventilator is that it may avoid intubation or tracheostomy. Because negative-pressure ventilation is provided without an artificial airway, it is sometimes referred to as noninvasive ventilation; however, it should be understood that all forms of mechanical ventilation provide ventilation in an "unnatural" form. In addition, both positive- and negative-pressure ventilation produce positive trans-respiratory pressures and may have similar complications as a result.

Time-cycled, pressure-limited ventilation (TCPV) has been the most common form of ventilation used in neonates and infants, mainly because it has been the traditional ventilation for that population. To define the inflation cycle of each breath, TCPV uses a preset (1) continuous flow during both inspiration and expiration, (2) inspiratory time, (3) frequency or inspiratory to expiratory (I:E) ratio, and (4) pressure setting.[8] Because flow is constant, pressure is variable throughout the inflation cycle.

Microprocessor ventilators are also capable of delivering preset pressure breaths and are useful for infant and pediatric ventilation. This form of pressure ventilation is pressure-controlled ventilation (PCV). PCV is fundamentally different from TCPV. Usually a preset inspiratory time and frequency or I:E ratio are set, and the ventilator up to a preset pressure level assists the patient's inspiratory effort. Flow, however, is a function of driving pressure and peaks almost instantly to attain the defined pressure level. Pressure is maintained constant throughout the inflation cycle, and flow decelerates rapidly.[9,10] The tidal volume is delivered early in the inflation stage, while pressure is held constant. When compared with other types of ventilation, the resulting distribution of alveolar pressures sustained by tidal volume may lead to a lower dead space to tidal volume (V_D:V_T) ratio, improved ventilation, and improved oxygenation.[11-17] Although the peak pressure level is constant or nearly constant, PCV results in a higher mean airway pressure ($\overline{Paw}$) than do other types of ventilation. The disadvantages of a higher $\overline{Paw}$ should be considered when instituting PCV. Another disadvantage is that when using any type of pressure ventilation, tidal volume will vary with changes in lung compliance.

Advances in ventilator and sensor technology have introduced new features into ventilators. The mode *pressure-regulated volume control* attempts to maintain a constant tidal volume with a constant pressure by manipulating the flow waveform. Another mode, *volume-assured pressure support,* uses pressure-support ventilation while maintaining a minimum tidal volume with each breath. If the patient does not receive the minimum tidal volume during a breath, the flow rate is constant and the pressure is increased until the volume is received.[18]

Many clinicians maintain that constant pressure ventilation is superior to other types of ventilation in neonates or pediatric patients who have leaks around a cuffless endotracheal tube. However, a leak around an endotracheal tube reduces ventilation during constant pressure ventilation just as it does with other types of ventilation.[19]

VOLUME VENTILATION

Volume ventilation is most often used in adult patients and is chosen when ventilating a pediatric patient. Because of improved sensor and ventilator technology, it is also possible to use volume ventilation in an infant.[5] A constant tidal volume characterizes volume ventilation, and the resulting peak inspiratory pressure varies with lung, airway, and ventilator compliance and resistance. A bellows or a flow-controlling valve usually controls tidal volume. When a flow-controlling valve is used, tidal volume is calculated by measuring the flow delivered over a preset inflation time.[7,20]

Volume ventilation with a constant flow has the advantage of a lower $\overline{Paw}$ when compared with pressure ventilation. This is often a critical factor after cardiac surgery in infants and children. In theory, tidal volume does not vary with changing lung compliance or airway resistance during volume ventilation. As lung impedance increases, however, tidal volume may decrease if the ventilator

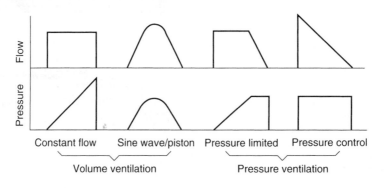

Fig. 19-1

Flow and pressure waveforms of four types of ventilation.

cannot correct for volume losses resulting from gas compression. When ventilating a larger patient, the volume loss may be negligible; however, in a small child or infant it may be a significant portion of the tidal volume. Failure to consider this volume loss may result in hypoventilation of the patient and may affect the calculations of thoracic compliance, oxygen consumption, carbon dioxide production, and dead space volume.[21] To account for this loss; an effective tidal volume should be calculated (Box 19-2).[22]

A piston-driven volume ventilator also delivers a constant volume with a variable peak pressure. Because of the piston action, flow peaks in the middle of the inflation when stroke speed is the greatest. Although piston ventilators are seldom used in the pediatric critical care setting, they become an inexpensive and practical choice for the non-acute care or home setting.

Many home ventilators also allow the use of pressure limiting by setting a desired maximum pressure level. Using this feature decreases tidal volume from the volume set on the ventilator, but exactly how it affects volume depends on the specific ventilator and inflation time settings. A piston-generated pressure preset mode is not appropriate for the pediatric or infant home setting. Using a microprocessor-based turbine-driven portable ventilator is a better home care choice in such a situation.

FLOW AND PRESSURE WAVEFORM PATTERNS

To fully understand mechanical ventilation, the clinician should relate each change in a ventilator setting with the effect it will have on respiratory variables. Using this approach helps the clinician to understand the relationship of each ventilator setting to the respiratory system, rather than memorizing a long list of cause-and-effect relationships.[7] The concepts of flow and pressure as they relate to time are helpful in relating ventilator settings to the goals of mechanical ventilation. The pressure and flow waveforms are altered each time a ventilator setting is changed. These waveforms can be viewed as two-dimensional pictures of the changes that occur in the lungs as the ventilator settings are adjusted. The relationship of tidal volume and Paw as they relate to a flow and pressure waveform is shown in Fig. 19-2. Assuming constant lung conditions and inflation time, an increase in the inspired volume per unit time results in an increase in peak pressure and an increase in both tidal volume and Paw. Similarly, if the tidal volume control on a ventilator increases, flow, peak pressure, and Paw also increase. Note that once a change occurs in one variable it results in changes in

---

BOX 19-2

CALCULATION OF EFFECTIVE TIDAL VOLUME

$$V_{Teff} = V_{Tset} - [(Pstatic^* - PEEP) \times Circuit]$$

DETERMINATION OF COMPLIANCE FACTOR OF CIRCUIT
1. With the circuit assembled and connected to the ventilator, the patient connection to the circuit is occluded.
2. A known volume of gas is delivered into the circuit through the ventilator, and the resulting peak inspiratory pressure is noted.
3. The resulting pressure is divided by the delivered volume to obtain the compliance factor of the circuit. This is generally 2 ml/cm H_2O for infant circuits and 3 to 4 ml/cm H_2O for larger circuits.

V_{Teff}, Effective tidal volume; V_{Tset}, tidal volume set on ventilator; *Pstatic,* static (plateau) pressure measured during inflation; *PEEP,* positive end-expiratory pressure set on ventilator; *circuit,* compliance or compression factor of circuit.

*If static or plateau pressure measurement cannot be obtained because of airway leaks, the peak inspiratory pressure may be used as an approximation.

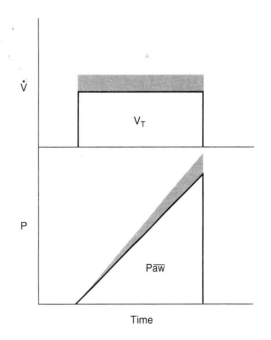

Fig. 19-2

Flow ($\dot{V}$) and pressure (P) waveforms during constant flow-volume ventilation. The unshaded area below each waveform represents tidal volume (V_T) and mean airway pressure (Paw). The shaded area represents the increase in V_T and Paw when flow is increased.

other variables. Two-dimensional images such as this help to illustrate concepts as they relate to ventilator management or other ventilator functions.

TIME CONSTANTS

The concept of a time constant in the lung represents how fast pressure equilibrates between the circuit and the alveoli. Conversely, it represents the maximum rate at which exhalation occurs. The time constant is a mathematic and physiologic concept that is not consistently applied clinically. Previously, accurately obtaining the values necessary for calculating a time constant was technically difficult. Recent advances in pulmonary function measurement techniques have made these data more available.

A time constant is the product of multiplying compliance and resistance. The time constant relates to both inspiratory filling and expiratory emptying of the lungs. Mouth pressure or proximal airway pressure equilibrates with alveolar pressure in three to five time constants.[23] In a healthy newborn this is 0.33 second. In severely premature infants with respiratory distress syndrome and decreased compliance, one time constant can be as short as 0.05 second.[24] This means that pressure equilibration will occur in 0.15 to 0.25 second, which is the minimum inspiratory time required to ensure complete delivery of the tidal volume. When airway resistance is high, such as in meconium aspiration syndrome, the time constant is longer. This would indicate using longer inspiratory times, lower inspiratory flows, and longer exhalation times to ventilate these infants.

Monitoring pulmonary mechanics to derive time constants assists in properly adjusting adequate inspiratory time and expiratory time. The time component is important when using rapid rates to allow adequate exhalation without developing breath stacking and automatic positive end-expiratory pressure (auto-PEEP) and to minimize iatrogenic lung damage. Using serial measurements of resistance and compliance directs the setting of ventilator parameters to match the changing physiology of the patient.[25]

TRIGGERING

Patient triggering is one of the most important links to the ventilator. Proper triggering can reduce work of breathing, allows a patient to be more comfortable, and reduces volutrauma. There are three types of sensing: pressure, flow, and motion (Table 19-1). Many ventilators can do one if not two of the types of sensing. When types of triggering are considered, the placement of the triggering device and its effects on the patient are evaluated. Flow and motion trig-

TABLE 19-1	SYNCHRONIZING SYSTEMS FOR MECHANICAL VENTILATORS	
Type	Source	Advantage/ Disadvantage
Pressure sensor	Proximal airway	Slow transit time Leaks cause autocycling Requires good patient effort
Flow sensor	Pneumotachometer (heated wire or differential pressure)	Fast response Adds dead space Affected by secretions Provides volume measurement
Motion sensor	Abdominal sensor (impedance electrode)	Requires correct placement False-positive measurements No volume measurement

gering are the most frequently used in the neonatal patient population.

PRESSURE SENSING

Some ventilators use a drop in the pressure signal sensed at the airway to trigger the ventilator with the patient's breath. Attempts to use esophageal pressure as the trigger source have not been well accepted clinically. For the pressure in the circuit to drop to less than the trigger level, or sensitivity setting, approximately 2 ml of volume must be displaced. This often accounts for a large portion of the neonatal tidal volume and thus is not well tolerated. A low-birth-weight infant may not consistently produce the level of effort necessary to trigger the ventilator. During pressure sensing, the response time tends to be slow because of delay from the progression of the pressure drop through the ventilator tubing. Because of this, synchronization is difficult to achieve at ventilator rates greater than 35 to 40 breaths per minute.

FLOW SENSING

A *pneumotachometer* between the circuit and the patient senses effort by measuring inspiratory flow. Two types of pneumotachometers used to sense flow are the heated-wire anemometer and the variable-orifice pneumotachometer. These units have fast response times, usually in the 30- to 70-msec range, and provide reliable synchronization at all rates.[26,27] However, flow sensors add dead space to the airway, and the potential increase in tidal volume associated with synchronized intermittent mandatory ventilation (SIMV) may be negated by an increase in carbon dioxide retention. Flow sensors may also be affected by secretions and require frequent cleaning.

MOTION SENSING

Two types of motion-sensing devices are used to detect patient effort and synchronize the ventilator. The first device incorporates a Graseby capsule taped to the infant's abdomen. Abdominal movement occurs 100 msec before air flow is initiated.[28] This movement compresses the capsule and sends a signal to the processing unit, which, in turn, triggers the ventilator. This system demonstrated slightly shorter response times than did flow sensors.[29] Another type of motion sensor uses impedance monitoring and receives the signal from the bedside cardiac and respiration monitor. The respiration signal is sent to a microprocessor in the ventilator, which triggers a mechanical breath. This system appears to have response times comparable to those of other systems and is successfully used in very low–birth-weight infants.[30]

Each of these systems accomplishes synchronization in different ways. Proper setting of the sensitivity and placement of the sensor are required to make the sensor work properly. Frequently, an infant may have abdominal movement not associated with a respiratory effort, which causes a false trigger. Impedance monitoring technology is prone to problems in the event of airway obstruction.

MODES OF VENTILATION

The mode of ventilation is defined by how a ventilator is going to interface with the patient's breathing efforts. These modes can use pressure, flow, or other signals to trigger. The main control variables may be volume, pressure, or flow and may use either positive or negative pressure as the driving force. Most ventilators are capable of providing multiple modes, and some even combine modes to enhance the patient-ventilator interface. Fig. 19-3 illustrates various modes of ventilation and how they interface with spontaneous breathing.

CONTROL MODE

The control mode is used when the clinician needs to maintain complete control over a patient's ventilation variables. To attain complete control, the patient-triggering mechanism is made inactive and all breaths are delivered at a preset volume or pressure, frequency, and inspiratory flow rate.[18] The patient should be sedated and paralyzed to avoid asynchrony between ventilator inflations and patient breathing efforts. Control ventilation may be

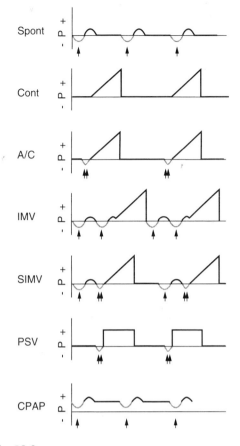

Fig. 19-3

Pressure waveforms of seven modes of ventilation. Single arrows note spontaneous inspiratory efforts. Double arrows note ventilator breaths triggered by inspiratory efforts. *Spont,* Spontaneous breathing; *Cont,* controlled ventilation; *A/C,* assist/control ventilation; *IMV,* intermittent mandatory ventilation; *SIMV,* synchronized intermittent mandatory ventilation; *PSV,* pressure support ventilation; *CPAP,* continuous positive airway pressure.

desirable when extreme ventilation variables are required, and asynchrony may result in complications such as pneumothorax. Such situations may occur during mechanical ventilation of the patient with severe acute respiratory distress syndrome (ARDS) or asthma.

ASSIST/CONTROL MODE

Like the control mode, the assist/control (A/C) mode allows the clinician control over most of the patient's ventilation variables except for rate. The volume or pressure, frequency, and inspiratory flow rate are preset, and the ventilator supports every breath. However, the patient is allowed to use his or her own ventilatory drive to trigger the ventilator and receive a breath at the preset volume or pressure. If the patient fails to take a breath during a specific period, the ventilator delivers the defined breath at a preset rate. The sensitivity of the triggering mechanism is set sufficiently low to be activated by any attempted breath. The sensitivity must also be set sufficiently high to prevent activation by artifacts (self-cycling), such as cardiac activity, airway leaks, or patient care procedures. The A/C mode may be useful for older children or adolescents. It is used less often in neonates and small children because of their higher respiratory rates. The advantage of the A/C mode is that every breath delivered to the patient, whether patient or machine triggered, has a guaranteed volume or pressure and flow rate. There are several disadvantages to this mode. In neonates, infants, or small children with high respiratory rates, hyperventilation and respiratory alkalosis may occur. The work of breathing may be increased, especially for patients who are not breathing in synchrony with the machine or who are "fighting the ventilator." Sedating the patient may alleviate this. If the peak flow or sensitivity is not set adequately, the patient's inspiratory effort may be increased and result in an increase in oxygen consumption.[6]

Because the operator controls the inflation variables during both the control and A/C modes, some ventilator classification systems include both of these as variations of one mode–continuous mandatory ventilation. Control and A/C are then defined as machine-triggered and patient-triggered continuous mandatory ventilation.[31] Some ventilators have control and A/C as the same mode, with the sensitivity setting being the only difference.

INTERMITTENT MANDATORY VENTILATION

During intermittent mandatory ventilation (IMV), spontaneous ventilation is allowed to occur between mandatory inflations that have a preset flow rate and pressure or volume. However, ventilator inflation occurs on spontaneous breathing efforts and results in breath-stacking or *patient-ventilator asynchrony*. This problem most often results in patient agitation, reduced tidal volume delivery, volutrauma, and the inability to ventilate. Because of the high spontaneous respiratory rate of a neonate, this mode has been the basis of neonatal ventilation.

SYNCHRONIZED INTERMITTENT MANDATORY VENTILATION

To avoid patient-ventilator asynchrony, a sensing mechanism is built into most modern ventilators. The ventilator presets a rate for the delivery of mandatory breaths (of preset volume or pressure and flow rate) and attempts to synchronize the breaths with the patient's spontaneous effort. If no patient effort is sensed within a specific window of time, a mandatory breath is given. Airway pressure or flow is the usual triggering mechanism for SIMV; however, a few designs incorporate abdominal motion or esophageal pressure as the triggering mechanism. Small volumes and rapid rates characterize an infant's spontaneous breathing effort, which makes synchronizing ventilator inflation difficult. With the latest advances in sensor technology, SIMV is now a feasible option in neonates and infants.[31-33] Advantages of this mode are that it allows the patient to perform part of the ventilatory work while maintaining a backup of mandatory ventilation and that it is useful in weaning the patient from mechanical ventilation (Box 19-3). Hyperventilation and respiratory alkalosis are risks just as with the A/C mode, but they are less likely to occur. Another risk associated with SIMV is increased work of breathing during spontaneous ventilation. This may be the result of inadequate inspiratory flow, ventilator response to the patient's inspiratory effort, ventilator circuitry, or endotracheal tube resistance.[6]

CONTINUOUS POSITIVE AIRWAY PRESSURE

During continuous positive airway pressure (CPAP), also termed *constant airway pressure,* a constant, above-ambient pressure is applied to the airways and maintained through the entire respiratory cycle.[34] Respiratory efforts are spontaneous and not supported by mandatory ventilator inflations.[18] In the pediatric setting, CPAP is applied to improve oxygenation by increasing the functional residual capacity, as in aspiration pneumonitis, or to stent floppy anatomic structures, as in tracheomalacia or disorders associated with sleep apnea.[26,35] CPAP should be considered as a primary mode to improve lung compliance and oxygenation in spontaneously

---

BOX 19-3

BENEFITS OF SYNCHRONIZED INTERMITTENT MANDATORY VENTILATION

Better distribution of ventilation by coordinating air flow with respiratory muscle effort

Improved oxygenation by reducing ventilation-perfusion mismatch

Better tidal volume at same positive inspiratory pressure

Improved minute ventilation through minimizing ineffective breaths

Reduced incidence of pneumothorax

Reduced incidence of intraventricular hemorrhage due to less variation in cerebral blood flow

Decreased use of sedation and paralysis

Reduced length of ventilation

breathing patients when the potential adverse effects of high peak airway pressures must be avoided.[27-29] It is frequently used when weaning from mechanical ventilation. High levels of CPAP may overdistend the lungs, increase the work of breathing, and reduce compliance (see Chapter 18 for a discussion of CPAP for the neonate).

AIRWAY PRESSURE RELEASE VENTILATION

Airway pressure release ventilation (APRV) is another form of CPAP in which a CPAP level and a pressure release level are set along with the frequency and time of the pressure release. The short intermittent decreases in the CPAP level allow alveolar emptying of gases. It is designed to assist spontaneously breathing patients. The advantages of APRV are similar to those of conventional CPAP in overcoming hypoxemia. Unlike conventional CPAP, however, the intermittent release of pressure augments ventilation and allows elimination of carbon dioxide.[6,36-38] The use of APRV for neonates and pediatrics is undocumented, but it may be considered for older pediatric patients who have the muscle and energy reserves to tolerate such a mode. APRV is referred to as *bilevel positive airway pressure* (BiPAP). In this mode, the pressure level changes between inspiration and expiration. Although its use in preventing sleep apnea is similar to that of conventional CPAP, it may be helpful in overcoming ventilation difficulties and avoiding tracheostomy in individuals afflicted with neuromuscular diseases, such as spinal muscular atrophy.[39]

PRESSURE-SUPPORT VENTILATION

Pressure-support ventilation (PSV) is a spontaneous ventilation mode in which each breath must be triggered by the patient. It incorporates a constant pressure inflation that is triggered by the patient and terminated when flow reaches a certain threshold (terminal flow or percentage of the peak flow). PSV improves the efficiency of inspiratory work of breathing, decreases the respiratory rate, and reduces the oxygen cost of breathing.[40,41] It may be associated with an improved sense of breathing comfort by the patient.[42,43] PSV is popularly used to augment breaths in conjunction with SIMV or as a mode for weaning patients from mechanical ventilation.[44] Combining PSV with SIMV may help reduce some of the work associated with demand valves and small endotracheal tubes, but it may also increase Paw. Caution should be used in clinical situations in which increased Paw may be harmful. PSV is useful as a stand-alone mode or for weaning patients receiving short- and long-term mechanical ventilation.

Managing the flow rate is critical to the successful use of PSV. If the flow rate is too high in patients with high airway resistance, the frequency and peak pressure increase and tidal volume and inspiratory time decrease. Reducing the flow rate or driving pressure to a level barely sufficient to maintain a constant pressure plateau may be necessary. When driving pressure controls the flow rate, a pressure gradient of 5 to 10 cm H_2O greater than the plateau pressure level may be sufficient to maintain the pressure waveform.[9,10] Ventilators have recently been introduced that allow the adjustment of flow rates, which may help alleviate this problem. Effective PSV results in adequate tidal volume and minute ventilation at a lower respiratory rate.[45] Fig. 19-4

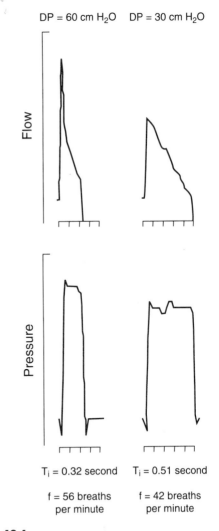

DP = 60 cm H_2O DP = 30 cm H_2O

Flow

Pressure

T_i = 0.32 second T_i = 0.51 second

f = 56 breaths per minute   f = 42 breaths per minute

Fig. 19-4

Waveforms and inflation variables comparing a high driving pressure (DP) (60 cm H_2O) and a low driving pressure (30 cm H_2O) to generate flow during pressure-support ventilation of an infant.

compares inflation variables when high and low driving pressures are used to generate flow during PSV in an infant. Other modes that adapt PSV to meet tidal volume or minute volume criteria are also available. Such modes provide true pressure-support inflation but then alter an inflation to meet a minimum condition if not met during the PSV inflation.[18]

INVERSE RATIO VENTILATION

Inverse ratio ventilation (IRV) is a nonconventional mode of ventilation in which an I:E ratio of greater than 1:1 is used during controlled ventilation. The patient is usually deeply sedated or paralyzed, or both, to avoid dyssynchrony with the ventilator. It is most often used in patients with ARDS. The major goals of IRV are to improve oxygenation by increasing the $\overline{Paw}$ and to allow recruitment of pulmonary units by increasing inspiratory time. Complications associated with IRV are pulmonary volutrauma and compromised cardiac output. There are currently very little data demonstrating the advantage of IRV over other more conventional modes of ventilation.[6]

Many types and modes of mechanical ventilation have been described, and each must be studied with its corresponding pressure and flow waveforms. Successful use of any type or mode of ventilation depends on gaining experience with it and understanding how inflation variables interact with each other and relate to the goals of mechanical ventilation, in addition to understanding the differences that exist among the various ventilators.

MANAGING VENTILATOR SETTINGS
MANIPULATING $Paco_2$

One of the main goals of mechanical ventilation is to manipulate the $Paco_2$, which is affected by changing the minute ventilation. The minute ventilation is directly related to ventilation frequency and tidal volume and is inversely related to the $Paco_2$.

Frequency. Frequency or rate is generally the first method used to increase minute ventilation. At low rates and conventional I:E ratios or during weaning, adjusting frequency is the most desirable option. Two disadvantages exist when manipulating frequency at higher rates or inverse I:E ratios. The first is that as frequency increases, air trapping is likely to occur.[46,47] Fig. 19-5 illustrates this on a flow/time scalar graphic. Notice flow does not come back to baseline. The second is that when the I:E ratio is kept constant, minute ventilation does not change.

Tidal Volume. An alternative to adjusting frequency is to change any variable that affects tidal volume and hence affects minute ventilation and $Paco_2$. The goal is to select a variable that will increase the area under the flow waveform. This is accomplished by increasing flow or inspiratory time. The tidal volume control on a microprocessor ventilator adjusts flow or times to derive an increase in tidal volume. Another variable that is available on some ventilators is the I:E ratio. Adjusting it to provide a longer inspiratory time may also improve elimination of carbon dioxide. Altering tidal volume variables is useful in

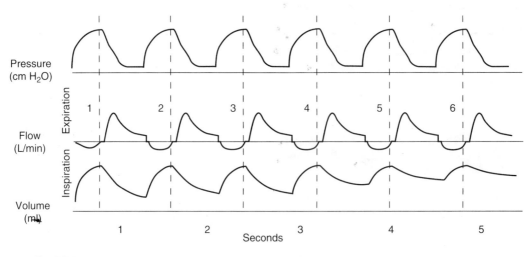

Fig. 19-5

Air trapping illustrated on a flow (lpm) over time scalar. Expiratory flow never returns to baseline before the ventilator cycles again.

situations such as severe asthma, in which the goal is to minimize the rate and air trapping while maximizing exhalation time and ventilation. Fig. 19-6 illustrates the three ways in which the flow waveform can

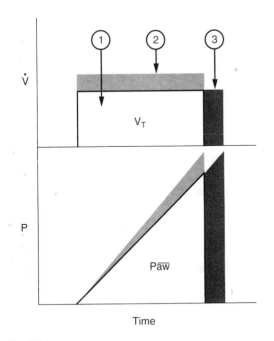

Fig. 19-6

Control variables that affect minute ventilation by increasing the area under the flow ($\dot{V}$) waveform to increase tidal volume (V_T). *1,* Increase V_T or rate. *2,* Increase inspiratory flow. *3,* Increase inspiratory time. Also shown is the associated change in mean airway pressure ($\overline{Paw}$). *P,* Pressure.

change to increase tidal volume and minute ventilation. The tidal volume in neonates varies from 4 to 8 ml/kg and from 8 to 10 ml/kg in pediatric patients, but lower tidal volumes should be accepted in ARDS.[48] Tidal volume should be corrected for compressible volume loss. Careful monitoring of breath sounds, chest expansion, arterial blood gas values, and chest radiographs is essential in determining adequate tidal volume.

During pressure ventilation, increasing the pressure limit may also increase tidal volume. The manner in which tidal volume increases during TCPV is different from that in PCV and PSV. Increasing the pressure limit during TCPV results in the pressure limit being reached later in the inspiratory cycle. When the pressure limit is reached, flow decelerates. The increase in tidal volume is the result of the delay in flow deceleration and widening of the area under the flow waveform. An increase in the pressure limit during PCV and PSV causes the initial flow to increase. The result is a larger decelerating flow waveform and larger tidal volume. Fig. 19-7 illustrates the way a change in the pressure limit affects both forms of pressure ventilation.

MANIPULATING PaO$_2$

Fraction of Inspired Oxygen. The most obvious way to improve oxygen delivery is to increase the alveolar oxygen tension by increasing the fraction of inspired oxygen (FIO$_2$). A simple method to determine the FIO$_2$ needed for a desired PaO$_2$ is derived from the arterial to alveolar oxygen tension

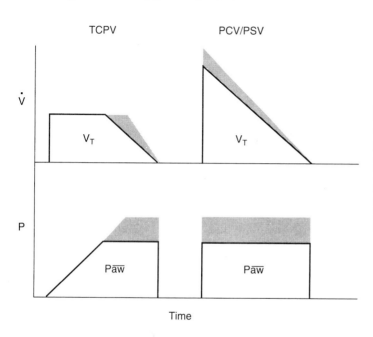

Fig. 19-7

Waveforms comparing the mechanism of increasing tidal volume (V_T) by adjusting pressure limit during time-cycled pressure-limited ventilation (TCPV) to pressure-control or pressure-support ventilation (PCV/PSV). Flow changes during PCV/PSV, but only the length of time changes before flow decelerates during TCPV.

ratio. Assuming constant barometric pressure, $PaCO_2$, and stable lung conditions, the equation simplifies to

$$FIO_2 \text{ desired} = PaO_2 \text{ desired} \times \frac{FIO_2 \text{ known}}{PaO_2 \text{ known}}$$

Because prolonged exposure to high levels of oxygen may be toxic, the lowest acceptable FIO_2 should be used.[49] However, high levels of oxygen may be necessary to correct hypoxemia when treating severe lung disease or persistent pulmonary hypertension of the newborn. To avoid these complications, other variables that relate to improving oxygenation must also be considered, such as $P\overline{aw}$, nitric oxide, and positive end-expiratory pressure (PEEP).

Mean Airway Pressure. Improvement in PaO_2 is directly related to an increase in $P\overline{aw}$. (It may have an inverse relationship in right-to-left cardiac shunts or in pulmonary volutrauma.[50-52]) This improvement is believed to be caused by recruitment of collapsed alveoli or the redistribution of lung fluid, or both.[21] $P\overline{aw}$ is the area under the pressure waveform from the beginning of inflation to the beginning of the

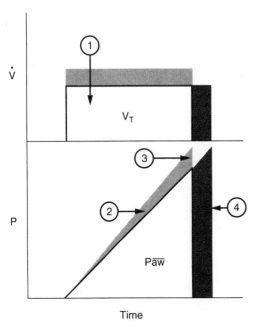

Fig. 19-8

Control variables that alter mean airway pressure ($P\overline{aw}$) by increasing the area under the pressure waveform. *1,* Increase tidal volume (V_T) or rate. *2,* Increase inspiratory flow. *3,* Increase peak pressure. *4,* Increase inspiratory time. Also shown is the associated change in V_T.

next inflation divided by the total cycle time. A simple equation for estimating $P\overline{aw}$ is as follows:

$$P\overline{aw} = \frac{1}{2} \times \text{peak pressure} \times \left(\frac{\text{inspiratory time}}{\text{inspiratory} + \text{expiratory times}} \right)$$

Several control variables affect the $P\overline{aw}$, including inspiratory time, peak pressure, frequency, flow, and PEEP. The denominator of the equation for $P\overline{aw}$ is cycle time or frequency. As frequency increases, cycle time decreases so that the result is an increase in the value of $P\overline{aw}$. Fig. 19-8 demonstrates how the pressure waveform can be altered by these variables to increase $P\overline{aw}$. The desired $P\overline{aw}$ is one in which both oxygenation and ventilation are optimized, and the risks of pulmonary volutrauma, impaired hemodynamics, and fluid retention are minimized.

Flow Rate. The flow rate will directly affect the $P\overline{aw}$. Ideally, inspiratory flow should be set to match the patient's peak inspiratory demands and depends largely on (1) the patient's spontaneous effort, (2) the work of breathing, and (3) patient-ventilator synchrony. Too much or not enough flow can increase the work of breathing or cause dyssynchrony.[53,54] Fig. 19-9 using a flow-volume loop illustrates when there is inadequate flow. The flow and pressure waveforms vary among ventilators. The flow required for spontaneous breathing is provided by means of continuous flow or a demand valve that is triggered by the patient's inspiratory effort.[6]

Inspiratory Time and I:E Ratio. The inspiratory time and I:E ratio also directly affect $P\overline{aw}$. Although there are little specific data regarding guidelines for inspiratory time and I:E ratio, it is suggested that the appropriate inspiratory time and I:E ratio depend on

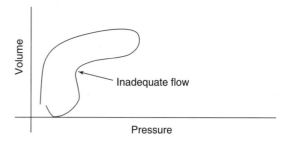

Fig. 19-9

Inadequate flow support on flow-volume loop. A normal loop should look like a football at a 45-degree angle. The inspiratory phase of this loop is concave, owing to inadequate flow.

the patient's ventilation and oxygenation status as well as on the level of spontaneous breathing. Ventilators are often set at an inspiratory time of 0.3 to 0.5 second for neonates, 0.5 to 0.75 second for toddlers/children, and 0.75 to 1.25 seconds for adolescents, with an I:E ratio of 1:2 to 1:3. Increasing the inspiratory time or I:E ratio is performed in an effort to increase Paw and improve oxygenation. When this is carried out, however, the impact on patient comfort, the need for sedation, the development of auto-PEEP, hemodynamic compromise, and breath stacking must be considered[6,55] (see discussion of IRV mode). Fig. 19-10 is what you will see on the ventilator graphics if the inspiratory time is excessive.

Positive End-Expiratory Pressure. The most significant variable affecting Paw is PEEP. Fig. 19-11 shows the relationship of PEEP to the pressure waveform and Paw. PEEP affects pressure throughout the entire respiratory cycle and alters the simple formula given previously for Paw to

$$Paw = \frac{1}{2} \times (Peak\ pressure - PEEP) \times$$
$$\left(\frac{Inspiratory\ time}{Inspiratory\ time + Expiratory\ time} \right) + PEEP$$

PEEP improves gas exchange by improving Pao_2, recruiting collapsed alveoli, increasing functional lung volume, decreasing intrapulmonary shunting, and improving lung compliance.[56-58] An adequate PEEP level is the amount of PEEP necessary to attain an acceptable Pao_2 at the lowest Fio_2, although avoidance of high PEEP levels is

desired.[59] It is determined by many physiologic factors, which may or may not be monitored in any given clinical situation. A conservative but acceptable Pao_2 is 40 to 60 mm Hg for neonates younger than 33 weeks' gestation and 60 to 80 mm Hg for pediatric patients at an Fio_2 of 0.4 to 0.5. PEEP usually begins at 3 to 5 cm H_2O, with increases made in increments of 2 cm H_2O.[60,61] A method of judging adequate PEEP levels is to monitor *static lung compliance* or calculate it by dividing the effective tidal volume formula by the end-inspiratory pause pressure minus PEEP. When the functional residual capacity is low, static compliance increases as PEEP increases because of shifting of the ventilating volume to the optimal point on the compliance curve. When optimal distention is reached, lung compliance is maximal. If PEEP is increased further, overdistention, reduced compliance, and decreased oxygen transport may result.[56] This concept is illustrated in Fig. 19-12. Static compliance can be hard to obtain in patients with cuffless endotracheal tubes if they have a leak.

Monitoring the $Paco_2$ to end-tidal carbon dioxide gradient may also be useful in judging PEEP levels (see Chapter 10). Overdistention and reduced cardiac output from excessive PEEP cause the gradient to widen. Caution must be used with this method because other abnormalities causing a low cardiac output may also increase this gradient.[17,62] Because excessive levels of PEEP affect cardiac function, monitoring mean blood pressure, mean pulmonary artery pressure, and other hemodynamic variables is also important while monitoring PEEP levels. When pulmonary artery catheters are used, cardiac output and the pulmonary shunt fraction are useful measures. A reduction of the shunt fraction, normally to less than 15%, is the goal when applying PEEP in patients with ARDS.[57] When using this variable to adjust PEEP and the shunt fraction is

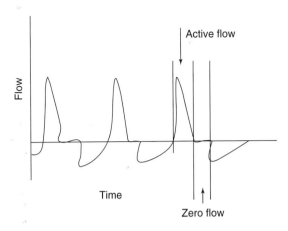

Fig. 19-10

Excessive inspiratory time on flow/time scalar. Flow returns to baseline before the ventilator cycles into expiration.

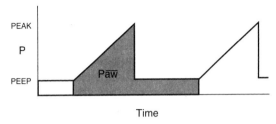

Fig. 19-11

The relationship of positive end-expiratory pressure (PEEP) to the pressure waveform. Note that mean airway pressure (Paw) is the area under the waveform during the entire respiratory cycle.

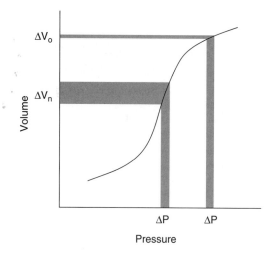

Fig 19-12

Compliance curve shows the effect of overdistention on tidal volume. ΔP is the same amount in each case. ΔV_n is normal compliance and tidal volume. Overdistention places the breath on the flat portion of the compliance curve, resulting in a smaller tidal volume, ΔV_o.

reduced to less than 15%, levels of PEEP in excess of 25 cm H_2O are usually required.[58] This aspect of using PEEP in the pediatric population is generally prohibited in patients with an uncuffed endotracheal tube because of the leak around the tube.

Not only can PEEP be applied as a ventilating variable, but it also can be present in the form of *auto-PEEP* (intrinsic, occult, or inadvertent PEEP).[63,64] Auto-PEEP is the difference between alveolar pressure and external airway pressure at end-expiration.[6] Causes include impedance to exhalation related to circuit or airway resistance, rapid breathing frequency, inverse I:E ratio, expiratory muscle activity, narrow endotracheal tube, water clogging the exhalation tube, an inadequate exhalation valve, or a malfunctioning PEEP regulator.[6] Auto-PEEP has the same clinical effects as therapeutically applied PEEP. The two possible goals to managing auto-PEEP are either (1) to minimize it or (2) to use it as a ventilation variable in manipulating $\overline{Paw}$. In either case, recognizing and monitoring auto-PEEP are clinically important and discussed later in this chapter. The use of PEEP in obstructive lung disease, such as asthma, is controversial, with some investigators reporting improved gas exchange and decreased airway resistance whereas others found increased air trapping and hemodynamic compromise.[65-67]

Multiple variables affect ventilation and oxygenation. It must be understood that manipulating a ventilator setting with the objective of improving one condition may result in undesirable effects on another.[6] Balancing these variables allows the clinician to meet the goals of mechanical ventilation, as well as optimize oxygen delivery, recruit lung volume, improve gas distribution, and alter minute ventilation.

PATIENT-VENTILATOR INTERFACE

Understanding the ventilator circuit is an integral aspect of ventilator management. The circuit is the interface between the ventilator and the patient system.[68] There are five major factors to consider when assessing the impact of the circuit on ventilation: (1) compressible volume, (2) air leak, (3) dead space, (4) resistance, and (5) humidification.

COMPRESSIBLE VOLUME

The influence of compressible volume on effective tidal volume during volume ventilation was discussed earlier. Ventilator circuit compression influences tidal volume during pressure ventilation as well.[19] When the ventilator delivers a breath, pressure inside the circuit increases and compresses the gas volume delivered. This compressed volume never reaches the patient, and the inspired volume is less than the set volume. During expiration, however, the compressed volume passes through the exhalation valve and is measured as part of the patient's exhaled volume. This results in the patient's actual inflation volumes being less than that recorded as exhaled volume. A circuit compliance or compression factor can be calculated, as illustrated in Box 19-2. Thus some clinicians describe this as volume "lost" in the tubing. The compressible volume of disposable tubing is generally greater than that of reusable tubing.[69] The humidifier also represents a source for gas compression and is included in calculating compressible volume. Using a constant-level self-feeding humidifier is necessary to minimize variations in compressible volume in all pediatric ventilation situations.[70]

AIR LEAK

In the pediatric clinical setting, it is important not to confuse compressible volume losses with air leaks. Air leaks are most notable around a cuffless endotracheal or tracheostomy tube. Accurately monitoring tidal volume is difficult in the presence of an air leak. An excessive air leak compromises tidal volume delivery, reduces lung-distending pressures, and may adversely affect the ventilator triggering mechanism. Generally, air leaks are monitored by the difference between the tidal volume delivered by the ventilator and the patient's exhaled tidal volume.[19] Another way to identify an air leak is via flow graphics. Fig. 19-13 illustrates an air leak on a volume/time scale. In most clinical situations, an air leak greater than 15% of the delivered tidal volume makes volume ventilation dif-

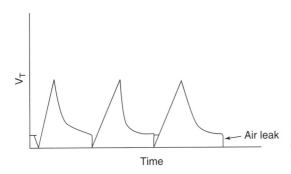

Fig. 19-13

Air leak shown on a volume/time scalar. Volume never returns to baseline before ventilator cycles again.

ficult. Even though the leak still occurs during constant pressure ventilation, switching to a higher flow rate and pressure setting may deliver a satisfactory tidal volume. Usually reintubation is necessary to maintain consistent volume ventilation and adequate triggering of the ventilator.

DEAD SPACE AND RESISTANCE

Dead space is the portion of the circuit distal to the main bias flow or circuit where gas can be rebreathed. This includes the volume of the circuit Y-connector, elbow, any monitoring device attached to the endotracheal tube connector, the endotracheal tube, and the conducting airways. The conducting airways are known as anatomic dead space and are not influenced by the circuit. However, the dead space added to the circuit is mechanical dead space. With smaller pediatric volumes, mechanical dead space may result in undesired rebreathing of carbon dioxide. Specially designed pediatric or infant monitoring devices and circuits help minimize this. Overzealous application of low dead space monitoring devices may result in increased resistance at the airway if the proper size is not used. Another component to evaluate as a choke point for gas flow is the adaptor connecting the tubing to the elbow or the endotracheal tube. A rule of thumb is that the endotracheal tube should be the point of highest circuit resistance. If a circuit component is smaller in cross-sectional area than the endotracheal tube, another circuit or component should be used.[71]

HUMIDIFICATION

The humidification system is an integral part of the patient-ventilator system. When the normal heating and humidification systems of the body are bypassed or are inadequate, it is necessary to artificially heat and humidify the inhaled gases. Optimal humidity and temperature are dependent on the clinical situation. Usually a temperature of 37° C and a water content of 44 mg/L are adequate.[72] Servo-controlled, heated humidifiers that possess a small compressible volume are used most often in pediatric patients who require mechanical ventilation. Complications associated with these humidifiers include overheating and nosocomial infection. Water condensation in the ventilator circuit may also lead to nosocomial infection as well as to the accidental drainage of water into the patient's lungs. With the use of a servo-controlled heated wire circuit, complications are not as frequent in the pediatric population as they once were. However, awareness of the operational characteristics of the humidifier and its controlling mechanisms is important in the ventilator management of the pediatric patient.

COMPLICATIONS OF MECHANICAL VENTILATION

Each of the physiologic effects of mechanical ventilation has an associated risk. Box 19-4 lists the complications associated with mechanical ventilation.[6]

OVERDISTENTION

Alveolar overdistention is a primary cause of complications encountered during mechanical ventilation and is a result of high ventilating pressures, large tidal volumes, and excessive PEEP. Extrapulmonary air leaks, or volutrauma, in the form of pneumothorax, pneumomediastinum, pneumoperitoneum, and subcutaneous emphysema are the most notable complications and are the result of overdistention of alveolar and peribronchial tissues.[5,73] Treatment consists of detecting the leak, decreasing tidal volume (if higher than 8 ml/kg), using PEEP, and relieving the leak with a chest tube if necessary. Permissive hypercapnia could also be a useful tool in the treatment of an air leak.[74] Overdistention also causes a decrease in static compliance as noted in Fig. 19-12, an increase in the work of breathing, an increase in anatomic dead space, an increase in the air leak around an endotracheal tube, and possible difficulties in weaning. As compliance diminishes, the $Paco_2$ may rise or fail to improve. To counter this, ventilation is increased, which may lead to further distention.

Because volumes are smaller in the neonatal and pediatric patient than in the adult, avoiding and detecting overdistention is a critical aspect of ventilator management. Alarms that may help detect this are indirect and can be activated by other problems. These alarms include high Paw; exhaled minute ventilation, which is useful during SIMV and other spontaneous modes; high peak pressure; high PEEP; high respiratory frequency; and inverse I:E ratio. Measures such as using an end-expiratory pause to

---

BOX 19-4

COMPLICATIONS OF MECHANICAL VENTILATION

BAROTRAUMA
Pneumothorax
Pneumomediastinum
Pneumopericardium
Pneumoperitoneum
Subcutaneous emphysema

NOSOCOMIAL INFECTION
ARDS
Pneumonia

PATIENT-VENTILATOR ASYNCHRONY
Auto-PEEP
Hyperventilation
Respiratory alkalosis
Increased work of breathing

NONCARDIOPULMONARY COMPLICATIONS
Psychologic distress
Renal dysfunction
  Fluid retention
Gastrointestinal dysfunction
  Vomiting
  Ulceration and bleeding
Increased intracranial pressure

AIRWAY COMPLICATIONS
Sinusitis
Vocal cord injury
Inadvertent extubation
Retention of secretions
Glottic injury
  Glottic edema
  Glottic stenosis
  Glottic erosion
Tracheal injury
  Tracheal erosion
  Tracheomalacia
  Tracheal dilation
  Tracheal–innominate artery fistula
Airway obstruction
  Main stem intubation
  Kinking of endotracheal tube
  Plugging of endotracheal-tracheostomy tube

CARDIOVASCULAR COMPROMISE
Decreased venous return
Decreased cardiac output

OXYGEN TOXICITY

ARDS, Adult respiratory distress syndrome; *PEEP,* positive end-expiratory pressure.

---

look for incomplete exhalation and an increase in PEEP or to detect auto-PEEP, measuring optimal static compliance, inspecting pressure-volume loops to determine overdistention or exhaled resistance, monitoring changes in $\overline{Paw}$, and obtaining a chest radiograph all help to detect overdistention.

The formation of a bronchopleural fistula presents an especially challenging clinical situation. Because the volume of gas delivered by the ventilator will follow the path of least resistance, a substantial part of the tidal volume will move into the pleural space during inspiration and escape through the chest tube. This volume is seen as the air bubbles through the water seal chamber of the chest tube drainage system, and the amount may be determined by noting the difference between the inspiratory and expiratory volumes. Although most bronchopleural fistulas are insignificant, if the leak is large enough it may result in inadequate ventilation and lead to ventilation-perfusion mismatch and further hypoxemia. Conventional treatment consisting of low pressures and volumes allowing permissive hypercapnia and allowing the patient to breathe spontaneously as much as possible may aid in decreasing flow through the fistula and facilitate its closure. When this is not possible in patients with severe ventilation problems, nonconventional modes of treatment may be needed. Independent lung ventilation or high-frequency ven-

tilation may be considered, as may using valves to occlude the chest tube during inspiration.[75-77]

CARDIOVASCULAR COMPLICATIONS

Reduced cardiac output from cardiac septal deviation, increased pulmonary vascular resistance, reduced venous return, and reduced myocardial blood flow is a complication of mechanical ventilation. In most cases, it is a result of increased intrathoracic pressures. In the neonatal and pediatric patient it can usually be prevented by increasing the circulating fluid volume.[58,78] Vasopressor drugs may also be used to maintain cardiac output during ventilation regimens that include high distending volumes.[50] An increase in intrathoracic pressure may be applied in some clinical situations to reduce left-to-right shunting, raise pulmonary vascular resistance, and impede pulmonary blood flow. However, other means such as nitrogen and oxygen gas mixtures with less than 21% oxygen may also accomplish this without risk of increasing intrathoracic pressures and reducing blood flow to other organ systems.

OXYGEN TOXICITY

Oxygen toxicity is another concern during mechanical ventilation. High FIO_2 levels that have been applied for an extended period may result in tissue injury that alters lung function and gas distribution.[49] Incorporating a high FIO_2 alarm

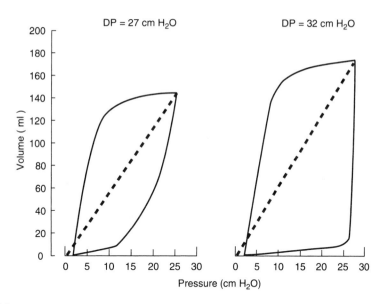

Fig. 19-14

An example of a pressure-volume loop demonstrating insufficient flow caused by setting the driving pressure (DP) too low during pressure-support ventilation of a child. With DP set at 27 cm H_2O, the peak pressure *(top right corner of the loop)* is reached at the end of inflation. With the DP set at 32 cm H_2O, the peak pressure is reached early during inflation *(lower right corner of the loop)*. Note the perpendicular right side of the loop.

and minimizing the F_{IO_2} to the level necessary to attain adequate tissue oxygenation, as well as using pulse oximetry and blood gas monitoring, are essential in attempting to prevent tissue damage.

HYPOVENTILATION/HYPERVENTILATION

The primary cause of hypoventilation during mechanical ventilation is disconnection from the ventilator and accidental extubation.[79,80] Care must be used when moving the patient connected to a ventilator, especially during transport and patient care procedures such as chest physiotherapy. A low-pressure or disconnect alarm is essential to alert the clinician when this occurs. Hypoventilation may also result from high impedance to inflation, which can be due to high resistance (resulting from anatomic, pathologic, or circuit design) or loss of pulmonary compliance.[81] A low-volume monitor will not detect these changes unless it is located at the airway connection. Underventilation can be avoided by calculating effective tidal volume or airway monitoring of ventilation variables, routinely monitoring or calculating compliance and resistance, monitoring pressure-volume and flow-volume loops, and using sufficient driving or working pressures to minimize attenuation of the inflating flow waveform. A chest radiograph also may be helpful in detecting underaeration.

Hypoventilation may also be related to "operator error" in establishing ventilation. Hypoventilation caused by minute ventilation, frequency, volume, or flow rate that is insufficient to meet inspiratory demand results in increased work of breathing and muscle fatigue. These conditions may also be present when weaning from the ventilator and may cause weaning failure. The alert patient may communicate feelings of respiratory distress. Retractions, use of accessory muscles, head bobbing, and a 10% to 20% increase in heart rate and spontaneous respiratory frequency are clinical signs of insufficient ventilation. In a sedated, paralyzed, or critically ill patient, however, this problem may not be as evident. Using pressure-volume and flow-volume loops, monitoring carbon dioxide production and oxygen consumption, and obtaining other measurements such as a diaphragm electromyogram may help detect this problem. Ensuring that the initial inspiratory flow rate meets the patient's inspiratory demand is usually the best method of avoidance.[41,82-84] An example of a pressure-volume loop demonstrating insufficient flow caused by insufficient driving pressure during PSV is shown in Fig. 19-14. Fig. 19-15 shows the effect of a faulty flow transducer on a diaphragm electromyogram tracing during PSV, leading to increased work of breathing.

Hyperventilation can also be a problem if the patient's lung compliance improves (i.e., surfactant administration or prone/supine positioning) in a pressure control or pressure support mode. Close monitoring of minute ventilation or tidal volume with alarms has proved to be useful in reducing this problem.

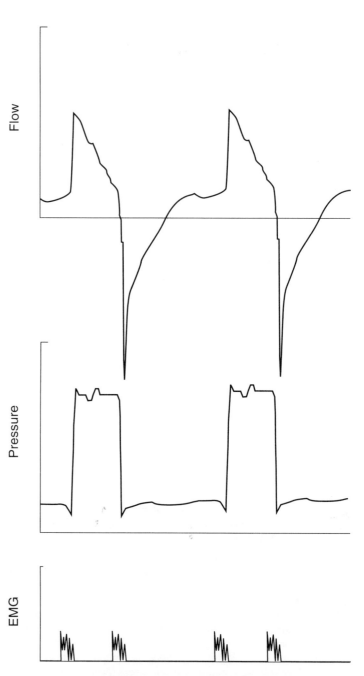

Fig. 19-15

A recording of the electromyographic (EMG) signal shows muscle activity to initiate inflation during pressure-support ventilation. The flow transducer on this ventilator is defective, and the electromyogram shows abnormal muscle activity, not seen by clinical observation, at the end of inflation to stop the breath. Transdiaphragmatic pressure measurements would also help detect this situation.

MONITORING DURING MECHANICAL VENTILATION

Monitoring effective ventilation is accomplished by using the techniques discussed previously. Box 19-5 lists monitoring applications as they apply to pediatric mechanical ventilation. Most ventilators monitor airway pressures, flow, ventilatory frequency, tidal volume, and minute volume. Essential aspects of monitoring include (1) calculation of effective tidal volume; (2) close observation of the patient for clinical signs of adequate ventilation as well as respiratory distress, such as chest expansion and retractions; (3) noninvasive methods of determining oxygenation and ventilation status, such as pulse oximetry, transcutaneous monitoring, and end-tidal carbon dioxide monitoring; and (4) direct measurement of blood gas values. Fig. 19-16 demonstrates possible problems detected using an end-tidal carbon dioxide monitor.[16,64,85]

BOX 19-5

MONITORING APPLICATIONS IN PEDIATRIC MECHANICAL VENTILATION

MEASURED VENTILATOR VARIABLES
Effective tidal volume
Minute ventilation
Mean airway pressure (P$\overline{aw}$)
Low-high positive end-expiratory
    pressure (PEEP)
High peak pressure
Fraction of inspired oxygen (FIO$_2$)
Pause pressure
Inspiratory:expiratory ratio
Pressure waveform
Flow waveform
Static compliance
Respiratory time fraction
Dynamic compliance
Airway resistance
Respiratory time constant

Maximal inspiratory occlusion pressure
Maximal expiratory occlusion pressure
Maximal minute ventilation
Vital capacity

SUPPLEMENTAL MONITORS
Pulse oximetry
End-tidal carbon dioxide
End-tidal carbon dioxide to PaCO$_2$ gradient
Pressure-volume loop
Esophageal pressure
Transpulmonary pressure
Dead space to tidal volume ratio
Ineffective to effective tidal volume ratio
Work of breathing
Pressure time product
Pressure time index

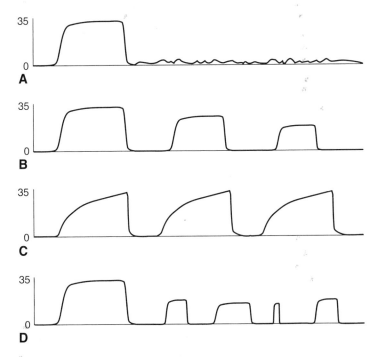

Fig. 19-16

End-tidal carbon dioxide recordings. **A,** Abrupt disconnection from the ventilator. **B,** Falling PETCO$_2$, possibly from an increase in tidal volume or, if PaCO$_2$ is unchanged, a reduction in pulmonary blood flow from overdistention or low cardiac output. **C,** Dampened waveform from severe air flow obstruction or side stream sampling tube obstruction. **D,** System leak or secretions in the sampling chamber. (Modified from Advanced Concepts in Capnography. Nellcor Inc., Hayward, Calif., 1988.)

WEANING FROM MECHANICAL VENTILATION

INITIATION

Weaning is the gradual process by which mechanical ventilation is discontinued and the patient resumes spontaneous breathing. The process may be rapid or slow, depending on the individual clinical situation. It is difficult to define at exactly what point during mechanical ventilation the weaning process should begin; however, most would agree that ideally it is after significant resolution or reversal of the pathologic condition for which it was initiated. Before weaning begins, the patient's condition should be stable and the patient should be receiving adequate nourishment and be able to breathe spontaneously and maintain a clinically acceptable PaCO$_2$. The ventilator should be on acceptable settings: usually PEEP less than 8 cm H$_2$O; peak pressure less than 30 cm H$_2$O; ventilator rate less than 20 breaths per minute for a neonate, 15 breaths per minute for an infant/toddler, and 10 breaths per minute for a child or adolescent; and FIO_2 less than 0.4 to 0.5.[3,10,81,85-87] Various methods exist for measuring respiratory muscle endurance and predicting successful weaning. Simple observations such as accessory or paradoxical muscle activity, respiratory rate, tidal volume, and minute ventilation are the first indicators of weaning readiness.[88,89] An increase in respiratory frequency of 15% to 20% or a reduction in tidal volume is associated with impending fatigue. Maintaining a normal or clinically acceptable $PaCO_2$ with a normal minute ventilation (0.5 to 1 L/min for an infant to 4 to 9 L/min for an adult) would indicate that the patient might tolerate weaning. Normal carbon dioxide production in an infant is 6 ml/kg/min, and it is 3 ml/kg/ min in an adult.[90] Excessive carbon dioxide production indicates a hypermetabolic state and may be corrected by adjusting nutritional elements to lower the respiratory quotient. Another helpful determinant of the ability to wean is the V_D:V_T ratio. The normal value is 0.3; however, intubation and mechanical ventilation may alter this. A value of less than 0.6 to 0.7 may predict successful weaning. Another clinically measurable variable that roughly approximates the V_D:V_T ratio is the ineffective to effective tidal volume ratio. Abnormal values may indicate continued pulmonary or cardiac dysfunction. Measurement of the end-tidal carbon dioxide to $PaCO_2$ gradient may also help detect continued pulmonary or cardiac dysfunction. In this case, cautious weaning may be indicated, although resolution of the clinical condition is most likely indicated.[86]

Other predicting factors may also be considered. A flow-volume loop may help discover impedance to inspiratory or expiratory flow that will precipitate fatigue. A pressure-volume loop may help determine work of breathing and evaluate various weaning modes. Measurements of dynamic and static compliance, resistance, transpulmonary pressure tracing, work of breathing, respiratory time fraction, the pressure time product (PTP), and the pressure time index (PTI) are useful variables in monitoring the course of weaning. PTP reflects the metabolic work of the respiratory system and is an electronically integrated value derived from tidal volume, compliance, esophageal pressure, and duration of the breath.[91] The PTI combines PTP and the respiratory time fraction and correlates directly with muscle fatigue and oxygen consumption.[92,93] Spontaneous maximum inspiratory and expiratory occlusion pressures may also be of value. These measurements are routine weaning values in many adult units, along with maximal spontaneous minute ventilation and vital capacity measurements. Unlike these measurements, however, occlusion pressure measurements do not require that a patient understand the breathing techniques necessary to effectively determine the values.

TECHNIQUES OF WEANING

The basic weaning techniques used in neonates and pediatric patients include CPAP, SIMV, and PSV. Using CPAP during weaning is common among pediatric patients. The positive airway pressure is used to provide the physiologic PEEP, which is bypassed when the patient is intubated.[30] Two techniques for using CPAP are practiced. The first is applied when there is sufficient respiratory drive and endurance but the physiologic effects of PEEP are still required. In this case, the CPAP is gradually reduced during the weaning process. The second technique is a postoperative weaning technique. The usefulness of this technique in pediatrics may be limited, however, because of the high resistance of the small-diameter airways. It may occasionally be employed to build respiratory muscle endurance by using a bias flow during short-duration exercises alternating with long periods of complete rest. The exercise periods are slowly increased as the resting periods are decreased. The process continues until the patient can breathe without support for a specified time. This technique is usually used only when the goal is to wean the patient to intermittent periods off the ventilator, such as with certain neuromuscular diseases or quadriplegia or in preparation for phrenic nerve pacing.

SIMV involves a gradual decrease in the ventilator frequency, usually in increments of 2 to 5 breaths per minute. As the ventilator rate is reduced, the patient is required to contribute more spontaneous efforts to the overall ventilation frequency. How quickly the SIMV rate is decreased depends on assessment of the patient's clinical status and blood gas values. The more slowly the process is performed, the more time the patient has to acclimate to less ventilator support. Factors such as ventilator system resistance, a sluggish demand valve, or insufficient inspiratory flow may affect the success of weaning with SIMV. If a bias flow is used during the spontaneous breathing periods, a reservoir is necessary to supply gas flow if inspiratory demand exceeds the bias flow. Weaning with SIMV is generally uncomplicated and is usually successful in older patients with endotracheal tube sizes large enough to minimize excessive inspiratory resistance. When weaning patients with smaller tube sizes, the goal is to wean to a rate of 20 breaths for an endotracheal tube less than 3.5 mm internal diameter, 15 breaths for endotracheal tube sizes

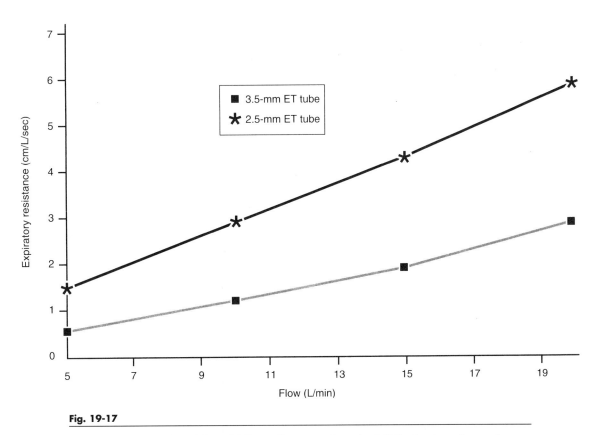

Fig. 19-17

Exhaled resistance using a 2.5- and 3.5-mm-diameter endotracheal (ET) tube at varying continuous-flow rates through the ventilator circuit.

4.0 to 5.0 mm internal diameter, and 10 breaths per minute for anything greater than a 5.0-mm tube, and then extubate. When using continuous flow, a common practice is to set a standard flow rate on all ventilators in the neonatal patient population. Fig. 19-17 shows the relationship of continuous flow to resistance. The smaller the diameter, the more likely that changes in flow rate influence exhaled resistance. Using a rate of less than just stated is thought to contribute to fatigue and unsuccessful weaning because of endotracheal resistance.

Weaning with PSV provides sufficient positive pressure to minimize the metabolic requirements for ventilation during weaning.[10,41,83,86,89] In addition, PSV allows the patient to initiate the breath, preventing atrophy of the inspiratory muscles. Fig. 19-18 illustrates a pressure-volume loop and other respiratory variables used to evaluate the effect of PSV and CPAP on an infant who is difficult to wean. Once weaning is indicated and PSV is selected, the pressure-support level should be adjusted to deliver the tidal volume of 5 to 7 ml/kg. Frequency should be monitored and the driving pressure adjusted to attain an appropriate flow rate. Once satisfactory volume, flow, and frequency are set, the pressure-support level can be reduced in increments of 2 to 5 cm H_2O. While on a higher pressure level, the patient contributes only the muscle work required to trigger the inflation. As the pressure is reduced, the patient progressively shares more of the work of breathing.[74] The pressure support should be weaned at a rate that is reasonable for each clinical situation. Endotracheal or tracheostomy tube leaks can hinder this progress. The patient who has been mechanically ventilated for only a short time, such as the stable postoperative patient, can be weaned at a rapid pace. The patient who has been on long-term mechanical ventilation requires patience and persistence in reducing the support level by only 1 or 2 cm H_2O over a longer period, such as a day or even a week. In these patients, weaning can be slowed by clinical events such as a viral illness or fluid and electrolyte imbalance. Once these clinical conditions are resolved, usually weaning can be continued with a successful outcome.[10]

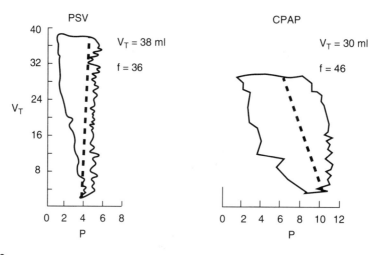

Fig. 19-18

Pressure-volume loops of an infant during weaning, demonstrating the effectiveness of using 5 cm H_2O of PEEP and 1 cm H_2O of pressure-support ventilation instead of using 10 cm H_2O of continuous positive airway pressure (CPAP).

ADVANCING CONCEPTS

Advances and improvements in technologies and practices such as high-frequency ventilation, nitric oxide, corticosteroids, prone positioning, permissive hypercapnia, extracorporeal membrane oxygenation, and surfactant replacement all influence future design and approaches to conventionally ventilating the neonate and pediatric patient. Now ventilators are becoming "partial support" in that they must work dynamically with the patient. New-generation ventilator companies are incorporating many modes, triggers, and graphics to help the clinician pick and choose what is best for that individual patient's needs. This fosters a dynamic relationship between the ventilator and patient. Liquid lung ventilation may be used by filling the lungs with a perfluorocarbon liquid that has a high oxygen solubility (see Chapter 22).[93] Initial studies used a lavage technique, but more recent studies have used an automated liquid breathing system. This device circulates the liquid and recycles it as necessary.[94] More studies are required to determine the safety and long-term outcomes of these techniques. Negative-pressure ventilation is also finding its way back into the critical care setting. Cardiopulmonary interactions are being investigated in children after simple cardiac surgery.[95]

REFERENCES

1. Mellins R et al: *Respiratory care in infants and children.* New York. American Lung Association, 1971; p 3.

2. Hess D: Pediatric and neonatal respiratory care: some implications for adult respiratory care practitioners. *Respir Care* 1991; 36:489-511.

3. Crowley CM, Marrow AI: A comprehensive approach to the child in respiratory failure. *Crit Care Q* 1980; 3:27-43.

4. Smith RA, Rasanen JO, Downs JB: Flow, pressure, and time modifications. *Contemp Management Crit Care* 1990; 1:15-28.

5. Chatburn R: Principles and practice of neonatal and pediatric mechanical ventilation. *Respir Care* 1991; 36:569-593.

6. American College of Chest Physicians: Consensus conference: mechanical ventilation. *Chest* 1993; 104:1835-1859.

7. Chatburn R: A new system for understanding mechanical ventilators. *Respir Care* 1991; 36:1123-1155.

8. Reynolds EO: Effect of alterations in mechanical ventilator settings on pulmonary gas exchange in hyaline membrane disease. *Arch Dis Child* 1971; 46:152-159.

9. Branson RD et al: Altering flow rate during maximum pressure support ventilation: effects on cardiorespiratory function. *Respir Care* 1990; 35:1056-1064.

10. Czervinske MP et al: Effects of working pressure on respiratory pattern and airway pressure during pressure support ventilation in infants with chronic lung disease. *Respir Care* 1988; 33:930.

11. Bergman NA: Effect of varying respiratory waveforms on distribution of inspired gas during artificial ventilation. *Am Rev Respir Dis* 1969; 100:518.

12. Boyson PG, McGough E: Pressure-control and pressure support ventilation: flow patterns, inspiratory time and gas distribution. *Respir Care* 1988; 33:126-134.

13. Abraham E, Yoshihara G: Cardiorespiratory effects of pressure control ventilation in severe respiratory failure. *Chest* 1990; 98:1445-1449.

14. Al Saady N, Bennet ED: Decelerating inspiratory flow improves lung mechanics and gas exchange in patients on intermittent positive pressure ventilation. *Intensive Care Med* 1985; 11:68-75.

15. Connors AF, McCaffree DR, Gray BA: Effect of inspiratory flow rate on gas exchange during mechanical ventilation. *Am Rev Respir Dis* 1981; 124:537-543.

16. Rau JL, Shelledy DC: The effect of varying inspiratory flow waveforms on peak and mean airway pressures with a time-cycled volume ventilator: a bench study. *Respir Care* 1991; 36:347-355.

17. Czervinske MP, Jiao JH, Teague WG: Improved effective to ineffective tidal volume ratio during pressure control ventilation of infant pigs. *Respir Care* 1989; 34:1067.

18. Branson RD, Chatburn RL: Technical description and classification of modes of ventilator operation. *Respir Care* 1992; 37:1026-1044.

19. Perez-Fontan JJ, Heldt GP, Gregory GG: The effect of a gas leak around the endotracheal tube on the mean tracheal pressure during mechanical ventilation. *Am Rev Respir Dis* 1985; 132:339-342.

20. Hakanson DO: Positive pressure ventilation: volume-cycled ventilators. In Goldsmith JP, Karrotkin EH, editors: *Assisted ventilation of the neonate.* Philadelphia. WB Saunders, 1981; pp 161-179.

21. Tobin MJ: Monitoring of pressure, flow, and volume during mechanical ventilation. *Respir Care* 1992; 37:1081-1096.

22. Demers RR, Pratter MR, Irwin RS: Use of the concept of ventilator compliance in the determination of static total compliance. *Respir Care* 1981; 26:644-648.

23. Boros SJ et al: The effect of independent variations in inspiratory-expiratory ratio and end expiratory pressure during mechanical ventilation in hyaline membrane disease: the significance of mean airway pressure. *J Pediatr* 1977; 91:794.

24. Carlo WA, Martin RJ: Principles of assisted ventilation. *Pediatr Clin North Am* 1986; 33:221.

25. Reynolds EOR: Pressure waveform and ventilator settings for mechanical ventilation in severe hyaline membrane disease. *Int Anesthesiol Clin* 1974; 12:259.

26. Abbey NC et al: Measurement of pharyngeal volume by digitized magnetic resonance imaging: effect of nasal continuous positive airway pressure. *Am Rev Respir Dis* 1989; 140:717.

27. Katz JA, Marks JD: Inspiratory work with and without continuous positive airway pressure in patients with acute respiratory failure. *Anesthesiology* 1985; 63:598-607.

28. Chatburn RL: Similarities and differences in the management of acute lung injury in neonates (IRDS) and in adults (ARDS). *Respir Care* 1988; 33:539-553.

29. Smith RA et al: Morphometric changes in a dog model of the adult respiratory distress syndrome after early therapy with continuous positive airway pressure. *Respir Care* 1987; 32:525-533.

30. Berman LS et al: Optimum levels of CPAP for tracheal extubation of newborn infants. *J Pediatr* 1976; 89:109-112.

31. Greenough A, Greenall F: Patient triggered ventilation in premature neonates. *Arch Dis Child* 1988; 63:77-78.

32. MacDonald K et al: Effect of patient flow-triggered ventilation pulmonary mechanics in neonates. *Respir Care* 1991; 36:1315.

33. Sassoon CSH: Mechanical ventilator design and function: the trigger variable. *Respir Care* 1992; 37:1056-1069.

34. American College of Chest Physicians-American Thoracic Society Joint Committee on Pulmonary Nomenclature: Pulmonary terms and symbols. *Chest* 1975; 67:583.

35. Waldhorn RE et al: Long-term compliance with nasal continuous positive airway pressure therapy of obstructive sleep apnea. *Chest* 1990; 97:33-37.

36. Stock MC, Downs JB: Airway pressure release ventilation: a new approach to ventilatory support during acute lung injury. *Respir Care* 1987; 32:517-521.

37. Garner W et al: Airway pressure release ventilation (APRV): a human trial. *Chest* 1988; 94:779-781.

38. Stock MC, Downs JB, Frolicher DA: Airway pressure release ventilation. *Crit Care Med* 1987; 15:426-466.

39. Bach JR, Alba AS: Management of chronic alveolar hypoventilation by nasal ventilation. *Chest* 1990; 97:52-56.

40. Kacmarek RM: The role of pressure support ventilation in reducing work of breathing. *Respir Care* 1988; 33:99-120.

41. MacIntyre NR: Weaning from mechanical ventilatory support: volume-assisting intermittent breaths versus pressure-assisting every breath. *Respir Care* 1988; 33:121-125.

42. MacIntyre NR: Pressure support ventilation. *Respir Care* 1986; 31:189-190.

43. Brochard L et al: Inspiratory pressure support prevents diaphragmatic fatigue during weaning from mechanical ventilation. *Am Rev Respir Dis* 1989; 139:513-521.

44. Brochard L et al: Inspiratory pressure support compensates for the additional work of breathing caused by the endotracheal tube. *Anesthesiology* 1991; 75:739-745.

45. Forrette TL et al: Changes in pediatric ventilatory dynamics during mechanical ventilation with PSV. *Respir Care* 1990; 35:1128.

46. Ramsden CA, Reynolds EOR: Ventilator settings for newborn infants. *Arch Dis Child* 1987; 62: 529-538.

47. Boros SJ et al: Using conventional ventilators at unconventional rates. *Pediatrics* 1984; 74:487-492.

48. Clark RH: Lung protective strategies of ventilation in the neonate: what are they? *Pediatrics* 2000; 105 (1).

49. Jenkinson SG: Oxygen toxicity in acute respiratory failure. *Respir Care* 1983; 28:614-617.

50. Ciszek TA et al: Mean airway pressure—significance during mechanical ventilation in neonates. *J Pediatr* 1981; 99: 121-126.

51. Boros SJ: Variations in inspiratory:expiratory ratio and airway pressure waveform during mechanical ventilation: the significance of mean airway pressure. *J Pediatr* 1979; 94:114-119.

52. Gallagher TJ, Banner MJ: Mean airway pressure as a determinant of oxygenation. *Crit Care Med* 1980; 8:244.

53. Kirby R: Improving ventilator patient interaction: reduction of flow dyssynchrony. *Crit Care Med* 1997; 25:10.

54. Amal J: Inspiratory flow rate: more may not be better. *Crit Care Med* 1999; 27:4.

55. Kacmarek RM: Essential gas delivery features of mechanical ventilators. *Respir Care* 1992; 37:1045-1055.

56. Suter PM, Fairley HB, Isenberg MD: Optimum end-expiratory pressure in patients with acute pulmonary failure. *N Engl J Med* 1975; 292:284-289.

57. Kirby RR et al: High level positive end-expiratory pressure in acute respiratory insufficiency. *Chest* 1977; 71:18-23.

58. Kirby RR: Best PEEP: issues and choices in the selection and monitoring of PEEP levels. *Respir Care* 1988; 33:569-576.

59. Witte MK et al: Optimal positive end-expiratory pressure therapy in infants and children with acute respiratory failure. *Pediatr Res* 1988; 24:217-221.

60. Carroll CG et al: Minimal positive end-expiratory pressure (PEEP) may be "best PEEP." *Chest* 1988; 93:1020-1025.

61. Nelson LD, Civetta JM, Hudson-Civetta J: Titrating positive end-expiratory pressure therapy in patients with early moderate arterial hypoxemia. *Crit Care Med* 1987; 15:14-19.

62. Bilen Z, Colhen IL: Auto-PEEP characterization and consequences. *Anesthesiol Rep* 1990; 3:255-261.

63. Benson MS, Pierson MD: Auto-PEEP during mechanical ventilation of adults. *Respir Care* 1988; 33:557-565.

64. Murray JP et al: Titration of PEEP by the arterial minus end tidal carbon dioxide gradient. *Chest* 1984; 85:100-104.

65. Marini JJ: Should PEEP be used in airflow obstruction? *Am Rev Respir Dis* 1989; 140:1-3.

66. Tuxen DV: Detrimental effects of positive end-expiratory pressure during controlled mechanical ventilation of

patients with severe airflow obstruction. *Am Rev Respir Dis* 1989; 140:5-9.

67. Smith PG, El-Khatib MF, Carlo WA: PEEP does not improve pulmonary mechanics in infants with bronchiolitis. *Am Rev Respir Dis* 1993; 147:1295-1298.

68. Czervinske MP: Mechanical ventilator: A life support system. *Crit Care Q* 1984; 7(1):1 (letter).

69. Hess D, McCurdy S, Simmons M: Compression volume in adult ventilator circuits: a comparison of five disposable circuits and nondisposable circuits. *Respir Care* 1991; 36:1113-1118.

70. Haddad C, Richards CC: Mechanical ventilation of infants: significance and elimination of ventilator compression volume. *Anesthesiology* 1968; 29:365-370.

71. Rasanen J, Leijala M: Breathing circuit respiratory work in infants recovering from respiratory failure. *Crit Care Med* 1991; 19:31-35.

72. Irlbeck D: Normal mechanisms of heat and moisture exchange in the respiratory tract. *Respir Care Clin North Am* 1998; 4:2.

73. Dreyfuss D et al: High inflation pressure pulmonary edema: respective effects of high airway pressure, high tidal volume, and positive end expiratory pressure. *Am Rev Respir Dis* 1988; 137:1159-1164.

74. MacIntyre NR: Pressure support ventilation: effects on ventilatory reflexes and ventilatory muscle workloads. *Respir Care* 1987; 32:447-453.

75. Gallagher TJ et al: Intermittent inspiratory chest tube occlusion to limit bronchopleural cutaneous airleaks. *Crit Care Med* 1976; 4:328-330.

76. Powner DJ, Grenvik AKE: Ventilatory management of life-threatening bronchopleural fistulae—a summary. *Crit Care Med* 1981; 9:54-58.

77. Bevelaqua FA, Kay S: A modified technique for the management of bronchopleural fistula in ventilator-dependent patients: a report of two cases. *Respir Care* 1986; 31: 904-908.

78. Walkinshaw M, Shoemaker WC: Use of volume loading to obtain preferred levels of PEEP. *Crit Care Med* 1980; 8:81-86.

79. Dellinger PR: Complications of mechanical ventilation. *Pulmonol Crit Care Update* 1989; 5:2-6.

80. Strieter RM, Lynch JP: Complications in the ventilated patient. *Clin Chest Med* 1988; 9:127-139.

81. Mathewson HS, Linn RC, Gish GB: Pediatric mechanical ventilators. *J Kansas Med Soc* 1983; 84:255-262.

82. Marini JJ, Capps JS, Culver BH: The inspiratory work of breathing during assisted mechanical ventilation. *Chest* 1985; 87:612-618.

83. Marini JJ: Strategies to minimize the work of breathing during assisted mechanical ventilation. *Crit Care Clin* 1990; 6:635-661.

84. Shannon DC: Rational monitoring of respiratory function during mechanical ventilation of infants and children. *Intensive Care Med* 1989; 15:S13-S16.

85. Harris K: Noninvasive monitoring of gas exchange. *Respir Care* 1987; 32:544-553.

86. Boyson PG: Respiratory muscle function and weaning from mechanical ventilation. *Respir Care* 1987; 32:572-581.

87. Pierson DJ: Weaning from mechanical ventilation in acute respiratory failure: concepts, indications, and techniques. *Respir Care* 1983; 28:646-660.

88. Venkataraman ST: Validation of predictors of extubation success and failure in mechanically ventilated infants and children. *Crit Care Med* 2000; 28(8).

89. Manczur TI: Comparison of predictors of extubation from mechanical ventilated in children. *Pediatric Crit Care Med* 2000; 1(1).

90. Doershuk CF, Orenstein DM: Pulmonary function and exercise testing. In Lough MD, Doershuk CF, Stern RC, editors: *Pediatric respiratory therapy.* Chicago, Year Book Medical, 1979; p 250.

91. Sassoon CSH et al: Pressure-time product during continuous positive airway pressure, pressure support ventilation, and t-piece during weaning from mechanical ventilation. *Am Rev Respir Dis* 1991; 143:469-470.

92. Grassino A, Macklem P: Respiratory muscle fatigue and ventilator failure. *Ann Rev Med* 1984; 35:625-647.

93. Greenspan JS, Wolfson MR, Rubenstein SD: Liquid ventilation of preterm neonates. *J Pediatr* 1990; 117:106.

94. Greenspan JS: Liquid ventilation: a developing technology. *Neonatal Network* 1993; 12(4):23.

95. Shekerdemian LS: Cardiopulmonary interactions in healthy children and children after simple cardiac surgery: the effects of positive and negative pressure ventilation. *Heart* 1997; 78(6):587-593.

CHAPTER 20

Noninvasive Mechanical Ventilation of the Infant and Child

W. Gerald Teague

Methods of respiratory assistance that do not require an indwelling artificial airway are termed *noninvasive.* Noninvasive positive-pressure ventilation (NPPV) systems include an external mask interface and positive-pressure mechanical ventilator. Negative-pressure–assisted ventilation, a second method of noninvasive ventilation, involves the intermittent application of subatmospheric pressure external to the rib cage by means of a tank or chest mold. Continuous positive airway pressure (CPAP) therapy is a third method of noninvasive ventilation. CPAP is administered through an external mask interface with a simple constant flow source or through a pressure-targeted bilevel ventilator in the CPAP mode. This chapter addresses noninvasive ventilation in children in general, but the focus is primarily on NPPV.

Starting in the early 1990s, NPPV has rapidly grown as a method of assisted ventilation in pediatric-age patients. This may be explained primarily by widespread commercial access to portable bilevel pressure ventilators and soft nasal masks. A second reason for the popularity of NPPV is growing dissatisfaction with standard methods of long-term mechanical ventilation. For example, positive-pressure–assisted ventilation by means of tracheotomy (TPPV) is considered standard therapy for the management of complicated pediatric respiratory disorders.[1] Although highly effective, TPPV can result in significant medical complications, loss of mobility, and social isolation. As a result, clinicians dissatisfied with TPPV look to NPPV as a less invasive alternative. A third factor promoting the use of NPPV in pediatric patients is improved survival of children with catastrophic lung injury. Owing in part to modern technologies such as extracorporeal membrane oxygenation and high-frequency oscillatory ventilation, children who survive are often left with significant chronic lung disease. Noninvasive modes of respiratory assistance are increasingly attempted in these children to facilitate early extubation and for long-term care.

Clinicians who attempt NPPV in pediatric-age patients should know that modern bilevel pressure ventilators were designed to treat adult and not pediatric patients. Common shortfalls in the implementation of NPPV in pediatric patients include poor mask fit, incorrect adjustment of the inspiratory and expiratory pressures, and failure of small infants to trigger many bilevel devices in the spontaneous mode. These issues must be resolved for NPPV to be effectively used in very small patients.

The respiratory clinician must carefully evaluate a number of variables before attempting NPPV. Foremost, the appropriate equipment and settings should be considered. After initiation of NPPV, the child must be assessed immediately to be certain that the work of breathing has decreased and there is sufficient improvement in respiratory gas exchange. The approach to these and other problems will be addressed in this chapter.

OBJECTIVES OF NONINVASIVE VENTILATION

NPPV AND NEGATIVE-PRESSURE–ASSISTED VENTILATION

The objective(s) of noninvasive ventilation are identical to those of invasive mechanical ventilation (see Chapter 19). The primary objectives are to decrease the work of breathing, restore adequate CO_2 elimination, improve oxygenation, maintain upper airway stability, and restore lung volume (Box 20-1). There are a number of methods to determine the effectiveness of noninvasive ventilation in meeting these goals in the clinical setting, each with advantages and disadvantages (Table 20-1). Whatever the method(s) used, each member of the respiratory team must carefully document in the medical record the patient's response to treatment. This requires the therapist to carefully evaluate the patient both before and after initiation of noninvasive ventilation to document that the goals of treatment have been achieved.

In the acute setting, an important goal of noninvasive ventilation is to decrease the patient's work of breathing. Children with acute respiratory distress typically breathe rapidly and shallowly, visibly recruit the accessory muscles of respiration, and have prolonged periods of paradoxical rib cage/abdominal motion, referred to as retractions. These symptoms manifest a high level of respiratory muscle work maintained by neural activation. However, children with neuromuscular disorders

---

BOX 20-1

OBJECTIVES OF NONINVASIVE VENTILATION IN PEDIATRIC PATIENTS WITH RESPIRATORY DISORDERS

- Decrease the work of breathing
  - Assist the respiratory muscles
  - Decrease the respiratory rate
  - Prevent retractions
  - Decrease oxygen consumption associated with breathing
- Increase alveolar ventilation
  - Increase tidal volume
  - Decrease arterial and end-tidal $PaCO_2$
- Increase functional residual capacity
  - Decrease the alveolar-arterial oxygen tension difference
  - Prevent atelectasis
  - Decrease auto-PEEP
- Maintain upper airway patency
  - Decrease the number and length of occlusive apneas and hypopneas

---

often do not demonstrate the classic signs and symptoms of respiratory distress despite severe derangement in respiratory gas exchange. In such patients and in young infants, arterial blood gas analysis is necessary to assess the degree of respiratory dysfunction and to determine the effectiveness of noninvasive ventilation.

In the chronic setting, the goals of noninvasive ventilation are often different than in the acute setting. In children with chronic disorders complicated by alveolar hypoventilation, intermittent NPPV at night can be offered as a clinical benefit as a means to improve the quality of sleep and to reduce the severity of daytime symptoms associated with hypercarbia—headache and fatigue.[2] Although the ultimate goal of NPPV in this setting is to increase CO_2 elimination, this goal may not be reached for a number of days to weeks while the patient may report significant subjective improvement.

The daytime $PaCO_2$ should decrease 1 to 2 weeks after initiation of intermittent NPPV treatment at night in patients with restrictive disorders and chronic hypercarbia.[2] The mechanism for this improvement is uncertain, but it is likely caused by restoration of the central ventilatory responsiveness to changes in pH as a result of increased nocturnal CO_2 elimination. We have found that intermittent NPPV treatment in pediatric patients with chronic hypoventilation disorders effectively improves daytime CO_2 elimination for at least a period of 1 year and that this improvement is associated with a decrease in total serum levels of bicarbonate.[3,4] Other improvements in respiratory function that

TABLE 20-1	METHODS TO DETERMINE THE CLINICAL EFFECTIVENESS OF NONINVASIVE VENTILATION	
Method	**Outcome Expected**	**Disadvantages**
DECREASE WORK OF BREATHING		
Physical examination	Acute decrease in respiratory rate, retractions, and use of accessory muscles	Not reliable in patients with neuromuscular and central disorders
IMPROVE RESPIRATORY GAS EXCHANGE		
Pulse oximetry	Acute improvement in SaO_2	Not reliable in the assessment of hypoventilation Interpretation obscured by concurrent O_2 treatment
Blood gas sampling	Increase in pH, decrease in $PaCO_2$, increase in PaO_2	Invasive; $PaCO_2$ may not decrease for hours
End-tidal CO_2 monitoring	Acute reduction in end-tidal CO_2	High background flow in NPPV circuit can wash out expired CO_2
Transcutaneous CO_2 monitoring	Subacute reduction in transcutaneous CO_2	Accuracy dependent on careful electrode placement, changes lag minutes behind change in actual $PaCO_2$
INCREASE FUNCTIONAL RESIDUAL CAPACITY		
Routine chest radiography	Increased lung expansion, decreased atelectasis	Difficult to accomplish while on therapy; changes can lag days behind
MAINTAIN UPPER AIRWAY PATENCY		
Sleep polysomnography	Subacute reductions in the number of airway occlusive episodes; decrease in the degree of thoracoabdominal asynchrony	Not amenable to acute clinical setting

might result from long-term NPPV treatment include prevention of atelectasis and maintenance of functional residual capacity, increased lung compliance, and increased endurance of the respiratory muscles as a result of periods of rest. However, none of these potential benefits has been conclusively found in clinical studies.

CONTINUOUS POSITIVE AIRWAY PRESSURE

The primary goal of CPAP therapy is to increase end-expiratory lung volume, thereby improving oxygenation. CPAP therapy may or may not improve tidal volume and alveolar ventilation. In children with restrictive respiratory dysfunction and decreased lung compliance, CPAP therapy can raise tidal volume. However, in children with lung overexpansion and increased compliance, CPAP therapy may actually decrease tidal volume. In clinical practice, the results of arterial or capillary

blood gas analysis in combination with the pattern of respiratory dysfunction and cardiovascular stability determine the mode of treatment (Fig. 20-1).

EXPERIENCE WITH NPPV IN PEDIATRIC PATIENTS

ACUTE RESPIRATORY DISTRESS

There are no clear clinical indications for NPPV in pediatric patients, in whom it has been shown conclusively that NPPV is superior to standard therapy (Table 20-2). This is particularly true in the setting of acute hypoxemic respiratory failure, in which the experience with NPPV in children, although promising,[5,6] has not been subjected to carefully controlled trials. In this setting, it is not known whether NPPV can avoid intubation altogether or simply delay intubation. This situation is in marked contrast to a growing body of evidence in support

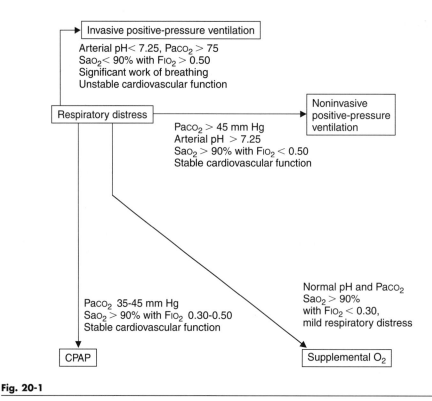

Fig. 20-1

Approach to the management of acute respiratory distress in pediatric-age patients.

of NPPV as superior to standard care in preventing intubation of adult patients with acute hypercarbic exacerbations of chronic obstructive lung disease.[7]

In pediatric-age patients admitted to an intensive care unit with acute hypoxemic respiratory failure associated with pneumonia, treatment with NPPV was safe and well tolerated, effectively improved oxygenation, and was associated with a relatively low incidence of endotracheal intubation.[8] In children with status asthmaticus complicated by acute hypoxemic respiratory failure, NPPV in the intensive care setting was effective in acutely improving oxygenation in most of the patients but did not prevent endotracheal intubation in a subset of children with hypercarbia on admission.[5,6] Furthermore, critically ill children treated with NPPV often require sedation, and in the latter study NPPV had to be withdrawn from nearly half of the patients as a result of agitation or deterioration of Sao_2. Controlled trials in children with specific categories of acute respiratory failure are indicated to best determine the role of NPPV in this challenging clinical setting.

CHRONIC RESPIRATORY DYSFUNCTION

In contrast to the acute setting, there is a better-defined role for NPPV in children with chronic disorders of the respiratory system complicated by alveolar hypoventilation (see Table 20-2). Children with chronic respiratory failure lead relatively normal lives for months to years as a result of the renal adaptation to hypercarbia. In the presence of lower respiratory tract infection or the stress of general anesthesia, the kidneys cannot compensate sufficiently, resulting in acute respiratory acidosis. In this setting, NPPV can be applied in the intensive care unit as a means to avoid endotracheal intubation. NPPV appears to work best when there is significant atelectasis and less so when the derangement in lung mechanical function is severe (see earlier). NPPV also shows promise as a weaning adjunct from invasive mechanical ventilation. In this role, NPPV has been used effectively in children with acute decompensation after adenotonsillar removal[9] and to stabilize airway function after laryngotracheoplasty.[10] Contraindications to a trial of NPPV include hemodynamic instability, significant upper airway obstruction (relative), inability to handle oral-pharyngeal secretions, and significant agitation.

Intermittent (nocturnal) NPPV has the potential to evolve as preferred therapy in pediatric patients with stable but chronic hypoventilation disorders.

TABLE 20-2	PUBLISHED CASE EXPERIENCE WITH NPPV IN PEDIATRIC PATIENTS WITH RESPIRATORY DISORDERS	
Disorder	**Published Outcomes***	**Reference**
ACUTE RESPIRATORY DISTRESS		
Pneumonia	Safe, well tolerated, low incidence of intubation	8
Status asthmaticus	Effectively improved oxygenation, but did not prevent intubation in children with hypercarbia on admission to the pediatric intensive care unit	5, 6
Decompensation after tonsillectomy	Effective in children with complicated sleep apnea syndrome after operation	9
Post laryngotracheoplasty	As a weaning step from invasive ventilation in the perioperative period	10
Weaning from invasive mechanical ventilation	NPPV immediate post extubation associated with need for reintubation in only two patients	21
CHRONIC RESTRICTIVE DISORDERS		
Neuromuscular disorders, spina bifida, scoliosis, cerebral palsy	Very effective in preventing sleep-associated hypoxemia associated with obstructive hypopnea	13
	Used as an alternate to tracheostomy and positive-pressure ventilation with improvement of daytime respiratory gas exchange	3, 4
CHRONIC OBSTRUCTIVE DISORDERS		
Cystic fibrosis	As a bridge therapy to lung transplantation in patients with advanced disease	22
	Prevented O_2-induced respiratory depression and improved CO_2 elimination during sleep	23
OBSTRUCTIVE HYPOVENTILATION SYNDROMES		
Obesity, complex anatomic upper airway obstruction	Improves oxygenation but less reliably improves ventilation with long-term nocturnal use. May prevent need for tracheostomy	4, 13

*All outcomes are based on published case reports and case series and not controlled trials.

Children with advanced neuromuscular disorders may go through an early stage of sleep disruption characterized by recurrent arousals and brief episodes of obstructive apnea/hypopnea with transient desaturation.[11,12] Rapid-eye-movement sleep in particular may be a relatively dangerous time for these patients because the upper airway muscle tone decreases, resulting in episodes of complete or partial airway occlusion. We have found that a long-term trial of NPPV administered at night in children with restrictive, obstructive hypoventilation and overlap (restrictive dysfunction with upper airway obstruction) disorders acutely improves sleep quality and reduces the number of occlusive events.[13] In a 1-year follow-up period, patient and family adherence to NPPV was better than expected and few patients required tracheostomy or died as a result of respiratory complications.[3,4]

NONINVASIVE VENTILATION WITH POSITIVE-PRESSURE DEVICES

BILEVEL PRESSURE-TARGETED VENTILATORS

In daily practice this type of ventilator is most often used for NPPV in pediatric patients. Bilevel devices set in the spontaneous mode respond to a step change in inspiratory flow rate by delivering a preset level of positive pressure, which is similar to the pressure-support function of contemporary ventilators designed for invasive mechanical ventilation. The result is an increase in tidal volume that is dependent on the compliance and resistance of the respiratory system and the gradient between the inspiratory and expiratory pressure adjustments.[14] Most bilevel ventilators available for commercial use are remarkably adept at delivering sufficient flow to reach the targeted level of inspiratory pressure.[15] These devices have a flow compensation feature so that leaks around the interface or through the mouth do not seriously impair performance. Other features standard on bilevel pressure-targeted ventilators include an expiratory positive airway pressure adjustment (EPAP), back-up ventilatory rate, and mode selection. Most do not have an independent oxygen blend feature.

The advantages of pressure-targeted ventilators designed for NPPV include ease of adjustment, portability, and relatively low cost. A significant disadvantage of these devices includes lack of a humidification system or independent oxygen blend adjustment. Furthermore, there is no U.S. Food and Drug Administration (FDA) approval for the first generation of bilevel ventilators for use as an invasive mode of mechanical ventilation in children with tracheostomies. Although this has not been an issue for inpatient application, it is a major impediment for outpatient use. Most home care companies require that physicians sign an indemnification agreement releasing them from liability should the device fail.

VOLUME-REGULATED VENTILATORS

NPPV can be accomplished through portable ventilators designed to cycle in the volume mode. The features of these ventilators are reviewed in Chapter 46. Most portable volume-regulated ventilators used in the home do not have a pressure support feature and must be adjusted carefully to ensure patient comfort. The potential advantages of volume-regulated devices for NPPV include superior performance when used in the synchronized intermittent mandatory ventilation mode in patients with significant neuromuscular weakness or central hypoventilation who may not trigger bilevel ventilators. Major drawbacks of portable volume-regulated ventilators for NPPV in pediatric patients include their relative size, their limited portability, and, most importantly, their limited attainment of high levels of inspiratory flow to support spontaneous respiratory efforts. Newer generations of portable ventilators are smaller and provide flow rates that support spontaneous breathing, including pressure support.

To appropriately adjust a volume-regulated ventilator for NPPV, the *delivered* tidal volume should be approximately twice that of the child's physiologic tidal volume to accommodate the dead space of the nasopharynx and conducting airways. Setting the tidal volume above the physiologic range and adjusting the peak inspiratory pressure until the required tidal volume is achieved can accomplish this. This method, often referred to as pressure plateau ventilation, is commonly used for

invasive long-term mechanical ventilation in pediatric patients.[16]

NONINVASIVE VENTILATION WITH NEGATIVE-PRESSURE DEVICES

Negative-pressure ventilation is a form of respiratory assistance in which subatmospheric pressure is applied intermittently through a cuirass or tank device external to the chest wall. This method of assisted ventilation is effective in pediatric patients with hypoventilation associated with acquired neurologic injury from trauma or infection and chronic restrictive lung disorders.[17,18] An advantage of negative-pressure ventilation is that it can improve CO_2 elimination without a tracheostomy. However, both the cuirass and tank devices require a fairly complete seal around the chest margins to be effective, and the tank device is large and difficult to move. Another important drawback of negative-pressure ventilation is significant disruption of sleep in patients with neuromuscular disorders and poor control of the muscle group supporting the upper airway. In these patients, treatment with negative-pressure ventilation can be complicated by recurrent episodes of obstructive apnea/hypopnea with desaturation.[11] Whereas NPPV is effective in preventing such episodes in children with unstable upper airway function, it is increasingly being used in lieu of a trial of negative-pressure ventilation for pediatric patients with chronic hypoventilation disorders.

NPPV MODES

Most bilevel pressure-targeted ventilators suitable for NPPV feature CPAP, spontaneous, timed, and spontaneous/timed operating modes. In the CPAP mode, these devices provide constant flow to maintain a target level of continuous positive airway pressure. Inspiratory pressure support is not provided. In the spontaneous mode, the ventilator responds to a threshold level of inspiratory flow that is initiated by the patient's spontaneous respiratory effort. At the inspiratory flow threshold, the ventilator delivers additional gas flow to reach the preset inspiratory positive airway pressure (IPAP). Exhalation occurs after the inspiratory flow peaks and then decreases to a threshold level. In the timed mode, the ventilator does not flow trigger but delivers intermittent pulses of positive airway pressure at a set rate. In the spontaneous/timed mode, the flow-trigger feature is activated. The ventilator cycles in the timed mode only in the event of prolonged apnea.

Pediatric patients are typically managed with NPPV in the spontaneous/timed mode. The chief advantage of this mode is patient comfort. This results when the child's inspiratory efforts are assisted with the inspiratory pressure support feature. A significant barrier to effective NPPV in young or very small patients is inability to achieve sufficient inspiratory flow to trigger the inspiratory pressure support feature. This problem may be solved by replacing the connector circuit between the mask interface and ventilator from standard tubing supplied by the manufacturer to shorter, less compliant tubing. However, this is clearly a departure from standard procedure that is not recommended by the manufacturer and should be attempted only in centers with experience in pediatric NPPV.

Another common problem with NPPV in the spontaneous mode in pediatric patients is the effects of significant gas leaks around the mask or through the mouth. In the presence of a significant leak, the inspiratory pressure target is never reached, resulting in a very long inflation time as the unit delivers massive amounts of inspiratory flow in an attempt to attain the preset inspiratory pressure. Some modern bilevel ventilators (VPAP II-ST, Res Med; BiPAP Vision, Respironics) designed for NPPV feature an adjustable inflation time that can be set to prevent this problem.

There is little published experience with pediatric patients treated with NPPV exclusively in the timed mode. In this mode the ventilator essentially functions as a time-cycled, pressure-limited device.

MONITORING THE PATIENT AND VENTILATOR CIRCUIT

Selection of patient and ventilator monitors with NPPV is based primarily on the clinical setting and the acuity of the patient.[19] In critically ill children with acute respiratory failure, NPPV is frequently attempted to prevent intubation. Under these conditions NPPV serves a life support function. Thus the child should be monitored in a setting appropriate to handle a child with an invasive airway with an electronic cardiorespiratory monitor, pulse oximeter, and airway disconnect alarm. Each monitor device should have alarm limits set by an experienced respiratory therapist and nurse.

Frequently, NPPV is used for stable patients with respiratory dysfunction as a clinical benefit. A hospital ward, sleep laboratory, or step-down unit is an appropriate setting for NPPV in this capacity. A pulse oximeter alone may be sufficient monitoring provided the child is clinically stable and not likely to decompensate in the event of equipment failure or removal of the interface. Intermittent NPPV can be accomplished safely at home without any patient or ventilator monitors.

However, children with limited capacity to spontaneously increase minute ventilation, such as an advanced neuromuscular disorder or congenital central hypoventilation syndrome, do require both a cardiorespiratory impedance monitor and pulse oximeter for NPPV in the outpatient setting.

PRESSURE TITRATION IN NONINVASIVE VENTILATION

With modern bilevel pressure ventilators, the IPAP adjustment determines the target distending airway pressure attained during flow-triggered or timed ventilator inflations. The IPAP should be set above the EPAP to raise the child's tidal volume, "unload" the respiratory muscles, and decrease respiratory distress. The differential between the IPAP and EPAP adjustment determines the tidal volume. Although second-generation bilevel devices are capable of achieving IPAP levels of 30 cm H_2O, children typically do not tolerate pressures higher than 20 cm H_2O without some type of sedation. There may be a delay of several hours before a step increase in IPAP achieves a reduction in arterial Paco$_2$. In this event, other factors can be used to determine the effectiveness in NPPV (see Table 20-1). In day-to-day clinical practice an IPAP setting of between 8 and 12 cm H_2O is typically sufficient to achieve the goals of NPPV in pediatric-age patients.

The EPAP adjustment with NPPV primarily determines the end-expiratory lung volume and maintains the stability of the upper airway. In a typical pediatric application of NPPV, EPAP levels of 6 to 8 cm H_2O are effective in improving oxygenation and preventing obstructive apnea. Most children regardless of the setting or indication poorly tolerate EPAP levels above 10 cm H_2O.

Overtitration of airway pressures is a common mistake when NPPV is attempted in pediatric patients (Figs. 20-2 to 20-4). In most patients, optimal results are seen at relatively low distending pressures. Raising the pressure to compensate for leaks around the nasal mask or through the mouth often is poorly tolerated in children and can lead to central hypoventilation. The mechanism behind this is uncertain, but it is also seen in adult patients with obesity hypoventilation syndrome treated with nasal CPAP.[20]

In negative-pressure–assisted ventilation the applied subatmospheric pressure is decreased incrementally to raise the tidal volume. A significant hazard in exposing patients with neuromuscular disorders to intermittent external subatmospheric pressures while leaving the head and neck exposed to ambient atmospheric pressure is episodic obstructive

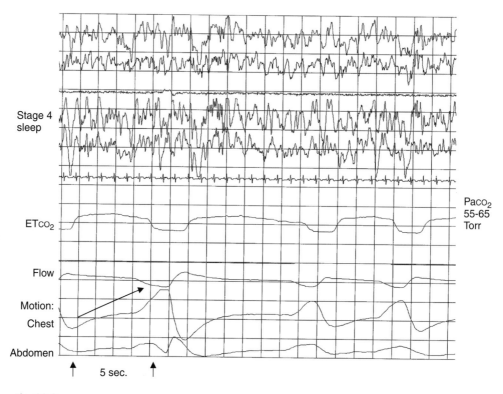

Fig. 20-2

"Loaded" inspiratory effort during sleep in a spontaneously breathing 3-year-old girl with obesity hypoventilation syndrome. With each inspiratory effort shown, there is a marked delay in the upstroke of the chest motion waveform before the onset of nasal air flow. The spontaneous respiratory rate was only 6 breaths per minute, end-tidal CO_2 ranged from 55 to 65 mm Hg, and the SaO_2 before application of low flow nasal oxygen was 80% to 83%.

apnea and hypopnea. In clinical practice this can be minimized by concomitant nasal CPAP therapy with negative-pressure–assisted ventilation.

INTERFACE SELECTION AND FIT

Interface devices appropriate for NPPV include nasal masks, nasal-oral masks, and nasal plugs or pillows.[21] In most clinical scenarios, the nasal mask is the preferred device. Nasal-oral masks do solve the problem of gas leak through the oral cavity, but they pose a significant risk of aspiration of gastric contents in the event of emesis. Nasal-oral masks should be considered for NPPV in the intensive care unit setting in children with significant respiratory distress. Under these conditions, sedation is often necessary and the child should not be fed. Nasal plugs or pillows can be substituted for nasal masks in children who complain of discomfort

with the nasal mask. Nasal plugs or pillows are not used very often because most children eventually adapt to the nasal mask very well.

Nasal masks are commercially available in a wide range of sizes and shapes to fit children and adolescents. Unfortunately, soft nasal masks are not widely available for small infants. Masks may be custom-molded to fit individual patients in specific circumstances such as in children with midfacial syndromes associated with maxillary hypoplasia. The nasal mask should fit snugly around the nasal margins. When the mask is too large, significant tension on the head straps is necessary to prevent mask leaks, thereby promoting dermal ulceration at the nasal bridge. Long-term intermittent NPPV by means of a nasal mask may impair maxillary bone growth. This concern, although theoretical, is considered significant by caregivers of children treated with NPPV.

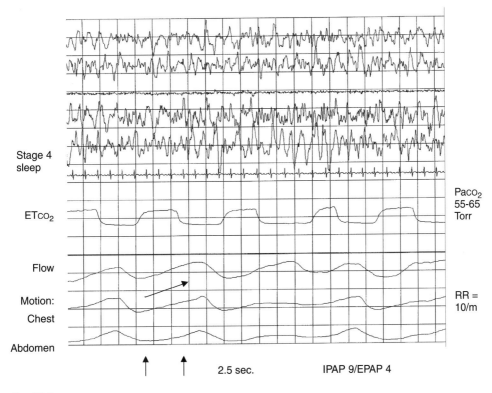

Fig. 20-3

Unloaded inspiratory effort with optimal NPPV in the same patient as in Fig. 20-2. With application of NPPV via nasal mask set at inspiratory positive airway pressure of 9 cm H_2O and expiratory positive airway pressure of 4 cm H_2O, there is a significant improvement of the respiratory pattern and a faster upstroke of the chest wall motion signal. Note that the end-tidal $PaCO_2$ has not decreased despite a demonstrable improvement in the work of breathing.

COMPLICATIONS AND CONTRAINDICATIONS TO NPPV

Pediatric-age patients are at relatively higher risk for complications to NPPV as a result of unique physiologic differences from adults (Table 20-3). However, in clinical experience, major complications to NPPV are unusual, while approximately 50% of children experience one or more minor complications. The most common minor complications reported include skin irritation due to the nasal mask, nasal dryness or discomfort, and eye irritation. Despite these complaints, preliminary reports of adherence to intermittent NPPV in children with chronic hypoventilation disorders are surprisingly good and better than those reported for adult patients treated with nasal CPAP.

The only absolute contraindication to a trial of NPPV in pediatric-age patients with acute respiratory distress is cardiovascular instability (see Fig. 20-1). Relative contraindications include nasopharyngeal obstruction, inability to handle oral secretions, and extreme agitation or anxiety.[21]

FUTURE OF NONINVASIVE VENTILATION

A major impediment to the future of NPPV in infants and children is the reluctance of companies that manufacture bilevel ventilators to seek FDA approval of their devices for pediatric-age patients. This is primarily because of the cost of FDA approval and the relatively low volume of units expected to be sold in the pediatric market. The result is that clinicians who care for children with chronic hypoventilation disorders that are attracted to NPPV as an alternative to TPPV get into funding disputes and legal conflicts with companies that dispense durable medical equipment.

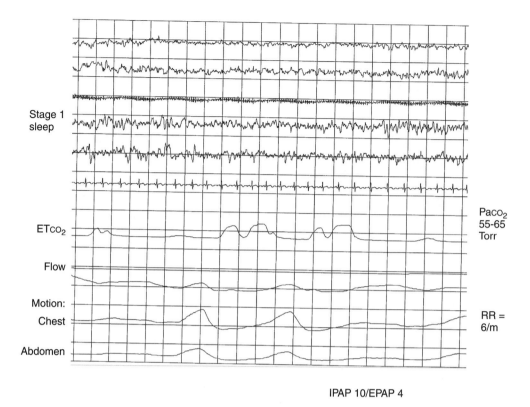

Stage 1
sleep

ET_{CO_2}

Flow

Motion:

Chest

Abdomen

Pa_{CO_2}
55-65
Torr

RR =
6/m

IPAP 10/EPAP 4

Fig. 20-4

Central hypoventilation with overadjustment of the inspiratory positive airway pressure in the same patient treated in Figs. 20-2 and 20-3. Note that with only a slight increase in the inspiratory positive airway pressure setting from 9 to 10 cm H_2O, the respiratory rate decreased to 6 breaths per minute and, as in Fig. 20-2, there is a relatively slow rise in the chest wall waveform.

TABLE 20-3	FACTORS UNIQUE TO PEDIATRIC PATIENTS PROMOTING COMPLICATIONS OF NPPV
Complication	**Factor Unique to Children**
Aspiration	Immaturity of airway reflexes
Exacerbation of gastroesophageal reflux	Impaired gastroesophageal sphincter function during infancy
Upper airway obstruction	Anatomic factors, difficulty clearing secretions
Large oral leak	Tendency to mouth breathe
Anxiety/need for sedation	Concern in new situations, developmental disorders

Despite these constraints, the future for NPPV in pediatric-age patients is very promising. Smaller interfaces and flow-triggered, pressure-targeted units suitable for small children are appearing for home use. Second-generation bilevel units already can achieve target inspiratory pressures of 30 cm H_2O and are equipped with independent oxygen adjustment settings. These units also come with a maximum inspiratory time setting so as to prevent prolonged inflations in the presence of uncompensated leaks. Proportion assist ventilation, a method of assisted ventilation that is responsive to the resistive and elastic properties of the respiratory system, can be administered by means of nasal mask. This method of assisted ventilation is well beyond preliminary trials in adults and may have significant advantages over NPPV with current bilevel devices.

REFERENCES

1. Make BJ et al: Management of pediatric patients requiring long-term ventilation. *Chest* 1998; 113:289S-344S.
2. Hill NS et al: Efficacy of nocturnal nasal ventilation in patients with restrictive thoracic disease. *Am Rev Respir Dis* 1992; 145:365-371.
3. Teague WG: Long term mechanical ventilation in infants and children. In Hill NS, editor: *Long-term mechanical ventilation.* New York. Marcel Dekker, 2001; pp 177-213.

4. Teague WG, Harsch A, Lesnick B: Non-invasive positive pressure ventilation as a long-term treatment for pediatric patients with chronic hypoventilation disorders. *Am J Respir Crit Care Med* 1999; 159:297a.

5. Teague WG: NPPV for acute respiratory failure in children. In *Proceedings of the 7th International Congress on Home Ventilation.* Orlando, Fla. American College of Chest Physicians, 1999.

6. Teague WG et al: Non-invasive positive pressure ventilation (NPPV) in critically ill children with status asthmaticus. *Am J Respir Crit Care Med* 1998; 1, 57:542a.

7. Brochard L et al: Reversal of acute exacerbations of chronic obstructive lung disease by inspiratory assistance with a face mask. *N Engl J Med* 1990; 323:1523-1530.

8. Fortenberry JD et al: Management of pediatric acute hypoxemic respiratory insufficiency with bilevel positive pressure (BiPAP) nasal mask ventilation. *Chest* 1995; 108:1059-1064.

9. Rosen GM et al: Postoperative respiratory compromise in children with obstructive sleep apnea syndrome: can it be anticipated? *Pediatrics* 1994; 93:784-788.

10. Hertzog JH et al: Noninvasive positive pressure ventilation facilitates tracheal extubation after laryngotracheal reconstruction in children. *Chest* 1999; 116:260-263.

11. Khan Y, Heckmatt JZ: Obstructive apnoeas in Duchenne muscular dystrophy. *Thorax* 1994; 49:157-161.

12. Khan Y et al: Effect of nasal ventilation on nocturnal hypoxaemia in neuromuscular patients. *Am Rev Respir Dis* 1992; 145:A863.

13. Teague WG et al: Nasal bi-level positive airway pressure acutely improves ventilation and oxygen saturation in children with upper airway obstruction. *Am Rev Respir Dis* 1991; 143:505A.

14. Strumpf DA et al: An evaluation of the Respironics BiPAP bi-level CPAP device for delivery of assisted ventilation. *Respir Care* 1990; 35:415-422.

15. Kacmarek RM: Characteristics of pressure-targeted ventilators used for noninvasive positive pressure ventilation. *Respir Care* 1997; 42:380-388.

16. Keens TG, Jansen MT, DeWitt PK: Home care for children with chronic respiratory failure. *Semin Respir Med* 1990; 11:269-281.

17. Frates RC et al: Outcome of home mechanical ventilation in children. *J Pediatr* 1985; 106:850-856.

18. Samuels MP, Southall DP: Negative extrathoracic pressure in the treatment of respiratory failure in infants and young children. *BMJ* 1989; 299:1253-1257.

19. Bach JR et al: Consensus statement: noninvasive positive pressure ventilation. *Respir Care* 1997; 42:364-369.

20. Piper AJ, Sullivan CE: Effects of short-term NIPPV in the treatment of patients with severe obstructive sleep apnea and hypercapnia. *Chest* 1994; 105:434-440.

21. Birnkrant DJ, Pope JF, Eiben RM: Pediatric noninvasive nasal ventilation. *J Child Neurol* 1997; 12:231-236.

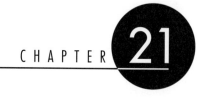

CHAPTER 21

High-frequency Ventilation

Keith S. Meredith

During the past decade we have witnessed the development and implementation of several exciting modalities for the respiratory care of newborns and pediatric patients. These new tools range from enhancements in the pharmacologic management of distinct cardiopulmonary disorders to tremendous strides in mechanical ventilation. Critical to the successful application of these new treatments, disease-specific strategies are being developed that also include ways in which some therapies may positively interact with others. High-frequency ventilation (HFV) continues to play an important role in this growth.[1-4]

The link between mechanical ventilation, oxygen, and subsequent acute and chronic lung disease was made in both pediatric and adult patients shortly after the introduction of conventional ventilation (CV) into clinical practice.[5,6] The various techniques of HFV emerged later from efforts to develop methods of managing respiratory failure that would minimize the negative pulmonary consequences of ventilatory support. At that time, our understanding of the mechanisms of these injuries was limited to the observed interactions between oxygen, pressure, and time.[7] Ironically, some of our early insights into the undesired interactions between the surfactant-deficient lung and mechanical ventilation occurred during experiments designed to determine if HFV would be beneficial at all.[8] This gap in the fundamental understanding of concepts of ventilator-induced lung injury explains both the early controversies regarding HFV strategies and the conflicting clinical reports.[9,10] The finding, at least in animal models, that a lung protective ventilator strategy is possible helped spawn a growing body of data describing lung-injury mechanisms and, therefore, prevention techniques.[8] These remain the focus of ongoing research and commentary.[11,12] Whereas initial clinical uses of HFV were in rescue situations, the primary focus of HFV research was to protect the lung from injury. This lung protection focus continues and should not be confused with rescue attempts to treat the already injured lung.

This chapter reviews (1) basic concepts of HFV, (2) current understanding of mechanisms of gas exchange during HFV, (3) basic approaches to the use of approved devices, (4) disease-specific HFV strategies, and (5) special patient care considerations. The chapter also introduces the emerging understanding of the interaction between new pharmacologic therapies and HFV.

DEFINITIONS

HFV is defined as mechanical ventilation using tidal volumes less than or equal to dead space delivered at supraphysiologic rates. Tidal volume, dead space volume, and breathing rate magnitude vary with patient age and size (tidal and dead space volumes vary inversely with increasing age, while rate varies directly). The U.S. Food and Drug Administration (FDA) has chosen to define HFV devices as those that provide breathing rates over 150 breaths per minute. This discussion is limited to those devices currently approved by the FDA for use in neonates and/or pediatric patients. These ventilators operate at breathing rates of 4 to 10 Hz (1 Hz = 60 breaths per minute, or 1 cycle per second) and deliver the requisite small tidal volumes. Several types of HFV devices have been tested and reported in the literature. They differ functionally by the way each breath is generated, their relationship to conventional ventilator settings (if any), the range of breathing rates, and the nature of the expiratory portion of the respiratory cycle (Table 21-1).

HIGH-FREQUENCY CONVENTIONAL AND POSITIVE-PRESSURE VENTILATION

High-frequency CV is a modification of conventional pressure-limited infant ventilators that provides breathing rates up to 150 breaths per minute (2.5 Hz).[13] The limitations of this approach include larger delivered tidal volumes than traditional HFV and the potential for intrapulmonary gas trapping. High-frequency positive-pressure ventilation (HFPPV)

was first described in the anesthesia literature as a tool for managing patients during bronchoscopic or laryngeal surgery.[14] HFPPV subsequently received brief exposure as a management tool for more chronic conditions in adults and underwent brief trials in a small series of infants with respiratory distress.[15,16] These definitions are included here for completeness only because the use of FDA-approved HFV devices has generally replaced the routine use of these techniques in infants.

HIGH-FREQUENCY FLOW INTERRUPTION

High-frequency flow interrupters (HFFI) deliver pressure-regulated, short-duration, low tidal volume breaths, frequently in conjunction with CV breaths. Each HFV breath is inserted proximal to the endotracheal tube (ETT), allowing the ETT to filter proximal pressures and minimize intratracheal and intrapulmonary pressure amplitudes. Exhalation of inspired gases takes place by passive chest recoil or by negative pressure assist at the exhalation valve. Continuous flow from CV provides the baseline pressure. This nomenclature may seem unnecessarily confusing because these devices are essentially hybrids of jet (passive exhalation) or oscillatory (assisted exhalation) ventilators.

HIGH-FREQUENCY JET VENTILATION

High-frequency jet ventilation (HFJV) devices deliver short pulsed jets distal to the proximal end of the ETT. Functional tidal volumes are a combination of the jet breath and entrainment volumes that are "dragged" along with each jet. Techniques using a modified triple-lumen ETT and those employing catheters placed in a standard ETT have been described.[17,18] These devices combine CV breaths with jet breaths and, like HFFI, rely on passive chest recoil for gas egress. Baseline pressures are provided by continuous flow from the CV. Initial difficulties with necrotizing tracheobronchitis have been overcome by unique design modifications that improved humidification of the jet breaths.[19] In tandem use with CV is usually required.

TABLE 21-1	FUNCTIONAL HIGH-FREQUENCY DEVICE CHARACTERISTICS		
Device Characteristic	**HFFI**	**HFJV**	**HFOV**
Breath generation	Interrupted variable flow	Pulsed high flow	Bias flow piston agitation
Relationship to conventional ventilator	In tandem or independent	In tandem (independent use on protocol)	Independent only
Operational frequencies	2-28 Hz	4-11 Hz	5-15 Hz
Expiratory flow	Passive or Venturi assisted	Passive	Active

HIGH-FREQUENCY OSCILLATORY VENTILATION

Of all HFV techniques, high-frequency oscillatory ventilation (HFOV) devices may be the most variable. Initial techniques included loudspeakers whose output was attached to the ETT and a host of piston pump devices with various performance characteristics.[20-23] Common to all of these devices is the provision of extremely small tidal volumes and very high rates of 8 to 30 Hz, as well as the presence of a continuous distending pressure (CDP) or mean airway pressure ($\overline{Paw}$). The outward flow of expiratory gases is enhanced by the active exhalation phase of the piston cycle. This last feature distinguishes HFOV from all other HFV methods. All current devices use standard ETT, allow precise control over $\overline{Paw}$ and pressure amplitude, and in general are not used in tandem with conventional ventilators. The ability to accurately adjust continuous (or mean) and phasic pressures and inspiratory:expiratory (I:E) ratio varies among devices. Ventilator output is delivered to the proximal ETT (at the ETT circuit connection). Because the ETT behaves as a low-pass filter at these rapid breathing rates, pulmonary structures "see" markedly dampened phasic pressures.

MECHANISMS OF GAS EXCHANGE

The HFV techniques previously described represent different locations on the mechanical ventilation spectrum. On this spectrum, CV occupies one extreme with relatively large tidal volumes and low breathing rates and HFOV resides on the other extreme with very small tidal volumes and high breathing rates. The techniques of HFCV, HFPPV, HFFI, and HFJV lie between. As one traverses this ventilatory spectrum, the classic roles of convection to deliver bulk gas to small airways and diffusion to distribute the gas among the gas-exchanging surfaces become blurred. Most of the research attempting to refine our understanding of gas transport and exchange during HFV has been accomplished in adult animal models with normal or injured lungs. At best, the injured states mimic secondary (not natural) surfactant deficiency, and adult pulmonary time constants and airway rigidity differ significantly from those of the neonatal lung.

Enhanced diffusion is found in large and medium airways in which alterations in gas flow velocity profiles occur. This is thought to be responsible for delivery of gas farther into the lung than can be explained by pure convection.[24] There is significant interdependence between adjacent alveolar units because the walls of any alveolar unit are shared with juxtaposed alveoli, each providing stability to the other. Once inflated, these units, which may have different time constants, can equilibrate gases by swinging ventilation between them. This phenomenon, called *pendelluft*, tends to equilibrate gas concentrations in conducting airways and serves to improve gas exchange from distal pulmonary units. Additionally, the impact of enhanced diffusion, the product of tidal volume and rate, and the relationship between pulmonary units may all vary depending on the HFV technique used, the settings chosen, the patient's lung size, and pathologic conditions.[25] Obviously, our understanding of this complex set of gas exchange dynamics remains incomplete.

VENTILATION

Classic physiology teaches that elimination of CO_2 is directly related to the product of breathing rate and tidal volume (minute ventilation, where $\dot{V}CO_2 = f \times V_T$); however, the volume that effectively removes CO_2 is alveolar volume, that is, the difference between tidal and dead space volumes. Based on this, if tidal volume is less than dead space, this difference, zero, and its product with breathing rate does not yield a meaningful number. Because all of the HFV methods described are effective means of ventilation, even with tidal volumes less than dead space, a new explanation is needed. Fredberg and co-workers provided insight into this apparent paradox by describing elimination of CO_2 as follows:

$$(\dot{V}CO_2) = (f)^x \times (V_T)^y$$

where x is 0.5 to 1 and y is 1.5 to 2.2 (depending on the device). From this relationship we see that tidal volume is more critical to ventilation than rate is during HFV, and HFV appears to reduce the impact of dead space volume on ventilation.[21]

Unlike oxygenation, in which the relationship of $\overline{Paw}$ to mean lung volume (MLV) and subsequent optimization of gas exchange is similar between CV and HFV, the elimination of CO_2 by CV and HFV is drastically different. This difference lies not only in the alterations to the minute ventilation equation just described but also in the nature of HFV devices themselves. In this regard, Fredberg and colleagues made several interesting observations during an evaluation of multiple neonatal HFV devices.[21] They noted that not only is CO_2 elimination during HFV more sensitive to changes in tidal volume than in rate but also the tidal volume output of HFV devices is sensitive to changes in ETT diameter and lung compliance. As ETT dimensions and compliance decreased so did tidal volume output from the HFV tested. This occurred in the presence of stable ventilator settings. Therefore any clinical change causing a decrease in ETT diameter, such as reintubation with a different-sized ETT or partial ETT obstruction with tracheal secretions, alters the delivered tidal volume. Furthermore, improvements in lung compliance (e.g., volume recruitment) and decrements in lung compliance (e.g., patent ductus arteriosus or alveolar derecruitment) have a direct effect on tidal volume.

In addition, the relationship between ventilator frequency and CO_2 elimination is nonintuitive. Changes in ventilator rate at a given pressure amplitude cause an inverse change in tidal volume. Thus, when ventilation must be improved, a reduction in breathing frequency improves ventilation because the increased volume output per stroke has a larger impact on ventilation than does the decrease in stroke frequency. The converse is also true. When less ventilation is needed and pressure amplitude is already minimized, increasing breathing frequency will further decrease tidal volume and allow weaning from ventilation. Fig. 21-1 depicts data collected during volume measurement experiments with the SensorMedics 3100A high-frequency oscillator. Observe that although varying $\overline{Paw}$ (10 and 20 cm H_2O) had no impact on tidal

volume output at any given oscillatory amplitude, there was a substantial difference in tidal volume with differing frequencies. Volumes at 10 Hz are much higher than those at 15 Hz for each oscillatory amplitude tested.

OXYGENATION

Although from a mechanistic perspective gas exchange remains complex, the clinical management of oxygenation is more straightforward. Excluding adjustments of FIO_2, oxygenation is improved during CV and HFV by recruiting or maintaining lung volume. In fact, there is a direct and linear relationship between lung volume and oxygenation (Fig. 21-2). This relationship is only nonlinear when the lung is underinflated with minimal alveolar recruitment, or overinflated when alveolar recruitment is maximized, but alveolar pressure exceeds pulmonary artery pressure and cardiac output begins to fall. Achieving an optimal MLV, then, optimizes ventilation-perfusion matching while avoiding impaired cardiac output. Adjusting several CV settings, such as tidal volume, peak pressure, inspiratory time, and end-expiratory pressure,

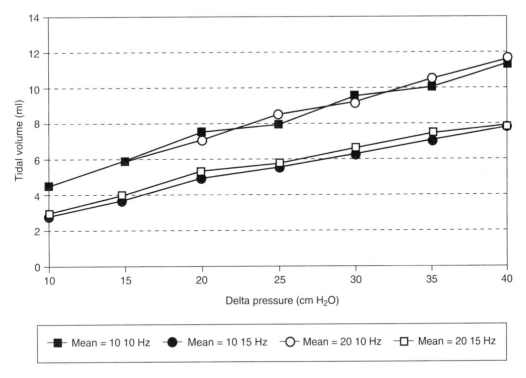

Fig. 21-1

Tidal volume output measured during high-frequency oscillatory ventilation (HFOV) with SensorMedics 3100A at mean airway pressure ($\overline{Paw}$) equal to 10 and 20 cm H_2O and frequency equal to 10 and 15 Hz. There is a nearly linear relationship between oscillatory amplitude and tidal volume. At each oscillatory amplitude tested, tidal volume at 10 Hz is higher than at 15 Hz. $\overline{Paw}$ has no effect.

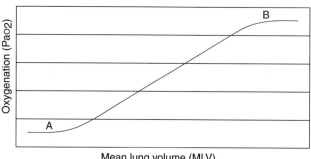

Fig. 21-2

Relationship between the mean lung volume and oxygenation (by inference—between P̄āw or CDP and MLV). **A,** Unopened lung. **B.** Over-inflated lung.

accomplishes this. The resulting P̄āw is an indirect expression of the pressure effort required to achieve and sustain the desired MLV. Phasic pressures delivered with CV during attempts to recruit lung volumes can damage the fragile, yet noncompliant, infant airways and lung parenchyma. Thus conventional tidal volume breathing applied to lungs with nonuniform compliances, as in the premature surfactant-deficient lung, results in non-homogeneous gas distribution, with overinflation of compliant areas and underinflation of noncompliant regions. During spontaneous or conventional mechanical breathing, the lung swings past the MLV and mean P̄āw during the cycles of inspiration and expiration, residing at the MLV (and P̄āw) for only brief periods. With normal lung mechanics, a stable functional residual capacity is maintained and oxygenation is not impaired. In the lung prone to atelectasis, however, residual lung volumes are dynamic. Although volume may seem adequate at peak inflation, stable lung volumes may not exist and oxygenation will be significantly impaired (even in the presence of positive end-expiratory pressures).[26,27]

The methods used to create and maintain P̄āw (or CDP during HFOV) therefore have a profound effect on the consequences of reaching the MLV. Conventional methods require the use of relatively high peak pressures to recruit collapsed noncompliant pulmonary units. The potential negative impact has already been described. The approach taken during HFV strategies, in contrast, is the application of a CDP without the use of high phasic pressures. In fact, direct control over CDP (P̄āw) is possible, with ventilation occurring around a relatively fixed intrapulmonary pressure and, therefore, relatively stable MLV. The danger of this technique, as mentioned earlier, is lung overdistention and resultant decreases in venous return and cardiac output. This can occur without changes in ventilation pressures during CV and HFOV when lung volume is silently recruited as compliance improves.

The optimal MLV, during high-volume strategies (see Ventilator Management section later), is reached when distending pressure exceeds alveolar opening pressures, and, as a result, the arterial to alveolar oxygen tension ratio (Pa/AO₂) is maximized. This measure of oxygenation is useful because it normalizes measured PaO₂ for delivered FIO₂.[28] Perfect oxygenation, unobtainable in nature, yields a ratio of 1:1. The safe application of pressures adequate to achieve a stable MLV during management of the uninjured, atelectasis-prone lung is the goal of mechanical ventilation. Recent data from both animal and human infant studies suggest that improved oxygenation, with acceptable ventilation, does occur safely with HFV techniques while using distending pressures that are initially higher than in CV controls.[10,29,30] Attempts to achieve improved oxygenation using mean pressures lower than those used in CV, although attractive in theory, have not proved fruitful except in short-term studies and in patients with pulmonary interstitial emphysema (PIE) in whom low-volume strategies are desired and intentional (see Ventilator Management section later). Experiments performed by McCulloch and co-workers using the surfactant-deficient rabbit model elegantly demonstrated the relationship between lung inflation strategy and resultant lung volume and gas exchange.[31] In this work, animals with similar pressure-volume relationships after lavage were managed for a 7-hour study period with conventional mechanical ventilation, HFOV with a low lung volume strategy, or HFOV with a high lung volume strategy. Fig. 21-3 graphically demonstrates the impact of these approaches on lung volumes. Note the significantly higher volumes obtained in the animals receiving HFOV and a high lung volume at an equivalent P̄āw. As anticipated, this group also had a fivefold higher PaO₂ and less evidence of significant bronchiolar epithelial injury.[31]

Fig. 21-3 also illustrates that an equivalent P̄āw does not imply equivalent lung volumes. As patient compliance changes, so does the P̄āw required to

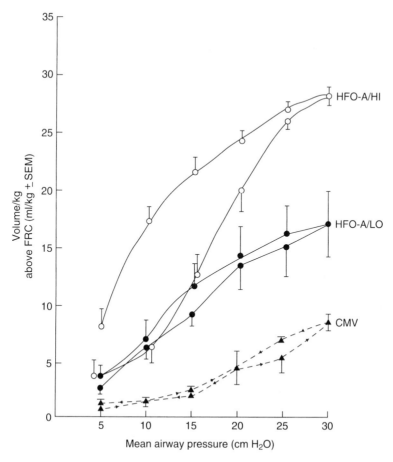

Fig. 21-3

Respiratory system pressure-volume curves obtained after 7 hours of ventilation in surfactant-depleted rabbits. Note the intergroup differences in total respiratory system compliance and lung volumes. The differences in hysteresis (inflation-deflation limb separation) are also significant between groups. (Modified from McCulloch PR, Forkert PG, Froese AB: Lung volume maintenance prevents lung injury during high-frequency oscillatory ventilation in surfactant deficient rabbits. *Am Rev Respir Dis* 1988; 137:1185.)

maintain optimal MLV. Obviously, a direct measure of MLV or compliance during HFV would be extremely useful; however, neither is currently available for routine bedside use. Clinical measures to properly wean patients and avoid inadvertent overdistention are discussed later in this chapter.

INDICATIONS

NEONATAL PATIENTS

The bulk of clinical data regarding appropriate application of HFV devices has been acquired from neonatal animals and humans. From these studies, two clear indications for HFV use during either routine or rescue circumstances have evolved. They are diffuse, homogeneous lung disease (or the atelectasis-prone lung), in which CV management is failing or may lead to increased risk of pulmonary morbidity, and existing pulmonary air leak syndromes (e.g., pneumothorax and PIE). Diffuse homogeneous lung disease includes natural surfactant deficiency (respiratory distress syndrome), shock lung in the newborn, and diffuse pneumonia. Other diagnoses, including congenital pulmonary hypoplasia (both the congenital diffuse variety and that associated with congenital diaphragmatic hernia), may be additional indications. The efficacy of HFV for pulmonary hypoplasia is promising but not yet clearly established.[32]

Each of the lung diseases just mentioned has been successfully managed with extracorporeal membrane oxygenation (ECMO).[33] The role of pre-ECMO HFV has been the subject of wide debate, with at least one published report describing a 50% reduction in the need for ECMO among infants referred to an ECMO center and meeting ECMO criteria who began HFOV on admission.[34] However, there are also data that imply an increased risk of pulmonary morbidity among infants avoiding ECMO with HFV. The timing of HFV intervention, the parameters determining HFV failure, and the decision for discontinuing HFV and initiating ECMO are currently empirical.[35]

There is no question that exogenous surfactant replacement is changing the course of respiratory distress syndrome (RDS) in affected infants. As a consequence, the role of HFV in patients treated with surfactant may differ from that in the pre-surfactant era. Proponents of early HFV for patients with RDS argue that tidal volume ventilation is damaging to immature lung structures after only a few minutes. In fact, there is no consensus regarding the timing of HFV initiation or surfactant administration in those treated with high-volume HFV. Encouraging, but not yet irrefutable, data are available regarding the early use of HFV in surfactant-treated infants.[36,37] Findings do show strong trends toward the need for fewer surfactant doses, less chronic lung disease and more pulmonary reserve at discharge, and decreased cost of hospitalization.

HFV continues to be indicated for infants in whom air leak syndromes develop, but, gratefully, the incidence of intractable air leak has decreased in recent years. This is probably the result of surfactant use, improved ventilatory techniques and devices, and better patient monitoring. Other conditions common to the neonate but not clearly benefited by HFV include particulate meconium aspiration, congenital lobar emphysema, bronchopulmonary dysplasia, and viral pneumonia. Further data from controlled trials with defined patient populations and treatment strategies are needed to offer clearer recommendations about HFV use in these conditions.

Pediatric Patients

Controlled trials in pediatric patients have been fairly limited.[38] However, as one would anticipate, proper strategic HFV use has had positive results in children with acute RDS and pulmonary air leak. Generally, HFOV (now approved in pediatric patients) is applied as a rescue therapy in those failing CV. (A more powerful HFOV device, SensorMedics 3100B, is being evaluated for approval use in larger pediatric patients.) An additional interesting HFV application is HFJV use during and after cardiac surgery, especially for children undergoing right ventricular outflow tract diversion or repair. At least two groups of investigators have reported improved hemodynamic measurements in children managed with the HFJV Bunnell Life Pulse both intraoperatively and postoperatively.[39,40] The ability to provide adequate ventilation with low mean and peak pressures in children with otherwise normal lungs offers a substantial advantage of HFJV over HFOV and CV. Furthermore, this feature makes HFJV a more efficacious method of treating traumatic or acquired bronchopleural fistulas than other forms of respiratory support.

VENTILATOR SETTINGS

Frequency

Breathing frequency ranges between 2 and 28 Hz, depending on the device. Rates lower than 4 Hz and greater than 15 Hz are rarely used. The impact of the breathing rate on ventilation during HFV is less than the impact of tidal volume. Frequency is therefore not usually changed, and management of ventilation occurs with changes in delivered volume. Changes in frequency are made when operating at machine limits of tidal volume (both low and high limits). Choices of breathing frequency depend on understanding optimal functional characteristics of each device and the nature of the patient and the disease treated. For example, with a similar disease, such as acute RDS, neonatal and pediatric patients are managed with different frequencies during HFOV. The smaller child requires a lower tidal volume and therefore a higher frequency. There are preliminary data in mature animals that suggest at an equivalent $Paco_2$ that higher frequencies during HFOV are less damaging to airways than lower ones.[41]

Oscillatory Amplitude or Peak Pressure

Each of the ventilators available in the United States is pressure limited. Changes in delivered pressure amplitude have a direct influence on tidal volume delivery. The purpose of measuring peak inspiratory pressure is to offer both patient safety and ease of adjustment of delivered tidal volume. Although HFJV provides separate control and display of distal ETT peak pressure, HFFI and HFOV do not. The latter two devices display oscillatory amplitude (the peak-to-trough pressure difference). Measurement of pressures (whether peak or peak-to-trough) distal to the insertion point of HFV breaths in the patient circuit is important to avoid underestimation of pressures seen by pulmonary structures. Transducers, amplifiers, and measuring circuit fidelity must be adequate and unfiltered to properly measure peak-to-peak pressures at these breathing frequencies.

During HFOV and HFFI, peak and trough pressures are measured, although they are not usually displayed. Because of the impact of the ETT on transmitted pressure, these values have only relative significance. Of more importance is the difference between peak and trough pressures, known as oscillatory amplitude or simply the delta P. Delivered volume is directly proportional to this peak-trough difference, and adjustments result in changes in tidal volume (see Fig. 21-1). During both HFOV and HFFI, the relationship between oscillatory amplitude and tidal volume actually delivered to the lung is subject to the same constraints as peak-to–end-expiratory pressure differences during pressure-limited CV. Changes in downstream compliance and impingement on the ETT lumen cause tidal volumes to vary without changes in displayed pressure amplitudes. Control over tidal volume during HFJV occurs by modifications in distally measured peak pressures. Although this measurement is less vulnerable to variations in the ETT lumen, total volume delivery during HFJV is a combination of jet pulse and gas entrained with each breath from the proximal ETT connection. This entrainment volume is vulnerable to reductions in the ETT lumen.

POSITIVE END-EXPIRATORY PRESSURE

Like peak pressure, the attempt to apply a conventional setting to an HFV technique can lead to confusion. One can easily measure trough pressures during HFV, but the meaning and value are unclear. With CV, we relate oxygenation to levels of end-expiratory pressure because this setting contributes so significantly to $\overline{Paw}$. With HFJV and HFFI this remains true because end-expiratory pressure is set by adding it from the CV. During HFOV, however, it is set directly, and true end-expiratory pressure (or trough pressure) is meaningless. In fact, to avoid confusion some authors suggest that CDP (rather than $\overline{Paw}$) be used to describe the constant pressure delivered during HFOV.

FRACTION OF INSPIRED OXYGEN

The principles for management of FIO_2 with CV also apply to HFV and are pulmonary disease dependent. There are no additional considerations for this setting during HFV.

MEAN AIRWAY PRESSURE OR CONTINUAL DISTENDING PRESSURE

Mean airway pressure or CDP controls MLV. During CV, this setting is the consequence of a combination of ventilator settings, and although it is a true mathematical average of pulmonary pressures, the lung maintains this pressure (and hence volume) for only brief periods. During HFV, especially HFOV, this pressure is directly controlled by the combination of bias flow and expiratory valve aperture. In this circumstance, the HFV static pressure (or CDP) truly creates a static lung volume, the magnitude of which depends on lung compliance. All the devices described provide a display of $\overline{Paw}$. During HFJV and HFFI, control over this parameter is achieved by changing the settings of the tandem CV. It cannot be overstated that as lung volume increases, so does compliance. In fact, at the very lung volume where oxygenation is optimized, compliance is as well. The importance of this concept is that ventilation is influenced if lung volume is too high, or too low, during HFV. Thus $\overline{Paw}$ facilitates oxygenation *and* permits optimal ventilation (see Fig. 21-2). Therefore using $\overline{Paw}$ to maintain the correct lung volume is doubly critical.

FLOW

The use of flow to control ventilator settings is variable among the devices described. During HFJV, jet pulses are delivered by means of a timing circuit with minimal control of flow. Pressures, and therefore volumes, are determined by variations of jet on-time and frequency. HFFI incorporates multiple solenoid technology to determine rate of pressure rise and end-expiratory pressures during CV, which has little impact on HFV functions. HFOV CDP is determined by the combination of circuit bias flow and the backpressure created by the expiratory valve opening. Even though desired CDP may be achieved with complete valve closure, care should be taken to avoid this because rapid rebreathing followed by circuit (and patient) overpressurization will occur.

INSPIRATORY TIME

Inspiratory time adjustments result in alterations in ventilator rate, I:E ratio, and tidal volume, all of which are significant, to differing degrees, for each type of HFV. Inspiratory time during HFJV is adjusted by changing jet on-time. Depending on ventilator frequency, this alters the I:E ratio and influences tidal volume output. Jet on-times of 20 to 34 msec are common. With HFOV, inspiratory time varies with ventilator rate but the I:E ratio is singularly meaningful. The recommendation is a 33% inspiratory time for the HFOV devices approved in the United States. The result is that for each completed respiratory cycle, one third is inspiratory and two thirds is expiratory. The importance of this lies in the enhancement of gas egress during exhalation because the 1:2 ratio favors the expiratory phase, thereby reducing inadvertent air trapping or breath stacking. This becomes a more significant factor as ventilator frequencies increase. Increases in inspiratory time at any given rate will increase tidal volume, but there is an obligatory reduction in I:E ratio that may offset any desirable effects. The inspiratory time during HFFI is fixed at 18 msec. Changes in ventilator rate are made with changes in expiratory time, and the I:E ratio varies with frequency. In comparison with the other ventilators, adjustments in tidal volume cannot be made by increasing inspiratory time, and I:E ratios will vary with frequency.

HIGH-FREQUENCY VENTILATORS ON THE U.S. MARKET

INFRASONIC INFANT STAR 950

The Infant Star 950 (Infrasonic) (Fig. 21-4) is a high-frequency flow interrupter (HFFI), approved by the FDA under the term *oscillator-like*. It was released in 1990 for use in the treatment of infants

with air leak and respiratory failure. This device is a modification of the Infant Star neonatal ventilator and has the advantage of offering both CV and HFV modes (individually or in combination). Multiple, rapidly responding, microprocessor-controlled solenoids permit an operating frequency range of 2 to 28 Hz. Frequency is adjusted by varying breath "off-times" with a fixed breath "on-time" of 18 msec. This yields HFV I:E ratios of 1:27 to 1:1. Pressure amplitudes are varied around conventional end-expiratory pressures, and P$\overline{aw}$ is determined by conventional, not HFV, settings. A Venturi jet placed at the exhalation valve assists the return of pressures to appropriate expiratory baselines.[42-44]

BUNNELL LIFE PULSE JET VENTILATOR

The Bunnell Life Pulse Jet ventilator (Bunnell) (Fig. 21-5) is the jet device approved by the FDA for use in infants. It was released in 1989 for rescue of air leak syndromes and respiratory failure after CV. Not intended as a stand-alone device, it is recommended for use with a conventional ventilator. Operational frequencies range from 4 to 11 Hz. Patients can now be managed with a high-low jet ETT (Fig. 21-6), with jet pulses delivered to the airways through a separate side lumen (the ETT is available in standard neonatal sizes) or through an ETT adapter (LifePort, Bunnell, Inc.). This latter feature mitigates the need for reintubation and facilitates a smooth transition to HFJV. The proximal lumen of the ETT is connected to the CV

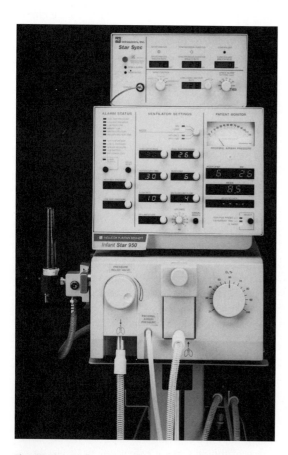

Fig. 21-4

High-frequency ventilation (HFV) Infant Star ventilator. (Courtesy Nellcor Puritan-Bennett, Pleasanton, Calif.)

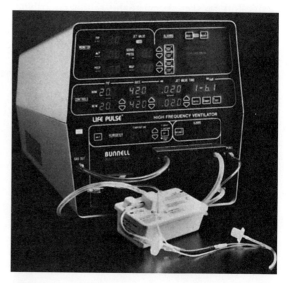

Fig. 21-5

Bunnell Life Pulse high-frequency jet ventilator. (Courtesy Bunnell, Salt Lake City, Utah.)

circuit, and a third (distal) lumen permits servo control of jet peak pressure. Inspiratory times are controllable from 20 to 34 msec, creating I:E ratios in excess of 1:6. This minimizes the possibility of intrapulmonary gas trapping. $\overline{Paw}$ is the consequence of both HFJV and CV settings. During a multicenter controlled trial comparing HFJV and CV in premature infants with PIE, significant improvements with greater survival and fewer treatment failures were seen in HFJV-treated patients.[45] Furthermore, a multicenter trial evaluating the use of HFJV compared with simple CV in uncomplicated RDS among preterm infants implied a clear benefit for HFV-managed patients, with less chronic lung disease and fewer patients requiring home O_2 at discharge.[46,47]

SensorMedics 3100A

The SensorMedics 3100A (SensorMedics) (Fig. 21-7) is the HFOV device approved by the FDA for general use in infants with respiratory failure and for pulmonary rescue. This device permits operator control over frequency, CDP (or $\overline{Paw}$), inspiratory time, and pressure amplitude. Frequencies range from 5 to 15 Hz, and inspiratory time ranges from 30% to 75% of the duty cycle. (The duty cycle is defined as one complete machine breath from the beginning of inspiration to end-expiration.) Pressure amplitude is adjusted by increasing electric power to the piston diaphragm (7 to 90 cm H_2O); peak and trough pressures are consequential. Varying the bias flow and expiratory valve aperture controls CDP (or $\overline{Paw}$). Data from two pre-surfactant studies in infants with RDS treated with this device and compared with controls treated with simple CV have shown reductions in both acute and chronic lung injury in HFOV-treated infants.[10,29] Subsequent publications that repeated these experiments in surfactant-treated patients showed benefit in residual lung disease and the cost of care in HFOV-treated patients.[36,48] Unfortunately, other authors have found mixed results.[9] Some, but not all, of these variations in findings can be attributed to differences between studies in devices used (data from institutions outside the United States may have been obtained with ventilators not available in the United States), nature of patient population (gestational age or birth weight), and duration of CV before surfactant administration and initiation of HFOV. A recent attempt to resolve this confusing data set was undertaken using a meta-analysis of HFOV clinical trials. The authors concluded that studies using HFOV strategies designed to optimize lung volume (high volume strategy) have consistently shown improvement in short-term indices of chronic lung disease without increases in morbidity.[37,49]

The SensorMedics 3100B is undergoing FDA evaluation as an oscillator capable of use in larger pediatric patients and adults. It has the ability to deliver high-frequency oscillations with a larger volume piston and to use higher distending pressure levels. Yet it maintains the ability to provide a protective low-stretch lung ventilation strategy.

Circuit Considerations

To achieve adequate gas exchange for both oxygenation and ventilation, high-frequency ventilators have unique design requirements. With the exception of HFCV, all HFV devices have special patient circuit considerations. Each of them must (1) use very low circuit compliance to reduce compressible volume and increase precision of control over the small volumes delivered; (2) have intrinsic timing mechanisms to allow breathing frequencies between 4 and 28 Hz (varying by device); (3) provide control over inspiratory times and circuit design to allow sufficient time for gas egress during exhalation; (4) adequately humidify gases; and (5) include alarms and fail-safe devices for patient safety. As a consequence of these considerations, circuit configurations cannot be altered without

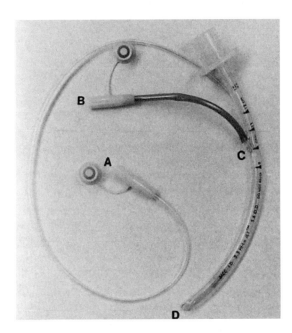

Fig. 21-6

Hi-Lo jet endotracheal tube for use with the Bunnell Life Pulse ventilator. **A,** Pressure monitoring port. **B,** Jet injector port. **C,** Insertion of jet injector into side of endotracheal tube wall. **D,** Distal end of endotracheal tube and site for pressure measuring from port A. (Courtesy Bunnell, Salt Lake City, Utah.)

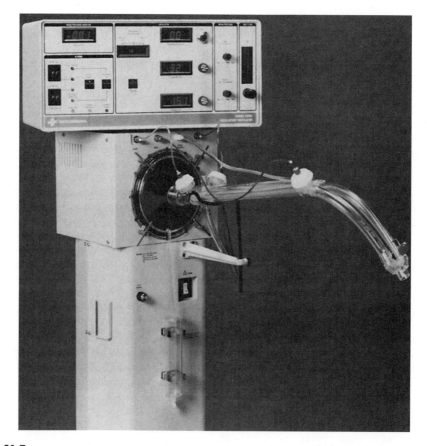

Fig. 21-7

SensorMedics 3100A high-frequency oscillatory ventilator. (Courtesy SensorMedics, Yorba Linda, Calif.)

careful investigation because function and safety are extremely sensitive to small changes in engineering.

A unique device-specific option is the use of the high-low jet ETT (see Fig. 21-6) with the Bunnell Life Pulse HFJV. This ETT was initially an integral feature of this device. Jet pulses are delivered through the side lumen of the ETT, and servo control over jet pressures is maintained by feedback from pressures sampled at the distal ETT lumen. Connection to a conventional ventilator is provided at the proximal ETT opening. An ETT adapter made specifically for this device now makes reintubation optional.

Originally the SensorMedics 3100A operated with a nonstandard semi-rigid circuit that required creative efforts on the part of caregivers to optimize patient positioning. Now a redesigned flexible circuit is also available and frees the infant from many of the position constraints of the older circuit design.

A thorough understanding of the limits of breathing frequency, tidal volume, P$\overline{aw}$ control, circuit design, ETT requirements, and specifics of ventilator design is critical to the safe and optimal use of each high-frequency ventilator.

VENTILATOR MANAGEMENT

Each HFV device was initially developed for specific lung disease states. Because of ethical, scientific, and legal constraints, use in human infants was at first confined to rescue patients in whom conventional methods were failing. With increasing anecdotal success noted by several groups, it became apparent that strategies applied to these infants were unique to each device. Subsequently, refinements in patient management led to tailoring device design, with a resultant narrowing of the spectrum of lung diseases to which they could be applied. For example, HFJV was directed toward air leak syndromes and HFOV toward diffuse alveolar disease. Studies have now shown that P$\overline{aw}$ recruitment of the atelectasis-prone lung can be accomplished with different HFV types with similar successes in gas exchange, histologic evidence of uniform gas distribution, and decreased hyaline membrane formation.[50,51] Conversely, Clark and associates reported successful treatment in a series of infants with PIE using HFOV and supported the value of HFOV use in patients with air leaks.[52] In another study of infants with PIE, Keszler and co-workers reported a clear superiority of HFJV over CV in a carefully controlled multicenter trial.[45] Keszler et al have subsequently had success managing infants with RDS with HFJV.[46] These findings imply that successful management of infants with significant pulmonary disorders is best accomplished by device-specific strategies directed toward specific lung pathophysiologic processes rather than by specific HFV types.

INITIAL SETTINGS

Clinical protocols guiding decisions to implement HFV techniques should be in place in each institution before these devices are used. Personnel involved in patient management must demonstrate proficiency in the use of the device and clinical expertise to ensure patient safety. Active training programs within each institution should be mandatory and include a demonstration by personnel that they understand ventilator controls and circuit design, basic troubleshooting, and management strategies. Before the initiation of HFV, each device and circuit should be inspected to ensure proper calibration and function. Specific care should be taken to ensure that (1) proper gas temperature and humidity are present, (2) ventilator and circuit position is such that a smooth transition can occur, and (3) initial settings are lower than anticipated requirements to allow a slow increase toward desired levels and prevent inadvertent injury. Finally, other appropriate primary therapies (e.g., surfactant replacement for surfactant deficiency and vasopressor support for impaired myocardial function) are not replaced by HFV and should be optimized along with ventilatory management.

Until recently, HFV use was limited to patients in whom CV was failing. Recent literature and experience with neonates are changing this impression so that HFV is increasingly being used before rescue situations develop. These developments are changing current protocols for changing patients from CV to HFV. Because of this, it is necessary to focus on the concepts that need to be considered when applying HFV to patients, rather than describing specific ventilator settings. The evolving literature and device-specific manufacturer's recommendations should be referred to for more details.

CLINICAL MANAGEMENT STRATEGIES

Successful application of any HFV device requires accurate comprehension of individual patient pulmonary pathophysiology and selection of an appropriate ventilatory strategy. Currently, there are two fundamentally differing strategies that are designed to approach contrasting pulmonary pathophysiologic processes.

HIGH-VOLUME STRATEGY

For the patient with an atelectasis-prone lung (e.g., natural or acquired surfactant deficiency), the primary therapeutic goal is to optimize lung inflation so that ventilation-perfusion mismatching is minimized while reducing inflation-deflation breathing patterns that initiate a cascade of events leading to lung tissue injury.[8,31] This has been termed the *high-volume strategy*. Two separate means of achieving this goal have evolved.

One method is increasing the distending pressures (P$\overline{\text{aw}}$ or CDP) in small increments (1 to 2 cm H_2O) while watching for improvement in oxygenation (arterial blood gas determinations, transcutaneous O_2 measurements, or pulse oximetry saturations) and MLV (chest radiograph). P$\overline{\text{aw}}$ is increased until oxygenation improves significantly or until MLV reaches desired levels, or both, which may be determined by the presence of a well-inflated lung on a radiograph (Fig. 21-8). While using this method, care must be taken to anticipate silent lung recruitment and to reduce P$\overline{\text{aw}}$ as appropriate to avoid serious impairment to venous return and reduction in cardiac output. Silent lung recruitment is gradual lung inflation taking place with static P$\overline{\text{aw}}$ settings (Fig. 21-9). Clinical clues heralding this include rapid improvements with subsequent unexplained decrements in oxygenation, decreasing Paco$_2$ without changes in oscillatory amplitude (improving compliance), and, finally, clinical changes in perfusion. These problems often can be avoided with diligence and anticipation. Silent recruitment, although more common during initial HFV management, can occur any time attempts are made to optimize MLV. Recent data confirm the pulmonary, central nervous system, and cardiovascular safety and efficacy of this technique.[10,29,30,53,54]

The other approach to recruiting the collapsed lung is the use of sustained inflations (SI), that is, applying plateau pressures at levels in excess of expected alveolar opening pressures for periods of 5 to 30 seconds. This technique should result in incremental improvement in oxygenation if pressure levels are adequate. Furthermore, because of lung hysteresis, the inter-SI P$\overline{\text{aw}}$ can frequently be reduced to levels slightly less than can be achieved with the other lung inflation method. SI are usually

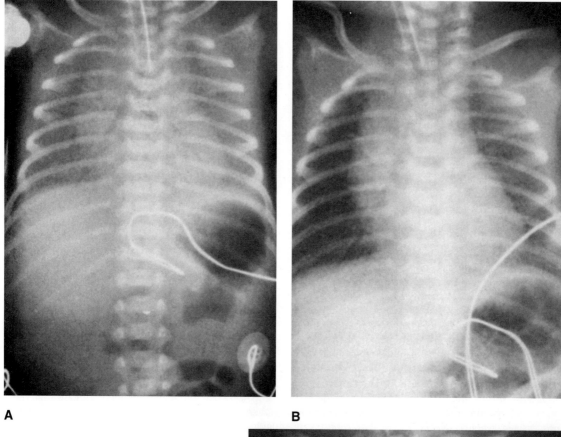

A

B

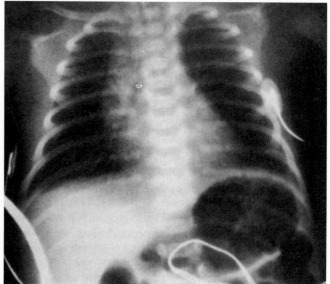

C

Fig. 21-8

Radiographs during the first day of life for a 30-week premature infant with respiratory distress syndrome (RDS) managed with HFOV to achieve optimal mean lung volume (MLV). **A,** Initial $\overline{Paw}$ equal to 10 cm H_2O, FIO_2 equal to 1. **B,** At 12 hours of age, with $\overline{Paw}$ equal to 15 cm H_2O and FIO_2 equal to 0.45. **C,** At 24 hours of age with $\overline{Paw}$ equal to 12 cm H_2O and FIO_2 equal to 0.28.

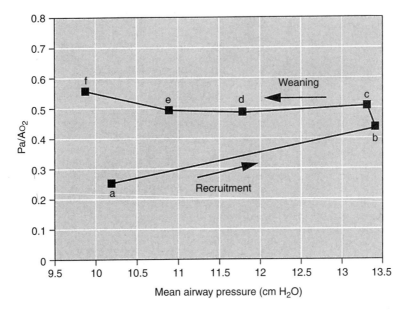

Fig. 21-9

Mean Pa/Ao$_2$ and P$\overline{\text{aw}}$ of 21 premature infants managed with HFOV immediately after surfactant replacement. Note that increasing P$\overline{\text{aw}}$ initially results in increased Pa/Ao$_2$ (alveolar recruitment); subsequent P$\overline{\text{aw}}$ weaning does not reduce oxygenation but is associated with gradual improvement in Pa/Ao$_2$. The line between points *b* and *c* represents silent lung recruitment as assessed by improving Pa/Ao$_2$ with essentially stable P$\overline{\text{aw}}$. Surfactant replacement (*a*); 12 hours later (*b*); 12 to 24 hours later (*c*); 24 to 48 hours later (*d*); 48 to 72 hours later (*e*); and 72 to 96 hours later (*f*).

repeated until no change in oxygenation is noted or until oxygenation decreases. Both imply that the lung is at the upper limits of lung capacity. The need for repeat SI maneuvers is determined by the level of inter-SI P$\overline{\text{aw}}$ used and the amount of subsequent alveolar de-recruitment. The SI method may achieve optimal MLV more rapidly and, because of the lower inter-SI P$\overline{\text{aw}}$, avoid silent recruitment. However, potential disadvantages include the risk of using too little pressure (minimal recruitment) or too much pressure (airway injury, air leak, and reductions in cardiac output). Data from excised baboon lungs suggest that lung recruitment responses to SI maneuvers are dependent on lung pathophysiology. Thus there is a difference in the response of surfactant-sufficient collapsed lungs and uninjured surfactant-deficient lungs.[3] This method has been used successfully in infants with minimal complications.[2,53] Definite superiority of one technique over the other has not been demonstrated.

Note the contrast between CV and HFV. With CV, lung recruitment is achieved by increasing inspiratory time, end-expiratory pressure, and the resultant mean airway pressure, whereas HFV uses P$\overline{\text{aw}}$ alone to achieve lung recruitment. Supplying adequate oscillatory amplitude around the baseline

P$\overline{\text{aw}}$ provides ventilation during HFFI and HFOV. With HFJV, ventilation is determined by changes in jet-pulse tidal volume delivery and by the amount of background CV used. It is critical to avoid the temptation to use HFV phasic pressure to recruit underinflated lung units. Table 21-2 suggests an algorithm for implementation of the high-volume strategy.

LOW-VOLUME STRATEGY

In distinction to the lung inflation strategies described, management of infants with PIE, pneumothorax, or air trapping requires the employment of alternative goals because attempts to achieve optimal MLV in these patients will exaggerate existing lung overinflation or serve to further damage injured lung. Here the primary objective should be to offer a ventilatory strategy that allows the lung to slowly deflate or one that minimizes ongoing air leakage while providing tolerable ventilation while accepting a higher FIO_2. This is accomplished with all HFV systems by using a lower P$\overline{\text{aw}}$ than that creating the problem. (These patients are usually on CV before switching to HFV.) This allows the lung to de-recruit and isolates damaged areas from inflation pressures. The consequence of this, however, is the frequent requirement for a higher FIO_2. Additionally, tidal volume delivery must be decreased to further reduce

TABLE 21-2	GENERIC OXYGENATION AND VENTILATION STRATEGIES FOR USE DURING HIGH-FREQUENCY VENTILATION IN PATIENTS WITH DIFFUSE LUNG DISEASE		
OXYGENATION STRATEGIES			
PaO2	Increased	Normal	Decreased
Lung inflation	Normal	Normal	Normal
Primary response	Decrease FIO2	None	Increase FIO2
Secondary response	None	None	None
PaO2	Increased	Normal	Decreased
Lung inflation	Decreased	Decreased	Decreased
Primary response	Increase Paw	Increase Paw	Increase Paw
Secondary response	Decrease FIO2	None	Increase FIO2
PaO2	Increased	Normal	Decreased
Lung inflation	Increased	Increased	Increased
Primary response	Decrease Paw	Decrease Paw	Decrease Paw
Secondary response	Decrease FIO2	None	Increase FIO2
VENTILATION STRATEGIES			
PaCO2	Increased	Normal	Decreased
Primary response	Increase OA	None	Decrease OA
Secondary response	Decrease frequency	None	Increase frequency

OA, Oscillatory amplitude.

tidal volume exposure while using I:E ratios and ventilatory frequencies that maximize gas egress. A PaCO2 between 50 and 60 mm Hg is frequently tolerated in these patients as long as the arterial pH exceeds 7.25 (these parameter limits will likely vary between institutions). Once there is radiographic evidence that the lung has adequately deflated and air leaks have resolved (for at least 12 to 24 hours), the lung is reinflated using one of the preceding lung inflation strategies. Air leak rarely recurs with this approach. This method is successful in at least 66% of infants with PIE. Those with PIE under tension and myocardial compromise are more difficult to manage and have poorer outcomes (Fig. 21-10).[10,52] This approach has been dubbed the *low-volume strategy.*

The choice of strategy is lung disease specific. Although simplistic, it is reasonable to try to inflate an underinflated lung and deflate an overinflated or air-trapped one.

WEANING

At this stage of HFV development, weaning remains a challenge. Weaning ventilation is for the most part simple. Minute ventilation can be weaned by reducing oscillatory amplitude during HFFI and HFOV and by decreasing peak pressure and on-time with HFJV. Changes in ventilation rarely have an impact on oxygenation because lung volume is preserved. Conversely, weaning Paw with improving compliance and increasing lung inflation is less straightforward. Radiographic assessment of lung volume and FIO2 may provide empirical information guiding management sufficiency. The well-inflated lung requires a reduction in mean pressure to avoid the negative consequences of excessive lung volumes. However, too rapid a reduction in distending pressures can cause alveolar de-recruitment in the unstable lung, and re-inflation will be necessary. In general, Paw should be reduced slowly (0.5 to 1 cm H2O) every 2 to 3 hours as long as there are no signs of overdistention (suggesting much more rapid decreases are necessary) or alveolar de-recruitment (decrements in oxygenation). By taking advantage of lung hysteresis, gradual reductions in mean pressure generally do not cause significant changes in oxygenation or, by inference, lung volume (see Fig. 21-9). Simple and reproducible bedside measures of lung volume are on the horizon. The application of these techniques to weaning may be useful in the future.[55]

Radiographic assessment of lung volume takes considerable practice. The novice is cautioned that although, in general, lung volume can be assessed by counting the number of posterior ribs seen above the diaphragm, radiographs of neonates are usually anterior to posterior views and counting ribs requires the juxtaposition of an anterior structure (the diaphragm) against a posterior structure (the rib interfacing with the diaphragm). This method assesses a three-dimensional object (the lung) with a two-dimensional picture (the radiograph) and is vulnerable to technician-selected focus angles. It is possible, then, to underestimate or overestimate inflation.

The present inability to routinely measure lung volume or compliance at the bedside and the ease with which acceptable oxygenation is achieved with relatively high Paw can confuse the clinician about the speed with which weaning should occur. Experience seems to be the best single teacher in this situation. The consequences of failing to wean the patient quickly enough are significant pulmonary

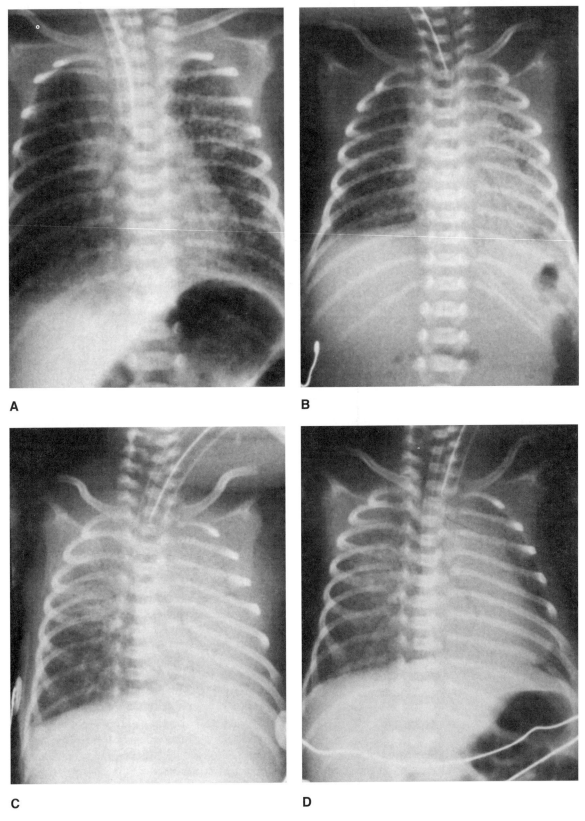

Fig. 21-10

Radiographs of a 2-day-old preterm infant with pulmonary interstitial emphysema (PIE). **A,** $P\overline{aw}$ equal to 16 cm H_2O and FIO_2 equal to 0.65. **B,** Six hours later, $P\overline{aw}$ equal to 8 cm H_2O and FIO_2 equal to 1. **C,** Twelve hours later, settings were unchanged, PIE was resolved, and lung was nearly totally deflated. **D,** Thirty-six hours later, reinflation was beginning, $P\overline{aw}$ was equal to 12 cm H_2O, and FIO_2 was equal to 0.45.

overdistention and impairment of cardiac output. In neonates, this complication can increase the risk of intracranial hemorrhage because venous return from vessels draining the head is impeded and venous hypertension and vessel rupture can ensue. Conversely, rapid weaning of $\overline{Paw}$ can result in alveolar de-recruitment requiring reinitiation of lung recruitment procedures. Efforts are currently underway to develop a simple, reproducible, safe, and inexpensive method to frequently estimate lung volumes at the bedside.[55]

CARE OF THE PATIENT

POSITIONING

As mentioned earlier, patient positioning is constrained with the use of the older SensorMedics HFOV circuits. The unique nature of the patient circuit challenges caregivers to ensure ETT stability. Positioning the patient appropriately by rotating among supine, prone, and left and right lateral decubitus positions remains as important during HFV as during CV. Protocols describing approaches to positioning have been described.[56] HFV devices using modifications of standard patient circuits, such as the HFV Infant Star and the HFJV Bunnell Life Pulse, impose few additional demands on caregivers attempting to optimize patient positioning.

ENDOTRACHEAL TUBE

The HFJV Bunnell Life Pulse requires the use of a triple-lumen high-low ETT (see Fig. 21-6). This is necessary for placement of jet breaths through a separate lumen located in the mid portion of the ETT, sampling of pressure at the distal ETT, and proximal ETT connection to the tandem CV. The HFV Infant Star and the HFOV SensorMedics do not require specific ETT. Care must be taken to ensure that the ETT bevel is not against the tracheal wall. This will decrease the functional opening of the ETT and impair volume transmission. The application of HFV techniques to the tracheotomized patient has not been extensively explored.

SUCTIONING

Suctioning techniques vary among institutions. One technique consists of quickly disconnecting the patient from the HFV circuit, performing suctioning, and reapplying HFV without bagging between disconnections. Because suctioning can reduce lung volume by the sudden drop in airway pressure at disconnection and by the negative pressures applied during the procedure, lung de-recruitment can occur. For some patients, this requires a temporary increase in $\overline{Paw}$ to regain baseline oxygenation. Closed tracheal suction systems with connections

appropriate for the ventilator circuit used may be utilized.

MONITORING

As during CV, the frequency of blood gas sampling is related to the patient's clinical status. Blood gas measurements should be obtained frequently during the early course of ventilatory management and in patients in extremis (e.g., every 1 to 4 hours). Intervals between samples should be increased as clinical conditions improve. For trending purposes, pulse oximetry and transcutaneous Po_2 and Pco_2 monitoring should be used. Because of rapid changes in $Paco_2$ noted especially during initial HFV management, transcutaneous monitoring is strongly recommended. There is no alteration in performance of these noninvasive gas exchange methods for patients receiving HFV.[57]

CIRCUITS AND HUMIDIFICATION

As implied earlier, the Infant Star 950 uses standard pressure ventilator circuits. The use of stiffer walled tubing reduces compressible volume. The Sensor-Medics circuit is constructed of smooth-walled semi-rigid tubing, unlike more flexible CV circuits. A larger-diameter tube provides the inspiratory gas flow, whereas a narrower length of tubing is used for exhalation. The circuit is constructed to minimize compressible volume losses and is specific to the ventilator (i.e., the ventilator cannot be used with conventional neonatal ventilator circuits). A standard mushroom valve controls pressures that develop in the circuit, whereas two additional valves provide a selectable upper $\overline{Paw}$ limit (usually 2 to 3 cm H_2O greater than the actual $\overline{Paw}$) and a preset high mean pressure limit (50 cm H_2O). Proximal airway pressure is monitored at the patient airway. An input distal to the ventilator and proximal to the patient conducts humidified bias flow with the selected Fio_2 into the inspiratory limb of the circuit. Airway temperature is monitored to control temperature and humidity. Each circuit is calibrated for each ventilator before use. The Bunnell Life Pulse uses regular pressure ventilator circuits, with the jet tubing attached to the patient via the middle port of the high-low jet ETT or the LifePort ETT adapter.

Humidification is provided via an integral metered system, and bias flow for volume entrainment is provided by the continuous flow of the tandem neonatal CV. Current departmental policies for conventional mechanical ventilator circuit changes may be followed when using HFV devices; these policies vary among institutions.

Early HFV rescue experiences noted the presence of necrotizing tracheobronchitis, and at least one group believed that poor humidification was in part responsible for this airway complication.[58] Manufacturers of all FDA-approved HFV devices have addressed this problem with specific instructions for the provision of gas humidification.

TROUBLESHOOTING

The approach to troubleshooting HFV devices should not be different from that during CV. Either deterioration of the patient's vital signs or a ventilator alarm may alert the clinician. In either circumstance, it is necessary to ensure that the patient is in no further jeopardy before proceeding with a detailed troubleshooting procedure. High-frequency ventilators are dependent on patient airway caliber for adequate volume delivery. A change in airway diameter (e.g., by accumulation of secretions or by migration of the tip of the ETT against the tracheal wall) may significantly reduce delivered volumes. The first step should be a quick assessment of chest wall movement to ensure unchanged ventilation. If chest wall motion is substantially decreased, a return to or increase in CV or hand bagging may dramatically improve the situation. Steps should be taken to correct any problems with the ETT lumen or position (i.e., suctioning, chest radiograph).

Like CV, there are conditions in which HFV techniques are not uniformly successful. HFV seems especially vulnerable to the state of myocardial performance. In patients with poor cardiac output (e.g., decreased intravascular volume or reduced contractility), lung inflation with high $P\overline{aw}$ can result in abrupt and serious cardiac output impairment. Ensuring the adequacy of cardiac output before initiating HFV can mitigate this. Low volume strategies will have less impact on cardiac output. For this reason, HFJV is very successful during cardiac surgery and in circumstances in which lung compliance is normal and cardiac output is reduced.[39,40]

Because a relatively high MLV is necessary for both HFFI and HFOV (when no SI or intermittent CV breaths are used), these two techniques are not optimal for use in normal lungs. Furthermore, in conditions in which airway resistance is increased, such as fresh particulate meconium aspiration, bronchopulmonary dysplasia, and reactive airway disease, HFOV and HFFI may not be optimal. Because of the tremendous impedance to flow created by reductions in airway lumen with these disorders (thus increasing pulmonary time constants), decreases in delivered tidal volume or gas trapping, or both, cause derangement in gas exchange. In contrast, HFJV using larger tidal volumes and lower breathing frequencies may be more efficacious in conditions in which airway time constants are

pathologically prolonged. These impressions are based on theoretical considerations and anecdotal experiences. Extensive controlled data supporting these contentions are not currently available.

Each ventilator manufacturer has developed detailed approaches to troubleshooting the mechanical problems of its own device, and these recommendations should be followed, tempered by actual clinical experience. A regular preventive maintenance program will help reduce mechanical failures.

EMERGING CLINICAL APPLICATIONS

The learning curve for these techniques continues to progress. Clinicians using HFV early in patients with respiratory distress syndrome believe that hospital courses are reduced and significant pulmonary morbidity is decreased.[10,29,48] The impact of HFJV on patients with PIE has been clearly demonstrated.[45] The precise role of HFV with respect to long-term outcome and cost of care continues to be defined. The availability of exogenous surfactant replacement, newer modes of CV for primary management, and ECMO and inhalational nitric oxide for patients with intractable respiratory failure continue to impact HFV use.[33,42,43,59,60] Ongoing investigations into the field of liquid ventilation, particularly partial liquid ventilation, are likely to stimulate new applications and enhance patient outcomes.

SURFACTANT REPLACEMENT

There remains little doubt that surfactant replacement therapy for immature infants with RDS is valuable. Issues that still confront surfactant replacement include the nature of the surfactant used, the timing of surfactant replacement (especially with HFV), and the method of delivery during HFV. As newer surfactants become available, the choice of surfactants increases and the determination of the best product to use becomes complex (see Chapter 16). Furthermore, the use of surfactants during HFV, which may permit uninterrupted and progressive lung recruitment, presents alternatives for timing and method of drug delivery. Many investigators, especially in European countries, prefer surfactant replacement once optimal lung volume is achieved, whereas others consider more traditional prophylactic treatment.[49] No data exist that confirm the value of one method over the other. However, bolus surfactant delivery, even during HFV, seems more effective in ensuring uniform drug distribution.

INHALED NITRIC OXIDE

The discovery that endothelial relaxing factor is nitric oxide has supplied medicine with a natural therapy for unwanted pulmonary vasoconstriction. Neonatal persistent pulmonary hypertension remains a problematic condition in critically ill near-term infants. Although it appears that inhaled nitric oxide is valuable in many circumstances, the delivery of this agent to the gas-exchanging surface is critical to its success. The uniform nature of gas delivery that occurs during HFV makes this method of ventilation an excellent delivery vehicle. Studies evaluating HFOV and CV with inhaled nitric oxide have convincingly supported the value of HFV for this indication.[60,61] This having been said, clear indications for inhaled nitric oxide therapy (with or without HFV) remain to be defined.

LIQUID VENTILATION

This clinical application relies on the concept that liquid perfluorocarbons carry much more oxygen than gases and can move carbon dioxide with ease (see Chapter 22).[62,63] Using liquid instead of gas to inflate the collapsed lung increases the uniformity of inflation with less injury. The addition of HFV to a liquid-filled lung permits ease of ventilation and may reduce lung injury.[64,65] This novel approach to RDS management is being evaluated.

REFERENCES

1. Bancalari E, Goldberg RN: High-frequency ventilation in the neonate. *Clin Perinatol* 1987; 14:581.
2. Froese AB, Bryan AC: High frequency ventilation. *Am Rev Respir Dis* 1987; 135:1363.
3. Gerstmann DR, deLemos RA: High-frequency ventilation: issues of strategy. *Clin Perinatol* 1991; 18:563.
4. Clark RH, Gerstmann DR: Controversies in high-frequency ventilation. *Clin Perinatol* 1998; 25:113.
5. Nash G, Blennerhassett JB, Pontoppidan H: Pulmonary lesions associated with oxygen therapy and artificial ventilation. *N Engl J Med* 1967; 276:368.
6. Northway WH, Rosan RC, Porter DY: Pulmonary disease following respirator therapy of hyaline membrane. *N Engl J Med* 1967; 276:357.
7. Taghizadeh A, Reynolds EOR: Pathogenesis of bronchopulmonary dysplasia following hyaline membrane disease. *Am J Pathol* 1976; 82:241.
8. Meredith KS et al: Role of lung injury in the pathogenesis of hyaline membrane disease in premature baboons. *J Appl Physiol* 1989; 66:2150.
9. HiFi Study Group: High-frequency oscillatory ventilation compared with conventional mechanical ventilation in the treatment of respiratory failure in preterm infants. *N Engl J Med* 1989; 320:88.
10. Clark RH et al: Prospective randomized comparison of high-frequency oscillatory and conventional ventilation in respiratory distress syndrome. *Pediatrics* 1992; 89:5.
11. Jobe AH: Too many unvalidated new therapies to prevent chronic lung disease in preterm infants. *J Pediatr* 1998; 132:200.
12. Clark RH, Slutsky AS, Gertsmann DR: Lung protective strategies of ventilation in the neonate: what are they? *Pediatrics* 2000; 105:112.
13. Bland RD et al: High frequency mechanical ventilation in severe hyaline membrane disease. *Crit Care Med* 1980; 8:275.
14. Borg U, Eriksson I, Sjostrand U: High-frequency positive pressure ventilation (HFPPV): A review based upon its use during bronchoscopy and for laryngoscopic and microlaryngeal surgery under general anesthesia. *Anesth Analg* 1980; 59:594.
15. Sjostrand U: High-frequency positive pressure ventilation (HFPPV): a review. *Crit Care Med* 1980; 8:345.
16. Heijman L, Sjostrand U: Treatment of the respiratory distress syndrome: preliminary report. *Opusc Med* 1974; 19:235.
17. Boros SJ et al: Neonatal high-frequency jet ventilation: four years' experience. *Pediatrics* 1985; 75:657.38.
18. Carlo WA et al: Decrease in airway pressure during high-frequency jet ventilation in infants with respiratory distress syndrome. *J Pediatr* 1984; 104:101.
19. Chatburn RL, McClellan LD: A heat and humidification system for high-frequency jet ventilation. *Respir Care* 1982; 27:1386.
20. Lunkenheimer et al: Intrapulmonaler Gasweschsel unter simulierter Apnoe durch transtrachealen, periodischen intrathorakalen Druckwechsel. *Anesthetist* 1973; 22:232.
21. Fredberg JJ et al: Factors influencing mechanical performance of neonatal high-frequency ventilators. *J Appl Physiol* 1987; 62:2485.
22. Jouvet P et al: Assessment of high-frequency neonatal ventilator performances. *Intensive Care Med* 1997; 23:208.
23. Hatcher D et al: Mechanical performances of clinically available, neonatal, high-frequency, oscillatory-type ventilators. *Crit Care Med* 1998; 26:1081.
24. Fredberg JJ: Augmented diffusion in the airways can support pulmonary gas exchange. *J Appl Physiol* 1980; 49:232.
25. Fredberg JJ et al: Alveolar pressure non-homogeneity during small amplitude high-frequency oscillation. *J Appl Physiol* 1984; 57:788.
26. Chang HK: Mechanisms of gas transport during ventilation by high-frequency oscillation. *J Appl Physiol* 1984; 56:553.
27. Robertson B: Pathology of neonatal surfactant deficiency. *Perspect Pediatr Pathol* 1987; 11:6.
28. Gilbert R, Keighley JF: The arterial/alveolar oxygen tension ratio: an index of gas exchange applicable to varying oxygen concentrations. *Am Rev Respir Dis* 1974; 142.38.
29. HiFO Study Group: Randomized study of high-frequency oscillatory ventilation in infants with severe respiratory distress syndrome. *J Pediatr* 1993; 122:609.
30. Kinsella JP et al: High-frequency ventilation versus intermittent mandatory ventilation: early hemodynamic effects in the premature baboon with hyaline membrane disease. *Pediatr Res* 1991; 29:160.
31. McCulloch PR, Forkert PG, Froese AB: Lung volume maintenance prevents lung injury during high-frequency oscillatory ventilation in surfactant deficient rabbits. *Am Rev Respir Dis* 1988; 137:1185.
32. Gerstmann DR et al: Treatment of congenital diaphragmatic hernia with high-frequency oscillatory ventilation. Presented at the Eleventh Conference on High-Frequency Ventilation of Infants. Snowbird, Utah, April 1994.
33. Bartlett RH et al: Extracorporeal circulatory support in neonatal respiratory failure: a prospective randomized study. *Pediatrics* 1985; 76:479.
34. Carter JM et al: High-frequency oscillatory ventilation and extracorporeal membrane oxygenation for the treatment of acute neonatal respiratory failure. *Pediatrics* 1990; 85:159.
35. Paranka MS et al: Predictors of failure of high-frequency ventilation in term infants with severe respiratory failure. *Pediatrics* 1995; 95:400.

36. Gerstmann DR et al: The Provo multicenter early high-frequency oscillatory ventilation trial: improved pulmonary and clinical outcome in respiratory distress syndrome. *Pediatrics* 1996; 98:1196.

37. Henderson-Smart DJ et al: Elective high frequency oscillatory ventilation versus conventional ventilation for acute pulmonary dysfunction in preterm infants. *Cochrane Database Syst Rev* 2000; 2:CD000104.

38. Duval EL et al: High-frequency ventilation in pediatric patients. *Neth J Med* 2000; 56:177.

39. Dekeon MK et al: High-frequency jet ventilation in postoperative Fontan patients. Presented at the Seventh Conference on High-Frequency Ventilation of Infants. Snowbird, Utah, April 1990.

40. Davis D et al: High-frequency jet ventilation: Intraoperative application during neonatal cardiac surgery. Presented at the Ninth Conference of High-Frequency Ventilation of Infants. Snowbird, Utah, April 1992.

41. Choong K: Low frequency oscillation is potentially more injurious than high frequency oscillatory ventilation. Presented at the Seventeenth Conference on High-Frequency Ventilation of Infants. Snowbird, Utah, April 2000.

42. Randel RC, Manning FL: One lung high-frequency ventilation in the management of an acquired neonatal pulmonary cyst. *J Perinatol* 1989; 9:66.

43. Bloom BT et al: Respiratory distress syndrome and tracheoesophageal fistula: management with high-frequency ventilation. *Crit Care Med* 1990; 18:447.

44. Cavanagh K, Bloom BT: Combined HFV and CMV for neonatal air leak. *Respir Manage* 1990; 20:43.

45. Keszler M et al: Multicenter controlled trial comparing high-frequency jet ventilation and conventional mechanical ventilation in newborns with pulmonary interstitial emphysema. *J Pediatr* 1991; 119:85.

46. Keszler M et al: Multicenter controlled trial of high-frequency jet ventilation in preterm infants with uncomplicated respiratory distress syndrome. *Pediatrics* 1997; 100:593.

47. Bhuta T, Henderson-Smart DJ: Elective high frequency jet ventilation versus conventional ventilation for respiratory distress syndrome in preterm infants. *Cochrane Database Syst Rev* 2000; (2):CD000104

48. Plavka R et al: A prospective randomized comparison of conventional mechanical ventilation and very early high frequency ventilation in extremely premature newborns with respiratory distress syndrome. *Intensive Care Med* 1999; 25:68.

49. Cools F, Offringa M: Meta-analysis of elective high frequency ventilation in preterm infants with respiratory distress syndrome. *Arch Dis Child Fetal Neonatal Ed* 1999; 80:F15.

50. Froese AB: High-frequency ventilation: strategy and device differences. Presented at the Seventh Conference on High-Frequency Ventilation of Infants. Snowbird, Utah, April 1990.

51. Hamm CR et al: High frequency jet ventilation preceded by lung volume recruitment decrease hyaline membrane formation in surfactant deficient lungs. *Pediatr Res* 1990; 27:305A.

52. Clark RH et al: Pulmonary interstitial emphysema treated by high-frequency oscillatory ventilation. *Crit Care Med* 1986; 14:926.

53. Ogawa Y et al: A multicenter randomized trial of high-frequency oscillatory ventilation as compared with conventional ventilation in preterm infants with respiratory failure. *Early Hum Dev* 1993; 32:1.

54. Clark RH et al: Intraventricular hemorrhage and high-frequency ventilation: A meta-analysis of prospective clinical trials. *Pediatrics* 1996; 98:1058.

55. Palmer C: Personal communication, August 2000.

56. Avila K et al: High-frequency oscillatory ventilation: a nursing approach to bedside care. *Neonatal Network* 1994; 13:23.

57. Meredith KS: Clinical evaluation of non-invasive blood gas monitoring. Presented at the Eighth Conference on High-Frequency Ventilation of Infants. Snowbird, Utah, April 1991

58. Ophoven JP et al: Tracheobronchial histopathology associated with high-frequency jet ventilation. *Crit Care Med* 1984; 12:829.

59. Fujiwara T et al: Artificial surfactant therapy in hyaline membrane disease. *Lancet* 1980; 1:55.

60. Kinsella JP et al: Randomized, multicenter trial of inhaled nitric oxide and high-frequency oscillatory ventilation in severe, persistent pulmonary hypertension of the newborn. *J Pediatr* 1997; 131:55.

61. Kinsella JP, Abman SH: High-frequency oscillatory ventilation augments the response to inhaled nitric oxide in persistent pulmonary hypertension of the newborn: Nitric Oxide Study Group. *Crit Care Med* 1998; 26:993.

62. Leach CL et al: Partial liquid ventilation with perflubron in premature infants with severe respiratory distress syndrome. The LiquiVent Study Group. *N Engl J Med* 1996; 335:761.

63. Weis CM, Wolfson MR, Shaffer TH: Liquid-assisted ventilation: physiology and clinical application. *Ann Med* 1997; 29:509.

64. Sukumar M et al: High-frequency partial liquid ventilation in respiratory distress syndrome: hemodynamics and gas exchange. *J Appl Physiol* 1998; 84:327.

65. Kinsella JP et al: Independent and combined effects of inhaled nitric oxide, liquid perfluorochemical, and high-frequency oscillatory ventilation in premature lambs with respiratory distress syndrome. *Am J Respir Crit Care Med* 1999; 159:1220.

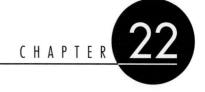

CHAPTER 22

Liquid Lung Ventilation

Jay S. Greenspan
Marla Wolfson

Respiratory insufficiency has many causes in the neonate, but the pathophysiologic end point is typically decreased lung compliance, decreased functional residual capacity, or increased lung debris. The traditional therapy for these problems has been conventional mechanical gas ventilation, in which high pulmonary inflation pressures are used to enhance tidal volume, recruit lung volume, and overcome lung stiffness, pulmonary debris, and atelectasis. Although conventional ventilators can maintain gas exchange, lung damage occurs from barotrauma and exacerbates the lung pathology, which delays or limits recovery.

Progress has been made over the past 2 decades to diminish the inflation pressures required to maintain pulmonary gas exchange. Such efforts focus on newer approaches to conventional gas ventilation, such as altering ventilation strategies using pulmonary function data, improving lung mechanics with new medications and therapies, and better ventilator designs. Nonconventional lung protection strategies have also been improved. These include high-frequency ventilation, extracorporeal life support (ECLS), and liquid breathing.

The concept of liquid breathing has evolved over the past century as a possible therapeutic approach to lung abnormalities that would minimize the inflation pressures required to move an adequate tidal volume. As first demonstrated in the 1920s, filling the lung with liquid can both remove debris and reduce the surface tension forces in the terminal lung units.[1,2] By filling the lungs with a liquid, the air-liquid interface is eliminated. Because surface tension is uniformly diminished throughout the lung fields, compliance improves and lower pressures are required to inflate the lungs. In addition, because aspiration is a frequent complication of many neonatal pulmonary pathologic processes, removal of this debris with liquid ventilation could prove advantageous in many clinical scenarios.

Saline and many other liquids can reduce surface tension and remove debris during lung insufflation.

However, breathable liquids must also be nontoxic, minimally absorbed, easily excreted, and able to dissolve adequate volumes of respiratory gases. Perfluorochemicals display these characteristics and have been proven to be effective as breathable agents.[3,4]

PROPERTIES OF PERFLUOROCHEMICALS

Perfluorochemicals are artificially derived from fluorinating organic compounds.[5] These newly formed carbon-fluorine bonds are exceptionally stable, and their physical properties vary with different carbon backbones. These liquids are insoluble in water, minimally soluble in lipid, and biologically inert. Whereas properties such as vapor pressure, density, and viscosity vary greatly between perfluorochemicals, all have a very high affinity for gases. Table 22-1 compares the chemical properties of water with five perfluorocompounds.

The feasibility of breathing perfluorochemicals during normobaric emersion was demonstrated in small animals in the late 1960s.[6] During breathing, very little perfluorochemical is absorbed into the pulmonary circulation. Once absorbed, these liquids are not metabolized and are excreted back through the lungs. The long-term toxicity of breathing, intravenously administering, or ingesting perfluorochemicals appears to be negligible.[7-9]

LIQUID VENTILATION TECHNIQUES

The physical characteristics of perfluorochemical liquids necessitate breathing strategies that differ from gas ventilation. Two categories of ventilating with liquid have been developed: tidal (TLV) and partial (PLV) liquid ventilation. TLV requires instilling a perfluorochemical into the lungs to replace the gas volume. During PLV the gas volume is only partially replaced with liquid and the infant is maintained on a conventional ventilator.

TIDAL LIQUID VENTILATION

TLV requires the instillation of a total lung volume of perfluorochemical, followed by tidal volumes of a perfluorochemical liquid. Because gases are dissolved in the liquid, all surface tension forces from a gas-liquid interface are eliminated. This provides maximal lung protection from inflation pressures. In addition, liquid is removed during exhalation and debris is washed from the lung with each breath. With TLV, lung volume is gently recruited, compliance is increased, and inflation pressures and pulmonary barotrauma are reduced.

During TLV, respiratory rate is slow, with rates generally 4 to 6 breaths per minute. Inspiratory and expiratory times must be prolonged, and an exchange period or "dwell" time is required for adequate gas exchange to occur.[1,2,4,10,11] Although simple gravity-assist ventilators are effective, more complex mechanical devices capable of ventilating liquids with precision control have been designed (Fig. 22-1).[12] These devices control ventilation through time cycling and regulating pressure, volume, or both. Tidal liquid ventilators perform much like a conventional gas mechanical ventilator. Tidal liquid ventilator designs include gravity-assist ventilators; manually controlled flow-assist pneumatic systems; roller pumps with pneumatic, fluidic, and electronic controls; and modified ECLS circuits that cycle liquid between a reservoir and the lungs.[1,2,13]

Unlike most forms of gas ventilation, TLV requires both active inspiration and active expiration to diminish the work of breathing and achieve adequate timing ratios. Preclinical animal studies demonstrated effective TLV with various oxygenated perfluorochemicals, successful recovery to gas breathing, and survival without long-term

TABLE 22-1	CHEMICAL PROPERTIES OF WATER AND FIVE PERFLUORO COMPOUNDS					
	Water	FC-77	RM-101	FC-75	Perfluorodecalin	Perflubron
Boiling point (° C)	100	97	101	102	140	143
Density at 25° C (g/ml)	1	1.78	1.77	1.78	1.95	1.93
Viscosity at 25° C (centistrokes)	1	0.8	0.82	0.82	2.9	1.1
Vapor pressure at 37° C (mm Hg)	47	85	64	63	14	11
Surface tension at 25° C (dynes/cm)	72	15	15	15	19	18
Oxygen solubility at 25° C (ml gas/100 ml liquid)	3	50	52	52	49	53
Carbon dioxide solubility at 25° C (ml gas/100 ml liquid)	57	198	160	160	140	210

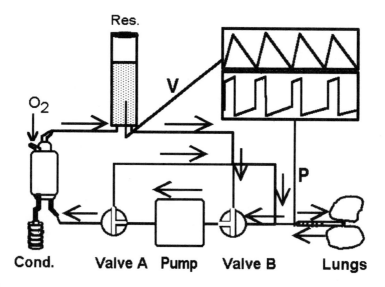

Fig. 22-1

Microprocessor-controlled tidal liquid ventilator. *Cond,* Condensor; *V,* volume; *P,* pressure signal; *Res,* reservoir. (From Heckman JL et al: Software for real-time control of a tidal liquid ventilator. *Biomed Instrum Technol* 1999; 33:268-276.)

compromise. Fig. 22-2 compares blood gas values before, during, and after TLV. Long-term stability has been demonstrated during TLV in term and preterm animals.

PARTIAL LIQUID VENTILATION

The successful recovery to gas ventilation after perfluorochemical liquid ventilation is associated with improved pulmonary function from preliquid ventilation values. This has led investigators to pursue partial liquid ventilation as a primary mode of liquid breathing.[14,15] PLV is performed by filling and maintaining the lung with a volume of perfluorochemical liquid equal to the functional residual capacity during mechanical gas ventilation (Fig. 22-3). Gas ventilation then continues on a liquid-filled lung with some adjustments to ventilator pressure and timing. Fluid must also be replaced as it evaporates out of the lungs. The rate of perfluorochemical loss is determined by the patient's minute ventilation, type of perfluorochemical used, lung function, distribution of the liquid within the lung, and volume of perfluorochemical in the lung.[14-16]

PLV eliminates the need for a liquid ventilator, yet takes advantage of some TLV aspects, such as homogeneous expansion of the lung and volume recruitment, thus lowering surface tension and resulting in a decrease in driving pressure and

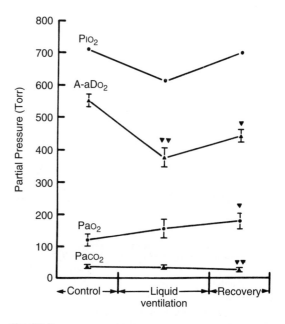

Fig. 22-2

Inspired-oxygen pressure (PIO_2), alveolar-arterial oxygen gradient ($A–aDO_2$), arterial oxygen pressure (PaO_2), and arterial carbon dioxide pressure ($PaCO_2$) during control, liquid ventilation, and recovery to gas ventilation after liquid ventilation. (From Shaffer TH et al: Liquid ventilation: improved gas exchange and lung compliance in pre-term lambs. *Pediatr Res* 1983; 17:303-306.)

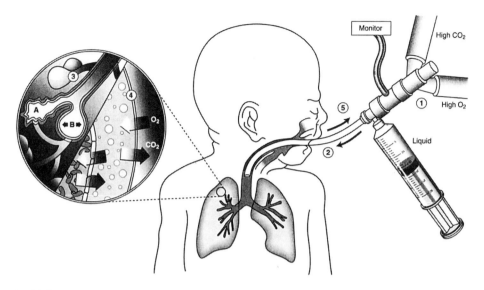

Fig. 22-3

A schematic representation of partial liquid ventilation. Conventional gas ventilation (1) is delivered on the liquid-filled lung. Perfluorochemical is instilled on inflation through a side-port adapter on the endotracheal tube (2). The liquid recruits potential air spaces (3), and gas exchange occurs through the liquid medium (4). Exhaled gases escape (5). (From Goldsmith IP, Karotkin BH, editors: *Assisted ventilation of the neonate,* ed 3. Philadelphia. WB Saunders, 1996.)

barotrauma. However, unlike TLV, during PLV gas-liquid interface tensions exist, both at the gas-lung interface during incomplete liquid fill and at the perfluorochemical-lung interface. With PLV the overall increase in compliance is between gas ventilation and TLV.[17] Surfactant-deficient animal studies demonstrate marked improvement in lung function with PLV, when compared with conventional gas ventilation.[18,19]

PULMONARY MECHANICS

The hypothesis that TLV could eliminate surface forces, recruit lung volume, improve gas exchange, and reduce required inflation pressures in the surfactant-deficient lung was first tested in 1976.[1,2,20,21] The initial study of preterm lambs of 135 to 138 days' gestation proceeded to include younger animals that were rescued from conventional mechanical ventilation. In all cases, inflation pressures and alveolar-arterial oxygen gradients were reduced and oxygenation and pulmonary compliance improved with TLV. Further evaluation of the extremely preterm animal demonstrated effective gas exchange during TLV at earlier stages of development than is possible with gas ventilation.[13,22] Additionally, pulmonary compliance in the liquid-ventilated lambs approximated that of gas-ventilated older lambs. When compared with the gas-ventilated

lungs during histomorphologic examination, the liquid-ventilated lungs had reduced pulmonary consolidation, atelectasis, and hemorrhage and showed less disruption of the alveolar-capillary membrane, as well as the absence of inflammatory infiltrates.

In addition to models of respiratory distress typical of a preterm infant, term infant lung model applications of TLV have been studied as well. In lung models of diseases typical of a term infant, results show improvements in lung mechanics, ventilation-perfusion matching, and cardiovascular stability.[1,2,23] During these studies, TLV was effective in removing caustic substances and improving pulmonary gas exchange by reducing surface tension, recruiting lung volume, and preserving lung architecture.

Preclinical studies of PLV in animals have shown adequate or improved gas exchange at reduced airway pressures compared with conventional gas ventilation in a wide range of animal models of respiratory failure.* Improvement in lung function and gas exchange with PLV is related to the type of perfluorochemical, underlying disease process, perfluorochemical dose, and pulmonary distribution. Several studies have investigated PLV for supporting gas exchange and lung mechanics in the presence of pulmonary hypoplasia. The low-pressure alveolar recruitment in models of

*References 1, 2, 14, 15, 18, 23.

congenital diaphragmatic hernia may effectively improve ventilation-perfusion matching and improve compliance but has little beneficial effect on lung histology.[24] In models of acute respiratory distress syndrome, when PLV is used, improvements in lung compliance are seen without changes in cardiac index.[25]

CLINICAL APPLICATION OF LIQUID VENTILATION

The clinical utility of perfluorochemical liquid ventilation has been explored for the past decade. The animal literature suggests that this technique would be most effective in the preterm neonate with respiratory distress syndrome. To the noninjured preterm lung, alveolar recruitment and reductions in surface tension and inflation pressure are potentially very beneficial. Debris removal may also contribute to clinical improvement in infants with lung injury from aspiration or pneumonia or in infants managed on ECLS. Whereas term animals with lung injury improve with liquid ventilation when compared with control groups on gas ventilation, these improvements are generally less dramatic than those observed in the preterm models. Models of pure pulmonary hypertension and lung injury caused by barotrauma are less well studied. However, our understanding of these pathophysiologic events suggests that liquid ventilation would have less use with these problems, unless combined with other therapies.

The initial clinical application of liquid ventilation in humans enrolled three premature human infants who were near death at the time of treatment.[26] A gravity-assisted lavage approach was used and tidal volumes of liquid were given to fill the lungs in two 5-minute cycles. The infants tolerated the procedure and showed improvement in several physiologic parameters, including lung compliance and gas exchange. Improvement was sustained after discontinuation of liquid ventilation, but eventually deterioration was evident. The ensuing protocol utilized a form of TLV but reported on the sustained benefit of gas ventilating the liquid-filled lung. Subsequent protocols have utilized a PLV technique.

Several studies of PLV have been completed in humans utilizing the perfluorochemical sterile perflubron (C8F17Br1, LiquiVent; Alliance Pharmaceutical). Thirteen premature infants with severe respiratory distress syndrome in whom conventional treatment had failed were treated with PLV for up to 96 hours.[27] The study was not randomized or blinded. The authors concluded that there was a clinical improvement and survival in some infants who were not predicted to survive.

PLV was also performed on term infants with respiratory failure from congenital diaphragmatic hernia and other causes who were being managed on ECLS.[28-30] Improvement in lung compliance and gas exchange was reported. The researchers concluded that this technique was safe and possibly effective in improving lung function and recruiting lung volume in these infants.

Three studies have evaluated PLV in children with acute respiratory failure.[30-32] They were treated with LiquiVent PLV up to 7 days. The investigators observed some improvement in gas exchange and pulmonary compliance without adverse events related to the LiquiVent or the technique. They concluded that PLV may be safe and efficacious in the treatment of pediatric acute respiratory failure.

There have also been several phase I/phase II studies of PLV with LiquiVent reported in adults with acute respiratory failure, some of whom were treated with ECLS.[30,33,34] The authors reported a decrease in the physiologic shunt ratio and an increase in pulmonary compliance. In a randomized study of PLV on adult patients, ventilator-free days and mortality did not differ between groups but the authors reported a statistically significant improvement in ventilator-free days in subjects treated with PLV who were younger than 55 years of age. These studies suggest that PLV can be accomplished safely in adults with acute respiratory failure and may be associated with improvement in lung function and gas exchange.

These initial studies of PLV in humans are encouraging and suggest the feasibility of this technique in the neonate with severe respiratory distress syndrome and acute respiratory failure. The response of the older, larger patient to PLV is frequently more gradual than is typically observed in the preterm infant with respiratory distress syndrome. The preterm infant often experiences improvement in lung compliance and gas exchange within hours of PLV initiation, most likely owing to reduction in surface tension and volume recruitment. Improving lung function in the term infant, child, and adult on PLV often requires debris removal, which occurs more gradually.

Several randomized clinical trials in infants, children, and adults are partially completed, and several are in the final planning stages. Whereas the results of the initial phase I and phase II trials demonstrate potential safety and efficacy, understanding the utility of ventilating with liquid awaits the results of ongoing studies.

OTHER APPLICATIONS OF LIQUID VENTILATION

The clinical application of perfluorochemical liquid instillation into the human lung is not limited to the treatment of respiratory failure. Studies indicate that

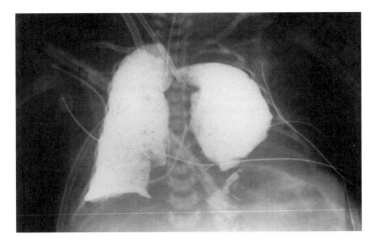

Fig. 22-4

A chest radiograph of lungs filled with the radiopaque perfluorochemical, LiquiVent. The infant was on extracorporeal life support for diaphragmatic hernia.

perfluorochemical liquids may modify biologic activity in the lung, which may reduce inflammation and injury.[2,35,36] In addition to preventing disruption and leakage of the alveolar lining during ventilation, perfluorochemicals may act directly on the pulmonary cellular elements to decrease the inflammatory response.

Because perfluorochemicals are inert and are slightly radiopaque, they provide a useful addition to diagnostic imaging to evaluate pulmonary structure (Fig. 22-4). This includes enhancement of plain films, computed tomography, and nuclear magnetic resonance imaging.[1,2,37,38]

Perfluorochemical pulmonary instillation may also be an effective means of delivering biologically active agents to the lung structures. The introduction of a therapeutic agent directly into the liquid-filled lung presents advantages for distribution and uptake of these agents. Several animal studies demonstrate the effective delivery of agents such as vasopressors, antibiotics, surfactant, adenovirus for gene transfer, and gases utilizing perfluorochemicals.[1,2,33,40]

SUMMARY

The concept of gently expanding and cleansing the lung with a breathable fluid has undergone nearly 8 decades of laboratory investigation, culminating in a decade of human work. Initial human trials appear to mimic the dramatic success seen in the many different animal models. Most of the clinical trials are demonstrating substantial improvement in both lung function and gas exchange and also some survival in patients not predicted to survive. The extraordinarily extensive amount of preclinical information has permitted safe, ongoing early human trials, which are proceeding in a very careful fashion. Although these clinical trials, and continued animal work, help to increase our ability to perform liquid ventilation more effectively, larger randomized studies are needed to prove the value of PLV. Once a perfluorochemical is approved for PLV use in humans, our capability of introducing TLV into the clinical setting will be explored and the clinical feasibility and application of liquid ventilation will be clarified.

REFERENCES

1. Shaffer TH, Wolfson MR, Clark LC: State-of-the-art: liquid ventilation. *Pediatr Pulmonol* 1992; 14:102-109.
2. Wolfson MR, Greenspan JS, Shaffer TH: Liquid-ASSISTED Ventilation: an alternative respiratory modality. *Pediatr Pulmonol* 1998; 26:42-63.
3. Modell JH, Calderwood HW, Ruiz BC: Long term survival of dogs after breathing oxygenated fluorocarbon liquid. *Fed Proc* 1970; 29:1731-1736.
4. Wolfson MR et al: A new experimental approach for the study of cardiopulmonary physiology during early development. *J Appl Physiol* 1988; 65:1436-1443.
5. Sargent JW, Seffl RI: Properties of perfluoronated liquid. *Fed Proc* 1970; 29:1699-1703.
6. Clark LC, Gollan F: Survival of mammals breathing organic liquids equilibrated with oxygen at atmosphere pressure. *Science* 1966; 152:1755-1756.
7. Shaffer TH et al: Liquid ventilation in premature lambs: uptake, biodistribution and elimination of perfluorodecalin liquid. *Reprod Fertil Dev* 1996; 8:409-416.
8. Holaday DA et al: Uptake, distribution and excretion of flurocarbon FX-80 (perflurobertyl perfluorotetrahydrafuon) during liquid breathing in the dog. *Anesthesiology* 1972; 37:387-394.
9. Modell JH et al: Liquid ventilation of primates. *Chest* 1976; 69:79-81.
10. Wolfson MR et al: Liquid ventilation equipment and methodology: a historical perspective. Presented before the 11th Annual CNMC ECMO Symposium, Keystone Colo, 1996.
11. Koen PA, Wolfson MR, Shaffer TH: Fluorocarbon ventilation: maximal expiratory flows and CO_2 elimination. *Pediatr Res* 1988; 24:291-296.
12. Heckman JL et al: Software for real-time control of a tidal liquid ventilator. *Biomed Instrum Technol* 1999; 33:268-276.

13. Wolfson MR, Shaffer TH: Liquid ventilation during early development: theory, physiologic processes and application. *J Dev Physiol* 1990; 13:1-12.

14. Curtis SB, Peek JT, Kelly DR: Partial liquid breathing with perflubron improves arterial oxygenation in acute canine lung injury. *J Appl Physiol* 1993; 75:2696-2702.

15. Fuhrman BP, Paczan PR, De Francisis M: Perfluorocarbon-associated gas exchange. *Crit Care Med* 1991; 19:712-722.

16. Miller TF, Shaffer TH, Wolfson MR: Effect of single vs. multiple dosing of perfluorochemical (PFC) elimination profile during partial liquid ventilation with LiquiVent. *Pediatr Res* 1996; 39:341A.

17. Tarczy-Hornoch P et al: Effects of exogenous surfactant on lung pressure-volume characteristics during liquid ventilation. *J Appl Physiol* 1996; 80:1764-1771.

18. Leach C et al: Perfluorocarbon associated gas exchange (partial liquid ventilation) in respiratory distress syndrome: a prospective randomized controlled study. *Crit Care Med* 1993; 21:1270-1278.

19. Curtis SB, Fuhrman BP, Howland DF: Airway and alveolar pressures during perfluorocarbon breathing in infant lambs. *J Appl Physiol* 1993; 75:2696-2702.

20. Shaffer TH et al: Gaseous exchange and acid-base balance in premature lambs during liquid ventilation since birth. *Pediatr Res* 1976; 10:227-231.

21. Shaffer TH et al: Liquid ventilation: improved gas exchange and lung compliance in pre-term lambs. *Pediatr Res* 1983; 17:303-306.

22. Wolfson MR et al: Comparison of gas and liquid ventilation: clinical, physiological, and histological correlates. *J Appl Physiol* 1992; 72:1024-1031.

23. Hirschl RB et al: Evaluation of gas exchange, pulmonary compliance, and lung injury during total and partial liquid ventilation in the acute respiratory distress syndrome. *Crit Care Med* 1996; 24:1001-1008.

24. Major D et al: Combined ventilation and perfluorochemical (PFC) tracheal instillation as an alternative treatment for near-death congenital diaphragmatic hernia. *J Pediatr Surg* 1995; 30:1178-1182.

25. Curtis SB, Peek JT, Kelly DR: Partial liquid breathing with perflubron improves arterial oxygenation in acute canine lung injury. *J Appl Physiol* 1993; 75:2696-2702.

26. Greenspan JS et al: Liquid ventilation of human pre-term neonates. *J Pediatr* 1990; 117:106-111.

27. Leach CL et al: Partial liquid ventilation with perflubron in premature infants with severe respiratory distress syndrome. *N Engl J Med* 1996; 335:761-767.

28. Pranikoff T, Gauger PG, Hirschl RB: Partial liquid ventilation in newborn patients with congenital diaphragmatic hernia. *J Pediatr Surg* 1996; 31:613-618.

29. Greenspan JS et al: Partial liquid ventilation in critically ill infants receiving extracorporeal life support. *Pediatrics* 1997; 99:E2.

30. Hirschl RB et al: Liquid ventilation in adults, children, and full-term neonates. *Lancet* 1995; 346:1201-1202.

31. Gauger PG et al: Initial experience with partial liquid ventilation in pediatric patients with the acute respiratory distress syndrome. *Crit Care Med* 1996; 24:16-22.

32. Toro-Figueroa LO et al: Perflubron partial liquid ventilation (PLV) in children with ARDS: a safety and efficacy pilot study. *Crit Care Med* 1996; 24(1):150A.

33. Barlett R et al: A phase II randomized controlled trial of partial liquid ventilation (PLV) in adult patients with acute hypoxemic respiratory failure (AHRF). *Crit Care Med* 1997; 25:A35.

34. Hirschl RB et al: Initial experience with partial liquid ventilation in adult patients with the acute respiratory distress syndrome. *JAMA* 1996; 275:383-389.

35. Cotton DM et al: Neutrophil infiltration is reduced during partial liquid ventilation in the setting of lung injury. *Surg Forum* 1994; 45:668-670.

36. Smith TM et al: A liquid perfluorochemical decreases the in vitro production of reactive oxygen species by alveolar macrophages. *Crit Care Med* 1996; 23:1533-1539.

37. Stern RG et al: High-resolution computed tomographic bronchiolography using perfluoroctylbromide (PFOB): An experimental model. *J Thorac Imaging* 1993; 8: 300-304.

38. Quintet M et al: Computer tomographic assessment of perfluorocarbon distribution and gas distribution during partial liquid ventilation for acute respiratory failure. *Am J Respir Crit Care Med* 1998; 58:249-255.

39. Wolfson MR, Greenspan JS, Shaffer TH: Pulmonary administration of vasoactive substances by perfluorochemical ventilation. *Pediatrics* 1996; 97:449-455.

40. Lisby DA et al: Enhanced distribution of adenovirus-mediated gene transfer to lung parenchyma by perfluorochemical liquid. *Hum Gene Ther* 1997; 8:919-928.

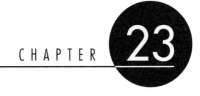

CHAPTER 23

Administration of Gas Mixtures

Mark Rogers

INHALED NITRIC OXIDE

Nitric oxide (NO), the 1992 *Science* magazine "Molecule of the Year," is a colorless, sweet-smelling, nonflammable toxic gas. Nitric oxide, not to be confused with *nitrous* oxide (N_2O, an anesthetic), is also an unstable, highly reactive, diatomic free radical. Commercially, NO is produced from the reaction of sulfuric acid and nitric acid.[1] NO also is produced by the oxidation of ammonia in the presence of a platinum catalyst at high temperatures.[2] Because of its high reactivity, NO is often combined with nitrogen in various concentrations and stored in aluminum alloy cylinders. The most common concentration available commercially is 800 ppm, although higher and lower concentrations are available as well.

PHYSIOLOGIC BASIS OF ACTION

Nitric oxide is a ubiquitous substance produced by nearly every cell and organ in the human body (Box 23-1). Directly or indirectly, NO performs numerous functions, including vasodilation, platelet inhibition, immune regulation, enzyme regulation, and neurotransmission.[3] This chapter, however, focuses on smooth muscle relaxation of the pulmonary vascular bed.

Pulmonary Smooth Muscle Relaxation and Contraction. An understanding of the mechanism of smooth muscle relaxation in the pulmonary vascular bed is based on the regulation of smooth muscle tone. In general, smooth muscle tone is regulated by chemical, hormonal, nervous, and physical interactions.[4] Current understanding suggests that vascular smooth muscle is largely dependent on intracellular calcium ion (Ca^{++}) concentration. Smooth muscle tissue comprises bundles of myofibrils, threadlike contractile fibers, encased by the sarcoplasmic reticulum, a network of tubes or channels that store Ca^{++}. Muscle contraction begins with the release of Ca^{++} from the sarcoplasmic reticulum. Calcium binds with the protein calmodulin. The calcium-calmodulin complex activates the enzyme myosin light-chain kinase, enabling phosphorylation of the myosin, resulting in contraction of the cell. Contraction continues until Ca^{++} is reabsorbed into the sarcoplasmic reticulum. Therefore any process that inhibits the release of Ca^{++} will interrupt smooth muscle contraction.

In the body the process of smooth muscle relaxation utilizes cyclic guanosine monophosphate (cGMP) to reduce Ca^{++} levels. In smooth muscle cells, cGMP activates cGMP-dependent kinase, preventing the release of Ca^{++} from the sarcoplasmic reticulum, resulting in smooth muscle relaxation. In the early 1980s, researchers reported a potent smooth muscle relaxing agent, *endothelium-derived relaxing factor* (EDRF),[5] now understood to be endogenous nitric oxide. Formation of EDRF results in increased levels of cGMP in smooth muscle cells. EDRF and cGMP are conceivably the two most important substances in regulating smooth muscle tone.[4,6]

Nitric Oxide Synthase and Endogenous Nitric Oxide Production. In the body, NO is produced by the combination of nitric oxide synthase (NOS) enzymes with the amino acid L-arginine and molecular oxygen. This combination results in the formation of the amino acid L-citrulline and NO (Fig. 23-1). The two types of NOS enzymes are constitutive and inducible. The *constitutive* NOS (cNOS) enzymes are normally expressed in tissues and consist of two isoforms: eNOS (endothelial in origin) and nNOS (neuronal in origin).[3] The one *inducible* NOS enzyme, iNOS, results from enzyme induction.[7] The cNOS, a calmodulin-dependent enzyme, produces relatively small amounts of NO (picomoles). The iNOS enzyme functions independently of calmodulin and produces relatively large amounts of NO (nanomoles). NO resulting from iNOS is most often produced in sepsis and is probably responsible for the pathologic decrease in systemic vascular resistance observed in septic shock.

Once NO is formed and bound to hemoglobin, guanylyl cyclase is activated, which converts cyclic guanidine triphosphate to cGMP. This increased cGMP results in reduced Ca^{++} and smooth muscle relaxation.

Exogenous Nitric Oxide. The underlying principle of *inhaled* nitric oxide (iNO) is its selectivity as a pulmonary vasodilator.[8] Inhaled NO will dilate only the pulmonary blood vessels adjacent to functioning alveoli. Atelectatic or fluid-filled lung units will not participate in iNO uptake. Therefore, if the pulmonary vasculature is constricted in

---

BOX 23-1

ORGANS AND CELLS IN ENDOGENOUS PRODUCTION OF NITRIC OXIDE

Brain
Peripheral nerves
Skeletal muscle
Liver
Myocytes
Epithelium
Platelets
Adrenals
Macrophages
Lungs

Fig. 23-1

Endogenous nitric oxide (NO) production. Under normal conditions, picomoles of NO are produced. When inducible nitric acid synthase (iNOS) is activated in conditions of sepsis or inflammation, nanomoles of NO are produced. *ATP,* Adenosine triphosphate; *ACh,* acetylcholine; *IL,* interleukin; *TNF,* tumor necrosis factor; *IFN,* interferon; *cNOS,* constitutive nitric oxide synthase; *eNOS,* endogenous nitric oxide synthase; *nNOS,* neuronal nitric oxide synthase; *iNOS,* induced nitric oxide synthase. (From Aranda A, Pearl RG: The biology of nitric oxide. *Respir Care* 1999; 44:157.)

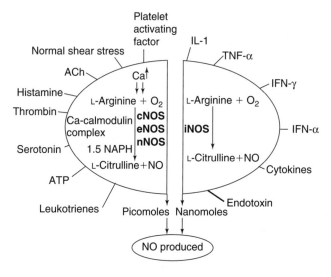

atelectatic regions of the lung, pulmonary blood flow will remain minimal in these regions, reducing intrapulmonary shunt (Fig. 23-2). This concept is in contrast to intravenous vasodilators such as nitroprusside or prostacyclin. These drugs will relax pulmonary vasculature globally, reducing pulmonary vascular resistance, but also increasing intrapulmonary right-to-left shunt. Ultimately, NO is excreted primarily by the kidneys as nitrates and nitrites.[9]

The concept of treating pulmonary hypertension with iNO has been advocated in many studies. In 2000, however, the first U.S. Food and Drug Administration (FDA) approval of iNO as a noninvestigative drug was in the treatment of primary pulmonary hypertension of the term or near-term newborn. Investigation is ongoing for iNO's approved use in other diseases. Current research is investigating its use in acute respiratory distress syndrome (ARDS). ARDS is a complex syndrome characterized by noncardiogenic pulmonary edema, diminished lung compliance, and pulmonary hypertension.

Current therapy for ARDS is primarily supportive, allowing time for the lung to heal. Although no definitive studies show improved outcomes, iNO has been suggested to improve oxygenation and ventilation-perfusion ($\dot{V}/\dot{Q}$) matching, consequently lowering airway pressure and oxygen concentration.

APPLICATION

Several methods have been advocated for the delivery of iNO.[10,11] Early systems were custom-built in-house and comprised two basic subsystems: delivery and monitoring. In these systems, NO is bled into the breathing circuit through a flowmeter or blender. NO and NO_2 levels are monitored with an NO/NO_2 analyzer (Fig. 23-3).

Now that the use of iNO has increased, several vendors have developed systems incorporating iNO delivery with NO and NO_2 monitoring. These devices come in a variety of designs. Some are large and designed for in-hospital use (Fig. 23-4). Others are small battery-operated devices for interfacility transport (Fig. 23-5). A recent FDA approval and subsequent patents led to the formation of INO Therapeutics, a for-profit company that currently holds the exclusive rights to market NO in the United States. Currently, iNO is only approved for use in persistent pulmonary hypertension in the newborn. These systems allow the quick and safe application of iNO to the patient.

SPECIAL CONSIDERATIONS

Nitrogen Dioxide. As discussed earlier, when combined with oxygen, NO produces NO_2, a toxic gas. Although rare, the patient as well as health care providers can be adversely affected. Factors influencing NO_2 production are oxygen concentration, NO concentration, and time of contact between NO and oxygen. Therefore the patients most at risk of NO_2 delivery include those receiving high oxygen concentrations and low ventilator flow rates.

Since decreasing the NO or oxygen concentration is usually not an option, to reduce NO_2 delivery to the patient, reduce the duration of contact between NO and oxygen. Two methods accomplish this: (1) increase the inspiratory flow or (2) add the NO as close to the patient as possible. Each of these methods has practical limitations. Increasing the ventilator flow will reduce the time of contact between NO and oxygen before reaching the

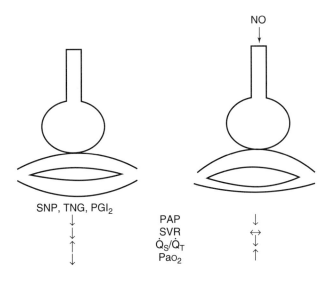

Fig. 23-2

Comparison of the vasodilator effects from systemic drugs and NO. Both reduce pulmonary artery pressure, but the systemic vasodilators also dilate the blood vessels not participating in gas exchange, thereby increasing the intrapulmonary shunt. *SNP*, Sodium nitroprusside; *TNG*, nitroglycerin; *PGI₂*, prostacyclin; *PAP*, pulmonary artery pressure; *SVR*, systemic vascular resistance; $\dot{Q}_S/\dot{Q}_T$, intrapulmonary shunt. (Redrawn from Hess D et al: Use of inhaled nitric oxide in patients with acute respiratory distress syndrome. *Respir Care* 1996; 41:428.)

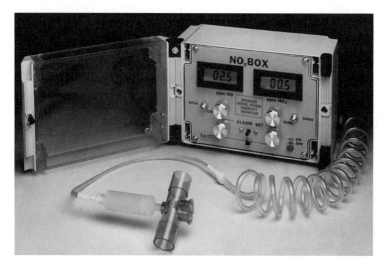

A

Fig. 23-3

Small, battery-operated, stand-alone NO/NO$_2$ monitors. **A,** NoxBox. **B,** Pulmonox IIRT. (**A** courtesy Bedfont Scientific, Rochester, Kent, UK; **B** courtesy Pulmonox, Tofield, Alberta, Canada.)

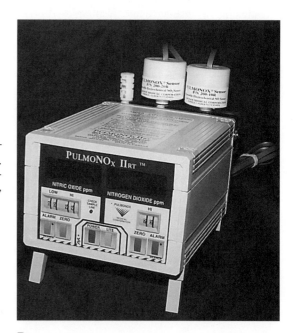

B

patient, but it may also affect inspiratory time, tidal volume, mean airway pressure, etc. Adding NO into the inspiratory limb of the ventilator circuit close to the patient will reduce contact time, but it also creates monitoring difficulties. The practitioner must allow an adequate distance for proper mixing to ensure an accurate NO measurement.

Additionally, the local atmosphere could become contaminated with NO and NO$_2$. Although this is rare, early systems included means for the scavenging of expiratory and wasted gases. Usually this was accomplished by the collection of gases into a gas evacuation system similar in design to those used in anesthesia. Gas was collected in a large reservoir and removed continuously through the hospital's vacuum system. Initially, scavenging was advocated to reduce the possible harmful inhalation of nitrogen dioxide by other personnel in the vicinity. Recent studies have shown this to be unnecessary due to the relatively small amounts of NO$_2$ present at the bedside. Most modern hospitals have adequate room air-exchange rates, and the chance of NO or NO$_2$ accumulation is remote. A possible caveat involves interfacility transport. Pressurized aircraft may not allow an adequate cabin air-exchange rate to ensure safety. The aircraft crew

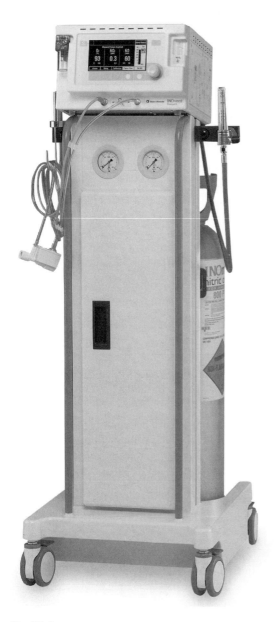

Fig. 23-4

INOVent, a stand-alone NO delivery and monitoring device. Versions are available for use in the operating room and for transport. (Courtesy Datex-Ohmeda, Helsinki, Finland.)

must be made aware of this so that proper measures are taken to reduce this risk.

Methemoglobin. The half-life of iNO is extremely short, about 5 seconds. Once NO crosses the vascular endothelium, it is rapidly bound by hemoglobin, forming nitrosyl-hemoglobin (methemoglobin). Methemoglobin production results from the oxida-

tion of the iron in the hemoglobin.[12] The quantity of methemoglobin depends on iNO concentration and concurrent nitrate-based drug therapy (e.g., nitroprusside, nitroglycerine). If the methemoglobin level is excessive, a reduction in iNO or other nitro-based vasodilators is warranted.

HELIUM-OXYGEN MIXTURES

Helium (He) was discovered in 1895 by Sir William Ramsay and independently by Langley and Cleve. Helium is one of the lightest elements, second only to hydrogen. It is a colorless, odorless, tasteless, and physiologically inert noble gas. Helium is present in dry air at a concentration of 0.0005%. Currently, the majority of helium comes from natural gas mines in the United States. The supply is limited, and until the Helium Privatization Act of 1996, production was under the control of the U.S. Government.

Physical properties of helium are remarkable for its low density and high viscosity. Pure helium gas has a density of 0.179 g/L, one-seventh the density of air. A common misconception is that because of its low density, helium has a low viscosity. Actually, helium is slightly more viscous than air. However, its *kinematic viscosity* (absolute viscosity divided by density) is almost seven times greater than air. Therefore, from the standpoint of fluid dynamics, helium is much more viscous than air.[13]

PHYSIOLOGIC BASIS OF ACTION

The use of helium-oxygen mixtures in treating airway obstruction was first described in 1934 by Barach.[14-17] Barach's studies reported a decrease in work of breathing in patients with both upper and lower airway obstruction. Helium is an inert gas, has no pharmacologic properties of its own, and does not participate or interfere with any biochemical activity in the body. Its sole purpose is to lower the total density of any gas mixture.

It is important to note that helium is not used to treat the underlying cause of increased airway resistance, but rather to decrease the work of breathing until more definitive therapies are effective. When helium is combined with oxygen, the resulting gas mixture density is one-third that of air. Given Poiseuille's law, if the diameter of a tube is reduced by half, the pressure gradient to achieve the same flow increases 16 times. Graham's law states that the flow of gas through an orifice is inversely proportional to the square root of its density.[18] In other words, if the driving pressure remains constant, a gas with lower density will have higher flow than a gas with higher density. Alternately, less pressure is required to maintain a given flow through a fixed orifice. Because of this physical property, helium

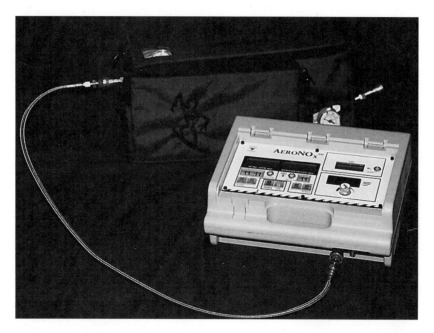

Fig. 23-5

Aeronox, a small stand-alone delivery and monitoring device designed for transport. (Courtesy Pulmonox, Tofield, Alberta, Canada.)

may be useful in overcoming airway resistance and obstruction.

In normal human anatomy, inspired gas is turbulent between the glottis and the tenth-generation airways, primarily because of the high gas flow and larger radii of the airways. Physics dictates that greater pressure is required to move gas through a tube (or airway) under turbulent conditions compared with the same volume of gas during laminar flow. A quick review of the Reynold's equation shows that decreasing density and increasing viscosity will reduce turbulent flow, decreasing the pressure and work required to move the gas (Fig. 23-6). Likewise, gas flow through a large, partially obstructed airway will create the same turbulent flow. Decreasing turbulent flow reduces the amount of pressure required to move the gas through the airways, decreasing the work required to breathe.

Aerosol Delivery. Two studies investigated the use of helium-oxygen mixtures and the deposition of aerosolized particles.[19,20] Anderson et al[19] studied patients with stable asthma. Ten patients inhaled radiolabeled particles of Teflon suspended in air or a helium-oxygen mixture. The study concluded there was more aerosol deposition in the lung and less deposition in the upper airways when breathing helium-oxygen mixtures. In a similar study, 42 patients were randomly assigned to

receive β-agonists with helium-oxygen mixtures or air.[21] Patients who used the helium-oxygen mixtures showed more improvement in expiratory peak flows than the group using air. These studies support the idea that medicated aerosol has better, deeper, and longer deposition in the lung.

Application

Helium must be combined with oxygen when used clinically, thus the term *heliox*. Several concentrations of medical-grade helium are available commercially: 80% helium/20% oxygen heliox mixture (80/20), 70% helium/30% oxygen (70/30), and 100% helium/0% oxygen (100%). The 80/20 mixture has essentially the same concentration of oxygen as air; the nitrogen and trace gases are replaced with helium. The 70/30 mixture is useful for patients with airway obstruction who require increased oxygen concentration. The 100% helium concentration is unique because it must be used with oxygen to be compatible with life. Extreme caution and close monitoring must be employed when using this concentration. It is possible to deliver a hypoxic gas mixture to the patient, possibly resulting in asphyxiation and death.

For the purposes of this chapter, only the use of nonhypoxic gas mixtures is discussed. Heliox cylinders containing at least 20% oxygen are brown and white (or brown and green) and use a CGA-280 fitting.

$$\text{Reynold's Number} = \frac{\text{Flow} \times \text{Diameter} \times \text{Density}}{\text{Viscosity}} \quad \text{Laminar} \leq 2000 \geq \text{Turbulent}$$

Fig. 23-6

Reynold's equation for turbulent flow. As density decreases or viscosity increases, flow becomes laminar.

Flowmeters. Because helium is less dense and therefore more diffusible than oxygen, standard oxygen flowmeters will indicate an incorrect flow when used with helium-containing mixtures. This error will cause the indicated flow to be erroneously low. An 80/20 heliox mixture is 1.8 times more diffusible than oxygen. To correct for the difference in gas density, the indicated flow on the flowmeter is multiplied by 1.8. A 70/30 heliox mixture is 1.6 times more diffusible than oxygen. To obtain the accurate flow rate for this mixture, the indicated flow is multiplied by 1.6. This error will be present in most gas-measuring devices (see later discussion in this section).

Spontaneously Breathing Patients. Spontaneously breathing patients with upper or lower airway obstruction can be given heliox via mask. Because the goal of heliox therapy is to reduce the density of the inspired gas, it is important to deliver the greatest concentration of helium. Therefore the patient must be able to tolerate the lowest fractional concentration of inspired oxygen (FIO_2) possible, and room-air entrainment must be minimized, resulting in a higher fractional concentration of inspired helium ($FIHe$). Because nasal cannulas and simple masks allow room-air entrainment, a close-fitting nonrebreathing mask should be used. This limitation makes treating young asthmatic patients difficult. Children in distress may not tolerate the tightly fitting mask required to minimize air entrainment.

Stillwell et al[22] investigated the use of heliox mixtures delivered through an infant hood. Not surprisingly, they found a greater concentration of helium at the top of the hood (due to its lower gas density), away from the infant's nose and mouth. This resulted in a lower $FIHe$ and therefore a denser gas being delivered to the infant.

Mechanically Ventilated Patients. Unfortunately, many patients with airway obstruction must be mechanically ventilated to manage respiratory failure and to reduce their work of breathing. This presents the practitioner with a new set of challenges. Patients with severe lower airway obstruction (as seen in status asthmaticus) have reduced expiratory flows. The resulting increased expiratory times could lead to air trapping, barotrauma, and hemodynamic compromise. The use of heliox mixtures has been advocated to minimize air trapping and reduce peak inspiratory pressures when mechanically ventilating a patient with severe lower airway obstruction.

The primary obstacle with heliox delivery via a mechanical ventilator is error in volume and flow measurement. Most mechanical ventilators rely on gas density to measure flows and volumes. Errors result from underestimation of flow due to the low-density characteristics of helium. These same characteristics result in a decreased work of breathing associated with airway obstruction. Because volume is a mathematic integration of flow and time, volumes are equally affected. In one study the Servo 900C (Siemens) demonstrated a statistically significant (approximately 10%) underestimation in volume measurement at a helium concentration of 50%, increasing to a 20% error at a helium concentration of 80%.[23] This error in flow and volume is also seen in external monitors as well. In the same study the Ventrak pulmonary monitor (Novametrix) underestimated volume by 20% at a helium concentration of 20%, increasing to a 40% error at a helium concentration of 80%.

The most popular method to deliver helium-oxygen mixtures via mechanical ventilation is to connect the heliox mixture to the air inlet of the mechanical ventilator. The practitioner then uses the ventilator's oxygen concentration control to adjust helium and oxygen to the desired mixture. This allows the practitioner to deliver a helium concentration up to the concentration of the heliox cylinder. It is important to note that some ventilators may not function properly with helium as a source gas. For example, the Puritan-Bennett 7200 will not function properly if 100% helium is connected to the air inlet, however, it will work if an 80/20 mixture is used. This anomaly appears to be related to the heated-wire flow anemometer on the gas inlets. The high thermal conductivity of helium rapidly cools the wires, simulating a high flow condition. The microprocessor responds by closing the gas inlet valve to such a degree that the ventilator will not function.

HYPOXIC AND HYPERCARBIC GAS MIXTURES

The primary goal of the practitioner is to maximize oxygen delivery to the tissues. To achieve this goal, hypoxic (less than 21% oxygen) or hypercarbic gas mixtures may be used. Oxygen is a potent pulmonary vasodilator, and conversely, carbon dioxide is an equally potent pulmonary vasoconstrictor. Knowing these effects allows the practitioner to alter pulmonary and systemic blood flow by manipulating pulmonary vascular resistance (PVR) in infants with congenital cardiac lesions.

PHYSIOLOGIC BASIS OF ACTION

Hypoxic or hypercarbic gas therapy may be beneficial in infants with certain lesions when pulmonary blood flow may be excessive through the ductus arteriosus, as in hypoplastic left-sided heart syndrome (HLHS) and single-ventricle syndromes. Because these cardiac lesions are addressed in Chapter 31, this section focuses on HLHS as representative physiology.

Infants with HLHS present with a constellation of cardiac disorders, including small or absent left ventricle, aortic and mitral stenosis, and hypoplasia of the ascending aorta. Because little or no blood is ejected from the left ventricle, pulmonary as well as systemic blood flow originates from the right ventricle. Blood returning from the lungs is shunted from the left atrium to the right atrium via an atrial septal defect. Systemic blood flow is supplied entirely from right-to-left flow through a patent ductus arteriosus (PDA). Preoperative survival of the patient depends on a PDA and an elevated PVR. Preoperatively the PDA is maintained with prostaglandin E_1 and judicious use of oxygen.

In these patients a delicate balance exists between pulmonary ($\dot{Q}p$) and systemic ($\dot{Q}s$) blood flow. This relationship can be expressed as the ratio between PVR and systemic vascular resistance (SVR). Changes in PVR and SVR affect $\dot{Q}p$ and $\dot{Q}s$ directly. A $\dot{Q}p/\dot{Q}s$ ratio greatly exceeding 1.0 results in systemic hypoperfusion, circulatory shock, decreased renal blood flow, and metabolic acidosis. A $\dot{Q}p/\dot{Q}s$ ratio much less than 1.0 results in pulmonary hypoperfusion leading to systemic oxygen debt.[24,25] Generally, $\dot{Q}p$ should be approximately one third to one half of $\dot{Q}s$.[26]

Supportive therapy before palliative or corrective surgery may require the use of hypoxic gas mixtures to increase PVR, thereby promoting systemic blood flow. Because PVR and SVR are not typically measured in infants, other means are needed to gauge the $\dot{Q}p/\dot{Q}s$ ratio. Typically, these patients are managed on an F_{IO_2} of 0.17 to 0.21, achieving an arterial oxygen saturation of 75% to 85%. Clinically, extremity temperature, color, and blood pressure are usually

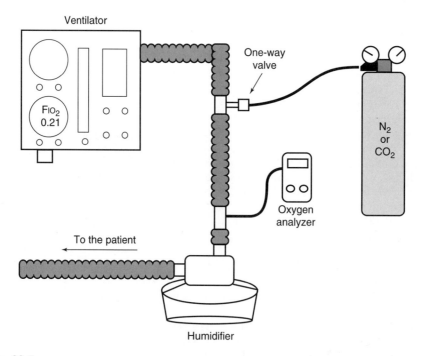

Fig. 23-7

Subambient oxygen therapy is achieved by introducing a flow of nitrogen (N_2) into the inspired gas stream of a ventilator circuit before it reaches the humidification system.

sufficient to assess systemic blood flow. If the patient has cool extremities but is pink, $\dot{Q}p/\dot{Q}s$ is probably too high. Conversely, if the patient has warm extremities but is cyanotic, $\dot{Q}p/\dot{Q}s$ is probably too low. Ongoing clinical examinations are required to assess the appropriateness of hypoxic gas mixture therapy.

At times the PVR cannot be increased without decreasing FIO_2 to precipitous levels. Increasing the infant's partial pressure of arterial carbon dioxide ($PaCO_2$) would be clinically advantageous. Although it is possible to allow the infant's $PaCO_2$ to increase secondary to alveolar hypoventilation, this technique may lead to atelectasis. The use of hypercarbic gas therapy has been advocated to increase PVR further while maintaining a safe FIO_2 and alveolar ventilation. These patients are typically managed on a fractional concentration of inspired carbon dioxide ($FICO_2$) of 0.02 to 0.05.

Extracorporeal Membrane Oxygenation. Some patients require extracorporeal membrane oxygenation (ECMO) to achieve adequate gas exchange (see Chapter 24). The membrane oxygenator in the ECMO circuit is very efficient, and sometimes too efficient, in exchanging gases with the blood. In cases when the "sweep gas" (usually 100% oxygen) through the oxygenator removes too much CO_2 from the blood, carbogen may be substituted as the sweep gas to inhibit excessive CO_2 removal. *Carbogen* is a mixture of 95% oxygen and 5% carbon dioxide.

APPLICATION

In principle the application of hypoxic gas therapy is straightforward. The gas delivery device (oxygen hood or mechanical ventilator) is set to deliver 21% oxygen. Nitrogen is then added to the gas flow before humidification (Fig. 23-7). Whenever hypoxic gas mixtures are used, extreme care must be used to monitor the gas delivered to reduce the chance of suffocation. The oxygen analyzer must be capable of measuring the lowest oxygen concentration to be used (17% to 18%). In addition, low oxygen alarms must be set at that low oxygen concentration. Because many commercially available oxygen analyzers limit the low oxygen alarm, the practitioner must ensure that the analyzer used is capable of monitoring (with alarms) at an oxygen concentration of 17% to 18%.

The delivery of hypercarbic gas mixtures follows the same procedure as for hypoxic gas mixtures. Carbon dioxide is added to the main gas flow of the device (oxygen hood or mechanical ventilator). The resulting mixture is analyzed for O_2 and CO_2. Hypoxic gas and hypercarbic gas can be combined for increased effect.

ANESTHETIC MIXTURES

Patients in status asthmaticus (SA) can be placed on helium-oxygen therapy as a temporizing measure to reduce work of breathing until other therapy (β-agonists, methylxanthines, corticosteroids) is effective. However, these patients frequently have bronchospasm that is refractory to conventional therapy. Certain volatile inhaled anesthetics are known for their bronchodilatory properties. Although no clinical trials have investigated the use of inhaled anesthetics (IAs) in the treatment of SA, several case reports exist.[27-31]

Of the several IAs used clinically for anesthesia, only a few have been widely reported as potential treatment for SA: halothane, isoflurane, enflurane, and sevoflurane. *Halothane* is an alkane derivative and has been the volatile anesthetic of choice in reducing bronchospasm in asthmatic patients. *Sevoflurane,* a methyl ethyl ether, has been shown to be as effective as halothane in reducing lung resistance; however, safety studies for its use in asthmatic children are needed.[28,32] *Isoflurane* and *enflurane* are also methyl ethyl ethers and are often used in the acute treatment of SA. As with halothane, each has advantages and disadvantages in treating bronchospasm (Table 23-1).

PHYSIOLOGIC BASIS OF ACTION

Volatile IAs reduce bronchospasm through a number of pathways: β-adrenergic receptor stimulation, direct smooth muscle relaxation, antagonism of acetylcholine and histamine, and inhibition of hypocapneic bronchoconstriction.[33] Therefore a patient receiving standard bronchodilators may see an additional response with the addition of an IA.[34]

TABLE 23-1	COMPARISON OF INHALED ANESTHETIC AGENTS		
	Halothane	**Isoflurane**	**Enflurane**
Mean arterial pressure	↓	↓↓↓	↓↓
Pulmonary vascular resistance	—	↓↓	↓
Heart rate	↓	↑	↑↑
Cardiac output	↓↓	—	↓↓↓
Airway irritant	—	↑↑	↑↑
Respiratory depression	↑	↑	↑↑
Myocardial sensitization to catecholamines	↑↑↑↑	—	—
Explosive risk	—	—	—

APPLICATION

The setup and delivery of IAs must be performed by qualified individuals, usually anesthesiologists. Most states expressly prohibit respiratory care practitioners from delivering anesthetic agents. In general, the anesthesiologist performs the initial setup and troubleshooting. Adjustments are usually done by the intensive care physician or anesthesiologist. The bedside caregiver handles routine monitoring procedures. All caregivers must understand the pharmacology of the IA being delivered and its side effect profile.

The two ways to deliver IAs are by face mask for the spontaneously breathing patient and through a mechanical ventilator. In either system the setup is similar to that used in the operating room. Both methods require similar equipment: vaporizers for the volatile anesthetic, scavenging devices, anesthetic gas analyzers, and vital signs monitoring.

Inhaled Anesthetics Via Face Mask. To avoid intubation and mechanical ventilation, treating the spontaneously breathing patient with an IA could be advantageous. The systems used for spontaneous breathing are very similar to continuous positive airway pressure (CPAP) circuits. The expiratory gases pass through a CO_2 absorber, then go into the inspiratory limb, creating a circle. A fresh gas supply (including the IA) is introduced after the CO_2 absorber. This design is called a *rebreathing circuit.*

The face mask must be tight fitting to prevent the leakage of the IA into the room and to ensure that the patient receives the IA. Because patients may be somewhat awake, they must be cooperative enough not to remove the mask. The IA must also be compatible with face mask administration. Enflurane and isoflurane are irritants to the upper airway and are unpleasant to breathe while conscious, especially for the pediatric patient. These vapors may produce laryngospasm and fighting. Isoflurane and enflurane are more suited for use with an intubated and mechanically ventilated patient. Conversely, halothane and sevoflurane are neutral-smelling vapors and may be taken more readily via mask.

Typically, halothane is the IA of choice when delivering to a conscious, spontaneously breathing patient. The dose range for halothane is approximately 0.25% to 0.5%. The patient usually is sufficiently awake to communicate in short sentences. Bronchodilation is usually rapid (15 to 20 minutes). The patient benefits by the reduced resistance as well as the sedative effect.

Inhaled Anesthetics Via Mechanical Ventilation. Almost universally, the Siemens Servo 900C is used to deliver IAs to mechanically ventilated patients. Although not the most modern pediatric ventilators, the 900C is designed for inhalation anesthesia. With a moderately priced conversion kit the 900C can easily be converted to a device with anesthesia capability. The ventilator itself is set up as normal. The outlet of the anesthesia vaporizer is connected to the low-pressure inlet of the 900C. Exhaled and waste gases are collected in a 2-L to 3-L anesthesia bag device connected to the hospital vacuum system. The bag fills, the suction system is activated, and the bag contents are emptied.

REFERENCES

1. Material safety data sheet: Nitric oxide in nitrogen. Murray Hill, NJ, Airco, 1993.
2. Braker W, Mossman A: *Matheson gas data book,* ed 6. Lundhurst, Matheson, 1980; p 514.
3. Hurford WE: The biological basis of inhaled nitric oxide. *Respir Care Clin North Am* 1997; 3:357-369.
4. Dagby RM, Corey-Kreyling MD: Structural aspects of the contractile machinery of smooth muscle. "Is the organization of contractile elements compatible with a sliding filament mechanism?" In Stephens NL, editor: *Smooth muscle contraction.* New York, Dekker, 1984; pp 47-74.
5. Furchgott RF, Zawadzki JV: The obligatory role of endothelial cells in the relaxation of arterial smooth muscle by acetylcholine. *Nature* 1980; 288:373-376.
6. Miller CC, Miller J: Pulmonary vascular smooth muscle regulation: the role of inhaled nitric oxide gas. *Respir Care* 1992; 37:1175-1185.
7. Aranda A, Pearl RG: The biology of nitric oxide. *Respir Care* 1999; 44:156-166.
8. Bigatello LM, Hurford WE, Hess D: Use of inhaled nitric oxide for ARDS. *Respir Care Clin North Am* 1997; 3: 437-458.
9. Jacob TD et al: Hemodynamic effects and metabolic fate of inhaled nitric oxide in hypoxic piglets. *J Appl Physiol* 1994; 76:1794.
10. Hess D, Ritz R, Branson RD: Delivery systems for inhaled nitric oxide. *Respir Care Clin North Am* 1997; 3:371-410.
11. Branson RD et al: Inhaled nitric oxide systems and monitoring. *Respir Care* 1999; 44:281-306.
12. Curry S: Methemoglobinemia. *Ann Emerg Med* 11:214, 1982.
13. Papamoschou D: Theoretical validation of the respiratory benefits of helium-oxygen mixtures. *Respir Physiol* 1995; 99:183-190.
14. Barach AL: Use of helium as a new therapeutic gas. *Proc Soc Exp Biol Med* 1934; 32:462-464.
15. Barach AL: The therapeutic use of helium. *JAMA* 1936; 107:1273-1275.
16. Barach AL: The use of helium in the treatment of asthma and obstructive lesions of the larynx and trachea. *Ann Intern Med* 1935; 9:739-765.
17. Barach AL: The use of helium as a new therapeutic gas. *Anesth Analg* 1935; 14:210-215.
18. Nunn JF: Diffusion and alveolar/capillary permeability. In *Applied respiratory physiology.* London, Butterworth, 1987; pp 184-206.
19. Anderson M et al: Deposition in asthmatics of particles inhaled in air or helium-oxygen. *Am Rev Respir Dis* 1993; 147:524-528.

20. Svartengren M et al: Human lung deposition of particles suspended in air or in helium/oxygen mixture. *Exp Lung Res* 1989; 15:575-585.
21. Melmed A et al: The use of heliox as a vehicle for beta-agonist nebulization in patients with severe asthma. *Am J Respir Crit Care Med* 1995 (abstract); 151:A269.
22. Stillwell PC et al: Effectiveness of open-circuit oxyhood delivery of helium-oxygen. *Chest* 1989; 95:1222-1224.
23. Rogers MS et al: Volume accuracy of the Siemens Servo 900C and Novametrix Ventrak when delivering helium oxygen mixtures. *Respir Care* 1995 (abstract); 40:1206.
24. El-Lessy HN: Pulmonary vascular control in hypoplastic left-heart syndrome: hypoxic- and hypercarbic-gas therapy. *Respir Care* 1995; 40:737-742.
25. Jobes DR et al: Carbon dioxide prevents pulmonary over-circulation in hypoplastic left heart syndrome. *Ann Thorac Surg* 1992; 54:150-151.
26. Mayer JE: Initial management of the single ventricle patient. *Semin Thorac Cardiovasc Surg* 1994; 6:2-7.
27. Bishop MJ, Rooke GA: Sevoflurane for patients with asthma. *Anesth Analg* 2000 (letter); 91:245-246.
28. Habre W et al: Respiratory mechanics during sevoflurane anesthesia in children with and without asthma. *Anesth Analg* 1999; 89:1177-1181.
29. Padkin AJ, Baigel G, Morgan GA: Halothane treatment of severe asthma to avoid mechanical ventilation. *Anesthesia* 1997; 52:994-997.
30. Miyagi T et al: Prolonged isoflurane anesthesia in a case of catastrophic asthma. *Acta Paediatr Jpn* 1997; 39: 375-378.
31. Rooke GA, Choi JH, Bishop MJ: The effect of isoflurane, halothane, sevoflurane, and thiopental/nitrous oxide on respiratory system resistance after trachea intubation. *Anesthesiology* 1997; 86:1294-1299.
32. Habre W, Wildhaber JH, Sly PD: Prevention of methacholine induced changes in respiratory mechanics in piglets with sevoflurane and halothane. *Anesthesiology* 1997; 87: 585-590.
33. Hirschman CA et al: Mechanism of action of inhalational anesthesia on airways. *Anesthesiology* 1982; 56:107-111.
34. Johnson RG et al: Isoflurane therapy for status asthmaticus in children and adults. *Chest* 1990; 97:698-701.

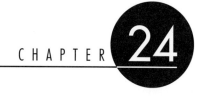

CHAPTER 24

Extracorporeal Life Support

Douglas R. Hansell

*E*xtracorporeal circulation is the technique of supporting the function of the heart or lungs, or both, with external artificial organs. This support was originally developed for use in the operating room during cardiac surgery and was limited to several hours' duration. In recent years, extracorporeal support has been applied in the intensive care unit in critically ill patients with pulmonary problems for days and even weeks. In this setting, extracorporeal circulation enables the practitioner to minimize the ventilator's support, thereby avoiding iatrogenic damage to the lungs and the problems associated with high mean airway pressures while allowing the disease process to run its natural course. This form of support is known as *extracorporeal membrane oxygenation* (ECMO), or *extracorporeal life support* (ECLS).

HISTORY

Hooke, writing of allowing "blood to circulate through a vessel, so as it may be openly exposed to air," recorded one of the earliest references to extracorporeal oxygenation in 1667.[1] His speculation, well ahead of its time, had no impact on medicine. In reality, the technique of ECLS evolved directly from the cardiopulmonary bypass procedure developed for cardiac surgery. Gibbon, the inventor of the mechanical oxygenator, is considered the "father" of extracorporeal circulation.[2] In 1937, he reported the use of cardiopulmonary bypass during pulmonary artery occlusion in animals.[3] It was not until 1953, however, that Gibbon first successfully performed extracorporeal circulation in a human. His invention substituted a roller pump for the heart. To achieve gas exchange, blood was distributed in a film along stainless steel screens vertically suspended in a plastic chamber. The thinness of the advancing blood film allowed uptake of oxygen and release of carbon dioxide by diffusion.

During the 1950s, studies in extracorporeal gas exchange involving cross-circulation in animals were performed using biologic lungs for gas exchange.

Lillehei and associates were the first to perform cross-circulation in humans. In 1955, they reported a series of eight pediatric patients in whom cardiac surgery was performed using the parent as the oxygenator.[4] All patients and donors survived, and no long-lasting donor morbidity was noted. Subsequently, a bubble oxygenator was designed and successfully used in seven patients.[5] With bubble oxygenators, however, the duration of bypass was limited to a few hours because the direct blood-gas interface resulted in hemolysis, denatured plasma proteins, and thrombus formation. Investigation continued for an extracorporeal circuit that was more biocompatible and capable of extended use.

The observation that blue venous blood entering a hemodialysis membrane turned red when the blood exited the membrane spurred interest in developing a membrane oxygenator.[6] In 1956, Clowes[7] reported the first clinical use of a membrane for gas exchange. The membrane oxygenator was constructed of polyethylene and Teflon and for the first time eliminated the direct blood-gas interface. Because gas exchange was inefficient, however, the membrane had to be very large, thus limiting its clinical application. Subsequently, silicone rubber was found to have gas transfer characteristics far superior to polyethylene, and in 1963 a silicone membrane similar to the one used today was developed.[8] With this device the first extended bypass procedure was performed in animals, which demonstrated minimal hematologic effect for up to 1 week.[9] This development paved the way for the successful application of long-term extracorporeal support.

In 1969, Dorsen et al[10] attempted to perfuse a 1.16-kg premature neonate with respiratory distress syndrome. The infant was supported with ECMO for 21 hours before death from intraventricular hemorrhage (IVH). Subsequently, 10 days of extracorporeal support in a 28-week premature neonate was reported.[11] Although this infant also died from IVH, the findings demonstrated that prolonged extracorporeal support was possible. The first successful use of ECMO was reported in 1972 in a 24-year-old man with multiple trauma and respiratory failure.[12] He was maintained on extracorporeal support for 75 hours, during which time his lung injury resolved.

Other trials in adults followed, with anecdotal reports of success. This prompted the National Institutes of Health (NIH) to sponsor a multicenter, randomized prospective study of ECMO in adults with acute respiratory failure, and a collaborative study was published in 1979.[13] Nine institutions randomized 90 adults with adult respiratory distress syndrome (ARDS) to either conventional mechanical ventilation (CMV) or ECMO. The results were dismal, with only eight survivors, four in the CMV group and four in the ECMO group. The authors were forced to conclude that although ECMO could support gas exchange, it could not improve survival in ARDS patients. Critics of the study have suggested that the results may be misleading.[14] Some of the centers involved had no experience with ECMO before the study. Additionally, because of the stringent entry criteria, a significant proportion of the patient population had irreversible lung injury that was subsequently noted at autopsy. Perhaps most important, although the purpose of ECMO was to allow resting of the lungs, most patients were still subjected to high ventilator settings and fractional concentration of inspired oxygen (FIO_2) while receiving ECMO. Bleeding complications were also significant, with an average blood loss of 2 L/day. Regardless of the shortcomings of the study, adult ECMO in the United States was virtually abandoned.

Despite these disappointing results, the search continued to identify a population with reversible lung disease that could potentially benefit from ECMO. In 1975, Bartlett and Harken[15] at the University of California–Irvine pioneered neonatal ECMO, developed the standard circuit, and successfully used ECMO in a neonate with meconium aspiration syndrome (MAS). Their success continued, and in 1982, Bartlett et al[16] reported 55% survival in a series of 45 neonates treated with ECMO. By the mid-1980s, two prospective randomized trials comparing ECMO to CMV were published. Bartlett's study reported a 100% survival of the 11 patients receiving ECMO and 0% survival in the control group.[17] This study was met with skepticism because only one patient constituted the control group. O'Rourke et al[18] subsequently reported 100% survival for nine ECMO patients compared with 33% for six CMV-treated newborns, but they too encountered criticism for the study design.

Meanwhile in Europe, interest in adult ECLS continued, and with the addition of several innovations, results improved. Gattinoni et al[19] believed that high airway pressures could cause progressive lung injury and that extracorporeal support could be employed to eliminate the need for high-pressure ventilator support. With an emphasis on carbon dioxide removal using a large membrane surface area and a venovenous route, they treated 43 adults selected by the same selection criteria used in the NIH adult ECMO study. They referred to this technique as "extracorporeal carbon dioxide removal" ($ECCO_2R$) and in 1986 reported an astounding 49% survival in adults.

Since Bartlett's first reported success with ECMO in neonates, the number of ECLS centers has continued to grow, with 114 active ECLS centers reported in 2002. In 1989 the ECLS centers formed a national organization known as the Extracorporeal Life Support Organization (ELSO). ELSO's purpose is to coordinate clinical research on extracorporeal support, develop ECLS guidelines, and maintain the ECMO National Registry data. This registry is a data bank of all reported ECLS cases from the active ELSO centers and contains information on more than 24,300 neonatal, pediatric, and adult cases to date.[20]

NEONATAL TREATMENT

The majority of the reported ECLS cases (76%) are neonates. In the 1990s, ECLS in this population became a standard mode of therapy for acute respiratory failure unresponsive to maximal medical therapy. This acceptance occurred despite the lack of a randomized controlled clinical trial proving the efficacy of ECMO in the treatment of ARDS. Finally, in 1996 the United Kingdom Collaborative ECMO Trial Group reported the results of a trial to assess whether a policy of referral for ECMO has a beneficial effect on survival to 1 year without severe disability in comparison with conventional management. Recruitment to the trial was stopped early (November 1995) because the data accumulated showed a clear advantage with ECMO. Of 185 infants in two groups, 81 (44%) died prior to leaving the hospital, and two died after discharge. Death rates differed between the two groups; 30 of 93 infants in the ECMO group died compared to 54 of 92 in the conventional care group. The results, reported in 1996, leave little doubt that ECMO is an effective lifesaving treatment for neonates with severe respiratory failure.[21]

PERSISTENT PULMONARY HYPERTENSION OF NEWBORN

Persistent pulmonary hypertension of the newborn (PPHN), the abnormal continuance of fetal circulation after birth, continues to be the major pathophysiologic condition treated with ECLS.[22]

There are two distinctive intracardiac structures in the fetus. The *ductus arteriosus* is a large vessel between the pulmonary artery and the aorta. The *foramen ovale* is a hole with a tissue flap, situated in the atrial septum. In utero, pulmonary vascular resistance (PVR) is greater than systemic vascular resistance (SVR), resulting in higher pressures in the right atrium than in the left atrium. Consequently, blood is diverted through the foramen ovale to the left atrium and through the ductus arteriosus to the aorta, thereby bypassing the pulmonary circulation. With the first breath, PVR is immediately reduced because of the effects of mechanical lung expansion and the increase in oxygenation. This reduction leads to an increase in pulmonary blood flow and a reversal in atrial pressures, resulting in a functional closure of the foramen ovale. Concurrently, an increased oxygen partial pressure (Po_2) causes constriction and functional closure of the ductus arteriosus, completing the transition to the postnatal circulatory pattern. A hypoxic state after birth can increase PVR, which in turn promotes the reinstitution of right-to-left shunting at both the atrial and the ductal levels, sustaining or reestablishing the fetal circulation.

PPHN can result from any underlying neonatal condition leading to hypoxia.[23] Most often it is associated with MAS, perinatal asphyxia, congenital diaphragmatic hernia (CDH), sepsis, and respiratory distress syndrome. The presentation and clinical course depend on the primary disease.[24] Immediate presentation of PPHN is the norm in perinatal asphyxia and CDH. Presentation at 4 to 12 hours of age is seen in the infant with MAS. Late presentation may be seen at 24 hours or more in the septic population. The majority of these neonates can be managed with pharmacologic and ventilatory support.[25,26] A small percentage are unresponsive to conventional therapy, however, and prior to ECLS, they would have died. Institution of ECLS interrupts the cycle of pulmonary hypertension, minimizes the need for escalating mechanical ventilation, and avoids barotrauma while the underlying condition resolves. Table 24-1 summarizes the survival of neonates treated with ECMO.[20]

MECONIUM ASPIRATION SYNDROME

The introduction of ECLS in neonates with MAS has resulted in the highest survival rate of all the

TABLE 24-1	NEONATAL EXTRACORPOREAL MEMBRANE OXYGENATION CASES BY DIAGNOSIS		
		Survivors	
Diagnosis	**Total**	**Number**	**Percent**
Meconium aspiration syndrome	5976	5612	94
Congenital diaphragmatic hernia	3816	2063	54
Sepsis/pneumonia	2475	1828	74
Persistent pulmonary hypertension of newborn	2471	1943	79
Respiratory distress syndrome	1333	1120	84
Air leak syndrome	87	60	69
Other	985	652	66

Data from ELSO National Registry Report. Ann Arbor. University of Michigan, 2002.

neonatal diseases commonly treated. Meconium is a sterile, dark-green substance that is normally present in the fetal colon. Meconium staining of amniotic fluid is common in 10% of all deliveries but is rare in neonates less than 37 weeks' gestation.[27] Premature passage of the meconium into the amniotic fluid may occur under several conditions, most notably fetal hypoxia.[27] Therefore the presence of meconium-stained fluid may indicate fetal distress.

The diagnosis of MAS is made if the infant has a history of meconium-stained fluid, the presence of meconium in the trachea at birth, and a variable radiographic pattern of patchy infiltrates with hyperinflation to consolidation.[28] The neonate's degree of respiratory distress may be mild to severe. The resulting hypoxia and acidosis can increase PVR, leading to right-to-left shunting and further hypoxia.

SEPSIS

The most common organism to cause sepsis in the neonate is *group B streptococcus*. The organism is found primarily in the intestinal tract, with colonization occurring in the mother's vagina.[29] Although sepsis is more often associated with early rupture of membranes, the fetus can still become infected with the membranes intact. This bacterial infection can be serious in the immediate newborn period, with mortality approaching 45%.[30] It can present as either pneumonia or overwhelming vascular collapse, referred to as *septic shock*. Other organisms such as *Escherichia coli* and *Listeria* can follow the same clinical course as group B streptococcus. The overall survival in this group is lower than in the group with MAS because cardiovascular instability and difficulties in coagulation management lead to a more complicated and prolonged course of ECLS.

CONGENITAL DIAPHRAGMATIC HERNIA

CDH occurs in approximately 1 in 2200 births.[31] It is characterized by the incomplete formation of the fetal diaphragm and usually occurs on the left side. The most common herniation is the posterolateral type known as *Bochdalek's hernia*. This defect allows herniation of the abdominal contents into the thoracic cavity, affecting fetal lung development. It compresses the lung on the affected side but also shifts the mediastinum to the opposite side and compresses the contralateral lung, resulting in varying degrees of bilateral pulmonary hypoplasia. Infants who are symptomatic within the first 6 hours of life have the highest mortality.[32] The distressed newborn has a scaphoid abdomen and diminished or no breath sounds on one side and has a chest radiograph that demonstrates gastrointestinal structures in the thorax.

CDH continues to have the lowest cure rate of all common neonatal diseases treated with ECLS. Before ECLS, identifying the infant who had such severe pulmonary hypoplasia as to be incompatible with survival had long been an elusive goal.[33] Since the introduction of ECLS, many predictors of mortality have been proposed; however, because of differences in clinical management, none has been reproducible from institution to institution.[34] Kays et al[35] found that infants who are maintained with "gentle ventilation" methods, including permissive hypercapnea, moderate hypoxemia, minimal use of sedatives, and minimal stimulation, are less likely to require ECMO and have significantly improved survival.

PATIENT SELECTION CRITERIA

The success of neonatal ECLS depends on the disease process. Most neonatal respiratory failure results in PPHN, which is completely reversible. However, the escalating ventilator pressures and FIO_2 used to treat PPHN can lead to secondary lung injury. Knowing the correct time to cease exposing the neonate's lungs to these iatrogenic complications becomes a concern for ensuring long-term survival and limiting morbidity.

In the early years of neonatal ECLS, deciding when to employ ECLS was purely subjective. Subsequently, several methods have been proposed to standardize ECLS criteria. Bartlett et al[36] developed the "neonatal pulmonary insufficiency index," which plotted pH and FIO_2 over time to a point where the risk of mortality exceeded 80%. However, the index became unsuitable for patients who had induced iatrogenic alkalosis as a treatment for PPHN.

Krummel et al[37] reported that an alveolar-arterial oxygen gradient ($PAO_2 - PaO_2$; also A-aDO_2) of greater than 620 mm Hg for 6 to 12 hours was indicative of an 80% mortality. However, this criterion was not useful in the neonate who failed rapidly. Ortega et al[38] proposed the *oxygenation index* (OI), a calculation based on mean airway pressure ($\overline{Paw}$), FIO_2, and arterial oxygenation (PaO_2), as follows:

$$OI = \overline{Paw} \times \frac{FIO_2}{PaO_2} \times 100$$

The authors found that when the OI exceeded 40, mortality exceeded 80%. Their results have been reproduced by other institutions, and OI is currently the most widely accepted predictor of mortality in neonates with respiratory failure on conventional ventilators. As experience with neonatal resuscitation improves, however, and as more institutions employ high-frequency ventilation as rescue therapy before ECLS, the value of OI and other guidelines will require constant reassessment.

In addition to statistical indicators for employing ECLS, other criteria need to be considered in the

---

BOX 24-1

NEONATAL EXTRACORPOREAL LIFE SUPPORT SELECTION CRITERIA

Oxygen index >40
No major cardiac defect
Reversible lung disease
Gestational age >33 weeks
Mechanical ventilation <14 days
No major intraventricular hemorrhage
No significant coagulopathy or bleeding
    complications (relative contraindication)

TABLE 24-2	**PEDIATRIC EXTRACORPOREAL MEMBRANE OXYGENATION CASES BY DIAGNOSIS**		
		Survivors	
Diagnosis	**Total**	**Number**	**Percent**
Viral pneumonia	622	381	61
Acute respiratory distress syndrome	288	155	54
Aspiration	160	103	64
Bacterial pneumonia	228	118	52
ARF, non-ARDS	563	268	48
Pneumocystis carinii infection	17	7	41
Other	374	193	52

Data from ELSO National Registry Report. Ann Arbor. University of Michigan, 2002.

candidate for ECLS. In early ECLS studies, IVH was a common complication among infants less than 35 weeks' gestation. They recommended that neonates younger than 35 weeks' gestation and those with preexisting IVH should be excluded from ECLS until anticoagulation management techniques used during ECLS are improved. Currently, several centers are reporting reduced extension of grade 1, 2, or 3 IVH with the use of antifibrinolytic therapy.[39] However, all candidates should have an ultrasound before initiation of ECLS. A "subependymal" or grade I bleed is currently considered only a relative contraindication. Because bleeding is the major complication of ECLS, active bleeding or uncorrectable coagulopathies are also considered relative contraindications.

Ultimately, the patient's pulmonary disease should be reversible; therefore prior mechanical ventilation for more than 14 days is considered a contraindication for ECLS because of the potential iatrogenic lung injury. Preexisting major cardiac defects should be ruled out before consideration of ECLS by performing an echocardiogram. If a major defect is detected, surgical intervention should be the first option. If lung disease prevents surgical correction, stabilization on ECLS before surgery for pulmonary resolvement is a valuable consideration. Other congenital and medical conditions associated with poor prognosis may be contraindications for ECLS. Box 24-1 summarizes current patient selection criteria.

PEDIATRIC TREATMENT

Beyond infancy, there is no pulmonary condition as completely reversible as PPHN. In older children, most conditions leading to respiratory failure involve pulmonary parenchymal injury, including posttraumatic respiratory failure, viral or bacterial pneumonia, and blood, gastric acid, and foreign substance aspiration. These conditions all present a picture more closely related to ARDS than to PPHN. In the mid-1970s, mortality from ARDS in children was 80%.[40] It continued to remain equally high in the late 1980s despite changes in ventilator strategies.[41]

Although interest in ECLS for the older patient population was virtually abandoned after the NIH study in the 1970s, the successful European ECLS experience in older patients, along with refinements in technology and coagulation control, has revitalized interest in using this technique in the pediatric population. Several small studies reported survival of nearly 50% with long ECLS runs and many complications.[42-44] Of particular note, one child cannulated via the right common carotid artery experienced left hemiparesis and seizures, suggesting an increased risk when using the carotid artery for cannulation in older patients.[44]

O'Rourke et al[45] reviewed the pediatric ECMO Registry of ELSO, which contained 285 cases in which ECLS was used for pediatric respiratory failure. Although 56 centers contributed at least one case, 50% of all the cases were contributed by only 7 centers, indicating that most neonatal centers had limited experience with pediatric ECLS. Despite concerns about carotid artery ligation in the older child, venoarterial ECLS via the right internal jugular vein and the right common carotid artery was employed in most cases. Traditional predictors of severity, such as those for neonatal ECLS, were not routinely used. The principal indication for ECLS in pediatric patients was based on the probability that the patient's condition was potentially reversible and that death was otherwise certain. Table 24-2 lists the principal diagnoses for which ECLS was employed, along with survival.

O'Rourke et al's report further noted that survivors were younger and had higher arterial pH values and lower peak and mean airway pressures

UNIVERSITY OF MICHIGAN PEDIATRIC AND ADULT EXTRACORPOREAL MEMBRANE OXYGENATION CRITERIA

INDICATIONS

Poor gas exchange despite "optimal" ventilator and pharmacologic therapy

Age <60 years

Ventilator support <6 days

Neurologic status responsive

Oxygenation decreased: shunt >30%

$Pao_2/Fio_2 \leq 100$

and/or

Carbon dioxide clearance decreased:
$Paco_2$ >45 mm Hg despite minute ventilation >0.2 L/kg

CONTRAINDICATIONS

RELATIVE

Ventilator support >6-10 days

Immunosuppression

Systemic sepsis

Active bleeding

ABSOLUTE

Septic shock

Cardiac arrest

Brain injury

Terminal disease

Metabolic acidosis (base deficit >5 mEq/L or 12 hours)

From Bartlett RH: *Extracorporeal life support manual for adult and pediatric patients.* Ann Arbor. University of Michigan Medical Center, 1993.

Pao_2, Arterial oxygen tension; *Fio_2,* fractional inspired oxygen concentration; *Paco_2,* arterial carbon dioxide tension.

before ECLS than did the nonsurvivors. The duration of pre-ECLS ventilatory support (0 to 129 days) and the mean duration of ECLS (10 days) were not significantly different between the neonatal and pediatric patients, although a higher incidence of complications was reported in the pediatric group. This may have been due to either longer ECLS runs that stressed the limits of the technology or the severity of illness in these patients. Finally, it was noted that death in this series occurred secondary to either progressive pulmonary failure or multisystem organ failure. The investigators suggested that selection criteria include reversibility indicators of both pulmonary and other organ dysfunction.[45] This recommendation was supported by Weber et al, who reported their ECLS experience in 32 pediatric patients. Overall survival was 41%, but 75% of the patients with isolated pulmonary disease survived, in contrast to only 8% of those with failure of even one other organ system.[46]

More recently, Swaniker et al[47] from the University of Michigan evaluated data from 128 pediatric patients with acute respiratory failure and found that overall survival to discharge was 71%.

Although it is impossible to provide specific recommendations for the institution of ECLS in postneonatal patients, some guidelines have been suggested. The University of Michigan has recently proposed a set of guidelines for patient selection (Box 24-2). Until a prospective randomized trial of ECLS in pediatric pulmonary failure can be undertaken, these guidelines are a reasonable attempt to bring some standardization to this area.[48]

EXTRACORPOREAL PHYSIOLOGY

VENOARTERIAL SYSTEM

Oxygen delivery in ECLS is provided by a combination of blood flow from the ECLS circuit and blood flow from the patient's own cardiopulmonary system.[48] The delivery of oxygen is a function of both the oxygen content of the blood and the cardiac output. Both variables (oxygenation and cardiac function) can be controlled by the venoarterial ECLS route. In this format a venous cannula, inserted via the right internal jugular vein, drains blood from the right atrium. An arterial cannula, inserted into the right common carotid artery, reinfuses the oxygenated blood into the aortic arch (Fig. 24-1).

By increasing the flow rate, blood is preferentially diverted into the circuit. At maximum performance, approximately 80% of the cardiac output can be replaced by the circuit, which is often reflected by a dampened pulse pressure. The oxygenated blood returning from the ECLS circuit combines in the aortic arch with the desaturated blood from the patient's native circulation. The oxygen content of the patient's blood therefore depends on the relative contributions of each system. For example, as more blood is diverted into the ECLS circuit, less blood is contributed by the native lungs, and Pao_2 increases. Because of this parallel circulation, an increase in systemic Pao_2 during ECLS may reflect either improving lung function (increased Pao_2 in the native circulation) or decreasing native cardiac output (less flow from the patient's circulation). Changes in tissue oxygen consumption and hemoglobin concentration will also alter oxygen content.

In ECLS the arterial carbon dioxide partial pressure ($Paco_2$) also reflects the combination of the perfusate blood mixing with the native cardiac output. Once adjusted, however, the $Paco_2$ remains relatively stable on ECLS, responding only slightly to large changes in pulmonary blood flow and carbon dioxide production.

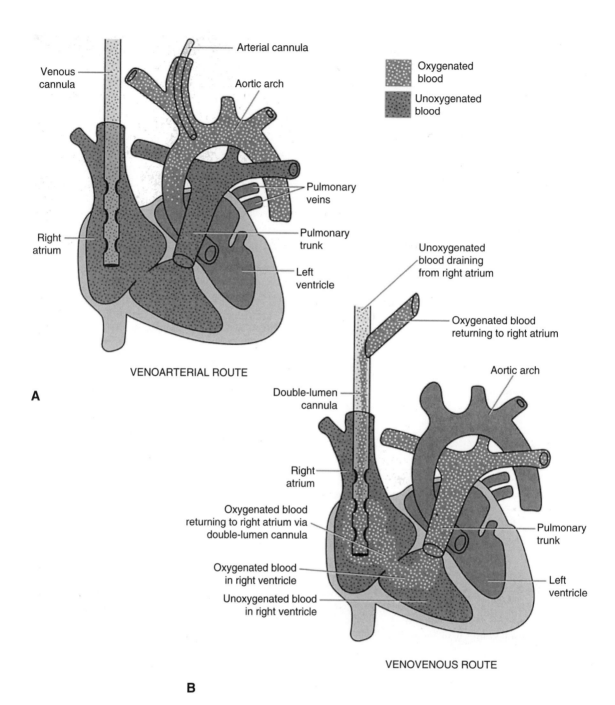

Fig. 24-1

Mechanisms of blood flow during extracorporeal membrane oxygenation (ECMO). **A,** In the veno-arterial route, blood is removed from the right atrium via a cannula inserted in the right internal jugu-lar vein. Oxygenated blood is returned to the aortic arch via a cannula in the right common carotid artery. The shaded area indicates unoxygenated blood. **B,** In the venovenous route, blood is also removed from the right atrium via a cannula inserted in the right internal jugular vein, but the oxy-genated blood is returned to the venous circulation. The shaded area indicates unoxygenated blood. Blood in the pulmonary trunk has been oxygenated via the cardiopulmonary bypass machine.

Although different vessels have been cannulated for venoarterial ECLS, the right internal jugular vein and right common carotid artery are the preferred vessels, especially in the neonate, in whom they are disproportionately large. This cannula orientation provides both pulmonary and cardiac support, a major advantage of this route.

The major disadvantage of the venoarterial approach is the need to ligate the right common carotid artery. In adults, acute disruption of the carotid artery results in strokes. In neonates, however, the risks remain unknown, although some suggest an increase in right-sided brain lesions.[49] Some patients have had the carotid artery reconstructed after ECLS, but the efficacy of this procedure is also unknown.[50]

Additional disadvantages, however, can also arise from the *efficiency* of venoarterial ECLS at diverting native flow. The ECLS circuit is nonpulsatile. Diverting blood away from the native cardiopulmonary system results in less pulsatile flow to the organs and disruption of the normal blood flow pattern.[51] The combination of the orientation of the reinfusion cannula (distant aortic arch) and poorly oxygenated blood leaving the left ventricle may potentiate lower oxygen delivery to the coronary arteries.[52] Another potential disadvantage to venoarterial support is that any particle or bubble in the circuit may be directly infused into the arterial circulation, leading to emboli formation.

VENOVENOUS SYSTEM

In venovenous support, blood is both drained and reinfused back into the venous circulation at the same rate, thereby providing only pulmonary support. The oxygenated perfusate mixes with the venous blood in the right atrium, raising the oxygen content and lowering the carbon dioxide content. Because both the drainage and the reinfusion cannulas are in the venous system, some of the perfusate blood returns to the circuit. This phenomenon, known as *recirculation,* decreases the efficiency of gas transfer between circuit and patient. Currently, the degree of recirculation is monitored by comparing the oxygen saturation of the venous drainage ($S\bar{v}O_2$) with the patient's arterial oxygen saturation (SaO_2).[53] If $S\bar{v}O_2$ is greater than SaO_2, the recirculation is excessive, and either blood flow rate or cannula placement requires adjustment.

Because venovenous ECLS is less efficient than venoarterial ECLS, the maximum SaO_2 achievable can be as low as 80% to 85%. As lung function improves, SaO_2 increases. Because venovenous ECLS is essentially operating in series with the native circulation, alterations in cardiac output will not have a significant effect on oxygenation. The volume of blood removed is equal to the volume reinfused, so there is also no effect on the patient's hemodynamics.

The advantages of venovenous support are that the carotid artery is spared, full pulsatile flow is maintained, and potential emboli from the circuit are trapped in the pulmonary vascular bed.[48] The major disadvantage is lack of cardiovascular support. The presence of mild to moderate myocardial dysfunction, however, should not discourage one from using the venovenous approach. The improved oxygenation and lower airway pressures achieved with implementation of ECLS often improve cardiac output substantially. If myocardial dysfunction worsens during ECLS, however, or if oxygen delivery is insufficient, the conversion to venoarterial support should be instituted by inserting an arterial cannula. Box 24-3 summarizes additional

---

BOX 24-3

ADVANTAGES AND DISADVANTAGES OF VENOVENOUS AND VENOARTERIAL EXTRACORPOREAL LIFE SUPPORT

VENOVENOUS EXTRACORPOREAL LIFE SUPPORT

ADVANTAGES
- Sparing of carotid artery
- Preservation of pulsatile flow
- Normal pulmonary blood flow
- Perfusion of lungs with oxygenated blood
- Perfusion of coronaries with oxygenated blood
- Avoidance of infusion of possible emboli directly into arterial circulation
- Central venous pressure accurate
- Selective limb perfusion does not occur

DISADVANTAGES
- No cardiac support
- Lower systemic PaO_2
- Recirculation issues

VENOARTERIAL EXTRACORPOREAL LIFE SUPPORT

ADVANTAGES
- Provides cardiac support
- Excellent gas exchange
- Rapid stabilization

DISADVANTAGES
- Carotid artery ligation
- Nonpulsatile flow
- Reduced pulmonary blood flow
- Lower myocardial oxygen delivery
- Direct infusion of possible emboli into arterial circulation
- Central venous pressure inaccurate

advantages and disadvantages of venoarterial and venovenous ECLS.

Venovenous ECLS can be performed using three different techniques: (1) the two-cannula system, (2) the tidal flow system, and (3) the double-lumen cannula.

Two-cannula System. The two-cannula system was the first design to be used. The circuit is identical to the one used for venoarterial support. Blood is drained from the right atrium and is reinfused into the femoral vein. Klein et al[54] compared their neonatal experience with this method and venoarterial support between 1981 and 1984. Venovenous support required a longer cannulation time and higher bypass flow rates to achieve a lower PaO_2. Complications included leg edema, frequent wound infections, and alterations in leg growth. Concerns about these issues have tempered enthusiasm for this route in the newborn. The two-cannula method is now most frequently used in pediatric and adult populations because no suitable equipment exists to provide other methods of venovenous support in these patients.

Tidal Flow System. The single-lumen tidal flow system, developed by Kolobow et al,[55] is a method currently available only in France. A single cannula is placed in the right internal jugular vein. Inflow and outflow are controlled by time-cycled valves that allow alternating drainage and infusion within the same cannula. The time-cycled valves have helped to minimize potential recirculation.[56] Despite reports of success, the introduction of the tidal flow system in the United States has been delayed by lack of Food and Drug Administration (FDA) approval.[57]

Double-lumen Cannula. The newest and most popular approach in the neonate is the double-lumen cannula. A single cannula is inserted into the right internal jugular vein, and blood is simultaneously drained and reinfused through the two lumens.[58] The larger lumen is used for drainage, and the smaller lumen is the reinfusion port. Although recirculation is also a problem with this method, it can be minimized by proper positioning of the cannula to direct the perfusate blood through the tricuspid valve into the right ventricle (see Fig. 24-1). Currently, four sizes are commercially available: the 12, 15, and 18 Fr Origen and the 14 Fr Kendal. Therefore application of this technique is limited to patients weighing 2 to 11 kg.

EXTRACORPOREAL LIFE SUPPORT CIRCUIT

The ECLS circuit is composed of several disposable and nondisposable components. The disposable components consist of the tubing and various connectors, bladder, membrane, heat exchanger, and cannulas. Preassembled sterile tubing packs simplify the setup. Currently the circuit is not standardized, leading most ECLS centers to customize their preassembled packs. The ideal design should promote laminar flow patterns, require minimum blood volume, be constructed for longevity, and be mobile for intrahospital transport. The nondisposable components include the pump, venous servoregulation system, water bath, coagulating timer, oxygen and carbon dioxide flowmeters, and portable ECLS cart.

With blood flow through a typical venoarterial circuit, blood is drained by gravity from the venous cannula to the bladder (Fig. 24-2). From there the blood is pumped through the membrane and the heat exchanger before it is reinfused via the arterial cannula. The bridge is located near the cannula section of the circuit. It allows the patient to be isolated from the circuit while a blood flow rate is maintained to prevent stagnation. The venovenous circuit follows the same pattern except that the reinfusion cannula is inserted into a vein.

CANNULAS

The ECLS circuit begins and ends with the cannulas. The cannulas chosen dictate the maximum flow rate that the system can achieve. The ideal cannula should be thin walled to achieve the largest internal diameter possible, stiff enough for insertion, kink resistant, and radiopaque. Wire-reinforced cannulas have many of these characteristics. A standardized rating system, the *M number,* has been developed to score different devices on their pressure to blood flow characteristic.[59] A device with a low M number indicates that a higher blood flow rate is possible at a lower pressure.

The arterial cannula is the source of highest resistance in the circuit because of its small diameter. Because hemolysis can occur at system pressures exceeding 350 mm Hg, it is important to select an arterial cannula large enough to handle the anticipated flow rates for a given patient.[60] The major differences between the venous and arterial cannulas are that the lower portion of the venous cannula has multiple side ports for optimal drainage, whereas the arterial cannula is shorter to reduce resistance. In addition to the diameter of the venous cannula, drainage depends on cannula position, right atrial pressure, and the height of the patient above the bladder. Subtle manipulations of these variables may be necessary to optimize flow. The most common causes of a decrease in venous return include malpositioning of the venous cannula, kinking of the cannula, shifting of the mediastinum, or a hypovolemic state.

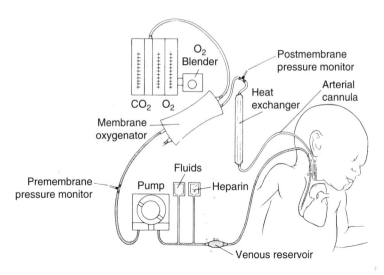

Fig. 24-2

Circuit for extracorporeal life support. (From Short BL: Physiology of extracorporeal membrane oxygenation. In Polin RA, Fox WW, editors: *Fetal and neonatal physiology.* Philadelphia. WB Saunders, 1992.)

PUMPS

Pumps are classified as either kinetic or positive displacement, depending on the way they exert energy to transport or compress fluid. The two pump systems employed with ECLS are the roller and centrifugal pumps.

Roller Pump. The roller pump, a positive displacement type, is most often used during ECLS. It functions on the principle of compression and displacement and is reliable and easy to operate. Flow is produced by compressing a segment of tubing between two roller heads, spaced 180 degrees apart, and a back plate. Volume is displaced as the rollers travel the length of the "raceway" (tubing contained within the pump's housing), delivering a forward force. The second roller begins compressing the tubing as the first roller is reaching the end. The output depends on the size of the tubing, the rotations per minute, and proper occlusion. *Occlusion* refers to the amount of pressure the roller heads exert on the tubing to prevent fluid from slipping backward. Most roller pumps require manual adjustment of the occlusion before each use.

One drawback to this device is that it is not pressure dependent and will pump to deliver the specified flow rate. Therefore, even if excessive pressure builds up within the system, the pump will continue to operate until the problem is recognized or rupture occurs. For safe operation, a roller pump requires the incorporation of a venous servo-regulation system, either a bladder box or a pressure monitoring system.

Bladder box system. The bladder is a small reservoir composed of thin, pliable silicone. Situated between the patient and the ECLS pump, the bladder allows the pump to pull from this reservoir instead of from the right atrium. If there is an acute decrease in venous drainage, the bladder will collapse on itself, preventing excessive negative pressure from being transmitted to the heart. The bladder section of the circuit is the site that is used most often for infusing fluids because of its ability to trap small amounts of air inadvertently administered with medications. Two vents for purging the inadvertent air and for continuous infusions are built into the top. The major complication associated with the bladder is the development of clots caused by the stagnant blood flow pattern near the bottom of the bladder. New streamlined designs, however, are reducing the occurrence of clots.

The bladder box assembly is the safety mechanism for the circuit. It is composed of two brackets to support the silicone bladder and a microswitch or plunger that rests on the bladder surface. When the bladder collapses, the microswitch is released and interrupts the electrical signal, stopping the pump and alerting the clinician with an audible alarm. When corrected, the bladder reexpands and depresses the microswitch, restoring the pump's electric current. The purpose of this bladder box assembly is to prevent the pump's flow rate from exceeding the venous drainage.

Pressure monitoring system. An alternative to the microswitch-operated bladder box is a servo-regulated pressure monitoring system. A pressure transducer is connected between the patient and the bladder. When flow diminishes, the pressure in the venous line decreases until a predetermined level is reached. At this point the pump is disengaged until adequate drainage is reestablished. This technology allows regulation thresholds as well as absolute limits, so the pump will actually slow down and speed up as the bladder pressure changes.

Centrifugal Pump. The centrifugal pump, a kinetic type, is also used by some centers. Energy is transferred to the blood by a rapidly rotating cone. Blood passes through a vortex created by the spinning motion of the cone and is forced out through the outlet. It automatically responds to the resistance against which it is pumping, resulting in changes in the delivered flow. As line pressure increases, flow decreases. This pressure-limited feature prevents pumping against a high-pressure head and ultimately eliminates potential system ruptures. Another advantage of this system is the elimination of the venous servo-regulating system and the raceway. If venous drainage is inadequate, however, significant negative pressure can be generated, which may cause hemolysis. This risk is why the centrifugal pump is still not universally accepted in the ECLS community.[54]

Collin Cardio Pump. Another unique pumping system is the Collin Cardio nonocclusive roller pump, which is currently available only in Europe.[57]

It incorporates a servo-regulated roller pump and distensible silicone rubber tubing stretched over the rollers. The silicone tubing resembles a long, thin chamber and fills passively, acting as a reservoir and limiting excessive pressure buildup.

MEMBRANE OXYGENATORS

Silicone Rubber Membrane. Most of the experience in ECLS has been with the Medtronic silicone rubber membrane (Medtronic Perfusion Systems), originally designed by Kolobow and Bowman.[8] It is a flat silicone membrane envelope wound in a spiral coil around a polycarbonate spool (Fig. 24-3). The two compartments in this membrane, for blood and for gas, are separated by the semipermeable silicone membrane. While the blood is pumped through its compartment in the membrane, a ventilating gas, the *sweep gas,* is flushed through the air compartment. Because this sweep gas is providing a constant fresh source of oxygen and is constantly flushing out diffused carbon dioxide, a gradient is established that optimizes transport of oxygen and carbon dioxide across the membrane. The efficiency of carbon dioxide removal is so high in this system that it is often necessary to use *carbogen* (95% oxygen, 5% carbon dioxide) as the sweep gas source. Carbogen prevents carbon dioxide partial pressure (Pco_2) from dropping to less than 37 mm Hg.

Microporous Membrane. Microporous hollow-fiber membranes have also been used in ECLS. The

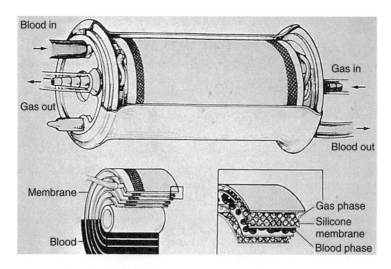

Fig. 24-3

Diagram of membrane oxygenator and the membrane unwound to demonstrate the large surface area used for gas exchange. (Courtesy Medtronic Perfusion Systems, Plymouth, Minn.)

hollow-fiber membrane is made of woven capillaries of microporous plastic. Gas passes through the capillaries while blood flows around them. The microporous membrane has excellent gas exchange capabilities and low resistance and is easy to prime. Over extended periods, however, condensation, wettability, and plasma leakage make it less desirable for long-term use. This type of membrane was used in the early clinical trials involving heparin-bonded circuits.[61]

Physiologic Basis. Membrane oxygenators are designed to eliminate direct contact between the blood and gas phases. This design avoids unnecessary trauma to the blood and makes membrane oxygenators more suitable than bubble oxygenators for long-term extracorporeal support. Gas transfer across the membrane depends on the nature of the gas, the thickness of the membrane, the surface area, and the difference in the partial pressure of the gases on each side of the membrane. This partial-pressure difference is referred to as the *driving pressure* or the *transmembrane pressure*. The characteristics of a membrane oxygenator that influence gas exchange can be simplified by describing the effect of the transfer rate and the blood film thickness.[48]

Transfer rate. The transfer rate is equal to the driving pressure times the permeability of the membrane. The driving pressure reflects the tendency of gases to diffuse from a high pressure to a low pressure. The greater this differential, the greater is the rate of exchange. The more permeable the membrane is for a particular gas, the greater the exchange of that gas.[62]

The driving pressure is different for each gas. If the sweep gas on the membrane is 100% oxygen, the gas-side P_{O_2} will be 760 mm Hg, and the venous P_{O_2} will be approximately 40 mm Hg. This difference results in an oxygen driving pressure of 720 mm Hg into the blood. Carbon dioxide's driving pressure is significantly less: zero on the gas side and 45 mm Hg in the blood. This results in only a 45-mm Hg force into the gas compartment (Fig. 24-4). Despite this small driving pressure, however, carbon dioxide exchange is very efficient because silicone rubber is six times more permeable to carbon dioxide than to oxygen. To enhance this gradient further, blood and gas flow in a countercurrent direction. This allows a consistently larger and extended gradient as the blood travels through the membrane.

Blood film thickness. The transfer rate of oxygen is limited by the thickness of the blood film between the membrane layers. As the blood film becomes thicker, the oxygenating efficiency decreases. In the human lung, this thickness is only one red cell, compared with a 20-cell to 60-cell layer in membrane oxygenators. The red cells closest to the membrane become saturated with oxygen first; with time, oxygen diffuses deeper into the blood, finally reaching the red cells in the innermost layer. The blood must remain in contact with the

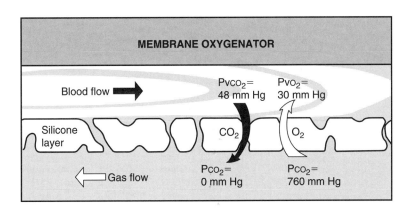

Fig. 24-4

Schematic drawing of the membrane lung illustrating separation of blood and gas compartments, with transfer of gases across the silicone membrane because of a pressure gradient. (Redrawn from Short BL: Physiology of extracorporeal membrane oxygenation. In Polin RA, Fox WW, editors: *Fetal and neonatal physiology.* Philadelphia. WB Saunders, 1992.)

membrane long enough for complete saturation to occur. If the blood moves too fast, this will not occur, and the blood leaving the membrane will be less than fully saturated. This limitation, the *rated flow,* is the flow rate at which venous blood leaves the oxygenator at 95% saturation.[63] Therefore oxygen transfer will continue to increase only until the rated flow is reached. If higher blood flow rates are required, a larger membrane with a larger surface area is needed.

Carbon dioxide transfer. Because of silicone's high permeability to carbon dioxide, the transfer of this gas is not dependent on the blood film thickness or blood flow rate. In practice, transfer depends more on the gas flow rate, the surface area of the membrane, and the driving pressure. Any situation that decreases the surface area (e.g., thrombus) will decrease carbon dioxide transfer. Increasing the sweep gas flow rate will lower the patient's $PaCO_2$, principally because it maintains a full driving pressure throughout the gas phase.

Carbon dioxide clearance decreases as water accumulates in the gas compartment of the membrane, because of the temperature difference between the two sides of the membrane. The warm blood and the cooler gas allow condensation to occur. A minimum fresh gas flow is required for continuous flushing of these water droplets. Unfortunately, the minimum flow rate required to remove condensation usually results in excessive elimination of carbon dioxide as well. To compensate for this, sweep gas is often blended to contain carbogen, which reduces the driving pressure across the membrane and maintains normocarbia.

Monitoring the difference between the premembrane PCO_2 and postmembrane PCO_2 is important because carbon dioxide transfer is more selectively sensitive than oxygen transfer. Changes in carbon dioxide can be an early indication of membrane malfunction. Box 24-4 summarizes the relationship between the artificial membrane and its effect on gas exchange.

Pressure drop. Each membrane oxygenator also has a rated pressure drop across the membrane. If this is exceeded, the membrane may rupture. *Pressure drop* is the resistance to blood flow produced by the membrane, obtained by subtracting the outlet pressure (postmembrane pressure) from the inlet pressure (premembrane pressure). The normal resistance within the membrane is usually fixed. This pressure difference can increase with internal clotting, higher flow rates, and an increase in blood viscosity. Monitoring of the premembrane and postmembrane pressures allows continuous assessment of the membrane's internal resistance.

> **BOX 24-4**
>
> ### GAS EXCHANGE OF THE MEMBRANE OXYGENATORS
>
> **CARBON DIOXIDE EXCHANGE**
> Independent of blood flow rate
> Dependent on driving pressure
> Dependent on sweep gas flow rate
> Increase sweep gas, decrease $PaCO_2$
> Dependent on membrane surface area
>
> **OXYGEN EXCHANGE**
> Dependent on blood flow rate
> Dependent on blood path thickness
> Independent of sweep gas flow rate
> Increase blood flow rate, increase PaO_2
> Dependent on membrane surface area

HEAT EXCHANGER

As blood travels through the ECLS circuit, heat is continually lost from the exposed surface of the tubing and through the oxygenator because of the cooling effects of the sweep gas and water evaporation. Therefore a disposable heat exchanger, which warms the blood and maintains the body temperature, is placed as the last component in the circuit before reinfusion into the patient. The heat exchanger is designed as a *countercurrent system* in which blood travels down stainless steel tubes in the center of the exchanger while warm water is pumped up the surrounding cylinders outside the tubes. In this manner the circulating water never has direct contact with the blood. The water itself is heated and pumped through a separate water pump and thermal regulator. To provide additional safety, the heat exchanger also acts as a bubble trap when mounted vertically so that blood enters the top and exits the bottom. In this design a small amount of air can be trapped at the top of the heat exchanger.

TUBING

The tubing used in the ECLS circuit is usually composed of $\frac{1}{4}$-, $\frac{3}{8}$-, or $\frac{1}{2}$-inch diameter polyvinyl chloride. The total length of tubing in the circuit varies from institution to institution. Most of the tubing is subjected to low stress, and component failure is rare. However, the section of tubing housed between the pump heads and the back plate, the raceway, is under continuous strain from the roller heads throughout the run. This has often resulted in rupture of the raceway tubing, which can be a catastrophic event. Therefore many techniques are employed to prevent undue stress on this tubing. The first method, "walking the raceway," involves advancing the tubing to a new section at predetermined intervals, thereby having each section of tubing in the raceway for a limited time only. Another approach is to use larger diameter tubing. Because larger tubing has a greater volume per unit length, the revolutions per minute necessary to generate a given flow rate are reduced. Finally, a new stronger polymer, known as "super Tygon tubing" (S-65-HL), has become available. It is ideally suited for the pump's raceway. Although its qualities would make it ideal for the entire ECLS circuit, because of its high cost it typically is used only for the raceway section.

The ECLS circuit also contains a variety of polycarbonate connectors in various configurations, allowing volume administration and blood sample withdrawing. An attempt is made to minimize the number of connectors because each connector can promote turbulent flow and thrombus formation and each is a potential source of disconnection and leak.

PRIMING

Before initiating ECLS, the circuit has to be prepared by the process of priming, which is divided into four stages: (1) carbon dioxide flush, (2) vacuum, (3) crystalloid prime, and (4) blood prime.[62]

Carbon dioxide is flushed through the circuit for a minimum of 2 minutes. This flushes out the air in the circuit and replaces it with carbon dioxide, which is highly soluble in blood, decreasing the risk of microbubbles.

A line vacuum is applied to the gas ports of the membrane for at least 5 minutes. The reservoirs will gradually collapse, removing the carbon dioxide from the blood partition of the membrane. This step opens the membrane, allowing more of its surface to be in full contact with the blood. The negative pressure also facilitates the subsequent filling of the circuit with fluid.

A crystalloid solution is added, and the circuit is filled systematically, expelling air as each section of the circuit is primed with fluid. Once completely filled, the vacuum is disconnected and the pump turned on to circulate the fluid. All air must be removed from the circuit. Special attention should be directed to the membrane and heat exchanger to ensure that they are free of bubbles. These components require aggressive shaking and slight tapping. Albumin is then added to the normal saline and circulated. Albumin coats and "pacifies" the internal surface of the circuit to minimize the blood–foreign surface interaction.

The crystalloid/albumin solution is then slowly drained from the priming bag and replaced with packed red blood cells. The blood is treated with heparin for anticoagulation, tromethamine (THAM) or sodium bicarbonate to adjust the pH, and calcium gluconate to reverse the citrate effect of stored blood. The blood is pumped into the circuit as the crystal-loid is "chased out," draining into a waste bag. Once the blood is circulating, gas flow is connected to the membrane, and a blood gas determination, activated clotting time, and ionized calcium level are obtained from the circuit. The water bath is also attached to the heat exchanger, and the circulating blood is warmed to 37° C before initiation of ECLS.

CANNULATION

Once ECLS criteria are met, parental consent is obtained, and blood products are ordered, it is critical that the team moves quickly, since candidates for ECLS are by definition critically ill. The patient is positioned with the head at the foot of an elevated bed in the intensive care unit or ECMO unit. The patient's head is then rotated to the left, and the right side of the neck and the chest are prepared in a sterile manner and draped. A small incision is made at the base of the neck, and the right common carotid artery and internal jugular vein are mobilized. The patient is then given 30 to 100 units/kg of heparin; when this has been circulating for several minutes, cannulation is begun.

Concurrently, the ECLS team assembles and primes the circuit at the bedside. While the surgeon is cannulating, it is the responsibility of the nursing team and associated physicians to monitor the patient's vital signs. With the vessels exposed, the artery and vein are distally ligated with absorbable sutures and controlled proximally by vascular clamps. The appropriate cannulas are selected for the patient size and anticipated flow rates. The venous cannula is introduced through the jugular vein into the right atrium. The arterial cannula is introduced into the distal aortic arch via the right carotid artery. Both cannulas are secured to vessels and to the patient's skin to avoid accidental decannulation. At this point the cannulas are connected to the ECLS circuit, avoiding any air bubbles in the system. Once connected, the circuit is turned on, and the flow is slowly increased while the ventilator settings are concomitantly decreased. This usually results in immediate stabilization of the patient's vital signs.

With VV ECMO via the double-lumen cannula, only the internal jugular vein is cannulated. This approach is often performed using a "semipercutaneous" technique that obviates the need to ligate the vessel.

MANAGEMENT AND MONITORING

CARDIOVASCULAR SYSTEM

The main goal of ECLS is to provide adequate oxygen delivery. This is assessed by monitoring $S\bar{v}O_2$, using a fiberoptic catheter inserted into the circuit.

An $S\bar{v}O_2$ of 75% is considered acceptable. On venovenous support, the $S\bar{v}O_2$ also reflects the recirculation and consequently cannot be used to assess oxygen delivery. Pulse oximetry provides continuous assessment of the patient's SaO_2, with 90% or greater being acceptable. On full venoarterial support, however, the pulse pressure is narrow and the oximeter may be inaccurate. Because of selective limb perfusion with venoarterial ECLS, the ideal sites for arterial blood gas monitoring are the lower extremities or the umbilical artery.

Once the cannulas are connected to the circuit, the pump's flow rate is slowly increased while the arterial pressure waveform is observed. With venoarterial support the arterial waveform decreases as flow is increased. The flow is increased to a goal of 100 to 120 ml/kg/min or until the $S\bar{v}O_2$ is 75%. This approximates 70% to 80% of total cardiac output and is usually sufficient to support gas exchange. In a hypermetabolic state, however, the flow requirement may exceed 150 ml/kg/min. When an adequate flow and $S\bar{v}O_2$ are established, ventilator settings are lowered, and subsequent adjustments in the PaO_2 are made by varying the FiO_2 of the sweep gas. Changes in $PaCO_2$ are accomplished by altering the flow rate of the sweep gas, including the carbogen flow rate.

The mean blood pressure range for neonates on ECLS is 40 to 65 mm Hg. If inotropic support was required during cannulation, it can often be rapidly weaned or discontinued, whereas in venovenous ECLS, inotropes are gradually decreased. Occasionally, hypertension will occur, requiring antihypertensive administration to maintain a mean blood pressure of less than 65 mm Hg. This is an essential precaution taken to reduce the incidence of IVH.

ANTICOAGULATION

Clotting will occur within the ECLS circuit unless the blood is anticoagulated. When blood is exposed to a foreign surface, several changes take place. A layer of protein adheres to the foreign surface instantly. Some of these proteins "pacify" the surface, whereas others activate platelets and the clotting and complement cascades, resulting in clot formation.

Preventing a thrombus during extracorporeal support requires administering an anticoagulant, such as heparin. The effect of heparin is immediate, and it produces no side effects. Heparin has no direct anticoagulant effect on the blood by itself but combines with a cofactor, antithrombin III, to prevent thrombi from forming. This stops the conversion of fibrinogen to fibrin and ultimately prevents blood from clotting. A deficiency in antithrombin III can cause heparin to be ineffective, resulting in excessive amounts of heparin use. If excessive clot-

ting in the circuit is noted, a deficiency in antithrombin III should be considered.

Activated clotting times are monitored to assess heparin administration. It is a simple whole-blood test performed at the bedside. A small quantity of blood is injected into a test tube containing a catalyst. The test tube is inserted into a spinning well. When a clot is detected, a timer stops. Generally, a continuous infusion of 20 to 60 units/kg/hr is required to sustain the activated clotting time at 180 to 200 seconds (normal 90 to 120 seconds). Once stable, the activated clotting times are measured at least hourly.

The amount of heparin required can be influenced by several factors. Because heparin binds to platelets, higher doses of heparin are required with platelet transfusions. Conversely, a lower level of heparin is needed when thrombocytopenia exists. Heparin is also excreted in the urine, so a higher dose may be required during significant diuresis.

HEMATOLOGIC SYSTEM

Of all the blood components, *platelets* are most affected by extracorporeal support. Platelets are continuously consumed on ECLS and are generally administered on a daily basis in concentrated form.[64,65] Platelets attach to areas in which fibrinogen is present, become activated, and attract more platelets. These platelet aggregates are continuously formed while the patient receives ECLS. Because platelets adhere to the silicone membrane, they are administered directly to the patient or into the circuit after the membrane. Other blood products also adhere to the circuit, but with less effect.[66]

Although protocols vary among institutions, platelets are generally administered when the count is less than 100,000/mm³, accompanied by additional heparin. The hematocrit, prothrombin time, and fibrinogen are also monitored. Box 24-5 provides an example of protocol guidelines.

If fluid administration is required and the hematocrit is acceptable, 5% albumin should be administered. Fresh frozen plasma or cryoprecipitate is

---

BOX 24-5

HEMATOLOGIC GUIDELINES FOR EXTRACORPOREAL LIFE SUPPORT

Hematocrit >35 ml/dl
Platelets >150,000/mm
Fibrinogen >150 g/dl
Prothrombin time <17 seconds
Activated clotting time = 180-220 seconds

Courtesy Wake Forest University Baptist Medical Center, Winston-Salem, NC.

considered if a bleeding complication occurs or factor replacements are necessary.

The effect of ECLS on the red blood cell is usually negligible if the roller pump is adjusted for proper occlusion. If dark plasma or hematuria occurs, however, hemolysis should be suspected. A plasma-free hemoglobin sample should be obtained and a search instituted for either a mechanical or a physiologic cause.

NEUROLOGIC SYSTEM

Paralysis during ECLS is usually avoided except during cannulation and decannulation procedures. The patients are sedated while on ECLS to prevent accidental decannulation or hypertension secondary to agitation and to provide comfort. Fentanyl, midazolam, and lorazepam are typically used. Studies have shown that fentanyl continues to bind to the membrane during ECLS, and increasing amounts are usually required.[67] Narcotic withdrawal can delay recovery after ECLS.[68]

Head ultrasounds are performed to rule out IVH. If IVH does occur, the mean blood pressure is decreased, the range of activated clotting times is lowered, coagulation values are optimized, and an antifibrinolytic drug may be given to avoid extension of the bleed. As with any complication, the risk versus benefit of continuing ECLS should be carefully considered.

Because of the ligation of the internal jugular vein and the right common carotid artery, the head is maintained in the midline position to ensure adequate cerebral drainage and perfusion. Some institutions also insert an additional cannula into the cephalad segment of the right jugular vein to avoid venous obstruction and to enhance drainage.[69]

PULMONARY SYSTEM

After the initiation of venoarterial ECLS, the ventilator is generally reduced to a FIO_2 of 0.21 to 0.3, a peak inspiratory pressure of 20 to 25 cm H_2O, a positive end-expiratory pressure of 4 to 10 cm H_2O, and a rate of 5 to 10 breaths per minute. These resting ventilator settings presumably allow the lung to heal. Pulmonary care should include chest vibrations, manual ventilation with an inspiratory hold, saline instillation, and suctioning. Chest radiographs are taken daily and often exhibit a generalized opacification within the first 24 hours.[70] This phenomenon has been attributed to an abrupt decrease in airway pressure and to the release of vasoactive substances from the blood-circuit interface.

Patients who continue to have persistent pulmonary air leaks while receiving ECLS may require low levels of continuous positive airway pressure for the lungs to heal. Keszler et al[71] have shown accelerated lung recovery by employing positive end-expiratory pressure levels of 12 to 14 cm H_2O. They found less opacification on chest x-ray films and a shorter duration of ECLS. In general, lung recovery usually occurs over 3 to 4 days, and it can be quantified by improvements in the chest radiograph, lung compliance, and gas exchange.[72]

FLUID BALANCE

Most patients receiving ECLS are edematous because of fluid resuscitation before ECLS. This edematous state can further compromise the lungs and impede lung recovery. Once capillary leak ceases, the goal of fluid management is to promote diuresis while maintaining adequate perfusion. Accordingly, fluid intake and output should be monitored for the duration of ECLS. Insensible water loss from the patient and the membrane cannot be measured but should not be forgotten. Although renal function is usually normal on ECLS, a decrease in urine output may be seen early in the run, especially if the patient sustained a prolonged period of hypoxia or hypotension before cannulation.

If oliguria or anuria occurs, ultrafiltration can be added to enhance output and manage fluid overload.[73] This is accomplished by connecting a hemofilter to the ECLS circuit, which allows a fraction of plasma water and dissolved solutes to pass through the filter's pores, while maintaining the cellular components and proteins. Nutrition is usually started on the third day of life; hyperalimentation and an intralipid infusion are usually initiated. However, transpyloric feeding can also be considered. In addition, most patients require calcium and potassium replacement while receiving ECLS.

WEANING

The amount of time a patient requires ECLS varies with the diagnosis. The average duration for a neonate is 4 to 6 days. Two approaches are used to wean patients from venoarterial ECLS. In the first approach, as lung function improves, ECLS is withdrawn slowly as ventilator support slowly increases. This is usually carried out over several days. Once the flow rate is decreased to 20 ml/kg/min, the patient is usually ready for decannulation.

In the second approach the patient is maintained on full flows of 100 ml/kg/min and minimal ventilator settings. At varying intervals the patient is weaned from the ECLS circuit over a few minutes while the ventilator settings are increased. The patient circuit is then clamped off, and blood gases are obtained to assess pulmonary function. The rationale for the second approach is that the longer period of low ventilator support maximizes the (resting) time for the lungs to heal. Both methods are used widely, and neither has been clearly shown to have any advantage over the other.

Weaning from venovenous ECLS is slightly different from weaning from venoarterial ECLS. After increasing the ventilator parameters, both the membrane's gas ports are isolated from the ambient air. Eventually the blood entering and exiting the membrane is in equilibrium and reflects typical venous values. This eliminates any issues associated with clamping of the cannulas, particularly thrombus formation, which allows a longer trial without any pulmonary support.

DECANNULATION

When the patient is ready to be removed from ECLS, the decannulation is performed at the bedside. Sedative and paralytic agents are administered, and all infusions are switched to a peripheral site. Heparin is discontinued; however, its anticoagulating effect is not pharmacologically reversed. In a mirror-image reversal of the original cannulation procedure, the cannulas are removed and the vessels either reconstructed or ligated. After the patient recovers from the paralysis, weaning from the ventilator can proceed. Before the patient is discharged from the hospital, it is essential that he or she be referred to a follow-up program within the hospital for further and future evaluations. Again, when the "semipercutaneous" method of cannulation is used, the cannula is simply pulled out and direct pressure held against the site until the bleeding stops.

COMPLICATIONS

Complications of ECLS can be divided into patient and technical issues. All patient complications may be caused by two physiologic alterations: alterations in the blood-surface interaction and changes in the blood flow pattern. Both these variables can have adverse effects on all the organ systems. As already stated, when blood comes into contact with a foreign surface, a chain of events results in thrombus formation and platelet consumption. This necessitates the use of heparin and consequently contributes to the bleeding complications of ECLS.

Systemic heparinization makes IVH the primary risk of ECLS. The central nervous system, therefore, becomes the major area of concern. The risk of IVH is compounded by blood flow changes from the ligation of both the right internal jugular vein and the right common carotid artery. The effect of this perfusion and drainage interruption to the right side of the brain has been documented by Schumacher et al,[49] who reported several occurrences of right-

TABLE 24-3	NEONATAL RESPIRATORY FAILURE: PATIENT COMPLICATIONS (TOTAL CASES: 17,143)
Complication	**Percent**
Dialysis-hemofiltration	16
Hemolysis	12.8
Hypertension	12.6
Seizures	12
Abnormal creatinine value	9.9
Hyperbilirubinemia	8.8
Infection	6.6
Surgical site bleeding	6.1
Pneumothorax	6.1
Myocardial stun	6.0
Cannula site bleeding	5.8
Intraventricular hemorrhage	5.2
Cardiac dysrhythmias	4.0

Data from ELSO National Registry Report. Ann Arbor. University of Michigan, 2002.

sided brain lesions after ECMO. Stolar et al,[74] in reviewing the experience of the Neonatal ECMO Registry, reported that neurologic complications were predominant, with a 24% occurrence. The incidence of IVH in the neonate receiving ECLS is approximately 14%. In early ECLS studies, Cilley et al[75] reported a series of eight infants less than 35 weeks' gestation who all experienced IVH while receiving ECLS. This finding has led to the recommendation that ECLS should not be offered to infants less than 36 weeks of gestation or until anticoagulation is minimized or eliminated.

Wilson et al[76] reported a different approach to this issue. They successfully employed an antifibrinolytic drug, *aminocaproic acid,* in infants considered at high risk for IVH and other types of hemorrhage. They reported a decrease in IVH from 18% to 0% with the use of this drug, along with a decrease in all postoperative bleeding. Circuit thrombotic complications, however, appeared to be greater with use of aminocaproic acid.

Venoarterial ECLS alters the blood flow pattern throughout the body, especially the cerebral and pulmonary perfusion. Diverting blood flow through a nonpulsatile pump contributes to the diminished pulse pressure. *Cardiac stun,* a term used to describe a dramatic decrease in the cardiac function of a patient receiving ECLS, is characterized by a minimum pulse pressure (<5 mm Hg).[77] This minimum pulse pressure infers nearly absent ventricular contribution, resulting in a PaO_2 almost equalizing the postmembrane PO_2. Cardiac stun occurs infrequently and lasts only transiently. Its exact mechanism is unknown, but cardiac stun is associated with increased mortality.

TABLE 24-4	NEONATAL RESPIRATORY FAILURE: MECHANICAL COMPLICATIONS (TOTAL CASES: 17,143)	
Complication	**Percent**	
Clots in circuit	18.6	
Cannula problems	11.1	
Oxygenator failure	5.7	
Air in circuit	5.5	
Pump malfunction	1.8	
Heat exchanger malfunction	0.9	
Tubing rupture	0.8	

Data from ELSO National Registry Report. Ann Arbor. University of Michigan, 2002.

The ELSO registry contains information from more than 17,000 cases and includes every reported occurrence of both physiologic and mechanical complications (Tables 24-3 and 24-4).

REFERENCES

1. Comroe JH Jr: *Retrospectroscope insights into medical discoveries.* Menlo Park, Calif. Von Gehr, 1983.
2. Gibbon JH: Application of a mechanical heart lung apparatus to cardiac surgery. *Minn Med* 1954; 37:171-185.
3. Gibbon JH: Artificial maintenance of circulation during experimental occlusion of pulmonary artery. *Arch Surg* 1937; 34:1105.
4. Lillehei CW et al: The results of direct vision closure of ventricular septal defects in 8 patients by means of controlled cross-circulation. *Surg Gynecol Obstet* 1955; 101:447.
5. Lillehei CW et al: Direct vision intracardiac surgery in man using a simple, disposable artificial oxygenator. *Dis Chest* 1956; 29:1-8.
6. Kolff WJ, Berk HT Jr: Artificial kidney: a dialyzer with a great area. *Acta Med Scand* 1944; 117:121.
7. Clowes GH: An artificial lung dependent upon diffusion of oxygen and carbon dioxide through plastic membranes. *J Thorac Surg* 1956; 32:630-637.
8. Kolobow T, Bowman RL: Construction and elimination of an alveolar membrane artificial heart-lung. *Trans Am Soc Artif Intern Organ* 1963; 9:238.
9. Kolobow T, Zapol WM, Pierce J: High survival and minimal blood damage in lambs exposed to long term venovenous pumping with a polyurethane chamber roller pump with and without a membrane oxygenator. *Trans Am Soc Artif Intern Organ* 1969; 15:172-177.
10. Dorson WJ et al: A perfusion system for infants. *Trans Am Soc Artif Intern Organ* 1969; 15:155-160.
11. White JJ et al: Prolonged respiratory support in newborn infants with a membrane oxygenator. *Surgery* 1971; 70: 288-296.
12. Hill JD: Prolonged extracorporeal oxygenation for acute post-traumatic respiratory failure: use of the Bramson membrane lung. *N Engl J Med* 1972; 286:629-634.
13. Zapol WM et al: Extracorporeal membrane oxygenation in severe respiratory failure: a randomized prospective study. *JAMA* 1979; 242:2193.
14. Hirschl RB, Bartlett RH: Extracorporeal membrane oxygenation (ECMO) support in cardio-respiratory failure. In Tompkins R, editor: *Advances in surgery.* Chicago. Year Book Medical, 1987; pp 189-211.
15. Bartlett RHL, Harken DE: Instrumentation for cardiopulmonary bypass: past, present, and future. *Assoc Adv Med Instr* 1976; 10:119-124.
16. Bartlett RH et al: Extracorporeal membrane oxygenation for newborn respiratory failure: 45 cases. *Surgery* 1982; 92:425-433.
17. Bartlett RH et al: Extracorporeal circulation in neonates with respiratory failure: a prospective randomized study. *Pediatrics* 1985; 4:479-487.
18. O'Rourke PP et al: Extracorporeal membrane oxygenation and conventional medical therapy in neonates with persistent pulmonary hypertension of the newborn: a prospective randomized study. *Pediatrics* 1989; 84:957-963.
19. Gattinoni L et al: Low frequency positive pressure ventilation with extracorporeal CO_2 removal in severe acute respiratory failure. *JAMA* 1986; 256:881-885.
20. ECMO National Registry. Ann Arbor. University of Michigan, 2002.
21. United Kingdom Collaborative ECMO Trial Group: The report of the UK collaborative randomised trial of neonatal extracorporeal membrane oxygenation. *Lancet* 1996; 348:75-82.
22. Fox W, Duara S: Persistent pulmonary hypertension in the neonate: diagnosis and management. *J Pediatr* 1983; 103:505.
23. Duara S, Fox W: Persistent pulmonary hypertension of the newborn. In Thibeault DW, Gregory GA, editors: *Neonatal pulmonary care,* ed 2, Menlo Park, Calif. Addison-Wesley, 1986.
24. Vacanti JP et al: The pulmonary hemodynamic response to perioperative anesthesia in the treatment of high risk infants with congenital diaphragmatic hernia. *J Pediatr Surg* 1984; 19:672.
25. Wung JT et al: Management of infants with severe respiratory failure and persistence of the fetal circulation without hyperventilation. *Pediatrics* 1985; 76:488-494.
26. Stahlman M: Acute respiratory disorders in the newborn. In Avery GB, editor: *Neonatology.* Philadelphia. Lippincott, 1981; p 390.
27. Miller FC et al: Significance of meconium during labor. *Am J Obstet Gynecol* 1975; 122:573.
28. Yeh TF et al: Roentgenographic findings in infants with meconium aspiration syndrome. *JAMA* 1979; 242:60.
29. Dillon HC Jr et al: Anorectal and vaginal carriage of group B streptococci in pregnant women. *J Infect Dis* 1984; 145:794.
30. Anthony BF, Okada DM: The emergence of group B streptococci in infections of the newborn infant. *Ann Rev Med* 1977; 28:355.
31. Puri P: Epidemiology of congenital diaphragmatic hernia. In Puri P, editor: *Modern problems in paediatrics,* New York. Karger, 1989.
32. Harrison MR, deLorimier AA: Congenital diaphragmatic hernia. *Surg Clin North Am* 1981; 61:1023.
33. Dibbins AW, Wiener ES: Mortality from diaphragmatic hernia. *J Pediatr Surg* 1974; 9:653-662.
34. Wilson JM et al: Congenital diaphragmatic hernia: predictors of severity in the ECMO era. *J Pediatr Surg* 1991; 26:1028-1033.
35. Kays DW et al: Detrimental effects of standard medical therapy in congenital diaphragmatic hernia. *Ann Surg* 1999; 230(3):340-351.
36. Bartlett RH et al: Extracorporeal circulation (ECMO) in neonatal respiratory failure. *J Thorac Cardiovasc Surg* 1977; 74:826-835.

37. Krummel TM et al: Alveolar-arterial oxygen gradients versus the neonatal pulmonary insufficiency index for prediction of mortality in ECMO candidates. *J Pediatr Surg* 1984; 19:380-384.

38. Ortega M et al: Oxygenation index can predict outcome in neonates who are candidates for extracorporeal membrane oxygenation. *Pediatr Res* 1987; 22:462A.

39. Muntean W: Coagulation and anticoagulation in extracorporeal membrane oxygenation. *Artif Organs* 1999; 23:979-983.

40. Conference report: Mechanisms of acute respiratory failure. *Am Rev Respir Dis* 1977; 115:1071-1078.

41. Bartlett RH et al: A prospective study of acute hypoxic respiratory failure. *Chest* 1986; 89:684-689.

42. Steinhorn RH, Green TP: Use of extracorporeal membrane oxygenation in the treatment of respiratory syncytial virus bronchiolitis: the national experience, 1983 to 1988. *J Pediatr* 1990; 116:338-341.

43. Adolph V et al: Extracorporeal membrane oxygenation for nonneonatal respiratory failure. *J Pediatr Surg* 1991; 26:326-332.

44. Scalzo AJ et al: Extracorporeal membrane oxygenation for hydrocarbon aspiration. *Am J Dis Child* 1990; 144:867-871.

45. O'Rourke PP et al: Extracorporeal membrane oxygenation: support for overwhelming pulmonary failure in the pediatric population. Experience from the Extracorporeal Life Support Organization. *J Pediatr Surg* 1993; 28:523-529.

46. Weber TR et al: Prolonged extracorporeal support for non-neonatal respiratory failure. *J Pediatr Surg* 1992; 27:1100-1104.

47. Swaniker F et al: Extracorporeal life support outcome for 128 pediatric patients with respiratory failure. *J Pediatr Surg* 2000; 35(2):197-202.

48. Bartlett RH: Extracorporeal life support for cardiopulmonary failure. *Curr Probl Surg* 1990; 27(10):261-705.

49. Schumacher RE et al: Rightsided brain lesions in infants following extracorporeal membrane oxygenation. *Pediatrics* 1988; 82:155-160.

50. Moulton SL et al: Carotid artery reconstruction following neonatal extracorporeal membrane oxygenation. *J Pediatr Surg* 1991; 26:794-799.

51. Hickey PR, Buckley MJ, Philbin DM: Pulsatile and nonpulsatile cardiopulmonary bypass: review of a counterproductive controversy. *Ann Thorac Surg* 1983; 36:720-737.

52. Gerstmann DR et al: Left carotid artery and coronary arterial flow partitioning during neonatal ECMO. *Pediatr Res* 1989; 25:37A.

53. Otsu T et al: Laboratory evaluation of a double lumen catheter for venovenous neonatal ECMO. *Trans Am Soc Artif Intern Organ* 1989; 35:647-650.

54. Klein MD et al: Venovenous perfusion in ECMO for newborn respiratory insufficiency: a clinical comparison with venoarterial perfusion. *Ann Surg* 1985; 201:520-526.

55. Kolobow T et al: Single catheter venovenous membrane lung bypass in the treatment of experimental ARDS. *Trans Am Soc Artif Intern Organ* 1988; 34:35-38.

56. Zwischenberger JB et al: Total respiratory support with single cannula venovenous ECMO: double lumen continuous flow vs. single lumen tidal flow. *Trans Am Soc Artif Intern Organ* 1985; 31:610-615.

57. Chevalier JY et al: Preliminary report: extracorporeal lung support for neonatal acute respiratory failure. *Lancet* 1990; 335:1364-1366.

58. Anderson HL et al: Venovenous extracorporeal life support in neonates using a double lumen catheter. *Trans Am Soc Artif Intern Organ* 1989; 35:650-653.

59. Montogia JP, Merz SI, Bartlett RH: A standardized system for describing flow/pressure relationships in vascular access devices. *Trans Am Soc Artif Intern Organ* 1991; 34:4-8.

60. Van Meurs KP et al: Maximum blood flow rates for arterial cannulae used in neonatal ECMO. *Trans Am Soc Artif Intern Organ* 1990; 36:679-681.

61. Toomasian JM et al: Evaluation of Duraflo II heparin coating in prolonged extracorporeal membrane oxygenation. *Trans Am Soc Artif Intern Organ* 1988; 34:410-414.

62. Bartlett RH: *Extracorporeal membrane oxygenation technical specialist manual,* ed 9. Ann Arbor. University of Michigan, 1988.

63. Galletti PM, Richardson PD, Snider MT: A standardized method for defining the overall gas transfer performance of artificial lungs. *Trans Am Soc Artif Intern Organ* 1972; 18:359.

64. Anderson HL et al: Thrombocytopenia in neonates after extracorporeal membrane oxygenation. *Trans Am Soc Artif Intern Organ* 1986; 32:534-537.

65. Moroff G et al: Reduction of the volume of stored platelet concentrates for neonatal use. *Transfusion* 1982; 22:125-127.

66. Zach TL et al: Leukopenia associated with extracorporeal membrane oxygenation in the newborn. *J Pediatr* 1990; 116:440-443.

67. Arnold JH et al: Tolerance and dependence in neonates sedated with fentanyl during extracorporeal membrane oxygenation. *Anesthesiology* 1990; 73:1136-1140.

68. Caron E, Maguie DP: Current management of pain, sedation, and narcotic physical dependency of the infant on ECMO. *J Perinatol Neonatal Nurs* 1990; 4:63-74.

69. Vogt JF et al: Cannulation of cephalad segment of internal jugular vein during extracorporeal membrane oxygenation in the neonate. Snowmass, Colo. Children's National Medical Center, 1989.

70. Taylor GA et al: Diffuse pulmonary opacification in infants undergoing extracorporeal membrane oxygenation: clinical and pathologic correlation. *Radiology* 1986; 161:347-350.

71. Keszler M et al: A prospective multicenter randomized study of high to low positive end-expiratory pressure during extracorporeal membrane oxygenation. *J Pediatr* 1992; 120:107-113.

72. Lotze A, Short BL, Taylor GA: The use of lung compliance as a parameter for improvement in lung function in newborns with respiratory failure requiring extracorporeal membrane oxygenation. *Crit Care Med* 1987; 15:226-229.

73. Heiss KF et al: Renal insufficiency and volume overload in neonatal ECMO managed by continuous ultrafiltration. *Trans Am Soc Artif Intern Organ* 1987; 33:557-560.

74. Stolar CJ, Snedecor SM, Bartlett RH: Extracorporeal membrane oxygenation and neonatal respiratory failure: experience from the Extracorporeal Life Support Organization. *J Pediatr Surg* 1991; 26:563-571.

75. Cilley RE et al: Intracranial hemorrhage during extracorporeal membrane oxygenation in neonates. *Pediatrics* 1986; 78:699-704.

76. Wilson JM et al: AMICAR decreases the incidence of intracranial hemorrhage and other hemorrhagic complications of ECMO. *J Pediatr Surg* 1993; 28:536-541.

77. Martin GR et al: Cardiac stun in infants undergoing extracorporeal membrane oxygenation. *J Thorac Cardiovasc Surg* 1991; 101:607-611.

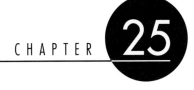

CHAPTER 25

Cardiopulmonary Resuscitation

Kathy Boyle

The causes of cardiac arrest in infant and pediatric patients are more diverse than those in adults. Special attention must be directed to related causes if resuscitation is to be successful. This chapter outlines the recommendations and procedures the respiratory care practitioner needs to resuscitate the pediatric patient. These recommendations are based on the *International Guidelines 2000 for Cardiopulmonary Resuscitation and Emergency Cardiovascular Care.*[1]

PHYSIOLOGY OF INFANT AND PEDIATRIC CPR

Cardiac arrest in the pediatric age groups is rarely of cardiac origin. More often it results from low oxygen levels secondary to respiratory difficulty or respiratory arrest. The resultant hypoxia and hypercapnia (respiratory acidosis) secondarily impair cardiac function, and cardiac arrest occurs. Because cardiac arrest is the result of a long period of hypoxemia, it is not surprising that outcomes of cardiopulmonary resuscitation (CPR) in children with cardiac arrest have been poor.[2-5] Conversely, the outcome of resuscitation after *respiratory* arrest, before the development of cardiac arrest, is considerably better.[6] In the arrest victim, basic life support (BLS) externally supports circulation and ventilation through the process of CPR.

Two theories postulate the mechanism of blood flow during CPR. The *cardiac pump theory* holds that direct compression of the heart between the sternum and the spine results in an increase in pressure within the ventricles, forcing blood out of the aorta and pulmonary artery. The *thoracic pump theory* holds that chest compressions increase intrathoracic pressures, resulting in blood flow through the great vessels.[7] The cardiac pump theory is believed to be more plausible in pediatric patients because of their small chests.[8] However, the mechanism for blood flow may change with prolonged arrest, during which changes occur in chest wall anatomy and chest compliance with changes in the force of chest compressions.

CHILDREN AT RISK

As stated, cardiopulmonary arrest is rarely an acute primary cardiac event in children. It usually follows a progressive deterioration of respiratory or cardiac function. Cardiac arrest most often is the end result of either profound hypoxemia and acidosis of respiratory origin or shock secondary to hypovolemia or infection. The causes of cardiopulmonary arrest in pediatric age groups are usually age related. Most arrests that occur in patients younger than 1 year are related to sudden infant death syndrome (SIDS), respiratory diseases, airway obstruction, submersion, sepsis, and neurologic disease, whereas those in patients older than 1 year are more often injury related[1,9-11] (Box 25-1).

With the exception of acute trauma, out-of-hospital arrests are uncommon in pediatric patients. In contrast to children who experience cardiac arrest outside the hospital, hospitalized pediatric arrest victims often have a chronic underlying disease, such as cancer or congenital heart disease, that predisposes them to arrest.[6,12] The role of CPR in the patient with chronic underlying disease is patient specific and must be constantly reevaluated in regard to its ethical implications and the parents' desires.

Another group of in-hospital patients are at risk of experiencing a cardiopulmonary arrest if not monitored closely. These patients include those with artificial airways, postoperative patients exposed to general anesthesia, patients who have had procedures that can cause bradycardia from Valsalva maneuvers (e.g., lumbar puncture), and those who have been sedated. Surveillance and proper monitoring of these patients will allow early intervention and reduce the incidence of cardiopulmonary arrest.

BASIC LIFE SUPPORT

For the purpose of BLS, an *infant* is defined as younger than 1 year of age, and a *child* is defined as between the ages of 1 and 8 years. The sequence of resuscitation in infants and children is the same; however, the technique of CPR varies with age. The sequence of initiating BLS is outlined in the following paragraphs. Table 25-1 outlines age-specific differences.

1. *Unresponsiveness or respiratory difficulty, or both, is determined.* The patient is tapped gently or spoken to in a loud voice to determine the level of consciousness or to assess for the degree of respiratory difficulty. Because movement may aggravate a spinal cord injury, the child who has sustained head or neck trauma should not be moved or shaken, and infants should never be shaken. Because most children experience arrest secondary to respiratory causes, at least 1 minute of CPR should be performed before calling local emergency medical services (EMS).

2. *Help is summoned.* This should be a call for help from those in the immediate area.

3. *The child is positioned.* The patient is moved gently to a hard, flat surface and positioned on the back while the head and neck are supported. Children with respiratory distress often position themselves to maintain patency of a partially obstructed airway. Children with stridor or signs of upper airway obstruction should be allowed to remain in the position that is most comfortable for them.

4. *The airway is assessed and opened.* The maintenance of a patent airway and support of adequate ventilation are essential in the successful resuscitation of a pediatric patient. Acute deterioration and cardiopulmonary arrest during childhood may be largely caused by hypoxemia and respiratory insufficiency. Whenever the patient is unconscious and not breathing, the airway should be opened immediately by the *head tilt–chin lift* maneuver (Fig. 25-1). This procedure will pull the tongue and soft

---

BOX 25-1

CAUSES OF CARDIOPULMONARY ARREST IN PEDIATRIC AGE GROUPS

UPPER AIRWAY OBSTRUCTION
  Croup
  Epiglottitis
  Foreign body
  Suffocation

LOWER AIRWAY OBSTRUCTION
  Aspiration
  Severe asthma
  Pneumonia
  Pneumothorax
  Pulmonary edema
  Smoke inhalation

UNSTABLE CARDIOVASCULAR STATUS
  Dysrhythmias/arrhythmias
  Hemorrhage
  Inflammatory cardiac disorders

CENTRAL NERVOUS SYSTEM DISORDERS
  Anoxia
  Encephalitis
  Meningitis
  "Near-miss" sudden infant death syndrome

TABLE 25-1	COMPARISON OF BASIC LIFE SUPPORT MANEUVERS IN INFANTS AND CHILDREN	
Maneuver	**Infant (<1 Year)**	**Child (1 to 8 Years)**
Check responsiveness	Gentle stimulation (never shake)	Shake and shout
Open airway	Head tilt–chin lift (if trauma, use jaw thrust)	Head tilt–chin lift (if trauma, use jaw thrust)
Initial breath	2 breaths at 1-1.5 sec/breath	2 breaths at 1-1.5 sec/breath
Subsequent breaths	20 breaths/min	20 breaths/min
Foreign body airway obstruction	Back blows and chest thrusts (no abdominal thrusts)	Abdominal thrusts
Check pulse	Brachial	Carotid
Compression landmarks	Lower half of sternum; one fingerbreadth below intermammary line	Lower half of sternum
Compression method	2 fingers (one rescuer) 2 thumbs, encircling hands (two rescuers)	Heel of one hand
Compression depth	About one-third depth of chest	About one-third to one-half depth of chest
Compression rate	100/min	100/min
Compression/ventilation ratio	5:1	5:1

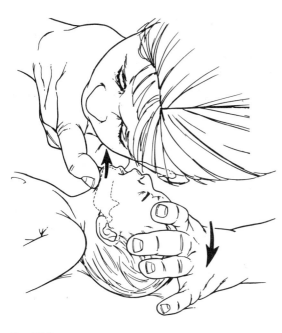

Fig. 25-1

Opening the airway with the head tilt–chin lift maneuver. One hand is used to tilt the head, extending the neck. The index finger of the rescuer's other hand lifts the mandible outward by lifting on the chin. Head tilt should not be performed if cervical spine injury is suspected. (From Guidelines for cardiopulmonary resuscitation and emergency cardiac care. *Resuscitation* 1992; 24(2):103-110.)

tissues away from the posterior pharynx, which may be the cause of airway obstruction in the unconscious patient. This procedure is performed by using the hand closest to the head to tilt the head back and, with the fingers of the other hand placed on the bony prominence of the lower jaw, lifting the chin upward. Care must be taken not to press on the soft tissues under the chin because this could obstruct the airway.

The *jaw thrust* is another method of opening an airway (Fig. 25-2). The rescuer places two or three fingers under each side of the lower jaw at its angle and lifts the jaw upward. The rescuer's elbow should rest on the surface on which the patient is lying. When there is no evidence of or concern for cervical spine injury, the jaw thrust may be accompanied by a slight head tilt when the jaw thrust alone does not open the airway. The jaw thrust, without head tilt, is the safest technique for opening the airway when neck injury is suspected.

5. *Breathing is assessed.* After the airway is opened by one of the preceding maneuvers, it must be determined if the patient is breathing. This can be accomplished by placing an ear close to the mouth and nose of the patient, observing for the chest or abdomen to rise and fall, and listening and feeling for expired air.

6. *Artificial ventilation is provided.* If there is no respiratory effort or if the respiratory effort is inadequate, the rescuer must maintain the head tilt–chin lift position and make a seal over the patient's mouth and/or nose. If ventilation is needed for an infant, a seal is made by placing the rescuer's

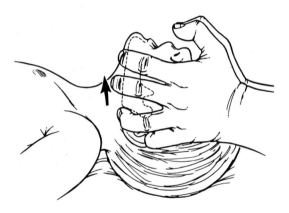

Fig. 25-2

Opening the airway with the jaw thrust maneuver. The airway is opened by lifting the angle of the mandible. The rescuer uses two or three fingers of each hand to lift the jaw while other fingers guide the jaw upward and outward. (From Guidelines for cardiopulmonary resuscitation and emergency cardiac care. *Resuscitation* 1992; 24(2):103-110.)

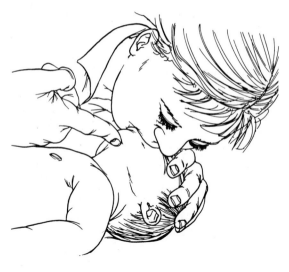

Fig. 25-3

Rescue breathing in an infant. The rescuer's mouth covers the infant's nose and mouth, creating a seal. One hand performs head tilt while the other hand lifts the infant's jaw. Avoid head tilt if the infant has sustained head or neck trauma. (From Guidelines for cardiopulmonary resuscitation and emergency cardiac care. *Resuscitation* 1992; 24(2):103-110.)

mouth over the infant's mouth and nose, or by providing mouth-to-nose ventilation if the infant's nose and mouth cannot be covered adequately (Fig. 25-3). A seal is made for a child by placing the rescuer's mouth over the child's mouth while pinching

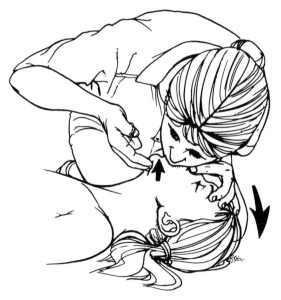

Fig. 25-4

Rescue breathing in a child. The rescuer's mouth covers the mouth of the child, creating a mouth-to-mouth seal. One hand maintains the head tilt; the thumb and forefinger of the same hand are used to pinch the child's nose. (From Guidelines for cardiopulmonary resuscitation and emergency cardiac care. *Resuscitation* 1992; 24(2):103-110.)

the nose shut (Fig. 25-4). Two slow breaths are then administered lasting 1 to 1.5 seconds each. A pause is allowed after each breath so that the rescuer can take a breath of fresh air.

The volume of air administered must be sufficient to make the chest rise. If immediately available, rescue breathing should be provided by a mask with a one-way valve or another mouth-to-mask barrier device. Face masks are available in a variety of sizes. The proper size is selected to provide an airtight seal on the face; the mask should extend from the bridge of the nose to the cleft of the chin (Figs. 25-5 and 25-6). Maintaining an adequate seal of the face mask to the face can be ensured if the rescuer remembers to create the seal by bringing the "face to the mask" rather than pushing the mask onto the face. This method allows the airway to be kept open by gentle pressure under the jaw while creating an adequate seal.

It is important that throughout rescue breathing the chest rises and falls with each breath. If this does not occur, air is not freely entering the airways. The most common causes of inadequate rise and fall of the chest are airway obstruction or insufficient breath volume or pressure. Repeated repositioning of the head or increasing the pressure of the rescuer's breath, or both, should be attempted until there is

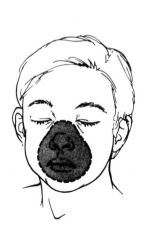

Fig. 25-5

Area of the face for a face mask. (From *Textbook of pediatric advanced life support.* 1988, American Heart Association.)

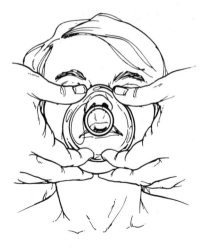

Fig. 25-6

Two-handed face mask application technique. A second person is needed to ventilate. (From *Textbook of pediatric advanced life support.* 1988, American Heart Association.)

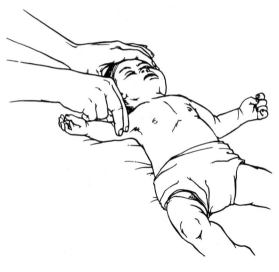

Fig. 25-7

Palpating the brachial artery pulse. (From Guidelines for cardiopulmonary resuscitation and emergency cardiac care. *Resuscitation* 1992; 24(2):103-110.)

adequate rise and fall of the chest. It is important to remember that rescue breathing, especially if performed rapidly, may cause gastric distention.[1,13,14] Excessive gastric distention in turn can interfere with rescue breathing by elevating the diaphragm and decreasing lung volume. Providing slow breaths during rescue breathing can minimize this problem.

7. *Circulation is assessed.* Once the airway is opened and two rescue breaths have been provided, the rescuer must assess the patient's cardiovascular status and the need for chest compressions. The optimal site to check the pulse in pediatric patients depends on the patient's age. In infants the *brachial pulse* is palpated on the arm nearest the rescuer (Fig. 25-7). The brachial pulse is located on the medial aspect of the upper arm between the elbow and shoulder. The pulse is palpated by placing the thumb on the outside of the arm and the index and middle fingers on the inside of the arm and gently pressing toward the bone.

In children older than 1 year the *carotid pulse* is palpated on the side of the neck nearest the rescuer (Fig. 25-8). In pediatric patients, the femoral artery is an alternative location to palpate for the presence or lack of a pulse. The precordial area is not a reliable site for assessing circulation. The presence or lack of the precordial impulse may be mistaken for the presence or lack of a pulse, and an erroneous decision may be made about the need for CPR.

Some studies show that lay people as well as health care professionals have difficulty correctly identifying the presence or absence of a pulse in 5 to 10 seconds.[15-17] Although the pulse check is still recommended in the sequence of BLS for the health care professional, the rescuer is instructed to take only a few seconds to palpate a pulse. Other signs of circulation should be used as well, including breathing, coughing, or movement in response to rescue breathing.[1] Because the reported complication rate from chest compressions is low in infants and children, if a pulse cannot be detected in a few seconds, cardiac compressions should be initiated.[1,18]

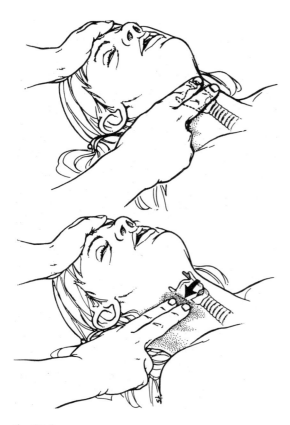

Fig. 25-8

Locating and palpating the carotid artery pulse in the child. (From Guidelines for cardiopulmonary resuscitation and emergency cardiac care. *Resuscitation* 1992; 24(2):103-110.)

8. *If a pulse is present and breathing is absent, rescue breathing is performed.* In both an infant and child, the rate is 20 times per minute, or one breath every 3 seconds.

9. *If no pulse is palpated, rescue breathing and external chest compressions are begun.* In infants and children, chest compressions should be performed if no pulse is detected or heart rate is less than 60 beats/min with signs of poor perfusion.

If there is no evidence of cervical spine injury, an infant is placed in a horizontal position on a firm surface. If the infant's shoulders lift off the surface when a head tilt is performed, a towel is placed under the shoulders to make a hard surface, or the hand not performing the compressions is placed under the shoulders. Head tilt is then maintained by the weight of the head and a slight lift of the shoulders. Rescue breaths should be given *slowly* (1 to 1.5 seconds' duration) to ensure adequate ventilation and reduce the likelihood of gastric distention.[1]

Unlike adult rescue, trained pediatric rescuers should provide approximately 1 minute of BLS

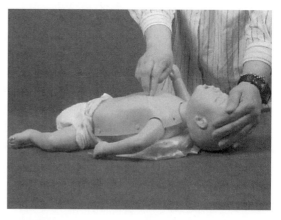

Fig. 25-9

Locating proper finger position for chest compression in an infant. Note that the rescuer's other hand is used to maintain head position to facilitate ventilation.

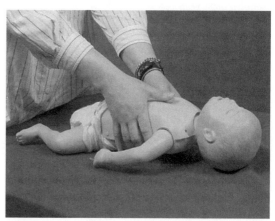

Fig. 25-10

Two thumb-encircling hands chest compression for infants.

before calling EMS. In the hospital setting a call for help or push of a "code blue" button would be done immediately on establishing unresponsiveness. To keep suggested numbers easy to recall, rescuers should provide 20 breaths or perform 20 cycles of five compressions and one ventilation before leaving the patient to call EMS.

The optimal rate and method of compression have not been determined. In an infant, the recommended location for chest compressions is the lower half of the sternum, approximately one fingerbreadth below the *intermammary line,* an imaginary line between the nipples. For one rescuer, the index and middle fingers are used to compress the chest (Fig. 25-9).[1] If two rescuers are present, the two thumb-encircling hands chest compression is preferred (Fig. 25-10).[1]

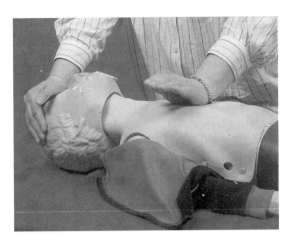

Fig. 25-11

Locating hand position for chest compression in the child. Note that the rescuer's other hand is used to maintain head position to facilitate ventilation.

Because of the difference in size of the hands and in each infant's chest, careful assessment must be made to avoid pressing the xiphoid process. In the very small infant, the thumbs may need to be placed on top of each other to avoid excessive pressure on the ribs. The depth of the compressions is approximately one-third the depth of the chest.[1] The rate of compressions is at least 100 times per minute.

For chest compressions in the child, the heel of one hand is placed over the lower half of the sternum (Fig. 25-11). Compressions are performed with the heel of one hand on the sternum while the other hand maintains head position. The depth of compressions is one-third to one-half the depth of the child's chest. The rate of the compressions is 100 times per minute.

External chest compressions must always be performed in combination with rescue breathing. In the infant and child, a ratio of five compressions to one breath is given. At the end of every fifth compression, the rescuer pauses to give slow ventilation, 1 to 1.5 seconds per breath. In the infant, after every fifth compression, the rescuer leaves the fingers in light contact with the chest while lowering his or her head to give a breath. The airway is maintained by a slight head tilt or by the weight of the head and slight lift of the shoulders. In the child, after every fifth compression, the rescuer lifts the heel of the hand from the chest and performs a head tilt–chin lift maneuver for ventilation. The hand closest to the feet is then visually placed in the proper location on the chest for each round of compressions. CPR is continued for 1 minute. The infant or child is reassessed for spontaneous breathing and a pulse. If

absent, CPR is continued, commencing with chest compressions.

AUTOMATED EXTERNAL DEFIBRILLATION

The previous BLS steps have been discussed in regard to infants and children up to age 8 years. It is difficult for pediatric health care providers to classify patients between ages 8 and 14 or 15 years as adults, but the strict definitions of the American Heart Association consider any child age 8 or older to be an adult. Since about 1997, use of the automated external defibrillator (AED) has been taught as a didactic portion of BLS courses. AEDs have improved out-of-hospital cardiac arrest outcomes in adults. The recommendation for use of AEDs now extends to the pediatric population who are age 8 (approximately 25 kg) or older. The current AEDs begin defibrillation at 200 J, which is a larger dose than would be required for most pediatric patients younger than 8 years. The other consideration is that most pediatric arrests are caused by bradyarrhythmias or asystole, not ventricular fibrillation or pulseless ventricular tachycardia.[1] Current research addresses the possibility of adapting AEDs to deliver charges in the infant and pediatric range.

PEDIATRIC ADVANCED LIFE SUPPORT

RHYTHM DISTURBANCES

The electrocardiogram (ECG) in all critically ill or injured children must be continuously monitored. In contrast to adults, whose rhythm disturbances are caused by intrinsic heart disease, pediatric patients have essentially normal hearts. Pediatric dysrhythmias are usually caused by prolonged exposure to hypoxia and acidosis as a complication of trauma or disease. Because of this commonality in origin, pediatric rhythms can be more easily categorized.

Pediatric dysrhythmias can be classified as *fast, slow,* or *absent.* Furthermore, these rhythms can be classified as to the patient's clinical condition: *stable* or *unstable.* A pediatric patient who is near death will have one of the following five common cardiac rhythms:

1. Bradycardia: slow, stable or unstable
2. Asystole: absent, unstable
3. Ventricular fibrillation (VF) or pulseless ventricular tachycardia (VT): fast, unstable
4. Supraventricular tachycardia (SVT): fast, stable or unstable
5. Electromechanical dissociation (EMD), or pulseless electrical activity (PEA): absent, unstable

Terminal rhythms in infants and children infrequently are ventricular in origin.[19,20] A study of terminal rhythms in this population found that ventricular rhythms accounted for only 6% of all rhythms, with all of the ventricular rhythms occurring in children with congenital heart disease.[21] Most often, cardiopulmonary collapse in infants and children is associated with *asystole* (absence of rhythm) or *idioventricular bradycardia.*

The maintenance of cardiac output is dependent on heart rate and stroke volume (the amount of blood volume ejected by the heart with each beat). Rhythm disturbances affect either heart rate or stroke volume, with a subsequent decrease in cardiac output. Any rhythm associated with a loss of palpable pulses or a substantial decrease in cardiac output requires maintenance of cardiac output with chest compressions, along with ventilation with a fractional concentration of inspired oxygen (FIO_2) of 1.0 to maintain tissue oxygen needs.

Bradyarrhythmias, Slow, Stable or Unstable. In bradyarrhythmias, cardiac output is compromised by a decreasing heart rate, whereas stroke volume is normal. Excessive vagal stimulation (e.g., suctioning) may produce bradycardia. In addition, conduction through and function of the sinus node are impaired by hypoxemia, acidosis, and hypotension. All slow rhythms that result in cardiovascular instability require immediate attention with reversal of the cause of hypoxemia, acidosis, hypotension, or increased vagal tone.

The approach to the bradycardic patient should include assessment of the airway, breathing, and circulation (ABCs), followed by securing an airway, administering 100% oxygen, and establishing vascular access (intraosseous or intravascular). Importantly, subsequent steps should not be delayed because of attempts to obtain vascular access. The bradycardic patient needs to be assessed in regard to the severity of cardiorespiratory compromise. Despite adequacy of oxygenation and ventilation, if the heart rate is less than 60 beats/min in an infant or child *and* the patient has poor perfusion (capillary refill of 3 seconds or longer), hypotension for age, or respiratory difficulties, chest compressions should be initiated. Pharmacologic therapy with epinephrine repeated every 3 to 5 minutes and atropine (two doses) may then be administered to reverse the bradycardia. If the patient with a bradycardic rhythm on assessment has no signs of cardiorespiratory compromise, only observation with frequent reassessments, continued support of the ABCs, and determination of cause are required.

Electromechanical Dissociation (Pulseless Electric Activity). In electromechanical dissociation, cardiac output is compromised because there is an electric signal but not a mechanical response. Thus both heart rate and stroke volume are compromised. Occasionally, cardiopulmonary collapse with no palpable pulses is observed in children with organized electrical activity on the ECG. Collapse may be caused by severe hypoxemia, acidosis, hypovolemia, tension pneumothorax, profound hypothermia, or pericardial tamponade. Therapy consists of assessment of the ABCs, with determination of pulselessness and institution of ventilation, oxygenation, and CPR. Vascular access should be obtained (intravascular or intraosseous), and epinephrine should be administered every 3 to 5 minutes. The cause must be investigated and resolved for patients with electromechanical dissociation to survive.

Pulseless Ventricular Tachycardia and Ventricular Fibrillation. When there is no congenital heart disease, VT and VF are rare in children. The pathophysiology of these rhythms is cardiac output compromised by a marked increase in heart rate with a marked decrease in stroke volume. Treatment involves first determining pulselessness and beginning CPR and then confirming cardiac rhythm in more than one lead. After establishment of an airway, CPR, and ventilation with an FIO_2 of 1.0, vascular access can be attempted. Any attempt at vascular access should not delay the definitive therapy of defibrillation. Defibrillation is administered with 2 J/kg followed by 4 J/kg, repeated twice if the first attempt is unsuccessful. If defibrillation is unsuccessful, epinephrine and lidocaine (or amiodarone[1]) are administered, and another 4-J/kg defibrillation is attempted 30 to 60 seconds after the medication is administered. If unsuccessful again, doses of epinephrine, lidocaine, and/or amiodarone are repeated, followed by another defibrillation with 4 J/kg 30 to 60 seconds after the medication is administered.

Because primary ventricular arrhythmias are rare in children, other causes of these dysrhythmias must be considered, including metabolic abnormalities (e.g., potassium, calcium, glucose, or magnesium imbalance), hypothermia, severe hypoxemia, acidosis, or drug toxicity (digitalis or tricyclic antidepressants).

Supraventricular Tachycardia: Fast, Stable or Unstable. SVT is a fast rhythm, with heart rates usually between 240 and 300 beats/min. This rhythm is most common during infancy. Unlike VT and VF, the SVT rhythm is not caused by hypoxemia, acidosis, or a complication of disease. SVT is caused by a reentrant mechanism by which an electrical impulse is abnormally propagated. The stability of the infant with SVT is related to the child's age, ventricular function, ventricular rate, and duration of the SVT. If SVT with high rates persists for a prolonged period, cardiac output is compromised because of the fast rate with decreased stroke volume. Clinically, the unstable SVT patient presents with signs of shock.

The treatment of SVT in an unstable patient is with synchronized cardioversion at a starting dose of 0.5 J/kg. If vascular access is available, adenosine may be administered (see later discussion). In the unstable patient, however, cardioversion must not be delayed to obtain vascular access. In the stable patient with SVT, adenosine is the drug of choice.[1,22,23]

EMERGENCY DRUGS

Even though most pediatric arrests are caused by respiratory problems, a knowledge of pharmacologic agents is essential to the successful resuscitation of a pediatric patient. Resuscitative drug administration in pediatric patients is considered a difficult part of advanced pediatric life support because drug dosages vary with the child's weight. To reduce errors in drug administration, a precalculated drug sheet should be generated for each patient admitted to the hospital, and a drug poster listing patient age, weight, and proper drug dosage should be available in the emergency department. If neither of these is available, a device such as a Broselow tape, which lists drug dosages by the length of the patient, should be available.

Epinephrine, atropine, and lidocaine can be given through the endotracheal tube (ETT) when vascular access is delayed.

Epinephrine is an endogenous catecholamine with α- and β-adrenergic properties used in asystole and pulseless arrest and profound bradycardia. The most important pharmacologic action in cardiac arrest is α-adrenergic–mediated vasoconstriction. This causes restoration of aortic diastolic pressure, which has been shown to be a critical determinant of success or failure in resuscitation.[24] During CPR, epinephrine has been shown to elevate perfusion pressure generated during cardiac compression, improve myocardial contractility, stimulate spontaneous contractions, and increase myocardial tone, enhancing the conversion of fine ventricular fibrillation to coarse ventricular fibrillation, which is more susceptible to cardioversion.[1,25,26] Epinephrine's vasoconstrictive properties increase perfusion pressure during chest compressions, which enhances delivery of oxygen to the heart. However, it is important to maintain adequate ventilation, oxygenation, and circulation in addition to the administration of epinephrine because the action of catecholamines can be depressed by acidosis or hypoxemia.[27] Dosage depends on the type of arrest. In asystolic or pulseless arrest the first intravenous (IV) or intraosseous (IO)

dose is 0.01 mg/kg (1:10,000); the first dose through the ETT is 0.1 mg/kg (1:1000). Doses as high as 0.2 mg/kg may be effective.[28] The results from other research using high-dose epinephrine have been disappointing.[29]

Although return of spontaneous circulation was improved with high-dose epinephrine, heart rate and blood pressure were elevated. Other costs of epinephrine administration are increased myocardial oxygen demand, reduced subendocardial vascular perfusion, systemic and intracranial hypertension, intracranial hemorrhage, myocardial hemorrhage, and necrosis.[1,28-31] The outcomes were no different in terms of survival.[28,29] Without further study, high-dose epinephrine cannot be confidently recommended.[1] For bradycardia the dose is 0.01 mg/kg (1:10,000) IV or IO or 0.1 mg/kg (1:1000) through ETT. Escalation of epinephrine doses is not recommended in bradyarrhythmias.

Atropine is the competitive antagonist of acetylcholine and is used to treat bradycardia accompanied by poor perfusion or hypotension. Again, bradycardia in infants and children usually reflects the adverse effects of a severe myocardial hypoxic-ischemic insult rather than the occurrence of heart block. Atropine may be useful to antagonize excess vagal activity during intubation. The dose is 0.02 mg/kg, with a minimum dose of 0.1 mg. A dose of less than 0.1 mg can cause paradoxical bradycardia. The dose can be repeated at 5-minute intervals. The maximum dose is 0.5 mg in a child and 1 mg in an adolescent.

Lidocaine reduces the automaticity and ectopic pacemakers of the ventricles and increases the fibrillation threshold. There are limited reports of lidocaine's effectiveness in children; it is recommended for VT and VF based on its extensive use in adults.[29] This drug is used in the treatment of ventricular ectopy; the dose is 1 mg/kg.[32]

Amiodarone is a highly lipid-soluble antiarrhythmic used for a wide range of both atrial and ventricular arrhythmias in adults and children. It is a noncompetitive inhibitor of both α- and β-adrenergic receptors. IV administration of amiodarone produces vasodilation and atrioventricular (AV) nodal suppression. For refractory pulseless VT or VF the dose is 5 mg/kg in rapid IV/IO bolus. For perfusing SVT or ventricular arrhythmias the loading dose is 5 mg/kg over 20 to 60 minutes, up to a maximum of 15 mg/kg/day.[1]

Adenosine is an endogenous nucleoside used in SVT that acutely slows AV nodal conduction, causing short-term asystole (10 to 15 seconds) to allow for conversion to a slower rhythm. Adenosine also causes arterial and coronary vasodilation.[33] The half-life of adenosine is approximately 10 seconds, so it must be rapidly administered via IV push followed immediately by a flush of normal saline. This rapid infusion will maximize the dose of the drug that reaches the heart. The initial dose should be 0.1 mg/kg; this can be doubled to 0.2 mg/kg if the first dose is not effective.[1]

Calcium chloride is no longer recommended in asystole or electromechanical dissociation. It is used in the treatment of documented hypocalcemia, hypermagnesemia, and overdose with calcium channel blocking agents. The dose is 20 mg/kg. The dose may be repeated one time in 10 minutes. Further doses must be based on calcium deficiencies.

Magnesium is a major intracellular cation and serves as a cofactor in more than 300 enzymatic reactions.[1] Magnesium can inhibit calcium channels, reducing intracellular calcium and causing smooth muscle relaxation. Magnesium has proven useful in the treatment of torsades de pointes VT with dosages of 25 to 50 mg/kg (maximum 2 g) IV over 10 to 20 minutes.[1]

Sodium bicarbonate is used in the treatment of metabolic acidosis accompanying cardiac arrest. During arrest, metabolic acidosis results from anaerobic metabolism that produces excess lactate and hydrogen ions. Anaerobic metabolism results from inadequate organ blood flow and is typically exacerbated by poor oxygenation. Because respiratory conditions are the most common cause of cardiac arrest in pediatric patients, ventilation is a prime consideration. Bicarbonate may be given in a dose of 1 mEq/kg in prolonged cardiac arrest once adequate ventilation has been established.

Glucose must be administered in the event of documented hypoglycemia. The recommended dose is 0.5 to 1 g/kg IV.

EQUIPMENT

Oxygen. In critically ill patients, oxygen delivery may be limited by inadequate circulatory volume or function or inadequate pulmonary gas exchange, or both; therefore oxygen should be administered immediately. Because oxygen delivery to the tissues may be compromised, oxygen should be administered to the patient even if measured arterial oxygen levels are high. In a spontaneously breathing patient, oxygen can be delivered by many different devices. In pediatric patients who are anxious, the best delivery device is the one the child will tolerate.

Airway Devices. If procedures to open the airway of an unconscious infant or child fail to provide a clear, unobstructed airway, an oropharyngeal airway is indicated. Oropharyngeal airways should never be used in conscious or semiconscious patients, how-

ever, because of the increased risk of vomiting caused by the patient's gagging on the airway.

Face Masks. For pediatric patients requiring ventilatory assistance, an age-appropriate face mask must be available. A properly fitting face mask is one that provides an airtight seal without excessive pressure on the eyes (see Fig. 25-5). In larger pediatric patients or in those with poorly compliant lungs, two hands may be required to maintain an airtight seal (see Fig. 25-6).

Resuscitation Bags. Resuscitation bags in children, as in infants, should have a minimum volume of 450 ml. Two types of resuscitation bags are available for the pediatric patient: the self-inflating bag and the non–self-inflating or anesthesia bag. To deliver oxygen concentrations of 60% to 95%, the self-inflating resuscitation bag requires an oxygen reservoir. The minimum flow rate for this type of pediatric bag is at least 10 to 15 L/min.[34] Successful use of the other type, the anesthesia bag, requires attention to the flow of gas, correct adjustment of the flow control valve, and careful attention to a tight seal at the face mask. To control all these factors, more training is required with the non–self-inflating than with the self-inflating bag. Appropriate use of the anesthesia bag requires constant monitoring of peak ventilatory pressures through a port with an attached pressure manometer. The anesthesia bag does offer the advantage of being able to provide more reliable control of oxygen concentration and a greater range of peak inspiratory pressures.

DEFIBRILLATION AND SYNCHRONIZED CARDIOVERSION

In pediatric patients with VF or pulseless VTs, untimed (asynchronous) depolarization of the myocardium is used to reestablish a normal rhythm. If the myocardium is oxygenated and acidosis is not excessive, defibrillation may produce a simultaneous depolarization of a critical mass of myocardial cells and allow the resumption of spontaneous depolarization. In the apneic and pulseless infant and child, ventilation, oxygenation, and chest compressions must be provided until a productive rhythm is reestablished. Defibrillation has not been shown to be effective in the treatment of asystolic arrest.[35] Although the optimal amount of electrical energy for the pediatric patient has not been conclusively established, data suggest an initial dose of 2 J/kg.[36] If this dose is unsuccessful, the energy dose should be doubled and repeated at 4 J/kg.

Synchronized cardioversion, in contrast to defibrillation, is the timed (synchronized) depolarization of myocardial cells. In symptomatic patients with SVT or VT, as well as poor perfusion, hypotension, or heart failure, synchronized cardioversion is used to produce a stable rhythm. The initial energy dose is usually 0.5 J/kg.

POSTRESUSCITATION STABILIZATION

The goal of care after resuscitation is to enable the patient to arrive at a tertiary care setting in the best possible physiologic state by avoiding exacerbation of the patient's primary problem and secondary organ injury. Postresuscitation stabilization should follow the ABCs of the initial resuscitation. During the postresuscitation period, deterioration often occurs after a brief period of stability; therefore frequent reassessments are necessary. Continuous monitoring of the patient's physiologic stability with a cardiorespiratory monitor, pulse oximetry, and end-tidal carbon dioxide determinations is recommended. During the reevaluation, attention should be paid not only to information obtained from monitors but also to the patient's clinical evaluation.

RISK OF INFECTION DURING CPR TRAINING AND RESCUE

Transmission of the hepatitis B virus (HBV) and human immunodeficiency virus (HIV) from patients to health care workers has been documented in cases of blood exchange or penetration of the skin by blood-contaminated instruments. Performance of mouth-to-mouth resuscitation or invasive procedures can result in exchange of blood between victim and rescuer if either has had breaks in the skin around the lips or soft tissues of the oral mucosa. The probability of a rescuer becoming infected with HBV or HIV as a result of performing CPR is minimal.[37] To date, transmission of HBV or HIV infection during mouth-to-mouth resuscitation has not been documented.[38]

Compared with HIV and HBV, the theoretic risk of infection is greater for salivary or aerosol transmission of herpes simplex and *Neisseria meningitidis* and for transmission of airborne diseases such as tuberculosis and respiratory infections. To minimize the risk of transmission of a variety of diseases, however, mechanical ventilation or barrier devices should be accessible to the health care worker, although their efficacy in preventing disease transmission has not been demonstrated conclusively. Early intubation should be encouraged when the equipment and trained professionals are available. Intubation obviates the need for mouth-to-mouth resuscitation and is more effective than the use of bag-mask devices.

BARRIERS TO EFFECTIVE CPR

The performance of CPR starts with the willingness of the rescuer to provide assistance. The first barrier to effective CPR involves the decision to perform mouth-to-mouth ventilation. In a survey of health care professionals, 57% would perform mouth-to-mouth ventilation on hospitalized children with an unknown HIV status, and 79% would perform mouth-to-mouth if the child was known to be HIV negative.[38] In general, as the level of familiarity with the victim decreased, so did the willingness to perform mouth-to-mouth ventilation.[39]

The second barrier to effective CPR is rescuer fatigue. One study using manikins showed that the quality of compressions decreased significantly within the first minute.[40] Decrease in compression quality preceded feelings of fatigue expressed by the participants.

The third potential barrier involves the rescuers doing the chest compressions and their level of training and experience. Pediatric arrests are an infrequent occurrence, even in pediatric hospitals, which means few people have much experience. The person with the extra set of hands does compressions and may be a student who has never done compressions on a person. Physicians rarely do compressions because they are usually managing the airway, starting IV lines, giving drugs, controlling traffic, and recording events.

In the hospital, barrier devices should be in every patient room, as well as waiting rooms and the cafeteria. This eliminates the need to make a decision about performing mouth-to-mouth ventilation. Bag-valve-masks and intubation equipment should be available on the crash cart. Even in the hospital, however, fatigue is a factor and affects the question of who should perform compressions. Regardless of who does compressions, someone must be constantly checking to ensure adequate compressions. Once compression quality diminishes, another person should take over. Without effective compressions, there is no blood flow to the essential organs, and drugs given to treat the arrest cannot be circulated.

REFERENCES

1. International Consensus on Science: Guidelines 2000 for cardiopulmonary resuscitation and emergency cardiovascular care. *Circulation* 2000; 102(suppl I):1-384.
2. Zaritsky A et al: CPR in children. *Ann Emerg Med* 1987; 16:1107-1111.
3. O'Rourke PP: Outcome of children who are apneic and pulseless in the emergency room. *Crit Care Med* 1986; 14:466-468.

4. Ronco R et al: Outcome and cost at a children's hospital following resuscitation for out-of-hospital cardiopulmonary arrest. *Arch Pediatr Adolesc Med* 1995; 149(2):210-214.

5. Torres A et al: Long-term functional outcome of inpatient pediatric cardiopulmonary resuscitation. *Pediatr Emerg Care* 1997; 13(6):369-373.

6. Lewis JK et al: Outcome of pediatric resuscitation. *Ann Emerg Med* 1983; 12:297-299.

7. Weisfeldt ML: Recent advances in cardiopulmonary resuscitation. *Jpn Circ J* 1985; 49:13-24.

8. Babbs CF et al: CPR with simultaneous compression and ventilation at high airway pressure in 4 animal models. *Crit Care Med* 1982; 10:501-504.

9. Eisenberg M, Bergner L, Hallstrom A: Epidemiology of cardiac arrest and resuscitation in children. *Ann Emerg Med* 1983; 12:672-674.

10. Centers for Disease Control, Division of Injury Control, Center for Environmental Health and Injury Control: Childhood injuries in the United States. *Am J Dis Child* 1990; 144:627-646.

11. Frei FJ et al: Respiratory and circulatory arrest in pediatric patients. *Acta Anaesth Scand Suppl* 1997; 111:200-201.

12. Gillis J et al: Results of inpatient pediatric resuscitation. *Crit Care Med* 1986; 14:469-471.

13. Wenzel V et al: Influence of tidal volume on the distribution of gas between the lungs and stomach in the nonintubated patient receiving positive-pressure ventilation. *Crit Care Med* 1998; 26(2):364-368.

14. A reappraisal of mouth-to-mouth ventilation during bystander-initiated cardiopulmonary resuscitation. A statement for healthcare professionals from the Ventilation Working Group of the Basic Life Support and Pediatric Life Support Subcommittees, American Heart Association. *Circulation* 1997; 96(6):2102-2112.

15. Cavallaro DL, Melker RJ: Comparison of two techniques for detecting cardiac activity in infants. *Crit Care Med* 1983; 11:189-190.

16. Lee CJ, Bullock LJ: Determining pulse for infant CPR: time for a change? *Milit Med* 1991; 156:190-191.

17. Flesche CW et al: The ability of health professionals to check the carotid pulse. *Circulation* 1994 (abstract); 90(suppl):1-288.

18. Hazinski MF: Basic life support: controversial and unresolved issues. *J Cardiovasc Nurs* 1996; 10(4):1-14.

19. Eisenberg M, Bergner L, Hallstrom A: Epidemiology of cardiac arrest and resuscitation in children. *Ann Emerg Med* 1983; 12:672-674.

20. Torphy DE, Minter MG, Thompson BM: Cardiorespiratory arrest and resuscitation of children. *Am J Dis Child* 1984; 138:1099-1102.

21. Walsh CK, Krongrad E: Terminal cardiac electrical activity in pediatric patients. *Am J Cardiol* 1983; 51:557-561.

22. Overholt ED et al: Usefulness of adenosine for arrhythmias in infants and children. *Am J Cardiol* 1988; 61:336-340.

23. Till J et al: Efficacy and safety of adenosine in the treatment of supraventricular tachycardia in infants and children. *Br Heart J* 1989; 62:204-211.

24. Sanders A, Ewy G, Taft T: Prognostic and therapeutic importance of the aortic diastolic pressure in resuscitation from cardiac arrest. *Crit Care Med* 1984; 12:871-878.

25. Zaritsky A, Chernow B: Use of catecholamines in pediatrics. *J Pediatr* 1984; 105:341-350.

26. Otto CW, Yakaitis RW, Blitt CS: Mechanism of action of epinephrine in resuscitation from asphyxial arrest. *Crit Care Med* 1981; 9:321-324.

27. Stokke DB et al: Acid-base interactions with noradrenaline-induced contractile response of the rabbit isolated aorta. *Anesthesia* 1984; 60:400-404.

28. Goetting MG, Paradis NA: High-dose epinephrine improves outcome from pediatric cardiac arrest. *Ann Emerg Med* 1991; 20:22-26.

29. Gelband H, Rosen M: Pharmacologic basis for treatment of cardiac arrhythmias. *Pediatrics* 1975; 55:59-67.

30. Berg RA et al: A randomized, blinded trial of high-dose epinephrine versus standard-dose epinephrine in a swine model of pediatric asphyxial cardiac arrest. *Crit Care Med* 1996; 24(10):1695-1700.

31. Thrush DN, Downs JB, Smith RA: Is epinephrine contraindicated during cardiopulmonary resuscitation? *Circulation* 1997; 96(8):2709-2714.

32. Ushay HM, Notterman DA: Pharmacology of pediatric resuscitation. *Pediatr Clin North Am* 1997; 44(1):207-233.

33. Frishman WH, Vahdat S, Bhatta S: Innovative pharmacologic approaches to cardiopulmonary resuscitation. *J Clin Pharmacol* 1998; 38:765–772.

34. Finer NN et al: Limitations of self-inflating resuscitators. *Pediatrics* 1986; 77:417-420.

35. Losek JD et al: Prehospital countershock treatment of pediatric asystole. *Am J Emerg Med* 1989; 7:571-575.

36. Gutgesell HP et al: Energy dose for ventricular defibrillation of children. *Pediatrics* 1976; 58:898-901.

37. Centers for Disease Control: Guidelines for prevention of transmission of human immunodeficiency virus and hepatitis B virus to health care and public safety workers. *MMWR* 1989; 38(6, suppl):1-37.

38. Sande MA: Transmissions of AIDS: the case against causal contagion. *N Engl J Med* 1986; 314:380-382.

39. Horowitz BZ, Matheny L: Health care professionals' willingness to do mouth-to-mouth resuscitation. *West J Med* 1997; 167:392-397.

40. Ochoa FJ et al: The effect of rescuer fatigue on the quality of chest compressions. *Resuscitation* 1998; 37:149-152.

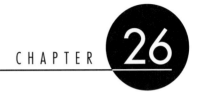

CHAPTER 26

Pharmacology

Robert G. Aucoin

Although most marketed drugs are used in pediatrics, only about one fourth of the drugs approved by the U.S. Food and Drug Administration (FDA) have a specific indication for use in neonatal and pediatric patients. Many differences exist among neonatal, pediatric, and adult patients with regard to a drug's pharmacokinetics, pharmacodynamics, and efficacy, and pediatric dosage regimens should not be simply extrapolated from adult data.[1]

Drug absorption, distribution, and metabolism vary greatly in neonatal and pediatric patients. Both physiochemical and physiologic factors affect drug distribution. Effects depend on the drug's specific pharmacologic properties. Clinically, this can lead to increased or decreased requirements for loading doses, dosing interval, metabolic rate, and time to excretion. Drug metabolism is slower in infants than in older children and adults, and even slower in premature infants. Between ages 1 and 9 years, metabolic rate increases to exceed that of the premature infant and the adult. Disease states may also alter drug dosing, metabolism, and elimination.[1]

Great progress has been made in the past few years in pediatric pharmacokinetics. The FDA Modernization Act of 1997, the 1998 Pediatric Final Rule, and the Children's Health Act of 2000 were designed to help increase pediatric studies of drugs. Together they provide increased support for pediatric clinical research and require pharmaceutical companies to conduct pediatric drug studies by allowing additional time for market exclusivity to designated drugs.[2]

β-ADRENERGIC AGONISTS

MECHANISM OF ACTION

β-Adrenergic agonists are the treatment of choice for managing acute exacerbations of asthma as well as acute episodes of bronchospasm. Activation of β-adrenergic receptor sites on airway smooth muscle results in activation of adenyl cyclase, which increases the production of cyclic

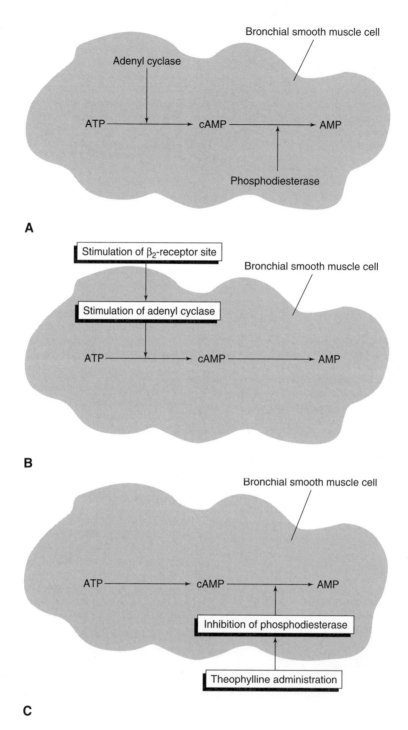

Fig. 26-1

A, Sympathetic mechanisms controlling bronchial muscle tone. The enzyme adenyl cyclase is the catalyst for the conversion of adenosine triphosphate *(ATP)* to cyclic adenosine monophosphate *(cAMP)*. The enzyme phosphodiesterase breaks down cAMP into adenosine monophosphate *(AMP)*. Increased levels of cAMP result in relaxation of bronchial smooth muscle. Decreased levels of cAMP lead to spasm of susceptible bronchial smooth muscle. **B,** Bronchial muscle receptors are called β_2-receptor sites. Stimulation of these sites results in stimulation of the enzyme adenyl cyclase, which produces an increased level of cAMP, resulting in bronchodilation. **C,** Administration of the methylxanthine theophylline inhibits the enzyme phosphodiesterase, which inhibits the breakdown of cAMP and results in increased levels of cAMP and bronchodilation.

adenosine monophosphate (cAMP). This increase results in bronchial smooth muscle relaxation and skeletal muscle stimulation and also inhibits the release of inflammatory mediators through stabilization of the mast cell membrane[3] (Fig. 26-1). This in turn slows progression of the inflammatory cascade.

ADVERSE EVENTS

Aerosol administration results in effective activation of bronchial β_2-receptors with minimal systemic adverse effects. Adverse effects occur through excessive activation of β-adrenergic receptors and are more common with the use of nonselective β-adrenergic agonists than with the selective β_2-adrenergic agonists given parenterally or orally.[4]

Stimulation of the β_2-receptors in skeletal muscle results in *tremor,* the most common adverse effect observed with the use of selective agents. Tolerance to the tremor generally develops over time. Vasodilation is observed when β_2-receptors in the peripheral vasculature are stimulated. Tachycardia is observed most often as a result of stimulation of the β_1-receptors of the heart. Direct stimulation of cardiac β_2-receptors and reflex mechanisms from the peripheral vasodilation also increase heart rate. Headache, nervousness, dizziness, palpitations, cough, nausea, vomiting, and throat irritation may also occur.[5] All these adverse effects are much less likely with inhalation therapy than with parenteral or oral therapy.[6-8] It has also been postulated that the (S)-isomers of the β-agonist are the culprits in the majority of side effects. When reviewing the side effect profile of levalbuterol it is possible to extend those same positive attributes to other β-agonists.[4]

Tolerance to the effects of β-adrenergic agonists has been extensively studied both in vitro and in vivo. Although long-term use of systemic β-agonists can lead to some tolerance, tolerance to the pulmonary effects of these drugs is probably not a major clinical problem for most asthmatic patients who do not exceed recommended dosages over a long period. Systemic tolerance occurs as a result of chronic administration, which decreases the number of β_2-receptors and decreases the binding affinity of the receptors.[3,5] A *subsensitivity* to allergen and methacholine in patients who regularly use β_2-agonists has been reported.[6,9] The subsensitivity was not overcome by high-dose albuterol. More studies are needed to determine the clinical importance of this phenomenon.

Overuse of inhaled β_2-agonists has been associated with increased mortality from asthma. This increased risk of sudden death was greater in patients using more than one canister of rescue inhaler each month. The cardiotoxic potential of β_2-agonists may increase mortality risk, as may overreliance on medication and the patient's comfort level with β_2-agonist use. Control of symptoms may postpone obtaining adequate medical care in the presence of worsening asthma. With use of a powerful bronchodilator the perceived need for corticosteroid therapy may not be realized. These patients also may have more severe disease. These concerns have led to the recommendation that when possible, these medications be used only on an "as needed" basis. Regular dosing schedules should be reserved for the management of acute episodes.[10-13]

SELECTIVE AGENTS

Selective agents have a more specific effect on β_2-receptors, with minimal effect on β_1-receptors, so that less stimulation of the heart rate is observed.[14] Several β-adrenergic agonists are available for the management of airway obstruction. These agents differ in β_2-selectivity, potency, elimination half-life, and availability of dosage formulations.

Albuterol (Proventil, Ventolin). Albuterol is the official generic name for this agent in the United States, although the World Health Organization's suggested name is *salbutamol.* Albuterol is indicated for the treatment and prevention of bronchospasm and is available in a variety of dosage forms. The recommended pediatric dosage for the metered-dose inhaler (MDI) is 1 or 2 inhalations every 4 to 6 hours as needed. Neonatal nebulization consists of 0.05 to 0.15 mg/kg/dose mixed with 2 to 3 ml of normal saline (NS) every 2 to 6 hours as needed. Pediatric nebulization doses range from 0.1 to 0.5 ml in 2 to 3 ml NS every 2 to 6 hours as needed. Nebulization treatments may be given as often as every 1 hour. In severe cases of status asthmaticus, continuous nebulization may be given. The normal oral dose in children less than 6 years of age is 0.1 mg/kg/dose every 8 hours, with a maximum dose of 12 mg/day. Dosages may be increased during acute exacerbation of the disease.[2] Table 26-1 lists the bronchodilators available in inhalation form that are commonly used with infant and pediatric patients.

Adverse reactions to albuterol are similar to those of other β_2-agonists. One of the documented side effects of albuterol therapy is *hypokalemia,* which may explain the increased mortality of patients using large doses of albuterol. The hypokalemia may predispose the heart to toxic effects by leading to arrhythmias.

Levalbuterol (Xopenex). Albuterol is composed of both R- and S-albuterol. The S-isomers

TABLE 26-1 INHALED BRONCHODILATORS

Agent	Availability	Dose	Adverse Events
Albuterol (Proventil, Ventolin)	MDI: 90 µg/puff Nebulized solution: 0.5% Unit-dose vial: 2.5 mg/3 ml	1-2 puffs q 4-6 hours Neonate: 0.05-0.15 mg/kg Pediatric: 0.1-0.5 ml in 2-2.25 ml saline q 1-6 hours 1 vial q 1-6 hours	Tachycardia, tremor, nervousness, headache, palpitations, dizziness, nausea, vomiting, hypokalemia (at high doses)
Levalbuterol (Xopenex)	Unit-dose vials: 0.63 mg/3 ml 1.25 mg/3 ml	1 vial q 6-8 hours (in patients 12 years and older)	Nervousness, tremor, dizziness, headache, tachycardia
Metaproterenol (Alupent, Metaprel)	MDI: 0.65 mg/puff Nebulized solution: 5% Unit-dose vials: (0.4%) 0.2 ml/2.5 ml saline (0.6%) 0.3 ml/2.5 ml saline	2-3 puffs q 3-4 hours (maximum 12 puffs in 24 hours) 0.1-0.3 ml/2-3 ml saline q 1-6 hours 1 vial q 1-6 hours	Tachycardia, tremor, nervousness, nausea, vomiting, headache, hypertension, dizziness
Terbutaline (Brethine, Brethaire)	Aqueous solution: 1 mg/ml	Nebulized: 0.5 mg or 1.5 mg/2-3 ml saline q 4-6 hours Subcutaneous: 0.01 mg/kg (maximum 0.4 mg) q 15-20 minutes times 3 doses	Tachycardia, tremor, nervousness, nausea, vomiting, headache, palpitations, dizziness
Pirbuterol (Maxair)	MDI: 200 µg/puff	2 puffs q 4-6 hours	Tachycardia, tremor, dizziness, nausea, vomiting, headache, nervousness, palpitations
Salmeterol (Serevent)	MDI: 21 µg/puff DPI (Discus): 50 µg/inhalation	2 puffs q 12 hours 1 inhalation q 12 hours (maximum 2 doses/day)	Tachycardia, tremor, headache, insomnia, nervousness, muscle cramps, palpitations, ECG changes
Formoterol (Foradil)	DPI (Aerolizer): 12 µg/25 mg lactose (carrier)	1 inhalation q 12 hours (maximum 2 doses/day)	Tachycardia, tremor, palpitations, angina, hypertension, nausea, nervousness, insomnia, headache, dizziness, muscle cramps, viral chest infection, fatigue, tonsillitis
Racemic epinephrine	Nebulized solution: 2.25%	0.05 ml/kg (maximum 0.5 ml) in 2 ml saline	Tachycardia, tremor, nervousness, nausea, headache, insomnia, palpitations
Ipratropium bromide (Atrovent)	MDI: 18 µg/puff Unit-dose vial: 500 µg/2.5 ml saline	1-2 puffs q 4-6 hours 125-250 µg, q 6-8 hours (<12 years old) 500 µg, q 6-8 hours (>12 years old) Can be mixed with albuterol solution in nebulizer	Dry mouth, headache, dizziness, cough, blurred vision, drying of secretions

MDI, Metered-dose inhaler; *DPI,* dry powder inhaler; *q,* every; *ECG,* electrocardiogram.

are not clinically beneficial and may worsen airway reactivity.[15,16] Levalbuterol is the modified name for R-albuterol hydrochloride and is the active component of albuterol. Most drugs are available in both dextro (*d-*) and levo (*l-*) isomers. Sepracor has tested both isomers and found that the *l*-isomer is the most active compound. It also possesses a longer duration of action and has a slightly better side effect profile.

Levalbuterol is indicated for the treatment or prevention of bronchospasm in adults and adolescents 12 years of age and older. In studies of asthma treatment in the pediatric patient, levalbuterol was compared to both racemic albuterol and placebo.[17] In doses of 0.31 and 0.63 mg, levalbuterol produced a greater degree of bronchodilation, as measured by percent change from predose forced expiratory volume at 1 second (FEV_1), than comparable doses of 1.25 and 2.5 mg of racemic albuterol. The study found that 0.63 mg levalbuterol was equipotent to 1.25 mg racemic albuterol, and 1.25 mg levalbuterol was equipotent to 2.5 mg racemic albuterol.

Levalbuterol is supplied in 3.0-ml unit-dose vials and requires no dilution before administration by nebulization.[18] Each unit-dose vial contains either 0.63 or 1.25 mg of levalbuterol. Suggested nebulization dosage for children over 12 years of age is 0.63 mg unit dose administered every 6 to 8 hours. Patients who do not respond adequately to a dose of 0.63 mg may benefit from a dosage of 1.25 mg administered every 6 to 8 hours. The solution is stored in a protective foil pouch and discarded if it is not colorless.

Adverse events reported in patients receiving levalbuterol are similar to those observed with racemic albuterol. However the incidence of tremor and nervousness is reported to be slightly less when using 0.63 mg levalbuterol.

Metaproterenol (Alupent, Metaprel). Metaproterenol is classified as a selective β_2-agonist, although it is less selective than albuterol. With the introduction of albuterol and other more specific agents, metaproterenol has fallen into disuse. It is indicated for the treatment of bronchospasm and is available as an oral syrup and tablet, MDI, and solution for nebulization.[3] The recommended dosing regimen for the MDI is 1 to 3 inhalations every 3 to 4 hours, up to a maximum dose of 12 inhalations/day. The recommended pediatric dosage for the 5% nebulized solution is 0.1 to 0.3 ml in 2 to 3 ml NS every 4 to 6 hours. The nebulized solution may be administered as frequently as every hour for severe bronchospasm. The medication may be administered orally at doses of 0.4 mg/kg/dose every 6 to 8 hours.[2,5]

Terbutaline (Brethine, Brethaire). Terbutaline is the only selective β_2-agonist available for parenteral administration in the emergency treatment of status asthmaticus. It is available as an oral tablet and a sterile aqueous solution for subcutaneous (SC) administration. The maximum pediatric oral dose recommended is 0.15 mg/kg/dose three times a day, not to exceed 5 mg/day. The aqueous solution is supplied in a 2-ml clear glass ampule containing 1 mg terbutaline per 1 ml of solution. Dosage for nebulization is 0.5 to 1.5 mg mixed with 2 to 3 ml NS every 4 to 6 hours. Two MDI inhalations every 4 to 6 hours is recommended. The SC dosage recommended for children is 0.01 mg/kg (0.4 mg maximum) every 15 to 20 minutes for three doses.[2]

Terbutaline may be administered intravenously (IV) as a continuous infusion to pediatric patients refractory to more common inhalation therapy. In most institutions, terbutaline is reserved for the management of acute episodes of severe asthma. Recommended dosing for continuous infusion begins at 0.4 µg/kg/min, increased as needed to a dose of 3 to 5 µg/kg/min. Tachycardia, often a dose-limiting adverse effect, is more frequently observed when using doses in the upper range.[2,5]

Pirbuterol (Maxair). Pirbuterol has a relatively fast onset of action, at 5 minutes or less, and a short duration of action at 5 hours. It is indicated for the prevention and reversal of bronchospasm in adults and children over 12 years old.[19] In many respects the adverse reaction profile of pirbuterol is better than for albuterol, with fewer incidences of tachycardia, palpitations, and tremor. Pirbuterol is available as an MDI and in an Autohaler formulation. The normal dose for adults and children over 12 years of age is 2 inhalations (0.4 mg) every 4 to 6 hours. One inhalation (0.2 mg) may be sufficient for some patients.[2,10]

Salmeterol (Serevent). Salmeterol is a long-acting β_2-agonist indicated for long-term maintenance treatment of asthma and prevention of bronchospasm in patients 4 years and older. It is also indicated for prevention of exercise-induced bronchospasm (EIB). Salmeterol has much the same profile for safety and adverse effects as albuterol. Long-acting β_2-agonists can be beneficial to patients when added to inhaled corticosteroid therapy, especially to control nighttime asthma symptoms.[12] They also attenuate EIB for longer time periods than do short-acting β_2-agonists. Studies suggest that for patients with inadequate symptom control who are receiving low-to-medium doses of inhaled corticosteroids, it may be more beneficial to add salmeterol than to increase the dose of inhaled corticosteroid.[20-22]

Salmeterol is available as an MDI that delivers 21 μg per inhalation and in a discus form that delivers 50 μg per inhalation. The normal dose for prevention of asthma symptoms is 2 inhalations of the MDI twice daily (12 hours apart) or 1 inhalation of the discus twice daily.[23] For the prevention of EIB, 42 μg (2 puffs) can be given 15 to 60 minutes before exercise. Patients using salmeterol twice a day for maintenance therapy do not take an additional dose before exercise.

Salmeterol is not used to treat acute asthma symptoms. The onset of action is not immediate and occurs approximately 30 minutes after intake.[22] Instead a short-acting β_2-agonist is used to relieve acute symptoms. When beginning treatment with salmeterol, instruct patients to discontinue any regular use of the short-acting β_2-agonist and to use the shorter-acting agent for symptomatic, quick relief during acute episodes only.

Adverse reactions to salmeterol are similar to those seen with other selective β_2-agonists, including tachycardia, palpitations, tremor, and nervousness. Although uncommon after administration at recommended doses, salmeterol can produce a clinically significant cardiovascular effect in some patients. Changes in the electrocardiogram (ECG) include flattening of the T wave, prolongation of the QT interval, and ST-segment depression. Fatalities have been reported in association with excessive use. Large doses (12 to 20 times the recommended dose) have been associated with ventricular arrhythmias. Therefore salmeterol is not given more frequently than twice daily at the recommended dosage.[2,8,10,23]

Formoterol (Foradil). Formoterol is a long-acting, highly β_2-selective bronchodilator. It is indicated for long-term, twice-daily (morning and evening) administration in the maintenance treatment of asthma and prevention of bronchospasm in adults and children 5 years of age and older.[24] Formoterol is also indicated for the acute prevention of EIB in adults and adolescents 12 years of age and older. It is inherently different from the short-acting inhaled β_2-agonists; formoterol is not used to treat acute symptoms and is not considered a substitute for inhaled or oral corticosteroids. When beginning treatment with formoterol, instruct patients to discontinue any regular use of the short-acting β_2-agonist and to use the shorter-acting agent for symptomatic, quick relief during acute episodes only.

Formoterol is available in a hard, gelatin capsule dosage form containing a dry powder blend of 12 μg of formoterol and 25 mg of lactose as a carrier. It is intended for oral inhalation only with the Aerolizer inhaler; the capsules are not swallowed.

The usual dosage is the inhalation of the contents of one 12-μg capsule every 12 hours, with a total daily dose not to exceed one capsule twice daily (24 μg total daily dose). If symptoms arise between doses, an inhaled short-acting β_2-agonist is taken for immediate relief. For the prevention of EIB, the usual dosage is the inhalation of the contents of one 12-μg capsule at least 15 minutes before exercise. Regular, twice-daily dosing in preventing EIB has not been studied. Patients who are receiving formoterol twice daily for maintenance treatment of their asthma do not use additional doses for prevention of EIB.

Adverse reactions to formoterol include tremor, tachycardia, arrhythmias, palpitation, nervousness, agitation, headache, muscle cramps, dizziness, fatigue, insomnia, dry mouth, nausea, hypokalemia, hyperglycemia, and metabolic acidosis. Adverse events occurring more frequently in children (ages 5 to 12 years) in need of daily bronchodilator and antiinflammatory treatment include viral infection, rhinitis, tonsillitis, gastroenteritis, abdominal pain, nausea, and dyspepsia. Clinical trials show no evidence of drug dependence with the use of formoterol.[24]

NONSELECTIVE AGENTS

Isoproterenol (Isuprel). The use of isoproterenol in the treatment of asthma has dramatically decreased with the introduction of more selective agents. Administration of isoproterenol results in relaxation of bronchial smooth muscle, cardiac stimulation, and peripheral vasodilation. It may be used intravenously in emergency situations to stimulate the heart rate in patients with bradycardia. Common adverse effects include palpitations, tachycardia, headache, nervousness, dizziness, nausea, vomiting, tremor, and cutaneous flushing.[3]

Isoproterenol is available as an injectable solution. Intravenous (IV) dosages range from 0.1 to 1.5 μg/kg/min and should be initiated at 0.1 μg/kg/min, with incremental increases until the desired effect is achieved.[2,16]

Ephedrine (Neo-Synephrine). Ephedrine is used primarily as a systemic decongestant. Its therapeutic index is low, with hypertension resulting from doses exceeding two to three times the normal dose. Ephedrine has a therapeutic half-life of 3 to 6 hours. Most excretion occurs through the kidney, with unchanged drug excreted in the urine. The most common adverse effect associated with ephedrine is hypertension. Tachycardia is another common side effect. Children with underlying vascular or cardiac problems should avoid the use of ephedrine if possible. The common pediatric dose for ephedrine is

2 to 3 mg/kg/day divided every 4 hours, with a maximum dose of 25 mg every 4 hours.[2]

RACEMIC EPINEPHRINE

Racemic epinephrine inhalant solution is a sympathomimetic that acts on both α-receptors and β-receptors of the respiratory tract. The α-adrenergic effects are thought to result from inhibition of the enzyme adenyl cyclase. Stimulation of the α-receptors results in vasoconstriction and a reduction of mucosal and submucosal congestion and edema. The β-adrenergic effects result from stimulation of adenyl cyclase and increased cAMP production, which results in reduction of airway smooth muscle spasm (see Fig. 26-1). Both actions work in concert to reduce airway swelling. In children, racemic epinephrine is used most often to treat postextubation edema and laryngotracheobronchitis (LTB).

The solution of racemic epinephrine, 2.25%, is an equal mixture of the *d-* and *l-*isomers of epinephrine. A plastic or glass dropper should be used to prepare the dose because the solution reacts on contact with metals.[2,25] Do not use the solution if the color is pinkish or darker than slightly yellow, or if it contains a precipitate. Refrigerate the solution once the bottle is opened. The recommended dose for LTB is 0.05 ml/kg (maximum 0.5 ml) in 2 ml NS nebulized every 1 to 4 hours as needed. Common adverse effects include tachycardia, palpitations, nervousness, tremor, insomnia, headache, loss of appetite, and nausea.[2,10,25]

ANTICHOLINERGICS

MECHANISM OF ACTION

The parasympathetic nervous system plays a major role in regulating airway homeostasis and bronchomotor tone. A variety of noxious stimuli have been demonstrated to increase parasympathetic activity with resultant bronchoconstriction. Vagal nerve fibers that end on muscarinic receptors innervate the larger airway smooth muscles. Cholinergic irritant receptors are also located in the junction between airway mucosal cells. Anticholinergic agents are competitive inhibitors of acetylcholine at the muscarinic receptors and are effective in relieving cholinergic-mediated bronchoconstriction (Fig. 26-2).[26] Increasing levels of acetylcholine can overcome this smooth muscle receptor blockade.

ATROPINE

Atropine, a potent bronchodilator, has been used in the short-term treatment and prevention of bronchospasm associated with chronic asthma, bronchitis, and chronic obstructive pulmonary disease (COPD).[27] Atropine is also used as an antidote for poisoning by cholinergic drugs or anticholinesterase agents (e.g., insecticides, "nerve gas"). Aerosol administration is more bronchoselective and results in fewer systemic adverse effects. The recommended pediatric dosage for bronchospasm is 0.05 mg/kg (minimum 0.25 mg, maximum 1.0 mg) in 2 to 3 ml NS every 6 to 8 hours by nebulization. Adverse effects include dry mouth, blurred vision, fever, bradycardia, tachycardia, urinary retention, central nervous system (CNS) excitement, fever, and mucus plugging caused by atropine's drying effect on secretions. Pupillary reflexes should be tested before atropine administration.[2,3,27]

IPRATROPIUM BROMIDE (ATROVENT)

Ipratropium bromide is an anticholinergic agent used in the treatment of bronchospasm associated with COPD, chronic bronchitis, and asthma.[2,10] It is a quaternary ammonium derivative of atropine. Ipratropium has little effect on mucociliary clearance and ciliary functions compared with atropine; use of ipratropium avoids accumulation of lower airway secretions.[26] Quaternary compounds are poorly absorbed across mucosal membranes and the blood-brain barrier. Inhalation of ipratropium therefore results in local airway effects with minimal systemic effects. Ipratropium inhalation is not sufficiently effective to be used as a single agent in the treatment of acute bronchospasm, but with salbutamol is often more effective than either agent alone.[28] This is often the case if the patient has no previous history of β-agonist use.

Although its use continues to increase, the role of ipratropium in childhood asthma is not completely understood. Studies favor its addition because of increased cholinergic tone.[5,11,29,30] Werner, in his review of the treatment of status asthmaticus, strongly recommended the incorporation of ipratropium in the emergency department treatment plan.[30] Craven et al found no significant difference between treatment groups when randomized to treatment with albuterol plus ipratropium versus albuterol alone. The study population included pediatric patients hospitalized with acute asthma. The end points studied included length of stay, asthma carepath progression, and requirement of additional therapy.[16] Safety and efficacy of ipratropium in children younger than 12 years of age have not been established.[31] However, ipratropium is routinely used in those patients greater than 3 months of age in many pediatric intensive care units.

Dosage and Administration. Ipratropium bromide is available as a nasal spray, an MDI, and a

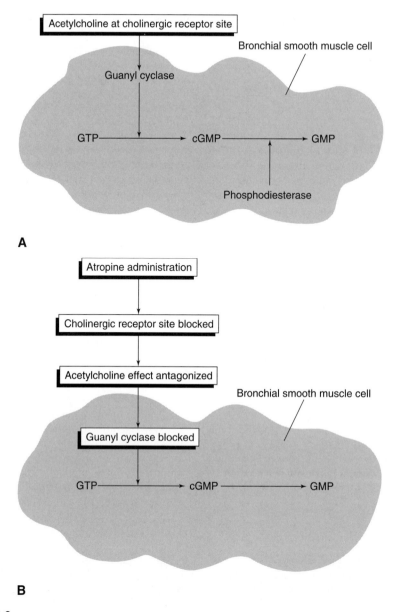

Fig. 26-2

A, Parasympathetic mechanisms controlling bronchial smooth muscle tone. Stimulation of the parasympathetic system causes the release of acetylcholine at the cholinergic receptor site. The acetylcholine stimulates the enzyme guanyl cyclase to convert guanosine triphospate *(GTP)* to cyclic guanosine monophosphate *(cGMP)*. Phosphodiesterase then breaks down cGMP to guanosine monophosphate *(GMP)*. High cGMP levels result in bronchoconstriction. **B,** Administration of an anticholinergic (atropine) antagonizes the acetylcholinergic effect and prevents cGMP from forming. This relieves the bronchoconstriction.

nebulization solution. The concentrations of the nasal spray are 0.03% and 0.06%. The dose for the nasal spray is 2 sprays in each nostril two or three times daily.[2,31] The nasal spray is used only for symptomatic relief of rhinorrhea associated with allergic and nonallergic perennial rhinitis; it does not relieve nasal congestion, sneezing, or postnasal drip.[32]

The inhalation solution is available in unit-dose vials containing 500 μg ipratropium in 2.5 ml NS.[31] The vials are packaged in a foil pouch and must be protected from light. The inhalation solution can be mixed in the nebulizer with albuterol or metaproterenol if used within 1 hour. Stability and safety of ipratropium when mixed with other drugs in a nebulizer have not been established. The usual dose for neonates by nebulization is 25 µg/kg/dose three times daily. For infants and children under 12 years the nebulization dose is 125 to 250 µg three times daily. For adults and children over 12 years the nebulization dose is 500 µg three or four times daily.

The MDI dose for children 3 to 12 years old is 1 or 2 inhalations every 4 to 6 hours as needed, with a maximum of 6 inhalations in a 24-hour period. The MDI dose for adults and children over 12 years of age is 2 inhalations every 4 to 6 hours, with a maximum of 12 inhalations in 24 hours. The most common adverse reactions are dry mouth, cough, headache, nausea, dizziness, blurred vision, and drying of secretions.[12,31] Ipratropium is also available mixed with albuterol (Combivent, DuoNeb), supplied as an MDI and in solution for nebulization. Dosage recommendations for this mixture follow those for ipratropium bromide alone.[33]

GLYCOPYRROLATE (ROBINUL)

Glycopyrrolate is a quaternary anticholinergic compound. This class of drugs is also known as *antimuscarinic* agents. These drugs are used to inhibit the muscarinic actions of acetylcholine at multiple sites. Glycopyrrolate is used specifically to inhibit salivation and excessive secretions of the respiratory tract. It is also used to counter the muscarinic effects of neostigmine and pyridostigmine during reversal of neuromuscular blockade.[34] Glycopyrrolate is contraindicated in patients with tachycardia, paralytic ileus, or myasthenia gravis. It is not recommended for use in children under 12 years of age.

The dose for control of secretions in children is 40 to 100 µg/kg three or four times daily. The intramuscular (IM) and IV dose is 4 to 10 µg/kg every 3 to 4 hours. Adverse reactions include tachycardia, ventricular fibrillation, and palpitations. Central effects include drowsiness, headache, and ataxia.[35]

METHYLXANTHINES

Methylxanthines relax smooth muscle, stimulate the central nervous system and cardiac muscle, increase mucociliary transport and diaphragmatic contractility, and act on the kidneys to promote diuresis. Their usefulness in promoting relaxation of bronchial smooth muscle is of benefit in the management of asthma.[4]

THEOPHYLLINE

Although no longer as widely used for the treatment of acute severe asthma, the methylxanthine theophylline is still considered as additive therapy when response to β-agonists is suboptimal.

The mechanism of action of theophylline is not completely understood, but it is known to competitively inhibit phosphodiesterase, the enzyme that degrades cAMP. Increased concentrations of cAMP may mediate the observed bronchodilation (see Fig. 26-1).[36] Other proposed mechanisms of action include inhibition of the release of intracellular calcium and competitive antagonism of the bronchoconstrictor adenosine.[5]

Dosage and Administration. Aerosol administration of theophylline is ineffective; it must be administered systemically. Theophylline is available in a multitude of dosage formulations and strengths, with great variation in the recommended dosing guidelines based on patient age. Sustained-release preparations generally provide more consistent drug levels and allow dosing once, twice, or three times daily, favoring patient compliance. However, the rate of absorption is variable between patients and is influenced by numerous medical interventions and conditions. Multiple factors increase the clearance rate of theophylline and result in higher dose requirements, including smoking, hyperthyroidism, and concurrent use of medications such as phenobarbital and rifampin. Factors that can decrease clearance and lead to toxicity include hypothyroidism, congestive heart failure, liver failure, and the use of oral contraceptives and various antibiotics, including ciprofloxacin and erythromycin.[37]

The therapeutic serum range for theophylline is 10 to 20 µg/ml. Blood levels are routinely monitored to avoid toxic levels, especially in patients requiring multiple medications. Many patients will respond to lower serum concentrations; 5 to 15 µg/ml is accepted as a safe and effective range.[2,5]

Adverse Events. The adverse gastrointestinal effects of theophylline include nausea, vomiting, abdominal pain, cramping, and diarrhea. Adverse CNS effects include insomnia, headache, dizziness, nervousness, and seizures, which are often more severe in children. Seizures may occur as the initial sign of theophylline toxicity without other preceding signs and symptoms of toxicity.[36] Increased tremor in the patient's dominant hand has been reported.[38] Cardiovascular and pulmonary adverse effects include tachycardia, arrhythmias, and tachypnea. Theophylline worsens gastroesophageal reflux disease (GERD), potentially resulting in an exacerbation of asthma. Because of these toxicities, theophylline is often used as a fourth-line asthma medication.

MAGNESIUM SULFATE

Magnesium is a cofactor in more than 300 enzymatic reactions in the body. In heart muscle, magnesium acts as a calcium channel blocker. In smooth muscle, it acts as a muscle relaxant. When given intravenously, magnesium promotes bronchodilation.[39] The use of magnesium sulfate ($MgSO_4$) in the treatment of moderate to severe exacerbations of asthma dates back more than 60 years.[40] Current evidence suggests that patients with severe asthma may benefit most from its use.[41-44]

The dose of $MgSO_4$ for bronchodilation is 25 mg/kg; doses as high as 75 mg/kg have been used to treat pediatric status asthmaticus. The literature reflects single doses of $MgSO_4$ as well as multidose schedules.[2] Standard dosage is 25 mg/kg every 4 hours, for a total of 4 doses. Monitor magnesium serum levels during administration. The normal serum value for magnesium is 1.5 to 2.5 mEq/L.[2]

Side effects include severe fatigue, somnolence, and pseudocoma.[16] Deep tendon reflexes are blunted with $MgSO_4$ injection. As magnesium action abates, deep tendon reflexes will return in reverse order of attenuation. Until further studies are completed in the pediatric population, controversy will remain regarding magnesium sulfate's place in therapy.

NONSTEROIDAL ANTIINFLAMMATORY DRUGS

CROMOLYN SODIUM (INTAL)

The Second Expert Panel on Asthma reports cromolyn sodium as a component of therapy in the treatment of mild and moderate persistent asthma.[12] Because it has no known long-term systemic effects, cromolyn is often used as first-line antiinflammatory therapy in children with mild or moderate persistent asthma. It is of little benefit during an acute exacerbation of asthma or to children with severe asthma.[5]

Cromolyn has been referred to as a mast cell stabilizer. Although the complete mechanism of action is unknown, it inhibits sensitized mast cell degranulation occurring after exposure to specific antigens. The drug also blocks the release of histamine and slow-reacting substance of anaphylaxis (SRS-A, a leukotriene) from the mast cell. These actions serve to inhibit the early asthmatic response through stabilization of the mast cell membrane. Cromolyn also inhibits the late asthmatic response. In some patients, cromolyn attenuates bronchospasm caused by exercise, aspirin, and cold air. Cromolyn has no intrinsic bronchodilator, antihistaminic, anticholinergic, or vasoconstrictor activity.[45]

Dosage and Administration. Cromolyn sodium is available as a nebulized solution and an MDI. The recommended dosage of the solution for nebulization in children older than 2 years is 20 mg (one 2-ml ampule) four times a day. Protect the ampule from light by storing it in a foil package, and do not use it if it contains a precipitate or becomes discolored. The recommended dosage of the MDI is 2 inhalations four times daily. For the prevention of bronchospasm after exercise or exposure to cold air, cromolyn is administered 10 to 15 minutes, but not more than 60 minutes, before exposure.[2,45] Long-term prophylaxis of 6 to 12 weeks is necessary to prevent the increased airway hyperreactivity associated with specific allergen exposure. Improvement in symptoms usually occurs within the first 4 weeks of administration. Cromolyn is extremely safe and is one of the most nontoxic drugs used in the management of asthma. However, the need for four-times-daily administration tends to decrease patient compliance.

NEDOCROMIL SODIUM (TILADE)

As with cromolyn sodium, nedocromil sodium is a nonsteroidal antiinflammatory drug indicated primarily for prevention of mild persistent to moderate persistent asthma. Although the exact mechanism of action has yet to be elucidated, clinical studies have reported that nedocromil inhibits the bronchoconstrictor response to several challenges, including various antigens, exercise, cold air, and fog. This inhibition is of both the early and the late phase bronchoconstriction. Nedocromil has no intrinsic bronchodilator, antihistamine, or corticosteroid action. It is not used for the reversal of acute bronchospasm, particularly during status asthmaticus.[46]

Dosage and Administration. Nedocromil is available as an MDI. The recommended dosage for children 6 years of age and older is 2 inhalations four times daily.[10,46,47] Twice-daily dosing may be effective in some patients. Some reports show nedocromil to have a modest effect in lowering the required dose of corticosteroids.[14] The most common adverse effect is a transient, mild, unpleasant taste. Nausea and headache have also been reported.

INHALED CORTICOSTEROIDS

MECHANISM OF ACTION

Corticosteroids are potent antiinflammatory agents used in the management of asthma. The mechanisms of action include (1) inhibition of the production of leukotrienes and prostaglandins through interference with arachidonic acid metabolism, (2) reduction of migration and inhibition of the activity of the inflammatory cells, (3) increase in the number of β-receptors, and (4) enhancement of the responsiveness of β-receptors in airway smooth muscle. Glucocorticoids act on mast cells by slowing the synthesis of histamines. This slowing of synthesis does not affect the rate of release of histamines.[5,22] The benefits of inhaled corticosteroids include a reduction in airway inflammation and hyperresponsiveness, as well as a decrease in mucus secretion and airway edema.

INDICATIONS

The Second Expert Panel on Asthma states that inhaled corticosteroids are the most effective long-term therapy available for mild, moderate, or severe persistent asthma and that in general they are well tolerated and safe at the recommended dosages.[12] Debate about the safety of long-term steroid use is ongoing. Again, the panel deems that risk of adverse effects is far outweighed by the benefit. When used at recommended dosages, corticosteroids are safe and have few untoward effects. Inhalation therapy allows the topical administration of potent antiinflammatory agents directly at the site of action in the airways. Administration directly to the site of action helps decrease the adverse effects observed with systemic corticosteroid therapy.

The five formulations for inhalation therapy currently available in the United States are *beclomethasone dipropionate* (Beclovent, QVAR, Vanceril), *budesonide* (Pulmicort), *flunisolide* (AeroBid), *fluticasone propionate* (Flovent), and *triamcinolone acetonide* (Azmacort). All five agents are available as dry powder and/or MDI formulations. Budesonide is also available in suspension for nebulization (Pulmicort Respules).[2]

DOSAGE AND ADMINISTRATION

Table 26-2 lists the antiinflammatory agents that are available for inhalation therapy in children and the recommended dosages. These dosages are often increased depending on the age of the patient and the response to therapy. Once asthma is under control, the initial dose is adjusted to the lowest effective dose to reduce the possibility of side effects. Maximum benefit may not be achieved for 1 to 2 weeks or longer after starting treatment.

ADVERSE EVENTS

The likelihood of systemic side effects increases when inhaled corticosteroids are used at higher doses and for long periods. Inhaled corticosteroids produce a dose-dependent suppression of the adrenal axis steroid production. Use of these agents may also impair growth and decrease bone forma-

tion.[48,49] The effects on linear growth are discussed extensively in the literature. Treatment with inhaled corticosteroids was associated with prepubertal growth impairment in one study using beclomethasone as the study drug. The suppression was limited to 1.5 cm/yr in children treated with 400 μg/day beclomethasone.[49] Many studies to determine the effects on growth have significant design limitations. Because delayed or impaired growth may be a result of asthma itself, the question remains as to whether the treatment or the underlying disease is the true determinant of linear growth reduction. Further studies have proved that even with this initial reduction in linear growth, the long-term effects do not last. In long-term follow-up, patients with a history of inhaled corticosteroid use achieved height that fell within the expectation based on hereditary models.[49]

The American College of Chest Physicians, along with four other national organizations, put forth a consensus statement in November 1998 in response to new FDA requirements.[50] Pharmaceutical companies that supply orally inhaled or intranasal corticosteroids must include new information on the potential effects of their use in children. The FDA also recommended using the lowest effective dose of these drugs and routine monitoring of patients' growth rates. The companion recommendation from the FDA was to advise parents not to stop current medication in their children before consulting their physician. Notably, in late 1998, a comparison of the effects on bone mineral density between fluticasone and beclomethasone was published.[51] Over a 20-month follow-up of users of both drugs, bone density increased significantly. The increase followed normal patterns of growth. Neither drug appeared to affect bone mineral density.

Dose-related local adverse effects include oropharyngeal candidiasis, dysphonia, cough, and dry throat. The dysphonia appears to be the result of a direct effect of the steroid on the musculature that controls the vocal cords. Proper inhalation technique, use of spacer or holding chamber devices, rinsing the mouth and gargling with water, and expectorating after inhalation may help decrease these local adverse effects. These techniques decrease drug deposition in the mouth. Increased wheezing has been reported infrequently.[5,11,52] Patients who have undergone long-term steroid therapy may experience hypertension when treatment levels are reduced.[53] Chickenpox and measles may lead to serious or even fatal complications in children taking immunosuppressant drugs. Therefore considerable care is taken to avoid exposure; if the child is exposed, immunoglobulin therapy may be indicated.[54,55] Development of cataracts and glaucoma caused by systemic

TABLE 26-2	INHALED ANTIINFLAMMATORY AGENTS		
Agent	**Availability**	**Dose**	**Adverse Events/Considerations**
Cromolyn sodium (Intal)	MDI: 800 µg/puff Unit-dose vial: 20 mg/2 ml	2 puffs, 4 times/day 1 vial per nebulizer, 4 times/day	Bad taste, nausea, cough, throat irritation
Nedocromil sodium (Tilade)	MDI: 1.75 mg/puff	2 puffs, 4 times/day	Bad taste, nausea, headache
Beclomethasone dipropionate (Beclovent, QVAR, Vanceril)	MDI: Beclovent: 42 µg/puff Vanceril: 42 µg/puff QVAR 40: 40 µg/puff QVAR 80: 80 µg/puff	1-4 puffs, 2-4 times/day, maximum 320 µg 2 times/day	Hoarseness, dry throat, dysphonia, cough, oropharyngeal candidiasis (thrush). Use a spacer or holding chamber with all MDIs.
Budesonide (Pulmicort Turbuhaler, Pulmicort Respules)	DPI: 200 µg/inhalation Unit-dose vials: 0.25 mg/2 ml 0.5 mg/2 ml	1-2 inhalations, 1-2 times/day 0.25-1.0 mg/day per nebulizer, 1-2 times/day	MDI cannisters should be at room temperature and shaken well before each actuation. Rinse mouth after use.
Flunisolide (Aerobid, Aerobid-M)	MDI: 250 µg/puff	1-4 puffs, q 12 hours	Aerobid-M contains menthol as a flavoring agent.
Fluticasone (Flovent, Advair)	MDI: 44 µg/puff 110 µg/puff 220 µg/puff DPI (Advair): Fluticasone/salmeterol 100 µg/50 µg 250 µg/50 µg 500 µg/50 µg	1-2 puffs, q 12 hours 1 inhalation, q 12 hours	Flovent will soon be available alone in the Discus form. Maximum frequency of Advair use is 1 inhalation q 12 hours.
Triamcinolone acetonide (Azmacort)	MDI: 100 µg/puff	2-4 puffs, 2-4 times/day	Azmacort is supplied with a white plastic spacer mouthpiece.

MDI, Metered-dose inhaler; *DPI,* dry powder inhaler; *q,* every.

absorption is associated with oral steroids, but no clear association exists with high doses of inhaled corticosteroids.[56]

LEUKOTRIENE MODIFIERS

Leukotrienes were initially known as "slow-reacting substances of anaphylaxis" (SRS-A). They are derived from the metabolism of *arachidonic acid,* a fatty acid found in cell membranes.[52,57] When sensitized mast cells are exposed to allergen triggers, there is synthesis and release of molecules, including histamine and leukotrienes. The leukotrienes work to constrict airway smooth muscle, increase vascular permeability that leads to airway edema, increase mucus production, and both attract and activate inflammatory cells in the airways of asthmatic patients.[58]

Leukotriene modifiers are the first new class of asthma medications to be introduced in the United States in more than 20 years. As clinical experience increases, the role of the antileukotrienes will most likely expand. Table 26-3 lists the leukotriene modifying agents currently available.

MECHANISM OF ACTION

Two approaches are available to prevent the action of leukotrienes: (1) antagonize or block leukotriene binding to its cellular receptor *(receptor antagonists)* and (2) inhibit the production of leukotrienes *(synthesis inhibitors).* The FDA has currently approved three oral leukotriene modifying drugs for use in the United States. *Zafirlukast* (Accolate) and *montelukast* (Singulair) are selective leukotriene receptor antagonists. *Zileuton* (Zyflo) is the only agent that inhibits 5-lipoxygenase, the enzyme

TABLE 26-3	LEUKOTRIENE MODIFYING AGENTS			
Agent	**Availability**	**Dosage**	**Population**	**Adverse Events**
SYNTHESIS INHIBITOR				
Zileuton (Zyflo)	600-mg tablet	1 tablet 4 times daily with or without food	Approved for patients 12 years and older	Abdominal pain, upset stomach, nausea, elevated liver enzymes; increased theophylline levels when added to existing theophylline regimen; increased level of propranolol when added to existing propranolol regimen; evaluation of liver function before beginning medication, monthly times 3, every 3 months for 1 year, then periodically
RECEPTOR ANTAGONISTS				
Zafirlukast (Accolate)	10-mg chewable tablet 20-mg tablet	1 tablet twice daily 1 hour before or 2 hours after eating	10 mg: 7-12 years old 20 mg: ≥12 years old	Headache, diarrhea, nausea, abdominal pain, dizziness, back pain, fever, muscle aches, elevated liver enzymes; report of Churg-Strauss syndrome when systemic steroids reduced; increased theophylline levels when added to existing theophylline regimen; periodic evaluation of liver function
Montelukast (Singulair)	4-mg chewable tablet 5-mg chewable tablet 10-mg tablet	1 tablet daily in the evening with or without food	4 mg: 2-4 years old 5 mg: >4-14 years old 10 mg: >14 years old	Headache (most common), heartburn, abdominal pain, rash, fatigue, dizziness, gastroenteritis, fever

responsible for converting arachidonic acid to the leukotrienes.[59,60]

INDICATIONS

The leukotriene modifiers are approved for prophylaxis and chronic treatment of asthma.[61] They are not an alternative to using β-adrenergic agonists during an acute asthma attack. However, they are continued during acute exacerbations of asthma. Treatment with leukotriene modifiers is associated with improved asthma symptoms and pulmonary function, including FEV_1 values. They are effective in preventing bronchospasm caused by exercise, cold air, aspirin ingestion, and aller-

gens. Leukotriene modifiers also reduce the severity of asthma and allow for a reduction in the dose of inhaled corticosteroids and the need for β-agonist therapy.[58] Potential candidates include patients with poor inhaler technique and those who are noncompliant in taking inhaled corticosteroids.

MONTELUKAST (SINGULAIR)

Montelukast is the most recent leukotriene modifier. It is an orally administered, selective cysteinyl leukotriene ($CysLT_1$) receptor antagonist.[62] The initial response after a single dose of montelukast occurs in 3 to 4 hours. The duration of action approaches 24 hours. In clinical studies, montelukast yielded significant improvement in parameters of asthma control, including improved FEV_1, daytime and nighttime symptoms, and a reduction in both as-needed β-agonist use and inhaled corticosteroid dose.[63] Montelukast also provides significant protection against EIB.[64] It is not a bronchodilator, however, and is not indicated for use in the reversal of bronchospasm in acute asthma attacks. Montelukast has also been shown to improve symptoms when used in combination with loratadine for the treatment of seasonal allergic rhinitis.[64]

Dosage and Administration. Montelukast is available in both a 4-mg and 5-mg chewable, cherry-flavored tablet, as well as a 10-mg film-coated tablet.[62] The dose for children 2 to 5 years old is one 4-mg tablet daily. The dose for children 6 to 14 years old is one 5-mg tablet daily. The dose for adolescents (15 years and older) and adults is one 10-mg tablet daily. The safety and efficacy of montelukast were demonstrated in clinical trials where it was administered in the evening without regard to the time of food ingestion. No clinical trials have evaluated the relative efficacy of morning versus evening dosing. Therefore it is recommended that the tablets be taken in the evening, with or without food.

Adverse Events. The most common side effect of montelukast is headache. Other side effects are usually mild and include fatigue, fever, abdominal pain, gastroenteritis, heartburn, dizziness, and rash. In rare cases, patients may present with clinical features of vasculitis consistent with *Churg-Strauss syndrome*. These events typically have occurred in patients undergoing a reduction in oral corticosteroid medication.[62]

ZAFIRLUKAST (ACCOLATE)

Zafirlukast is a leukotriene receptor antagonist of leukotrienes D_4 and E_4, components of SRS-A. These leukotrienes are associated with airway edema, smooth muscle constriction, and altered cellular activity associated with the inflammatory process. Zafirlukast is rapidly absorbed after oral administration, with response 3 hours after dosing. The duration of action is approximately 10 hours. Clinical trials demonstrated that zafirlukast improved daytime asthma symptoms, nighttime awakenings, rescue β-agonist use, FEV_1, and morning peak expiratory flow rate.[65] Zafirlukast is not a bronchodilator and is not used to treat acute episodes of asthma.

Dosage and Administration. Zafirlukast is available in a 10-mg chewable tablet and a 20-mg coated tablet.[65] The recommended dose for children 7 to 12 years of age is 10 mg twice daily. The dose for adults and children 12 years and older is 20 mg twice daily. Because food reduces its bioavailability, zafirlukast should be taken at least 1 hour before or 2 hours after meals.[60] Zafirlukast has been reported to inhibit the metabolism of warfarin, resulting in an increased prothrombin time (PT). Patients receiving oral warfarin anticoagulant therapy and zafirlukast should have their PT closely monitored and anticoagulant dose adjusted accordingly.

Adverse Events. Initially it was believed that zafirlukast was relatively free of adverse events. With increasing use, however, side effects have become evident. Headache, nausea, diarrhea, abdominal pain, dizziness, fever, back pain, and vomiting have been reported.[65] Elevation of liver enzymes, progressing to hepatitis and hepatic failure, has occurred in patients using zafirlukast. Although most incidents occurred while using doses four times higher than the recommend dose, cases have occurred in patients receiving the recommended daily dose. In most patients the clinical symptoms abated and the enzyme levels returned to normal after discontinuing zafirlukast.

In rare cases, patients had increased theophylline levels, with or without clinical symptoms of theophylline toxicity, after zafirlukast had been added to the existing theophylline regimen.[65] The mechanism of the interaction between zafirlukast and theophylline in these patients is currently unknown.

At least eight patients given zafirlukast presented with systemic eosinophilia, pulmonary infiltrates, cardiomyopathy, and clinical features of vasculitis similar to Churg-Strauss syndrome.[66-68] The patients had severe asthma and were reducing or discontinuing oral corticosteroids after beginning zafirlukast therapy, during which time the reactions occurred. The symptoms reversed when zafirlukast was discontinued and corticosteroid therapy resumed. Although further studies are needed to determine the extent of the association, many believe that the syndrome was unmasked after corticosteroid withdrawal and was not a direct effect of zafirlukast.

ZILEUTON (ZYFLO)

Zileuton inhibits 5-lipoxygenase, the enzyme that catalyzes the formation of leukotrienes from arachidonic acid, and thus inhibits leukotriene formation.[14,69] It is the only member of the leukotriene-synthesis inhibitors currently approved for use. Zileuton has been shown to be effective in the treatment of cold air, aspirin-intolerant, exercise-induced, and nocturnal asthma.[61] Zileuton reduces asthma symptoms and the supplemental use of β-agonists, improves FEV_1 values, and may have an additive effect with inhaled steroids.[70,71] It is not indicated for use in the reversal of bronchospasm in acute asthma attacks, although its use can be continued during an acute exacerbation.

Zileuton is a cytochrome P-450 enzyme substrate and as such will affect plasma concentration of other such substrates. Caution should be used when dosing zileuton with theophylline, propranolol, warfarin, and terfenadine.[2,14]

Dosage and Administration. Zileuton is available as a 600-mg tablet. The recommended dosage in adults and children 12 years and older is one 600-mg tablet four times a day for a total daily dose of 2400 mg.[69] It can be taken with or without food, although for ease of administration, zileuton should be taken with meals and at bedtime.

Adverse Events. The most common side effects are abdominal pain, upset stomach, and nausea. Zileuton is associated with threefold or greater elevations of liver enzymes (serum aminotransferase) in 2% to 4% of patients. The elevations usually occur during the first 3 months of treatment and return to normal when zileuton is discontinued. Therefore liver function should be evaluated before starting zileuton, monthly for the first 3 months of treatment, then every 3 months of the first year, and periodically thereafter.[58] The inconvenient, four-times-daily dosing, incidence of elevated liver transaminases, and need for frequent liver function studies have limited the use of zileuton.

MUCOLYTIC AGENTS

N-ACETYLCYSTEINE (MUCOMYST)

N-acetylcysteine is an aerosolized mucolytic agent often used as adjunctive therapy for pulmonary complications of cystic fibrosis (CF) in combination with vigorous chest physiotherapy. The viscosity of mucous secretions in the lungs depends on the concentrations of mucoprotein and the presence of disulfide bonds between these macromolecules and DNA. N-acetylcysteine acts to split the sulfide bonds in the macromolecules, thereby decreasing viscosity, allowing for their removal by normal chest physiotherapy. The action of N-acetylcysteine is pH dependent, with mucolytic action significant at pH ranges of 7.0 to 9.0.[72] N-acetylcysteine is also used as an antidote in acetaminophen overdose to prevent or lessen hepatic injury.

Dosage and Administration. The recommended dose of N-acetylcysteine in children is 3 to 5 ml of the 20% solution diluted with an equal volume of water or saline (or 6 to 10 ml of a 10% solution) administered by nebulization three or four times a day.[2]

Adverse Events. Adverse effects reported with N-acetylcysteine include stomatitis, vomiting, hemoptysis, and severe rhinorrhea. It has an unpleasant, pungent odor that may lead to an increased incidence of nausea. Bronchospasm has also been reported with N-acetylcysteine therapy.[73]

RECOMBINANT HUMAN DNASE (PULMOZYME)

An additional factor that contributes to viscous mucus in CF patients is extracellular DNA. Bacterial cell death and subsequent cell lysis release DNA into the extracellular environment. This high extracellular DNA content works to thicken airway secretions further.[74] DNase is a highly purified solution of recombinant human deoxyribonuclease I (rhDNase), an enzyme that selectively cleaves DNA.[72] rhDNase has been demonstrated to reduce the viscosity of sputum in CF patients by hydrolyzing the extracellular DNA. Studies have shown that daily administration of rhDNase results in a definite improvement in the outcome of pulmonary function, as assessed by improved FEV_1 above baseline. Using rhDNase also resulted in a significant reduction in the number of patients experiencing respiratory tract infections requiring parenteral antibiotics.[75,76]

Dosage and Administration. Recombinant human DNase was approved by the FDA in 1993 and currently is indicated in the management of patients with CF to improve pulmonary function and decrease the frequency of respiratory infections. The recommended dose for most patients with CF is 2.5 mg by nebulization once daily. Some patients may benefit from twice-daily treatments. Safety and efficacy have not been demonstrated in children less than 5 years of age.

Adverse Events. Adverse effects are minimal and include voice alteration, pharyngitis, laryngitis, rash, and chest pain. To date there have been no case reports of anaphylaxis.[72,76] rhDNase should be kept refrigerated and not exposed to room temperature for a total time exceeding 24 hours. Discolored and cloudy solutions of rhDNase should be discarded.[76]

PARALYTICS (NEUROMUSCULAR BLOCKADE OR CHEMICAL PARALYSIS)

PANCURONIUM (PAVULON)

Pancuronium is a nondepolarizing neuromuscular blocking agent. It is nearly five times as potent as tubocurarine and one-third less potent than vecuronium. Pancuronium has little effect on the circulatory system. A small rise in heart rate may be associated with a small rise in peripheral vascular resistance and mean airway pressure. Pancuronium is not associated with histamine release.[77] The initial IV dose for endotracheal intubation is 0.06 to 0.1 mg/kg. Time of onset of action may take several minutes, requiring bag-mask ventilation to maintain oxygenation. Doubling the dose will shorten this time, but the drug effect will last longer. Patients with myasthenia gravis may have profound effects from small doses of pancuronium. Pancuronium is excreted primarily through the kidneys, so caution should be used in dosing patients with renal problems.

VECURONIUM (NORCURON)

Vecuronium, a nondepolarizing neuromuscular blocker, is nearly one-third as potent as pancuronium and does not have the cardioactive or histaminic actions of rocuronium. Vecuronium is highly protein bound (60% to 80%) and therefore over time moves into adipose tissue. For this reason, reversal of the paralytic effects may be prolonged after a course of continuous IV therapy.[77] An initial IV dose of 0.1 mg/kg immediately before intubation is suggested. The continuous IV dose is 0.08 to 0.1 mg/kg/hr. A peripheral nerve stimulator should be used in monitoring all patients on continuous infusions of neuromuscular blockers. Patients with myasthenia gravis will be profoundly affected by small doses of vecuronium.

Prolonged use of neuromuscular blocking agents may result in peripheral neuropathy, thus prolonging the effects of chemical paralysis and slowing recovery. It is difficult to distinguish the cause for the delay in reversal of neuromuscular blockade. Recovery may be hampered by recirculation of paralytic agents from adipose tissue or third spacing. It may also be due to peripheral neuropathy associated with the underlying disease process, as in severe sepsis, or secondary iatrogenic effect of the neuromuscular blockade combined with corticosteroid use.

ROCURONIUM (ZEMURON)

Rocuronium injection is a nondepolarizing neuromuscular blocking agent with a rapid to intermediate onset and intermediate duration of action. It acts by competing for cholinergic receptors at the motor end plate. Acetylcholinesterase inhibitors such as neostigmine and edrophonium antagonize this action. Rocuronium is used in rapid-sequence intubations and when a quick-acting, short-duration paralytic agent is needed. Other indications are the need for skeletal muscle relaxation or

increased pulmonary compliance, especially in trauma patients. The recommended dose for continuous infusion is 0.01 to 0.012 mg/kg/min and titrated to effect. The time to complete recovery after discontinuation of the infusion is proportional to the total dose given.[77] Rocuronium has the capacity to release clinically significant concentrations of plasma histamines. Cardiogenic effects may occur, including tachycardia and increases or decreases in mean arterial pressure. It may be associated with increased pulmonary vascular resistance, so caution is appropriate in patients with pulmonary hypertension or valvular heart disease. In patients with myasthenia gravis, small doses of rocuronium may have a profound effect.

KETAMINE

Ketamine is an anesthetic agent that produces anesthesia, sedation, and amnesia without significant respiratory depression. Because of its bronchodilating effects, ketamine has been used as part of rapid-sequence intubation in the pediatric patient with status asthmaticus. It has also been used as a combined bronchodilator and sedative in patients with asthma requiring mechanical ventilation.[78,79] The mechanism of action appears to be a selective interruption of the association pathways of the brain. The resulting bronchodilation may be of sympathetic origin. There is also a parasympathetic limb of action whereby ketamine diminishes acetylcholine activity on the bronchial smooth muscle, resulting in bronchodilation.

Ketamine is given through a central venous catheter as a continuous infusion. The normal sedation dose is listed as 5 to 20 μg/kg/min. For bronchodilation, the starting dose may be as small as 2 μg/kg/min and titrated to effect.[80,81] For sedation or minor procedures, the dose is 0.5 to 1 mg/kg.[82] Duration of action of a single dose is 10 to 20 minutes. State laws vary as to who is allowed to administer and titrate ketamine.

Adverse effects seen with ketamine include increased sympathomimetic activity, seizures, delirium, increased laryngeal secretions, and respiratory depression. During the recovery phase, unusual dreams and hallucinations have been reported. Premedication with midazolam (less than 0.1 mg/kg) can attenuate this effect. Intubation equipment must be readily available before administering ketamine, because the sedative effects may result in respiratory failure and the need for emergency intubation. Epinephrine should also be available for possible bradycardia.

NARCOTIC ANTAGONISTS

FLUMAZENIL (ROMAZICON)

Flumazenil, a benzodiazepine antagonist, is effective in reversing benzodiazepine-induced sedation. Flumazenil is indicated for the complete or partial reversal of the sedative effects of benzodiazepines used for general sedation or anesthesia and for the management of benzodiazepine overdose.[83] The ability of flumazenil to reverse benzodiazepine-induced respiratory depression remains controversial. This parameter is difficult to assess because respiration is both automatic and voluntary. Increased alertness may result in improved respiration even though central respiratory drive remains depressed.[84]

The antagonistic effects of flumazenil are both competitive and dose dependent. A higher relative concentration of the antagonist near the receptor site will result in a reversal of the benzodiazepine action.[85] The use of flumazenil does not preclude the need for observation and prompt recognition of hypoventilation, along with intervention by establishing an airway and assisting ventilation.[83]

Dosage and Administration. Flumazenil is recommended for IV administration only and is most often used for the reversal of conscious sedation. The recommended initial dose is 0.2 mg over 15 seconds. A second dose of 0.2 mg may be given after waiting 45 seconds if the desired level of consciousness is not achieved. Repeated doses of 0.2 mg may be administered every 60 seconds to a maximum total dose of 1 mg. This initial dosing regimen may be repeated every 20 minutes for control of resedation, up to a maximum of 3 mg in a 1-hour period. Dosing regimens vary slightly for the management of suspected benzodiazepine overdose.[2,83] The half-life of flumazenil is often less than that of the offending benzodiazepine, so multiple doses may be needed before the effects of the initial drug have worn off. Patients should be monitored for resedation.

Adverse Events. Adverse effects attributed to flumazenil include injection site pain, nausea, vomiting, and dizziness. Seizures are the most frequently reported serious adverse event, most often occurring (1) in patients receiving benzodiazepines for anticonvulsant therapy, (2) in patients physically dependent on benzodiazepines, and (3) in the presence of mixed ingestion of cyclic antidepressants.[2,83]

NALOXONE (NARCAN)

Naloxone is a pure opiate antagonist with little or no agonist action. In the absence of narcotics, it exhibits no detectable pharmacologic activity. Naloxone appears to work by competing for opiate receptor binding sites and reversing or antagonizing most of the opiate effects. It antagonizes the respiratory depression, hypotension, and sedation observed with opiate administration. Naloxone's duration of action is often shorter than that of the opiate. Therefore close observation of the patient is necessary because repeat dosing may be required.[86] Naloxone is indicated for the treatment of opiate-induced respiratory depression and acute opiate overdose. It is often used in neonates to aid in the management of hypoxia resulting from the administration of opiates to the mother during delivery.[87]

Dosage and Administration. Naloxone is available as an IV, IM, or SC injection. It may also be administered through an endotracheal tube in emergency situations when IV access cannot be established. The recommended dose for children weighing less than 20 kg is 0.01 to 0.1 mg/kg, with repeat doses as needed every 3 to 5 minutes. Dosage for children weighing 20 kg or greater, or children 5 years of age or older, is 2 mg every 3 to 5 minutes as needed.[2,86]

Adverse Events. Abrupt reversal of narcotic depression may result in nausea, vomiting, diaphoresis, tachycardia, hypertension, and tremors. Postoperative naloxone use has been associated with hypotension, hypertension, ventricular tachycardia, and pulmonary edema.[86]

AEROSOLIZED ANTIBIOTICS

AMINOGLYCOSIDES, β-LACTAMS, AND COLISTIN

Direct aerosol delivery of antibiotics reduces systemic adverse effects and is often used for targeted drug delivery. Aminoglycosides (e.g., tobramycin), β-lactams (e.g., ceftazidime), and colistin have all been used with varying degrees of success.[74] Preliminary analysis of a study evaluating inhalation of 600 mg of tobramycin every 8 hours has reported a positive response, as demonstrated by favorable improvement in pulmonary status and reduction in *Pseudomonas* sputum density.

Doses currently used for nebulization of colistin (Coly-Mycin) is 150 mg/day divided every 6 to 12 hours. Recommended dose for tobramycin is 40 to 80 mg two or three times daily. High-dose regimen for adults and children older than 6 years of age is 300 mg every 12 hours. Colistin is administered in repeated cycles of 28 days "on" the drug followed by 28 days "off" the drug.[72,88]

PENTAMIDINE (NEBUPENT)

Pneumocystis carinii pneumonia (PCP) is one of the most common opportunistic infections in patients with acquired immunodeficiency syndrome (AIDS). Mortality for adults approaches 50% in severe cases of PCP in patients requiring mechanical ventilation. PCP is associated with even higher mortality in children. Effective PCP prophylaxis improved the quality of life and reduced mortality among patients with AIDS.[89,90] Prophylaxis has not, however, removed the threat of PCP. There are still treatment failures, persons who are not aware of their disease, and lack of compliance with prophylactic treatment.

The Centers for Disease Control and Prevention (CDC) recommends aerosolized pentamidine as an effective agent for PCP prophylaxis. Although the mechanism of action is not completely understood, pentamidine inhibits protein and nucleic acid synthesis.[91] The role of aerosolized pentamidine for PCP prophylaxis in children has not been completely evaluated. However, pentamidine may be an effective option in children who are old enough to comply with aerosol administration.

Dosage and Administration. The recommended dose is 300 mg of pentamidine given by nebulization every 4 weeks. This is shown to be more effective than a dosing regimen of 30 mg given every 2 weeks or 150 mg given every 2 weeks. Pentamidine in doses of 300 mg every 28 days has been shown to prevent first episodes of PCP in 60% to 70% of patients.[90] The nebulizer used to administer pentamidine should include a one-way valve assembly.

Adverse Events. Aerosol administration of pentamidine is associated with fewer systemic adverse effects than is oral administration of prophylactic agents. Common side effects include cough, rash, dizziness, nausea, and gagging. Reversible bronchospasm is also a frequent adverse effect. A common practice is to pretreat patients with an inhaled β-agonist to reduce the occurrence of bronchospasm.[91]

ANTIVIRAL AGENTS

RESPIRATORY SYNCYTIAL VIRUS INFECTIONS

Respiratory syncytial virus (RSV) is a frequent cause of lower respiratory tract infection in infants and young children. More than 50% of infants experience RSV infections during their first year of life, with virtually all children experiencing a RSV infection during the first 3 years of life. Outbreaks are seasonal and most common during the fall and winter months.[92] In the Northern Hemisphere, RSV season is usually designated as October through March or April. Approximately 0.5% to 2% of infants with severe lower respiratory tract disease require hospitalization and medical intervention, with most of these infants less than 6 months of age.[93]

Children most susceptible to serious or even fatal disease include those with a history of congenital heart disease, bronchopulmonary dysplasia (BPD), pulmonary hypertension, premature birth (gestational age less than 34 weeks), and immunodeficiency. Patients with severe illness are typically younger than 3 months of age and present with an oxygen saturation less than 95%, respiratory rates greater than 70 breaths per minute, and atelectasis. These patients often require intensive respiratory support that includes mechanical ventilation.[93]

RIBAVIRIN (VIRAZOLE)

Ribavirin is a synthetic nucleoside with broad-spectrum antiviral activity. It appears to disrupt viral protein synthesis through inhibition of messenger ribonucleic acid (mRNA) expression.[94] Ribavirin is approved for the treatment of hospitalized children with severe, lower respiratory tract disease caused by RSV. The American Academy of Pediatrics (AAP) guidelines for ribavirin therapy are stringent because of concerns about cost, benefit, safety, and variable clinical efficacy.[92]

Dosage and Administration. Ribavirin is recommended for continuous aerosol administration through an oxygen hood, tent, or face mask for 12 to 20 hours daily for a mean of 4 days.[95] Aerosolized ribavirin should be administered only with the Viratek SPAG-2 aerosol-generating device (ICN Pharmaceuticals). A 20-mg/ml ribavirin solution is the recommended treatment regimen. Special precautions are essential in mechanically ventilated patients to prevent complications and reduce the risk of crystalline precipitation in the circuit, with subsequent ventilator dysfunction.[95]

Adverse Events. Adverse events attributed to ribavirin are infrequent but include worsening respiratory function and cardiovascular effects. The most common adverse effects reported by health care personnel exposed to the aerosolized ribavirin include eye irritation (especially in those wearing contact lenses) and headache. Because ribavirin can precipitate on contact lenses, protective goggles or glasses are recommended. Teratogenic toxicities have been observed in animal models. These effects have not been reported in humans.[96]

RESPIRATORY SYNCYTIAL VIRUS IMMUNE GLOBULIN INTRAVENOUS (RESPIGAM)

Respiratory syncytial virus immune globulin IV (RSV-IGIV) is sterile, liquid immunoglobulin G (IgG) containing neutralizing antibody to RSV. It is used for RSV prophylaxis. Released in 1996, RespiGam was the first antiviral agent approved for the prevention and amelioration of RSV disease. RespiGam contains IgG antibodies representative of the large number of normal, healthy persons who contributed to the plasma pools from which the product was derived. The immune globulin contains a high concentration of neutralizing and protective antibodies directed against RSV.[97] According to the AAP, RespiGam is considered an *immunoprophylaxis* agent.

Dosage and Administration. RespiGam is approved for use in children less than 24 months of age. It is administered once per month for 4 to 5 months, at the height of RSV season. The AAP reports the following factors and recommendations in the use of RespiGam:

1. RSV-IGIV prophylaxis should be considered for infants and children younger than 2 years of age with BPD who are currently receiving or have received oxygen therapy within the 6 months before the anticipated RSV season.
2. Infants with a gestational age of 32 weeks or less who do not have BPD may benefit from RSV-IGIV prophylaxis.
3. The FDA has not approved RSV-IGIV for patients with congenital heart disease.
4. RSV-IGIV use, either prophylactically or therapeutically, has not been evaluated in randomized trials in immunocompromised infants and children.
5. The need for and efficacy of RSV-IGIV prophylaxis in an RSV outbreak in a high-risk hospital unit (e.g., pediatric intensive care unit) has not been documented.
6. RSV-IGIV prophylaxis should be initiated before the onset of RSV season and terminated at the end of the season.
7. In infants and children receiving RSV-IGIV prophylaxis, immunization with measles-mumps-rubella (MMR) and varicella vaccines should be deferred for 9 months after the last dose.[92]

Adverse Events. The most common adverse effects of RespiGam are fever, fluid overload, and decreased oxygen saturation. The decision to initiate RSV-IGIV prophylaxis should be patient specific. Considerations include underlying disease, chance of therapy completion, cost of administration, and socioeconomic environment.[98]

PALIVIZUMAB (SYNAGIS)

In 1998, the FDA approved palivizumab (Synagis), the latest drug in MedImmune's quest for a RSV vaccine or prophylactic agent.[99] Palivizumab is a humanized monoclonal antibody for the prevention of disease caused by RSV. In Phase III trials, 1502 high-risk infants were treated with palivizumab. The hospitalization rate was 55% less in the palivizumab group than in the placebo-controlled group. Unlike its predecessor RespiGam, which must be administered as an IV infusion, palivizumab is an IM formulation. It still must be given for the 5 months of RSV season. Studies have found palivizumab to be safe and well tolerated in the high-risk pediatric population targeted for this product.[100,101] This group includes infants born prematurely (less than 35 weeks' gestation), those less than 6 months of age, and infants with BPD who are less than 24 months of age. Doses of 15 mg/kg given once monthly maintain serum concentrations of greater than 40 µg/ml for most patients.

TROMETHAMINE (THAM)

Tromethamine is a sodium-free alkalinizing agent that acts as a hydrogen ion (proton) acceptor. THAM is a weak base that combines with hydrogen ions from carbonic acid to form bicarbonate and cationic buffer. Administration of tromethamine decreases pH, which results in a decrease in carbon dioxide concentrations and an increase in bicarbonate concentrations. Decreased carbon dioxide removes a potent respiratory stimulus and may result in hypoxia. The administration of tromethamine also increases urine output through osmotic diuresis. Excretion of electrolytes and carbon dioxide is also increased. Urine pH increases with excretion of electrolytes.[102,103]

Tromethamine is indicated for the correction of metabolic acidosis. It may be preferable to sodium bicarbonate for the management of metabolic acidosis in patients with restricted sodium or carbon dioxide elimination.[104] Tromethamine is administered as a slow infusion. The dosage is based on the severity of the metabolic acidosis and is the minimal amount required to return the pH to within normal limits. The equation for estimating tromethamine infusion is as follows:

$$0.3M \text{ Tromethamine (ml)} = 1.1 \times \text{Body weight (kg)} \times (\text{Normal HCO}_3 - \text{Patient's HCO}_3)$$

Subsequent doses are based on additional laboratory values and the patient's overall condition.

Adverse effects are infrequent with THAM but include transient hypoglycemia, respiratory depression, and hemorrhagic hepatic necrosis. Most reported side effects are local and occur from the administration of an alkaline solution. Local adverse effects include irritation at the injection site, chemical phlebitis, and venous thrombosis.[104]

REFERENCES

1. Nahata MC: Pediatrics. In DiPiro JT et al, editors: *Pharmacotherapy: a pathophysiologic approach.* Norwalk, Conn, Appleton & Lange, 1997; pp 77-85.
2. Taketomo CK, Hodding JH, Kraus DM, editors: *Pediatric dosage handbook,* ed 8. Cleveland, Lexi-Comp, 2001-2002; pp 3-5.
3. Hoffman BB, Lefkowitz RJ: Catecholamines, sympathomimetic drugs, and adrenergic receptor antagonists. In Hardman JG et al, editors: *Goodman and Gilman's the pharmacological basis of therapeutics,* ed 9. New York, McGraw-Hill, 1996; pp 199-248.
4. Serafin WE: Drugs used in the treatment of asthma. In Hardman JG et al, editors: *Goodman and Gilman's the pharmacological basis of therapeutics,* ed 9. New York, McGraw-Hill, 1996; pp 659-682.
5. Kelly HW, Kamada AK: Asthma. In DiPiro JT et al, editors: *Pharmacotherapy: a pathophysiologic approach,* ed 3. Norwalk, Conn, Appleton & Lange, 1997, pp 653-688.
6. Cockcroft DW: Inhaled B$_2$-agonist and airway responses to allergen. *J Allergy Clin Immunol* 1998; 102(5):S96-S97.
7. Everard ML, LeSouef PN: Aerosol therapy and delivery systems. In Taussig LM, Landau LI, editors: *Pediatric respiratory medicine.* St Louis, Mosby, 1999; pp 286-299.
8. Dolovich M: Aerosol delivery to children: what to use, how to choose. *Pediatr Pulmonol Suppl* 1999; 18:79-82.
9. Lipworth BJ, Aziz I: A high dose of albuterol does not overcome bronchoprotective subsensitivity in asthmatic subjects receiving regular salmeterol or formoterol. *J Allergy Clin Immunol* 1999; 103:88-92.
10. Spitzer WO et al: The use of beta agonists and the risk of death and near death from asthma. *N Engl J Med* 1992; 326:501-506.
11. Smith L: Childhood asthma: diagnosis and treatment. *Curr Probl Pediatr* 1993; 23:271-305.
12. Second Expert Panel on Asthma: *Guidelines for the diagnosis and management of asthma.* Bethesda, Md, National Asthma Education and Prevention Program, National Heart, Lung and Blood Institute, 1997.
13. Kornecki A, Shemie SD: Bronchodilators and RSV-induced respiratory failure: agonizing about β$_2$-agonists. *Pediatr Pulmonol* 1998; 26:4-5.
14. Kastrup EK et al, editors: Respiratory drugs. In *Drug facts and comparisons.* St Louis, Facts and Comparisons, 1997; pp 1095-1336.
15. Handley D: The asthma-like pharmacology and toxicology of (S)-isomers of beta-agonists. *J Allergy Clin Immunol* 1999; 104(suppl):S69.
16. Spagnolo SV: Status asthmaticus and hospital management of asthma. *Immun Allergy Clin North Am* 2001; 21: 503-533.
17. Gawchik SM et al: The safety and efficacy of nebulized levalbuterol compared with racemic albuterol and placebo in the treatment of asthma in pediatric patients. *J Allergy Clin Immunol* 1999; 103:615-621.
18. Xopenex inhalation solution package insert. Marlborough, Mass, Sepracor, 1999.
19. Maxair Autohaler package insert. Northridge, Calif, 3M Pharmaceuticals, 1999.
20. Condemi JJ et al: The addition of salmeterol to fluticasone propionate versus increasing the dose of fluticasone propionate in patients with persistent asthma: Salmeterol Study Group. *Ann Allergy Asthma Immunol* 1999; 82:383-389.
21. Murray JJ et al: Concurrent use of salmeterol with inhaled corticosteroids is more effective than inhaled corticosteroid dose increases. *Allergy Asthma Proc* 1999; 20: 173-180.
22. Pearlman DS et al: A comparison of salmeterol with albuterol in the treatment of mild-to-moderate asthma. *N Engl J Med* 1992; 327:1420.
23. Serevent Discus package insert. Research Triangle Park, NC, Glaxo Wellcome, 1999.
24. Foradil Aerolizer package insert. East Hanover, NJ, Novartis Pharmaceuticals, 2001.
25. Racepinephrine inhalation solution package insert. Orlando, Fla, Nephron Pharmaceuticals, 1996.
26. Brown JH, Taylor P: Atropine, scopolamine, and related antimuscarinic drugs. In Hardman JG et al, editors: *Goodman and Gilman's the pharmacological basis of therapeutics,* ed 9. New York, McGraw-Hill, 1996; pp 149-154.
27. Atropine sulfate package insert. Cherry Hill, NJ, Elkins-Sinn, 1989.
28. Garrett JE et al: Nebulized salbutamol with and without ipratropium bromide in the treatment of acute asthma. *J Allergy Clin Immunol* 1997; 100(2):165-170.
29. Qureshi F et al: Effect of nebulized ipratropium on the hospitalization rates of children with asthma. *N Engl J Med* 1998; 339:1030.
30. Schuh S et al: Efficacy of frequent nebulized ipratropium bromide added to frequent high-dose albuterol therapy in severe childhood asthma. *J Pediatr* 1995; 126:639.
31. Atrovent Inhaler package insert. Ridgefield, Conn, Boehringer Ingelheim Pharmaceuticals, 1999.
32. May JR, Feger TA, Guill MF: Allergic rhinitis. In DiPiro JT et al, editors: *Pharmacotherapy: a pathophysiologic approach.* Norwalk, Conn, Appleton & Lange, 1997; pp 1801-1813.
33. Combivent Inhaler package insert. Ridgefield, Conn, Boehringer Ingelheim Pharmaceuticals, 1999.
34. McEvoy GK: Respiratory smooth muscle relaxants. In McEvoy GK, editor: *American Hospital Formulary Service drug information.* Bethesda, Md, American Society of Hospital Pharmacists, 1993; pp 2278-2285.
35. Kastrup EKM et al, editors: Gastrointestinal anticholinergics/antispasmodics. In *Drug facts and comparisons.* St Louis, Facts and Comparisons, 1997; pp 2024-2037.
36. Theophylline extended-release tablets package insert. Kenilworth, NJ, Key Pharmaceuticals, 1989.
37. Joint Task Force on Practice Parameters: Practice parameters for the diagnosis and treatment of asthma. *J Allergy Clin Immunol* 1995; 96(suppl):707-870.
38. Bender B, Milgrom HA: Theophylline-induced behavior change in children: an objective evaluation of parent's perceptions. *JAMA* 1992; 267:1621-1624.
39. Skobeloff EM et al: Effect of magnesium chloride on rabbit bronchial smooth muscle. *Ann Emerg Med* 1990; 19:1107.
40. Haury VG: Blood serum magnesium in bronchial asthma and its treatment by administration of magnesium sulfate. *J Lab Clin Med* 1940; 26:340.
41. McNamera RM et al: Intravenous magnesium sulfate in the management of acute respiratory failure complicating asthma. *Ann Emerg Med* 1989; 18:197.
42. Noppen M et al: Bronchodilating effect of intravenous magnesium sulfate in acute severe bronchial asthma. *Chest* 1990; 97:373-377.
43. Okayama H et al: Treatment of status asthmaticus with intravenous magnesium sulfate. *J Asthma* 1991; 28:11-17.
44. Ciarallo L, Sauer AH, Shannon MW: Intravenous magnesium therapy for moderate to severe pediatric asthma: results of a randomized placebo-controlled trial. *J Pediatr* 1996; 129(6):809-814.
45. Intal Inhaler package insert. Collegeville, Pa, Rhone-Poulenc Rorer Pharmaceuticals, 1997.
46. Tilade Inhaler package insert. Collegeville, Pa, Rhone-Poulenc Rorer Pharmaceuticals, 1998.

47. Kemp JP: Nedocromil sodium, a new bronchial anti-inflammatory agent. *Today Ther Trends* 1992; 10:39-48.

48. Wolthers OD, Pedersen S: Controlled study of linear growth in asthmatic children during treatment with inhaled glucocorticosteroids. *Pediatrics* 1992; 89:839-842.

49. Tinkelman DG et al: Aerosol beclomethasone dipropionate compared with theophylline as primary treatment of chronic, mild to moderately severe asthma in children. *Pediatrics* 1993; 9264-9277.

50. American College of Chest Physicians Consensus Statement: Medscape.com/other/guidelines/ACCP/accp.fda/accp.fda.html.

51. Gregson RK et al: Effect of inhaled corticosteroids on bone mineral density in childhood asthma: comparison of fluticasone propionate with beclomethasone dipropionate. *Osteoporos Int* 1998; 8:418-422.

52. Wenzel SE: New approaches to anti-inflammatory therapy for asthma. *Am J Med* 1998; 104:287-300.

53. Sanders P et al: Hypertension during reduction of long-term steroid therapy in young subjects with asthma. *J Allergy Clin Immunol* 1992; 89:816-821.

54. Flovent package insert. Research Triangle Park, NC, Glaxo Wellcome, 1999.

55. Aerobid package insert. St Louis, Forest Pharmaceuticals, 1996.

56. Hanania NA, Chapman KR, Kesten S: Adverse effects of inhaled corticosteroids. *Am J Med* 1995; 98:196-208.

57. Horwitz RJ, McGill KA, Busse WW: The role of leukotriene modifiers in the treatment of asthma. *Am J Respir Crit Care Med* 1998; 157:1363-1371.

58. Drazen J: Clinical pharmacology of leukotriene receptor antagonists and 5-antagonists. *Am J Respir Crit Care Med* 1998; 157:S233-S237.

59. Bernstein PR: Chemistry and structure-activity relationships of leukotriene receptor antagonists. *Am J Respir Crit Care Med* 1998; 157:S220-S226.

60. Aharony D: Pharmacology of leukotriene receptor antagonists. *Am J Respir Crit Care Med* 1998; 157:S214-S219.

61. Chung KF: Leukotriene receptor antagonists and biosynthesis inhibitors: potential breakthrough in asthma therapy. *Eur Respir J* 1995; 8:1203-1213.

62. Singulair package insert. Whitehouse Station, NJ, Merck, 1999.

63. Knorr B et al: Montelukast for chronic asthma in 6- to 14-year-old children. *JAMA* 1998; 279:1181-1186.

64. Leff JA et al: Montelukast, a leukotriene-receptor antagonist, for the treatment of mild asthma and exercise-induced bronchoconstriction. *N Engl J Med* 1998; 339(3):147-152.

65. Accolate package insert. Wilmington, Del, Zeneca Pharmaceuticals, 1999.

66. Wechsler ME et al: Pulmonary infiltrates, eosinophilia, and cardiomyopathy following corticosteroid withdrawal in patients with asthma receiving zafirlukast. *JAMA* 1998; 279:455-457.

67. Holloway J et al: Churg-Strauss syndrome associated with zafirlukast. *J Am Osteopath Assoc* 1998; 98(5):275-278.

68. Knoell DL et al: Churg-Strauss syndrome associated with zafirlukast. *Chest* 1998; 114(1):332-334.

69. Zyflo package insert. Chicago, Abbott Laboratories, 1998.

70. Isreal E et al: The effect of inhibition of 5-lipoxygenase by zileuton in mild-to-moderate asthma. *Ann Intern Med* 1993; 119:1059-1066.

71. Liu MC et al: Acute and chronic effects of a 5-lipoxygenase inhibitor in asthma: a 6-month randomized multicenter trial. *J Allergy Clin Immunol* 1996; 98:859-871.

72. Kastrup EK et al, editors: Respiratory inhalant products. In *Drug facts and comparisons.* St Louis, Facts and Comparisons, 1997; pp 1141-1163.

73. McEvoy GK: Mucolytic agents. In McEvoy GK, editor: *American Hospital Formulary Service drug information.* Bethesda, Md, American Society of Hospital Pharmacists, 1993; pp 1680-1682.

74. Duplantier D, McWaters DS: Cystic fibrosis: progress against a childhood killer. *US Pharm* 1992; 17:34-52.

75. Ranasinha C et al: Efficacy and safety of short-term administration of aerosolized recombinant human DNase I in adults with stable stage cystic fibrosis. *Lancet* 1993; 342:199-202.

76. Pulmozyme package insert. San Francisco, Calif, Genentech, 1993.

77. Kastrup EK et al, editors: Muscle relaxants: adjuncts to anesthesia; Nondepolarizing neuromuscular blockers. In *Drug facts and comparisons.* St Louis, Facts and Comparisons, 1997; pp 1901-1943.

78. Strube PJ, Hallam PL: Ketamine by continuous infusion in status asthmaticus. *Anesthesia* 1986; 41:1017.

79. Sarma VJ: Use of ketamine in acute severe asthma. *Acta Anaesthesiol Scand* 1992; 36:106.

80. Howton JC et al: Randomized, double-blind, placebo-controlled trial of intravenous ketamine in acute asthma. *Ann Emerg Med* 1996; 27:170-175.

81. Hemming A, MacKenzie I, Finfer S: Response to ketamine in status asthmaticus resistant to maximal medical treatment. *Thorax* 1994; 49:90-91.

82. Nehama J et al: Continuous ketamine infusion for the treatment of refractory asthma in a mechanically ventilated infant: case report and review of the pediatric literature. *Pediatr Emerg Care* 1996; 12:294-297.

83. Romazicon package insert. Nutley, NJ, Roche Laboratories, 1993.

84. Shalansky SJ, Naumann TL, Englander FA: Effect of flumazenil on benzodiazepine-induced respiratory depression. *Clin Pharm* 1993; 12:483-487.

85. Smith RC: Flumazenil: a novel benzodiazepine antagonist. *OR Pharm* 1990; V(2):1-5.

86. Naloxone package insert. Westborough, Mass, Astra Pharmaceutical Products, 1991.

87. McEvoy GK: Opiate antagonists. In McEvoy GK, editor: *American Hospital Formulary Service drug information.* Bethesda, Md, American Society of Hospital Pharmacists, 1993; pp 1257-1259.

88. Bosso JA: Cystic fibrosis. In DiPiro JT et al, editors: *Pharmacotherapy: a pathophysiologic approach.* Norwalk, Conn, Appleton & Lange, 1997; pp 649-662.

89. Paar DP, Walker RE: PCP prophylaxis in patients with HIV infection. *Pharm Ther* September 1992; pp 429-438.

90. Fletcher CV, Collier AC, editors: Principles and management of human immunodeficiency virus infection. In DiPiro JT et al, editors: Pharmacotherapy: a pathophysiologic approach. Norwalk, Conn, Appleton & Lange, 1997; pp 2353-2386.

91. McEvoy GK: Miscellaneous anti-infectives. In McEvoy GK, editor: *American Hospital Formulary Service drug information.* Bethesda, Md, American Society of Hospital Pharmacists, 1993; pp 493-520.

92. Peter G et al: *Report of the Committee on Infectious Disease (1997 Red Book),* ed 24. Elk Grove, Ill, American Academy of Pediatrics, 1997; pp 683-690.

93. Christenson JC: Respiratory syncytial virus infections in the young infant: new developments in the treatment and prevention. *Neonatal Pharmacol Q* 1992; 1:39-45.

94. Virazole package insert. Costa Mesa, Calif, ICN Pharmaceuticals, 1993.

95. Committee on Infectious Diseases: Use of ribavirin in the treatment of respiratory syncytial virus infection. *Pediatrics* 1993; 92:501-504.

96. McEvoy GK: Antivirals. In McEvoy GK, editors: *American Hospital Formulary Service drug information.* Bethesda, Md, American Society of Hospital Pharmacists, 1993; pp 365-424.

97. RespiGam package insert. Gaithersburg, Md, MedImmune, 1993.

98. Sandritter TL, Kraus DM: Respiratory syncytial virus-immunoglobulin intravenous (RSV-IGIV) for respiratory syncytial viral infections. Part II. *J Pediatr Health Care* 1998; 12:85-92.

99. MedImmune: Press release. Gaithersburg, Md, 1998.

100. Welliver RC: Respiratory syncytial virus immunoglobulin and monoclonal antibodies in the prevention and treatment of respiratory syncytial virus infections. *Semin Perinatol* 1998; 22:87-95.

101. Subramanian KN et al: Safety, tolerance and pharmacokinetics of a humanized monoclonal antibody to respiratory syncytial virus in premature infants and infants with bronchopulmonary dysplasia. *Pediatr Infect Dis J* 1998; 17(2): 110-115.

102. Kilroy RA: Acid-base disorders. In DiPiro JT et al, editors: *Pharmacotherapy: a pathophysiologic approach.* Norwalk, Conn, Appleton & Lange, 1997; pp 1139-1159.

103. Nahas GG et al: Guidelines for the treatment of acidemia with THAM. *Drugs* 1998; 55:191-224.

104. McEvoy GK: Alkalinizing agents. In McEvoy GK, editors: *American Hospital Formulary Service drug information.* Bethesda, Md, American Society of Hospital Pharmacists, 1993, pp 1559-1566.

CHAPTER

Thoracic Organ Transplantation

Paul C. Stillwell
George B. Mallory, Jr.

Although the surgical techniques for thoracic organ transplantation have been available since the 1960s, it was not until more effective immunosuppression regimens became available in the late 1970s and early 1980s that there was a significant increase in the number of successful thoracic organ transplantations (Fig. 27-1).[1,2] Between 1984 and 1993, there were approximately 1970 heart transplants done in children younger than 19 years of age; more than half of these were between 1990 and 1993.[1] In contrast, only approximately 189 lung transplants were done in children between 1987 and 1993.[1] Between 1993 and 2000 annually there were about 350 pediatric heart transplants performed and about 65 to 85 pediatric lung and heart-lung transplants, respectively.[1] In the mid 1980s, heart-lung transplantation was employed for end-stage pulmonary disease because of the difficulty of maintaining the tracheal or bronchial anastomosis with lung transplantation alone. With improvement in surgical technique, as well as recognition that a single-lung transplant was effective for many disease states, it is now unusual to consider heart-lung transplantation for isolated pulmonary disease.[2,3] Therefore the practice is to provide heart transplantation for primary cardiac insufficiency and either single- or double-lung transplantation for end-stage pulmonary disease, reserving heart-lung transplantation for the infrequent circumstance of combined left ventricular heart failure with pulmonary disease or combined congenital defects of both the heart and lung (Table 27-1).[1-3]

The number of children waiting for thoracic organ transplantation is fewer than those waiting for kidney or liver transplantation (Fig. 27-2). There has been a steady increase in the number of transplantation candidates, but unfortunately there has been no increase in the number of donors. It is estimated that only 30% to 50% of potential organ donors consent

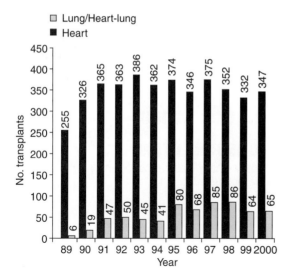

Fig. 27-1

The frequency of transplantation per year by type of transplant in children younger than 17 years of age. The number of pediatric heart, heart-lung, and lung transplants has remained stable over recent years after increases year by year in the early days of thoracic organ transplantation. (Redrawn from Hosenpud JD et al: The registry of the International Society for Heart and Lung Transplantation: eighteenth official report—2001. *J Heart Lung Transplant* 2001; 20:805-815.)

to donation. In patients who do consent to donate, it is common for the heart, kidney, and liver to be suitable for transplantation but not the lungs. This is because the lungs are frequently infected or damaged by prolonged intubation and ventilation, pulmonary edema, trauma, or aspiration. Until recently, clinicians managed potential donors with liberal fluid administration to optimize perfusion of abdominal organs, often with little regard to the condition of the lungs. A standardized clinical protocol for the management of patients meeting brain death criteria who may be potential organ donors has yet to be developed and circulated within the medical community. There is a critical need to increase awareness among health care professionals and the public of the need for organ procurement, but this alone will not meet the needs of all potential transplant recipients. One innovative solution to the donor shortage is the utilization of living lobar donation for lung transplantation (using a lower lobe of a living relative, usually a parent, rather than a whole lung from a brain-dead, size-matched donor).[4] Xenotransplantation, the transplantation of organs from an animal into a human, is another potential option to address donor organ shortages, but this option appears to be years away from implementation.[5]

TABLE 27-1	PEDIATRIC THORACIC ORGAN TRANSPLANTATION
Transplant Type	**Clinical Indication**
Heart	Cardiomyopathy
	Isolated congenital heart disease (irreparable)
Single lung*	Pulmonary fibrosis
	Pulmonary hypoplasia
	Bronchopulmonary dysplasia
	Idiopathic pulmonary hypertension
Double lung†	Bronchiectasis
	Cystic fibrosis
Single lung plus heart repair*	Pulmonary hypertension with atrial septal defect, ventricular septal defect, and patent ductus arteriosus
Heart-lung	Lung disease or pulmonary vascular disease with left ventricular dysfunction

*Some centers prefer to use two lungs in prepubertal children because of the uncertainties of potential growth in the remaining native lung.
†Many centers are now performing double-lung transplantation for pulmonary hypertension.

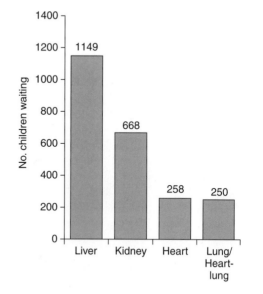

Fig. 27-2

The number of children awaiting solid organ transplantation by organ type as of June 30, 2000. There are a relatively large number of children awaiting kidney or liver transplantation compared with those waiting for heart, lung, or heart-lung transplantation. (Data from United Network for Organ Sharing, http://www.UNOS. org. October 2001.)

For children who undergo successful thoracic organ transplantation, the quality of life usually returns to normal.[6,7] Within weeks after the operation, depending on their pretransplantation nutritional and physical state, most patients are able to resume age-appropriate activities with improving exercise tolerance. Cardiac function is generally normal in heart transplant patients.[8] Gas exchange and pulmonary function rapidly return to near normal in the first months after lung transplantation.[6,7] Minor childhood illnesses appear to be well tolerated, although it is frequently difficult to ascertain in its initial stage whether a febrile illness represents a minor infection or a life-threatening infection in the immunocompromised host. Growth delay often remains a problem, at least in part resulting from the prednisone immunosuppression. However, subsequent growth of the patient as well as of the allograft is possible, and it is unlikely that the subject will outgrow the transplanted organ.[9]

HEART TRANSPLANTATION

In the 1980s, the primary indication for heart transplantation was cardiomyopathy; however, in recent years the proportion of transplantations for congenital heart defects has been increasing (Table 27-2).[1] Congenital lesions are the predominant problem leading to heart transplantation in children younger than 1 year of age, and cardiomyopathy is predominant in older children.[1] The early posttransplant mortality rate after transplantation is higher in younger children, as evidenced by the 25% mortality rate in the birth to 4-year age-group compared with 12% for the 10- to 18-year age-group.[1] The majority of early deaths in the posttransplantation period are directly related to intrinsic cardiovascular complications such as dysrhythmia or myocardial failure, with relatively fewer problems from infections and acute rejection. Late deaths, however, are primarily caused by rejection or infection. A small number of deaths in the early and late groups have been related to central nervous system complications such as stroke. There is approximately a 4% late death rate from malignancy (i.e., lymphoproliferative disease) as a result of chronic immunosuppression.[10] Other morbidities from heart transplantation have included hypertension in approximately 40% of individuals, renal insufficiency in 20%, and seizures in 25%.[8,11]

A troublesome problem in long-term heart transplant survivors, regardless of age, is the development of premature coronary artery disease, also known as graft atherosclerosis.[8,10,12] This condition may be asymptomatic and may be discovered only at the time of surveillance coronary angiography.

TABLE 27-2	INDICATIONS FOR HEART TRANSPLANTATION BY PERCENTAGE OF FREQUENCY IN EACH AGE-GROUP		
	<1 Yr (%)	1-10 Yr (%)	11-17 Yr (%)
Myopathy	19.7	52.4	65.4
Congenital	76.5	37.3	25
Other	2.6	5.0	6.3
Retransplantation	1.2	5.3	3.4

Modified from Hosenpud JD et al: The Registry of the International Society for Heart and Lung Transplantation: eighteenth official report—2001. *J Heart Lung Transplant* 2001; 20:805-815.

In some patients, the disease can be significant enough to cause myocardial ischemia and may contribute to dysrhythmias or sudden death. There is speculation that this premature coronary artery disease is immunologically mediated as a manifestation of chronic graft rejection and therefore may decrease in prevalence with improvements in immunosuppressive regimens.[12]

Neonatal heart transplantation has been successful at some centers. This has been used almost exclusively for hypoplastic left-heart syndrome, which is uniformly fatal if surgical correction or transplantation is not offered. The current experience with either surgical correction or transplantation does not clearly indicate which is more appropriate to optimize survival.[13] A controversial ethical issue in recent years involves the potential use of anencephalic infants as donors of hearts and other organs.[14] There are some suggestions that neonates are less sophisticated hosts by virtue of their relatively immature immune response and therefore might tolerate transplantation more readily than older subjects. The survival rate and duration of survival with good cardiac function appear to be the same for children as for adult heart transplant recipients.[1,13]

HEART-LUNG TRANSPLANTATION

Before the surgical technique for successful lung transplantation was developed, heart-lung transplantation was offered for end-stage pulmonary disease as well as for the unusual situation in which left-sided cardiac disease and pulmonary disease coexisted. With the ability to successfully transplant a single lung or two lungs, the use of heart-lung transplantation for pulmonary disease has been decreasing.[1,3] There are multiple reasons for this, including (1) the limited availability of satisfactory coupled heart-lung donations from a single donor (governed in part by the distribution algorithm unique to each country), (2) the practical advantage of utilizing the heart-lung block for three separate donations (one heart and two single lungs), (3) the decreased risk of cardiac rejection, (4) the decreased risk of premature coronary artery disease, and (5) perhaps a decreased risk of bronchiolitis obliterans. Despite concerns about the degree of right ventricular dysfunction commonly associated with chronic pulmonary disease, there has generally been an excellent improvement in right ventricular function with single- or double-lung transplantation, so severe right-sided cardiac dysfunction is rarely an indication for heart-lung transplantation.[2,3] For patients with congenital heart defects such as atrial septal defect, ventricular septal defect, or patent ductus arteriosus, as well as pulmonary hypertension from Eisenmenger's disease, the currently preferred surgery is lung transplantation (single or double) with repair of the congenital heart defect.[15] The volume of heart-lung transplantation has decreased by more than half over the past decade, from a peak of 240 transplants per year in 1989 to 104 per year in 2000.[1] The decrease in utilization of heart-lung transplantation is most dramatic in the United States compared with other countries, notably the United Kingdom.

LUNG TRANSPLANTATION

Once the problem of tracheal and bronchial anastomosis failure was overcome in the late 1980s, single- and double-lung transplantation became an option for adult patients with chronic pulmonary disease. Table 27-1 also lists the diseases appropriate for single- or double-lung transplantation. Fig. 27-3 shows which chronic lung diseases in children lead to transplantation. As can be seen in this figure, cystic fibrosis is the most common indication for bilateral lung transplantation.[1] Enthusiasm for lung transplantation has been somewhat tempered by the low survival rate; the initial 1-year survival rate was only 54% at 12 months (all patients, all ages).[16] This compares with early survival rates after heart-lung or double-lung transplants in patients with cystic fibrosis of 60% to 70% at 1 year.[1,17] As overall experience has increased, survival after lung transplantation has improved; the most recent actuarial survival at 1 year after transplant is 75%,[1] with some individual centers reporting even better survival.[18] Longer-term survival rates remain disappointing, however, with a 5-year survival of just below 50%.[1,16] Recent United Network for Organ Sharing (UNOS) data indicate a 1-year survival of 75.1% and a 5-year survival rate of 41.1%.[16] Lung transplant survival rates have a long way to go to be comparable with the successes

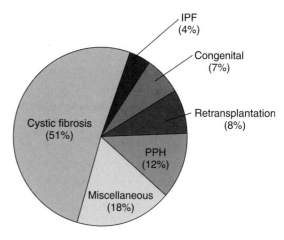

Fig. 27-3

The frequency of primary diseases leading to lung transplantation in children. Cystic fibrosis accounts for the majority of cases. The category "miscellaneous" is primarily made up of bronchopulmonary dysplasia or congenital lung defects. *IPF,* Idiopathic pulmonary fibrosis; *PPH,* primary pulmonary hypertension. (Redrawn from Hosenpud JD et al: The Registry of the International Society for Heart and Lung Transplantation: eighteenth official report—2001. *J Heart Lung Transplant* 2001; 20:805-815.)

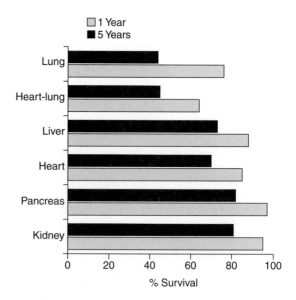

Fig. 27-4

The overall 1-year and 5-year survival rate for solid organ transplantations as reported by the United Network for Organ Sharing. Although improved from early experience, lung and heart-lung transplantations are not yet as successful as other solid organ transplantations, particularly long-term.

of kidney, heart, pancreas, and liver transplantation (Fig. 27-4).[16]

Deaths within the first 90 days after lung transplantation (early deaths) usually result from surgical difficulty such as airway anastomotic dehiscence or massive hemorrhage, acute graft failure, overwhelming infection with multiple organ failure, or acute rejection. Late deaths are generally related to infection or bronchiolitis obliterans, which is a form of chronic rejection.[6,7]

A particular concern in pediatric lung transplantation is the problem of donor-recipient size matching. In addition to the problems of donor availability among all transplantation candidates, the thoracic dimensions of infants and small children add another obstacle, so that size-appropriate donors are even less frequently available than for adolescents or adults.[19] A potential solution to this problem is reduced-size transplantation, often from a living donor (e.g., transplanting an adult lower lobe to a pediatric patient to replace the recipient's entire lung[20]). Although initial attempts at living-related donation were disappointing, more recent experience suggests that living-related lobar transplantation can be as successful as cadaveric transplantation with only minimal risk to the donor.[19,20] Therefore living donor lobar transplantation can help overcome the obstacles of donor waiting time, size limitation, and organ availability.[20,21]

IMMUNOSUPPRESSIVE REGIMENS

Although children frequently resume normal activity within weeks after transplantation, the medical regimen after thoracic transplantation is extensive, especially in the first year. In addition to a vast new pharmacologic program, there are frequent routine office visits, multiple blood tests, repeated radiographs, and, in most centers, surveillance biopsies. Even a minor illness can lead to hospitalization to rule out graft rejection or serious infection. With increasing time after transplantation and successful graft function, there are fewer impositions on the lives of the child and family. In another sense, the transplant patient trades one set of problems (the burdens of living with a terminal disease) for another (the long-term immunosuppression and lifelong awareness of potential life-threatening complications).

Most immunosuppressive regimens for organ transplantations (thoracic and other solid organs) include the combined use of cyclosporine or tacrolimus, azathioprine or mycophenolate mofetil, and prednisone.[1] The administration of cyclosporine or tacrolimus and azathioprine or mycophenolate mofetil is generally needed for the life of the transplant recipient. There has been an increasing trend to embrace a corticosteroid-free immunosuppres-

TABLE 27-3	COMMON SIDE EFFECTS OF IMMUNOSUPPRESSIVE DRUGS
Drug	**Side Effect**
Cyclosporine, tacrolimus	Headache
	Seizures
	Hirsutism (cyclosporine)
	Hypertension
	Hyperlipidemia
	Hypomagnesemia
	Hepatotoxicity
	Glucose intolerance
	Nephrotoxicity
	Lymphoproliferative disease
Azathioprine, mycophenolate mofetil	Neutropenia
	Nausea and vomiting
	Bone marrow suppression
	Hepatotoxicity
Prednisone	Cataract
	Acne
	Diabetes
	Psychosis
	Thin skin
	Hypokalemia
	Osteoporosis
	Fluid retention
	Growth impairment
	Cushingoid appearance
	Moon face
	Central obesity
	Ruddy complexion

sant program in pediatric heart transplant centers. Many other heart centers wean or attempt to discontinue prednisone within weeks to months after the transplantation. Because lung allografts are more susceptible to both acute and chronic rejection, immunosuppressant dosing is generally higher and more prolonged compared with that in heart transplant recipients. Fewer lung transplant centers attempt to wean patients off prednisone completely, opting for alternate-day dosing instead.

Immunosuppressive drugs are given intravenously in the immediate period after transplantation but are then changed to the oral route as patients recover from surgery. There are serious potential side effects from these medications (Table 27-3) as well as a multitude of drug interactions, of which all prescribing physicians need to be aware. Episodes of acute rejection are treated with augmented immunosuppression, generally with 3 days of high-dose intravenous steroid pulse. The clinical response is usually favorable and prompt. Occasionally, with repeated episodes of acute rejection or the appearance of chronic rejection, additional immunosuppressive agents may be required, such as antilymphocyte globulin, antithymocyte globulin, or monoclonal antibodies such as muromonab-CD3 (Orthoclone OKT3).[3] Although chronic rejection is also treated with augmented immunosuppression, the response is less often favorable than with acute rejection.[22,23]

COMPLICATIONS

The complications of thoracic organ transplantation can be grouped into the following major categories: (1) respiratory failure and related problems, (2) acute rejection, (3) infection, (4) chronic rejection or bronchiolitis obliterans, (5) drug toxicity, and (6) other complications.[3]

RESPIRATORY PROBLEMS

All thoracic transplantation patients return to the intensive care unit with an endotracheal tube in place and receiving mechanical ventilatory support. Most heart transplant patients who have good cardiac contractility in the immediate postoperative period can be weaned from mechanical ventilation within the first hours. The surgical incision and thoracostomy tube will result in reduced thoracic compliance, and both deep inspiration and cough will likely be compromised. With the judicious use of intravenous analgesics and chest physiotherapy, and occasionally regional nerve block or epidural anesthesia, most heart transplant patients, like their counterparts who undergo other cardiac surgical procedures, do well. A subset of heart transplant patients experience severe myocardial failure postoperatively. Extracorporeal membrane oxygenation may be required with or without mechanical ventilatory support for several days. Other patients require aggressive intravenous cardiotonic and diuretic medications. Oxygen supplementation is almost always used in these patients. More rarely, a relatively large heart graft that is placed in a smaller child may compress the intrathoracic airways, the left mainstem bronchus being most vulnerable to such compression. With compression, consolidation with absent breath sounds over the left lower lobe or low-pitched expiratory wheezing with a variable degree of dyspnea may result. Bronchodilators and vigorous chest physiotherapy are usually employed to maintain maximum airway patency and minimize atelectasis and retained secretions.

Heart-lung and lung transplant patients are more vulnerable to respiratory complications than are heart transplant patients. The thoracic incision is more extensive when lungs are transplanted. Allograft dysfunction after lung transplantation is common but highly variable. The delicate pulmonary capillary bed appears to be more susceptible to ischemic injury than is the myocardium, liver, or kidney; and capillary leak is common after lung transplantation.

This reperfusion injury, which occurs in 10% to 20% of lung transplants, mimics the acute respiratory distress syndrome clinically and radiographically. On chest radiography, pulmonary edema, either immediately after transplantation or within the first 72 hours, is usually a sign of ischemic injury or reperfusion injury (Fig. 27-5).[24,25] Interruption of the pulmonary lymphatics, which are cut during the surgery, may also contribute to the alveolar and interstitial fluid accumulation. On rare occasions, reperfusion injury is especially severe and progresses to a clinical and radiographic picture compatible with adult respiratory distress syndrome, which carries significant mortality.[25] Another complication occurring in a small subset of patients in the first week after lung transplantation is the overproduction of mucus (bronchorrhea). Signs and symptoms of abundant lower airway secretions without fever or leukocytosis will often lead to emergent bronchoscopy in which abundant thick mucus is found. With isolated bronchorrhea, cultures are sterile and Gram's stains demonstrate mucus, polymorphonuclear leukocytes, and no bacterial organisms. Vigorous chest physiotherapy and the addition of aerosolized atropine can be helpful. Bronchorrhea slowly subsides over several days to weeks. The cause is unknown, although it may be the result of autonomic imbalance related to vagotomy from the transplantation surgery.

Subacute respiratory failure requiring ventilatory support for 1 to 2 weeks without severe parenchymal disease is seen in some patients who had significant preoperative hypercapnia. Respiratory control mechanisms may require many days to reset after lung or heart-lung transplantation.[26] The keys to management are to avoid oversedation and provide adequate nutrition and ventilatory support until weaning can be achieved. Noninvasive ventilatory support with bilevel positive airway pressure (BiPAP) may help make the transition from the pretransplant hypercarbic state to the posttransplant normocarbic state.

Significant bronchial obstruction may develop after lung or heart-lung transplantation because of stricture or dehiscence at the site of the bronchial anastomosis. Most airway complications will present within 3 months of transplantation, and although a few can be fatal if severe and early, most are treatable with bronchoscopic dilation, laser resection of granulation tissue, or the placement of airway stents.[27,28]

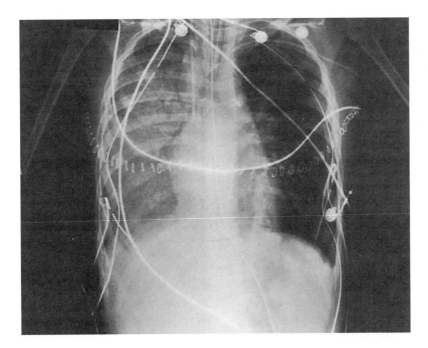

Fig. 27-5

This chest radiograph demonstrates reperfusion injury to the right lung immediately after double-lung transplantation in an 11-year-old girl with cystic fibrosis. There is a ground-glass haziness with air bronchograms over the right lung field. The staples across the chest are external and used for surgical skin closure. There are surgical clips in each hilar region where the vascular anastomoses were performed. There is also an endotracheal tube, a nasogastric tube, a left subclavian vein catheter, a right internal jugular vein catheter, bilateral chest tubes, and surface electrodes.

ORGAN REJECTION

The clinical signs and symptoms of organ rejection may be minimal or subtle. Acute rejection of the transplanted heart, if clinically apparent, results in decreased cardiac contractility with signs and symptoms of congestive heart failure. Tachycardia, tachypnea, and malaise may be noted. Echocardiography is the noninvasive diagnostic mode of choice to ascertain the physiologic signs of cardiac rejection. In the lung transplant patient, tachypnea, bibasilar inspiratory crackles on auscultation, increased interstitial infiltrates on chest radiography, and oxygen desaturation are often associated with acute rejection (Fig. 27-6). For older patients who can perform spirometry, a drop in pulmonary function, either restrictive or obstructive, is often the most sensitive indicator of acute rejection. Many transplantation centers perform routine surveillance biopsies of the transplanted tissue in an effort to identify and treat early rejection before permanent organ damage occurs.[29] When clinically suspected, the diagnosis of rejection is also usually confirmed by biopsy.[8,29] Endomyocardial biopsy by means of biopsy forceps passed through a vascular-accessed catheter is the method of choice in heart transplant patients. Flexible bronchoscopy with transbronchial biopsy in children and adolescents is used to obtain multiple pieces of tissue for histopathologic examination in lung transplant patients. For infants and young children, rigid bronchoscopy or open-lung biopsy may be required, although recently developed tiny biopsy forceps may allow biopsy through the flexible bronchoscope even in very small children. Most transplantation centers are uncomfortable augmenting immunosuppression without tissue confirmation of rejection.

INFECTION

It can be difficult to separate rejection from infection, especially on a clinical diagnostic basis, and in some cases they may coexist.[25] Although pulmonary infections are common because of the immunosuppression required with any solid organ transplant, the pulmonary infection rate for lung transplantation appears to be particularly high.[30] This may be partially explained by the fact that the lung is the only solid organ that after

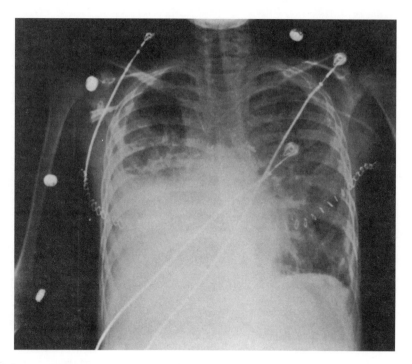

Fig. 27-6

The same patient in Fig. 27-5 seen 3 weeks later during an episode of acute lung rejection. A large right pleural effusion obscures the right hemidiaphragm and the border of the right side of the heart. There is an extensive increase in the peribronchial markings in both lungs and a blunted left costophrenic angle. All chest tubes and the endotracheal tube have been removed. A right subclavian vein catheter has been added.

transplantation is regularly in direct contact with the external environment and multiple potential pathogens. Many pulmonary bacterial infections are readily identified and easily treated with antibiotics. Pulmonary viral infections are less frequent but more often fatal, especially if cytomegalovirus is involved.[3,30] Fungal infections are particularly troublesome in terms of both identification and treatment. Because the transplant patient with cystic fibrosis retains the native trachea and sinuses, there is a potential increase in infections from chronic colonization of the respiratory epithelia in the trachea and the frank infection within the paranasal sinuses.[31] This can be particularly serious if the colonizing organisms have multiple antibiotic resistances.[32] In fact, some centers consider infection with *Pseudomonas* species that have no antibiotic sensitivity a contraindication to transplantation.[3] The highly antibiotic-resistant *Burkholderia cepacia* has been associated with significant morbidity and mortality in patients with cystic fibrosis.[32] These resistant organisms are found most often in the older patient with advanced

lung disease, and this is the cystic fibrosis patient who most likely needs transplantation. Of recent concern is the report that *B. cepacia* is particularly lethal to transplant patients with cystic fibrosis who acquire it after transplantation.[32,33] The role of antibiotic prophylaxis in patients with cystic fibrosis who undergo lung transplantation remains to be clarified. A common and potentially effective prophylaxis for transplant patients with cystic fibrosis uses inhaled antibiotics, usually an aminoglycoside such as tobramycin.[34]

BRONCHIOLITIS OBLITERANS

Bronchiolitis obliterans is unfortunately a common late complication in both heart-lung and lung transplant recipients.[1,22,23] The exact cause is unknown, but it most likely represents the common pathway for different insults such as chronic rejection, infection, and aspiration.[22] Bronchiolitis obliterans can be initially identified by a decrease in flow rates at low lung volumes during surveillance pulmonary function testing and can be confirmed by transbronchial biopsy or open-lung biopsy

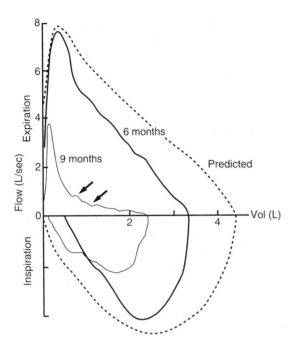

Fig. 27-7

These curves represent serial flow-volume pulmonary function tests in a patient with cystic fibrosis after sequential double-lung transplantation. Flow is on the vertical axis, with volume on the horizontal axis. The *dashed line* represents the predicted value for the patient's age, sex, and height. Six months after transplantation, the pulmonary function is nearly normal, with no suggestion of significant air flow limitation. The *curve* at 9 months demonstrates the changes associated with the development of bronchiolitis obliterans; the *arrows* demonstrate the marked flow limitation at mid and low lung volumes characteristic of this condition. (From Moodie DS, Stillwell PC: Thoracic organ transplantation in children: the state of heart, heart-lung, and lung transplantation. *Clin Pediatr* 1993; 32:322-328.)

(Fig. 27-7). Because of the high frequency of false-negative transbronchial biopsies, most clinicians use the clinical definition of bronchiolitis obliterans syndrome for both diagnosis and treatment decisions.[33] In the majority of patients, bronchiolitis obliterans is a progressive disease manifested by increasing dyspnea, increased coughing with sputum production, colonization with *Pseudomonas* species, and eventual respiratory failure and death. A small minority of patients respond favorably to augmented immunosuppression, with reversal or stabilization of their airway dysfunction.[23] Bronchiolitis obliterans remains a major obstacle to the success of lung and heart-lung transplantation.

DRUG TOXICITY

All immunosuppressive regimens place the patient at risk for infection. In addition, each arm of the regimen may cause other complications from side effects or drug toxicity.[1] Cyclosporine and tacrolimus can have multiple side effects (see Table 27-3). Hypertension and nephrotoxicity are the most common. Fortunately, these are usually manageable. Some experienced heart transplant physicians expect the incidence of renal failure to increase with increasing survivors and prolonged exposure to immunosuppressive agents. The major complication from azathioprine and mycophenolate mofetil is a decreased white blood cell count caused by bone marrow suppression. This improves with temporary discontinuation of the medicine or a decrease in its dose. There may be more symptoms of gastrointestinal disturbance with mycophenolate mofetil compared with azathioprine. The complications of prednisone are quite common in the immediate post-transplantation period when high doses are used, but complications become minimal with decreasing dosages after several months. Some children and adolescents will experience little or no skeletal growth until the prednisone can be decreased to low daily doses (0.1 to 0.15 mg/kg/day) or an alternate-day dosage schedule. It is common for patients to assume a cushingoid appearance. Many become glucose intolerant, particularly patients with cystic fibrosis who may have partial glucose intolerance because of pancreatic involvement by the disease.

OTHER COMPLICATIONS

There is a broad spectrum of other complications that occur infrequently after transplantation. For patients receiving heart or heart-lung transplants, accelerated coronary artery disease may be a problem.[12] Other potential complications include obstructive sleep apnea, cerebrovascular accidents, and aspiration of gastric contents. Epstein-Barr virus–related lymphoproliferative disease is a neoplastic disorder that occurs in relation to the intensity and duration of immunosuppression. The incidence in pediatric thoracic transplantation varies from 1% to 10%.[35,36] It may regress with decreased levels of immunosuppression or progress to fatal malignancy.[36] Other fairly common medical complications include generalized seizures, aggravated acne, and mild suppression of maximal exercise performance. Up to 25% of lung transplant recipients may experience unilateral vocal cord or hemidiaphragm paralysis, which may recover 3 to 6 months after transplant. Equally important are the psychosocial adjustments to the emotional "roller coaster" of thoracic organ transplantation.[37] Although almost all patients can benefit from extensive psychosocial support, occasionally some will require pharmacologic assistance to deal with either anxiety or depression.[37,38] These psychologic or psychiatric complications are quite common, and they are potentially very serious. Nonadherence to the medical regimen is often fatal. The entire transplantation team must be alert for any psychologic or psychiatric complications in the hope of either their prevention or their early detection and treatment.

ROLE OF THE RESPIRATORY CARE PRACTITIONER

There are multiple areas of interaction between the respiratory care practitioner (RCP) and the transplant patient. Care of the patient who undergoes thoracic transplantation always involves teamwork from a variety of health care professionals. The child who receives a lung or heart-lung transplant is especially likely to require an RCP on the team. Familiarity with the diseases leading to transplantation, as well as the transplantation process, will help the practitioner provide more comprehensive care to the patients as well as improve interaction with the health care team. Many RCPs will already be familiar with the transplant candidate because of their role in providing routine care for the primary disease process, particularly for chronic pulmonary diseases such as cystic fibrosis. The RCP may become the true contact with the transplantation candidate in the initial evaluation process or during pulmonary function testing. After the patient has been accepted to the transplantation list, the RCP may be involved in providing an exercise evaluation or a rehabilitation program, or both, in an effort to optimize the patient's condition while he or she is awaiting transplantation. Immediately after the transplantation procedure, the RCP will be involved with the patient in the intensive care unit, primarily providing mechanical ventilatory support. Because of the temporary interruption of ciliary function, the RCP may be asked to provide aerosolized bronchodilators and bronchopulmonary hygiene. For most patients, this therapy is not required on a long-term basis. Shortly after the patient is taken off mechanical ventilation, the RCP may be involved in reinstituting the exercise and rehabilitation program that had been initiated before the procedure. Lastly, the RCP may be involved in the transplant patient's care by assisting with follow-up pulmonary function tests, instructing the patient in the use of home spirometry, and assisting with bronchoscopies.

REFERENCES

1. Hosenpud JD et al: The Registry of the International Society for Heart and Lung Transplantation: eighteenth official report—2001. *J Heart Lung Transplant* 2001; 20:805-815.
2. Cooper JD: The evolution of techniques and indications for lung transplantation. *Ann Surg* 1990; 212:249-256.
3. Trulock EP: Lung transplantation. *Am J Respir Crit Care Med* 1997; 155:789-818.
4. Starnes VA et al: Living-donor lobar lung transplantation experience: immediate results. *J Thorac Cardiovasc Surg* 1996; 112:1284-1291.
5. Cooper DK et al: Report of the Xenotransplantation Advisory Committee of the International Society for Heart And Lung Transplantation: potential role in the treatment of end-stage cardiac and pulmonary diseases. *J Heart Lung Transplant* 2000; 19:1125-1165.
6. Sweet SC et al: Pediatric lung transplantation at St Louis Children's Hospital, 1990-1995. *Am J Respir Crit Care Med* 1997; 155:1027-1035.
7. Noyes BE, Kurland G, Orenstein DM: Lung and heart-lung transplantation in children. *Pediatr Pulmonol* 1997; 23:39-48.
8. Baum D et al: Pediatric heart transplantation at Stanford: Results of a 15 year experience. *Pediatrics* 1991; 88: 203-214.
9. Cohen AH et al: Growth of lungs after transplantation in infants and in children younger than age. *Am J Respir Crit Care Med* 1999; 159:1747-1751.
10. Houcek MM et al: The registry of the International Society of Heart and Lung Transplantation: first official pediatric report—1997. *J Heart Lung Transplant* 1997; 16: 1189-206.
11. Pennington DG et al: Heart transplantation in children: an international survey. *Ann Thorac Surg* 1991; 52:710-715.
12. Pahl E et al: Coronary arteriosclerosis in pediatric heart transplant survivors: limitation of long-term survival. *J Pediatr* 1990; 116:177-183.
13. Boucek MM et al: Cardiac transplantation in infancy: donors and recipients. *J Pediatr* 1990; 116:171-176.
14. Shewmon DA et al: The use of anencephalic infants as organ sources: a critique. *JAMA* 1989; 261:1173-1178.
15. Spray TL et al: Pediatric lung transplantation for pulmonary hypertension and congenital heart disease. *Ann Thorac Surg* 1992; 54:216-225.
16. United Network for Organ Sharing: Available at www.unos.org.
17. Ramirez JC et al: Bilateral lung transplantation for cystic fibrosis. *J Thorac Cardiovasc Surg* 1991; 103:287-294.
18. Mendeloff EM et al: Pediatric and adult lung transplantation for cystic fibrosis. *J Thorac Cardiovasc Surg* 1998; 115:404-113.
19. Noirclerc M et al: Size matching in lung transplantation. *J Heart Lung Transplant* 1992; 11:S203-S208.
20. Starnes VA et al: Current trends in lung transplantation: lobar transplantation and expanded use of single lungs. *J Thorac Cardiovasc Surg* 1992; 104:1060-1066.
21. Starnes VA et al: Comparison of outcomes between living donor and cadaveric lung transplant children. *Ann Thorac Surg* 1999; 68:2279-2283.
22. Boehler A et al: Bronchiolitis obliterans after lung transplantation: a review. *Chest* 1998; 114:1411-1426.
23. Date H et al: The impact of cytolytic therapy on bronchiolitis obliterans syndrome. *J Heart Lung Transplant* 1998; 17:869-885.
24. Jurmann MJ et al: Pulmonary reperfusion injury: evidence for oxygen-derived free radical mediated damage and effects of different free radical scavengers. *Eur J Cardiothorac Surg* 1990; 4:665-670.

25. Paradis JL et al: Distinguishing between infection, rejection, and the adult respiratory distress syndrome after human lung transplantation. *J Heart Lung Transplant* 1992; 11:S232-S236.

26. Trachiotis GD et al: Carbon dioxide response in lung transplant recipients. *Am Rev Respir Dis* 1992; 145:A702.

27. Patterson GA et al: Airway complications after double lung transplantation. *J Thorac Cardiovasc Surg* 1990; 99:14-21.

28. Kaditis AG et al: Airway complications following pediatric lung and heart-lung transplantation. *Am J Respir Crit Care Med* 2000; 162:301-309.

29. Trulock EP et al: The role of trans-bronchial lung biopsy in the treatment of lung transplant recipients: an analysis of 200 consecutive procedures. *Chest* 1992; 102:1049-1054.

30. Mauer JR et al: Infectious complications following isolated lung transplantation. *Chest* 1992; 101:1056-1059.

31. Nunley DR et al: Allograft colonization and infections with *Pseudomonas* in cystic fibrosis lung transplant recipients. *Chest* 1998; 113:1235-1243.

32. Chaparro C et al: Infection with *Burkholderia cepacia* in cystic fibrosis: outcome following lung transplantation. *Am J Respir Crit Care Med* 2001; 163:43-48.

33. Cooper JD et al: A working formulation for the standardization of nomenclature and for clinical staging of chronic dysfunction in lung allografts. International Society for Heart and Lung Transplantation. *J Heart Lung Transplant* 1993; 12:713-716

34. Snell GI et al: *Pseudomonas cepacia* in lung transplant recipients with cystic fibrosis. *Chest* 1993; 103:466-471.

35. Stillwell PC, Mallory GB Jr: Pediatric lung transplantation. *Clin Chest Med* 1997; 18:405-414.

36. Cohen AH et al: High incidence of posttransplant lymphoproliferative disease in pediatric patients with cystic fibrosis. *Am J Respir Crit Care Med* 2000; 161:1252-1255.

37. Kurland G, Orenstein DM: Lung transplantation and cystic fibrosis: the psychosocial toll. *Pediatrics* 2001; 107:1419-1421.

38. Craven JL, Bright J, Dear CL: Psychiatric, psychosocial and rehabilitative aspects of lung transplantation. *Clin Chest Med* 1990; 11:247-257.

Neonatal and Pediatric Disorders: Presentation, Diagnosis, and Treatment

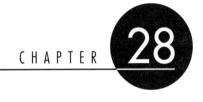

CHAPTER 28

Neonatal Pulmonary Disorders

David L. Ellwanger
Lorilie A. Weber-Hardy

Most infants are admitted to a neonatal intensive care unit because of respiratory distress.[1] The more premature the neonate is, the more likely that respiratory complications will exist at presentation. However, term and postmature infants can also experience respiratory difficulty resulting from pulmonary as well as nonpulmonary conditions (Table 28-1). Whatever the cause, disorders that result in respiratory distress remain a major reason for morbidity and mortality in the neonate. The more common neonatal pulmonary disorders are addressed in this chapter.

RESPIRATORY DISTRESS SYNDROME

INCIDENCE

First described in 1903, respiratory distress syndrome (RDS), also referred to as hyaline membrane disease, usually affects premature infants with inadequate lung development. Each year approximately 250,000 premature infants are born in the United States, up to 50,000 of whom are born with RDS. Of those with RDS, nearly 10% die of it.[2] It occurs more often in boys than in girls and more often in whites than in nonwhites.[3-6] There is a higher incidence of RDS, with a greater clinical impact, in infants with very low birth weights. It is most often associated with infants born at less than 37 weeks' gestation, in infants of diabetic mothers, in multiple births, when cesarean section is performed before the onset of labor, in asphyxia, in cold stress, and in infants of mothers who have previously had infants with RDS.[4,5,7,8]

ETIOLOGY AND PATHOPHYSIOLOGY

In 1959, Avery and Mead reported that RDS was associated with a deficiency of pulmonary surfactant and abnormal lung surface tension properties.[9] Since that time, it has been widely accepted that the

TABLE 28-1 CLUES TO DIAGNOSIS OF TYPES OF RESPIRATORY DISTRESS	
Information from Maternal History	**Most Probable Condition in Infant**
Peripartum fever	Pneumonia
Foul-smelling amniotic fluid	Pneumonia
Excessive obstetric manipulation at delivery	Pneumonia
Infection	Pneumonia
Premature rupture of membranes	Pneumonia
Prolonged labor	Pneumonia
Prematurity	Hyaline membrane disease (RDS)
Diabetes	Hyaline membrane disease
Hemorrhage in days before delivery	Hyaline membrane disease
Meconium-stained amniotic fluid	Meconium aspiration syndrome
Hydramnios	Tracheoesophageal fistula
Excessive medications	Central nervous system depression
Reserpine	Stuffy nose
Traumatic or breech delivery	Central nervous system hemorrhage; phrenic nerve paralysis
Fetal tachycardia or bradycardia	Asphyxia
Prolapsed cord or entanglements	Asphyxia
Postmaturity	Asphyxia
Amniotic fluid loss	Hypoplastic lungs
Signs in the Infant	**Most Probable Associated Condition**
Single umbilical artery	Congenital anomalies
Other congenital anomalies	Associated cardiopulmonary anomalies
Situs inversus	Kartagener's syndrome
Scaphoid abdomen	Diaphragmatic hernia
Erb's palsy	Phrenic nerve palsy
Cannot breathe with mouth closed	Choanal atresia; stuffy nose
Gasping with little air exchange	Upper airway obstruction
Overdistention of lungs	Aspiration, lobar emphysema, or pneumothorax
Shift of apical pulse	Pneumothorax, chylothorax, hypoplastic lung
Fever or rise in temperature in a constant-temperature environment	Pneumonia
Shrill cry, hypertonia, or flaccidity	Central nervous system disorder
Atonia	Trauma, myasthenia, poliomyelitis, amyotonia
Frothy blood from larynx	Pulmonary hemorrhage
Head extended in the absence of neurologic findings	Tracheoesophageal fistula or pharyngeal incoordination
Plethora	Transient tachypnea

From Avery ME, Fletcher BD, Williams RG: *The lung and its disorders in the newborn infant.* Philadelphia. WB Saunders, 1981.

pathophysiology of RDS is the result of an insufficient amount of surfactant as well as immature cell and vascular development of the lungs.[10,11] Disturbances in the normal progression of postnatal circulatory changes may also play an important role in the pathogenesis of RDS.[12]

At approximately 16 weeks of gestation, the alveolar type II cells synthesize and store surfactant. Increasing amounts are produced as the fetus approaches term. Between the 28th and 38th weeks of gestation, surfactant is secreted into the alveoli and eventually migrates into the amniotic fluid through the trachea and esophagus. With its release into the alveoli, surfactant reduces the surface tension and helps to maintain alveolar stability[13-15] (see Chapters 1 and 16). Primitive alveoli form between the 27th and 35th weeks of gestation, with true alveoli forming between the 30th and 36th weeks of gestation.[16,17] Infants born before 28 weeks' gestation have structural underdevelopment of the terminal air spaces with little or no surfactant, leading to a susceptibility to RDS.

Deficient surfactant production or deficient release of surfactant into the immature respiratory alveoli, along with the extremely compliant chest wall of the preterm infant, results in an increase in surface forces and lung elastic recoil. This leads to atelectasis, which is characterized by decreased functional residual capacity (FRC), decreased pulmonary compliance, increased pulmonary resistance, and ventilation-perfusion mismatch.[18] The resulting hypoxia, hypercarbia, and respiratory acidosis cause constriction of the pulmonary arteries and a reduction in pulmonary blood flow. This results in damage to the cells lining the alveoli.[19] The pulmonary hypertension can lead to increased right-to-left shunting through a patent ductus arteriosus (PDA) and the foramen ovale (extrapulmonary), as well as within the lung itself (intrapulmonary).[20] The shunting of blood results in greater hypoxemia and possibly metabolic acidosis, which increases the pulmonary vascular resistance (PVR) even more. This vicious cycle continues and may even lead to further suppression of surfactant synthesis.

Other pathophysiologic processes are present that contribute to the clinical picture. They include poor gas exchange secondary to inadequate surface area, a compliant chest wall that reduces effectiveness of ventilation, a thickened alveolar-capillary membrane and insufficient vascularization, and poor clearance of lung fluid, which may produce pulmonary edema.[21]

Within 2 days of birth, immature lungs begin to mature while true alveoli and an increased number of capillaries continue to develop in the lung. If lung damage does not occur, the signs and symptoms of respiratory distress should subside.

Chronic stress seems to protect infants at risk for the development of RDS. Conditions associated with chronic stress include maternal heroin addiction, which is thought to induce surfactant synthesis, and maternal toxemia. Premature rupture of membranes (PROM) for duration of more than 24 hours preceding birth may also have a sparing effect on the incidence of RDS.[4]

CLINICAL PRESENTATION

The clinical features of RDS include a manifestation of the surfactant deficiency and a highly compliant chest wall. Infants with RDS are usually preterm and exhibit tachypnea or labored breathing, or both, beginning at or immediately after birth. A decrease in the respiratory rate may indicate impending respiratory failure. A characteristic grunt during expiration (which is an attempt to maintain the FRC) and nasal flaring are also present.[22] Intercostal and subcostal retractions are apparent and occur when the high inspiratory pressures distort the chest wall instead of inflating the stiff lungs.[18] The retractions may have a "seesaw" appearance,

with the abdomen protruding as the chest pulls in. Infants frequently look distressed, and the very premature infant may be hypotonic and unresponsive. Chest auscultation reveals diminished air in the alveoli in spite of the increased work of breathing.

Without stabilization of the alveoli, infants with RDS have increasing cyanosis that is relatively unresponsive to oxygen therapy. Larger infants may need minimal oxygen initially but require more as atelectasis becomes progressively worse. Some may have a decrease in oxygen requirements as acidosis and hypothermia (a result of delivery) are corrected but then have an increased need after 3 to 6 hours of life.

Arterial blood gas (ABG) analysis reveals moderate to severe hypoxemia, varying degrees of hypercarbia, and mixed acidosis (owing to respiratory failure and lactic acid accumulation). The $Paco_2$ may initially be normal or low, but as the work of breathing increases and the infant begins to fail, there is resulting hypercarbia.

The chest radiograph typically reveals diffuse, fine, granular (reticulogranular) densities, which give a ground-glass appearance. The heart may be slightly enlarged, and the thymus is nearly always present radiographically. The appearance of the chest radiograph in RDS can be described as stages representing increasing severity of the disease. Stage I is described as a fine, diffuse reticulogranular pattern over the lung fields. Stage II reveals a more dense lung, with the presence of air bronchograms within the heart border. Stage III is increasing density and the presence of air bronchograms beyond the heart border. Stage IV is termed "white out," used to describe the radiograph of the infant with severe disease that is complicated by pulmonary edema.[23] The view of the heart border and edge of the diaphragm may be obliterated in this stage. The disease may progress from one stage to the next, but the severity of the disease is initially described as the stage of RDS on the first chest film.[24]

DISEASE PROGRESSION

In milder cases, the signs and symptoms reach a peak within 72 hours, followed by gradual improvement. Spontaneous diuresis with an increased ability to oxygenate the infant are the first signs of improvement. Severely affected infants may die, usually between days 2 and 7, with death most often associated with pulmonary interstitial emphysema, pneumothorax, or intraventricular hemorrhage (IVH). Surfactant and early use of nasal continuous positive airway pressure (NCPAP) have altered the classic presentation of the progression of RDS. Rapid weaning of ventilator settings and stabilization with low Fio_2 can be observed in a matter of hours. Extremely premature infants (23 to 25 weeks' gestation) may have an initial "honeymoon" period in which the patient has stable ventilator settings but will exhibit increased oxygen and ventilator demands as time progresses. These extremely low–birth-weight infants not only have immature lungs but their extreme prematurity also presents challenges because metabolic and cardiac functions are affected.

DIAGNOSIS

Diagnosis is based on the history, clinical assessment, chest radiograph, and laboratory evaluation. Acute respiratory distress in the newborn is fairly common and may be caused by a multitude of pathophysiologic conditions. Box 28-1 lists some of the more common neonatal problems that may present as respiratory distress.

Infants at risk for RDS may be identified by several laboratory tests that have been developed to

---

BOX 28-1

NEONATAL DISORDERS THAT MAY PRESENT AS RESPIRATORY DISTRESS

AIRWAY DISORDERS
  Pneumonia
  Pulmonary hypoplasia
  Air leaks
  Pulmonary edema
  Pulmonary hemorrhage
  Pleural effusion
  Vascular ring
  Choanal atresia
  Macroglossia
  Micrognathia
  Cysts and tumors
  Laryngomalacia-atresia
  Tracheomalacia-atresia
  Tracheoesophageal fistula
  Wilson-Mikity syndrome
  Respiratory distress syndrome
  Meconium aspiration syndrome
  Transient tachypnea of the newborn

THORACIC DISORDERS
  Thoracic dystrophy
  Osteogenesis imperfecta
  Cysts and tumors

DIAPHRAGM DISORDERS
  Diaphragmatic hernia
  Phrenic nerve paralysis
  Eventration

CARDIOVASCULAR DISORDERS
  Persistent pulmonary hypertension
  Congenital heart disease

---

estimate lung maturity. Lung maturity may be determined by assessing the amniotic fluid lecithin-to-sphingomyelin (L:S) ratio. Lecithin, also known as dipalmitoyl phosphatidylcholine, is the most abundant phospholipid found in surfactant. When the lung is mature, there is twice as much lecithin as sphingomyelin. Thus an L:S ratio of more than 2:1 is considered evidence of lung maturity. Nearly 100% of the infants with an L:S ratio less than 1:1 tend to acquire RDS, whereas those with a ratio greater than 2:1 do not. The L:S ratio is unreliable in pregnancies characterized by diabetes and Rh isoimmunization.[24,25] Levels of phosphatidylglycerol (PG), the second most abundant phospholipid in surfactant, increase toward term. The presence of PG in amniotic fluid indicates a low risk for RDS. A patient with an L:S ratio less than 2:1 and a lack of PG has more than an 80% risk for the development of RDS. However, with the presence of PG and an L:S ratio greater than 2:1, the risk drops to nearly 0%.[4,26] In the foam stability test, amniotic fluid is mixed with different volumes of 95% ethanol. When this mixture is shaken with air, a foam develops that can be seen for several hours at room temperature. If no surfactant is present, the foam will not appear or will appear only briefly, indicating the strong possibility of immature lungs. The shake test is not as specific as a low L:S ratio.[27]

TREATMENT

Prevention. Because RDS is associated with incomplete development of the lung at birth, the first line of treatment is prevention. If predictive tests indicate that the infant is at high risk for the development of RDS, elective cesarean section should not be performed. Premature delivery should be delayed, when possible, and glucocorticoids given for at least 2 days before delivery.[2] Antenatal corticosteroid therapy may accelerate lung development and promote pulmonary surfactant secretion.

Surfactant Replacement. Prophylactic and therapeutic surfactant replacement therapy has been shown to reduce morbidity and mortality in infants with RDS (see Chapter 16). Although studies have not found that it decreases the incidence of bronchopulmonary dysplasia (BPD) in RDS survivors, it does seem to reduce the severity of the chronic condition.[29,30] Combined therapy with antenatal corticosteroids and surfactant has been shown to reduce the time of mechanical ventilation. This improves survival and neurodevelopment outcome in those preterm infants who require mechanical ventilation.[31]

Oxygen Therapy. Treatment of the infant with RDS centers around providing adequate oxygenation, preventing atelectasis, and reducing the risk of complications. Oxygen therapy begins with delivery of oxygen via an oxygen hood in an attempt to maintain the PaO_2 between 50 and 80 mm Hg. The FIO_2 may be increased in increments of 0.10 and oxygenation assessed by means of either ABG analysis or pulse oximetry until the appropriate oxygen level is obtained. Use of the oxygen hood as an initial therapy for mild respiratory distress symptoms should be reserved for those larger infants who require above ambient FIO_2. Increases in FIO_2 greater than 0.40 with further signs of distress may be a sign of loss of lung volume. If surfactant deficiency is determined to be a likely cause of distress, continuous positive airway pressure (CPAP) should be applied to prevent further loss of FRC.

Continuous Positive Airway Pressure. If oxygenation fails to improve with the oxygen hood, CPAP via nasal prongs may be instituted (see Chapter 20). A CPAP of 4 to 6 cm H_2O is the usual starting point in these infants. In infants weighing more than 1500 g, CPAP levels of 7 to 8 cm H_2O may be needed. As CPAP levels are increased, or when pulmonary compliance improves, alveoli may become overdistended, with impairment of ventilation and pulmonary circulation. Continuous pulse oximetry is imperative to wean oxygen and CPAP to minimally acceptable levels. Frequent ABG analysis should be provided for early detection of respiratory failure.

Early NCPAP in the moderately preterm newborn of 28 to 32 weeks' gestation can reduce the need for intubation.[32,33] Stabilization of the alveoli in this gestational age may allow surfactant production to occur without further intervention. During this time, if the infant requires an FIO_2 of more than 0.40 on NCPAP, it is an indication for intubation and exogenous surfactant treatment. Early intubation and prophylactic administration of surfactant with subsequent extubation within 10 minutes of administration to NCPAP may be effective in reducing the need for prolonged intubation and mechanical ventilation.[34,35] Treatment of the very low–birth-weight infant is often more assertive. In many patient care protocols, management of the newborn younger than 28 weeks' gestation can begin with intubation and prophylactic use of surfactant. Moderately aggressive treatment with these smaller infants can improve clinical outcome in the form of lower risk of pneumothorax, pulmonary interstitial emphysema, and mortality[36] (see Chapter 16).

Mechanical Ventilation. Classic indications for endotracheal intubation and mechanical ventilation occur if the infant requires greater than 80% oxygen

with a CPAP of 10 cm H_2O, if there is increasing hypercarbia with respiratory acidosis, or if apneic episodes become prolonged. Some patient care protocols are less tolerant, with intubation, surfactant, and subsequent ventilation occurring at a much lower threshold. In the very low–birth-weight infant (<1000 g), intubation and positive-pressure ventilation may be necessary immediately after birth while the infant is still in the delivery room. Intubation may also be indicated in larger infants with severe respiratory distress or asphyxia. Once the infant is stabilized and in the intensive care unit, a pressure-limited ventilator utilizing a sinusoidal flow pattern is used. Peak inspiratory pressures (PIPs) generally begin at 15 to 25 cm H_2O, depending on the size of the infant and the severity of the disease. Special care must be given to observing chest rise. Chest rise is a reliable indication of appropriate tidal volume. The chest rise should appear to be as if the patient were taking an easy breath, with a minimal or excessive chest rise corrected by altering the pressure to maintain an appropriate tidal volume. Positive end-expiratory pressure (PEEP) levels of 3 to 6 cm H_2O are used to prevent further alveolar collapse, and rates of 20 to 50 breaths per minute are used to treat hypercapnia. Inspiratory times should be initiated at 0.3 to 0.4 second. If a longer inspiratory time is required before surfactant administration, it should be lowered to 0.3 second after surfactant is administered.

Current technology allows for a greater range of ventilator modes and options for the neonatal patient. If available, measured exhaled tidal volume should be between 3 and 5 ml/kg. Synchronous intermittent mandatory ventilation or assist-control modes can reduce work of breathing and blood pressure fluctuations if sensitivities are set properly.[37] Modes that maintain a consistent tidal volume reduce the risk of volutrauma, particularly after the administration of surfactant (see Chapter 19). High-frequency ventilation (HFV) may be indicated in infants who cannot be ventilated with the usually effective FIO_2 levels, ventilator pressures, and rates (see Chapter 21).

Minimizing Oxygen Consumption. Because cold stress can increase oxygen consumption and suppress surfactant synthesis, infants with RDS should be kept in a warm environment to maintain oxygen consumption at a normal level. Patient stimulation and pain may also increase oxygen consumption and should be kept to a minimum. PaO_2 values have been noted to decrease during arterial and capillary punctures, tracheal suctioning, diaper changes, and weighing of the infant. Developmental care protocols that emphasize positioning, minimal stimulation, and sedation are included in the care of low-birth-weight infants with respiratory distress.

Pharmacologic Support. Infusion of saline or blood is used to treat hypovolemia, whereas low-dose dopamine is used to increase arterial blood pressure not associated with hypovolemia. Bicarbonate should be given sparingly, respiratory acidosis treated with increased ventilation, and metabolic acidosis treated with increased oxygenation and maintenance of adequate perfusion. Some infants may need to be sedated before adequate ventilation can be obtained. PDA increases oxygen requirements and interferes with ventilation, prolonging the need for mechanical ventilation. Treatment with indomethacin (Indocin) may be indicated if a PDA is diagnosed.

Monitoring. When RDS is characterized by both high surface tension and high-permeability pulmonary edema, fluid input and output should be closely monitored. Excess fluids may contribute to more difficult ventilatory management and to the development of a PDA. Although diuresis has been tried clinically, the results are inconclusive.[4,5,38] Umbilical or peripheral arterial lines should be used initially for ABG measurements. Transcutaneous oxygen and CO_2 monitors, end-tidal CO_2, pulse oximetry, cardiopulmonary monitors, and Doppler flow studies can be used to monitor the infant's progress. Routine daily chest radiographs may be useful in managing the very low–birth-weight infant who is mechanically ventilated. Abnormalities ranging from malposition of the endotracheal tube to pulmonary interstitial emphysema can occur from one day to the next.[39]

LARGE INFANTS WITH RESPIRATORY DISTRESS SYNDROME

Beware the large infant with respiratory distress.
Old Neonatology Proverb

One group of patients commonly overlooked are the term or near-term infants in whom RDS develops. These infants are typically 34 to 37 weeks' gestational age and are born to diabetic mothers or to mothers with a history of late-gestational infants with RDS. Because of their strength and pulmonary reserve, they may be able to cope with RDS for a longer period; however, they will demonstrate increasing oxygen demands requiring an FIO_2 greater than 0.6. These infants often have borderline hypovolemia, blood pressure, and oxygenation and persistent metabolic acidosis. If the condition remains unrecognized, they often experience a sudden, and at times catastrophic, deterioration requiring maximum support before stabilization occurs. It

often takes more than 12 hours of mechanical ventilation with high FIO_2 levels before ABG values begin to improve.[40]

COMPLICATIONS

The clinical outcome in preterm infants surviving RDS is often associated with chronic lung disease in the form of BPD, reactive airway disease, and an increase in and vulnerability to respiratory disorders.[41] Pulmonary function testing frequently demonstrates increased pulmonary resistance and work of breathing as well as decreased lung compliance and a tendency toward oxygen desaturation.[42,43] Other complications encountered include IVH, retinopathy of prematurity, infection, air leaks, and necrotizing enterocolitis (NEC). Management of RDS with surfactant replacement therapy and HFV may limit the complications that have plagued these infants in the past. Current research in developmental care and nutrition also may play a role in improving the outcome of these patients.

TRANSIENT TACHYPNEA OF THE NEWBORN

INCIDENCE

First described by Avery and colleagues in 1966, transient tachypnea of the newborn (TTN) is a relatively benign, self-limited disease.[44] Also known as RDS type II and wet lung syndrome, it occurs in approximately 11 of every 1000 live births. It is more common in boys and in infants with perinatal asphyxia.[45] The incidence after elective cesarean section delivery without labor is as high as 23%. Although TTN does appear in infants born prematurely, it occurs more frequently in term infants. Box 28-2 lists factors that are associated with the occurrence of TTN.[46]

BOX 28-2

FACTORS ASSOCIATED WITH TRANSIENT TACHYPNEA OF THE NEWBORN

Cesarean section delivery
Term or preterm infant
Maternal analgesia during labor
Maternal anesthesia during labor
Maternal fluid administration
Maternal asthma
Maternal diabetes
Maternal bleeding
Perinatal asphyxia
Prolapsed umbilical cord

ETIOLOGY AND PATHOPHYSIOLOGY

Although the precise cause is unknown, TTN is believed to be due to delayed resorption of fetal lung fluid and may be caused by any condition that elevates central venous pressure and delays the clearance of pulmonary liquid by the lymphatics. This delay in pulmonary fluid absorption by the lymphatics and pulmonary capillaries results in a decrease in pulmonary compliance, a decreased tidal volume, and an increase in dead space.[47]

CLINICAL PRESENTATION

The infant with TTN may be mildly depressed at birth with fairly good Apgar scores. Tachypnea (60 to 150 breaths per minute), cyanosis, grunting, retractions, and nasal flaring begin within a few hours. ABG analysis reveals mild to moderate hypoxemia, hypercapnia, and respiratory acidosis. These symptoms are nearly identical to RDS, hence the term RDS type II. Some have referred to TTN as "persistent postnatal pulmonary edema" because tachypnea is not a consistent finding (it is often masked by drugs given to the mother during labor) and also because some of the fluid may enter the lungs postnatally from the pulmonary circulation.

The chest radiograph shows pulmonary vascular congestion, prominent perihilar streaking, fluid in the interlobular fissures, hyperexpansion, and a flat diaphragm, which is why it is sometimes referred to as wet lung syndrome. Mild cardiomegaly and pleural effusions may also be present. Pulmonary function studies reveal that pulmonary function in infants with TTN is compatible with airway obstruction and gas trapping. The FRC is normal or reduced, and thoracic gas volumes are usually increased, suggesting that some of the gas in the lungs is not in communication with the airways.

DIAGNOSIS

Because TTN is similar in initial clinical presentation to conditions such as RDS, group B streptococcal pneumonia, and persistent pulmonary hypertension of the newborn (PPHN), it is usually diagnosed after these disorders have been ruled out. The respiratory distress seen with TTN usually resolves after 24 hours of oxygen therapy, whereas in RDS the infant generally requires longer support. Although the chest radiograph of an infant with RDS will demonstrate hypoaeration and a reticulogranular pattern, that of an infant with TTN may appear as a flattened diaphragm, bulging intercostal spaces, and perihilar streaking. Because the symptoms and radiographs of an infant with TTN are also similar to those of an infant with neonatal sepsis and pneumonia, the infant should

be evaluated for infection, which would include looking for an elevated white blood cell count. A broad-spectrum antibiotic may be administered until a differential diagnosis is made.[44]

TREATMENT

Oxygen Therapy and Continuous Positive Airway Pressure. The objectives of treatment of TTN are to maintain adequate oxygenation and ventilation.[44] Supplemental oxygen via oxygen hood (usually <40%) is indicated when signs of respiratory distress are present.[48] The distress, hypoxemia, and mild respiratory acidosis usually resolve within 12 to 24 hours, with the infant frequently breathing room air by 48 hours of age. CPAP levels of 3 to 5 cm H_2O may be needed when higher FIO_2 levels are required. The infant's position is changed frequently to prevent further retention of pulmonary fluid. Bottle feedings are postponed until the tachypnea resolves to prevent aspiration.

Mechanical Ventilation. Occasionally an infant with TTN will require mechanical ventilation for respiratory failure. This usually occurs in the preterm infant who is unable to exert sufficient transpleural pressure to clear the alveoli of fluid. Low ventilator settings are used with a minimal pressure or normal tidal volume of 3 to 4 ml/kg to maintain adequate ventilation, PEEP of 3 to 4 cm H_2O, and intermittent mandatory ventilation of 15 to 20 breaths per minute. Weaning is fairly rapid, with ventilatory support rarely needed for more than 24 hours.

COMPLICATIONS

Although air leaks occur in some infants requiring NCPAP or mechanical ventilation, complications are rarely encountered with TTN, and no permanent pulmonary damage has been reported.[49]

NEONATAL PNEUMONIA

Pneumonia presents one of the most serious challenges in neonatal care, with the tiny immature lung being a common site of infection. Infections may be acquired in utero (transplacental), during delivery (perinatal), or postnatally in the nursery.[45] The severity of the disease course and subsequent level of treatment vary widely and are often dependent on the particular organism responsible for infection. Pneumonias are classified as either early-onset (infants <7 days of age) or late-onset infections (infants >7 days of age), based on the manifestation and clinical symptoms. Late-onset infections are often easier to treat and are usually less devastating to the infant.[50-52]

INCIDENCE

Pneumonia occurs in greater than 10% of the infants in a neonatal intensive care unit, with premature infants affected more often than term infants.[45] Certain groups of mothers seem to have a higher incidence of infection, including those of lower socioeconomic status, those who are teenagers, and those who are sexually active. Group B streptococcal pneumonia causes sepsis in 1 to 8 of every 1000 live births.

ETIOLOGY AND PATHOPHYSIOLOGY

Pneumonia in the newborn is often associated with the development of hyaline membranes.[45] Atelectasis is a result of damage to the alveolar capillary membrane and leakage of proteins into the alveolus. This effluent disturbs the surface properties of pulmonary surfactant, which is why neonatal pneumonia is often indistinguishable from surfactant-deficient RDS.[53] An inflammatory response may occur, followed by partial obstruction of terminal bronchioles and even pneumothorax. An interstitial pneumonitis may develop, as may necrosis of the lung and pulmonary hemorrhage.

Transplacental Pneumonia. Transplacental or congenital pneumonia involves widespread infection that is transmitted to the fetus across the placenta, causing significant distress or even death either in utero or at birth. It is more often a result of a maternal viral infection than of a maternal bacterial infection during pregnancy. Box 28-3 lists organisms that are generally associated with transplacental and congenital pneumonias.

Perinatal Pneumonia. Most pneumonias seen in the newborn are a result of infection acquired during labor and delivery. The infant can contract pneumonia through contaminated amniotic fluid, which may be aspirated, or by extended exposure to bacteria that may be in the vaginal tract. This type of "ascending vertical transmission" of bacteria is a result of heavy colonization of the maternal genitourinary tract. PROM greater than 12 to 24 hours before delivery poses a significant chance of the infant's contracting bacteria and is thought to be one of the greatest predisposing factors to neonatal pneumonia.[54-57] Box 28-3 lists organisms that are often responsible for early-onset pneumonia.

Group B *Streptococcus* has emerged as a predominant pathogen in neonatal pneumonia and presents a serious threat to the newborn. Obstetric complications have been implicated in 50% to 80% of infants with early onset of group B streptococcal pneumonia, indicating intrauterine infection; this infection occurs most often in very low–birth-weight infants. Early-onset pneumonia from group B *Streptococcus* may progress rapidly to shock or death, and mortality is high (20% to 50%) regardless of treatment. When the onset of group B streptococcal disease is later (2 to 3 weeks after birth), (1) the infant may present with meningitis rather than pneumonia, (2) the pathogen is usually a different strain of the organism, and (3) there is a more optimistic prognosis.[50,54-57]

Postnatal Pneumonia. Nosocomial pneumonia acquired in the postnatal period, also known as horizontal transmission, can be caused by numerous sources. In the treatment of neonates, certain invasive lines (e.g., umbilical catheters, intravenous lines) as well as intubation and respiratory equipment can be avenues for infection. Cross-contamination of bacteria or viruses within the hospital setting is unfortunately a risk with the neonatal patient, especially if there is a large patient-to-caregiver ratio. Careful

---

BOX 28-3

PATHOGENS OFTEN RESPONSIBLE FOR PNEUMONIA IN NEONATES

PNEUMONIA ACQUIRED TRANSPLACENTALLY
Listeria monocytogenes
Haemophilus influenzae
Mycobacterium tuberculosis
Treponema pallidum
Toxoplasma
Syphilis
Rubella
Varicella zoster
Cytomegalovirus
Herpes simplex virus
Human immunodeficiency virus

PNEUMONIA ACQUIRED DURING LABOR AND DELIVERY
Group B β-hemolytic *Streptococcus*
Klebsiella
Escherichia coli
Chlamydia trachomatis

NOSOCOMIAL PNEUMONIA ACQUIRED AFTER DELIVERY
Pseudomonas
Serratia marcescens
Staphylococcus aureus
Staphylococcus epidermidis
Klebsiella
Candida albicans
Respiratory syncytial virus
Cytomegalovirus
Herpes simplex virus

screening of visitors and extensive care in hand washing and other protective infection control measures should be undertaken to protect these particularly susceptible neonates. Box 28-3 lists some of the pathogens that often cause nosocomial pneumonias. Some of these organisms are airborne, whereas others are spread by contact. Many can be fatal to the neonate whose immune system is not fully developed.

CLINICAL PRESENTATION

The infant who has acquired transplacental pneumonia may be in noticeable distress at birth or within 6 to 12 hours later. If the infant has aspirated bacteria or otherwise acquired pneumonia during delivery or in the postnatal period, the initial symptoms may not be present until several days later. The infant may have a history of fetal tachycardia with low Apgar scores and often requires some type of supplemental oxygen or even resuscitation at birth.

BOX 28-4

CLINICAL MANIFESTATIONS AND COMPLICATIONS OF NEONATAL PNEUMONIA

Respiratory distress
   Tachypnea
   Cyanosis
   Grunting
   Nasal flaring
   Retractions
Apnea
Poor peripheral perfusion
Tachycardia
Lethargy
Temperature instability
Abdominal distention
Excessive jaundice
Asphyxia
Septic shock
Persistent fetal circulation
Pulmonary hemorrhage
Pulmonary edema
Myocardial insufficiency
Pleural effusion
Hypotension
Disseminating intravascular coagulation
Hypoxemia
Hypercarbia
Respiratory acidosis
Metabolic acidosis
Barotrauma
Intraventricular hemorrhage
Bronchopulmonary dysplasia
Necrotizing enterocolitis

The chest radiograph may show a diffuse granular pattern with widespread bilateral involvement, especially if the infant acquired the infection in utero. If aspiration of contaminated amniotic fluid has occurred, the chest radiograph may appear as an aspiration pneumonitis with patchy infiltrates. When an infection is acquired postnatally, the radiographic findings often change from normal to severely abnormal over the first few days. Depending on the severity of the disease process and required treatment, pleural effusions, pulmonary edema, pneumatoceles, cardiomegaly, and evidence of barotrauma may be seen. ABG values reveal hypoxemia that is refractory to oxygen therapy and hypercarbia that responds poorly to ventilatory efforts. Metabolic acidosis may develop as infection becomes more severe. Box 28-4 lists clinical signs and symptoms in the infant with neonatal pneumonia.

DIAGNOSIS

Several factors should alert the health care provider to the possibility of neonatal pneumonia, namely, a history of maternal infection or fever, toxemia, premature labor, PROM, malodorous or stained amniotic fluid, lesions of the vagina or placenta, and frequent digital examinations of the cervix.[42] Anytime neonatal pneumonia is suspected, appropriate laboratory diagnostic tests should be performed, such as cultures of blood, urine, and cerebrospinal fluid. Newborns with pneumonia often have an abnormal white blood cell count along with tracheal or gastric aspirates that provide evidence of infection. These test results can help in making a definitive diagnosis of pneumonia.

TREATMENT

The normal course of treatment in neonatal pneumonia is relatively straightforward, regardless of the pathogen, and includes appropriate antibiotic or antiviral therapy, oxygenation, adequate ventilation, and pharmacologic support. To prevent rapid deterioration, early intervention, aggressive management, and continuous monitoring are required, especially in the infant with early-onset group B streptococcal disease.

Pharmacologic Support. Many physicians believe that PROM, or the onset of premature labor in and of itself, is often the first sign of infection and should be treated as such, with broad-spectrum antibiotic therapy instituted immediately. This has been shown to be effective in improving the outcome in certain disease processes, especially infection with group B *Streptococcus*. Whenever neonatal pneumonia is suspected, broad-spectrum antibiotics are given for at least 72 hours, or until definitive culture results are obtained. If results prove that infection is present, antibiotics are continued for 14 to 21 days. It is often thought that the bacteria itself may be the cause of prematurity that leads to RDS, which is why the infant with RDS is often treated empirically with antibiotics. Infants with pneumonia may require vasopressor support and intravascular volume replacement to maintain circulation. Blood transfusions may also be necessary in the course of treatment, especially if the infant is having frequent ABG and laboratory assessments.

Antiviral agents (e.g., ribavirin, acyclovir) may be administered in infants with pneumonia of viral origin. In the case of some viral pathogens that are congenitally transmitted, such as cytomegalovirus and rubella, irreversible damage to the central nervous system has already occurred and there is little therapy available to reverse it.

Mechanical Ventilation. The infant with cyanosis, hypoxemia, and hypercarbia may require mechanical ventilation to maintain oxygenation. The most critically ill infants may need extreme ventilator settings with high PIP, rate, and oxygen levels. ABG values and transcutaneous monitors, or pulse oximetry, or both, are used to monitor the patient's respiratory status.

Extracorporeal Membrane Oxygenation. Near-term and term infants who are unresponsive to conventional ventilation and other supportive measures may benefit from extracorporeal membrane oxygenation (ECMO).[58] Improved rates of survival have been reported in this group.

COMPLICATIONS

Careful management requires frequent assessment for signs of complications that may accompany prematurity, sepsis, and treatment interventions. These include the risk of IVH, air leaks, and necrotizing enterocolitis, as well as the development of BPD if mechanical ventilation is required for extended periods. These infants can suffer significant neurologic damage and developmental delay, or they may have totally normal capabilities. In some cases, however, the impairment may have occurred in utero, and severe neurologic problems or even death may be imminent.

Morbidity and mortality associated with neonatal pneumonia are dependent on the organism and the ability to successfully treat the infant and keep complications to a minimum. The key to treatment in these infants would seem to be early intervention and aggressive therapy; however, in some infants, especially those with early-onset group B strepto-

coccal pneumonia, the disease process is often fulminative and unresponsive to therapy.

MECONIUM ASPIRATION SYNDROME

Meconium is the green-tinged bowel content of an infant, which is usually passed within 48 hours after delivery. Although it seems impossible, this substance of tarry consistency is sterile and composed of swallowed amniotic fluid, salts, mucus, bile, and other cellular debris.[59] In and of itself, meconium is harmless; however, if in utero the infant passes meconium into the amniotic fluid, it may cause serious airway obstruction, air trapping, and enhanced growth of bacteria. Thus it becomes a life-threatening entity that must be dealt with immediately.

INCIDENCE

Meconium staining of the amniotic fluid at the time of delivery occurs in 8% to 15% of all infants delivered, with approximately 5% of these infants acquiring meconium aspiration syndrome (MAS). Approximately 30% of the infants in whom MAS develops will require mechanical ventilation, at least 11% will experience pneumothorax, and more than 4% will die.[60] Because meconium passage into the amniotic fluid requires strong peristalsis and anal sphincter tone, which is not common in preterm infants, MAS rarely occurs in infants of less than 36 weeks' gestational age.[61] The longer a pregnancy is allowed to continue past 42 weeks, the greater the chances are of the passage of meconium.

ETIOLOGY AND PATHOPHYSIOLOGY

Fetal passage of meconium has long been accepted as a sign of intrauterine stress or hypoxia. Theoretically, the infant becomes hypoxic in utero (possibly because of cord or fetal head compression or prolonged labor), which exhausts oxygen reserves, causing a vagal response, relaxed anal sphincter tone, and passage of meconium into the amniotic fluid. The normal intrauterine activity of the neonate involves the movement of small amounts (1 to 5 ml) of amniotic fluid into and out of the upper airways. The potential of aspiration is always present, but chances are increased with hypoxia or stress because of greater respiratory effort and possibly gasping respirations in utero. Even more damaging is the aspiration that occurs after delivery of the chest when expansion allows the fluid or meconium, or both, to be dispersed even farther into the infant's lungs.[62]

After delivery, the normal pulmonary mechanisms are hindered and the clinical picture varies drastically. The amount and viscosity or dilution of the meconium present may significantly affect the degree of obstruction that occurs. If the infant has a large amount of thick meconium within the airways at the time of delivery, complete bronchiole obstruction with subsequent alveolar collapse will result. The more typical picture, however, is that of smaller amounts of meconium within amniotic fluid, causing a ball-valve effect because of partial obstruction of the airways. The airways dilate on inspiration, whereas air remains trapped behind the obstruction during expiration, causing hyperinflation and greatly predisposing the infant to air leaks. Inflammation of the airways and secretion production (a normal body response to a foreign substance within the lungs) also occurs, and a chemical pneumonitis often develops.[63,64] Studies have also suggested that meconium hinders surfactant, which may lead to atelectasis and decreased pulmonary compliance.[65]

It has been suggested that intrauterine hypoxia not only stimulates the passage of meconium but also causes restructuring of the pulmonary vascular bed. The profound hypoxia may result in pulmonary vasoconstriction, which may be the reason that many infants with MAS quickly develop PPHN.[66] Fig. 28-1 summarizes the pathophysiologic events that occur with the passage of meconium and MAS.

CLINICAL PRESENTATION

The infant with MAS is usually a term or postterm infant who has been delivered through meconium-stained fluid (often referred to as pea soup) and has already experienced significant intrauterine stress or hypoxia. The history may include prolonged labor, breech delivery, and ominous fetal heart rate monitor tracings such as late decelerations or nonvariability.

On completion of delivery, the physical examination often reveals a mature infant with yellowish skin, nails, and cord, as well as the postmature signs of peeling skin and long fingernails. The umbilical cord may lack or have very little Wharton's jelly. Depending on the extent of stress or hypoxia, the infant is depressed at birth with low Apgar scores; however, some infants have 1-minute Apgar scores of 5 or more. The infant quickly exhibits signs of respiratory distress, including cyanosis, gasping respirations, grunting, retractions, nasal flaring, and tachypnea. The respiratory distress is often related to the viscosity of the meconium, with a thicker meconium causing more respiratory symptoms.[62,67] Auscultation of the chest reveals rales as well as areas of significantly diminished aeration, with the anteroposterior diameter of the chest often increased. The infant may or may not appear to need immediate intervention,

depending on the severity of the aspiration and the degree of hypoxia.

ABG analysis indicates hypoxemia in infants with mild MAS having a normal pH and normal or decreased $PaCO_2$ resulting from the increased respiratory effort. The infant may also have significant metabolic acidosis depending on the severity of the hypoxia before birth. The infant with moderate to severe MAS has increasing hypoxemia and hypercarbia. A combination of respiratory and metabolic acidosis eventually develops as the infant is unable to overcome the obstructive and inflammatory processes. This progresses to the point of respiratory failure and severe hypoxemia, which alerts the physician to the probability of PPHN.[68]

The radiographic appearance varies according to the severity of the disease and complications. The typical chest radiograph shows patchy areas of atelectasis due to obstruction, as well as hyperexpansion from air trapping. There is usually widespread involvement, with no particular area of the lungs being affected more. The radiograph of the infant with severe MAS may reveal total bilateral opacity with only large bronchi distinguishable. Pulmonary air leaks, including pulmonary interstitial emphysema, pneumothorax, and pneumomediastinum, may also be found. The chest radiograph of the infant with MAS is similar to that of an infant with pneumonia, especially when a bacterial infection develops.[69]

DIAGNOSIS

Although the majority of infants are normal, MAS is suggested whenever there is meconium staining of the amniotic fluid. The diagnosis of MAS is generally made whenever meconium is visualized at the vocal cords and the infant has clinical signs of respiratory distress, including hypoxemia, hypercarbia, and a characteristic chest radiographic pattern.

TREATMENT

Intrapartum Intervention. Some fetuses may be assessed as "at risk" for MAS, including those with oligohydramnios, abnormal fetal heart rate tracings, and thick, meconium-stained amniotic fluids.[61] A promising intrapartum intervention for these infants is amnioinfusion.[70,71] It is believed that by infusing fluid into the mother's uterus, the uterine fluid volume may either dilute the meconium or alleviate compression of the cord and prevent gasping.

Suctioning. Although no prevention has been found for MAS, prompt intervention in the delivery room can make a drastic difference in the outcome. To prevent aspiration into the lungs, pharyngeal

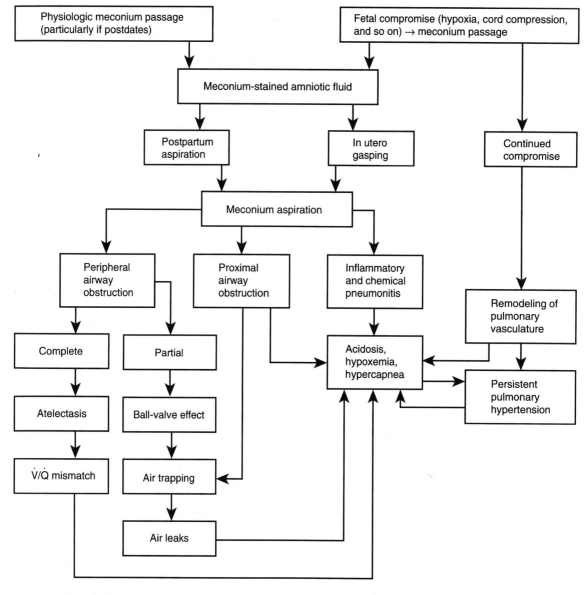

Fig. 28-1

Pathophysiology of the passage of meconium and the meconium aspiration syndrome. (Redrawn from Wiswell TE, Bent RC: Meconium staining and the meconium aspiration syndrome. *Pediatr Clin North Am* 1993; 40:957; modified from Bacsik RD: Meconium aspiration system. *Pediatr Clin North Am* 1977; 24:467.)

suction should be performed when the infant's head is delivered and before delivery of the thorax (before the first breath is taken). A bulb syringe may be used; however, a No. 8 or 10 French flexible suction catheter may be more effective in removing thick meconium. Regardless of the thickness of meconium, infants who are vigorous at birth with adequate tone and respiratory effort and heart rate greater than 100 beats per minute may not require immediate intubation. These infants should be observed for signs of respiratory distress before deciding on intubation.[71] Infants who are depressed at birth with poor tone and absent or gasping respirations should have the trachea cleared of meconium. Once the infant is intubated, the endotracheal tube should be used as a suction catheter with

80 to 100 cm H_2O negative pressure applied as the tube is withdrawn. Suction catheters inserted into the endotracheal tube are too small to aspirate thick meconium and may become clogged, delaying removal. More than one pass may be needed to clear the trachea of meconium. Ventilation and oxygenation according to established neonatal resuscitation guidelines should be carried out after suctioning. Saline lavage may be used to dilute the meconium while the infant continues to be intubated. All infants born with meconium-stained amniotic fluid should be closely monitored.[72-75]

Mechanical Ventilation. In spite of early intervention with thorough suctioning, some infants will still acquire MAS.[76] The infant who presents with meconium-stained amniotic fluid and progresses to a state of worsening respiratory distress and hypoxemia should be intubated and mechanically ventilated. This infant is a management challenge. Sedation and paralysis are often required for effective ventilation. Optimal ventilator parameters are a combination of PIP, PEEP, inspiratory time, and flow rates that result in the lowest mean airway pressure possible to provide adequate oxygenation and ventilation. Ventilator parameters range from a gentle ventilation with higher $Paco_2$s and lower Pao_2s to more aggressive techniques with the $Paco_2$ at 25 to 30 mm Hg and a "high normal" Pao_2.[77] Aggressive ventilation may affect hemodynamics, prompting worsening of blood gases. This may lead to higher ventilator settings with little clinical improvement.

Other therapies associated with the treatment of neonates with MAS include sedation, alkalosis with bicarbonate or tromethamine (Tham), paralytic agents, minimal stimulation, and chest physiotherapy and suctioning.[78]

High-frequency Ventilation. HFV has been used in MAS in the hope that the lower pressures and higher frequencies will prove advantageous.[79] Benefits may include less barotrauma, increased mobilization of secretions, maintenance of respiratory alkalosis, and fewer chronic changes. However, the high airway resistance and obstructive nature of MAS may hinder the effectiveness of HFOV. Oxygenation is not necessarily improved with the use of either conventional ventilation or HFV.

Emerging Clinical Treatments. Because surfactant within the lung may be hindered by the presence of meconium, surfactant replacement therapy is currently being studied as an effective treatment for MAS (see Chapter 16).[79] Surfactant administration seems to reduce severity of respiratory symptoms and reduces progression of the disease and

may reduce the need for ECMO.[80] Some infants with MAS will progress to the point of developing severe hypoxemia and respiratory failure, exacerbating pulmonary hypertension.[81] Liquid ventilation with perfluorocarbon may be beneficial in MAS by washing out meconium, improving surface tension and ventilation-perfusion mismatch (see Chapter 22). Animal models have shown some promising results.[82,83]

COMPLICATIONS

Complications of MAS are widespread and are dependent on the severity of the disease and the level of treatment necessary for survival. Barotrauma or air leak syndrome is always a risk with positive-pressure ventilation, especially in the infant with MAS in which the ball-valve effect produces air trapping. Because the infant is at significant risk for air leaks, frequent chest films should be obtained so that prompt treatment can be instituted. The patient should be closely monitored for sudden deterioration, which could be indicative of tension pneumothorax. Immediate needle aspiration of the air or insertion of a chest tube, or both, may be indicated.

Another serious complication in MAS is increased intracranial pressure. Because the cranium is a fixed cavity, volume capacity is limited. Venous drainage is inhibited by the increased intrathoracic pressures, creating a potential for elevated intracranial pressure. The neonate with unstable vasculature who is already compromised may be predisposed to a higher incidence of IVH, and frequent ultrasonography of the head is performed to monitor for this complication.

OUTCOME

The outcome in infants with MAS has drastically changed over the past 25 years.[84] Passage of meconium was previously associated with imminent fetal mortality. However, with new techniques at delivery aimed at prevention of further aspiration, as well as the careful administration of resuscitative measures, many more infants survive today and do well. Some infants with MAS experience delayed neurologic function and cerebral palsy.[85,86] When managed properly, however, the majority of these infants do mature with normal neurologic development. Survivors of MAS often acquire chronic respiratory disease, including BPD.[84,87] Another common occurrence is spontaneous wheezing or exercise-induced bronchospasm, with a large component of obstructive airway disease found years later. As technology expands and new modalities are more accessible, the outcome of long-term chronic problems may be diminished.

PERSISTENT PULMONARY HYPERTENSION OF THE NEWBORN

PPHN is a clinical syndrome characterized by severely increased PVR with right-to-left shunting and alterations in pulmonary vasoreactivity. It occurs most often in infants who are term or postterm and is associated with several underlying neonatal clinical conditions, including MAS, RDS, and birth asphyxia; however, it may also be idiopathic with no known cause. Because of the persistent right-to-left fetal shunts (i.e., PDA, foramen ovale) and lack of a known cause, idiopathic pulmonary hypertension of the newborn was formerly known as persistent fetal circulation. The term *persistent* was added to reflect the pathophysiology of the disease.[47,88]

ETIOLOGY AND PATHOPHYSIOLOGY

PPHN may be caused by many factors that are classified as primary or secondary. Primary causes deal with anatomic malformation (e.g., alveolar capillary dysplasia, pulmonary hypoplasia), genetic differences in pulmonary smooth muscle development, chronic intrauterine stress, intrauterine closure of the ductus arteriosus, and abnormal levels of vasoactive agents (i.e., increased vasoconstrictors, decreased vasodilators). Secondary causes are associated with underlying disease processes, such as MAS, congenital heart disease, infection, polycythemia, and upper airway obstruction.[47] Box 28-5 lists factors frequently associated with PPHN.

In fetal life, the placenta functions as the organ for gas exchange. This function is facilitated by both the shunting of the blood through the foramen ovale and the hypoxic pulmonary arteriole vasoconstriction, which causes the blood to bypass the lungs and move toward the placenta. At birth, the umbilical cord is cut and the lungs make the transition to becoming the organ for gas exchange. With the first postnatal breaths, PVR decreases dramatically. By 24 hours of life, 80% of the total decrease in PVR has occurred, with the remaining reduction taking place over the next 2 weeks of life. The reduction in PVR is in response to (1) increases in PaO_2 and pH, (2) air expanding the lung, and (3) release of vasoactive substances, including prostaglandins, bradykinin, and endothelium-derived relaxing factor.[89] In infants with PPHN, this decrease in PVR either fails to occur or is reversed by pulmonary vascular hyperreactivity to irritating stimuli. However, pulmonary hypertension caused by irritating stimuli is not reversed simply by removing the stimulus. Infants with PPHN may have a muscular thickening of the small pulmonary arteries, which results in increased stiffness of the vascular bed and reduced alveolar expansion.[90,91]

BOX 28-5

FACTORS ASSOCIATED WITH PERSISTENT PULMONARY HYPERTENSION OF THE NEWBORN

FETAL FACTORS
Intrauterine stress
   Hypoxia
   Acidosis
Placental vascular abnormalities

MATERNAL FACTORS
Diabetes
Hypoxia
Cesarean section

PHARMACOLOGIC FACTORS
Prostaglandins
Indomethacin
Salicylate
Phenytoin

PULMONARY FACTORS
Pneumonia
Meconium aspiration
Pulmonary hypoplasia
Diaphragmatic hernia
Respiratory distress syndrome
Transient tachypnea of the newborn
Lobar emphysema

HEMATOLOGIC FACTORS
Increased hematocrit
Maternal-fetal blood loss
Abruptio placentae
Placenta previa
Acute blood loss
Polycythemia

CARDIOVASCULAR FACTORS
Systemic hypotension
Congenital heart disease
Shock

OTHER FACTORS
Central nervous system disorders
Neuromuscular disease
Hypoglycemia
Hypocalcemia
Septicemia

CLINICAL PRESENTATION

The infant with PPHN usually presents within the first 12 hours of life with cyanosis, tachypnea, hypoxia that is refractory to oxygen therapy, and signs of respiratory distress, including retractions, grunting, and nasal flaring.[88,92] ABG assessment reveals hypoxemia. Infants may hyperventilate owing to the persistent hypoxemia. Hypocalcemia and hypoglycemia may develop rapidly as well. A right-to-left shunt through a PDA or the foramen ovale, or both, may be present, along with tricuspid and pulmonic valve regurgitation.[93]

The chest radiograph varies depending on the associated disorder. Early chest radiographs are often clear, with minimal evidence of respiratory involvement, which is often perplexing in light of the severe cyanosis and respiratory distress the infant exhibits. Idiopathic and asphyxic PPHN may show well-expanded or hyperexpanded lungs with diminished vascularity, whereas PPHN resulting from pulmonary disorders (e.g., MAS, RDS, TTN) reveals abnormal pulmonary findings characteristic of that particular disorder. Cardiomegaly may be evident and develops as a result of the increased right ventricular afterload caused by the pulmonary hypertension.

DIAGNOSIS

The differential diagnosis of PPHN includes RDS, lung disease, and congenital heart disease. Various tests may be used to assist in the diagnosis.

Hyperoxia Test. The Pa_{O_2} is evaluated on room air and after administering 100% oxygen for 20 minutes. A minimal increase or no increase in the Pa_{O_2} indicates a right-to-left shunt, which may be caused by PPHN or congenital heart disease.

Preductal-Postductal Pa_{O_2} Comparison. A Pa_{O_2} measurement from the right radial artery is compared with that from the umbilical artery, *or* a transcutaneous Pa_{O_2} measurement from the right arm is compared with that from the abdomen. Right-to-left shunting is demonstrated if the preductal sample is more than 20 mm Hg greater than the simultaneous postductal sample. However, a normal test result (difference in preductal and postductal samples <20 mm Hg) does not rule out PPHN. An abnormal test result can also occur in infants with some congenital heart defects.

Hyperoxia-Hyperventilation Test. In the hyperoxia-hyperventilation test, the infant is hyperventilated until a Pa_{CO_2} of 20 to 25 mm Hg is attained. PPHN is nearly always confirmed if the Pa_{O_2} rises to greater than 100 mm Hg after hyperventilation. Pa_{CO_2} levels should not remain that low for long periods owing to a potential reduction in cerebral blood flow.

Doppler Flow Studies and Cardiac Catheterization. Shunts through the foramen ovale and a PDA can be observed with cardiac ultrasound studies. Pulmonary artery pressure may be measured by means of pulmonary artery catheterization, with infants having PPHN demonstrating elevated pressures.[94]

TREATMENT

Oxygen Therapy. Oxygen therapy at high F_{IO_2} levels is administered to help vasodilate the pulmonary vasculature and reduce the PVR. Because of the extreme sensitivity of the pulmonary circulation to oxygen tension changes, however, the optimal Pa_{O_2} is a point of debate. Some investigators prefer to keep the Pa_{O_2} at 80 to 100 mm Hg, whereas others attempt to maintain it between 50 and 70 mm Hg in an effort to minimize damage that may result from prolonged hyperoxia (i.e., surfactant disruption, destruction of alveolar type II cells). Initial relative hyperoxia is likely to aid in further reduction of pulmonary vasoconstriction. This may be of less long-term risk than the long-term concerns of oxygen toxicity. Retinopathy of prematurity is not generally a significant concern in this population because most patients with PPHN are term or near term.

Mechanical Ventilation. If the infant does not respond well to higher oxygen concentrations, mechanical ventilation is implemented. The infant is hyperventilated to maintain the Pa_{CO_2} values between 25 and 35 mm Hg. The respiratory alkalosis that is produced reduces PVR, which induces an elevated systemic oxygenation and decreases the pulmonary artery pressure. Because vasodilation of the pulmonary vasculature is brought about by an alkaline pH (7.45 to 7.5) and not hypocarbia, infusions of bicarbonate and tromethamine have been used to produce alkalosis.[95]

A conservative ventilatory scheme has been proposed, with the goal being to maintain the Pa_{O_2} at 60 to 80 mm Hg, the Pa_{CO_2} at 35 to 45 mm Hg, and the pH at 7.45 to 7.5. Hyperventilation, however, is associated with an increased incidence of barotrauma and gas trapping, with Pa_{CO_2} levels less than 25 mm Hg associated with severely decreased cerebral blood flow.[96] Some infants may require sedation or muscle paralysis to effectively control ventilation.

High-frequency Ventilation. HFV has been used to ventilate infants with PPHN. Retrospective studies indicate that there is no difference in mortality, incidence of air leaks, or BPD between high-frequency jet ventilation and conventionally ventilated groups. Some reports suggest, however, that high-frequency oscillatory ventilation may improve the outcome in PPHN.[93,97,98]

Pharmacologic Support. Infusion of the vasodilator tolazoline has been recommended to dilate the pulmonary vasculature and decrease PVR. Although tolazoline may rapidly improve the PaO_2, its effect can be inconsistent, and systemic hypotension, gastric and pulmonary hemorrhage, and decreased platelet counts may occur. Agents to support systemic blood pressure, such as dopamine, should be given simultaneously with tolazoline.[99] Prostaglandin I_2 improves oxygenation in PPHN but is also associated with systemic hypotension, prolonged bleeding times, and myocardial infarction. Sodium nitroprusside and nitroglycerin, both nonspecific vasodilators, have also been used. Exogenous surfactant may be useful in PPHN, when meconium aspiration or diaphragmatic hernia is also present.[100]

Extracorporeal Membrane Oxygenation. ECMO is being used in some centers for neonates with PPHN who are not responding to other conventional therapies, with studies indicating an increase in survival from 20% to 83%[101,102] (see Chapter 24).

Nitric Oxide Therapy. Nitric oxide has been successfully used in the treatment of PPHN.[103-108] Nitric oxide was thought of simply as an air pollutant; however, that view changed in the late 1980s when research proved that it was produced endogenously in the body and that two forms were released.[109]

Nitric oxide is provided via the mechanical ventilator for inhalation by the infant. Low-dose therapy of 20 ppm for 4 hours and 6 ppm for 20 hours has been reported to possibly eliminate the need for ECMO in the severely ill infant with PPHN.[104] Some infants have benefited from a combination of high-frequency oscillatory ventilation and nitric oxide.[110] Echocardiographic measurements have shown a decrease in PVR, in right-to-left shunting, and in tricuspid insufficiency and an increase in pulmonary blood flow and PaO_2.[108] Nitric oxide has been used for 23 days (median, 20 ppm) without tachyphylaxis or increased methemoglobin concentrations.

There are many factors that must be considered with nitric oxide therapy. In the presence of oxygen, nitric oxide can oxidize to form nitrogen dioxide, which is capable of producing acute respiratory distress even at very low levels. The actual speed of this conversion in the ventilator patient system is unknown; therefore both nitric oxide and nitrogen dioxide should be analyzed during nitric oxide inhalation. Acute cyanosis and pulmonary edema have been associated with extremely high dosages of nitric oxide administration.[111] Although no large controlled studies have been published to establish firm guidelines for safe levels and time spans of nitric oxide use, most studies suggest that low doses (5 to 80 ppm) are safe. Box 28-6 lists clinical conditions that may benefit from nitric oxide therapy (see Chapter 23).[112-117]

COMPLICATIONS AND OUTCOME

The mortality rate for infants with PPHN ranges from 20% to 40%, with an increase in survival seen when nitric oxide or ECMO is used. Approximately 12% to 32% of patients with PPHN suffer from neurologic problems, including impaired neurologic development and neurosensory hearing loss. Seizures, cerebral infarction, and IVH have all been documented in PPHN survivors. BPD is also a risk in patients who require ventilatory assistance with high FIO_2 levels, high rates, and high pressures. The underlying disorder, as well as the management of the patient, contributes to patient outcome.[118]

APNEA OF PREMATURITY

Apnea of prematurity is defined as a cessation of breathing effort greater than 20 seconds in duration, or any respiratory pause that is long enough for signs of bradycardia or cyanosis, or both, to appear in an infant younger than 37 weeks' gestation.[119] Periodic breathing, which is benign, is frequently seen in young infants and may be distinguished from apnea by its characteristic cycle of short pauses in respiration followed by an increased respiratory rate.[120]

INCIDENCE

Apnea of prematurity is perhaps the most common form of infant apnea and is a significant cause of morbidity and mortality in premature infants.[121] Approximately 75% of premature infants weighing less than 1250 g and more than 25% of those weighing more than 1500 g suffer from severe apnea. The incidence of apneic episodes is related to the degree of infant immaturity. Neurologic immaturity and the degree of maturity of pulmonary stretch reflexes and the ventilatory response to carbon dioxide may be better predictors of the risk for apneic spells than chronologic age.[122]

BOX 28-6

CONDITIONS THAT MAY BENEFIT FROM NITRIC OXIDE THERAPY

Persistent pulmonary hypertension of the newborn
Hypoxic pulmonary hypertension
Methacholine-induced bronchoconstriction
Septic shock
Pulmonary hypertension before and after cardiac surgery
Adult respiratory distress syndrome
High-altitude pulmonary edema

ETIOLOGY AND PATHOPHYSIOLOGY

There are two types of apnea related to the degree of asphyxia. Primary apnea occurs after a rapid increase in respiratory rate and depth. The infant can usually be manually stimulated to begin breathing again. If allowed to continue, the infant then suffers approximately 1 minute of apnea followed by several minutes of gasping. This apneic episode can progress to a secondary stage in which resuscitation is required to reestablish respiration. Approximately 30% of all premature infants suffer from this secondary form, which lasts for more than 30 seconds and is associated with a drop in oxygen saturation. Secondary apnea may also be accompanied by bradycardia and hypotension.

Premature infants are believed to be susceptible to apneic episodes because of immature afferent input from chemoreceptors, lung and airway receptors, and the central nervous system. Sleep may be a factor in apnea and periodic breathing. Nearly 80% of a preterm infant's time is spent sleeping, with approximately 90% of a sleep cycle spent in rapid-eye-movement (REM) sleep in which there is respiratory depression. However, only 50% of a full-term infant's sleep is spent in REM sleep. Also, the infant's very compliant rib cage is less compliant during REM sleep, which may result in decreased lung volumes. Box 28-7 lists factors that are believed to trigger apneic spells in infants.[123-127]

CLINICAL PRESENTATION

Infants with apnea invariably respond with bradycardia. Other initial symptoms include snoring, choking, and mouth breathing, although some infants exhibit no signs of respiratory distress. There may be changes in muscle tone, skin color (cyanosis or pallor), and respiratory pattern.

DIAGNOSIS

Infants with frequent apnea should have routine screening tests that include a chest radiograph, ABG analysis, electrocardiogram and Holter monitoring, complete blood cell count, and electrolyte

---

BOX 28-7

FACTORS ASSOCIATED WITH APNEA IN INFANTS

SYSTEMIC PROCESSES
Sepsis
    Group B *Streptococcus*
Respiratory syncytial virus
Hypothermia
Hypoglycemia
Hyponatremia
Hypocalcemia

PULMONARY DISEASE
Pneumonia
Respiratory distress syndrome

CARDIAC DISEASE
Left-to-right shunt
Congestive heart failure
Patent ductus arteriosus closure

NEUROLOGIC DISEASE
Seizures
Meningitis
Intracranial hemorrhage

GASTROINTESTINAL DISEASE
Botulism
Gastroesophageal reflux
Abnormal coordination of
    swallowing

REFLEXES
Hiccups
Vagal response to bowel movement
Suctioning of nasopharynx and trachea
Stimulation of laryngeal chemoreceptors

CONTROL OF VENTILATION
Rapid-eye-movement sleep
Depressed response to hypoxia
Depressed response to hypercarbia
Congenital central hypoventilation (Ondine's curse)

ENVIRONMENTAL CONDITIONS
Ambient temperature changes

POSITION
Head flexion

DRUG DEPRESSION
Sedatives
Analgesics
Prostaglandins

ANATOMIC ABNORMALITIES
Micrognathia
Macroglossia
Choanal atresia
Temporomandibular ankylosis

Modified from Leistner HL: Apnea in infants and children. In Zimmerman SS, Gildea J, editors: *Critical care pediatrics.* Philadelphia. WB Saunders, 1985.

determination. Blood, urine, and cerebrospinal fluid cultures should be performed if infection is believed to be a contributing factor and all other causes are ruled out. Close monitoring to evaluate possible causes of the apnea should include respiratory rate and pattern, heart rate, circumstances preceding the apneic episode, associated bradycardia, skin color, muscle tone, and termination of the episode (whether spontaneous, with stimulation, or with resuscitation).

TREATMENT

Once the underlying cause for the apnea has been determined, the treatment focuses on preventing further episodes from occurring. This begins with monitoring and treatment of ineffective respiration before it degenerates to apnea. The infant may benefit from tactile stimulation only; however, if the apnea persists, ventilation with oxygen is initiated with bag and mask. To reduce the risk of retinopathy of prematurity, the infant should be ventilated only with the FIO_2 needed to maintain adequate oxygen saturation. Upright positioning; small, frequent feedings of thickened formula; temperature stability; or a combination of these factors may be helpful in prevention. Frequently, a low FIO_2 of 0.23 to 0.25 is effective in decreasing apneic episodes. With prolonged episodes, a low dose of a methylxanthine derivative, such as caffeine, theophylline, or doxapram, has been initiated to stimulate respiration.[128] Because gastroesophageal reflux may be exacerbated by xanthine therapy, it should be ruled out before xanthines are administered. Oscillating water beds or "bump" beds may be used to stimulate respiration in the infant. A bump bed can be constructed by connecting a rubber glove to a pressure ventilator or intermittent positive-pressure breathing machine with a respiratory rate and inspiratory pressure set. The glove is placed under the infant's mattress pad, and the periodic inflation-deflation of the glove will bump the infant and, it is hoped, stimulate respirations. Current studies have not been adequate to determine the effectiveness of kinesthetic stimulation compared with other treatments.[129] With current minimal stimulation and developmental care guidelines for premature infants, this method is discouraged in most nurseries.

OUTCOME

Although in most infants with apnea the episodes gradually decrease in both frequency and severity as the infants mature, there is a questionably higher incidence of sudden infant death syndrome associated with neonatal apnea. If results from polysomnography or sleep testing show persistent abnormalities of respiration, the infant may be discharged on a home apnea-bradycardia monitor (see Chapters 11, 32, and 46).

REFERENCES

1. Miller JM, Fanaroff AA, Martin RJ: Other pulmonary problems. In Fanaroff AA, Martin RJ, editors: *Neonatal-perinatal medicine diseases of the fetus and infant,* ed 5, vol II. St Louis. Mosby, 1992; pp 834-861.
2. U.S. Department of Health and Human Services: Press release (P10-33). Washington, DC, July 26, 1989.
3. Farrell PM, Wood RE: Epidemiology of hyaline membrane disease in the United States: analysis of national mortality statistics. *Pediatrics* 1976; 58:167.
4. Hansen T, Corbert A: Disorders of the transition. In Taeusch HW, Ballard RA, Avery ME, editors: *Schaffer and Avery's diseases of the newborn,* ed 6. Philadelphia. WB Saunders, 1991.
5. Kliegman RM, Behrman RE: Disturbances of organ systems. In Behrman RE et al, editors: *Textbook of pediatrics,* ed 14. Philadelphia. WB Saunders, 1992.
6. Hulsey TC, Alexander GR, Robilland PY: Hyaline membrane disease: the role of ethnicity and maternal risk characteristics. *Am J Obstet Gynecol* 1993; 168:572.
7. Graven SN, Misenheimer HR: Respiratory distress syndrome and the high risk mother. *Am J Dis Child* 1965; 109:489.
8. Usher RH, Allen AC, McLean FH: Risk of respiratory distress syndrome related to gestational age, route of delivery and maternal diabetes. *Am J Obstet Gynecol* 1971; 111:826.
9. Avery ME, Mead J: Surface properties in relation to atelectasis and hyaline membrane disease. *Am J Dis Child* 1959; 97:517.
10. Stahlman M et al: Six-year follow-up of clinical hyaline membrane disease. *Pediatr Clin North Am* 1973; 20:433.
11. Rooney SA: The surfactant system and lung phospholipid biochemistry. *Am Rev Respir Dis* 1985; 131:439.
12. Seppanen MP et al: Doppler-derived systolic pulmonary artery pressure in acute neonatal respiratory distress syndrome. *Pediatrics* 1994; 93:769.
13. Meyrick B, Reid L: Ultrastructure of alveolar lining and its development. In Hodson WA, editor: *Development of the lung.* New York. Marcel Dekker, 1977; pp 135-214.
14. Clements JA, King RJ: Composition of surface-active material. In Crystal RG, editor: *The biochemical basis of pulmonary function.* New York. Marcel Dekker, 1976; pp 363-387.
15. Hawgood S, Clements JA: Pulmonary surfactant and its apoproteins. *J Clin Invest* 1990; 86:1.
16. Boyden EA: Development and growth of the airways. In Hodson WA, editor: *Development of the lung.* New York. Marcel Dekker, 1972; pp 3-36.
17. Hislop AA, Wigglesworth JS, Desai R: Alveolar development in the human fetus and infant. *Early Hum Dev* 1986; 13:1.
18. Stark AR, Frantz ID III: Respiratory distress syndrome. *Pediatr Clin North Am* 1986; 33:533.
19. Nelson NM et al: Pulmonary function in the newborn infant, the alveolar-arterial oxygen gradient. *J Appl Physiol* 1963; 18:534.
20. Murdock AI, Swyer PR: The contribution to venous admixture by shunting through the ductus arteriosus in infants with respiratory distress syndrome of the newborn. *Biol Neonate* 1968; 13:194.
21. Verma RP: Respiratory distress syndrome of the newborn infant. *Obstet Gynecol Surv* 1995; 50:542-555.
22. Davis GM, Bureau MA: Pulmonary and chest wall mechanics in the control of respiration in the newborn. *Clin Perinatol* 1987; 14:551.

23. Escobedo MB: Hyaline membrane disease. In Schreiner RL, Kisling JA, editors: *Practical neonatal respiratory care.* New York. Raven Press, 1982; pp 87-103.

24. Whitfield CR, Sproule WD: Prediction of neonatal respiratory distress. *Lancet* 1972; 1:382.

25. Lemons JA, Jaffe RB: Amniotic fluid lecithin/sphingomyelin ratio in the diagnosis of hyaline membrane disease. *Am J Obstet Gynecol* 1973; 115:233.

26. Hallman M et al: Phosphatidylinositol and phosphatidylglycerol in amniotic fluid: indices of lung maturity. *Am J Obstet Gynecol* 1976; 125:613.

27. Clements JA et al: Assessment of the risk of the respiratory distress syndrome by a rapid test for surfactant in amniotic fluid. *N Engl J Med* 1972; 286:1077.

28. Ballard PL: Hormonal regulation of pulmonary surfactant. *Endocr Rev* 1989; 10:165.

29. Pramanik AK, Holtzman RB, Merritt TA: Surfactant replacement therapy for pulmonary diseases. *Pediatr Clin North Am* 1993; 40:913.

30. Long W et al: Effects of two rescue doses of a synthetic surfactant on mortality rate and survival without bronchopulmonary dysplasia in 700- to 1350-gram infants with respiratory distress syndrome. *J Pediatr* 1991; 118:595.

31. Gaillard EA, Cooke RW, Shaw NJ: Improved survival and neurodevelopmental outcome after prolonged ventilation in preterm neonates who have received antenatal steroids and surfactant. *Arch Dis Child Fetal Neonatal* 2001; 84(3):F194-F196.

32. Gittermann MK et al: Early nasal continuous positive airway pressure treatment reduces the need for intubation in very low birth weight infants. *Eur J Pediatr* 1996; 56:384-388.

33. Kamper J: Early nasal continuous positive airway pressure and minimal handling in the treatment of very-low birthweight infants. *Biol Neonate* 1999; 76(suppl 1):22-28.

34. Alba J et al: Efficacy of surfactant therapy in infants managed with CPAP. *Pediatr Pulmonol* 1995; 20:172-176.

35. Schimmel MS, Hammerman C: Early nasal continuous positive airway pressure with or without prophylactic surfactant therapy in the premature infant with respiratory distress syndrome. *Pediatr Radiol* 2000; 30:713-714.

36. Soll RF, Morley CJ: Prophylactic versus selective use of surfactant in preventing morbidity and mortality in preterm infants (Cochrane Review). *Cochrane Database Syst Rev* 2001; 2:CD000510.

37. Hummler H et al: Influence of different methods of synchronized mechanical ventilation on ventilation, gas exchange, patient effort, and blood pressure fluctuations in premature neonates. *Pediatr Pulmonol* 1996; 22:305-313.

38. Green TP et al: Prophylactic furosemide in severe respiratory distress syndrome: blinded prospective study. *J Pediatr* 1988; 112:605.

39. Greenough A et al: Routine daily chest radiographs in ventilated, very low birthweight infants. *Eur J Pediatr* 2001; 160: 147-149.

40. Mannino FL, Gluck L: The management of respiratory distress syndrome. In Thibeault DW, Gregoary GA, editors: *Neonatal pulmonary care.* Reading, Mass. Addison-Wesley, 1979; pp 261-276.

41. Avery ME et al: Is chronic lung disease in low birthweight infants preventable? A survey of eight centers. *Pediatrics* 1987; 79:26.

42. Lebourges F et al: Pulmonary function in infancy and in childhood following mechanical ventilation in the neonatal period. *Pediatr Pulmonol* 1990; 9:34.

43. Bhutani VK et al: Pulmonary mechanics and energetics in preterm infants who had respiratory distress syndrome treated with synthetic surfactant. *J Pediatr* 1992; 120:S18.

44. Avery ME, Gatewood OB, Brumley G: Transient tachypnea of the newborn. *Am J Dis Child* 1966; 111:380.

45. Whitsett JA et al: Acute respiratory disorders. In Avery GE, Fletcher MA, MacDonald MG, editors: *Neonatology,* ed 4. Philadelphia. JB Lippincott, 1994.

46. Tudehope DI, Smith MH: Is transient tachypnoea of the newborn always a benign condition? *Aust Paediatr J* 1979; 15:160.

47. Levin DL: Idiopathic persistent pulmonary hypertension of the newborn. In Rudolph AM, Hoffman JIE, Rudolph CD, editors: *Rudolph's pediatrics,* ed 19. Norwalk, Conn. Appleton & Lange, 1991.

48. Bucciarelli RL et al: Persistence of fetal cardiopulmonary circulation: manifestation of transient tachypnea of the newborn. *Pediatrics* 1976; 58:192.

49. Gross TL, Sokol RJ, Kwong MS: Transient tachypnea of the newborn: the relationship to preterm delivery and significant neonatal morbidity. *Am J Obstet Gynecol* 1983; 14:236.

50. Battaglia FC, Rosenberg AA: The newborn infant. In Groothuis JR et al, editors: *Current pediatric diagnosis & treatment.* Norwalk, Conn. Appleton & Lange, 1993.

51. Durand DJ, Gleason CA: Respiratory complications. In Keith LG, Witter FR, editors: *Textbook of prematurity.* Boston, Little, Brown, 1993.

52. Pursley DM, Richardson DK: Management of the sick newborn. In Graef JW, editor: *Manual of pediatric therapeutics,* ed 5. Boston, Little Brown, 1994.

53. Rudiger M et al: Disturbed surface properties in preterm infants with pneumonia. *Biol Neonate* 2001; 79:73-78.

54. Corbet A, Hansen T: Neonatal pneumonias. In Avery ME, Ballard RA, Taeusch AW: *Schaffer and Avery's diseases of the newborn,* ed 6. Philadelphia. WB Saunders, 1991.

55. Nelson RM: Group B *Streptococcus* (GBS). In Behrman RE, et al, editors: *Textbook of pediatrics,* ed 14. Philadelphia, WB Saunders, 1992.

56. Adams WG et al: Outbreak of early onset group B streptococcal sepsis. *Pediatr Infect Dis J* 1993; 12:565.

57. Tooley WH: Neonatal pneumonia due to beta-hemolytic *Streptococcus* group B. In Rudolph AM, editor: *Rudolph's pediatrics,* ed 19. Norwalk, Conn. Appleton & Lange, 1991.

58. Hocker JR, Simpson PM, Rabalais GP: Extracorporeal membrane oxygenation and early-onset group B streptococcal sepsis. *Pediatrics* 1992; 89:1.

59. Goetzman BW: Meconium aspiration. *Am J Dis Child* 1992; 146:1282.

60. Wiswell TE, Tuggle JM, Turner BS: Meconium aspiration syndrome: have we made a difference? *Pediatrics* 1990; 85:715.

61. Wiswell TE, Bent RC: Meconium staining and the meconium aspiration syndrome. *Pediatr Clin North Am* 1993; 40:955.

62. Rossi EM et al: Meconium aspiration syndrome: intrapartum and neonatal attributes. *Am J Obstet Gynecol* 1989; 161:1106.

63. Tyler DC, Murphy J, Cheney FW: Mechanical and chemical damage to lung tissue caused by meconium aspiration. *Pediatrics* 1978; 62:454.

64. Wiswell TE et al: Management of a piglet model of the meconium aspiration syndrome with high frequency or conventional ventilation. *Am J Dis Child* 1992; 146:1287.

65. Moses D et al: Inhibition of pulmonary surfactant by meconium. *Am J Obstet Gynecol* 1991; 104:758.

66. Perlman EJ, Moore GW, Hutchins GM: The pulmonary vasculature in meconium aspiration. *Hum Pathol* 1989; 20:701.

67. Dooley SL et al: Meconium below the vocal cords at delivery: correlation with intrapartum events. *Am J Obstet Gynecol* 1985; 153:767.

68. Mitchell J et al: Meconium aspiration and fetal acidosis. *Obstet Gynecol* 1985; 65:352.

69. Yeh TF et al: Roentgenographic findings in infants with meconium aspiration syndrome. *JAMA* 1979; 242:60.

70. Henleigh P, Loots M: Complications associated with amnioinfusion for meconium. *Am J Obstet Gynecol* 1991; 164:317.

71. Wiswell TE et al: Delivery room management of the apparently vigorous meconium-stained neonates: results of the multi-center, international collaborative trial. *Pediatrics* 2000; 105:1-17.

72. American Academy of Pediatrics and American College of Obstetricians and Gynecologists: *Guidelines for perinatal care.* Evanston, Ill. AAP/ACOG, 1983; p 69.

73. Hageman JR et al: Delivery room management of meconium staining of the amniotic fluid and the development of meconium aspiration syndrome. *J Perinatol* 1988; 8:127.

74. Linder N et al: Need for endotracheal intubation and suction in meconium-stained neonates. *J Pediatr* 1988; 112:613.

75. Kresch MJ, Brion LP, Fleischman AR: Delivery room management of meconium-stained neonates. *J Perinatol* 1991; 11:46.

76. Davis RO et al: Fatal meconium aspiration syndrome despite airway management considered appropriate. *Am J Obstet Gynecol* 1985; 151:731.

77. Vidyasagar D et al: Assisted ventilation in infants with meconium aspiration syndrome. *Pediatrics* 1975; 56:208.

78. Wiswell TE: Advances in the treatment of the meconium aspiration syndrome. *Acta Paediatr Suppl* 2001; 436:28-30.

79. Wiswell TE, Davis JM, Merritt TA: Surfactant therapy and high frequency jet ventilation in the management of a piglet model of the meconium aspiration syndrome. *Pediatr Res* 1993; 33:350A.

80. Soll RF, Dargaville P: Surfactant for meconium aspiration syndrome in full term infants. *Cochrane Database Syst Rev* 2000; (2):CD002054

81. Koumbourlis C, Moyoyama EK, Mutich RL: Airway reactivity in neonates after extracorporeal membrane oxygenation (ECMO) for meconium aspiration syndrome (MAS). *Pediatr Res* 1992; 31:322A.

82. Barrington KJ et al: Partial liquid ventilation with and without inhaled nitric oxide in a newborn piglet model of meconium aspiration. *Am J Respir Crit Care Med* 1999; 160:1922-1927.

83. Shaffer TH et al: Liquid ventilation: effects on pulmonary function in distressed meconium-stained lambs. *Pediatr Res* 1984; 18:47.

84. Swaminathan S et al: Long-term pulmonary sequelae of meconium aspiration syndrome. *J Pediatr* 1989; 114:356.

85. Nelson KB: Relationship of intrapartum and delivery room events to long-term neurologic outcome. *Clin Perinatol* 1989; 16:995.

86. Altshuler G, Hyde S: Meconium-induced vasocontraction: a potential cause of cerebral and other fetal hypoperfusion and of poor pregnancy outcome. *J Child Neurol* 1989; 4:137.

87. MacFarlane PI, Heaf DP: Pulmonary function in children after neonatal meconium aspiration syndrome. *Arch Dis Child* 1988; 63:368.

88. Levin DL et al: Persistent pulmonary hypertension of the newborn infant. *J Pediatr* 1976; 89:626.

89. Loeb AL et al: Endothelium-derived relaxing factor in cultured cells. *Hypertension* 1987; 9:186.

90. Stevens DC, Schreiner RL: Persistent fetal circulation. In Schreiner RL, Kisling JA, editors: *Practical neonatal respiratory care.* New York. Raven Press, 1982.

91. Geggel RL, Reid L: The structural basis of PPHN. *Clin Perinatol* 1984; 11:525.

92. Drummond WH, Peckham GJ, Fox WW: The clinical profile of the newborn with persistent pulmonary hypertension: observations in 19 affected neonates. *Clin Pediatr* 1977; 16:335.

93. Walsh-Sukys MC: Persistent pulmonary hypertension of the newborn: The black box revisited. *Clin Perinatol* 1993; 20:127.

94. Peckman GJ, Fox WW: Physiologic factors affecting pulmonary artery pressure in infants with persistent pulmonary hypertension. *J Pediatr* 1978; 93:1005.

95. Schreiber MD, Heymann MA, Soifer SJ: Increased arterial pH, not decreased Paco$_2$ attenuates hypoxia-induced pulmonary vasoconstriction in newborn lambs. *Pediatr Res* 1986; 20:113.

96. Bifano EM, Pfannenstiel A: Duration of hyperventilation and outcome in infants with persistent pulmonary hypertension. *Pediatrics* 1988; 81:657.

97. Kohelet D et al: High-frequency oscillation in the rescue of infants with persistent pulmonary hypertension. *Crit Care Med* 1988; 16:510.

98. Carlo WA et al: High-frequency jet ventilation in neonatal pulmonary hypertension. *Am J Dis Child* 1989; 143:233.

99. Drummond WH et al: The independent effects of hyperventilation, tolazoline, and dopamine on infants with persistent pulmonary hypertension. *J Pediatr* 1981; 98:603.

100. Weinberger B et al: Pharmacologic therapy of persistent pulmonary hypertension of the newborn. *Pharmacol Ther* 2001; 89:67-79.

101. O'Rourke PP et al: Extracorporeal membrane oxygenation and conventional medical therapy in neonates with persistent pulmonary hypertension of the newborn: a prospective randomized study. *Pediatrics* 1989; 84:957.

102. Roberts JD, Shaul PW: Advances in the treatment of persistent pulmonary hypertension of the newborn. *Pediatr Clin North Am* 1993; 40:983.

103. Roberts JD: Inhaled nitric oxide for treatment of pulmonary hypertension in the newborn and infant. *Crit Care Med* 1993; 21:S374.

104. Oriot D et al: Paradoxical effect of inhaled nitric oxide in a newborn with pulmonary hypertension. *Lancet* 1993; 342:364.

105. Davidson D: NO bandwagon, yet: inhaled nitric oxide (NO) for neonatal pulmonary hypertension. *Am Rev Respir Dis* 1993; 147:1078.

106. Kinsella JP, Abman SH: Inhalational nitric oxide therapy for persistent pulmonary hypertension of the newborn. *Pediatrics* 1993; 91:997.

107. Kinsella JP et al: Selective and sustained pulmonary vasodilation with inhaled nitric oxide therapy in a child with idiopathic pulmonary hypertension. *J Pediatr* 1993; 122:803.

108. Roberts JD Jr et al: Inhaled nitric oxide reverses pulmonary vasoconstriction in the hypoxic and acidotic newborn. *Circ Res* 1993; 72:246.

109. Moncada S et al: Nitric oxide: physiology, pathophysiology, and pharmacology. *Pharmacol Rev* 1991; 43:109.

110. Kinsella JP, Neish SR, Ivy DD: Clinical responses to prolonged treatment of persistent pulmonary hypertension of the newborn with low-doses of inhaled nitric oxide. *J Pediatr* 1993; 123:103.

111. Greenbaum R et al: Effects of higher oxides of nitrogen on the anaesthetized dog. *Br J Anaesth* 1967; 39:393.

112. Wessel DL: Inhaled nitric oxide for the treatment of pulmonary hypertension before and after cardiopulmonary bypass. *Crit Care Med* 1993; 21:S344.

113. Rich GF et al: Inhaled nitric oxide: selective pulmonary vasodilation in cardiac surgical patients. *Anesthesiology* 1993; 78:1028.

114. Gibaldi M: What is nitric oxide and why are so many people studying it? *J Clin Pharmacol* 1993; 33:488.

115. Weitzberg E et al: Nitric oxide inhalation attenuates pulmonary hypertension and improves gas exchange in endotoxin shock. *Eur J Pharmacol* 1993; 233:85.

116. Bone RC: A new therapy for the adult respiratory distress syndrome. *N Engl J Med* 1993; 328:431.

117. Bouchet M et al: Safety requirements for use of inhaled nitric oxide in neonates. *Lancet* 1993; 341:968.

118. Dworetz AR et al: Survival of infants with persistent pulmonary hypertension without extracorporeal membrane oxygenation. *Pediatrics* 1989; 84:1.

119. Keens TG, Ward SLD: Apnea spells, sudden death, and the role of the apnea monitor. *Pediatr Clin North Am* 1993; 40:897.

120. Toney SB: Apnea. In Fleischer GR, Ludwig S, editors: *Textbook of pediatric emergency medicine,* ed 3. Baltimore. Williams & Wilkins, 1993.

121. Thach BT: Apnea and the sudden infant death syndrome. In Saunders NA, Sullivan CE, editors: *Sleep and breathing,* ed 2. New York. Marcel Dekker, 1994; pp 649-671.

122. Gerhardt T, Banclari E: Apnea of prematurity: lung function and regulation of breathing. *Pediatrics* 1984; 74:58.

123. Leistner HL: Apnea in infants and children. In Zimmerman S, Gildea J, editors: *Critical care pediatrics.* Philadelphia. WB Saunders, 1985.

124. Martin RJ, Miller MB, Carlo WA: Pathogenesis of apnea in preterm infants. *J Pediatr* 1986; 109:733.

125. Rigatto H, Brady JP: Periodic breathing and apnea in preterm infants: I. Hypoxia as a primary event. *Pediatrics* 1972; 50:219.

126. Brouillette RT et al: Hiccups in infants: characteristics and effects on ventilation. *J Pediatr* 1980; 96:219.

127. Menon A, Schefft G, Thach BT: Apnea associated with regurgitation in infants. *J Pediatr* 1985; 106:625.

128. Aranda JV, Thurman T: Methylxanthines in apnea of prematurity. *Clin Perinatol* 1979; 6:87.

129. Osborn DA, Henderson-Smart DJ: Kinesthetic stimulation versus theophylline for apnea in preterm infants. (Cochrane Review). In The Cochrane Library, Issue 2. Oxford. Update Software, 2001.

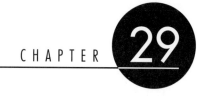

CHAPTER 29

Congenital and Surgical Disorders That Affect Respiratory Care

Roberta E. Sonnino

Numerous congenital anomalies and surgical disorders in children have a direct or indirect effect on the respiratory system, often with serious consequences. Some anomalies are corrected electively, whereas others require immediate recognition and emergency intervention. Knowledge of the most common surgical disorders of infancy and childhood and any intervention they may require helps the clinician successfully manage the respiratory status of an infant or child presenting with these or similar disorders. The respiratory care practitioner is often asked to assist in the management of these patients. Patients with such conditions often need ventilator support and respiratory therapy in the preoperative and postoperative periods. In this chapter, the focus of the discussion is on the most common surgical conditions that can significantly affect respiratory function. Points of pathology and physiology that are important in the respiratory care of these children are examined.

CONGENITAL DIAPHRAGMATIC HERNIA

The diaphragm arises from the fusion of the pleura in the chest and the peritoneum in the abdomen. Closure is completed between the sixth and eighth weeks of intrauterine life. The intestine returns to the abdomen from the yolk sac during the 10th week. During this time, if the pleuroperitoneal canal of the diaphragm, most commonly in the posterolateral location (Bochdalek's hernia), fails to close, the abdominal viscera herniate into the pleural cavity. Congenital diaphragmatic hernias (CDHs) are more common on the left side (L:R ratio = 9:1). Bilateral defects are rare. The defect may be as small as 2 to 3 cm in diameter, or it may involve the entire diaphragm. There is little relationship between size of the defect and the amount of herniated viscera. Fig. 29-1 shows the typical physical appearance and radiographic course of a patient with CDH.

Survival of a newborn with CDH depends on the degree of lung maturity and the presence and reversibility of pulmonary hypertension. Normal lung volumes may be reduced by as much as 50%. In the majority of cases, the ipsilateral lung is small because of compression of the pulmonary parenchyma during lung development in utero. The contralateral lung can also be compressed by the heart and mediastinum, which have been displaced to the opposite side. In addition to pulmonary hypoplasia, histologic studies have demonstrated muscular hypertrophy in the media of the pulmonary arteries with abnormal muscularization of the acinar spaces at the alveoli.[1] Muscular hypertrophy of the pulmonary vasculature makes the infant with a CDH particularly susceptible to decreased pulmonary blood flow from pulmonary artery vasoconstriction and hypertension.

Hypoxia, hypercapnia, acidosis, and hypothermia precipitate pulmonary hypertension. Preventing these "triggers" during the immediate newborn period is crucial if an infant with a CDH is to survive.[2] The immediate resuscitation of a dyspneic infant with a CDH should include the following steps:

1. A large nasogastric or orogastric sump tube (No. 10 F Replogle) is inserted to remove swallowed air and avoid further pressure caused by a distended gastrointestinal tract in the chest.

2. An endotracheal tube is inserted, and the patient is ventilated *very gently.* Mask ventilation introduces large amounts of gas into the stomach and is contraindicated. Aggressive (high pressure) ventilation is to be avoided at all cost.

3. Barotrauma is avoided by using a high-frequency oscillator or a ventilation strategy that is compatible with reduced lung volumes, such as a high rate, short inspiratory time, and low peak pressure.

4. Strategies to decrease pulmonary vasoconstriction include maintenance of a Pao_2 greater than or equal to 150 mm Hg and a relative alkalosis with pH greater than or equal to 7.44. Adequate alkalosis can usually be maintained with $Paco_2$ levels between 25 and 30 mm Hg. The pulmonary vasculature of infants with CDH appears particularly sensitive to changes in Pao_2 and pH. Pharmacologic measures may also be used to raise serum pH.

5. Chest tubes are used only for contralateral pneumothoraces. The pneumothorax is usually the result of excessive ventilating pressures.

Positive-pressure ventilation can rapidly enlarge the pneumothorax and compress the functioning lung unless a chest tube is in place. Chest tubes on the side of the CDH before repair are contraindicated.[3]

Operative repair of the CDH does not reverse pulmonary hypertension or hypoplasia. Several studies since the mid 1980s have shown that allowing the infant to adjust to postnatal life and stabilize before surgical correction enhances outcomes.[4] In addition, it appears that pulmonary function deteriorates transiently after CDH repair. Improved survival has been documented by delaying repair to allow a period for postnatal increases in lung compliance and tidal volume. Stabilization periods of 8 hours to 11 days have been of benefit.[5,6]

Operative repair, usually through an abdominal approach, reduces the abdominal viscera from the chest cavity with closure of the defect, either primarily or with a prosthetic patch. The mediastinum is allowed to gradually return to the midline, permitting the contralateral lung to expand and work at optimal efficiency. Residual air in the ipsilateral chest after repair is a result of the hypoplastic lung being unable to occupy the entire hemithorax. It is not technically a pneumothorax, and there is no advantage to placement of a chest tube postoperatively. A chest tube may actually cause too rapid shift of the mediastinum to the center, with acute displacement and obstruction of major vascular structures and overexpansion of either the ipsilateral or the contralateral lung. Gentle, spontaneous return of the mediastinum to the midline is preferred, and chest tubes are no longer routinely used.

Endotracheal intubation is usually maintained for several days or more. Low levels of positive end-expiratory pressure (0 to 3 cm H_2O) may be necessary to prevent microatelectasis. Higher values may result in decreased pulmonary blood flow and increased right-to-left shunting. Low lung volume ventilation strategies are continued postoperatively. In general, if the peak intratracheal pressure has to be maintained at greater than 35 cm H_2O, or other abnormally high ventilator settings are necessary to maintain adequate pH and Pao_2, the prognosis is grave. This clinical situation, preoperatively or postoperatively, is an indication for more advanced life support measures, such as high-frequency ventilation (now frequently used from the onset), nitric oxide, and extracorporeal membrane oxygenation (ECMO), today used mostly as a last resort.

Many infants do well for the first 8 to 24 hours after repair ("honeymoon period"), but increasing hypoxia and acidosis may develop and can be difficult to treat. An infant's survival depends on being able to reverse pulmonary artery vasospasm,

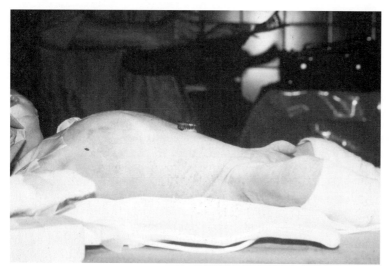

A

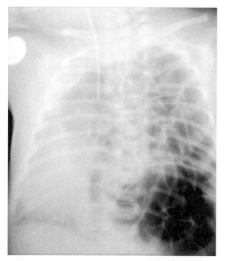

B

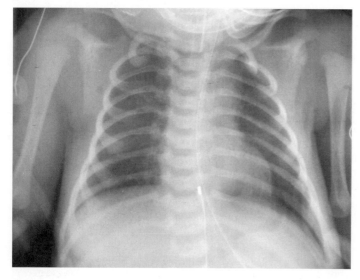

C

Fig. 29-1

A, Newborn with congenital diaphragmatic hernia. Note large chest and scaphoid abdomen caused by presence of abdominal viscera in chest. **B,** A chest radiograph of an infant with congenital diaphragmatic hernia. Note gas-filled loops of bowel in the left hemithorax. The heart and mediastinal contents are shifted to the right, compressing the right lung. **C,** Chest radiograph after repair of the hernia. (Photographs courtesy Roberta E. Sonnino, MD.)

right-to-left shunting, and a failing myocardium. When desaturated venous blood enters the systemic arterial system through shunting, generalized tissue hypoxia and increasing metabolic acidosis develop. As a result, cardiac output is diminished and right-to-left shunting increases.

The primary stimuli for pulmonary artery vasospasm are combinations of hypoxemia, acidosis, and, to a lesser degree, hypercarbia. Stimuli that might contribute to pulmonary vasoconstriction are pain, endotracheal tube suctioning, loud noises, and persistent atelectasis.[7] An environment with minimal stimulation is mandatory. Pulmonary vasospasm, right-to-left shunting, and acidosis after a successful operation are particularly troublesome in the care of newborns with CDH. This sequence of events is more common for infants diagnosed and treated within the first 6 hours of life and affects 20% to 80% of patients.

Tolazoline and dopamine were used in the past to treat the pulmonary vasoconstriction that may develop after repair of a CDH.[8] Tolazoline is an adrenergic blocking agent with histamine-releasing properties. Fluid retention, gastric hypersecretion and bleeding, seizures, and systemic hypotension are serious side effects of tolazoline and have virtually eliminated its use. Other methods have been sought to reduce or reverse the pulmonary artery to aortic pressure gradient or right-to-left shunt. The adrenergic effect of dopamine in doses greater than 10 mg/kg/hr raises aortic blood pressure and decreases the right-to-left shunting. Dopamine also has inotropic effects that strengthen cardiac contraction secondary to the release of myocardial norepinephrine. However, the concomitant vasoconstriction of the splanchnic vasculature induced by high-dose dopamine puts an already compromised gut at severe risk of ischemia, and therefore limits its use.

Today, the most common forms of treatment of CDH-associated pulmonary hypertension are high-frequency ventilation, permissive hypercapnia, nitric oxide, and ECMO. Although nitric oxide has not been uniformly as successful in infants with CDH as compared with its use in infants with pulmonary hypertension from other causes, it has provided beneficial results in several infants with CDH and warrants a trial of use before committing the infant to a course of ECMO.

Extracorporeal respiratory and circulatory support through ECMO, once thought to provide the ideal treatment for CDH-associated pulmonary hypertension, is now considered the treatment of last resort.[9,10] (The actual technique of ECMO is discussed in Chapter 24.) If used, to reduce barotrauma during ECMO, the ventilator settings are reduced to minimal values: inspiratory pressure, 18 to 20 cm H_2O; FIO_2, 0.3; rate, 15 to 20 breaths per minute. Because the membrane oxygenator is also very efficient at removing CO_2, respiratory alkalosis can easily be induced by increasing the "sweep" of gases through the oxygenator.

As pulmonary vascular resistance improves, ECMO is decreased by reducing the flow rate to allow more blood to enter the right atrium and pulmonary circulation. Continued pulmonary vascular dilatation will eventually allow reduction of ECMO to the point that therapy can be discontinued. To prevent recurrent pulmonary hypertension, all of the precautions outlined previously (maintaining relative alkalosis and normal oxygenation, avoiding noxious stimuli) are important in the immediate period after ECMO. This treatment can also be used preoperatively in the moribund infant who in all likelihood would not survive repair.[11]

Prenatal ultrasound can accurately diagnose a CDH. Attempts at primary repair in utero have been accompanied by high morbidity and mortality and have been abandoned.[12] More recently, several centers have advocated tracheal ligation in utero, which "forces" growth of the hypoplastic lung by trapping respiratory secretions in the airway and expanding the alveolar spaces. These procedures are still experimental and continue to raise technical and ethical issues beyond the scope of this chapter.[13,14] In-utero procedures for CDH are not yet accepted as mainstream treatment.

ESOPHAGEAL ATRESIA AND TRACHEOESOPHAGEAL FISTULA

Esophageal atresia and tracheoesophageal fistula represent a clinical spectrum of malformations. The essential elements of their pathophysiology are the child's inability to swallow saliva or food owing to the esophageal atresia and the potential aspiration of saliva or gastric secretions through a fistula between the esophagus and trachea.

Esophageal atresia and associated tracheoesophageal fistula result from an in-utero malformation that is one of the better-characterized embryologic foregut anomalies. Separation of the foregut (dorsal) from the trachea (ventral) begins distally at the carina and progresses proximally. If these two structures fail to separate during this process, tracheoesophageal anomalies occur in the form of atresias, fistulas, or laryngotracheal clefts. Different embryonic studies have focused on the "ingrowth" of the epithelial ridge in this area, which must be uninterrupted for complete tracheoesophageal formation. For unknown reasons, this constellation of tracheal and esophageal abnormalities may be associated with other midline vertebral, anal, cardiac, and renal or peripheral limb anomalies, which are known by the acronym

VACTERL (vertebral, anal, cardiac, tracheal, esophageal, renal, limb) association.[15]

Tracheoesophageal fistula and esophageal atresia have been classified to describe anatomically the presence or absence of esophageal atresia and whether there is an associated fistula (Fig. 29-2). This has important management, as well as operative, significance.[16] The most common combination of lesions is esophageal atresia associated with a distal tracheoesophageal fistula. Over 85% of patients present with this anomaly, which results in a blind-ending upper esophageal pouch of variable length associated with a fistula between the lower trachea (or rarely the right mainstem bronchus) and the distal esophagus. The second most common anomaly, occurring in 5% of patients, is an isolated

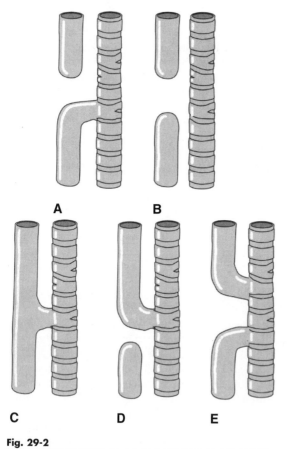

Fig. 29-2

Five anatomic classifications describing tracheoesophageal fistula and esophageal atresia. **A,** Esophageal atresia with a distal tracheoesophageal fistula. **B,** Isolated esophageal atresia with a long gap of missing esophagus between proximal and distal esophageal pouches. **C,** Tracheoesophageal fistula without esophageal atresia, "H-type." **D,** Esophageal atresia with proximal fistula. **E,** Esophageal atresia with both proximal and distal tracheoesophageal fistulas.

esophageal atresia with a proximal blind-ending pouch and a long gap of missing esophagus, with a very small distal esophageal pouch. In 3% of patients, esophageal atresia may be associated with both a proximal and a distal tracheoesophageal fistula. The H-type fistula is an isolated tracheoesophageal fistula without atresia that usually occurs in the lower cervical or upper thoracic area. Finally, 1% of patients have an esophageal atresia with a proximal fistula, a long gap, and a small blind distal esophageal pouch.

Excessive salivation with drooling is the first symptom in the majority of newborns with esophageal atresia. The infant is unable to handle its own saliva, and the first feedings result in choking, coughing, and episodes of cyanosis. The respiratory distress may be severe and progressive, which should prompt an immediate workup for esophageal atresia. If esophageal atresia is suspected, a nasogastric 10 F Replogle tube is introduced until resistance is met. The tube is connected to constant suction and irrigated with 1 to 2 ml of air at frequent intervals. A chest radiograph showing the tube coiled in the upper pouch is diagnostic.

Esophageal atresia with tracheoesophageal fistula occurs in 1 in 3000 births with an equal male and female distribution. Because of the obstruction to swallowing amniotic fluid during fetal life, polyhydramnios may be present prenatally.[17] The postnatal presentation of each type of anomaly varies with the lesion and the consequences of obstruction or aspiration. Tracheoesophageal fistula without atresia (H-type) may present as late as early adulthood with subtle symptoms of wheezing and recurrent respiratory infections. Infants with larger fistulas may have frequent choking and coughing episodes. Significant abdominal distention caused by excessive air passing from the respiratory tract directly to the gastrointestinal tract through a patent fistula may also be a presenting symptom. Auscultation of the chest may reveal a murmur from concomitant congenital heart disease or decreased breath sounds caused by atelectasis or pneumonitis. The physical examination must include a careful search for other components of the VACTERL association, such as imperforate anus or limb abnormalities, before surgical correction is undertaken.[18]

Chest and abdominal radiographs are critical to the diagnosis, as illustrated in Fig. 29-3. Several important radiographic findings are specific for esophageal atresia. The course of the Replogle tube, coiled or ending in the cervical esophagus, confirms obstruction of the proximal esophagus (atresia) and suggests the relative position of the upper esophageal pouch. The lung fields must be examined to determine the presence of parenchymal changes

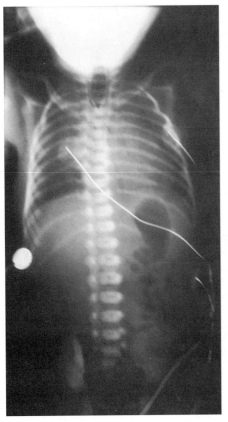

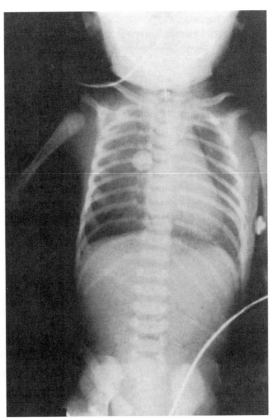

A

C

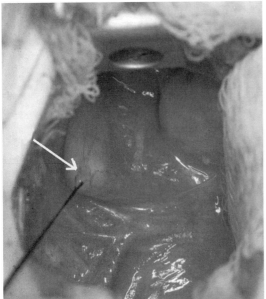

Fig. 29-3

A, Chest and abdominal radiograph of a newborn with esophageal atresia and a distal tracheoesophageal fistula. Note the Replogle tube in the proximal esophagus and gas in the intestinal loops, indicating the presence of a fistula. **B,** Intraoperative photograph of tracheoesophageal fistula/esophageal atresia repair. Note blind proximal esophageal pouch *(arrow)*. **C,** Chest and abdominal radiograph of a newborn with isolated esophageal atresia. Despite the fairly long upper pouch, a long gap of esophagus is missing. The lack of abdominal gas indicates that no fistula is present. (**B** courtesy Roberta E. Sonnino, MD.)

B

resulting from aspiration. The configuration of the mediastinal structures may give an early indication of congenital heart disease, and a careful search must be made for the aortic arch to determine its left-or right-sided position. This is extremely important for surgical management because it directs the surgeon to a thoracotomy on the side away from the aortic arch. The next most important finding is the presence or absence of a gastric bubble. A proximal esophageal atresia with air in the gastrointestinal tract indicates the presence of a distal tracheoesophageal fistula, the most common form of the anomaly. Injecting 5 to 10 ml of air through the Replogle tube will clearly outline the blind pouch. Never use other contrast media due to the possibility of it being aspirated. A proximal obstruction without evidence of gas distally suggests an isolated esophageal atresia without fistula. Other studies that aid in the diagnosis of related congenital anomalies include an echocardiogram, renal ultrasonography, and vertebral spine films.

Once the diagnosis is made, the overall clinical condition of the infant dictates the timing of repair. For patients who present with severe respiratory distress and low birth weight, mechanical ventilation is essential.[19] It may be necessary to perform an emergency procedure to place a gastrostomy tube and divide the distal tracheoesophageal fistula if delivered tidal volume is compromised by losses through the fistula and respiratory failure progresses. This approach commits the infant to a second operative procedure to repair the esophageal atresia at a later date. Operative maneuvers to place balloon catheters in the fistula or staple the distal esophagus may be employed for emergency, life-threatening situations. The preferred elective approach is through a right thoracotomy with extrapleural dissection for division and closure of the fistula and primary anastomosis of the esophagus.

The most significant complications of a primary repair are leaks from the esophageal anastomosis, strictures, or recurrent fistula formation. These complications have important implications for postoperative respiratory care. Even infants with successful anastomoses often have persistent respiratory problems. Premature postoperative extubation is to be avoided because reintubation could cause direct injury to either the esophageal anastomosis or the fistula repair. With or without complications, postoperative respiratory symptoms have been noted in up to 50% of patients. Complications range from apnea and bradycardia to aspiration, recurrent pneumonia, and even respiratory arrest.[20] The largest single cause of persistent respiratory disease is gastroesophageal reflux from either esophageal dysmotility or an abnormal lower esophageal sphincter. Infants with reflux have recurrent aspiration pneumonias that must be treated medically; however, many of these infants require further operative management with a gastroesophageal fundoplication.

The majority of infants with esophageal atresia, with or without tracheoesophageal fistula, have variable degrees of persistent tracheomalacia.[21] This may be a difficult group of patients to manage. In some infants, even the slightest esophageal anastomotic stricture may affect the respiratory status with compression of the trachea by a distended pre-stricture esophagus during feedings. Dilatation of the stricture may alleviate much of the respiratory compromise. In selected cases, an aortopexy may be necessary. By suspending the aorta from the sternum, the trachea is no longer compressed between the esophagus and the pulsating aorta. Recurrent fistulas or an undiscovered proximal fistula may be the cause of persistent wheezing and respiratory difficulty. These fistulas can be diagnosed and defined by bronchoscopy or a contrast esophagogram with direct pressure injection at different levels of the esophagus.

With precise preoperative, perioperative, and postoperative management, the survival rate in infants with esophageal atresia is now greater than 95%. The respiratory care during each phase must be tailored with an understanding of the pathophysiology of each malformation and its related complications.

OMPHALOCELE AND GASTROSCHISIS

Three distinct embryonic folds—cephalic, caudal, and lateral—composed of somatic and splanchnic tissues eventually become the body walls and gastrointestinal tract. Failure in the development of these structures in the fetus results in the persistence of an extracoelomic cavity and a defect in the abdominal or chest wall. A classic omphalocele represents a failure of the normal fusion of the lateral embryonic folds, with a resultant midline defect at the umbilical opening (Fig. 29-4). Abdominal viscera protrude through this defect within the umbilical cord, covered by amnion and peritoneum. Omphaloceles are commonly accompanied by other anomalies of the sternum, heart, diaphragm, hindgut, and bladder as a result of splanchnic layer deficiencies in these same folds.[22]

A gastroschisis is a full-thickness defect of the abdominal wall, lateral and almost always to the right of the umbilicus. The protruding small intestine is not covered by a sac (Fig. 29-5). The definitive embryologic explanation for gastroschisis remains controversial. Proposed explanations include developmental arrest or injury to the mesenchymal elements responsible for forming the abdominal wall,

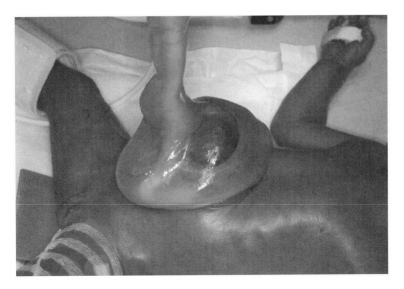

Fig. 29-4

Classic omphalocele with defect in the umbilical ring and protrusion of intraabdominal viscera within the cord. The viscera remain covered by a sac. (Photograph courtesy Roberta E. Sonnino, MD.)

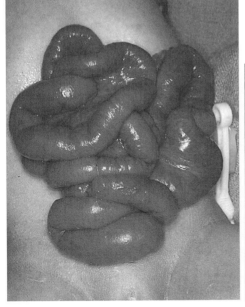

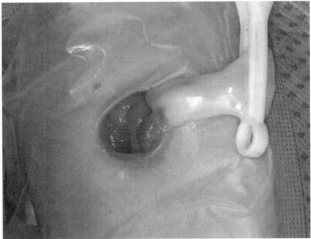

A **B**

Fig. 29-5

Gastroschisis. **A,** Note the bowel exposed with no covering sac. **B,** Bowel has been reduced into the abdomen. The lesion is to the right of the umbilicus. (Photographs courtesy Roberta E. Sonnino, MD.)

resulting in injury and involution of the right umbilical vein. This may explain the right-sided predominance of this lesion.[23] Another theory suggests that gastroschisis is an in-utero rupture of a minor omphalocele.[24]

The diagnosis of gastroschisis or omphalocele is usually established by prenatal ultrasonography. Elevations of maternal serum α-fetoprotein are seen in gastroschisis and omphalocele and may be a useful screening tool for the detection of these lesions early during pregnancy.[25] There is early evidence that biochemical mediators of ischemia may be detectable in the amniotic fluid as well.[26] No important differential diagnosis exists for either lesion, and inspection alone is generally sufficient to secure the diagnosis. Gastroschisis is usually an isolated lesion, whereas omphalocele is associated with other significant anomalies in approximately 50% of cases. The combined incidence of the two lesions is approximately 1 in 4000 live births[27] but appears to be on the rise.

Radiographic evaluation is generally useful only to search for associated anomalies in infants with omphalocele. One in three patients with omphalocele will have a chromosomal abnormality such as trisomy 13, 18, or 21. Omphalocele in association with macroglossia suggests Beckwith-Wiedemann syndrome, whereas cryptorchism and an abnormal lateral abdominal wall suggest the prune-belly syndrome. In addition, both lesions are consistently accompanied by rotational abnormalities of the intestine. Twenty percent of patients with omphalocele have congenital heart disease. Tetralogy of Fallot is the most common congenital cardiac lesion seen in these patients.[28]

Repair of the fascial defect in the abdominal wall and skin closure are the main aspects of surgical management of these lesions. Primary closure is preferred if technically feasible.[29] The major obstacle to successful primary repair is the diminished size of the peritoneal cavity secondary to the absence of intraabdominal viscera during growth of the abdominal cavity, with resultant loss of domain. Pulmonary complications may result from placing the viscera back into the abdominal cavity with consequent increased pressure on the diaphragm. Reducing the viscera too quickly may result in restrictive pulmonary insufficiency as well as ischemic injury to the viscera themselves. Several authors have defined pressure parameters for successful closure of abdominal wall defects.[30] Measuring intragastric, central venous, and intravesical pressures has been proposed in managing the successful closure of these defects.[31] Hypertension in any of these variables correlates with elevated intraperitoneal pressure, decreased renal perfusion, and significant restrictive respiratory insufficiency. In these cases, a staged reduction using a prosthetic silo (or the sac itself used as a silo in an intact omphalocele) may be necessary.[32-34] Sequential silo ligation gradually reduces the viscera into the abdominal cavity. The protruding viscera are wrapped and shielded to maintain moisture and prevent infection. The silo is suspended from a support hanging over the abdomen.

Respiratory and cardiovascular complications in patients undergoing tension-free primary repair are uncommon. The mortality seen in this group is generally related to the associated congenital anomalies and not to the abdominal wall defect or complications of its surgical repair.[35,36] Patients with larger defects requiring staged procedures have added mortality related to infectious complications.

LUNG BUD ANOMALIES

The term *lung bud anomaly* broadly describes four pathologic entities in a spectrum of parenchymal disease: bronchogenic cyst, congenital cystic adenomatoid malformation, pulmonary sequestration, and congenital lobar emphysema. The pathogenesis of these anomalies is poorly understood, but some speculation can be made based on known embryologic sequences.[37,38] In early fetal development a tube of endodermal epithelium, the cellular covering of all body cavities, is present along the entire longitudinal axis of the fetus. This tube, the primordial gastrointestinal tract, is referred to as the primitive foregut. At approximately 3 weeks of gestation, a small groove appears in the floor of the primitive foregut, near the oral end of the fetus (Fig. 29-6). The groove develops into a ridge, and the ridge branches into two blind pouches at its distal end. This ridge eventually develops into the trachea, and the thickenings are referred to as lung buds; the entire ridge with the lung buds will eventually migrate away from the main epithelial tube, thus separating the early pulmonary system from the esophagus.

As these endodermal structures develop, their blood supply is formed from primitive tributaries to the aorta—the fourth and sixth aortic arches. The lung derives its blood supply from two distinct sources: (1) the pulmonary artery (sixth arch), which brings oxygen-poor blood from systemic veins for oxygenation, and (2) the bronchial arteries (direct branches of the arch), which bring oxygen-rich blood to the parenchyma of the lung for nutritive purposes.

The budding part of the tube is composed of endoderm, a multipotential tissue in the embryo that forms the "business end" of each organ (e.g., the alveoli of the lungs, the mucosa of the gastrointestinal tract, the nephron of the kidney). The lung buds grow into the mesoderm, which is also a multipotential tissue that forms, in each organ, the connective tissue and the important supporting framework, including the blood vessels.

The interaction between these tissues is important in the development of each organ. In the primitive pulmonary system, the bud-forming endoderm induces important changes in the surrounding mesoderm that lead to a cohesive, functioning organ. Knowledge of these processes may help to

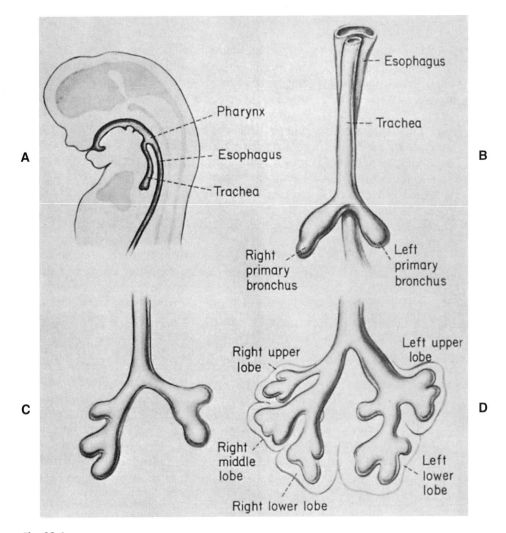

Fig. 29-6

Developmental anatomy of the lung. The pulmonary tree develops from a common tube with the esophagus **(A).** By 3 weeks of gestation, the trachea (anterior) is separate from the esophagus. Two blind pouches that represent the left and right lung buds have appeared at the distal end of the primitive pulmonary system **(B).** Further dichotomous branching of the main bronchi results in the main lobes of each lung **(C and D).** (From Doty DB: Thoracic surgery in infants. In Sabiston DC, Spencer FC, editors: *Gibbon's surgery of the chest,* ed 4. Philadelphia. WB Saunders, 1983.)

explain how each anomaly occurs. For example, if both lung buds fail to form, the fetus would have bilateral pulmonary agenesis, which is incompatible with life; however, unilateral pulmonary agenesis is survivable. If the longitudinal groove with its attached buds fails to completely separate from the epithelial tube, a laryngoesophageal cleft or tracheoesophageal fistula may result. Although the exact nature of the developmental cause behind each anomaly is unclear, I will speculate as to the embryologic defect underlying the four lesions that

compose lung bud anomalies as each anomaly is discussed.

INCIDENCE

As a group, these entities are considered uncommon but not rare. Many factors make a precise assessment of the incidence extremely difficult. Some cystic pulmonary disease may result from barotrauma, not representing a congenital origin. Asymptomatic patients may be uncounted because sequestrations may be silent for many years and become evident only during clinical investigation for unrelated complaints. Congenital lobar emphysema has been thought to resolve spontaneously, which may result in an underestimate of its true incidence.

CLINICAL CORRELATION

Although these lung bud anomalies have very different histopathology, there are patterns in clinical presentation common to all. The presentation seems to follow two distinct patterns: (1) the condition becomes obvious in the early newborn period and is manifested by respiratory distress and (2) the condition occurs later in childhood and is characterized by repeated infections.

Newborns may be identified in the delivery room if the lesion is so large that immediate respiratory distress and circulatory compromise result. A cyst or emphysematous lobe can obstruct blood flow to the right side of the heart, causing edema that results in a "hydropic" appearance.

In many cases, the distress is not readily apparent but is characterized by a progressive course of intermittent tachypnea over the first few days or weeks. It is during this period that a chest radiograph may be taken and the diagnosis suggested, based on location and character of the lesion. In lobar emphysema, there is a hyperlucent lobe with a surrounding zone of atelectasis. The atelectasis may be interpreted as pneumonia, and the hyperlucent abnormal lung is accordingly misinterpreted as normal compensatory hyperinflation. Intubation and hyperventilation in this situation could be disastrous: the emphysematous lobe will expand preferentially according to the law of Laplace. As this lobe enlarges and pressure in the chest rises from the expanding mass, blood return to the thoracic cavity is impaired. As the infant's condition worsens, the clinician may mistake the emphysematous lobe for a pneumothorax because of its similar clinical behavior—a shift of the mediastinum to the opposite side and hyperresonance on the affected side. A chest tube inserted into this lobe may considerably worsen the situation.

An important aspect of the differential diagnosis includes a consideration that a "multilocular cyst" may actually be air-filled loops of bowel from a CDH. Auscultation for bowel sounds may help to differentiate these two problems, as will decompression of the bowel loops with a nasogastric tube: pulmonary cysts will not decompress. In some cases, an upper gastrointestinal series may be necessary to differentiate these conditions.

Presentation in the newborn is due to a mass effect in the small thoracic space. Bronchogenic cysts and cystic adenomatoid malformations do not have direct communications with the bronchial tree, but air can still enter these cysts through the pores of Kohn. Some cysts contain tissue so immature that they lack these pores, and air entry is not possible. These lesions, lacking a way for air to enter, are not likely to expand abruptly in the newborn period. Cysts with pores or emphysematous lobes, however, will enlarge with ventilation and can present under tension. Should a cyst rupture, the lesion may present mimicking a pneumothorax. This is rare and less frequent than a pneumothorax caused by insertion of a chest tube into an intact cyst. As a cyst or lobe progressively enlarges, it may directly compress the trachea, a major bronchus, or the vena cava. Even without direct compression of these structures, the pressure rise within the thorax can cause mediastinal deviation with its attendant consequences of decreased venous return. Presentation in the newborn period with tension may require emergency thoracotomy and resection.

After infancy, the most common presentation is with repeated or prolonged episodes of pneumonia despite adequate antibiotic coverage. The infectious course arises because the contents of the cyst do not communicate with the tracheobronchial tree, allowing bacteria and debris to accumulate in the cyst. This material cannot be cleared and acts as a nidus for infection, which often spreads to adjacent healthy tissue and lymph nodes in the hilum of the involved lung. Thus, a small infected cyst can result in pneumonia with fever and purulent cough. Although antibiotics are helpful, they are not curative and the underlying cause, that is, the cyst, must be resected to prevent recurrence of pulmonary infections.

The indolent course of this process may result in these children undergoing extensive diagnostic evaluation before reaching the correct diagnosis. There are usually numerous radiographs that, in retrospect, implicate a particular lobe. An ultrasound may have been obtained to evaluate cystic-appearing structures. Computed tomography or magnetic resonance imaging may have been used to elucidate airway anatomy and tissue density in the hope of securing a cause for frequent pneumonias. A child may have also undergone bronchoscopy to rule out aspiration of a foreign body. Bronchoscopy, however, has a limited role in the patient in whom a lung bud anomaly has already been diagnosed and could be dangerous if it causes complete obstruction of a lobe that previously was only partially obstructed. The diagnosis should be suspected when a febrile, septic child has a tube thoracostomy performed for drainage of a postpneumonic empyema and the cavity occupied by the now-drained fluid does not collapse: an infected cyst, rather than an empyema, is the likely diagnosis.

Serial chest radiographs are the most valuable source of information in reaching the diagnosis.

Resection of the infected cyst is curative. Preoperative treatment with antibiotics is important. In patients with severe sepsis, initial simple drainage of the cavity may be required for temporary palliation, allowing time for optimal preparation of the patient before definitive surgery.

BRONCHOGENIC CYST

The bronchogenic cyst may be thought of as a lung bud cyst, with endoderm that differentiates into respiratory epithelium but without normal bronchial components. It is therefore nonfunctional. These cysts can be located either within the thoracic cavity or outside it. When intrathoracic, the cyst can be in the bronchial wall, the pleura, the mediastinum, or the parenchyma of the lung itself. Ten percent of mediastinal masses are bronchogenic cysts. They are commonly located in the retrocarinal region (Fig. 29-7, *A*). When intrapulmonary, they are usually on the right and may be multiple or multilocular (Fig. 29-7, *B*).

The diagnosis of a bronchogenic cyst may be apparent radiologically in the newborn with respiratory distress where the radiograph reveals a circular or ovoid mass with smooth edges. Similarly, the radiograph can suggest the diagnosis in an older child who presents with stridor, wheezing, or recurrent pneumonia.

Treatment of bronchogenic cysts is surgical excision. The extent of resection will depend on the location of the cyst and any associated inflammatory conditions. A unilocular cyst can usually be enucleated or removed by wedge resection. Lobectomy is performed in the exceptional case. A pneumonectomy is rarely needed.[39]

CONGENITAL CYSTIC ADENOMATOID MALFORMATION

Congenital cystic adenomatoid malformation (CCAM), originally described in 1949,[39] has been recognized more frequently in recent years. In this lesion, differentiation of mesenchymal tissue appears to stop at the bronchial stage, before cartilage develops. The lesion is a hamartoma, that is, a disorganized overgrowth of embryonal tissue. This lesion reflects a failure of the inductive process, discussed earlier.

The morphologic appearance of this lesion (Fig. 29-8) may be of a single large cavitary cyst (type I), multiple small cysts (type II), or a solid mass (type III). The CCAM may be multilobular and bilateral, but it is most commonly located in the left lung. The clinical presentation and radiographic diagnosis are similar to those of a bronchogenic cyst. The surgical treatment usually requires a lobectomy and occasionally a pneumonectomy. Unlike a bronchogenic cyst, this lesion cannot usually be enucleated. Unless there is unusually extensive or bilateral disease, the postoperative course is smooth and the prognosis is excellent. Larger lesions, however, may be associated with pulmonary hypoplasia, hypertension, hydrops fetalis, and myocardiopathy. These features, depending on their magnitude, are associated with a severe prognosis.

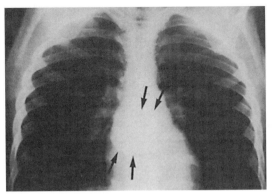
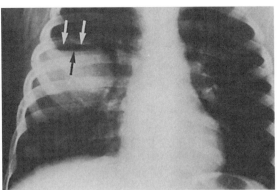

A   B

Fig. 29-7

Bronchogenic cysts. **A,** Note the smooth border of the round, retrocarinal mass on this radiograph *(arrows).* **B,** Chest radiograph demonstrates an intraparenchymal mass that has become infected. Note the air-fluid level *(arrows).* This cyst is located on the right, which is typical of intraparenchymal bronchogenic cysts.

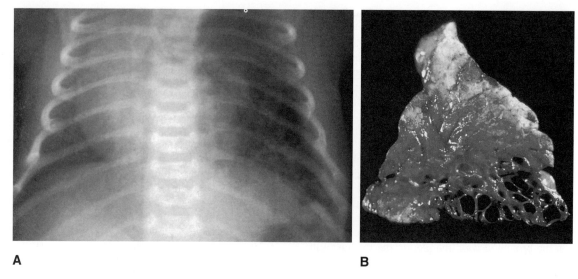

A   **B**

Fig. 29-8

Cystic adenomatoid malformation. **A,** Chest radiograph demonstrating the type I left lower lobe lesion. **B,** Gross appearance of lesion after resection. (Photograph courtesy Roberta E. Sonnino, MD.)

PULMONARY SEQUESTRATION

Sequestrations are foci of mature lung tissue separate from the rest of the tracheobronchial tree, with concomitant failure of separation of the pulmonary and systemic circulations. The tissue may be either nonaerated or aerated through collateral channels (i.e., pores of Kohn), albeit with poor gas exchange. The sequestration typically has a systemic arterial blood supply (Fig. 29-9). The venous drainage is usually into the pulmonary veins in intrapulmonary sequestrations and into systemic veins (azygos or hemiazygos vein, inferior vena cava, or right atrium) in extrapulmonary sequestrations. The extrapulmonary variety has a separate pleural envelope and may lie below the diaphragm. The defect in development may be caused by migration of an accessory lung bud before separation of the systemic and pulmonary circulations. Sequestrations are most commonly located in the left lower lobe region.

The patient with a sequestration may present with a variety of clinical symptoms, including a large shunt, a heart murmur, and heart failure.[40] A large, nonfunctional intrathoracic mass can present as obstructive respiratory signs such as wheezing and tachypnea. A common presentation is a recurrent febrile course with an occult infected sequestration.

The diagnosis of pulmonary sequestration can be elusive. A space-occupying lesion with or without an air-fluid level is often seen on a plain chest radiograph.[41] If a sequestration is suspected, an arteriogram can be diagnostic and helpful to define the arterial anatomy, which is crucial to successful resection. The systemic arterial supply may arise directly from the aorta, at times even through the diaphragm from the intraabdominal aorta. Injury or inadvertent division of this vessel without proper control may result in a hemorrhagic catastrophe. An upper gastrointestinal contrast study may reveal a fistulous connection to the intestinal tract. Radionuclide lung scanning may reveal an unventilated but perfused mass in the chest. Finally, computed tomography can demonstrate extrathoracic lesions, and magnetic resonance imaging can visualize any abnormal blood supply. Resection of the mass is curative.

CONGENITAL LOBAR EMPHYSEMA

Congenital lobar emphysema is an overdistention of one lobe of the lung, usually one of the upper lobes.[42] The lobe becomes distended because air enters but cannot exit, often owing to obstruction of a segmental or lobar bronchus. Alternatively, there may be a defect in the cartilage so that increases in parenchymal pressure during expiration cause the bronchus to collapse.[43] This results in airway obstruction and air trapping. Additionally, an aberrant artery or vascular ring may compress the bronchus during expiration. Regardless of the cause, the lobe becomes progressively more distended, eventually causing obstruction to air entry at the main bronchus or trachea and obstruction of venous return to the right atrium. These two conditions, separately or together, may constitute a surgical emergency.

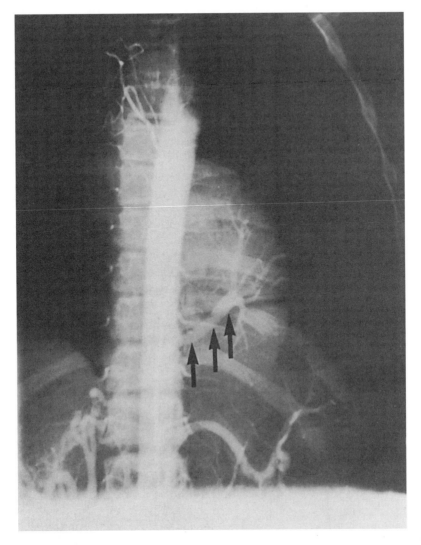

Fig. 29-9

Sequestration. This aortic angiogram shows the segment of lung above the diaphragm that is supplied by a vessel from below the diaphragm *(arrows)*. The splenic and hepatic branches of the celiac axis are seen below.

The radiographic appearance may be confusing. Normal lung in proximity to the diseased lung tissue may be collapsed and appear atelectatic or consolidated (Fig. 29-10). Thus, the child with respiratory distress and such a radiograph may be thought to have pneumonia, with the real diagnosis unsuspected. Recognition of this lesion is critical early in the symptomatic course because of the general tendency to hyperventilate a child in respiratory distress. In the case of lobar emphysema, such a maneuver would hasten circulatory collapse by rapidly overdistending the affected lobe. Without a confirmatory radiograph, a chest tube may be inadvertently inserted into the emphysematous lobe

with disastrous consequences. Resection of the lobe is curative.

FOLLOW-UP OF PATIENTS WITH LUNG BUD ANOMALIES

Children tolerate thoracotomies remarkably well. Postoperatively, the patient will have a chest tube that is usually removed within a few days of the operation. Analgesics are important so that the child will breathe deeply and open atelectatic areas. For children too young to understand the use of incentive spirometry, the deep breath required before blowing soap bubbles or spinning a windmill will achieve the same effect. Patient-controlled

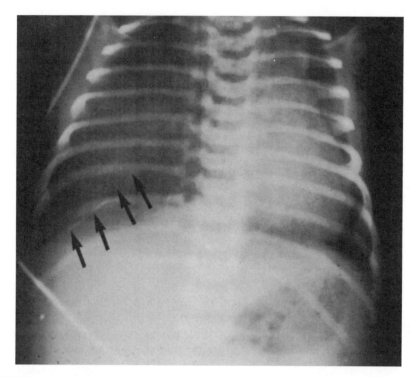

Fig. 29-10

Congenital lobar emphysema. The hyperexpanded right upper lobe pushes the fissure inferiorly, compressing the normal right lower lobe *(arrows)*. The mediastinum is shifted to the left, compressing the normal left lung.

anesthesia in the older child, intrapleural or epidural anesthesia, intercostal blocks, and intravenous morphine are all important postoperative pain control strategies. Adequate analgesia also permits chest physical therapy, which is crucial in the recovery process.[44] Recovery is usually rapid, and normal growth is to be expected. When the child has an isolated lung bud anomaly, the prognosis is excellent. For bilateral or extensive disease, or when there are associated cardiac or genetic anomalies, the prognosis may be worse and is related mostly to the degree of parenchymal involvement or the associated anomaly.

MANDIBULAR HYPOPLASIA

Mandibular hypoplasia, or micrognathia, is generally found in conjunction with various other anomalies in conditions such as Pierre Robin or Treacher Collins syndrome. Pierre Robin syndrome is the most common of these associations, but the pathophysiology of respiratory distress associated with micrognathia is identical in the other disorders.

The primary features of Pierre Robin syndrome include micrognathia, glossoptosis or posterior dis-placement of the tongue, and cleft palate.[45] These features result in pharyngeal obstruction and respiratory distress. If left untreated, infants with respiratory complications such as airway obstruction, cor pulmonale, and pulmonary hypertension have a mortality rate approaching 30%. Other complications of Pierre Robin syndrome are failure to thrive, malnutrition, chronic hypoxia, and pneumonia. Polysomnographic studies using oximetry have demonstrated that hypoxia and carbon dioxide retention can occur without overt signs of airway obstruction.[46] Close monitoring and a complete evaluation must be performed before therapy has been instituted and for some time thereafter.

Treatment for patients with micrognathia includes positioning, insertion of an intraoral or nasopharyngeal airway, and surgical procedures. Prone positioning combined with supplemental oxygen administration and carefully supervised feedings has been useful in treating mild forms of micrognathia. Intraoral and nasopharyngeal tubes or prostheses have been used in treating mild to moderate forms of micrognathia, but feeding difficulties limit the usefulness of these techniques. Surgical procedures designed to hold the tongue forward have been advocated for symptomatic and severe forms of the disorder. These procedures include suture transfixion, creation of lip-tongue adhesion with sutures, and various sling procedures. The most severe cases may require tracheostomy. All of these treatments are designed to "buy time" because these disorders gradually improve with facial growth.

MACROGLOSSIA

Macroglossia, or a greatly enlarged tongue, causes respiratory distress by direct pharyngeal obstruction. Macroglossia can be associated with other disorders such as Beckwith-Wiedemann and Down syndromes, or it may be the result of congenital lymphangioma or hemangioma. The diagnosis is relatively straightforward, and polysomnography and pulse oximetry are used to evaluate the extent to which macroglossia affects respiratory function.

Treatment of macroglossia should be individualized, depending on the severity of respiratory obstruction. For isolated macroglossia, prone positioning usually relieves mild cases, whereas more severe cases may require surgical reduction of tongue size. Lymphangiomas and small hemangiomas of the tongue may require excision, and large congenital hemangiomas frequently respond to systemic corticosteroid or interferon therapy. Chronic hypoxia and carbon dioxide retention are frequent sequelae of macroglossia and require close follow-up.

CHOANAL ATRESIA

Most newborns are obligate nose breathers. The presence of complete nasal obstruction by choanal atresia therefore results in immediate respiratory distress and possible death by asphyxia. During the newborn's first breaths, the tongue comes in direct contact with the hard and soft palates, creating a vacuum. An oral airway should be inserted and maintained to relieve the airway obstruction. Mouth breathing is a learned response that develops within 1 to 6 weeks after birth.

The exact embryologic malformation is unknown; some theories implicate abnormalities in the direction of mesodermal flow to reach preordained positions in the facial process. Any abnormalities in this flow would affect the normal penetration of the nasal pits and the thinning that allows breakthrough at the anterior choana.[47]

Choanal atresia occurs in approximately 1 in 700 live births, with females affected at a ratio of 2:1 over males. Unilateral choanal atresia is twice as common as bilateral choanal atresia. The majority of these atresias are caused by bony obstruction or obliteration of the nasal apertures at either the anterior or posterior nasal choana. Fifty percent of patients with choanal atresia have associated congenital anomalies that are either craniofacial or a cluster of defects known by the acronym CHARGE (colobomas, congenital heart defects, choanal atresia, retarded development, genital hyperplasia, and ear anomalies). Choanal atresia may frequently be associated with isolated congenital heart defects.

The clinical presentation of choanal atresia may be severe, with immediate respiratory distress that requires intubation or an oral airway. Unilateral atresia may not cause acute respiratory distress and may present as unilateral mucoid discharge. Alternatively, bilateral atresia or a secondarily obstructed unilateral atresia may present as cyanosis cycling with momentary relief from obstruction. The neonate struggles to breathe normally and creates a vacuum between the tongue and the palate, resulting in obstruction and cyanosis. At the point of complete obstruction there is a cry of distress and the mouth opens, relieving the symptoms.

A 6 French catheter is the best diagnostic tool for choanal atresia in the newborn intensive care unit. If the catheter fails to pass through the nose into the oropharynx, choanal atresia should be suspected. The neonate is stabilized by immediately inserting an oral airway. Secondary anomalies should be sought, and facial computed tomography with coronal projections, and possibly endoscopy, should be performed to delineate the anomaly. The ultimate management is surgical correction. However, appropriate respiratory care must be provided preoperatively to ensure that the oral or orotracheal airway is maintained until the infant can be brought to the operating room.

The surgical procedure involves perforation of the atresia to establish and maintain adequate choanae. The timing and surgical approach are dependent on other medical problems; infants weighing more than 1.5 kg may be operated on by either the transpalatal or the transnasal route. There are risks and benefits with each procedure; however, the direct visualization afforded by the transpalatal route is preferred by many surgeons.[48] Once the repair is performed, a standard folded endotracheal tube is used to stent the choanae in a U-shaped configuration. A 4-mm tube is usually selected for a full-term neonate, and a 3.5-mm tube is used for a premature infant.[49] A suction catheter is measured so that it passes through the end of the stent into the nasopharynx. The catheter is passed through each side of the stent to prevent obstruction. The stent is mobilized every 4 hours to reduce the risk of stenosis and delay or minimize granulation tissue formation. Prophylactic antibiotics are given, and the stent is usually removed with the patient under general anesthesia. Continuing respiratory problems caused by nasal congestion may be expected for 3 to 4 weeks postoperatively.

The prognosis after reconstruction is excellent and generally without complication; the most significant complication is restenosis of the choanae. This is managed by repeated dilatations of the choanae under endoscopic visualization with replacement of the stent. Rarely, tracheostomy or long-term intubation may be required when choanal atresia is complicated by reconstructive maneuvers for other craniofacial abnormalities.

NECROTIZING ENTEROCOLITIS

Necrotizing enterocolitis (NEC) of the newborn remains a common but poorly understood illness. The incidence has been estimated at 2.4 cases in 1000 live births but varies significantly by location and over time. These infants represented 2.1% of all admissions to neonatal intensive care units in one large study.[50] NEC mainly affects premature infants and those who are small for gestational age.

Intestinal ischemia is the pathologic end point of NEC. Animal models have identified platelet-activating factor, lipopolysaccharide, and tumor necrosis factor as likely mediators of intestinal ischemia and NEC.[51,52] Platelet-activating factor, intestinal fatty acid binding protein, and tumor necrosis factor have also been identified in the serum of infants with NEC.[53,54] Secretory phospholipase A_2 is speculated to be a common inciting pathway for the release of all these mediators.[55] If confirmed, its early detection and inhibition could lead to prevention or treatment of the ischemic consequences of NEC. The risk factors implicated in the development of NEC are descriptive of the newborn population at risk rather than being specific for NEC.

Infants generally present with abdominal distention, ileus, and bloody stools, usually associated with dilated loops of bowel. Physical findings on examination of the abdomen, including abdominal wall erythema and mass effect, depend on the presence or absence of peritoneal irritation or perforation. The diagnosis of NEC is established radiographically.[56] The classic finding is of distended loops of bowel with areas of intramural gas. The presence of pneumatosis intestinalis in this clinical setting is pathognomonic for NEC. Portal venous gas[57] and ascites may also be present. Pneumoperitoneum is diagnostic of a perforation. Metabolic acidosis may be present along with less specific laboratory findings such as leukocytosis or, more commonly, leukopenia and thrombocytopenia. The combination of metabolic acidosis and abdominal distention may result in respiratory insufficiency and usually requires intubation and mechanical ventilation. The respiratory status may be further compromised by injury mediated by neutrophils activated by the cytokines released by the ischemic bowel.[58]

The majority of NEC cases can be managed nonoperatively with intravenous fluid resuscitation, broad-spectrum antibiotics, and nasogastric decompression. Twenty percent of these patients will require surgical intervention as the NEC progresses to full-thickness necrosis with gangrene or perforation. Placement of drains in very low–birth-weight premature infants[59] or conservative resection with construction of an intestinal stoma and evacuation of the peritoneal fluid in larger infants generally diminishes the restrictive component of respiratory insufficiency.[60] Resection of gangrenous tissue allows correction of the acid-base balance. Because the disease may be progressive, second-look explorations after 24 to 48 hours with further bowel resection may be indicated. These infants usually have a history of respiratory distress syndrome before or coincidental with the development of NEC. This may result in prolonged intubation and difficulty weaning from mechanical ventilation postoperatively.[61] The reported survival is now in the range of 60% to 70%, with long-term outcome depending almost entirely on the presence or absence of other serious organic disease and on the magnitude of the intestinal resection required for cure and survival.

CHEST WALL MALFORMATIONS

The pathogenesis of chest wall malformations involves both lung growth and lung function. The most striking example affecting lung growth is thoracic dystrophy. In this entity, the chest wall has not developed sufficiently to permit adequate lung growth, and infants born with this anomaly usually die within hours of birth.

Less striking are mild degrees of sternal or rib cage deformity, which may include congenitally missing ribs, deformed ribs, lack of chest wall muscles, and sternal clefts. In these cases, pulmonary function is usually sufficient to allow normal growth and development without symptoms. Increasingly severe deformities may produce no symptoms at rest but may cause a reduced capacity for exercise, especially with paradoxical chest wall movement. Some children avoid exercise entirely and thus report no symptoms. In these children, repair of the deformity can result in increased activity. In severe deformities, dyspnea at rest may be present.

Pulmonary complaints are not the only potential problems with chest wall malformations. If the deformity displaces the heart significantly, cardiac filling may be altered by ventricular compression or distorted relationships to the great vessels. If any intrathoracic structure impinges on the atria, arrhythmias may result. Thus the patient may present with atrial fibrillation or syncope from a severely deformed chest wall.

Lastly, one cannot ignore the cosmetic implications and impact on psychosocial development of chest wall deformities. Because progressive distortion of the chest may cause compensatory scoliosis, the child's entire posture can be affected. The distorted appearance of the chest wall and overall posture are distressing to the child and his or her parents and are often the presenting complaints.

THORACIC DYSTROPHY

Thoracic dystrophy, also known as asphyxiating thoracic dystrophy, is a rare genetic disorder with few survivors.[62] It is apparent at birth because of the obvious small chest, respiratory distress, and other associated birth defects, such as pelvic bone malformations, short extremities, and polydactyly.[63] The chest is small in the transverse and anteroposterior dimensions, which constricts the space available for lung growth throughout the fetal period. The chest wall does not expand to permit ventilation, and the lungs are structurally immature, with fewer generations of bronchioles available to participate in air exchange.[64] Thus there are decreased vital and functional capacities. Patients with thoracic dystrophy may behave like patients with CDH, but with bilateral, severe hypoplasia.

Surgical procedures designed to modify the chest wall by stenting it open to permit ventilation have met with little success. A similar picture may occur after early repair of pectus excavatum.[65] The inability to ventilate a small, stiff chest represents only the most obvious problem. The lungs, constrained throughout the fetal period, are structurally immature. Therefore restoring volume by modifying the chest wall in the postnatal period is ineffective in the short term to augment the hypoplastic lungs. Work with neonatal piglets does suggest, however, that some postnatal pulmonary growth may be affected by thoracic volume restoration.[66] In the few infants who can be ventilated and supported throughout the early course, there may be reason to attempt stenting the chest wall to increase the volume available to the lungs for postnatal growth.

PECTUS EXCAVATUM

Pectus excavatum is a common disorder without a known cause representing close to 90% of the chest wall deformities seen by the pediatrician. Although there are some familial cases, most are sporadic.[67] There is an occasional association with Marfan syndrome and congenital heart disease, but this occurs in a minority of cases. The rich surgical history in the United States largely consists of the 40-year experience of Ravitch,[68] who defined the surgical approach to this problem. More recently a minimally invasive technique has been described by Nuss.[69]

The defect is primarily caused by a deformity of the cartilaginous ends of the ribs at the costosternal junction. The affected cartilages are curved inward, causing a depression of the sternum that may secondarily become deformed as well. Patients with this deformity have an obvious depression of the chest wall ranging from a mild "dent" to a cavity that is aesthetically unappealing. The disorder is sometimes known as funnel chest; with the patient in the supine position, the more severe defects can hold water. In fact, the volume that the funnel can hold is one measure of the severity of the defect. Children often hide small toys in the depressed area.

The anteroposterior diameter of the chest is significantly decreased, and the sternum may be in close proximity to the anterior border of the vertebral column. In the most severe cases, the sternum may come to lie in the paravertebral gutter. Overall, there is decreased volume available for pulmonary expansion, especially during periods of increased demand such as exercise. Furthermore, there is altered airway flow as the bronchi are distorted. This can compromise both air exchange and clearance of secretions. Pneumonia may result from these changes. A study of Air Force basic trainees demonstrated an 850-fold increase in the incidence of pneumonia among individuals with pectus excavatum when compared with control subjects.[70]

The existence of a true associated pulmonary function deficit has been debated for many years. Many authors report no alteration in pulmonary function testing. However, these studies were often performed at rest, with the patient in the recumbent position. Under exercise conditions, with increased blood flow and air movement, mild to moderate obstructive and restrictive patterns can appear. The reduced capacity for exercise is now well accepted.[71] The variable results of laboratory evaluations are not surprising given the variable clinical presentation of patients with pectus excavatum. Some patients offer no complaints, but after repair of the defect they notice a remarkable improvement in their breathing at rest and during exercise. These patients may represent those who subconsciously limited their activity to avoid discomfort and thus remained symptom free or may have failed to recognize any limitations of their activity until after repair. Other patients, however, report reduced exercise tolerance or even shortness of breath at rest. These patients are more acceptable candidates for surgery.

Pulmonary complaints are often the dominant but not sole component of the clinical picture. As the sternum is displaced posteriorly, the heart is rotated in relation to the great vessels and is forced into the left side of the chest, sharing this space with the left lung.[72] This causes a reduction in the amount of blood able to fill the heart and may contribute to the decreased exercise tolerance experienced by these patients. The traction and kinking of the great vessels can lead to venous hypertension because blood is unable to enter the heart on the right side. The compression of the heart into the left side of the chest can irritate the atria and precipitate rhythm irregularities, such as atrial fibrillation. This can be incapacitating for some patients, especially if there are already problems with ventricular filling.

Most pectus excavatum patients are referred to the pediatric surgeon not because of arrhythmias or reduced exercise tolerance but because of the cosmetic deformity. The altered thoracic cage also causes secondary changes in the spine, with a compensatory kyphoscoliosis. The typical appearance of a patient with a long-standing pectus excavatum deformity is lanky, with shoulders rounded forward and the upper spine curved to the right (Fig. 29-11). The neck is pushed forward and there is often an abdominal protrusion secondary to the overall postural changes. There may be breast asymmetry, which is more noticeable in adolescent girls. These changes may cause embarrassment during play or when the child changes clothes in front of others, such as in gym class. The psychological impact can be as great as the physical deformity if the child becomes withdrawn and afraid of social contact.

The physical appearance of the deformity throughout the growth of a particular child may vary. Some cases are noticeable at birth. One must beware, however, of "pseudopectus excavatum." This is seen frequently in neonates, especially when they cry. The neonatal chest wall is very pliant, and the sternum may retract during vigorous breathing. This usually disappears by 6 months of age, and pectus excavatum repair before this age is not recommended in any case.[73] Other children appear normal at birth, and as they grow the deformity appears and progressively worsens. Scoliosis becomes pronounced during the pubertal growth spurt. Finally, the sternum twists to the right because the heart thrusts the left edge of the sternum upward. The right side of the chest becomes relatively depressed and may cause hypoplasia of

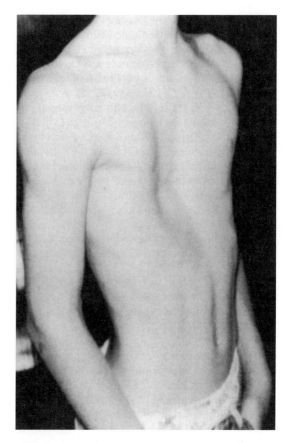

Fig. 29-11

A 15-year-old boy with pectus excavatum. Note the concave deformity and the hypoplastic right nipple. The patient is thin and has a slight, typical kyphoscoliosis.

the right breast, which becomes more noticeable in adolescence.

Indices of severity have been developed in an attempt to objectively determine indications to repair the defect. They include the funnel index, which rates deformities based on the volume of the funnel, as well as the pectus index, which relates the anteroposterior diameter to the transverse diameter. These indices are interesting and help to monitor progression of a given patient's deformity; however, they are not predictive of disability and therefore cannot guide the surgeon. The symptomatic patient, regardless of any such indices, should undergo repair; opinions differ on whether the lesion should be repaired solely for cosmetic purposes. One view is that defects severe enough to cause physiologic impairment are often cosmetically the worst; conversely, the less cosmetically severe defects probably do not impair exercise tolerance to a significant degree. Another opinion is that some of the broader, flatter defects are not as noticeable but actually represent greater pulmonary volume encroachment than do the strikingly deep but narrow lesions.

The age at which to undertake repair has also been an issue of debate. Few would advocate repair in the infant because one would obviously like to avoid unnecessary procedures such as the repair of pseudopectus conditions. Cases identified in infancy should be followed until the child is older. Waiting until puberty, however, increases the likelihood of secondary scoliosis and permanent chest wall changes. These changes, which include bony segments of ribs rather than cartilage alone requiring resection, usually result in more complex operative procedures. In addition, most of the psychological impact of the deformity occurs before puberty. Thus the time between ages 4 to 7 years appears to be optimal for repair. These children are old enough to understand parts of the hospital experience and cooperate with the postoperative care but are not yet extremely self-conscious about the defect. After the age of 7 years, the defect should be repaired if it is symptomatic or progressive. Repair in the older adolescent and young adult is more complicated and may involve major chest wall reconstruction.

Pectus repair techniques have undergone significant changes in recent years.[67-75] The traditional, "open" repair as described by Ravitch requires a large horizontal incision with subperichondrial resection of the involved cartilages. The perichondrium is left in place to allow regrowth of normal cartilage. Intercostal muscle bundles are separated from the sternum, and the sternum is brought to a more normal anterior location. Osteotomies on the sternum may be necessary to facilitate complete correction. Retrosternal struts may be used to keep the sternum in place, but complications related to the struts themselves, such as infection, are fairly common. More recently, Nuss and colleagues described a "minimally invasive" approach, in which a retrosternal bar is placed through two small lateral incisions.[69] The bar forces the sternum into a raised position, without cartilage resection or osteotomies. The bar is left in place for approximately 2 years or until the correction has stabilized. This procedure is rapidly gaining popularity, although the long-term results and full extent of potential complications are not yet known.[74,75]

Complications of both forms of repair may include infection, dislodged strut or bar resulting in lung and heart injury, cardiac tamponade, and pneumothorax. If unrecognized, these complications may be fatal. In general, however, the results are excellent, with rapid recovery. Most children breathe more easily postoperatively. Contact sports should be limited for several months. The condition can recur, especially in patients with Marfan syndrome. In this condition, a biochemically abnormal cartilage may continue to grow improperly despite surgical correction.

PECTUS CARINATUM AND OTHER STERNAL DISORDERS

Pectus carinatum is essentially the opposite of pectus excavatum. Also known as pigeon breast, patients with pectus carinatum have a significant protrusion of the sternum. The physiologic defects are much less pronounced, and this is most often a cosmetic problem rather than one of heart and lung compression. Repair is similar to the Ravitch approach for pectus excavatum and has given good results.[76]

There are a variety of other sternal disorders that produce a spectrum of morbidity for the patient. In some patients, the sternum may have a congenital cleft throughout all or part of its length, leaving the heart unprotected by bony covering. The pulmonary and ventilatory problems are not major in these patients until the sternum is closed and the vital capacity is temporarily lowered. These are rare conditions.

SCOLIOSIS AND KYPHOSCOLIOSIS

Severe forms of scoliosis (lateral spine curvature) and kyphoscoliosis (combined anteroposterior and lateral curvature) often lead to secondary chest wall deformities.[77] These deformities are often more severe than with primary chest wall defects, particularly in neurologically impaired children. Respiratory function may be significantly impaired with decreased vital capacity and residual lung volumes. These pulmonary function parameters may be unchanged even after surgical correction of the spinal deformity, owing to the persistence of the secondary chest wall deformity. In addition, the surgical procedure itself can transiently affect pulmonary function, particularly if the anterior approach to the spine through a thoracotomy has been used. Respiratory support with positive-pressure ventilation and aggressive postoperative analgesia are often needed for these patients. Kyphosis alone does not usually cause respiratory dysfunction.

REFERENCES

1. Geggel RL et al: Congenital diaphragmatic hernia: arterial structural changes and persistent pulmonary hypertension after surgical repair. *J Pediatr* 1985; 107:457.
2. Cartlidge PHT, Mann NP, Kapila L: Preoperative stabilization in congenital diaphragmatic hernia. *Arch Dis Child* 1986; 61:1226.
3. Wung JT et al: Congenital diaphragmatic hernia: survival treated with very delayed surgery, spontaneous respiration and no chest tube. *J Pediatr Surg* 1995;30:406-409.

4. Langer JC et al: Timing of surgery for congenital diaphragmatic hernia: is emergency operation necessary? *J Pediatr Surg* 1988; 23:731-734.

5. Breaux CW et al: Improvement in survival of patients with congenital diaphragmatic hernia utilizing a strategy of delayed repair after medical and/or extracorporeal membrane oxygenation stabilization. *J Pediatr Surg* 1991; 26:333.

6. Nakayama DK, Motoyama EK, Tagge EM: Effect of preoperative stabilization on respiratory system compliance and outcome in newborn infants with congenital diaphragmatic hernia. *J Pediatr* 1991; 118:793.

7. Peckham GJ, Fox WW: Physiologic factors affecting pulmonary artery pressure in infants with persistent pulmonary hypertension. *J Pediatr* 1978; 93:1005.

8. Cloutier R, Fournier L, Levasseur L: Reversion to fetal circulation in congenital diaphragmatic hernia: a preventable postoperative complication. *J Pediatr Surg* 1983; 18:551.

9. Muratore CS et al: Pulmonary morbidity in 100 survivors of congenital diaphragmatic hernia in a multidisciplinary clinic. *J Pediatr Surg* 2001; 36:133-140.

10. Bailey PV et al: A critical analysis of extracorporeal membrane oxygenation for congenital diaphragmatic hernia. *Surgery* 1989; 106:611.

11. Muratore CS, Wilson JM: Congenital diaphragmatic hernia: where are we and where do we go from here? *Semin Perinatol* 2000; 24:418-428.

12. Harrison MR et al: Successful repair in utero of a fetal diaphragmatic hernia after removal of herniated viscera from the left thorax. *N Engl J Med* 1990; 322:1582.

13. Kitano Y et al: Lung growth induced by prenatal tracheal occlusion and its modifying factors: a study in the rat model of congenital diaphragmatic hernia. *J Pediatr Surg* 2000; 36:251-259.

14. Bratu I et al: Pulmonary structural maturation and pulmonary artery remodeling after reversible fetal ovine tracheal occlusion in diaphragmatic hernia. *J Pediatr Surg* 2001; 36:739-744.

15. Quan L, Smith DW: The VATER association: vertebral defects, anal atresia, T-E fistula with esophageal atresia, radial and renal dysplasia: a spectrum of associated defects. *J Pediatr* 1973; 104:7.

16. Aschcraft KW, Holder TM: The story of esophageal atresia and tracheoesophageal fistula. *Surgery* 1969; 65:332-340.

17. Langer JC et al: Prenatal diagnosis of esophageal atresia using sonography and magnetic resonance imaging. *J Pediatr Surg* 2001; 36:804-807.

18. Weber TR, Smith W, Grosfeld JL: Surgical experience in infants with the VATER association. *J Pediatr Surg* 1980; 15:849.

19. Templeton JM et al: Management of esophageal atresia and tracheoesophageal fistula in the neonate with severe respiratory distress syndrome. *J Pediatr Surg* 1985; 20:394.

20. Delius RE, Wheatly MJ, Coran AG: Etiology and management of respiratory complications after repair of esophageal atresia with tracheoesophageal fistula. *Surgery* 1992; 112:527.

21. Davies MRQ, Cywes S: The flaccid trachea and tracheoesophageal congenital anomalies. *J Pediatr Surg* 1978; 13:363.

22. Schuster SR: Omphalocele and gastroschisis. *J Pediatr Surg* 2:740-763.

23. deVries PA: The pathogenesis of gastroschisis and omphalocele. *J Pediatr Surg* 1980; 15:245.

24. Glick PL et al: The missing link in the pathogenesis of gastroschisis. *J Pediatr Surg* 1985; 20:406.

25. Touloukian RJ, Hobbins JC: Maternal ultrasonography in the antenatal diagnosis of surgically correctable fetal abnormalities. *J Pediatr Surg* 1980; 15:373.

26. Sonnino RE et al: Intestinal fatty acid binding protein in peritoneal fluid is a marker of intestinal ischemia. *Transplant Proc* 2000; 32:1280.

27. Baird PA, MacDonald EC: An epidemiologic study of congenital malformations of the anterior abdominal wall in more than half a million consecutive live births. *Am J Hum Genet* 1981; 33:470.

28. Lynch FP et al: Cardiovascular effects of increased intraabdominal pressure in newborn piglets. *J Pediatr Surg* 1974; 9:621.

29. Haynes JH et al: Is primary repair preferable to the use of a pouch for gastroschisis? Resident Debate. *Perspect Gen-Laparosc Surg* 1993; 4:89-102.

30. Yaster M et al: Prediction of successful primary closure of congenital abdominal wall defects using intraoperative measurements. *J Pediatr Surg* 1989; 24:1217.

31. Lacey SR et al: The relative merits of various methods of indirect measurement of intraabdominal pressure as a guide to closure of abdominal wall defects. *J Pediatr Surg* 1987; 22:1207.

32. Fisher JD et al: Gastroschisis: a simple technique for staged silo closure. *J Pediatr Surg* 1995; 30:1169-1171.

33. Hong AR et al: Sequential sac ligation for giant omphalocele. *J Pediatr Surg* 1994; 29:413-415.

34. Dolgin SE, Midulla P, Shlasko E: Unsatisfactory experience with "minimal intervention management" for gastroschisis. *J Pediatr Surg* 2000; 35:1437-1439.

35. Driver CP et al: The contemporary outcome of gastroschisis. *J Pediatr Surg* 2000; 35:1719-1723.

36. Molik KA et al: Gastroschisis: a plea for risk categorization. *J Pediatr Surg* 2001; 36:51-55.

37. Ferguson TB: Congenital lesions of the lungs and emphysema. In Sabiston DC, Spencer FC, editors: *Gibbon's surgery of the chest*, ed 4. Philadelphia. WB Saunders, 1983.

38. Skandalakis JE, Gray SW, editors: *Embryology for surgeons: the embryological basis for the treatment of congenital defects*. Baltimore. Williams & Wilkins, 1994.

39. Haller JA Jr et al: Surgical management of lung bud anomalies: lobar emphysema, bronchogenic cyst, cystic adenomatoid malformation, and intralobar pulmonary sequestration. *Ann Thorac Surg* 1979; 28:33.

40. Levine MM et al: Pulmonary sequestration causing congestive heart failure in infancy: a report of two cases and review of the literature. *Ann Thorac Surg* 1982; 34:581.

41. John PR, Beasley SW, Mayne V: Pulmonary sequestration and related disorders: a clinico-radiological review of 41 cases. *Pediatr Radiol* 1989; 20:4.

42. Hendren HW, McKee D: Lobar emphysema of infancy. *J Pediatr Surg* 1966; 1:24.

43. Murray GF: Congenital lobar emphysema (collective review). *Surg Gynecol Obstet* 1967; 124:611.

44. McIlvaine WB, Chang JHT, Jones M: The effective use of intrapleural bupivacaine for analgesia after thoracic and subcostal incisions in children. *J Pediatr Surg* 1988, 23: 1184-1187.

45. Bull M et al: Improved outcome in Pierre Robin sequence: effect of multidisciplinary evaluation and management. *Pediatrics* 1990; 86:294.

46. Freed G et al: Polysomnographic indications for surgical intervention in Pierre Robin sequence: acute airway management and follow-up studies after repair and take-down of tongue-lip adhesion. *Cleft Palate J* 1988; 25:151.

47. Hengerer AS, Strome M: Choanal atresia: a new embryologic theory and its influence in surgical management. *Laryngoscope* 1982; 92:913.

48. Tneogaray T, Dawson S: Practical management of congenital choanal atresia. *Plast Reconstr Surg* 1981; 72:634.

49. Cotton RT, Stith JA: Choanal atresia in current therapy in otolaryngology. In Gates GA, editor: *Head and neck surgery,* vol 3. Philadelphia. BC Decker, 1987.

50. Ryder RW, Shelton JD, Guinan ME: Necrotizing enterocolitis: a prospective multicenter investigation. *Am J Epidemiol* 1980; 112:113.

51. Hsueh W et al: Platelet activating factor–induced ischemic bowel necrosis: the effect of PAF antagonists. *Eur J Pharm* 1986; 123:79.

52. Sun XM, Hsueh W: Bowel necrosis induced by tumor necrosis factor in rats as mediated by platelet-activating factor. *J Clin Invest* 1988; 81:1328.

53. Caplan MS et al: Role of platelet activating factor and tumor necrosis factor-alpha in neonatal necrotizing enterocolitis. *Pediatrics* 1990; 116:960.

54. Edelson MB et al: Plasma intestinal fatty acid binding protein in neonates with necrotizing enterocolitis: a pilot study. *J Pediatr Surg* 1999; 34:1453-1457.

55. Arcuni J et al: Secretory event in intestinal grafts during preservation ischemia. *J Surg Res* 1999; 84:233-239.

56. Berdon WE et al: Necrotizing enterocolitis in the premature infant. *Radiology* 1964; 83:879.

57. Molik KA et al: Portal venous air: the poor prognosis persists. *J Pediatr Surg* 2001; 36:1143-1145.

58. Brus F et al: Number and activation of circulating polymorphonuclear leukocytes and platelets are associated with neonatal respiratory distress syndrome severity. *Pediatrics* 1997; 99:672-680.

59. Cass DL et al: Peritoneal drainage as definitive treatment for neonates with isolated intestinal perforation. *J Pediatr Surg* 2000; 35:1531-1536.

60. Dzakovic A et al: Primary peritoneal drainage for increasing ventilatory requirements in critically ill neonates with necrotizing enterocolitis. *J Pediatr Surg* 2001; 36:730-732.

61. Moss RL et al: A meta-analysis of peritoneal drainage versus laparotomy for perforated necrotizing enterocolitis. *J Pediatr Surg* 2001; 1210-1213.

62. Finegold MJ et al: Lung structure in thoracic dystrophy. *Am J Dis Child* 1971; 122:152.

63. Ravitch MM: Disorders of the sternum and the chest wall. In Sabiston DC, Spencer FC, editors: *Gibbon's surgery of the chest,* ed 4. Philadelphia. WB Saunders, 1983.

64. Haller JA Jr, Turner CS: Diagnosis and operative management of chest wall deformities in children. *Surg Clin North Am* 1981; 61:1199.

65. Weber TR, Kurkchubasche AG: Operative management of asphyxiating thoracic dystrophy after pectus repair. *J Pediatr Surg* 1998; 33:262-265.

66. Price MR, Galantowicz ME, Stolar CJH: Mechanical forces contribute to neonatal lung growth: the influence of altered diaphragm function in piglets. *J Pediatr Surg* 1992; 27:376.

67. Ravitch MM: *Congenital deformities of the chest wall and their operative correction.* Philadelphia. WB Saunders, 1977.

68. Ravitch MM: The operative treatment of pectus excavatum. *Ann Surg* 1949; 129:429.

69. Nuss D et al: A 10-year review of a minimally invasive technique for the correction of pectus excavatum. *J Pediatr Surg* 1998; 33:545-552.

70. Weg JG, Krumholz RA, Harkleroad LE: Pulmonary dysfunction in pectus excavatum. *Am Rev Respir Dis* 1967; 96:936.

71. Morshuis W, Folgering H, Barentsz J: Pulmonary function before surgery for pectus excavatum and at long-term follow-up. *Chest* 1994; 105:1646-1652.

72. Quigley PM, Haller JA, Laughlin GM: Cardiorespiratory function before and after corrective surgery in pectus excavatum. *J Pediatr* 1996, 178:638.

73. Haller JA Jr, Colombani PM, Humphries CT: Chest wall constriction after too extensive and too early operations for pectus excavatum. *Ann Thorac Surg* 1996, 61:1618-1625.

74. Molik KA et al: Pectus excavatum repair: experience with standard and minimal invasive techniques. *J Pediatr Surg* 2001; 36:324-328.

75. Moss RL, Albanese CT, Reynolds M: Major complications after minimally invasive repair of pectus excavatum: case reports. *J Pediatr Surg* 2001; 36:155-158.

76. Shamberger RC, Welch KJ: Surgical correction of pectus carinatum. *J Pediatr Surg* 1987; 22:48-53.

77. Edmonson AS: Scoliosis. In Crenshaw AH, editor: *Campbell's operative orthopedics,* ed 8. St Louis. Mosby, 1992; pp 3605-3654.

CHAPTER **30**

Neonatal Complications of Respiratory Care

Donald W. Thibeault
Perry L. Clark

O f the numerous complications of respiratory care, barotrauma and various types of chronic lung disease are the focus of the discussion in this chapter. In addition, special conditions often associated with the care of the very low–birth-weight infant, that is, retinopathy of prematurity and intracranial hemorrhage, are addressed.

PULMONARY BAROTRAUMA

Barotrauma is a nonspecific term and without further qualification, as will be shown, it tells very little about the type of pressure trauma. The same pressure or volume applied to the same lung under different conditions will cause different degrees and locations of trauma. The severity and type of damage depend on the stage of lung development and surfactant maturation, as well as on the magnitude of the applied force.

LUNG OVERDISTENTION WITH ADEQUATE SURFACTANT IN PRETERM AND TERM INFANTS

In the normal term infant lung (Fig. 30-1), with each inspiration the pressure applied to the intraacinar walls is balanced by the pressure in the open alveoli that surround the airways. Surfactant lines the alveoli, alveolar ducts, and respiratory bronchioles; therefore the inspiratory pressure required to deliver a normal tidal volume is low. With each breath, the site of the major stress is in the concentration of elastic tissue in the alveolar ducts, where they interface with the mouths of the alveoli.[1] The alveolar walls or septa need little elastic tissue, because the pressure applied to one alveolar wall is balanced by the neighboring pressurized alveolus. Therefore the transseptal pressure is essentially zero. Surfactant has the unique property of resisting lung inflation at high pressures, so that stress to the delicate alveolar wall connective

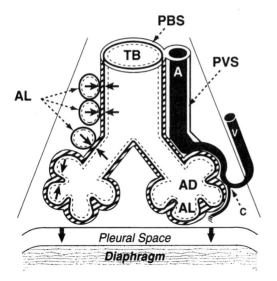

Fig. 30-1

A normal acinus. Surfactant *(broken lines)* lines the alveoli *(AL)*, alveolar ducts *(AD)*, and respiratory bronchioles. Alveoli are open and have a pressure equal and opposite to the airway pressure *(small arrows)*. The transseptal pressure in the alveoli is zero, with equal pressures on both sides of the septa *(small arrows)*. The pulmonary artery *(A)* runs with the airway and ends in capillaries *(C)* before continuing as a vein *(V)* in the periacinar connective tissue. The terminal bronchiole *(TB)* is surrounded by a peribronchiolar space *(PBS)*, and the artery is surrounded by a perivascular space *(PVS)*.

tissues is minimized at end inspiration, provided that the applied pressure and volume are not excessive. At end inspiration, the energy stored in the stressed lung elastic tissue and the increased alveolar surface tension cause the lung to recoil to its resting volume.

Most animal models have employed lung overdistention in mature lungs to create barotrauma. Macklin and Macklin,[2] in 1944, and others[3] noted that overdistention led to rupture of the alveolar walls and small airways, with the air tracking directly into the pleural space (Fig. 30-2) or into the perivascular and peribronchial spaces. In a normal lung with surfactant, the sites of rupture occur at alveolar bases, next to vascular structures or atelectatic alveoli, or at sites where the pressure is imbalanced (i.e., higher in alveoli or airways), rather than in the juxtaposed low-pressure tissues. Locally, at the site of rupture there is atelectasis, edema, and extravasated blood. The interstitial and perivascular air can cause marked splinting of the lung and compression of blood vessels by the air collection, and this causes the so-called air-block syndrome. With lung overdistention, the alveolar

capillaries may be compressed without lung rupture, causing ventilation-perfusion problems. Perivascular air is freely transported along the sheaths of pulmonary blood vessels to the mediastinum in mature lungs. The most striking accumulations of air are seen at the roots of the lungs in the hilar regions, where the converged airstreams merge into large blebs. Air apparently does not move easily in the sheaths of bronchi. The air can track distally along the trabeculae of the intralobular septal connective tissue to the pleura to form blebs. Pneumomediastinal air can track to the contralateral lungs or break into a pleural cavity to form a pneumothorax or move to extrathoracic areas. The movement of air away from the mediastinum is related to the connective tissue planes, degree of lung development, and status of surfactant. Preterm infants rarely develop a pneumomediastinum, and this occurrence is even more rare if the infants have surfactant deficiency. Pneumothoraces appear to arise from air leaks through tears in the walls of the mediastinal blebs or by rupture of hilar or subpleural blebs.

Barotrauma in the preterm infant, with adequate surfactant or following surfactant treatment, has some similarities to that in term humans and animals, but there are notable differences. The majority of preterm infants of less than 30 weeks' gestation are born with less than adequate surfactant. The lungs have a very small end-expiratory lung volume because of the increased elastic recoil associated with the increased surface tension forces (Fig. 30-3, *A*). Surfactant should be administered during the first minutes of life to these infants with surfactant deficiency. The effect of surfactant is to reduce the alveolar and small airway surface tension forces to levels found in term infants. This reduces the need for peak inspiratory pressure (PIP) and for positive end-expiratory pressure (PEEP). The same 23-week gestation infant shown in Fig. 30-3, *A,* after receiving surfactant, needed only a PIP of 10 cm H_2O and a PEEP of 2 cm H_2O (Fig. 30-3, *B*). The lungs are excessively inflated during inspiration with this low PIP, but with further reduction of pressure the lungs become atelectatic, which indicates a low, sharp critical closing pressure. This overinflation is associated with marked hypercarbia, most likely related to the compression of capillaries and increased alveolar dead space. The cause of this problem is overdistention in surfactant-treated lungs that have small amounts of elastic tissue in the alveoli, alveolar ducts, and pleura. This overdistention can lead to alveolar rupture and pneumothorax or to pulmonary interstitial emphysema (PIE) and air-block syndrome acutely or to chronic distal acinar deformation and altered lung development.

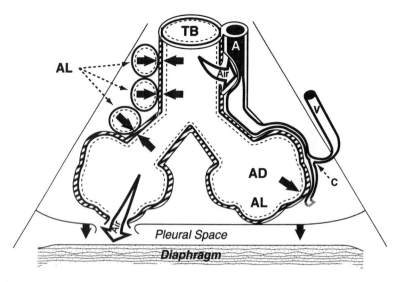

Fig. 30-2

Lung overdistention and volutrauma in a lung with adequate surfactant. The excessive inspiratory volume has overdistended the small airway and alveoli. The larger acinar airway is protected by an equally large pressure and volume in the surrounding alveoli *(AL, solid arrows)*. However, in areas where the alveolar and bronchiolar pressures are not balanced there is a rupture of the wall *(open large arrows)*. The interstitial air can compress arteries *(A)* and lead to the air-block syndrome with decreased perfusion to the capillaries *(C)* and veins *(V)*. Air can move in the perivascular space to the mediastinum or break into the pleural space to form a pneumothorax.

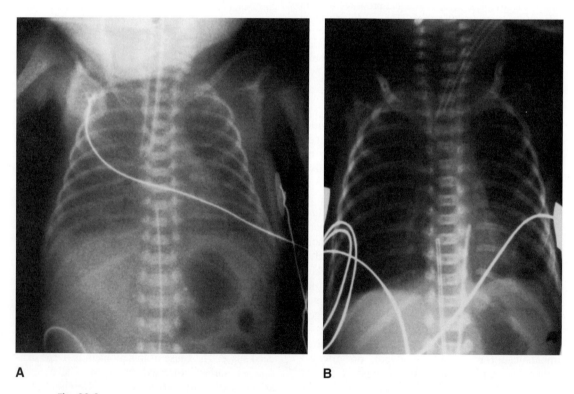

A   B

Fig. 30-3

A, Chest radiograph of a 23-week-old infant with respiratory distress syndrome showing ground-glass appearance and air bronchogram. **B,** Twenty-four hours after the patient received a second dose of surfactant, the chest radiograph shows hyperinflation while on a low ventilator pressure of PIP 10 cm H_2O and PEEP 2 cm H_2O.

LUNG OVERDISTENTION WITH INADEQUATE SURFACTANT

Surfactant deficiency has a profound influence on the severity and type of barotrauma. Surfactant deficiency causes atelectasis of the alveoli (saccules) and alveolar ducts. These structures fill with fluid because of the increased surface tension forces that pull fluid and protein from the vascular space during inflation. The opening pressure of surfactant-deficient ducts and alveoli exceeds 25 cm H$_2$O. In the immature lung, this inspiratory pressure causes a ballooning of the respiratory bronchioles, with damage to the epithelial lining layer and basement membranes. The airway wall pressure is not balanced by an equal and opposing pressure in the surrounding alveoli because they are atelectatic. Increasing the inspiratory pressure or tidal volume will eventually rupture the wall of airways, causing PIE that dissects through the tissues.[4] These blebs of air can compress vessels, causing air-block syndrome (Fig. 30-4). PIE may dissect to the pleura to cause subpleural and intralobular blebs, and a pneumothorax may occur. This PIE is space occupying and splints the lung by increasing the interstitial pressure, which decreases the lung compliance and necessitates higher and higher PIPs to maintain gas exchange.

In more mature preterm and term infants, that is, infants of 30 to 40 weeks' gestation, PIE is less common because the small airway connective tissues elastin and collagen are much better developed. These more mature infants with surfactant deficiency who do not respond to surfactant treatment are placed on high-frequency ventilation (HFV) or extracorporeal membrane oxygenation (ECMO), and the lung damage is interrupted and healing can occur.

CLINICAL CHARACTERISTICS AND TREATMENT OF BAROTRAUMA

Lung Overdistention, Acinar Deformation, and Epithelial Damage of Small Airways. Necrosis and exfoliation of the epithelium of the small intraacinar airways are constant findings at postmortem examination in infants receiving high tidal volumes or with lung overdistention. The more immature the infant, the greater the surfactant deficiency, and the more severe the problem. This epithelial damage takes days to weeks to repair and places the lungs at risk for problems, such as increased airway secretions, infections, lung

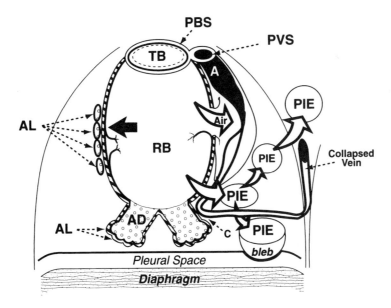

Fig. 30-4

Surfactant deficiency and barotrauma. The pressure waveform reaches the respiratory bronchiole *(RB),* but the high surface tension forces in the alveolar ducts *(AD)* and alveoli *(AL)* do not allow expansion. These alveoli and ducts are collapsed and filled with fluid. The RB balloons out during inspiration because the surrounding alveolar pressure is low. With expiration, the RB slams shut. These shear forces occur with each breath, eventually causing severe damage of the epithelium (frayed ends) and rupturing the RB wall *(arrows with air).* The interstitial air (pulmonary interstitial emphysema) obstructs the blood supply and splints the interstitial space so that lung volume is severely restricted.

inflammation, bronchospasm, and the need for increased inspired oxygen concentrations. In small immature infants, the airways are ballooned out and are deformed by the increased PIP, which damages the elastic and collagen templates that are necessary for normal lung development and also are at risk for wall rupture and PIE. Early surfactant treatment, low ventilator pressures, and HFV can ameliorate this epithelial wall damage and barotrauma. Infants with prolonged rupture of fetal membranes and oligohydramnios, because of their deficient elastic tissue, develop severe deformation with a cystic pattern seen histologically and radiographically.[5] HFV and nitric oxide are highly effective therapies for this condition.

Pulmonary Interstitial Emphysema. Widespread bilateral PIE is primarily a problem of surfactant deficiency. The interstitial air splints the lung and compresses neighboring alveoli and vessels, causing decreased compliance, hypoxemia, and hypercarbia. With the early use of surfactant therapy, and gentle ventilation, severe PIE in infants older than 30 weeks' gestation has been substantially decreased in recent years. Ironically, however, with the use of surfactant, smaller infants, down to 23 weeks' gestation, are surviving and these infants are at greatest risk to develop PIE. Diffuse bilateral PIE in preterm infants younger than 32 weeks' gestation is associated with greater than 70% mortality.[6-9] PIE usually has its onset within the first 24 hours of life, but it can occur later.[10] The treatment of established PIE is to avoid a generalized body edema that is associated with increased lung water by maintaining a good urine output and systemic blood pressure and by keeping the ductus arteriosus closed by early treatment with indomethacin. HFV significantly improves the outcome of infants with PIE compared with conventional ventilation.[11] A short 3-day course of systemic dexamethasone has been shown to clinically improve lung function in infants with PIE.[10] This suggests that inflammation plays a role in aggravating the effects of PIE.

Pneumomediastinum. A pneumomediastinum is always preceded by a rupture of the intraacinar airway walls or alveoli except in the rare instance of a perforated trachea or esophagus, where air can be directly admitted to the mediastinum. A pneumomediastinum is rare in preterm infants younger than 34 weeks' gestation. The incidence of pneumomediastinum before the era of assisted ventilation was greater than 2.5 per 1000 live births.[12] A so-called silent pneumomediastinum may also form in mature infants for no apparent reason and may only be detected if a chest radiograph is taken.[12] Silent pneumomediastinum may be caused by the enormous negative pressures generated by an infant with the first breath. Interestingly, postmature infants also have a high incidence of pneumomediastinum, possibly related to their increased incidence of meconium aspiration. At one time, it was thought that the pressure in the mediastinum could be elevated significantly by a pneumomediastinum and cause inhibition of venous return. However, this is no longer thought to occur, and a pneumomediastinum does not appear to be functionally significant and needs no treatment. Pneumomediastinal air is usually confined anterior to the heart.[13,14] The interesting radiologic sign of a windblown spinnaker sail with pneumomediastinum is caused by the peculiar fascia planes and large thymuses of infants.[14] Abnormal air collections can also rarely be seen in the posterior mediastinum surrounding the esophagus and extending between the hemidiaphragm and the parietal pleura in the subpulmonic area.[15,16] In contrast with the anterior pneumomediastinum, enough gas can collect within the posterior mediastinum to compress the lung and impair lung function. A pneumomediastinum is diagnosed radiographically by the typical air collections in the anterior mediastinum[14] or in the inferior pulmonary ligament with air dissecting above the hemidiaphragm below the parietal pleura.[15,16] On physical examination there is a barrel configuration to the chest, with an increased anteroposterior diameter, and the heart sounds are muffled by the air collection. The air collection spontaneously disappears in 1 to 2 days. Subcutaneous emphysema with air tracking up into the subcutaneous tissue of the neck is a rare occurrence in newborns, but it is easily detected by ballooning of the skin with a crepitant feel. No treatment is required, but a pneumothorax should be anticipated.

Pneumothorax. There is a tendency to equate air leak syndrome with a pneumothorax; however, it is the severity of PIE and not the associated pneumothorax that is the most devastating air leak. Having said this, it should be clear that death can follow pneumothorax if it is not properly treated. A pneumothorax may occur spontaneously in the first minutes[17,18] to hours of life. The cause is thought to be the large pressure generated by the first breath of life; however, the incidence of spontaneous pneumothorax is less than 0.05% of live-born infants. Spontaneous pneumothoraces are more likely to occur in the wet lung of those infants with transient tachypnea of the newborn and with meconium aspiration syndrome or after in utero asphyxia, in which amniotic fluid contents are aspirated, and the partially obstructed small airways act as ball valves, permitting gas trapping and lung rupture. Any positive pressure applied to the lungs, no matter how brief, may cause a pneumothorax.

Clinically, tachypnea, desaturation, and a rising $Paco_2$ should lead to a suspicion of a pneumothorax. The onset may be slow or occur with devastating rapidity. With a tension pneumothorax, the venous return to the heart is blocked by a kinking of the inferior and superior vena cava with a shift of the heart to the contralateral side by the air collection. Clinically, the apical pulse and the heart sounds are shifted away from the side of the pneumothorax. This can be associated with hypotension and bradycardia. A chest radiograph is the definitive diagnostic test. All nurseries have a focused bright light, where the point of light is placed on the chest in a darkened room, and the air collection will glow red, indicating a pneumothorax. The new ventilators also show a decrease in the compliance and tidal volume at a given set pressure. Usually, there is time to obtain a chest radiograph to confirm the clinical diagnosis. However, if severe cardiopulmonary collapse or death is imminent, treatment cannot await the results of chest radiography. Sticking needles into the pleural space should be avoided because it may puncture the lungs and cause or aggravate a pneumothorax. In emergency situations, an 18-gauge plastic catheter with a stylet can be inserted into the pleural cavity and the stylet quickly removed. If the infant is receiving assisted ventilation, the catheter can be left open to air pressure until a chest tube is placed. For definitive treatment of a pneumothorax we use a percutaneous placement of a small-bore pigtail 8.5 French catheter (see Chapter 43).[19,20]

Pneumopericardium and Pneumoperitoneum. A pneumopericardium is a rare sequela of pulmonary barotrauma, occurring virtually always as a complication of high-pressure ventilation in preterm infants who have respiratory distress syndrome (RDS).[21-23] PIE usually precedes a pneumopericardium. A pneumopericardium may rarely occur if the trachea is perforated during intubation and the pericardium is entered directly. A pneumopericardium is related to lung overdistention with high PIPs, lung volumes, PEEP, and prolonged inspiratory times.[24,25] Pneumopericardium is rare since the use of surfactant and ECMO; however, it does occur and demands rapid diagnosis and treatment to prevent a high mortality. A tension pneumopericardium that tamponades the heart may be confused clinically with a tension pneumothorax, but the breath sounds should be normal with a tension pneumopericardium.

Sudden onset of bradycardia and muffled heart sounds, cyanosis, and hypotension are the cardinal signs of cardiac tamponade. Chest radiographs show gas surrounding the heart on the anterior and lateral views, but gas under the inferior surface of the heart is the diagnostic radiographic sign.[26] Some patients are asymptomatic or just have a tachycardia, and the diagnosis is first made by chance from a chest radiograph. However, most asymptomatic patients with pneumopericardium go on to develop symptoms; indeed, 40% die.[27] Cardiac tamponade may rapidly cause death unless immediate cardiac decompression is achieved.[28] Therefore it is wise to treat asymptomatic patients with a pneumopericardium if they are being mechanically ventilated. The treatment is to evacuate the gas around the heart initially by needle aspiration. After this, continuous drainage is recommended if the infant has been symptomatic.[29] Before inserting a needle the infant should receive a systemic analgesic as well as a local anesthetic. A 5 French arterial line catheter attached to a syringe is inserted through the skin at the right of the xyphoid process. The syringe and needle are maintained at 30 to 50 degrees above the plane of the abdomen and advanced toward the tip of the left scaphoid. Gentle suction is applied to the syringe. After removal of the air, the needle is removed and the plastic catheter is passed over the guide wire into the pericardial sac. The catheter is sutured to the skin, and the catheter is attached to a chest tube drainage system at 20 cm H_2O suction for continuous drainage. An echocardiogram should be obtained to confirm the placement of the catheter. If the air reaccumulates, a pericardial drainage tube is placed surgically in the pericardial sac under direct vision.[30] There are serious complications to placing needles or catheters in the pericardial sac. These include a pneumothorax, hemopericardium, or lacerated heart.

A pneumoperitoneum, which is free air in the peritoneal cavity, is an unusual but serious complication of pulmonary barotrauma. It must be differentiated from a pneumoperitoneum associated with a perforation of the gastrointestinal tract from various causes.[31] Differentiation of the two causes of pneumoperitoneum is difficult, particularly in the presence of severe respiratory insufficiency. Delayed gastric emptying, bile-stained vomitus, bloody stools, signs of sepsis, necrotizing enterocolitis, and absence of lung disease point strongly toward gastrointestinal perforation. Instillation of water-soluble contrast medium in the stomach by nasogastric tube may give a definitive answer. It has been shown that the measurement of the oxygen concentration of gas aspirated from the peritoneal cavity will differentiate a pneumoperitoneum of gastrointestinal origin from a ventilator-induced pneumoperitoneum.[32] At the time of aspiration, the stomach should be under constant suction with a nasogastric tube. If the peritoneal oxygen tension is greater than room air, then the source of the gas is most likely from a lung leak, provided that an elevated F_{IO_2} is being breathed.

BRONCHOPULMONARY DYSPLASIA AND CHRONIC LUNG DISEASE OF PREMATURITY

Some degree of lung disease occurs in all preterm infants younger than 30 weeks' gestation, with or without ventilator assistance. These lung conditions are labeled pulmonary insufficiency in prematurity,[33] chronic pulmonary insufficiency of prematurity[34] (CPIP), Wilson-Mikity syndrome,[35] chronic lung disease of prematurity[36] (CLD), and bronchopulmonary dysplasia[37] (BPD) and appear to be part of a spectrum of varying degrees of disturbances of lung function. The variation in the clinical picture of these lung disturbances is primarily a function of the stage of lung development, type of barotrauma, adequacy of lung surfactant, oxygen exposure, and inflammatory response of the lung immune system to these insults.

PULMONARY INSUFFICIENCY IN PREMATURITY

Many preterm infants of 26 to 30 weeks' gestation with minimal assisted ventilation and minimal hyperoxia undergo a deterioration of lung function in the first week of life. This has been attributed to ventilation-perfusion problems secondary to mechanical immaturity of the thorax and airway. This condition was described by Burnard and colleagues in 1965 before the use of ventilators.[33] The quantity of positive-pressure ventilation by bag and mask and amount of hyperoxia exposure were not measured or mentioned in their article.

Similar deterioration of lung function at 4 to 7 days of life has been shown to occur in preterm infants weighing less than 1200 g who had normal lung function in the first 2 days. This condition has been labeled CPIP.[34] These infants become apneic and require supplemental oxygen, but the chest radiographs are within normal limits. In 1975, this condition was associated with a 10% to 20% mortality rate, but now all are expected to survive. Recovery is complete by 2 months of age.

WILSON-MIKITY SYNDROME

Wilson and Mikity, in 1960, described five preterm infants with a new form of respiratory disease.[35] At that time ventilators were not used and the toxicity of inspired oxygen was only vaguely appreciated. Virtually all preterm infants with severe RDS died.

Many centers would hand-ventilate infants with respiratory distress for days on end, if necessary. To understand this syndrome it is important to understand the state of respiratory care in that era. These five preterm infants had respiratory distress in the first few days of life, which then subsided. However, at 1 to 5 weeks after birth there was progressive onset of cyanosis and tachypnea, which increased for up to 3 months of age, at which time either death occurred or there was a slow return to normal function. In the sickest infants, cor pulmonale and heart failure occurred. Radiologically, there were bilateral diffuse pulmonary infiltrates of a coarse, nodular, or reticular pattern usually first seen between 10 and 30 days of life. Later, this picture changed to a cystic emphysematous pattern. In survivors, the radiographs became normal, but this often took a year or more. Numerous cases were published between 1960 and 1968.[38-40] Oxygen toxicity and abnormal lung development after birth in the immature lungs were believed to be the etiology of this syndrome.[40] In long-term survivors, pulmonary function testing showed flow rates to be significantly lower in infants with this syndrome compared with preterm infants who did not have the syndrome.[41] This suggests persistent ventilatory disturbances perhaps related to the residue of the cystic changes that occurred early in life.

CLASSIC BRONCHOPULMONARY DYSPLASIA

With the widespread use of ventilators in preterm infants the clinical diagnosis and expression of the Wilson-Mikity syndrome were hidden within, and superseded in 1967 by, the condition referred to as BPD.[37] At that time there was quantitation of ventilatory pressures and inspired oxygen concentrations. In addition, there were smaller and sicker infants who were surviving because of the use of ventilators.

Etiology and Pathophysiology. As described by Northway and colleagues,[37] BPD is inextricably intertwined with the surfactant deficiency syndrome called RDS. Classic BPD has four stages, with each stage having an identifiable clinical, radiologic, and pathologic pattern (Table 30-1).[37,42] The four stages are infrequently seen since the use of surfactant in small preterm infants and since the use of ECMO and HFV in larger infants. The first stage has the typical radiographic pattern of RDS with small lung volumes and air bronchograms (see Fig. 30-3, *A*).[42] The second stage, at 4 to 10 days, shows opacification on the chest radiograph (Fig. 30-5, *A*). Pathologically, there is hyaline membrane disease formation, necrosis and repair of alveolar epithelium, and thickening of the

TABLE 30-1	RADIOLOGIC STAGING OF CLASSIC BRONCHOPULMONARY DYSPLASIA, WITH PATHOLOGIC CORRELATES		
Radiologic Stage	**Patient Age (Days)**	**Radiologic Description**	**Pathologic Description**
I	2-3	Granular pattern Air bronchograms Small lung volume	Atelectasis Hyaline membranes Lymphatic dilation
II	4-10	Opacification	Necrosis and repair of alveolar epithelium Persistent hyaline membranes Emphysematous coalescence of alveoli and bronchiolar necrosis
III	10-20	Small areas of lucency alternating with areas of irregular density	Persisting airway injury to alveolar epithelium Groups of emphysematous alveoli with atelectasis of surrounding alveoli Interstitial edema and septal thickening Bronchiolar mucosal metaplasia and hyperplasia with marked mucus secretions
IV	Beyond 30 days	Enlargement of lucent areas alternating with thinner strands of radiodensity	Emphysematous alveoli, next to atelectatic and normal alveolus Septal fibrosis Perimucosal fibrosis and metaplasia Medial hypertrophy of arterioles

Data from Northway WH, Rosan RC, Porter DY: Pulmonary disease following respiratory therapy of hyaline membrane disease. *N Engl J Med* 1967; 276:357-368; and Edwards DK, Colby TV, Northway WH: Radiographic-pathologic correlation in bronchopulmonary dysplasia. *J Pediatr* 1979; 95:835-846.

alveolar septa. If the infant survives at 10 to 20 days, a chest radiograph shows small areas of lucencies alternating with areas of irregular density (Fig. 30-5, *B*). Pathologically, there is persistent damage to the airway epithelium with bronchiolar mucosa metaplasia. The septa are thickened, with groups of emphysematous alveoli interspersed with atelectasis. The fourth stage occurs after 30 days and shows large cystic areas on the chest radiograph with adjacent strands of radiodense material (Fig. 30-5, *C*). Pathologically, there are cystic areas, septal fibrosis, atelectasis, and hypertrophy of the media of small arteries. At the time BPD was first described, PIE was not recognized as a major source of lung damage in mechanically ventilated preterm infants.[4,43] PIE is an important contributor to the pathology of BPD and is often recognized radiographically between the second and third stages in BPD.[43]

Diagnosis, Clinical Presentation, and Treatment. BPD begins as a severe form of RDS, and the high ventilator settings required for oxygenation persist into the first week of life. In the surfactant era, the syndrome is seen when RDS is unresponsive to multiple doses of surfactant or with severe bilateral PIE. In the near-term infant unresponsive to surfactant, HFV is used if the lung disease fails to respond to surfactant. ECMO, which essentially cures the condition in 4 to 5 days, is also used. In preterm infants, HFV and surfactant are the primary therapeutic agents. A patent ductus arteriosus may complicate the early course of BPD in infants and should be suspected when the lung chest radiograph does not improve after surfactant administration. A patent ductus arteriosus is treated with indomethacin after confirming the diagnosis with an echocardiogram. In those infants in whom the lungs do not clear, after 10 days the condition becomes chronic.

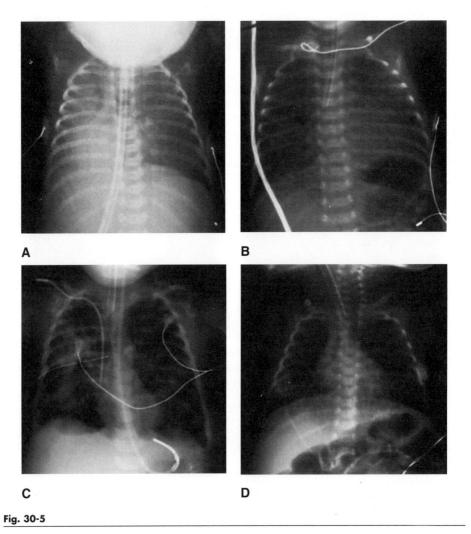

Fig. 30-5

A, Chest radiograph of 24-week-gestation infant at 6 days old showing opacified lung fields with streaky densities in right lung, which is stage 2 classic bronchopulmonary dysplasia (BPD). Note the radiograph is reversed in comparison to other three films. **B,** Radiograph of same infant, at 15 days of age, showing small areas of lucency alternating with areas of irregular densities. **C,** Cystic stage of classic BPD. **D,** Note the bubbly pseudocystic pattern of infants with chronic lung disease.

The treatment at that stage is to maintain the lowest ventilatory support and FIO_2 to permit lung healing. After 10 days there is hypertrophy of the small airway wall muscle, which may result in bronchospasm and is treated with bronchodilators.[44] Good nutrition and lung growth eventually lead to adequate lung function and the opportunity to extubate these infants. This may take weeks to months, depending on the severity of the BPD. These infants, after extubation, all require nasal oxygen to maintain an arterial saturation greater than 90%. They have severe ventilation-perfusion mismatching, secondary to the cystic lung disease and atelectasis. In addition, they have pulmonary hypertension and

some go on to develop cor pulmonale. It is common for these infants to have a $Paco_2$ in the 60s and 70s for some months. The pulmonary hypertension leads to water retention and pulmonary edema, which requires daily or frequent use of diuretics. To improve growth and restrict water intake a high-calorie diet of 24 to 28 calories per ounce is used. Most infants recover from their lung disease within a year. There are, however, long-term effects on lung function in infants with moderate BPD. In infants with moderate BPD, the arterial blood gases become normal during the first year. BPD infants continue to have increased airway resistance and are prone to severe pulmonary insufficiency after upper respiratory viral or bacterial infections. Although the pulmonary function remains abnormal for a year in moderate BPD, only in the severest cases is there exercise intolerance into the late years of childhood.[45]

Classic BPD fulfilling all the criteria of Northway and co-workers[37] is infrequent. The condition may still occur if surfactant treatment is delayed and especially if severe RDS is complicated by severe bilateral PIE. A similar condition also occurs in infants with congenital diaphragmatic hernias who receive high concentrations of oxygen and volutrauma for prolonged periods. Their lungs are hypoplastic, which predisposes to BPD even though these infants are term.[46] Also, infants with prolonged ruptured fetal membranes have severe lung hypoplasia with very little lung elastic tissue.[5] This lack of elastic tissue leads to cystic lung changes and gives a pulmonary insufficiency picture similar to that of BPD. The mortality rate is much higher than that of BPD.

CHRONIC LUNG DISEASE OR NONCLASSIC BPD

After the liberal use of surfactant in the first minutes of life in infants with RDS, the lung disorder called classic BPD (the four stages described by Northway and co-workers[37]) has virtually disappeared. However, classic BPD has been replaced by another lung disorder variably called CLD, BPD, atypical BPD,[47,48] or nonclassic BPD. This new lung disorder of CLD is much milder than classic BPD. This favorable change has occurred even though immature infants as young as 23 weeks' gestation are surviving. The current definition of BPD or CLD is vague. One definition is the need for supplemental oxygen for 28 days or longer during the first 2 months of life in association with chest radiographic changes of opacification, cystlike changes, or alternating patterns of density or lucency.[48] Another definition is oxygen need at 28 days of life with at least 21 days of oxygen supplementation and a compatible chest radiograph. Another definition is the need for oxygen at 36 weeks' corrected gestational age with no requirement for radiographic changes.[36] At the present time, neonatologists use the terms *BPD* and *CLD* interchangeably. The need for supplemental oxygen at 36 weeks' corrected gestational age is most often the definition used for nonclassic BPD or CLD. Henceforth, we will use the term *CLD* for this nonclassic form of BPD.

Incidence, Etiology, and Pathophysiology. The incidence of CLD in infants weighing less than 1500 g is difficult to obtain because of the variation in diagnostic criteria and of the confusion with classic BPD. Ogawa and associates have shown

BOX 30-1
FACTORS ASSOCIATED WITH THE DEVELOPMENT OF CHRONIC LUNG DISEASE OF PREMATURITY
Prematurity Prolonged rupture of fetal membranes Low birth weight Cardiac failure Pulmonary barotrauma Apnea of prematurity Mechanical ventilation Pulmonary hypoplasia Prolonged exposure to high FIO_2 levels Aspiration Surfactant deficiency Respiratory distress syndrome Sepsis Endotracheal intubation Pulmonary dysmaturity

that 23% of infants weighing less than 1500 g will develop CLD and 48% of those weighing less than 1000 g will be affected.[49] There are a number of risk factors associated with development of CLD.[50,51] Low gestational age and high ventilatory support and hyperoxia are accepted by all to be fundamental etiologic factors. The low gestational lung is at a mechanical disadvantage by its immature elastic recoil[52] (Box 30-1). Therefore volutrauma before 30 weeks' gestation leads to lung structural changes, such as severe deformation of airways and saccules, as well as to damage to the epithelium. These effects are compounded by hyperoxia, lack of surfactant, and ongoing lung inflammation. Tracheal aspirates have been shown repeatedly to have elevated proteins, elastases, and various cytokines, all of which indicate ongoing inflammation.[53,54] This is supported by the rapid beneficial clinical response to treatment with corticosteroids.

Clinical Presentation and Treatment. CLD can present in the immediate newborn in a number of ways. The most common is to have surfactant deficiency and increasing respiratory failure in the first minutes or hours of life. The chest radiograph shows typical low lung volume and ground-glass appearance associated with atelectasis and air bronchograms (see Fig. 30-3, *A*). These infants are treated with surfactant as near in time to delivery as possible and with low ventilatory settings. By the second day of life, the ventilator settings and oxygen requirements are minimal and the chest radiograph becomes nearly normal. Extubation at the earliest possible time should be the goal. However, in infants younger than 28 weeks' gestation, low ventilatory settings or continuous positive airway pressure may be needed to prevent apnea, bradycardia, and arterial desaturation. Caffeine lessens the severity of apnea and bradycardic spells. To avoid reintubation, nasal cannula with oxygen, nasal continuous positive airway pressure, or nasal pharyngeal cannula with low ventilator rate are often successful. Many of these infants develop large, but hazy, lung fields radiographically at 7 to 14 days of age.[55] During this period, the FIO_2 increases sometimes to 1.0. If the newborn is not on the ventilator, one may be needed to prevent hypercarbia and apnea. Most infants continue this course for 2 to 4 weeks with this typical radiographic picture of hazy lung fields. A 3- to 7-day regimen of dexamethasone may be needed. Marked improvement of lung function is usual in the 24 to 48 hours after corticosteroid treatment, with better aeration of the lungs clinically and radiographically. Many infants can be extubated after corticosteroid therapy. However, corticosteroids have many deleterious effects on the growing brain and other organs, so their use should be a last resort.[56] These infants with hazy lung fields are very sensitive to fluid retention, and diuretics may be needed once or twice per week. A patent ductus arteriosus with a left-to-right shunt may lead to lung flooding, but this is usually a problem within the first 2 to 3 days of life.[57] This condition is treated medically with indomethacin. The ductus arteriosus may reopen after stopping therapy with indomethacin, and a second course may be required. Very few infants need surgical ligation of the ductus, perhaps 1% to 5% of infants weighing less than 1000 g.

After corticosteroid treatment or just letting time pass, the CLD resolves in most infants. However, some of the infants do not significantly improve with corticosteroids and by the third to fourth week the hazy radiograph evolves into a bubbly pattern (Fig. 30-5, *D*).[55] Histologically, the alveoli are immature with poor septation. The alveoli or saccules have a large diameter with thickened interstitium, which gives the bubbly appearance. These infants have hypercarbia and need supplemental oxygen, corticosteroids, and diuretics. They may go home on supplemental oxygen. They almost never develop the fourth stage of cystic lung disease of classic BPD. These infants, after they go home, are at high risk for readmission to the hospital with viral pneumonia. Therefore they are treated before discharge with antibodies against respiratory syncytial virus. Within 6 to 8 months of life, these infants are usually asymptomatic.

The second most common clinical presentation of CLD is that of having essentially clear lung fields with minimal RDS from birth. These infants, depending on their maturity, may need low oxygen or just room air in the first week of life. Respiratory assistance in the form of ventilator or nasal continuous positive airway pressure may be required to control apnea. After 1 week, these infants develop hazy lung fields on a chest radiograph and blend into the clinical course as described previously.

The third most common course, but fortunately infrequent, follows the four stages of classic BPD as described earlier. These infants do not respond to surfactant and can go on to develop cystic lung disease.

Complications. The complications of CLD are nonspecific and related to barotrauma, ventilatory care, endotracheal intubation, infection, and corticosteroids. There are also extrapulmonary complications, which include retinopathy of prematurity, intracranial hemorrhage, and sepsis.

The palate may be grooved by long-term oral intubation. This can be prevented by having a plastic palatal prosthesis molded to the infant's palate. The intubation tube then abuts against this prosthesis and the groove is prevented. Nasotracheal intubation can result in nostril inflammation and narrowing of the nasal passages. Oral tubes can also damage the alveolar ridge and lead to abnormal dental development. Subglottic edema and subglottic stenosis, although less frequent than in the 1980s, are still important, often unrecognized, serious complications. In infants with CLD in which there is difficulty in maintaining extubation, subglottic narrowing should be suspected and a flexible bronchoscopic examination should be performed. Necrotizing tracheobronchitis is rarely seen in the present era, and this decline is related to better humidification and gentler ventilatory strategies. Infants with CLD who require assisted ventilation are retarded in developing alveolar septation and normal lung growth. The elastic tissue of the lungs acts as a template for lung structural growth. The combination of ventilator therapy, hyperoxia, and immaturity leads to overgrowth of elastic tissue, but in a bizarre fashion that is also associated with retardation of alveolarization.[52,58] This maldevelopment is compounded by the use of corticosteroids.[59,60] The benefits of corticosteroids are clearly evident by their antiinflammatory properties, but their use also permanently retards alveolarization. Infants with CLD have increased airway muscle, which leads to bronchospasm.[44] Preterm infants with CLD have recurrent bouts of sepsis, sometimes associated with pneumonia and more often with systemic infections. This is related to the immaturity of the immune system of preterm infants as well as to indwelling central line catheters, intubation tubes, intralipid therapy, and the frequent use of antibiotics.

Infections are usually bacterial, but fungal infections are increasingly common, promoted by the use of corticosteroids and antibiotics.

Outcome. The short- and long-term pulmonary outcomes of infants with CLD (nonclassic BPD) are generally very favorable. However, infants with classic BPD and CLD are still lumped together, so it is nearly impossible to separate the effects of CLD from those of classic BPD. Corticosteroids have a profound effect on long-term lung growth, and this is usually not factored into the long-term pulmonary function testing.[61-63] These infants with CLD have long-term airway obstructions assessed by expiratory air flow studies but with a normal lung volume that indicates a compensatory growth of the parenchyma but not of the airway size. The more severe the early lung disease, the worse the air flow obstruction and wheezing. Patients with more severe cases of BPD have gas trapping and hyperinflation as late as 11 years of age.

Infants with nonclassic BPD clearly have short-term problems such as oxygen requirements at home, and they also have frequent readmissions to the hospital for upper respiratory tract infections.

LARYNGOMALACIA AND TRACHEOBRONCHOMALACIA

LARYNGOMALACIA

The term *laryngomalacia* refers to a larynx that collapses during inspiration. The arytenoids, epiglottis, and aryepiglottic folds are individually or all too soft. Laryngomalacia is the most common cause of congenital laryngeal anomalies and neonatal stridors. Clinically, an inspiratory stridor is heard and there may be significant intercostal retractions.[64] The symptoms usually appear from birth, but they may be mild initially and get worse in the first 6 months and then resolve by 24 months. The stridor can be frightening to see and hear, but the infant is usually pink and not concerned. The obstruction is made worse by crying, feeding, and being in a supine position. Rarely, infants may choke or asphyxiate with feeding. The diagnosis is by direct vision of the larynx with flexible bronchoscopy.[65] If there are feeding problems, motility studies of the pharynx and swallowing mechanism are required as well as studies for gastroesophageal reflux. Laryngomalacia is relatively a benign condition of unknown cause. However, other conditions must be ruled out, such as central nervous system, brain stem, and neuromuscular disorders. There also may be other problems in the respiratory tract.[66]

The treatment in most cases is reassurance of the parents and just observation. The rare patient may develop cor pulmonale and the inability to thrive because of the associated feeding problem. A tracheostomy is the usual treatment in severe cases; however, alternative surgical procedures are now being described.

TRACHEOMALACIA

Tracheomalacia is the condition in which the structural integrity of the trachea is lost and the cartilaginous rings are not rigid enough to prevent collapse during inspiration and especially on expiration.[67] This is a developmental problem, but, as is shown here, tracheomalacia can also be acquired. Clinically, there may be no other abnormalities and this condition usually improves or disappears within months. However, this condition may be associated with other anomalies such as esophageal atresia, tracheoesophageal fistula, vascular rings, and so on. Diagnosis of tracheomalacia is by rigid bronchoscopy. If the condition is very severe or associated with other conditions, the infant may have severe apnea, sudden death spells, or respiratory failure. A tracheostomy may be needed. There are other innovative surgical procedures that are being developed.[68]

TRACHEOBRONCHIAL INJURY AND MECHANICAL VENTILATION

Prolonged mechanical ventilation can result in chronic injury to the large upper airways.[69] The proximal airways are very compliant in preterm infants, and prolonged high-pressure ventilation can result in acquired tracheomegaly.[70] This injury is relatively common and can lead to respiratory symptoms after extubation or during weaning from continuous positive airway pressure. Tracheomegaly leads to increased dead space and collapse of the upper airways during expiration. After extubation there may be wheezing and cyanosis. The diagnosis can initially be made on the chest radiograph, which shows the enlarged diameter of the trachea. Flexible endoscopy is then performed.[71-73] The flow-volume loop will demonstrate dynamic airway collapse.[74] A tracheostomy may be needed in severe conditions. PEEP is important to support the upper airway during expiration. It may take many months for these lesions to recover. Long-term studies over a period of years are not yet available.

RETINOPATHY OF PREMATURITY

Retinopathy of prematurity (ROP) is quite similar to a disease first described in 1942 called retrolental fibroplasia (RLF). After the RLF epidemic of the 1940s and 1950s was linked to the use of high inspired oxygen concentrations and oxygen use in nurseries subsequently curtailed, it was said that RLF was "eliminated" by the 1970s. By the late 1980s, the term RLF gave way to the current term, ROP, when it was realized that the disease had just changed slightly and was occurring in the increasing number of surviving premature infants. The disease in its present form is seen as various degrees of disordered vascularization and fibrovascular changes limited almost exclusively to the retinas of premature infants, occurring during the time of retinal vessel development. The overall incidence of ROP in the CRYO-ROP study in infants weighing less than 1250 g was 66%. In infants weighing less than 750 g, the incidence was 90%, illustrating that the risk of development of the disease increases dramatically with increasing immaturity.[17] The same study also found that black infants seem less likely to develop ROP.[75]

PATHOPHYSIOLOGY

The eye undergoes rapid development starting in the middle of the second trimester. Retinal vascularization of a normal eye begins as growth of vessels from the optic disc, extending peripherally over time until complete retinal vessel development is attained at 40 to 42 weeks after conception. ROP is a disruption of this normal vascularization process.

Originally it was thought that RLF/ROP was caused by excessive oxygen administration. Although hyperoxia can indeed injure the retina, hyperoxia is not the sole cause of ROP. In fact, infants with cyanotic congenital heart disease with relative hypoxemia may develop ROP.[18] Other fac-

tors, such as immature antioxidant systems, exposure to reactive oxygen species, hypercarbia,[76,77] hypocarbia,[78] light exposure,[79-82] blood transfusions,[83,84] and magnesium and copper deficiency[85] have been suggested to have roles (Box 30-2).

Currently the most excitement in the ROP field relates to control of vascular growth factors. There is evidence indicating that highly fluctuating oxygen levels, or tissue hypoxia occurring after vasoconstrictive injury perhaps itself secondary to prior hyperoxia, may dispose to overexpression of various growth factors and/or their receptors, and the most conspicuous of these is vascular endothelial growth factor (VEGF).[86-88] Overabundance of VEGF stimulus is believed to produce an uncontrolled neovascularization in the affected area, sometimes leading to scarring and retinal retraction and perhaps retinal detachment, the most severe complication of ROP.

CLINICAL PRESENTATION

In most cases, ROP is now detected during screening examinations of preterm infants done by pediatric ophthalmologists. Screening criteria may vary, but the goal is to identify those patients with ROP who will require treatment so that treatment can be undertaken at the most appropriate time. Screening is usually done in infants born at less than 32 weeks' gestation who have lived 4 to 6 weeks. Earlier examinations only identify immature retinas that will need repeat examinations. Ophthalmologic screening for ROP is repeated every 1 to 2 weeks until the retinal vascularization has extended well into zone 3 (see Fig. 30-6, *A*) and the risk for "threshold disease" is gone. So-called threshold disease is that degree of ROP for which intervention is generally performed.

ROP is diagnosed on the basis of the description of retinal fibrovascular changes as outlined by international conference (ICROP) criteria.[89,90] Disease changes are described by location (e.g., zone 1, 2, or 3), extent (number of clock hours involved, either total or contiguous), and severity. Stage 1 is minimal severity, whereas stage 4, the most serious, includes at least partial retinal detachment (Figs. 30-6 and 30-7). Sometimes confusing words are used in describing details of the disease, such as "plus" and "rush." "Plus disease" is a phrase used to denote a case with particularly severe vessel engorgement and tortuosity, which are signs of a poor prognosis. "Rush disease" stems from Japan, where the phrase describes rapidly progressive, severe disease, hence the "rush" to treat, if possible.

The disease generally develops in the several weeks before term and reaches its peak severity at about the time equivalent of term gestation. Most cases of ROP regress over time, with scarring and

---

BOX 30-2

RISK FACTORS ASSOCIATED WITH RETINOPATHY OF PREMATURITY

Prematurity
Low birth weight
Oxygen therapy
Bradycardia
Heart disease
Blood transfusions
Magnesium and copper deficiencies
Bronchopulmonary dysplasia
Intraventricular hemorrhage
Apnea
Hypoxia
Acidosis
Hypercarbia
Infection
Respiratory distress syndrome
Multiple births
Anemia

remodeling of the retina, resulting in minimal to severe visual acuity deficits. Cases that fail to regress, however, may finally result in severe, permanent retinal scarring, with cicatricial retraction leading to retinal detachment.

TREATMENT

Therapy for eyes that have reached "threshold" (generally defined as disease in either zone 1 or 2, stage 3 or greater, covering 5 contiguous or 8 total clock hours) is operative treatment with either cryotherapy

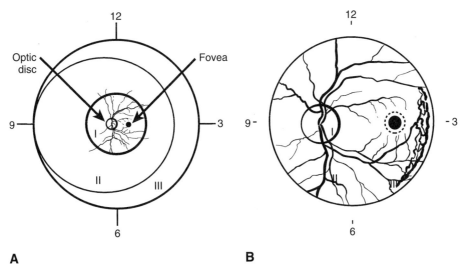

A **B**

Fig. 30-6

A, Chart illustrating zones and clock hour orientation used in describing the location and extent of retinopathy of prematurity (ROP) lesions. **B,** Diagrammatic representation of early ROP lesion with line of demarcation. This lesion could be described as zone 1, stage 1, extending 3 clock hours (2 to 5 o'clock). The vessels are usually not significantly tortuous nor increased in stage 1 lesions.

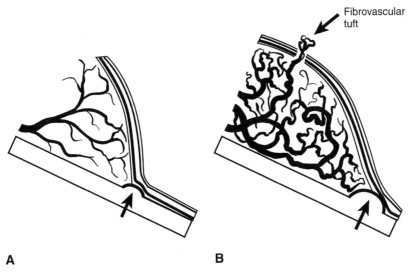

A **B**

Fig. 30-7

A, Three-dimensional diagrammatic sketch of stage 2 retinopathy of prematurity (ROP). Line of demarcation of stage 1 has progressed to a raised ridge, with increased vessel tortuosity. **B,** A sketch similar to that in **A,** representing stage 3 ROP, with dilated, tortuous vessels, a prominently raised fibrous ridge, and an extraretinal fibrovascular tuft. Stage 4 disease would include the preceding, plus some degree of retinal detachment. Stage 5 ROP is complete retinal detachment as the result of the disease.

or laser ablation of diseased portions of the retina to halt the disease progress and, it is hoped, allow regression to occur. Indirect laser therapy, apparently less traumatic, is currently preferred.

There are other interventions that have been proposed to possibly prevent, or limit the severity and extent of, the disease. These include light reduction,[82] vitamin E supplementation,[91-95] and, most recently, oxygen supplementation.[96-100] The light reduction trial failed to show any benefit for ROP.[82] The studies on vitamin E are mixed; the meta-analysis by Raju and associates[94] suggests that a proper, randomized controlled trial should be performed. Although it may seem paradoxical to suggest oxygen supplementation for treatment of ROP, it may improve the outcome by keeping oxygen delivery adequate—but not too high—to the injured areas of retina, thereby limiting the overproduction of VEGF or other growth factors that would otherwise stimulate further disordered neovascularization and disease progression.[86-88, 98-100] A randomized, controlled trial testing this hypothesis—the STOP-ROP trial—found a modest reduction in progression of ROP from prethreshold to threshold in infants whose Spo_2 was maintained at 96% to 99% versus those in whom Spo_2 of 89% to 94% was accepted. (The effect was larger, however, in the group of infants without plus disease.) This modest effect failed to reach statistical significance, and came at the expense of a modest increase in exacerbations of pulmonary disease, especially in the group with the worst lung disease at study entry.[101] Previous trials evaluating the use of transcutaneous oxygen monitoring failed to find benefit from continuous transcutaneous oxygen monitoring.[100] Based on the parsed results of the STOP-ROP trial, it may be reasonable to consider the use of supplemental oxygen if necessary to maintain Spo_2 in the higher range during the time when ROP development is most likely (i.e., beyond about 32 weeks' postconception), although such decisions must be individualized for each patient.[102,103]

The complications of the disease process are those stemming from various degrees of visual loss to total blindness. Given the potential of ROP for producing severe, permanent sequelae, preventive treatment is preferred over ameliorative therapy; however, given our current understanding and technical limitations, our ability to prevent ROP is limited.

INTRAVENTRICULAR HEMORRHAGE

Among the myriad potential problems facing a newborn premature infant is that of intraventricular/germinal matrix hemorrhage (IVH). Almost exclusively a problem for preterm infants, IVH almost always occurs in the subependymal areas along the bases of the lateral ventricles of the brain just above the basal ganglia, in an area called the germinal matrix.

Infants at greatest risk for suffering IVH are younger than 32 weeks' gestational age at birth; most at risk are those younger than 29 weeks' gestation. The hazard increases with decreasing gestational age and brain maturity. The risk also increases concomitantly with increased overall severity of illness. The tiniest, sickest infants are at the greatest peril of suffering IVH and the potentially severe long-term sequelae. Incidence of IVH among infants weighing less than 1500 g is 20% to 25%.[104,105]

PATHOPHYSIOLOGY

The germinal matrix, a site of neural and glial cell development for the brain, contains a rich web of fragile blood vessels in a gelatinous matrix, and it is at the site of these vessels that bleeding may occur. Extremely thin vessel walls and vascular immaturity,[106] an absence of usual vascular connective tissue structure in the region,[107] and contorted venous drainage through the thalamostriate vein contribute to susceptibility of bleeding in the area.[108] Hemorrhage at this site is almost exclusively a problem for significantly premature infants because the germinal matrix and its network of tiny vessels involute by about 36 weeks' gestational age.[109]

Factors adversely affecting cerebral blood flow velocity and pressure in neonates contribute to the genesis of IVH. Under normal circumstances, the cerebral vasculature autoregulates blood flow in spite of variation in systemic blood pressure. Sick premature infants have quite poor autoregulation of cerebral blood flow,[110] leading to pressure-passive blood flow[111] that may fluctuate with arterial blood pressure and venous pressure, producing similar fluctuations in cerebral blood flow that predispose to IVH.[112,115] Elevated and/or abrupt increases in systemic blood pressure are particularly stressful.[114,116] Sampling from umbilical artery catheters may affect cerebral blood flow.[117] Significant patent ductus arteriosus may also contribute to the causation of IVH.[118,119] Thrombocytopenia contributes to IVH as well.[120,121]

Extravascular factors also influence systemic and cerebral perfusion pressure. Hypoxemia and hypercarbia greatly increase cerebral blood flow. Swings in $Paco_2$ may effect large fluctuations in cerebral blood flow, and thus hyperventilation and severe hypoventilation should be avoided. Sodium bicarbonate infusions have been associated with IVH, possibly owing to the increased CO_2 load or because of the hyperosmolar nature of the infusion.[122] The occurrence of pneumothorax has been strongly associated with subsequent IVH,[123-125] thought owing to abrupt, dramatic changes in cerebral perfusion. Positive-pressure ventilation itself increases cerebral venous pressure and may decrease systemic blood pressure if cardiac blood return is diminished.

Special mention should be made of HFV. The use of high-frequency oscillatory ventilation was associated with a significant risk of IVH in the HIFI study[126]; however, other studies,[127-130] including meta-analyses by Clark and colleagues[131] and Bhuta and associates,[132] suggest that there is no relationship between the use of HFV per se and IVH.

CLINICAL PRESENTATION

The occurrence of intraventricular/germinal matrix hemorrhage may be a catastrophic event, with the dramatic onset of severe neurologic, respiratory, and cardiovascular compromise, or, in contrast, it may be a nearly silent one, heralded by minimal changes in amount and types of patient movement, tone, and responsiveness to stimuli. The single most helpful sign of significant IVH may be an abrupt drop in hematocrit.[133] Failure of hemoglobin levels to rise in response to a packed red cell transfusion may also be worrisome. In catastrophic presentations, severe hypoxemia and bradycardia may be life threatening.

DIAGNOSIS

IVH is most frequently diagnosed by cranial ultrasound examination, which may be performed at the patient's bedside in the intensive care nursery. Less commonly, computed tomography is used. The lesion is usually described by laterality (i.e., which hemisphere is involved) and graded according to a standard system. The scale most commonly used grades intraventricular/germinal matrix hemorrhages from 1 (least severe) to 4 (most severe).[134] Grade 1 lesions represent only blood within the germinal matrix/subependyma. Grade 4 hemorrhages include extension of blood into the ventricle, distorting ventricular anatomy and extending into brain parenchyma. Because the vast majority of IVH occur in the first 3 days of life, head ultrasound examinations are usually performed during the latter part of the first week.[135,136]

TREATMENT

Care of patients with IVH is centered on supportive care of the patient and family, stabilization in attempts to limit extension of the lesion, and such therapies as are needed for long-term sequelae, such as ventriculoperitoneal shunting for posthemorrhagic hydrocephalus.

COMPLICATIONS

Prognosis after IVH correlates roughly with the extent of the primary lesion,[134] but it is also affected by the presence or absence of other illness or injury. For patients with only a grade 1 or 2 IVH, the prognosis appears to be essentially the same as for patients without IVH and the same degree of underlying illness; approximately 10% will have neurodevelopmental disability noted during long-term follow-up.[137] Infants with grade 3 hemorrhage as a group have approximately a 40% incidence of significant neurologic sequelae.[138] Grade 4 intraventricular/periventricular hemorrhage carries the worst prognosis: up to 80% to 90% of these patients will have severe neurodevelopmental disability.[139] Those with the most extensive intraparenchymal involvement have the greatest severity of sequelae. The most common form of disability is a hemiparesis involving the contralateral side, or other forms of paresis and spasticity eventually earning the poorly named diagnosis of cerebral palsy. Visual difficulties and learning disabilities may occur as well. Mortality also corresponds roughly with the grade and extent of the lesion. Approximately 50% of those with a grade 4 hemorrhage may die in the short term.[106]

The course of a given patient with IVH may be complicated by other problems. The most common of these is posthemorrhagic hydrocephalus, occurring after intraventricular blood blocks cerebrospinal fluid flow through the aqueduct of Sylvius, or, more commonly, as a result of arachnoiditis causing obliteration of arachnoid villi and ensuing communicating hydrocephalus. Progressive ventricular dilatation is occasionally amenable to observation and/or medical treatment, but it often requires placement of a ventriculoperitoneal shunt. When complicating factors preclude definitive shunt placement (e.g., infection), sometimes the shunt is externalized or brought to a small reservoir at the subcutaneous level under the scalp, where it can be tapped under sterile conditions with a needle and fluid withdrawn. When a ventricular shunt is externalized, it is mandatory that the patient's head be kept in proper relation to the reservoir bag and the rest of the body, usually under specific instructions from the neurosurgeon.

Periventricular leukomalacia and periventricular echodensity are two other entities that may arise in conjunction with IVH. Periventricular leukomalacia occurs possibly as a result of venous infarction of periventricular white matter. Intraparenchymal echodensities, or periventricular echodensities, may arise from the same or other factors, such as ischemia arising from hypocarbia- and hypoventilation-induced reductions in cerebral blood flow.

Both are associated with significant, often severe, neurodevelopmental disability. Periventricular leukomalacia and intraparenchymal echodensities may arise in the absence of IVH, although about 80% of cases of intraparenchymal echodensities are associated with severe IVH.[139]

PREVENTION

Efforts to prevent IVH may be made either prenatally or after delivery of the premature infant. Antenatal interventions evaluated have included phenobarbital, magnesium sulfate, and corticosteroids. Of these, only antenatal corticosteroids have been shown to clearly reduce the incidence and severity of IVH, and thus are recommended.[140]

Postnatal therapies that have been investigated as means of reducing IVH incidence/severity include phenobarbital, indomethacin, ethamsylate, and vitamin E. Of the therapies mentioned, only indomethacin has been shown to be of probable value in reducing the rate and severity of IVH.[141]

Pulmonary and respiratory care factors can, as discussed earlier, contribute to causation of IVH. Particular care should be taken to avoid factors producing fluctuations in cerebral blood flow, such as hypoxemia, hypercarbia and hypocarbia, and pneumothorax. Careful attention to assisted ventilation of premature infants may have long-lasting effects on their brain development.

REFERENCES

1. Stamenovic D: Micromechanical foundations of pulmonary elasticity. *Physiol Rev* 1990; 70:1117-1134.
2. Macklin MT, Macklin CC: Malignant interstitial emphysema of the lungs and mediastinum as an important occult complication in many respiratory diseases and other conditions: an interpretation of the clinical literature in the light of laboratory experiment. *Medicine* 1944; 23:281-358.
3. Ovenfors CO: Pulmonary interstitial emphysema: an experimental roentgen-diagnostic study. *Acta Radiol Suppl* 1964; 224:7-131.
4. Thibeault DW et al: Pulmonary interstitial emphysema, pneumomediastinum and pneumothorax. *Am J Dis Child* 1973; 126:611-614.
5. Kilbride HW, Thibeault DW: Neonatal complications of preterm premature rupture of membranes: pathophysiology and management. *Clin Perinatol* 2001; 28(4):761-785.
6. Gaylord MS et al: Predicting mortality in low birth weight infants with pulmonary interstitial emphysema. *Pediatrics* 1985; 76:219-224.
7. Hart SM et al: Pulmonary interstitial emphysema in very low birth weight infants. *Arch Dis Child* 1983; 58:612-615.
8. Watts JL et al: Chronic pulmonary disease in neonates after artificial ventilation: distribution of ventilation and pulmonary interstitial emphysema. *Pediatrics* 1977; 60: 273-281.
9. Morisot C et al: Risk factors for fatal pulmonary interstitial emphysema in neonates. *Eur J Pediatr* 1990; 149: 493-495.
10. Fitzgerald D et al: Dexamethasone for pulmonary interstitial emphysema in preterm infants. *Biol Neonate* 1998; 73:34-39.
11. Keszler M et al: Multicentre controlled trial comparing high-frequency jet ventilation and conventional mechanical ventilation in newborn infants with pulmonary interstitial emphysema. *J Pediatr* 1991; 119:85-93.
12. Morrow G, Hope JW, Boggs TR: Pneumomediastinum, a silent lesion in the newborn. *J Pediatr* 1967; 70:554-560.
13. Marchand P: The anatomy and applied anatomy of mediastinal fascia. *Thorax* 1951; 6:359-368.
14. Quattromani FL et al: Fascial relationship of thymus: radiologic-pathologic correlation in neonatal pneumomediastinum. *AJR Am J Roentgenol* 1981; 137:1209-1211.
15. Volberg FM Jr, Everett CJ, Brill PW: Radiologic features of inferior pulmonary ligament air collections in neonates with respiratory distress. *Radiology* 1979; 130: 357-360.
16. Rabinowitz JG, Wolf BS: Roentgen significance of the pulmonary ligament. *Radiology* 1966; 87:1013-1020.
17. Palmer EA et al: Incidence and early course of retinopathy of prematurity: the Cryotherapy for Retinopathy of Prematurity Cooperative Group. *Ophthalmology* 1991; 98:1628-1640.
18. Johns KJ et al: Retinopathy of prematurity in infants with cyanotic congenital heart disease. *Am J Dis Child* 1991; 145:200-203.
19. Lawless S et al: New pigtail catheter for pleural drainage in pediatric patients. *Crit Care Med* 1989; 17:173-175.
20. Wood B, Dubik M: A new device for pleural drainage in newborn infants. *Pediatrics* 1995; 96:955-956.
21. Nostrand CV, Beamish WE, Schiff D: Neonatal pneumopericardium. *Can Med Assoc J* 1975; 112:186-189.
22. Cimmino CV: Some radio-diagnostic notes on pneumomediastinum, pneumothorax, and pneumopericardium (Editorial). *Va Med Mon* 1973; 94:205-212.
23. Mansfield PB et al: Pneumopericardium and pneumomediastinum in infants and children. *J Pediatr Surg* 1973; 8:691-699.
24. Pomerance JJ et al: Pneumopericardium complicating respiratory distress syndrome: role of conservative management. *J Pediatr* 1974; 84:883-886.
25. Glenski JA, Hall RT: Neonatal pneumopericardium: analysis of ventilatory variables. *Crit Care Med* 1984; 12:439-444.
26. Burt T, Lester P: Neonatal pericardium. *Radiology* 1982; 142:81-84.
27. Emery RW et al: Surgical treatment of pneumopericardium in the neonate. *World J Surg* 1978; 2:631-638.
28. Emery RW, Foker J, Thompson TR: Neonatal pneumopericardium: a surgical emergency. *Ann Thorac Surg* 1984; 37:128-132.
29. Emery RW, Lindsay WG, Nicoloff DM: Placement of pericardial drainage tube for the treatment of pneumopericardium in the neonate. *Am Thorac Surg* 1978; 26:84-85.
30. Emery RW: Surgical treatment of pneumopericardium in the neonate. *World J Surg* 1978; 2:631-637.
31. Leonides JC et al: Pneumoperitoneum in ventilated newborns: a medical or a surgical problem? *Am J Dis Child* 1974; 128:677-681.
32. Chang JHT, Hernandez J: Ventilator-induced pneumoperitoneum—a rapid diagnosis. *Pediatrics* 1980; 66:135-136.
33. Burnard ED et al: Pulmonary insufficiency in prematurity. *Aust Paediatr J* 1965; 1:12-38.
34. Krauss AN, Klain DB, Auld PAM: Chronic pulmonary insufficiency of prematurity. *Pediatrics* 1975; 55:55-58.
35. Wilson G, Mikity VG: A new form of respiratory disease in premature infants. *Am J Dis Child* 1960; 99:489-499.

36. Shennan A et al: Abnormal pulmonary outcomes in premature infants: prediction from oxygen requirement in the neonatal period. *Pediatrics* 1988; 82:527-532.

37. Northway WH, Rosan RC, Porter DY: Pulmonary disease following respiratory therapy of hyaline membrane disease. *N Engl J Med* 1967; 276:357-368.

38. Hodgman JE et al: Chronic respiratory distress in the premature infant. *Pediatrics* 1969; 44:179-195.

39. Swyer PR et al: The pulmonary syndrome of Wilson and Mikity. *Pediatrics* 1965; 36:374-383.

40. Thibeault DW et al: Radiologic findings in the lungs of premature infants. *J Pediatr* 1969; 74:1-10.

41. Coates AL et al: Long-term sequelae of the Wilson-Mikity syndrome. *J Pediatr* 1978; 92:247-252.

42. Edwards DK, Colby TV, Northway WH: Radiographic-pathologic correlation in bronchopulmonary dysplasia. *J Pediatr* 1979; 95:835-836.

43. Campbell RE: Intrapulmonary interstitial emphysema: a complication of hyaline membrane disease. *AJR* 1970; 110:449-456.

44. Sward-Comunelli SL et al: Airway muscle in preterm infants: changes during development. *J Pediatr* 1997; 130:570-576.

45. Jacob SV et al: Long-term pulmonary sequelae of severe bronchopulmonary dysplasia. *J Pediatr* 1998; 133: 193-200.

46. Broughton AR et al: Airway muscle in infants with congenital diaphragmatic hernia: response to treatment. *J Pediatr Surg* 1988; 33:1471-1475.

47. Charafeddine L, D'Angio CT, Phelps DL: Atypical chronic lung disease patterns in neonates. *Pediatrics* 1999; 103:759-765.

48. Rojas AM et al: Changing trends in the epidemiology and pathogenesis of neonatal chronic lung disease. *J Pediatr* 1995; 126:605-610.

49. Ogawa Y et al: Epidemiology and classification of chronic lung disease. *Pediatr Pulmonol* 1997; 16:25-26.

50. Kraybill EN et al: Risk factors for chronic lung disease in infants with birthweights of 751 to 1000 grams. *J Pediatr* 1989; 115:115-120.

51. Cooke RWI: Factors associated with chronic lung disease in preterm infants. *Arch Dis Child* 1991; 66:776-779.

52. Thibeault DW et al: Lung elastic tissue maturation and perturbations during evolution of chronic lung disease (CLD). *Pediatrics* 2000; 106:1452-1459.

53. Merritt TA et al: Elastase and alpha-1-proteinase inhibitor activity in tracheal aspirates during RDS. *J Clin Invest* 1983; 72:656-662.

54. Pierce MR, Bancalari E: The role of inflammation in the pathogenesis of bronchopulmonary dysplasia. *Pediatr Pulmonol* 1995; 19:371-378.

55. Swischuk LE, Shetty BP, John SD: The lungs in immature infants: how important is surfactant therapy in preventing chronic lung problems? *Pediatr Radiol* 1996; 26:508-511.

56. Thebaud B, Lacaze-Masmonteil T, Watterberg K: Postnatal glucocorticoids in very preterm infants: "The good, the bad, and the ugly"? *Pediatrics* 2001; 107(2):413-415.

57. Thibeault DW et al: Patent ductus arteriosus complicating the respiratory distress syndrome in preterm infants. *J Pediatr* 1975; 86:120.

58. Albertine KH et al: Chronic lung injury in preterm lambs: disordered respiratory tract development. *Am J Respir Crit Care Med* 1999; 159:945-958.

59. Thibeault DW et al: Chronic modifications of lung and heart development in glucocorticoid-treated newborn rats exposed to hyperoxia or room air. *Pediatr Pulmonol* 1993; 16:81-88.

60. Burri PH, Tschanz SA, Damke BM: Influence of postnatally administered glucocorticoids on rat lung growth. *Biol Neonate* 1995; 68:229-245.

61. Gross SJ et al: Effect of preterm birth on pulmonary function at school age: a prospective controlled study. *J Pediatr* 1998; 133:188-192.

62. Doyle LW et al: Bronchopulmonary dysplasia and very low birthweight: lung function at 11 years of age. *J Paediatr Child Health* 1996; 32:339-343.

63. Chernick V: Long-term pulmonary function studies in children with bronchopulmonary dysplasia: an ever-changing saga. *J Pediatr* 1998; 133:171-172.

64. Holinger L: Congenital laryngeal anomalies. In Holinger L, Lusk R, Green C, editors: *Pediatric laryngology and bronchoesophagology.* New York. Lippincott-Raven, 1997; pp 139–142.

65. de Blic J, Delacourt C, Scheinmann P: Ultrathin flexible bronchoscopy in neonatal intensive care units. *Arch Dis Child* 1991; 66:1383-1385.

66. Gonzalez C, Reilly JS, Bluestone CD: Synchronous airway lesions in infancy. *Ann Otol Rhinol Laryngol* 1987; 96:77-85.

67. Othersen B, Filler R: Tracheomalacia. In Othersen HB, editor: *The pediatric airway.* Philadelphia. WB Saunders, 1991; pp 97–106.

68. Cacciaguerra S, Bianchi A: Tracheal ring-graft reinforcement in lieu of tracheostomy for tracheomalacia. *Pediatr Surg Int* 1998; 13:556-559.

69. Schelhase DE et al: Diagnosis of tracheal injury in mechanically ventilated premature infants by flexible bronchoscopy: a pilot study. *Chest* 1990; 98:1219-1225.

70. Bhutani VK, Ritchie WG, Shaffer TH: Acquired tracheomegaly in very preterm neonates. *Am J Dis Child* 1986; 140:449-452.

71. Engle WA et al: Neonatal tracheobronchomegaly. *Am J Perinatol* 1987; 4:81-85.

72. Sotomayor JL et al: Large-airway collapse due to acquired tracheobronchomalacia in infancy. *Am J Dis Child* 1986; 140:367-371.

73. Cohn RC, Kercsmar C, Dearborn D: Safety and efficacy of flexible bronchoscopy in children with bronchopulmonary dysplasia. *Am J Dis Child* 1998; 142:1225-1228.

74. DeKeon M, Mosca R: Application of pulmonary graphics to congenital heart disease. In Dunn E, editor: *Neonatal and pediatric pulmonary graphics.* Armonk, NY. Futura, 1988; p 355.

75. Saunders RA et al: Racial variation in retinopathy of prematurity: the Cryotherapy for Retinopathy of Prematurity Cooperative Group. *Arch Ophthalmol* 1997; 115: 604-608.

76. Holmes JM et al: Carbon dioxide–induced retinopathy in the neonatal rat. *Curr Eye Res* 1998; 17:608-616.

77. Holmes JM, Duffner LA, Kappil JC: The effect of raised inspired carbon dioxide on developing rat retinal vasculature exposed to elevated oxygen. *Curr Eye Res* 1994; 13:779-782.

78. Shohat M et al: Retinopathy of prematurity: Incidence and risk factors. *Pediatrics* 1983; 72:159-163.

79. Organisciak DT et al: Retinal light damage in rats exposed to intermittent light: comparison with continuous light exposure. *Invest Ophthalmol Vis Sci* 1989; 30:795-805.

80. Glass P: Light and the developing retina. *Doc Ophthalmol* 1990; 74:195-203.

81. Fielder AR et al: Light and retinopathy of prematurity: does retinal location offer a clue? *Pediatrics* 1992; 89: 648-653.

82. Reynolds JD et al: Lack of efficacy of light reduction in preventing retinopathy of prematurity: Light Reduction

in Retinopathy of Prematurity (LIGHT-ROP) Cooperative Group. *N Engl J Med* 1998; 338:1572-1576.

83. Hesse L et al: Blood transfusion: iron load and retinopathy of prematurity. *Eur J Pediatr* 1997; 156:465-470.

84. Teoh SL et al: Duration of oxygen therapy and exchange transfusion as risk factors associated with retinopathy of prematurity in very low birthweight infants. *Eye* 1997; 9:733-737.

85. Caddell JL: Hypothesis: the possible role of magnesium and copper deficiency in retinopathy of prematurity. *Magnes Res* 1995; 8:261-270.

86. Alon T et al: Vascular endothelial growth factor acts as a survival factor for newly formed retinal vessels and has implications for retinopathy of prematurity. *Nat Med* 1995; 1:1024-1028.

87. Pierce EA, Foley ED, Smith LE: Regulation of vascular endothelial growth factor by oxygen in a model of retinopathy of prematurity [see comments] [published erratum appears in *Arch Ophthalmol* 1997; 115:427]. *Arch Ophthalmol* 1996; 114:1219-1228.

88. Robbins SG, Rajaratnam VS, Penn JS: Evidence for upregulation and redistribution of vascular endothelial growth factor (VEGF) receptors flt-1 and flk-1 in the oxygen-injured rat retina. *Growth Factors* 1998; 16:1-9.

89. An international classification of retinopathy of prematurity: the Committee for the Classification of Retinopathy of Prematurity. *Arch Ophthalmol* 1984; 102:1130-1134.

90. An international classification of retinopathy of prematurity: II. The classification of retinal detachment. The International Committee for the Classification of the Late Stages of Retinopathy of Prematurity [published erratum appears in *Arch Ophthalmol* 1987; 105:1498]. *Arch Ophthalmol* 1987; 105:906-912.

91. Johnson L et al: Vitamin E supplementation and the retinopathy of prematurity. *Ann N Y Acad Sci* 1982; 393:473-495.

92. Kretzer FL et al: Vitamin E protects against retinopathy of prematurity through action on spindle cells. *Nature* 1995; 309:793-795.

93. Johnson L et al: Effect of sustained pharmacologic vitamin E levels on incidence and severity of retinopathy of prematurity: a controlled clinical trial. *J Pediatr* 1989; 114:827-838.

94. Raju TN et al: Vitamin E prophylaxis to reduce retinopathy of prematurity: a reappraisal of published trials. *J Pediatr* 1997; 131:844-850.

95. Hittner HM, Rudolph AJ, Kretzer FL: Suppression of severe retinopathy of prematurity with vitamin E supplementation: Ultrastructural mechanism of clinical efficacy. *Ophthalmology* 1984; 91:1512-1523.

96. Tailoi CL, Gock B, Stone J: Supplemental oxygen therapy: basis for noninvasive treatment of retinopathy of prematurity. *Invest Ophthalmol Vis Sci* 1995; 36:1215-1230.

97. Gaynon MW et al: Supplemental oxygen may decrease progression of prethreshold disease to threshold retinopathy of prematurity. *J Perinatol* 1997; 17:434-438.

98. Stone J et al: Roles of vascular endothelial growth factor and astrocyte degeneration in the genesis of retinopathy of prematurity. *Invest Ophthalmol Vis Sci* 1996; 37:290-299.

99. Penn JS, Tolman BL, Lowery LA: Variable oxygen exposure causes preretinal neovascularization in the newborn rat. *Invest Ophthalmol Vis Sci* 1993; 34:576-585.

100. Bancalari E et al: Transcutaneous oxygen monitoring and retinopathy of prematurity. *Adv Exp Med Biol* 1987; 220:109-113.

101. Supplemental therapeutic oxygen for prethreshold retinopathy of prematurity (STOP-ROP), randomized controlled trial. I: primary outcomes. *Pediatrics* 2000; 105(2):295-310.

102. Flynn JT, Bancalari E: On "supplemental therapeutic oxygen for prethreshold retinopathy of prematurity (STOP-ROP), a randomized, control trial. I: primary outcomes." *J AAPOS* 2000; 4(2):65-66.

103. Hay WW Jr, Bell EF: Oxygen therapy, oxygen toxicity, and the STOP-ROP trial. *Pediatrics* 2000; 105(2):424-425.

104. Paneth N et al: Incidence and timing of germinal matrix/intraventricular hemorrhage in low birth weight infants. *Am J Epidemiol* 1993; 137:1167-1176.

105. Volpe JJ: *Neurology of the newborn,* ed 3. Philadelphia. WB Saunders, 1995.

106. Ment LR et al: Germinal matrix microvascular maturation correlates inversely with the risk period for neonatal intraventricular hemorrhage. *Brain Res Dev Brain Res* 1995; 84:142-149.

107. Kamei A et al: Developmental change in type VI collagen in human cerebral vessels. *Pediatr Neurol* 1992; 8:183-186.

108. Pape KE, Wigglesworth JS: *Haemorrhage, ischaemia and the perinatal brain.* Philadelphia. JB Lippincott, 1979.

109. Kuban KC, Gilles FH: Human telencephalic angiogenesis. *Ann Neurol* 1985; 17:539-548.

110. Lou HC, Lassen NA, Friis-Hansen B: Impaired autoregulation of cerebral blood flow in the distressed newborn infant. *J Pediatr* 1979; 94:118-121.

111. Lou HC et al: Pressure passive cerebral blood flow and breakdown of the blood-brain barrier in experimental fetal asphyxia. *Acta Paediatr Scand* 1979; 68:57-63.

112. Pryds O: Control of cerebral circulation in the high-risk neonate. *Ann Neurol* 1991; 30:321-329.

113. Greisen G: Cerebral blood flow in preterm infants during the first week of life. *Acta Paediatr Scand* 1986; 75:43-51.

114. Miall-Allen VM et al: Blood pressure fluctuation and intraventricular hemorrhage in the preterm infant of less than 31 weeks' gestation [see comments]. *Pediatrics* 1989; 83:657-661.

115. Milligan DW: Failure of autoregulation and intraventricular haemorrhage in preterm infants. *Lancet* 1980; 1:896-898.

116. Perlman JM, McMenamin JB, Volpe JJ: Fluctuating cerebral blood-flow velocity in respiratory-distress syndrome: relation to the development of intraventricular hemorrhage. *N Engl J Med* 1983; 309:204-209.

117. Lott JW, Conner GK, Phillips JB: Umbilical artery catheter blood sampling alters cerebral blood flow velocity in preterm infants. *J Perinatol* 1996; 16:341-345.

118. Perlman JM, Hill A, Volpe JJ: The effect of patent ductus arteriosus on flow velocity in the anterior cerebral arteries: ductal steal in the premature newborn infant. *J Pediatr* 1981; 99:767-771.

119. Evans N, Kluckow M: Early ductal shunting and intraventricular haemorrhage in ventilated preterm infants. *Arch Dis Child Fetal Neonatal Ed* 1996; 75:F183-186.

120. Amato M, Fauchere JC, Hermann U Jr: Coagulation abnormalities in low birth weight infants with peri-intraventricular hemorrhage. *Neuropediatrics* 1988; 19:154-157.

121. Andrew M et al: Clinical impact of neonatal thrombocytopenia. *J Pediatr* 1987; 110:457-464.

122. Papile LA et al: Relationship of intravenous sodium bicarbonate infusions and cerebral intraventricular hemorrhage. *J Pediatr* 1978; 93:834-836.

123. Wallin LA et al: Neonatal intracranial hemorrhage: II. Risk factor analysis in an inborn population. *Early Hum Dev* 1990; 23:129-137.

124. O'Shea TM et al: Perinatal events and the risk of intra-parenchymal echodensity in very-low-birthweight neonates. *Paediatr Perinatal Epidemiol* 1998; 12:408-421.

125. Hill A, Perlman JM, Volpe JJ: Relationship of pneumothorax to occurrence of intraventricular hemorrhage in the premature newborn. *Pediatrics* 1982; 69:144-149.

126. High-frequency oscillatory ventilation compared with conventional intermittent mechanical ventilation in the treatment of respiratory failure in preterm infants: neurodevelopmental status at 16 to 24 months of postterm age. The HIFI Study Group. *J Pediatr* 1990; 117:939-946.

127. Tamura M et al: Comparison of the incidence of intracranial hemorrhage following conventional mechanical ventilation and high frequency oscillation in beagle puppies. *Acta Paediatr Jpn* 1992; 34:398-403.

128. Ogawa Y et al: A multicenter randomized trial of high frequency oscillatory ventilation as compared with conventional mechanical ventilation in preterm infants with respiratory failure. *Early Hum Dev* 1993; 32:1-10.

129. Cheung PY et al: Rescue high frequency oscillatory ventilation for preterm infants: neurodevelopmental outcome and its prediction. *Biol Neon* 1997; 71:282-291.

130. Gerstmann DR et al: The Provo multicenter early high-frequency oscillatory ventilation trial: Improved pulmonary and clinical outcome in respiratory distress syndrome [see comments]. *Pediatrics* 1996; 98:1044-1057.

131. Clark RH et al: Intraventricular hemorrhage and high-frequency ventilation: a meta-analysis of prospective clinical trials. *Pediatrics* 1996; 98:1058-1061.

132. Bhuta T, Henderson-Smart DJ: Elective high-frequency oscillatory ventilation versus conventional ventilation in preterm infants with pulmonary dysfunction: systematic review and meta-analyses. *Pediatrics* 1997; 100:E6.

133. Lazzara A et al: Clinical predictability of intraventricular hemorrhage in preterm infants. *Pediatrics* 1980; 65:30-34.

134. Papile LA et al: Incidence and evolution of subependymal and intraventricular hemorrhage: a study of infants with birth weights less than 1,500 gm. *J Pediatr* 1978; 92:529-534.

135. Dolfin T et al: Incidence, severity, and timing of subependymal and intraventricular hemorrhages in preterm infants born in a perinatal unit as detected by serial real-time ultrasound. *Pediatrics* 1983; 71:541-546.

136. Perlman JM, Volpe JJ: Intraventricular hemorrhage in extremely small premature infants. *Am J Dis Child* 1986; 140:1122-1124.

137. Lowe J, Papile L: Neurodevelopmental performance of very-low-birth-weight infants with mild periventricular, intraventricular hemorrhage: outcome at 5 to 6 years of age. *Am J Dis Child* 1990; 144:1242-1245.

138. Papile LA, Munsick-Bruno G, Schaefer A: Relationship of cerebral intraventricular hemorrhage and early childhood neurologic handicaps. *J Pediatr* 1983; 103:273-277.

139. Guzzetta F et al: Periventricular intraparenchymal echodensities in the premature newborn: critical determinant of neurologic outcome. *Pediatrics* 1986; 78:995-1006.

140. Effect of corticosteroids for fetal maturation on perinatal outcomes. *NIH Consensus Statement* 1994; 12:1-24.

141. Ment LR et al: Low-dose indomethacin and prevention of intraventricular hemorrhage: a multicenter randomized trial. *Pediatrics* 1994; 93:543-550.

CHAPTER 31

Congenital Cardiac Defects

James P. Keenan
John W. Salyer

It has been suggested that congenital cardiac anomalies are the most common cardiac conditions of childhood in industrialized nations.[1] As recently as the turn of the twentieth century, conventional medical wisdom held that many congenital cardiac anomalies were incompatible with life and that little could be done to ameliorate their effects.[2] Congenital heart disease occurs in about 10 in 1000 live births.[3] Advances in the identification and treatment of these conditions have been no less than revolutionary, and improved pharmacologic and surgical interventions have contributed to a dramatic drop in infant mortality.

CARDIOPULMONARY ANATOMY AND PHYSIOLOGY

Knowledge of blood flow during fetal circulation, changes that occur at birth (see Chapter 2), circulation of a normal heart, persistent fetal circulation, and the importance of the ductus arteriosus are essential to understanding the treatment and management of congenital cardiac anomalies.

ANATOMY AND BLOOD FLOW OF THE NORMAL HEART

The normal heart can be thought of conceptually as a pump consisting of four chambers (Figs. 31-1 and 31-2). The right atrium (RA) receives blood from all parts of the body (except the lungs) through three veins: (1) the superior vena cava brings blood from parts of the body superior to the heart; (2) the inferior vena cava brings blood from parts of the body inferior to the heart; and (3) the coronary sinus drains blood from most of the vessels supplying the walls of the heart. The RA then delivers the blood into the right ventricle (RV), which pumps it into the main pulmonary artery. This artery divides into a right and a left pulmonary artery, each of which carries blood to the lungs. In the lungs, carbon dioxide diffuses out of the blood and oxygen diffuses in. This oxygenated blood is then returned to the heart

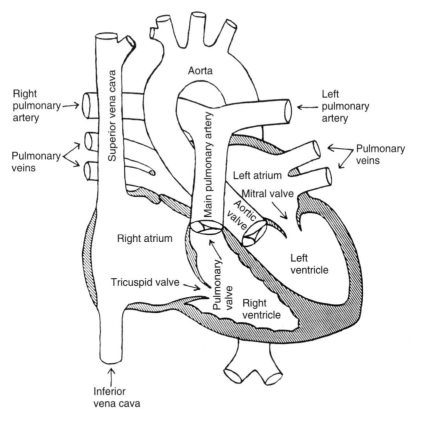

Fig. 31-1

Anatomy of the normal heart and great vessels. (From Mullin CE, Mayer DC: *Congenital heart disease: a diagrammatic atlas.* New York. John Wiley & Sons, 1988.)

through four pulmonary veins that empty into the left atrium (LA), from which the blood is pumped into the left ventricle (LV). The blood is then pumped from the LV into the aorta and from there to all other parts of the systemic circulation.

The size of each chamber of the heart varies according to its function. The RA, which must collect blood coming from nearly all parts of the body, is slightly larger than the LA, which receives blood only from the lungs. The thickness of the chamber walls varies, too. The atria are thin walled because they need only enough cardiac muscle to create pressure adequate to deliver the blood into the ventricles. This is relatively easy because at the same time that the atria contract, the ventricles relax (diastole). The RV has a thicker layer of myocardium than does the atria because it must overcome pulmonary vascular resistance (PVR). The LV has the thickest walls because it must pump blood at higher pressures through thousands of miles of vessels in the head, trunk, and extremities. Atrioventricular (AV) valves lie between the atria and the ventricles. The right AV valve is also called

the tricuspid valve because it consists of three flaps, or cusps. The left AV valve has two flaps and is called the bicuspid or mitral valve. Both arteries that exit the heart have a semilunar valve that prevents blood from flowing back into the heart. The pulmonary semilunar valve lies in the opening where the pulmonary artery leaves the RV. The aortic semilunar valve is situated at the opening between the LV and the aorta. Like the AV valves, the semilunar valves permit blood to flow in one direction only, in this case from the ventricles into the arteries.

ADAPTATION TO EXTRAUTERINE LIFE

Once the umbilical vessels are clamped, the low-pressure system of the placenta is removed from the fetal circulation. As the lungs inflate and gas exchange occurs, the increase in Pao_2 causes dilatation of the pulmonary artery bed, resulting in a reduction in PVR. Pressures in the right side of the heart decrease and pressures in the left side increase. During this time, the pressure in the aorta increases and becomes greater than the pressure in

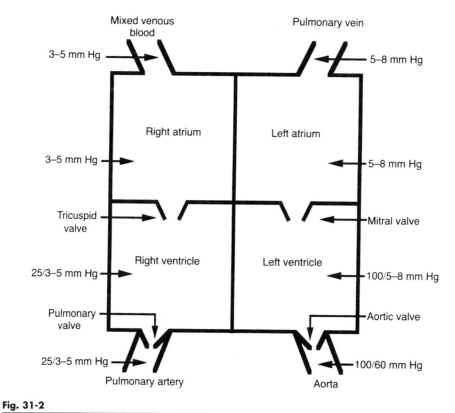

Fig. 31-2

Pressures of the normal heart and great vessels of the older child.

the pulmonary artery, thus decreasing the amount of shunting through the ductus arteriosus and foramen ovale. During the immediate postnatal period, these two shunts may not close completely. Closure of the ductus arteriosus usually occurs within the first 24 hours to 2 weeks of life, except in the premature infant in whom musculature of the ductus arteriosus may not be well developed and its ability to constrict is limited. In these infants, the PVR will be lower than the systemic vascular resistance (SVR) and blood will flow into the lungs from the systemic circulation (left to right). The ductus arteriosus may not close completely in some postterm infants (e.g., in meconium aspiration). These patients may experience very high PVR, and blood will then flow from right to left through the ductus arteriosus from the pulmonary circulation to the systemic circulation, bypassing the lungs. Because the foramen ovale flap allows blood to flow only from right to left, it closes when the pressures in the LA become greater than those in the RA. If the foramen ovale lacks a flaplike structure or has a defective one, the opening begins to function as an atrial septal defect (ASD).

CLASSIFICATION OF CARDIAC ANOMALIES

When discussing congenital cardiac anomalies, two categories have typically been used to classify these lesions—cyanotic and acyanotic—referring to whether the principal direction of extrapulmonary shunting is right to left (cyanotic) or left to right (acyanotic). However, patients with right-to-left shunting do not always actually manifest cyanosis, whereas some patients with left-to-right shunting may well be cyanotic. Within these two categories, numerous subcategories have been recognized: cyanosis as the outstanding physical feature, cyanosis with moderate respiratory distress, and cyanosis with low cardiac output. For simplicity, this chapter separates the anomalies into the two categories describing the shunting of blood: left-to-right shunts (increased pulmonary blood flow) and right-to-left shunts (decreased pulmonary blood flow). When possible, the description, radiographic findings, presurgical management, surgical repair, and postsurgical management are discussed for each cardiac anomaly.

In congenital cardiac disease with a right-to-left shunt (often termed *cyanotic cardiac defect*), desaturated systemic venous blood is shunted from right to left within the heart (extrapulmonary), bypassing the lungs and entering the systemic arterial circulation. Acrocyanosis and central cyanosis are frequent findings and lead to the early diagnosis of most of these lesions. In congenital cardiac disease with a left-to-right shunt (often termed *acyanotic cardiac defect*), oxygenated blood is shunted from left to right within the heart, mixing with deoxygenated blood. Even though there is a mixing of oxygenated and deoxygenated blood, these infants often appear pink and healthy. The left-to-right shunt often results in increased pulmonary blood flow as well as increased PVR. With both types of shunts, there are several lesions that depend on a patent ductus arteriosus (PDA) for adequate pulmonary blood flow. These anomalies are also called ductal-dependent lesions because spontaneous closure of the ductus arteriosus can prove catastrophic (e.g., coarctation of the aorta, tetralogy of Fallot). Often, acyanotic infants are discharged home with their condition undiagnosed, with symptoms developing as the ductus arteriosus begins to close 12 to 48 hours later.

CONGENITAL CARDIAC ANOMALIES

PATENT DUCTUS ARTERIOSUS AND PERSISTENT PULMONARY HYPERTENSION

During fetal life, the ductus arteriosus allows most of the right ventricular output to bypass the lungs and be shunted from right-to-left from the pulmonary artery to the aorta. Within hours to days after birth, the ductus arteriosus closes spontaneously as a result of hormonal, chemical, and blood gas changes. However, it does not constrict but remains open in some infants, especially those born prematurely, resulting in a persistent fetal circulation. The term *persistent pulmonary hypertension of the newborn* (PPHN) is replacing *persistent fetal circulation* in recent literature. PPHN can also refer to the combination of a PDA and some left-to-right shunting that may also occur through the foramen ovale. After birth, as the PVR falls, the pressure in the aorta is higher than that in the pulmonary artery and the direction of blood flow through the PDA reverses. The blood flow is now from left-to-right from the aorta to the pulmonary artery, causing an increase in pulmonary blood flow (Fig. 31-3). The constrictor response of the ductus arteriosus to oxygen and the dilator effect of prostaglandin E_2 are functions of gestational age; hence, the greater the prematurity, the more delayed the ductal closure.[4-7] Because delayed closure of the ductus arteriosus is associated with respiratory distress syndrome and prematurity, PDA is the most common cardiac defect seen in neonatal intensive care units. Precise statistics on the incidence of this condition are not available, but it has been reported that approximately 45% of infants weighing less than 1750 g and approximately 80% of those weighing less than 1250 g have some clinical evidence of a PDA.[8] If both PPHN and a PDA are suggested, the presence of ductal shunting can be confirmed by obtaining preductal (right radial or temporal artery) and postductal (umbilical artery) blood samples with the infant breathing 100% oxygen. A differential of greater than 15 mm Hg is considered indicative of ductal shunting of some kind.[9,10]

In numerous congenital cardiac defects it is imperative for survival that a PDA is present to provide either systemic or pulmonary blood flow. In these defects all attempts, pharmacologic or surgical, will be made to maintain its patency.

A persistent PDA that is not associated with a congenital cardiac defect can eventually lead to congestive heart failure and pulmonary hypertension. Although a PDA may close spontaneously at any time, it is unlikely that this will occur after the patient is 1 year of age; therefore, surgical repair is required. Chest radiographic findings are usually normal, but in extreme cases in which congestive heart failure develops, there may be enlarged pulmonary vascular markings. The definitive diagnosis of PDA is typically made with echocardiography.

Medical management of the PDA includes close scrutiny of fluid and electrolyte balance and, if necessary, treatment with indomethacin, which results in a gradual closing of the ductus arteriosus over 24 to 48 hours.[11] The use of indomethacin is most successful when it is administered to infants younger than 10 days of age.[12] Also important is the maintenance of adequate hematocrit and hemoglobin values. Failure to maintain these values may require an increase in cardiac output to sustain peripheral oxygenation, thus imposing additional work on an already stressed myocardium. The decision to treat a PDA is usually a complex one and is often preceded by an inability to wean the infant from ventilatory support. If evidence of congestive heart failure develops, digoxin and diuretics can be used to improve cardiac function and limit vascular engorgement, respectively, although digoxin in extremely small preterm infants has been described as relatively ineffective and potentially toxic.[8] The Pao_2 and Sao_2 can be normal to low, depending on the degree of venous admixing.

Surgical repair of a PDA before the tenth day of life has been reported to reduce the duration of ventilatory support and hospital stays and result in

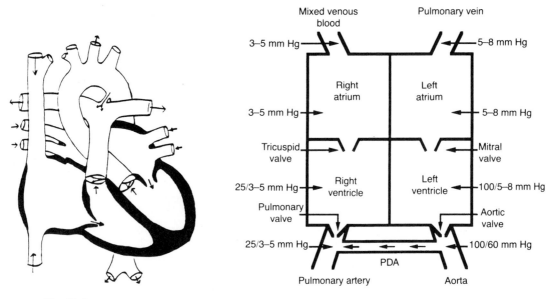

Fig. 31-3

Patent ductus arteriosus. Communication between the pulmonary artery and the aorta. (From *Congenital heart abnormalities.* Clinical Education Aid No. 7. Columbus, OH. Ross Products Division, Abbott Laboratories, 1970.)

lower morbidity.[13] Practice varies considerably, but the most common approach involves a trial of indomethacin followed within a few days by surgical repair if symptoms persist. The surgery can now be performed with minimal morbidity and mortality and indeed is often carried out without anesthetic gases in the intensive care unit.[14] The surgery for neonates is ligation of the ductus arteriosus with a heavy suture through a lateral chest wall incision; in older children the ductus arteriosus is cut and separated and the ends are sutured. Postoperative ventilatory support is not often necessary except in those patients who required it preoperatively. Normal arterial blood gas and pulse oximetry measurements can be expected.

ATRIAL SEPTAL DEFECT

An ASD is a communication between the right and left atria (Fig. 31-4). Several anatomic types result in a defect of the lower or upper sections of the septum, including (1) an incompetent foramen ovale that allows regurgitation between the atria, (2) a developmental defect in the septum itself, or (3) failure of development in the endocardial cushion area. Blood flow is usually shunted from left to right through the ASD, with an increase in pulmonary blood flow occurring. This rarely produces congestive heart failure in children, although the RV may hypertrophy because of the increased blood flow.[15] Although symptoms have been reported in the neonatal period,

most of these patients remain asymptomatic until school age, with only approximately 8% having their conditions identified before they are 2 years old.[16,17] For cosmetic reasons, minimally invasive surgical repairs are now being done successfully, replacing full sternotomies that were previously necessary for ASDs and ventricular septal defects (VSDs).[18,19] Chest radiographic findings are usually normal, but in extreme cases in which congestive heart failure develops there may be enlarged pulmonary vascular markings and cardiomegaly.

If congestive heart failure is present, surgical repair is indicated and the defect is closed during cardiopulmonary bypass, usually by a simple suture. If the defect is large enough, a tailored patch, usually of polyester, is sewn into the septum. Postsurgical management often includes mechanical ventilation, during which blood gas and pulse oximetry measurements can be expected to be normal.

VENTRICULAR SEPTAL DEFECT

A VSD is a communication between the right and left ventricles (Fig. 31-5). It may be as small as a pinhole or large enough to make the ventricular septum almost completely absent. The location can be anywhere along the ventricular septum. In about 10% of infants with VSD, other anomalies are also present. Approximately 20% of all patients with congenital cardiac anomalies have a VSD as the only lesion.[20,21] The majority of the blood flow is

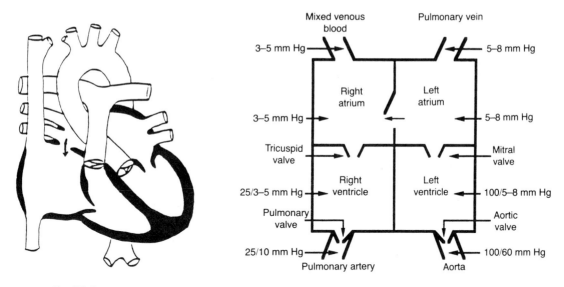

Fig. 31-4

Atrial septal defect. Communication between the right and left atria through the septum. (From Mullin CE, Mayer DC: *Congenital heart disease: a diagrammatic atlas.* New York. John Wiley & Sons, 1988.)

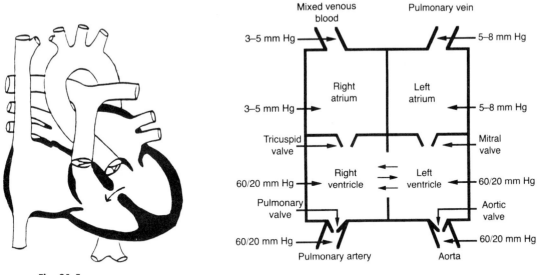

Fig. 31-5

Ventricular septal defect. Communication between the right and left ventricles through the septum. (From *Congenital heart abnormalities.* Clinical Education Aid No. 7. Columbus, OH. Ross Products Division, Abbott Laboratories, 1970.)

shunted from left to right, because the resistance of the pulmonary vascular bed is relatively low and shunting occurs during ventricular systole.

The shunt may be large and result in congestive heart failure. If the VSD is small, the heart may appear normal on the chest radiograph. If the VSD is large, the cardiac silhouette will be enlarged and the pulmonary vascular markings increased, as is seen in infants with congestive heart failure. A left-to-right shunt may increase pulmonary blood flow to the point that the increased pressure and volume result in thickening and fibrosis of the pulmonary arterioles. This causes permanent damage to the pulmonary vascular bed, resulting in irreversible pulmonary hypertension and/or congestive heart failure.[22] Resistance in the pulmonary system may become greater than that in the systemic circulation, and the left-to-right shunt is reversed to a right-to-left shunt. This is called Eisenmenger's syndrome and is rarely seen in children today because most defects are corrected before irreversible damage can occur. These patients have noncompliant lungs and experience difficulty breathing.

The majority of VSDs close spontaneously within the first and second years of life, and in most cases no intervention is necessary. If medical management is mandated, it usually includes digoxin and furosemide. The decision to proceed from medical management to surgical repair is difficult and varies considerably among patients. Typically, patients in whom medical management fails exhibit poor growth, repeated pulmonary infections, and pulmonary hypertension.[23] The PaO_2 and SaO_2 will be low to normal, depending on the degree of mixing across the ventricular wall.

Pulmonary banding is sometimes performed to help direct the cardiac blood flow by narrowing the diameter of the pulmonary artery and thus increasing resistance to blood flow. It consists of tightly wrapping a Dacron or polytetrafluoroethylene (Teflon) strip around the pulmonary artery and decreasing the degree of left-to-right shunting. This is a relatively simple palliative procedure that does not correct the defect itself. It is often performed when an infant or child's condition is too unstable for the corrective repair to be undertaken; the banding allows the child to grow and the condition to stabilize before open-heart surgery is performed. If total repair is indicated, the defect is closed during cardiopulmonary bypass, usually by suturing. If the defect is large, a tailored patch (usually Dacron) is sewn to the septum. If the patient has undergone previous pulmonary banding, the band is removed at this time as well. Brief postoperative mechanical ventilation is used in most patients. Normal arterial blood gas and pulse oximetry measurements can be expected.

ATRIOVENTRICULAR CANAL DEFECT

The term *AV canal* refers to an anomaly in which there is incomplete development of the septa between both the atria and the ventricles and a common AV valve that takes origin from both atria (Fig. 31-6). Simply stated, there is a large ASD and a VSD with deformed mitral and tricuspid valves, resulting in a large "hole" that allows the blood to flow within any of the heart chambers. The defect has a "scooped-out" appearance, hence the term *canal*. There are varying degrees of AV canal, but all involve a mixing of atrial and ventricular blood. There is a large left-to-right shunt, resulting in increased pulmonary

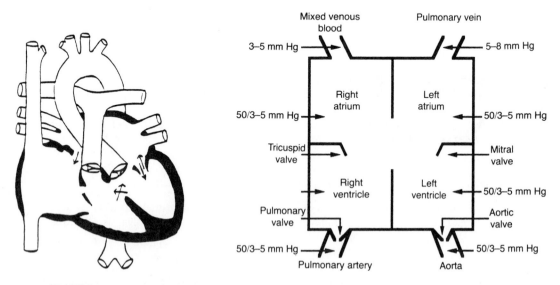

Fig. 31-6

Atrioventricular canal defect. Incomplete development of the atrial and ventricular septa, which allows complete cardiac mixing of blood. (From Mullin CE, Mayer DC: *Congenital heart disease: a diagrammatic atlas.* New York. John Wiley & Sons, 1988.)

blood flow. AV canal anomalies are the most common type of heart disease present in infants with Down syndrome.[24]

Chest radiography usually reveals cardiomegaly with increased pulmonary vascular markings and congestive heart failure. Although a mechanism by which lung overinflation is associated with increased pulmonary blood flow has not been identified, it has been suggested that pulmonary hyperinflation is often present secondary to increased pulmonary blood flow.[25] The presurgical management of a newborn with an AV canal defect is designed to ameliorate the effects of volume overloading and includes the administration of digoxin and diuretics. This is often sufficient for many months before surgery is required. Pulse oximetry values often remain low because of venous admixing and left-to-right shunting. Supplemental oxygen may be given, but this should be carried out judiciously to minimize pulmonary vascular dilatation, which might increase pulmonary vascular engorgement.

There are divergent opinions regarding the best surgical approach to managing AV canal defects. Banding of the pulmonary artery to increase PVR and thus decrease pulmonary blood flow has been the procedure of choice because of its simplicity. This procedure lessens congestive heart failure but does nothing for the defect itself (i.e., it is palliative), giving the infant time to become stabilized and gain weight before future repairs are undertaken. A complete surgical repair is sometimes performed without banding of the pulmonary artery. The atrial and ventricular septa are closed with a patch or with whatever part of the septum is available. The common AV valve (tricuspid and mitral) is divided and reconstructed on the newly constructed septum. An abnormal mitral valve is reported in most all AV canal malformations.[26] Rebuilding the common valve and making two valves tend to be the most difficult parts of the procedure and frequently result in a leaky or deformed mitral valve. Although this is a significant undertaking, especially in infants at risk, the overall outcome is generally better than banding of the pulmonary artery alone.[27]

Postoperative management varies, depending on the surgical procedure performed. If pulmonary artery banding is performed, the mixing of oxygenated and deoxygenated blood will continue; therefore, lower PaO_2 and SaO_2 values should be expected. If a complete repair is performed, normal arterial oxygenation can be anticipated. Because of the complexity of the septal repairs performed, leaking sometimes occurs within the heart (between the pulmonary and systemic circulations), with the direction of shunting usually being from left to right. Whenever the septa are surgically repaired, there can be an interference of the conductive system; therefore, these patients have pacing wires placed to treat emergent arrhythmias.

AORTIC STENOSIS

Left ventricular outflow obstructions include a number of conditions that cause a physical impediment to the ejection of blood from the left ventricle. They include valvular aortic stenosis, coarctation of the aorta, obstructed aortic arch, and aortic atresia or hypoplastic left-heart syndrome.[28] Valvular aortic stenosis is a narrowing located below (subvalvular), at (valvular), or above (supravalvular) the aortic valve (Fig. 31-7). The degree of clinical manifestation of impaired cardiac function is related to the position of the stenosis, with valvular stenosis usually constituting the worst presentation. The myocardium is always hypertrophied, with the ventricle overdistended to varying degrees. If left ventricular pressures are great enough, congestive heart failure may result. Occasionally, left atrial pressures and the resulting distention can cause blood to flow from left to right through the foramen ovale.

The chest radiograph reveals findings similar to those of an infant in congestive heart failure. The heart is usually enlarged and may be massive. The pulmonary vessels are distinct because of pulmonary venous congestion. Infants with aortic stenosis are rarely symptomatic in the first month of life. If they are symptomatic, it generally indicates that they are critically ill and that cardiac output is extremely low. These infants are likely to die unless surgery is performed rapidly.[28] Ventilatory support is necessary to relieve acidosis, cyanosis, and the respiratory distress that often accompanies this defect. These patients are often ductal dependent, with systemic circulation depending on blood flow through the ductus arteriosus. Although supplemental oxygen is most likely indicated, it should be given judiciously to limit the vasodilatory effects of oxygen on the pulmonary vasculature and the constricting effect on the ductus arteriosus. The most important aspect of presurgical management of symptomatic aortic stenosis is the use of prostaglandin E_1 to minimize ductal constriction.[29] Dosages range from 0.05 to 0.1 µg/kg/min.[28] Diuretics and digoxin are sometimes given because treatment parallels that of congestive heart failure.

A variety of procedures have been reported for correcting aortic stenosis.[30-33] Current surgical techniques for correction of valvular stenosis include (1) removal of the stenotic area of the aortic valve (usually a complete aortic valvotomy), (2) repair of the supravalvular area with a patch to widen the stenosis, and (3) balloon dilation or valvuloplasty of the aortic valve. Balloon valvuloplasty is the most widely used procedure in the

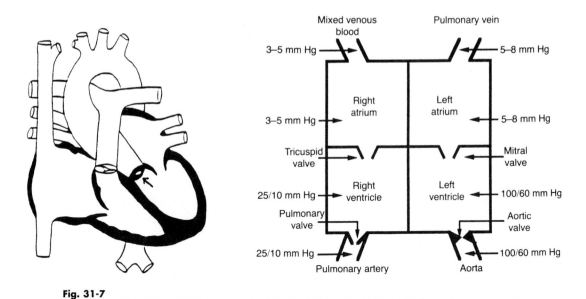

Fig. 31-7

Aortic stenosis. Outflow obstruction of the aorta, impeding blood flow from the left ventricle. (From *Congenital heart abnormalities.* Clinical Education Aid No. 7. Columbus, OH. Ross Products Division, Abbott Laboratories, 1970.)

treatment of aortic stenosis if there are no other extenuating circumstances.[34] If valvotomy is performed, it may be carried out by employing either open or closed techniques, that is, placing the patient on cardiopulmonary bypass and opening the heart or performing the surgery blindly through an opening made in the ventricular wall without the benefit of bypass. Normal arterial blood and pulse oximetry values can be expected. Derangements in cardiac output are sometimes encountered secondary to the combined effects of the patient's having to adjust to considerable alterations in cardiac anatomy and physiology and having to recover from the gross physiologic insult of thoracic surgery. Because some of the surgical repairs involve inducing hypothermia, careful attention to temperature stability should be considered.

COARCTATION OF THE AORTA

Coarctation of the aorta is defined as severe narrowing of the aortic lumen resulting in decreased blood flow through the aorta (Fig. 31-8). This narrowing causes an increased left ventricular pressure and workload. As an isolated anomaly, this defect is the fifth or sixth most commonly occurring congenital cardiac anomaly.[35] The hospital mortality rate is 3% to 4% for infants with this defect alone but 24% to 32% for those who also have the often-associated

anomalies, such as VSD.[36] During fetal life, coarctation results in an increase in left ventricular outflow resistance compared with right ventricular outflow resistance. Thus the RV assumes the preponderance of work with regard to systemic circulation. Ultimately, the RV becomes hypertrophic as a result.

The location of the coarctation may be either preductal or postductal. A preductal narrowing (the more serious defect) is frequently associated with other cardiac anomalies such as VSD, PDA, and transposition of the great arteries. In the postductal type, there is a pressure gradient between the proximal and distal (with respect to the coarctation) portions of the aorta during fetal life, which is a strong stimulus for the development of collateral circulation. This allows continued systemic blood flow even after ductal closure. Such a pressure gradient is absent in the preductal type of coarctation. In fetal life, the descending aorta is perfused by the RV at systemic pressure through the ductal right-to-left shunt. When the ductus arteriosus begins to constrict after birth, there is a sudden decrease in perfusion of the descending aorta, with possible resulting circulatory shock and renal shutdown.

Radiographically, the heart is enlarged and there is pulmonary vascular congestion secondary to left-to-right shunting, owing to a distended foramen

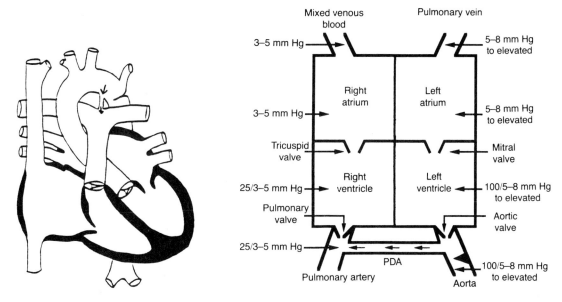

Fig. 31-8

Coarctation of the aorta. Severe narrowing of the aortic lumen, which decreases blood flow through the aorta. A patent ductus arteriosus is often present to allow pulmonary blood flow when the coarctation is severe. *PDA,* Patent ductus arteriosus. (Modified from Mullin CE, Mayer DC: *Congenital heart disease: a diagrammatic atlas.* New York. John Wiley & Sons, 1988.)

ovale. These patients often present with dyspnea, tachypnea, and irritability. Hypertension is often seen in the upper extremities; thus, blood pressure should be measured in both upper limbs and one leg. Systolic gradients may range between 20 and 140 mm Hg.[37]

The presurgical management of a newborn with coarctation may include digoxin administration to treat mild cardiac failure and inotropic agents, such as dopamine or dobutamine, for more severe presentations.[38] Diuretics are used to limit vascular engorgement. The use of prostaglandin E_1 to minimize ductal constriction until surgical correction can be achieved has drastically improved the outcome in these patients.[39] Ventilator management with oxygen therapy is often, but not always, necessary to treat cyanosis, respiratory distress, and acidosis secondary to systemic lactic acidemia from circulatory insufficiency. Surgery is usually postponed until later in the first year of life if cardiac failure can be controlled medically and an adequate weight gain sustained.[37]

The goal of surgical repair is twofold. First, the obstruction must be relieved and, second, restenosis, or recoarctation, must be avoided. A variety of procedures are used, including (1) excision of the coarctated segment of aorta with an end-to-end anastomosis of the cut ends, (2) tubular graft bypass of

the coarctation, and (3) patch aortoplasty (to enlarge the area) using a longitudinal incision through the coarctation with a patch on the open vessel. This patch is either synthetic (polyester) or fashioned from an excised portion of the patient's subclavian artery (subclavian flap procedure).[40] It is believed that the chance of recoarctation is lessened when a patch aortoplasty is used. Postoperative management usually includes a period of mechanical ventilation. Normal blood gas and pulse oximetry values can be expected. Rebound hypertension is sometimes present and may require treatment.

HYPOPLASTIC LEFT-HEART SYNDROME

Hypoplastic left-heart syndrome describes a number of conditions including mitral or aortic atresia, or both, a small left ventricular cavity, and marked hypoplasia of the ascending aorta (Fig. 31-9). However, the principal functional defect is the hypoplastic LV. Because there is little or no output from the LV, the pulmonary venous blood returning to the LA must pass through the septum to the RA. The entire systemic output is supplied by means of right-to-left flow through the PDA. As the ductus arteriosus narrows postnatally, there is severe impairment of cardiac output, producing circulatory shock and metabolic acidosis. The flow through the foramen ovale usually provides sufficient pulmonary blood

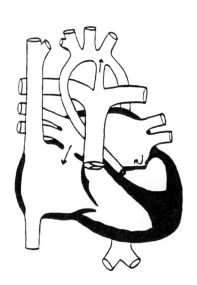
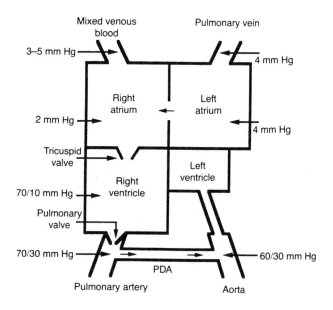

Fig. 31-9

Hypoplastic left ventricle. Underdeveloped left ventricle and severe narrowing of the ascending aorta. It may include mitral atresia *(pictured here),* lack of the mitral valve, aortic atresia, or lack of the aorta, or a combination. A patent ductus arteriosus is necessary for systemic blood flow. *PDA,* Patent ductus arteriosus. (From Mullin CE, Mayer DC: *Congenital heart disease: a diagrammatic atlas.* New York, John Wiley & Sons, 1988.)

flow to prevent obvious cyanosis. Because the overall direction of shunting is from left to right, this anomaly is often classified as acyanotic. The average age at death in these patients is usually younger than 1 week of age. Occasionally, the infants live for many weeks if the PDA and atrial septal opening are large. Chest radiography reveals a moderately to markedly enlarged heart with increased pulmonary vascular markings. The heart may also have a globular shape.[41]

Because a hypoplastic LV is incompatible with life and most often fatal, treatment is frequently terminated at the time of a definitive diagnosis. As recently as 1986 this defect was not considered reparable and the only treatment offered was comfort care.[10] Currently, there is reported success because of the advancements with transplantation and the Norwood procedure. Prostaglandin E_1 is given immediately to maintain ductal patency, and the infants are usually intubated. Because this is a ductal-dependent lesion, care must be used in the administration of oxygen, and subambient oxygen concentrations are sometimes administered to keep systemic oxygen saturations in a range of 70% to 80%.[42]

Surgical management of a hypoplastic LV is accomplished in phases by redirecting systemic venous drainage directly into the pulmonary arteries

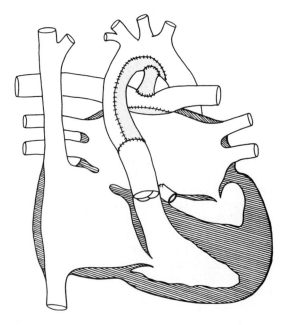

Fig. 31-10

Norwood procedure, stage 1. The main pulmonary artery is transected and attached to the aorta. A patent ductus arteriosus is created, and the atrial septum is removed to allow pulmonary venous return to flow easily into the right atrium.

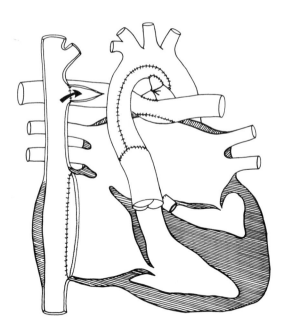

Fig. 31-11

Norwood procedure, stage 2. The ductus arteriosus is ligated, the connection between the vena cava and the right atrium is closed, and a communication is created between the superior vena cava and the pulmonary artery.

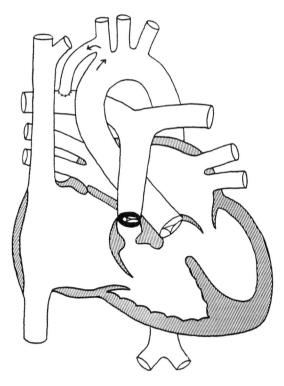

Fig. 31-12

A Blalock-Taussig shunt. Anastomosis of a subclavian artery to the pulmonary artery, shown here with pulmonary valve stenosis and a ventricular septal defect. (From Mullin CE, Mayer DC: *Congenital heart disease: a diagrammatic atlas.* New York. John Wiley & Sons, 1988.)

and redirecting pulmonary venous return into the RV, where the outflow is then routed into the aorta. The initial management is carried out using the Norwood procedure (Figs. 31-10 and 31-11). The exact description of this procedure may vary among surgeons but generally includes (1) attachment of the main pulmonary artery to the enlarged aorta with the distal end of the pulmonary artery patched closed, (2) removal of the atrial septum to relieve any pulmonary venous obstruction, and (3) a systemic to pulmonary connection to increase blood flow to the lungs (usually a Blalock-Taussig shunt from the subclavian artery to the pulmonary artery).

Postoperative management of patients who have had the Norwood procedure is often difficult because of the extensive nature of the repair. There is often profound hemodynamic instability requiring numerous cardiovascular supportive drugs. Ventilatory management is an important aspect of care, and the FIO_2 may be kept at less than or equal to 0.21. The Blalock-Taussig shunt acts as a man-made PDA and is the only blood supplier to the pulmonary system (Fig. 31-12). If oxygen is given, it may decrease PVR and allow large amounts of blood to flow from the aorta through the Blalock-Taussig shunt to the lungs, diverting systemic circulation. Thus the lungs can become easily "flooded." A helpful convention

is the "rule of forties," which seeks to keep arterial blood gases in the following range: pH greater than 7.40, PaO_2 nearly equal to 40 mm Hg, and $PaCO_2$ nearly equal to 40 mm Hg. Because suctioning changes hemodynamics and PVR and may even cause an irreversible decline in the patient's condition, it is performed sparingly, if at all.

The second phase of surgical management of a hypoplastic LV is the Fontan procedure (Fig. 31-13). It is generally performed when the patient is between 6 months and 4 years of age, when PVR has reached its lowest point. In the Fontan procedure, systemic venous blood is routed directly from the vena cava or the RA to the pulmonary artery through a fenestrated conduit. The ASD is closed, and the Blalock-Taussig shunt is ligated. The PVR must now be kept low to allow deoxygenated blood to flow freely to the lungs. If the PVR becomes too high, this fenestration is used to allow a pop-off action, with some blood escaping into the RA to prevent systemic venous congestion. The heart is now operational as a single-ventricle pump. These patients are normally unstable and require numerous

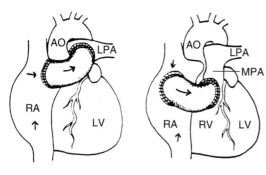

Fig. 31-13

Fontan procedure. Blood from the right atrium is routed to the left or main pulmonary artery using a baffle, which may contain a fenestration or pop-off valve to allow blood flow to enter the ventricle in the presence of high pulmonary artery pressures. *AO,* Aorta; *LPA,* left pulmonary artery; *RA,* right atrium; *LV,* left ventricle; *MPA,* main pulmonary artery; *RV,* right ventricle.

cardiovascular supportive drugs. The patient often returns from surgery with shock trousers (or abdominal waste cuffs) in place, which are used to increase preload and assist systemic venous blood to pass through the "Fontan" into the pulmonary system.

If hemodynamics and PVR are stable, normal arterial blood gas and pulse oximetry measurements can be expected. Oxygen can now be used more conventionally to lower PVR. Because positive-pressure ventilation can increase PVR, weaning from the ventilator is carried out as quickly as possible. The extubated patient's negative intrathoracic pressures during spontaneous inhalation enhance blood flow through the "Fontan"; however, extubation is often difficult because of patient instability.

TOTAL ANOMALOUS PULMONARY VENOUS RETURN

Anomalies involving aberrant connections between the pulmonary venous drainage and the systemic circulation have been described in every conceivable variety.[43] Simply stated, this lesion is defined as one in which the pulmonary veins have no connection with the LA and drain either directly or indirectly into the RA (Fig. 31-14). This results in mixing of pulmonary and systemic blood returning to the RA as well as increased pressures and volume in the right side of the heart. A simplified convention of classification of total anomalous pulmonary venous return (TAPVR) lists the four common anomalies as (1) supracardiac, in which the common pulmonary vein drains into the superior vena cava through a vertical vein that runs above the heart; (2) cardiac, in which the common pulmonary vein either drains into the coronary sinus or

is routed through the heart to the RA; (3) infracardiac, in which the common pulmonary vein drains to the portal vein, ductus venosus, hepatic vein, or inferior vena cava; and (4) subdiaphragmatic, in which the common pulmonary vein penetrates the diaphragm through the esophageal hiatus.

The chest radiograph in TAPVR is relatively normal, although there can be increased pulmonary vascular markings in infants with severe obstruction. Occasionally, the dilated accessory venous channels to the superior vena cava can be seen on the anteroposterior film. Intubation and mechanical ventilation for acidosis, cyanosis, and ventilatory failure are not uncommon. PEEP is often used for the management of pulmonary edema. Because of the venous admixture and the right-to-left shunt across the ASD, the PaO_2 and $PaCO_2$ will be nearly equal to 40 mm Hg (rule of forties) and oxygen saturations are typically 75%. Symptoms of congestive heart failure are treated with digoxin and diuretics. Balloon atrial septostomy may be performed at the time of cardiac catheterization to enlarge the ASD.

In the surgical management of supracardiac TAPVR, the vertical vein that runs above the heart and drains the pulmonary vein into the RA is ligated and anastomosed into the LA. The ASD is then closed to allow normal cardiac circulation. When the common pulmonary vein drains into the coronary sinus (cardiac TAPVR), a communication is made between the coronary sinus and the LA. Both the coronary sinus blood and pulmonary venous blood now drain into the LA. The ASD is then closed. When the common pulmonary vein is routed through the heart to the RA, the vein is ligated and tied off. The atrial septum is excised and a patch is sewn in such a way that pulmonary venous return is diverted to the LA. In infracardiac TAPVR, an anastomosis between the common pulmonary vein and the LA is performed. The common pulmonary vein that descends into the abdominal cavity is dissected and removed. Extensive hepatic and diaphragmatic repairs may be needed. The ASD is then closed to allow normal cardiac circulation.

Postoperative mechanical ventilation is universally indicated in all of the preceding repairs. The infracardiac repair requires extensive revision and is the most unstable of all repairs because of the hepatic and diaphragmatic involvement. Normal arterial blood gas and pulse oximetry values can be expected after all repairs. Pulmonary edema may occur, requiring prolonged ventilatory support with PEEP. There are considerable fluctuations in pulmonary artery pressure in some patients in the immediate postoperative period.[44] If these fluctuations include severe pulmonary artery hypertension,

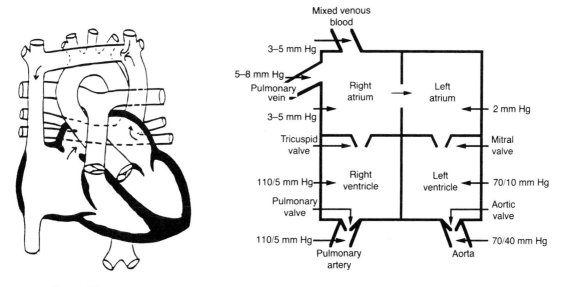

Fig. 31-14

Total anomalous pulmonary venous return. Pulmonary venous return is routed to the right atrium instead of the left atrium. Pulmonary drainage can be routed (1) above the heart (supracardiac), as pictured here; (2) through the heart (cardiac); (3) through the portal vein, ductus venosus, hepatic vein, or inferior vena cava (infracardiac); or (4) through the diaphragm or esophageal hiatus (subdiaphragmatic). (From Mullin CE, Mayer DC: *Congenital heart disease: a diagrammatic atlas.* New York. John Wiley & Sons, 1988.)

paroxysmal right ventricular failure and death may result.

TETRALOGY OF FALLOT

Tetralogy of Fallot is one of a class of anomalies called *conotruncal,* a term referring to the site of the developmental derangement that leads to the lesion. Others in this family of anomalies include truncus arteriosus and transposition of the great arteries. Tetralogy of Fallot consists of four concomitant conditions: (1) overriding aorta, (2) pulmonary stenosis, (3) VSD, and (4) right ventricular hypertrophy (Fig. 31-15). Depending on the severity of the pulmonary stenosis, the magnitude of the shunt through the VSD will vary. With mild stenosis, the shunt may be from left to right, with the infant being acyanotic. However, the majority of infants with tetralogy of Fallot present with pronounced pulmonary stenosis, resulting in a right-to-left shunt that produces significant cyanosis and oxygen saturations as low as 60%. The infant may be mildly cyanotic at birth while the ductus arteriosus is open; however, after the ductus arteriosus constricts and the child grows, the stenosis becomes more severe and the child becomes more cyanotic and hypoxemic.[45] Infants with extreme cases of tetralogy of Fallot may present with pulmonary atresia or pulmonary stenosis that is so severe that they are totally dependent on blood flow through the PDA. These infants are severely cyanotic at birth and require emergency surgery to provide pulmonary blood flow once the ductus arteriosus closes. Prostaglandin E_1 is administered to maintain a PDA until surgery or cardiac catheterization can be performed.[45] Chest radiography often reveals a classic boot-shape appearance of the heart if the patient has been sufficiently hypoxemic. This is caused by a narrow mediastinum and the effect of sustained increases in PVR, which result in ventricular engorgement and right ventricular hypertrophy. A right aortic arch is visible in many cases.

Because the VSD equalizes pressure in both ventricles, the heart of the infant with tetralogy of Fallot may be treated as a single chamber. The relative amounts of blood flow to the pulmonary versus systemic vasculatures are directly related to the degree of pulmonary stenosis and SVR. A slight change in any of these factors can dramatically change the hemodynamics and constrict the pulmonary outflow tract. These changes are sometimes manifested in spells of profound cyanosis, often referred to as "Tet" spells. Tet spells occur most commonly in infants 2 to 4 months of age and are characterized by (1) hyperpnea or exaggerated, deep spontaneous breathing; (2) irritability and prolonged crying; (3) increasing cyanosis; (4) decreased intensity of

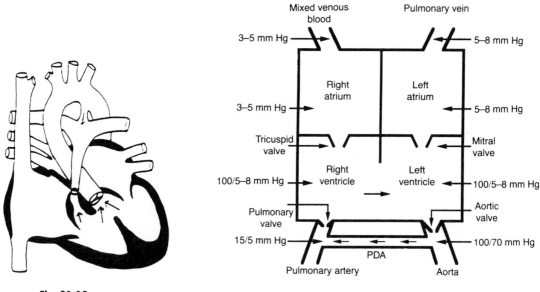

Fig. 31-15

Tetralogy of Fallot. Overriding aorta, pulmonary artery stenosis, right atrial hypertrophy, and a ventricular septal defect. A patent ductus arteriosus is often present to allow pulmonary blood flow if pulmonary stenosis is severe. *PDA,* Patent ductus arteriosus. (From Mullin CE, Mayer DC: *Congenital heart disease: a diagrammatic atlas.* New York. John Wiley & Sons, 1988.)

the heart murmur; and (5) fainting. Otherwise benign phenomena such as difficulty defecating or any event that causes a sudden increase in systemic venous return or a sudden drop in SVR and results in a large right-to-left shunt can precipitate Tet spells. In the presence of the fixed opening (pulmonary stenosis) and fixed resistance at the pulmonary artery, the systemic venous return flows out the aorta without being oxygenated. A vicious cycle of hypoxemic spells from which escape may not be possible can thus be engaged. Patients with tetralogy of Fallot are often slow to recover from these potentially catastrophic events, which should be avoided by minimizing interventions such as suctioning, handling, and manipulating the ventilatory circuit or airway. Box 31-1 lists steps that may be used to break the cycle of a Tet spell.

Intubation and assisted mechanical ventilation are usually necessary because of the degree of cyanosis, acidosis, and recurring Tet spells. Prostaglandin E_1 is given to minimize PDA closure and to ensure adequate pulmonary blood flow by reducing PVR. Because of the venous admixture, the PaO_2 values will be nearly equal to 40 mm Hg and the SaO_2 will be nearly equal to 75%.

Surgical repair involves a number of procedures. If the pulmonary stenosis or the right ventricular outflow tract is severely impaired, a systemic to pul-

monary connection is accomplished to increase blood flow to the lungs (palliative). This is usually a Blalock-Taussig shunt from the subclavian artery to the pulmonary artery. There are several variations of shunts that allow systemic arterial blood to flow to the lungs (e.g., central shunt, Waterston, Potts); however, it is beyond the scope of this chapter to offer detailed description of these variations.[46,47] Open-heart surgery is required for corrective repair of tetralogy of Fallot and consists of enlarging the right ventricular outflow tract through dilation of the pulmonary stenosis and closing the VSD. Widening of the right ventricular outflow tract can also be performed by resection of the infundibular tissue and placement of a polyester patch.

Ventilatory support is indicated in any repair of tetralogy of Fallot. It is particularly important for the clinician to know which particular repair is used when caring for these patients postoperatively. If the pulmonary stenosis is repaired through dilation or reconstruction of the infundibular tissue and the VSD is closed, normal arterial blood gas and saturation values can be expected. If the pulmonary stenosis is so severe that a systemic to pulmonary shunt is performed, ventilatory and hemodynamic management is much more tenuous. The VSD is usually not closed to allow blood to be shunted from right to left. In such cases, the FIO_2 may be

TREATMENT OF TET SPELLS

- *Hold the child in the knee-chest position.* This may trap venous blood in the legs and decrease the systemic venous return as well as calm the child.
- *Administer morphine sulfate.* This will suppress the respiratory center and abolish hyperpnea. (The hyperpnea causes a decrease in intrathoracic pressure and may increase venous return to the chest.) It will also chemically mediate pulmonary artery dilation directly, which allows more blood flow through the patent ductus arteriosus and increases pulmonary blood flow and oxygenation.
- *Administer oxygen.* This will improve oxygenation and decrease pulmonary vascular resistance.
- *Administer sodium bicarbonate for acidosis.* This will minimize the resultant pulmonary artery constriction.
- *Administer propranolol (Inderal).* Although the mechanism of action is not clear, this may reduce pulmonary artery spasms or act peripherally by stabilizing vascular reactivity of the systemic arteries, thereby preventing a sudden decrease in systemic vascular resistance.
- *Administer vasoconstrictors.* These may raise systemic vascular resistance should it suddenly drop.

maintained at less than or equal to 0.21. If oxygen is given in a cavalier fashion, it may decrease PVR and allow large amounts of blood to flow from the aorta through the shunt to the lungs, thus diverting systemic circulation and ultimately leading to pulmonary vascular congestion. Once again, the rule of forties applies so that blood gases are maintained in a fairly hypoxemic range. Cardiovascular and hemodynamic instability are often encountered in infants requiring systemic pulmonary shunts, and inotropic drips may be necessary postoperatively. When the septum is repaired, there may be a derangement of the conductive system. Therefore these infants have pacing wires placed in the event arrhythmias occur.

TRUNCUS ARTERIOSUS

Truncus arteriosus is a defect in which a single great artery arises from the ventricles of the heart supplying the coronary, pulmonary, and systemic arteries (Fig. 31-16). A large VSD allows total mixing of blood from the two ventricles, making the heart function as a single ventricle. The truncal valve usually resembles a normal aortic valve. This defect occurs in about 1.5% of all critically ill infants with congenital cardiac disease.[48] PVR and SVR mediate oxygenation and cardiac output. If PVR decreases, there is an increase in blood flow to the lungs through the truncus, decreasing cardiac output. Pulmonary vascular engorgement may

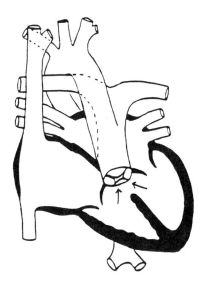
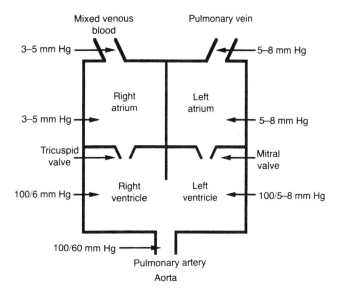

Fig. 31-16

Truncus arteriosus. A single great artery arises from the ventricles carrying both pulmonary and systemic blood flow. (From Mullin CE, Mayer DC: *Congenital heart disease: a diagrammatic atlas.* New York. John Wiley & Sons, 1988.)

then occur. If SVR decreases, blood flow will be shunted from right to left and bypass the lungs, resulting in severe hypoxemia and acidosis.

The heart is enlarged on chest radiography because of dilatation of the LA and LV. The pulmonary vascular markings are increased, and there may be symptoms of congestive heart failure. A right aortic arch is present in about one fourth of the cases. Intubation and ventilation are usually required because of the unstable hemodynamics of the pulmonary and systemic vascular circulation, which causes hypoxemia and acidosis. Because of the degree of venous admixture, the rule of forties is also used for blood gas management. Like the other conotruncal anomalies described, extreme care must be used with oxygen therapy, and subambient FIO_2 may be employed. The symptoms of congestive heart failure are treated with digoxin and diuretics.

Palliative pulmonary artery banding may be performed in newborns presenting with congestive heart failure or in infants who might not survive the surgical procedure required for total repair. To minimize pulmonary blood flow, the banding may be performed to the right or left pulmonary artery, or both. Unfortunately, banding of these arteries has been associated with high mortality and may also deform the pulmonary artery so that later correction is difficult if not impossible.

Corrective (total) repair can be performed and is sometimes referred to as a modified Rastelli procedure, with "modified" meaning the use of only one conduit (Fig. 31-17). The right and left pulmonary arteries are separated off the main truncus along with a cuff of tissue. The truncus is patched in the places from which the arteries have been removed. A valve-bearing conduit is attached from the RV to the separated pulmonary arteries. The VSD is then closed; the truncus will then act as the aorta. In both types of repair, postoperative mechanical ventilation is always required. If pulmonary banding is performed, mixing of deoxygenated and oxygenated blood will continue. PaO_2 is acceptable at 40 mm Hg, and SaO_2 should be at approximately 75%. If corrective repair is performed, normal and arterial blood gas and pulse oximetry values can be expected. Because of the extensive repair, there are often problems with hemodynamic instability that require inotropic support.

TRANSPOSITION OF THE GREAT ARTERIES

In transposition of the great arteries, the positions of the aorta and the pulmonary artery are reversed. The aorta arises from the RV, and the pulmonary artery arises from the LV (Fig. 31-18). Basically, the two circulations are in parallel instead of in series with each other. The systemic venous blood passes

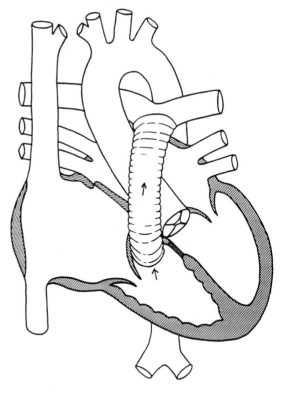

Fig. 31-17

Modified Rastelli procedure. Blood is routed from the right ventricle to the pulmonary artery using a conduit, and the ventricular septal defect is closed. (From Mullin CE, Mayer DC: *Congenital heart disease: a diagrammatic atlas.* New York. John Wiley & Sons, 1988.)

through the heart chambers on the right and then back out to the body without flowing through the lungs. The pulmonary venous blood traverses the left side of the heart and then returns to the lungs. Survival depends on mixing between the two circuits. In the immediate postnatal period, shunting through a PDA and the foramen ovale is usually sufficient. This bidirectional shunting from aorta to pulmonary artery and LA to RA improves mixing and prevents severe cyanosis. However, as the ductus arteriosus closes, the shunting is eliminated and the only site of mixing becomes the foramen ovale. This mixing is usually inadequate, resulting in severe hypoxemia, acidosis, and eventually death if it is not corrected. Approximately 10% of all infants born with congenital cardiac disease have transposition of the great arteries.[48] The chest radiograph is usually normal for a newborn except that the malposition of the great arteries is seen. This malposition is often described as egg-shaped or egg-on-side. After a few hours to days, pulmonary vascular enlargement and cardiomegaly may be seen.

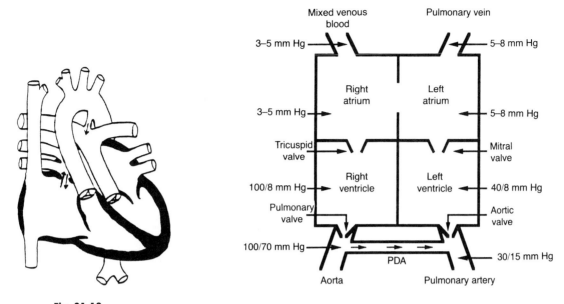

Fig. 31-18

Transposition of the great arteries. The aorta arises from the right ventricle, and the pulmonary artery arises from the left ventricle. A patent ductus arteriosus is necessary to allow pulmonary blood flow. *PDA,* Patent ductus arteriosus. (From Mullin CE, Mayer DC: *Congenital heart disease: a diagrammatic atlas.* New York. John Wiley & Sons, 1988.)

Prostaglandin E_1 is used immediately after diagnosis to maintain ductal patency because continued survival is dependent on it. Intubation and ventilation are usually required because of hypoxemia, acidosis, and apnea that may arise from the prostaglandin infusions. Oxygen is given judiciously so as not to decrease PVR. Because there is considerable venous admixture, the rule of forties is used for oxygenation management. These patients usually have a small ASD; however, in some cases it needs to be larger, and a Rashkind procedure, also called a balloon atrial septostomy, is performed during cardiac catheterization. Advancing a balloon-tipped catheter from the RA through the foramen ovale into the LA carries this out. The balloon is inflated and rapidly and forcefully withdrawn to create a large ASD. This ensures adequate mixing between the two atria until corrective surgery can be performed.

Three surgical repairs are currently being performed in patients with transposition of the great arteries: (1) Mustard, (2) Rastelli, and (3) arterial switch. In the Mustard procedure, blood is routed from the RA to the left side of the heart using the atrial septum. Pulmonary venous blood is routed to the right side of the heart using a baffle (Fig. 31-19). Both of the baffles are sutured in place, thus hindering blood flow from the RA into the RV and flow from the LA into the LV. Therefore, no mixing occurs.

In the Rastelli procedure, redirection of the pulmonary and systemic blood flow is carried out at the ventricular level, in comparison with the atrial level in the Mustard procedure (Fig. 31-20). This procedure is selected if the infant also has a VSD because left ventricular output is tunneled through the VSD to the aorta. The conduit allows deoxygenated blood to enter the pulmonary system. The pulmonary venous blood flows from the LA into the LV, as in a normal heart, and is then diverted through a conduit from the VSD into the aorta, providing systemic circulation. Both conduits are sutured directly to the pulmonary and aortic valves, respectively, thus preventing mixing.

The arterial switch, sometimes called the Jatene operation, is the latest corrective procedure for transposition of the great arteries (Fig. 31-21). It is indicated in infants with good left ventricular function, enabling them to have normal systemic output.[49] This is opposed to those patients whose RV is actually the more efficient of the two ventricles and thus are not candidates for the arterial switch. The main trunks of the pulmonary artery and the aorta are cut (transected) just above their respective origins on the heart. The portion of the pulmonary artery still attached to the LV is now anastomosed to the cut section of the aorta. The portion of the aorta still attached to the RV is anastomosed to the cut section of the pulmonary artery. Because

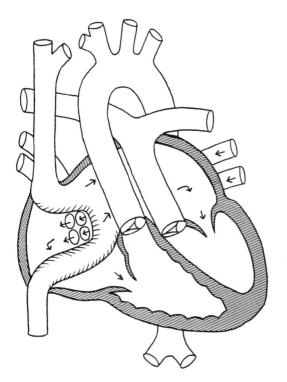

Fig. 31-19

Mustard procedure. The atrial septum is removed, and a conduit is placed inside the atria. Blood from the right atrium is directed to the mitral valve, into the left ventricle, out the pulmonary artery, and then to the lungs. Blood from the pulmonary veins is directed from the left atrium by a baffle to the tricuspid valve. It then flows into the right ventricle and out the aorta. (From Mullin CE, Mayer DC: *Congenital heart disease: a diagrammatic atlas.* New York. John Wiley & Sons, 1988.)

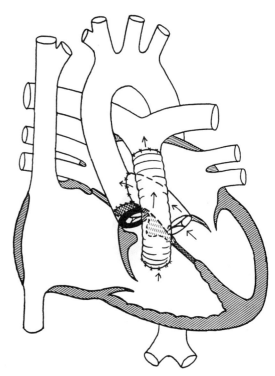

Fig. 31-20

Rastelli procedure. Blood is routed from the right ventricle to the pulmonary artery through the ventricular septal defect using a conduit. The pulmonary artery is separated and is anastomosed to the aorta. (From Mullin CE, Mayer DC: *Congenital heart disease: a diagrammatic atlas.* New York. John Wiley & Sons, 1988.)

the coronary arteries arise off the section of the aorta remaining attached to the RV, they must be excised from the aorta and implanted into the section of the pulmonary artery that remains attached to the LV so that they may carry oxygenated blood to the myocardium.

Because of the obvious hemodynamic problems associated with transposition of the great arteries, these patients will likely be unstable and require inotropic support and mechanical ventilation. Normal arterial blood gas and pulse oximetry values can be expected postoperatively.

HYPOPLASTIC RIGHT VENTRICLE

Two anomalies, tricuspid atresia and pulmonary atresia, both of which cause the right ventricle to be hypoplastic (Fig. 31-22), can cause a hypoplastic RV. With tricuspid atresia, there is a lack of forma-

tion of the tricuspid valve. There is no blood flow between the RA and RV. The only way for blood to leave the RA is through an ASD or patent foramen ovale. The systemic and pulmonary venous blood enters and mixes in the LA, then empties into the LV. A VSD allows blood to flow back into the RV, but only a small amount, if any, is pumped to the pulmonary system. A PDA must be present to facilitate additional pulmonary blood flow.

Pulmonary atresia obstructs the outflow of the RV and may be located at, or slightly distal to, the pulmonary valve. The left side of the heart receives blood from the right side of the heart through an ASD or patent foramen ovale. There may be a VSD, although it is unusual because of the hypoplastic nature of the RV. There is no blood flow from the RV to the pulmonary system; thus, a PDA must be present to support life.

The chest radiograph reveals a heart that may be normal to slightly enlarged. There are decreased

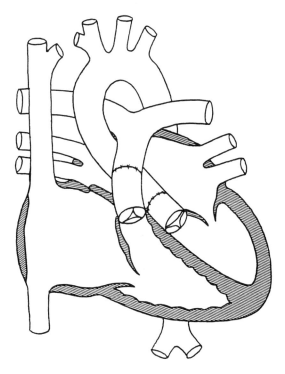

Fig. 31-21

Arterial switch. The pulmonary artery and aorta are separated from their respective origins and reattached to provide normal pulmonary and aortic blood flow. (From Mullin CE, Mayer DC: *Congenital heart disease: a diagrammatic atlas.* New York. John Wiley & Sons, 1988.)

pulmonary vascular markings and a concave main pulmonary artery. The LV can be slightly enlarged, giving the overall heart a boot-shaped appearance. An enlarged RA may also be noted.

Preoperative management includes the administration of prostaglandin E_1, given immediately to maintain ductal patency. Mechanical ventilation is usually required for hypoxemia, acidosis, and prostaglandin-induced apneic episodes. Oxygen therapy depends on the need for increasing or decreasing PVR. Because there is total venous admixing present, PaO_2 and $PaCO_2$ values are kept near 40 mm Hg and SaO_2 is maintained at 75%. A balloon atrial septostomy may be performed during cardiac catheterization if there is the need to improve the right-to-left shunt.

A variety of surgical repairs can be performed, depending on the severity of the hypoplastic RV and whether tricuspid or pulmonary atresia is involved. These repairs are performed in stages to allow patient growth and stability between them.

In the first stage, a Blalock-Taussig shunt is performed to create a systemic to pulmonary commu-

nication used to offset the effect of ductal closure. In the second stage, a Glenn procedure is performed to enhance pulmonary blood flow and reduce hypoxemia (Fig. 31-23). In this procedure, the superior vena cava is separated from the RA and is anastomosed to the right pulmonary artery, which is separated from the main pulmonary artery, so it receives only systemic venous blood flow from the superior vena cava through the Glenn shunt. This procedure allows the venous return from the head and upper extremities to flow directly into the right pulmonary circulation. As a result, only venous return from the inferior vena cava will enter the RA and flow to the LA to mix with oxygenated pulmonary venous return. After the initial surgical correction, the Fontan procedure is performed.

Postoperative management of the first stage of surgical repair includes limiting oxygen administration, instituting the rule of forties for blood gas measurement, and providing inotropic support for cardiovascular instability. Management after the Fontan procedure was discussed earlier.

CLINICAL MONITORING OF PATIENTS WITH CARDIAC ANOMALIES

BLOOD PRESSURE

There is a wide array of physiologic monitoring capabilities available to the clinician caring for the patient with congenital cardiac anomalies. The development of indwelling plastic catheters, combined with computerized signal processing, has made sophisticated monitoring of hemodynamic variables commonplace. The systemic arterial, central venous, pulmonary arterial, and left atrial blood pressures are typically monitored.[50,51]

The measurement of systemic arterial blood pressure offers a generally reliable estimation of various aspects of cardiac function. Systolic pressure measurements are useful in assessment of systemic afterload, whereas diastolic pressure relates more to supply. Mean arterial pressure probably best estimates total perfusion and can be estimated as one third of the difference between the systolic and diastolic pressures if the shape of the arterial waveform is normal. Pulse pressure (the difference between systolic and diastolic pressures) generally narrows in the presence of hypovolemia and when increased can open collapsed capillary beds.[52]

Central venous pressure has historically been considered indicative of preload, although this relationship is often tenuous. Preload is better assessed through the measurement of pulmonary artery and capillary wedge pressures through flow-directed Swan-Ganz catheters.[53] These catheters

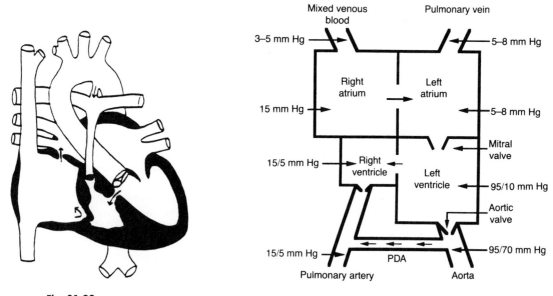

Fig. 31-22

Hypoplastic right ventricle. This results from either lack of a tricuspid valve, as pictured here, or pulmonary atresia. An atrial septal defect or patent foramen ovale is necessary for right atrial outflow of blood. A patent ductus arteriosus is necessary to allow pulmonary blood flow. *PDA,* Patent ductus arteriosus. (From Mullin CE, Mayer DC: *Congenital heart disease: a diagrammatic atlas.* New York. John Wiley & Sons, 1988.)

also allow reliable sampling of true mixed venous blood. Samples of venous blood from the superior and inferior vena cava have had differing amounts of oxygen extracted from them because they have circulated through parts of the body with widely different oxygen demands. The theory is that blood sampled from the vena cava has been insufficiently mixed to be considered "true" mixed venous blood. The insertion of a Swan-Ganz catheter into the pulmonary artery (as opposed to a central venous line) is required to compute certain cardiovascular variables using mixed venous blood.

Auscultated Heart Sounds

When listening to the heart with a stethoscope, one does not hear the opening of the valves because this slow process makes no noise. When the valves close, however, the veins of the valves and the surrounding fluids vibrate under the influence of the sudden pressure differentials that develop, giving off sound that travels in all directions through the chest. When the ventricles first contract, one hears a sound that is caused by closure of the AV valves, the so-called *lub.* This low-pitch, comparatively long vibration is known as the first heart sound. When the aortic and pulmonary valves close, one hears a short sound, owing to the rapid closure of

the valves, and the surroundings vibrate for only a short time. This sound is known as the second heart sound, termed the *dub.* Occasionally, one hears an atrial sound because vibrations associated with the flow of blood into the ventricles occur when the atria beat. Also, a third heart sound sometimes occurs at about the end of the first third of diastole and is believed to be caused by blood flowing with a rumbling motion into the nearly filled ventricles.

Pulse Oximetry

Pulse oximetry has become a de facto standard for noninvasive monitoring of oxygenation in intensive care patients, including those with congenital cardiac anomalies. Applications include the ongoing monitoring of systemic oxygenation and assessment of the degree of right-to-left shunting. In the presence of such shunting, there can be significant differences in oxygen saturation in the preductal and postductal arterial circulation. Placing one pulse oximeter probe (or transcutaneous oxygen electrode) on a right upper extremity (preductal) and concomitantly placing a probe on any other extremity (postductal) can assess this. A difference between preductal and postductal oxygen saturation, with saturation in the legs 5% to 10% lower

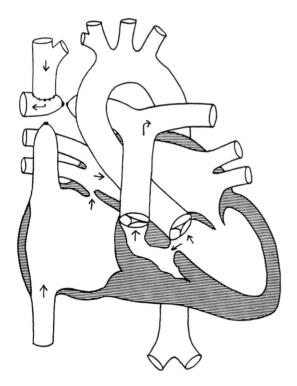

Fig. 31-23

Glenn procedure. Note the hypoplastic right. ventricle. The superior vena cava is separated from the right atrium, and the proximal end of the superior vena cava is sewn to the right pulmonary artery. The right pulmonary artery is separated from the main pulmonary artery. (From Mullin CE, Mayer DC: *Congenital heart disease: a diagrammatic atlas.* New York. John Wiley & Sons, 1988.)

than in the right arm shunting, should be suspected.[42] Some clinicians do not support measurement of postductal blood in the left arm, believing that there may be incomplete mixing of preductal and postductal blood by the time the flow traverses the origin of the left subclavian artery. Hence, there may be a disproportionately large amount of preductal (e.g., oxygenated) blood in the left upper extremity. In such a case, a significant shunt may be masked. An oxygen saturation difference of greater than 10% is usually indicative of a significant right-to-left shunt. There is some concern that the accuracy of pulse oximetry deteriorates as patients become progressively more desaturated.[54] There is, however, a divergence of data and opinions regarding these findings.[55-59] In general, it is believed that oximeter performance less than 75% is sometimes unreliable. Thus, in patients with target ranges of approximately 75%, clinicians should be fairly skeptical when evaluating pulse oximeter readings.

OXYGEN AND VASCULAR RESISTANCE

The pulmonary and systemic vasculatures are defined as low- and high-resistance systems, respectively. In congenital cardiac anomalies, the PVR and SVR heavily influence oxygenation, cardiac output, and patient survival. Abnormal shunting of blood between the pulmonary and vascular systems occurs from the system with the highest resistance to the system with the lowest. Because oxygen can act as a pulmonary vasodilator, supplemental oxygen administration can significantly decrease PVR, thus allowing more blood flow to the lungs. However, if the LA and LV have insufficient pumping capacities, as occurs in many cardiac anomalies, the pulmonary vasculature can become engorged with blood, resulting in pulmonary vascular congestion. This congestion and fluid overload are sometimes referred to as "flooding of the lungs." Box 31-2 describes the effects of various interventions on pulmonary and vascular resistance including respiratory and ventilatory manipulations. The effects of certain agents and conditions on the pulmonary artery and ductus arteriosus are described in Table 31-1.

RESPIRATORY CARE OF PATIENTS WITH CARDIAC ANOMALIES

VENTILATOR MANAGEMENT

In general, the preoperative and postoperative ventilator management of patients with congenital cardiac anomalies is not demonstrably different from that in most other ventilated populations, with some important exceptions. A postoperative goal of ventilatory support is to minimize variations in oxygenation and acid-base status that might otherwise cause fluctuations in PVR and SVR. Such swings in pressure can impede healing and cause the operative sites to leak within the myocardium and great vessels.

Although debate will continue about the utility of volume versus pressure modes of ventilation, knowledge of the tidal volume being delivered in this patient population is the essential ingredient in ventilator management, regardless of whether it is delivered in a volume or a pressure mode.[60-68] This is particularly true because infants and children with congenital cardiac anomalies usually do not have a great deal of pulmonary disease or a large derangement in ventilation. Their airway resistance is typically normal, although they may exhibit some decreased compliance that is usually secondary to increased pulmonary vascular blood volumes. In the presence of rapidly changing time constants in the lung (due to reactive airway disease or accumulation of secretions), tidal volumes may vary considerably

---

BOX 31-2

FACTORS INFLUENCING SYSTEMIC AND PULMONARY VASCULAR RESISTANCE

RESPIRATORY MANIPULATIONS TO INCREASE PULMONARY VASCULAR RESISTANCE
Increase tidal volume
Decrease ventilatory rate
Decrease pH (<7.35)
Decrease FIO_2 (subambient if necessary)
Increase positive end-expiratory pressure (>6 cm H_2O)
Increase $PaCO_2$ (>45 mm Hg)
Increase mean arterial pressure (>10 cm H_2O)

RESPIRATORY MANIPULATIONS TO DECREASE PULMONARY VASCULAR RESISTANCE
Increase FIO_2
Increase ventilatory rate
Increase pH (>7.45)
Decrease tidal volume
Decrease positive end-expiratory pressure (<4 cm H_2O)
Decrease $PaCO_2$ (<35 mm Hg)
Decrease mean arterial pressure (<10 cm H_2O)

FACTORS INCREASING SYSTEMIC VASCULAR RESISTANCE
Dopamine
Epinephrine
Hypovolemia
Hypocarbia
Norepinephrine (Levarterenol, Levophed)
Phenylephrine (Neo-Synephrine)
Septic shock (late stages)

FACTORS DECREASING SYSTEMIC VASCULAR RESISTANCE
Nitroglycerin
Morphine
Hypercarbia
Nitroprusside (Nipride)
Septic shock (early stages)

FACTORS INCREASING PULMONARY VASCULAR RESISTANCE
Hypoxia
Acidosis
Endarteritis
Hemothorax
Tumor mass
Pulmonary emboli
Sclerosis
Epinephrine
Norepinephrine (Levarterenol, Levophed)
Phenylephrine (Neo-Synephrine)
Histamine
Dopamine
Prostaglandin F_3

FACTORS DECREASING PULMONARY VASCULAR RESISTANCE
Oxygen
Nitric oxide
Aminophylline
Isoproterenol (Isuprel)

TABLE 31-1	**FACTORS INFLUENCING THE PULMONARY ARTERY AND THE DUCTUS ARTERIOSUS**	
Factor	**Effect on Pulmonary Artery**	**Effect on Ductus Arteriosus**
Oxygen	Dilate	Constrict
Hypoxia	Constrict	Dilate
Acidosis	Constrict	Dilate
α-Adrenergic agents (epinephrine, norepinephrine)	Constrict	Unknown
Vagal stimulation	Dilate	Unknown
Prostaglandin E_1	Dilate	Dilate
Prostaglandin E_2	Constrict	Constrict

when pressure-control modes are used. In such cases, volume-controlled intermittent mandatory ventilation is a preferred mode. Animal studies indicate that when pressure and volume are controlled independently, it is volumetric overdistention of the lung that causes ventilator-induced pulmonary injury.[69-71] When volume-controlled ventilatory modes are used, tidal volumes are typically kept in the range of 8 to 15 ml/kg. Ventilator frequency and thus minute volume are adjusted to achieve the desired range of $PaCO_2$.

When ventilating patients with congenital cardiac disease postoperatively, efforts are made to minimize airway pressures, particularly mean airway pressure of less than 10 cm H_2O.[72] The rationale is that pressures created within the thorax through the airways can be transmitted to the alveolar capillaries, causing a mechanical impediment to blood flow through the capillary bed with the resultant increase in PVR. With this in mind, positive end-expiratory pressure is also kept at a minimum. These concerns are largely theoretical and have not been well documented empirically.

Extubation criteria for the postsurgical management of most cardiac surgery patients include (1) intact cough, (2) ability to clear the airway, (3) adequate oxygenation with the FIO_2 less than or equal to 0.4, (4) normalized $Paco_2$ in the presence of age-adjusted normal spontaneous respiratory rates, (5) cardiovascular stability, and (6) adequate cardiac output.[28]

Fio_2 management is sometimes driven by the concern to avoid overoxygenating a patient. The term *overoxygenate* here is a relative one. Because oxygen can act as a pulmonary vasodilator, the Fio_2 must be carefully considered. What might be acceptable levels of oxygenation in healthy infants might indeed be unacceptably high in patients with ductal-dependent lesions in whom the systemic circulation is dependent on maintaining an elevated PVR. Indeed, at times technical modifications are made to administer subambient levels of Fio_2.

SUBAMBIENT OXYGEN THERAPY

The preoperative survival of patients with certain types of cardiac lesions is often partially dependent on maintaining an elevated PVR. An Fio_2 of less than 0.21 may be administered to patients with ductal-dependent lesions to limit the pulmonary vasodilatory effect of oxygen. One technical limitation with this technique is that it is possible to measure only an Fio_2 of greater than 0.17 on most commercially available clinical oxygen analyzers, thus limiting how much the Fio_2 can be lowered and still be monitored. Care must be taken to diligently monitor the patient and the function of such a setup because there is the potential for a mechanical malfunction or misapplication that could result in the patient's receiving an Fio_2 outside the desired range, which is typically 0.17 to 0.21. Also, because the routine bedside measurement of PVR is not common in neonates, other means must be used to guide this therapy, for example, by titrating the Fio_2 to less than 0.21 to achieve an oxygen saturation of less than 80% to 85%.

One method in decreasing the Fio_2 less than 21% is the use of nitrogen. It is a relatively safe gas because atmospheric air already contains approximately 79% nitrogen. As greater than 79% nitrogen is added to the system, it will begin to replace, or drive down, the 21% O_2 to subambient levels. The theory of using nitrogen is to reduce oxygen in the lungs, thereby lowering PVR. Normal gas exchange will occur in the lungs, but hypoxia should be expected. An acceptable Pao_2 will have to be established. The use of nitrogen has little effect on $Paco_2$, and its regulation will be the same using ventilator manipulations.

A variation to subambient Fio_2 therapy for increasing PVR is the use of CO_2. Whereas nitrogen reduces available oxygen, CO_2 directly affects $Paco_2$ blood levels and only 2% to 6% is needed. Increasing inspired CO_2 results in acidosis and will

assist in increasing PVR.[42,73,74] If CO_2 is selected as the desired gas to increase PVR, extreme caution must be used. If excess gas is given, or a system failure occurs, the patient or caregiver may suffer from CO_2 poisoning. Scavenger systems are often used to evacuate excess CO_2 from the expiratory limb of the ventilator to prevent CO_2 from entering the room.

REFERENCES

1. Daniels SR: Epidemiology: Cardiovascular disorders of the term neonate. In Long WA, editor: *Fetal and neonatal cardiology*. Philadelphia. WB Saunders, 1990; pp 425-438.
2. Osler W: *The principles and practice of medicine*. New York. D Appleton, 1990; p 765.
3. Halliday HL, McClure BG, Reid M: Cardiovascular problems. In Halliday HL, editor: *Handbook of neonatal intensive care*. Philadelphia. WB Saunders, 1998; pp 277-297.
4. Kitterman JA et al: The patent ductus arteriosus in premature infants. *N Engl J Med* 1972; 287:473.
5. Clyman RI: Ontogeny of the ductus arteriosus response to prostaglandins and inhibitors of the synthesis. *Semin Perinatol* 1980; 4:115.
6. Clyman RI, Heymann MA: Pharmacology of the ductus arteriosus. *Pediatr Clin North Am* 1981; 28:77.
7. McMurphy DM et al: Developmental change in constriction of the ductus arteriosus: response to oxygen and vasoactive substances in the isolated ductus arteriosus of the fetal lamb. *Pediatr Res* 1972; 6:231.
8. Heyman MA: Patent ductus arteriosus. In Adams FH, Emmanouilides, GC, editors: *Moss' heart disease in infants, children, and adolescents*. Baltimore. Williams & Wilkins, 1983; pp 158-171.
9. Schumacher RE, Donn SM: Persistent pulmonary hypertension of the newborn. In Sinha SK, Donn SM, editors: *Manual of neonatal respiratory care*. Armonk, NY. Futura, 1999; pp 281-287.
10. Fluck RR: Congenital cardiovascular disorders. In Aloan CA, Hill TV, editors: *Respiratory care of the newborn and child*. Philadelphia. Lippincott-Raven, 1997; pp 223-249.
11. Peckman GJ et al: Clinical course to 1 year of age in premature infants with patent ductus arteriosus: results of a multi-centered randomized trial of indomethacin. *Pediatrics* 1984; 105:285.
12. McCarthy JS, Zies LG, Gelbank J: Age dependent closure of the patent ductus arteriosus by indomethacin. *Pediatrics* 1978; 62:706.
13. Cotton RB et al: Randomized trial of early closure of symptomatic patent ductus arteriosus in small preterm infants. *Pediatrics* 1978; 93:647.
14. Edmonds LJ et al: Surgical closure of the ductus arteriosus in premature infants. *Circulation* 1973; 48:856.
15. Robbins RC: Atrial septal and ventricular septal defects. In Nichols DG, editor: *Critical heart disease in infants and children*. St Louis. Mosby, 1995; pp 553-579.
16. Wyler F, Rutishauser M: Symptomatic atrial septal defect in the neonate and infant. *Helv Paediatr Acta* 1976; 30:399.
17. Spangler JG, Feldt RH, Danielson GK: Secundum atrial septal defect encountered in infancy. *Thorac Cardiovasc Surg* 1976; 71:398.
18. Black MD: Minimally invasive repair of atrial septal defects. *Ann Thorac Surg* 1998; 65:765-767.

19. Burke RP: Minimally invasive techniques for congenital heart surgery. *Semin ThoracCardiovasc Surg* 1997; 9: 337-344.

20. Keith JD, Rowe RD, Vlad P: *Heart disease in infancy and childhood.* New York. Macmillan, 1967.

21. Nadas AS, Fyler DC: *Pediatric cardiology.* Philadelphia. WB Saunders, 1972; p 348.

22. Jarmakani JM: The effect of corrective surgery on left heart volume and mass in children with ventricular septal defect. *Am J Cardiol* 1971; 27:254-258.

23. Graham TP, Bender HW, Spach MS: Ventricular septal defect. In Adams FH, Emmanouilides GC, editors: *Moss' heart disease in infants, children, and adolescents.* Baltimore. Williams & Wilkins, 1983; pp 134-154.

24. Rastelli GC: Surgical repair of the partial form of persistent common atrioventricular canal, with specific reference to the problem of mitral valve incompetence. *Circulation* 1965; 31/32(suppl I):I-31.

25. Barber G, Chin AJ: Volume loads except TAPVD. In Long WA, editor: *Fetal and neonatal cardiology.* Philadelphia. WB Saunders, 1990; pp 452-464.

26. Ungerleider RM: Atroventricular canal defects. In Nichols DG, editor: *Critical heart disease in infants and children.* St Louis. Mosby, 1995; pp 601-622.

27. Feldt RH: Atrial septal defects and atrioventricular canal. In Adams FH, Emmanouilides GC, editors: *Moss' heart disease in infants, children, and adolescents.* Baltimore. Williams & Wilkins, 1983; pp 118-134.

28. Young TE, Mangum B: A manual of drugs used in the neonatal care. *Neofax,* ed 13. North Carolina Acorn Publishing, 2000; p 108.

29. Radford DJ et al: Prostaglandin E₁ for interrupted aortic arch in the neonate. *Lancet* 1976; 2:95.

30. Bailey CP: Surgical treatment of aortic stenosis. *JAMA* 1952; 150:1647.

31. Ellis FH, Kirklin JW: Congenital valvular aortic stenosis: anatomic findings and surgical technique. *Thorac Cardiovasc Surg* 1962; 43:199.

32. Lewis FJ : Aortic valvulotomy under direct vision during hypothermia. *Thorac Surg* 1956; 32:481.

33. Spencer FC, Neill CA, Bahnson HT: The treatment of congenital aortic stenosis with valvotomy during cardiopulmonary bypass. *Surgery* 1958; 44:109.

34. Zeevi B: Invasive catheter techniques in the management of critical aortic stenosis in infants. In Jacobs ML, editor: *Pediatric cardiac surgery.* Boston. Butterworth-Heinemann, 1992; pp 115-122.

35. Keith JD, Rowe RD, Vlad P: Coarctation of the aorta. In Keith JD, Rowe RD, Vlad P, editors: *Heart disease in infancy and childhood,* ed 3. New York. Macmillan, 1978; p 226.

36. Williams WG et al: Results of repair of coarctation of the aorta during infancy. *Thorac Cardiovasc Surg* 1980; 79:603.

37. Gersony WM: Coarctation of the aorta. In Adams FH, Emmanouilides GC, editors: *Moss' heart disease in infants, children, and adolescents.* Baltimore. Williams & Wilkins, 1983; pp 188-199.

38. Whitley HG, Perry LW: Coarctation. In Long WA, editor: *Fetal and neonatal cardiology.* Philadelphia. WB Saunders, 1990; pp 477-486.

39. Leoni F et al: Effect of prostaglandin on early surgical mortality in obstructive lesions of the systemic circulation. *Br Heart J* 1984; 52:654.

40. Hesslein PS et al: Comparison of resection versus patch aortoplasty for repair of coarctation in infants and children. *Circulation* 1981; 64:164.

41. Freedom RM: Hypoplastic left heart. In Adams FH, Emmanouilides GC, editors: *Moss' heart disease in infants,* children, and adolescents. Baltimore. Williams & Wilkins, 1983; pp 411-422.

42. Schamberger MS: Congenital heart diseases/arrhythmias. In Tobias JD, editor: *Pediatric critical care: the essentials.* Armonk, NY. Futura, 1999; pp 155-180.

43. Lucas RV: Anomalous venous connections, pulmonary and systemic. In Adams FH, Emmanouilides GC, editors: *Moss' heart disease in infants, children, and adolescents.* Baltimore. Williams & Wilkins, 1983; pp 458-491.

44. Bull C: Total anomalous pulmonary venous drainage. In Long WA, editor: *Fetal and neonatal cardiology.* Philadelphia. WB Saunders, 1990; pp 439-451.

45. Hazinski MF: Congenital heart disease: II. Cyanotic and aortic obstructive heart lesions. *Life Support Nurs* 1982; 2:7.

46. Long WA: Fetal and neonatal cardiology. Philadelphia. WB Saunders, 1990.

47. Adams FH, Emmanouilides GC: *Moss' heart disease in infants, children, and adolescents.* Baltimore. Williams & Wilkins, 1983.

48. Fyler DC: Report of the New England regional cardiac program. *Pediatrics* 1980; 65(suppl):375.

49. Planch C: Arterial switch. *Pediatric Cardiol* 1998; 19: 297-307.

50. Gardner PE: Hemodynamic pressure monitoring. Clinical Application Series. Redmond, WA. Spacelabs Medical, 1992.

51. Slye DA, Nara AR: Cardiac output and hemodynamic calculations. Clinical Application Series. Redmond, WA. Spacelabs Medical, 1992.

52. Lake CL: Monitoring of arterial pressure. *Clin Monitoring* 1990; 115-146.

53. Schwenzer KJ: Venous and pulmonary pressures. *Clin Monitoring* 1990; 147-197.

54. Severinghaus JW, Naifeh KH, Koh SO: Errors in 14 pulse oximeters during profound hypoxia. *Clin Monitoring* 1989; 5:72.

55. Miyasaka K, Katayama M, Kusakawa I, et al: Use of pulse oximetry in neonatal anesthesia. *Perinatology* 1987; 7:343.

56. Jones J: Continuous emergency department monitoring of arterial saturation in adult patients with respiratory distress. *Ann Emerg Med* 1988; 17:463.

57. Sendak MJ, Harris AP, Donham RT: Accuracy of pulse oximetry during arterial oxyhemoglobin desaturation in dogs. *Anesthesiology* 1988; 68:111.

58. Mihm FG, Halperin DH: Noninvasive detection of profound arterial desaturations using a pulse oximetry device. *Anesthesiology* 1985; 62:85.

59. Lazzell VA, Jopling MW: Accuracy of pulse oximetry in cyanotic congenital heart disease. *Anesthesiology* 1987; 67:A169.

60. Abubakar KM, Keszler M: Patient-ventilator interactions in new modes of patient-triggered ventilation. *Pediatr Pulmonol* 2001; 32(1):71-75.

61. McIntyre NR: Pressure-limited versus volume-cycled breath delivery strategies. *Crit Care Med* 1994; 22:4.

62. Rappaport SH et al: Randomized, prospective trial of pressure-limited versus volume-controlled ventilation in severe respiratory failure. *Crit Care Med* 1994; 22:22.

63. El-Khatib MF: Volume controlled ventilation is superior to pressure controlled ventilation in a model of restrictive lung disease. *Respir Care* 1993 (abstract).; 38:1242.

64. El-Khatib MF: Pressure controlled ventilation is superior to volume controlled ventilation in a model of obstructive lung disease. *Respir Care* 1993 (abstract); 38:1241.

65. Reynolds R: Pressure control ventilation: another view. *Respir Care* 1992; 37:83.

66. Jones MR: PIP and barotrauma: a response to Chatburn. (Letter.) *Respir Care* 1992; 37:84.

67. Chatburn RL: Letter to the editor. *Respir Care* 1992; 37:86.
68. Chatburn RL: Some misconceptions about peak airway pressure. (Letter.) *Respir Care* 1991; 36:872.
69. Caldwell EJ, Powell RD, Mullooly JP: Interstitial emphysema: a study of physiologic factors involved in experimental induction of the lesion. *Am Rev Respir Dis* 1970; 102:516.
70. Hernandez LA et al: Chest wall restriction limits high airway pressure-induced lung injury in rabbits. *Appl Physiol* 1989; 66:2364.
71. Dreyfuss D et al: High inflation pressure pulmonary edema: respective effects of high airway pressure, high tidal volume, and positive end-expiratory pressure. *Am Rev Respir Dis* 1988; 137:1159.

72. Meliones JN: Perioperative management of patients with congenital heart disease: a multidisciplinary approach. In Nichols DG, editor: *Critical heart disease in infants and children.* St Louis. Mosby, 1995; pp 553-579.
73. Kulik TJ: Pulmonary hypertension. In Chang AC, editor: *Pediatric cardiac intensive care.* Baltimore. Williams & Wilkins, 1998; pp 497-506.
74. Jobes DR: Carbon dioxide prevents pulmonary overcirculation in hypoplastic left heart syndrome. *Ann Thorac Surg* 1992; 54:150-151.

CHAPTER 32

Sudden Infant Death Syndrome and Pediatric Sleep Disorders

Patrick Sorenson
Ronald E. Becker

Sudden infant death syndrome (SIDS), also referred to as "crib death," is a major disorder associated with sleep during the first year of life. It is the leading cause of death in infants between 1 week and 1 year of age, affecting more than 5000 infants in the United States each year. SIDS is best defined as the sudden and unexpected death of an infant for which sufficient cause cannot be found by a death scene investigation, review of the history, and a postmortem examination. As this definition implies, it is a diagnosis of exclusion; there are no findings on autopsy that are entirely specific for SIDS. Because of the breadth of the definition and the lack of specific postmortem lesions, it is probable that SIDS has multiple causes.[1]

Closely linked to any discussion of SIDS is that of apparent life-threatening events. An apparent life-threatening event (ALTE) is defined by the American Thoracic Society as "an episode of apnea, color change (pallor, cyanosis or erythema), and hypotonia that the observer believes to be life-threatening to the infant and for which some intervention (stimulation, shaking, and/or cardiorespiratory resuscitation) is felt to be required."[2] Although the relationship between ALTE and SIDS is poorly understood, many believe that ALTE may indicate a risk for cardiorespiratory instability, which could lead to death.

SIDS almost always takes place when the infant is presumed to have been asleep, either during the day or night. However, more than 70% of its victims are found in the early morning hours after the nighttime sleep.[3] SIDS is widely considered to have a developmental component because infants in the first month of life are generally spared. The incidence then peaks in infants from 2 to 4 months of life, which coincides with significant changes known to

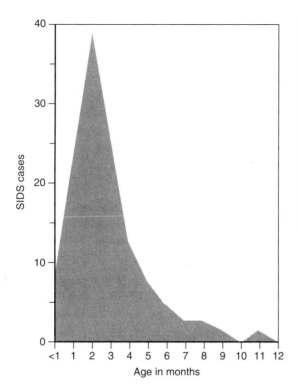

Fig. 32-1

Sudden infant death syndrome (SIDS) deaths in Maryland in 1985. Note the peak at 2 months of age and a decrease after 6 months of age.

occur in sleep organization and in the modulation of brain-stem centers involved in respiratory and arousal state control by the forebrain.[4] Crib death is uncommon after infants are 6 months old, with 90% of SIDS victims affected in the first 6 months of life. It is rare after the first birthday. This particular pattern of incidence is unique to SIDS (Fig. 32-1).

There are many risk factors for SIDS, most of which cannot be easily eliminated (Box 32-1). However, there are several risk factors that lend themselves to intervention. They are (1) prone positioning, (2) maternal smoking, and (3) bottle-feeding.

Historically, numerous international epidemiologic studies pointed to an increased risk of SIDS when infants are put to sleep in the prone position.[5-7] A U.S. study confirmed this relationship, although the relative risk of prone versus supine posture in this study was lower than it had been in the foreign studies. Many mechanisms have been proposed to explain the relationship to sleep position, but most have not been tested or have not withstood critical examination. One hypothesis is that a subgroup of prone-positioned infants actually "burrow" their faces into their bedding rather than keep their heads

turned to one side. These infants are theorized to die because of suffocation or rebreathing of carbon dioxide.[8] An analysis of one supine-sleeping campaign in Norway published in 1998 showed that the SIDS rate dropped from 3.5 deaths per 1000 live births to 0.3 deaths per 1000 live births 4 years after an intervention program designed to avoid prone sleeping.[5] Similar public education campaigns to inform parents about the risk factors associated with SIDS in the United States have yielded a clear decline in the incidence of SIDS. These risk factors include prone and side infant sleeping positions, exposure of infants to cigarette smoke, and potentially hazardous crib-related sleeping environments.[9]

Maternal cigarette smoking during pregnancy is associated with increased risk in a dose-dependent fashion: the more cigarettes smoked, the greater the risk.[10] This dose dependency suggests a relationship between a factor that may be causing SIDS and prenatal maternal cigarette smoking. In addition, there is evidence that postnatal exposure to cigarette smoke (passive smoking) further increases the risk. Some studies have found breast-feeding to be partly protective against SIDS, but other studies have found no effect. Any beneficial effect may be related to the fact that breast-fed babies have fewer infections than do bottle-fed babies because infections may increase the risk for SIDS.

NORMAL CONTROL OF BREATHING AND HEART RATE

Much of the control of breathing resides in the most primitive part of the brain, the brain stem. It is there that the central rhythm generator (CRG) is postulated to exist, and information flows from the peripheral chemoreceptors and the mechanoreceptors to the brain stem, modulating the output from the CRG. The presence of an "off switch" mechanism is also postulated because phrenic nerve output to the diaphragm is absent during expiration. The off switch terminates inspiration by inhibition of the CRG. Input from higher centers of the brain, such as the cortex, is also integrated within the brain stem. Hence, the ability to voluntarily control breathing also exists.

Control of the heart rate occurs primarily through the autonomic nervous system, which is divided into sympathetic and parasympathetic branches. Sympathetic stimulation of the heart increases heart rate, whereas parasympathetic stimulation acts to decrease the heart rate. The vagus nerve is the parasympathetic conduit from nuclei (ambiguous nuclei and tractus solitarius) in the brain stem to the heart. "Vagal" stimuli such as coughing, choking, or expiring against a closed glottis (the Valsalva maneuver) can induce bradycardia. The bradycardia that follows obstructive apnea may also be vagally mediated.

ETIOLOGY

The importance of the brain stem in the control of breathing and possibly SIDS is further supported by the fact that apnea in premature infants is associated with immaturity of the brain stem. Premature infants with apnea have prolonged brain-stem conduction times for auditory evoked responses compared with premature infants without apnea. Also, some SIDS victims have gliosis (representing scarring) of cellular bodies in the medulla oblongata, specifically in the area of the arcuate nucleus that controls respiratory and cardiac function.[11,12]

Although the specific neuronal dysfunction that leads to both central apnea and periodic breathing has yet to be determined, it appears as though factors in the maturation of central chemoreceptors and mechanoreceptors play a pivotal role in the alterations of respiratory drive in preterm infants. Some preterm infants exhibit an unexpected and paradoxical decrease in ventilatory response to increases in carbon dioxide values. Also, preterm infants often respond to a fall in inspired oxygen concentrations with a transient increase in ventilation followed by a return to baseline or even a depression of ventilation. The diminution of respiratory drive during hypercarbia and the biphasic response to hypoxia can potentially predispose a vulnerable child to apnea and its sequelae.[13]

As intriguing as these hypotheses may be, the precise cause of SIDS is not known. SIDS may have several causes, but all are likely to be related to a developmental immaturity or malfunction of the brain leading to either cardiac or respiratory death.

TESTS TO ASSESS RISK OF SUDDEN INFANT DEATH SYNDROME

There is no test that accurately predicts risk for SIDS, perhaps because it has multiple causes and because most tests are performed weeks or months before death, during a period of life in which the infant is undergoing rapid change. The pneumocardiogram is a two- to four-channel recording usually consisting of transthoracic impedance (chest movements) and heart rate, as well as oxygen saturation data and an air flow channel in the more sophisticated models (Fig. 32-2). It is usually performed overnight in a controlled but unattended setting. Its value is markedly diminished because it provides limited ability to differentiate between central and obstructive apnea and does not provide thorough information regarding the severity and physiologic consequences of the breathing disturbance. It is widely accepted that the pneumocardiogram is not effective at screening for risk of SIDS.[14]

Polysomnography (PSG) performed according to the standards accepted by the American Thoracic Society[2] provides the clinician with a more thorough evaluation of pediatric sleep and breathing disorders than a pneumocardiogram. PSG for cardiopulmonary indications includes simultaneous recording of physiologic variables, including sleep state, respiration, cardiac rhythm, muscle activity, gas exchange, and snoring data (Fig. 32-3). The personnel in attendance during PSG are trained to evaluate and document behavioral and physiologic changes as well as quality of sleep. Thus a more accurate diagnosis of obstructive sleep apnea is possible with PSG, in contrast to the lack of this capability in the limited-channel pneumocardiogram (Fig. 32-4).

Although PSG is not always indicated after an uncomplicated ALTE, it may be helpful to define the frequency of type of apnea and the extent of cardiac, blood gas, and sleep alterations in certain infants with apnea or an ALTE. PSG is especially useful for the detection of occult hypoxemia. Test results may also suggest the further direction of the workup; for example, if abnormal amounts of obstructive apnea are noted, consultation with an otolaryngologist may be indicated. In addition, data acquired from these studies are often helpful in the later interpretation of waveforms from home memory monitors. However, the major concern after an ALTE episode is the related risk of recurrent events or death.

POLYSOMNOGRAPHIC PARAMETERS

Data used for the staging of infant sleep include the combined measurement of the electroencephalogram (EEG) to record brain activity, the electrooculogram

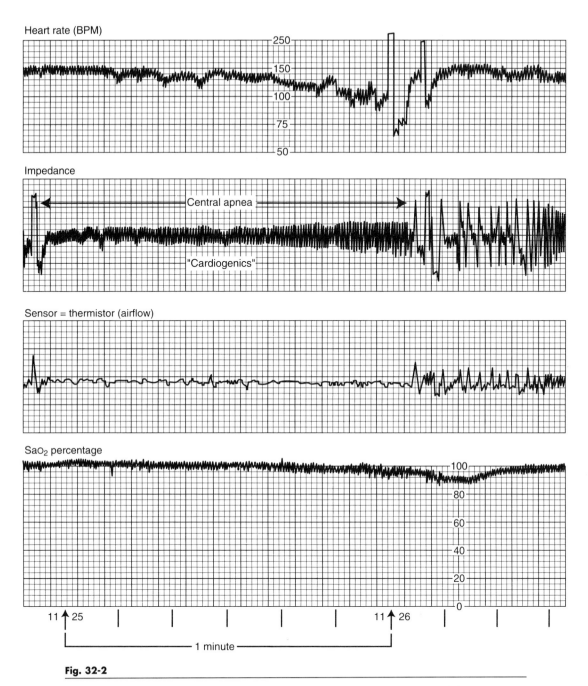

Fig. 32-2

Four-channel Edentec study that captured a 1-minute-long central apneic episode in a premature infant. Cardiogenics refers to the artifactual detection of heart beats by the impedance channel; these signals occur with each heart beat and thus are not breaths. The SaO₂ percentage channel displays oxygen saturation data with a superimposed pulse waveform. *BPM,* Beats per minute.

(EOG) to record bilateral eye movements, and the electromyogram (EMG) to record facial and inter-costal muscle tone. The placement of the EEG leads is based on the international "10-20" electrode place-ment system. EEG placement for scoring sleep in children is similar to that used in an adult population. Electrodes are placed at A1, A2, O1, O2, C3, and C4, and sleep stage is determined by the monopolar derivation C3/A2 or C4/A1. However, because of the special criteria used to define sleep states in infants

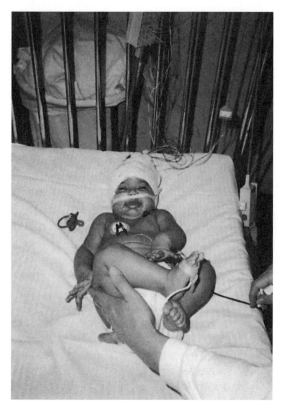

Fig. 32-3

This patient is nearly ready for polysomnography. The head is wrapped with gauze to protect the scalp electroencephalogram (EEG) electrodes. An electrode to detect movements of the left eye is also covered by gauze, although monitoring bilateral eye movements using two separate electrodes is standard. Tape below the nostrils will hold the thermistor and the CO_2 cannula in place. A transcutaneous oxygen electrode sits on the right side of the upper chest, and an electrocardiographic electrode is opposite it. Stretching across the abdomen is a strain gauge to detect breathing efforts. An oxygen saturation sensor is attached to the left foot.

younger than 6 months old and the unique EEG features for this population, an extended EEG montage, or PSG channel derivation, is preferred. This extended montage should include bilateral EEG electrodes utilizing bipolar channels to more accurately evaluate the EEG of the two hemispheres of the brain. EEG features specific to infants, such as tracé alternant and "brushes," as well as certain epileptiform activity can provide useful information regarding the maturity of the brain and alert clinicians to potential problems in brain activity. Additionally, certain normal features of the infant EEG, such as rudimentary sleep spindles, are better seen using an extended EEG montage that includes frontal leads.

The accurate scoring of sleep stages also requires bilateral EOG sensors to monitor the rapid eye movements that normally occur in rapid-eye-movement (REM) sleep and the slow eye movements that occur with the onset of sleep. An EMG recording of facial muscle tone assists the clinician in more accurately determining the presence of REM sleep when skeletal muscle tone, particularly the muscles of the face, is normally inhibited.

To comprehensively assess the adequacy of ventilation and identify and differentiate between central and obstructive apnea and its severity, PSGs should also include movements of the chest wall and abdomen, air flow at the nose and mouth, transcutaneous oxygen saturation data (with validating pulse wave from the monitor), and end-tidal carbon dioxide ($ETCO_2$) measures. A pulse waveform is necessary to assess the reliability of oxygenation data because oxygen saturation monitors can yield artifactual data at times when the infant is feeding or moving. Capnography, a graphic representation of $ETCO_2$, is recommended because it can assess both air flow and ventilation simultaneously. Calibrated $ETCO_2$ measurements can effectively detect possible CO_2 retention associated with apnea or prolonged hypoventilation.

Standard PSG also includes additional parameters that can provide important information relevant to the patient's electrophysiologic status. An electrocardiogram (ECG) monitors cardiac rate and rhythm and is useful in evaluating the consequences of breathing disorders on the heart. An EMG recording of the intercostal muscles detects expansion of the chest wall to assess for the presence of respiratory effort to help differentiate between central versus obstructive apnea. A PSG can include EMG of the anterior tibialis muscles to identify periodic leg movement disorders, although these disorders are rare in infants and leg EMGs are not routinely monitored in children younger than 6 months old.

To assess for the presence of gastroesophageal reflux, and its potential cardiorespiratory consequences, continuous esophageal pH measurement can be done in conjunction with PSG. Video recording with sound is recommended because it provides invaluable information on sleep behavior, snoring, respiratory effort, and sleep positions associated with a particular respiratory pattern. Finally, PSG on infants is attended by a trained technologist who ensures the integrity of the recording, provides descriptions regarding unusual events or behaviors, and makes notations on the recording regarding physiologic changes such as snoring and color changes such as cyanosis, pallor, and erythema. Polysomnographic technologists working with this

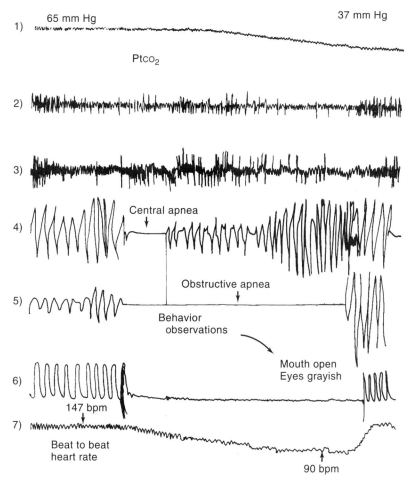

65 mm Hg

37 mm Hg

1)

PtcO$_2$

2)

3)

4)

Central apnea

Obstructive apnea

5)

Behavior
observations

Mouth open
Eyes grayish

6)

147 bpm

7)

Beat to beat
heart rate

90 bpm

Fig. 32-4

Thirty-seven-second mixed apnea recorded during polysomnography. Channel 1 shows a drop in transcutaneous oxygen tension from 65 to 37 mm Hg over the 1 minute of this recording. Channel 4 depicts breathing movements, and channels 5 and 6 depict nasal air flow. Note the onset of central apnea, as indicated on channel 4, followed by obstructive apnea, as channels 5 and 6 show no air flow despite breathing movements in channel 4. *PtcO$_2$*, Transcutaneous oxygen; *bpm*, beats per minute.

age group must be certified in pediatric cardiopulmonary resuscitation (CPR).

LABORATORY SUPERVISION

A pediatrician with training and experience in pediatric respiratory disorders and/or sleep medicine should be responsible for supervision of a sleep laboratory whose primary activity is performing PSG in infants and children with cardiorespiratory disorders. If this is not possible, owing to limited PSG resources, it is recommended that a pediatrician with expertise in pediatric pulmonology, neonatology, neurology, or pediatric sleep medicine oversee laboratory operations related to children.

A pediatric specialist can ensure that the PSG is performed, scored, and interpreted appropriately for the age and condition of the child.

SETTING

Children should be studied in a dedicated pediatric facility with a laboratory decor that is both age appropriate and nonthreatening. If a separate pediatric laboratory is not available, an area of the laboratory should be dedicated for children. Accommodations for a parent to sleep near the child are recommended because immediate parental access to the child is often necessary to reduce fear and anxiety and provide ordinary child care while the study is in progress. It is sometimes helpful to use videocassette recorders and provide stickers to toddlers and older children for distraction and to obtain compliance during the setup. Safe and comfortable bedding is necessary when performing PSG on infants and children. Mattresses should be made of material that is easy to clean and disinfect if soiled.

PERSONNEL

A pediatric sleep laboratory should be staffed with personnel trained to deal with children and their parents or guardians. Because PSG evaluation can be seen as stressful, particularly in this age group, laboratory personnel should have knowledge of childhood behavior and developmental stages to effectively deal with children and provide medical information in a nonthreatening manner. Because of the differences in the sleep characteristics of children as compared with adolescents and adults, only qualified individuals who know the unique characteristics of sleep breathing in children of different ages should evaluate the PSG.[2]

NORMAL SLEEP DEVELOPMENT

Neonates cycle through REM and non-REM (NREM) sleep differently than an older child or adult.[15] In the first few months of life they have not yet become fully entrained on a day-night cycle and more of the control of sleep is internal. Full-term infants can spend as much as 50% of their total sleep time in REM sleep. At this age, this is referred to as "active sleep."[16] The infant often enters the sleep cycle in REM. By about 4 months of age, as sleep cycling approaches the adult mode, sleep state progression matures and NREM sleep typically precedes REM sleep. Breathing abnormalities, including obstructive sleep apnea syndrome (OSAS), may be exacerbated or only seen in REM sleep. For this reason, sleep staging is an important aspect of PSG evaluation to assess the sleep-state dependence of breathing abnormalities and to ensure that all stages have been documented during the study.[2]

Normally, brief arousals occur as the sleeper transitions between each stage of sleep, usually without a return to full wakefulness.[17,18] These endogenous transitional arousals are common as sleep begins to differentiate in the REM and NREM progression of the infant both quantitatively and qualitatively as the child matures. As an individual transitions to REM through the lighter phases of NREM sleep during the night, a continuum of behaviors including stretching, brief vocalizing, crying, or changing of position is common. Arousals during PSG are scored because these may

also be consequences of abnormal breathing events during sleep. However, there is the suggestion that apnea in children may not always be terminated with frank cortical arousal.[2]

APNEA

Apnea is best defined as the absence of air flow at the nostrils and mouth. The three main categories of apnea are central, obstructive, and mixed. Central apnea occurs when respiratory effort ceases; there is no chest movement and hence no air flow (Fig. 32-5). Diagnosis of central apnea must take into account a multitude of factors. It is ordinarily significant when it exceeds 20 seconds in duration. Because infants normally have a more rapid baseline respiratory rate and a reduced respiratory reserve, and therefore less protection from hypoxia, shorter central events can be more clinically significant in this age group. Central apnea can yield significant physiologic compromise such as bradycardia or color change associated with declining oxyhemoglobin levels.

For infants, central sleep apnea must be distinguished from other causes for respiratory pauses, including the more common periodic breathing pattern and the obligatory respiratory pauses that follow a deep yawn or sigh. Although a rare cause of central apnea, seizures will also change the respiratory pattern seen on a tracing. In the more severe cases, central apneas can be treated with medication. The presence of frequent central sleep apnea is a usual cause for respiratory monitoring during sleep. Premature infants are at increased risk for central apneas. Central apnea accounts for 10% to 25% of all apnea in premature infants.[13]

In children, OSAS is a disorder of breathing during sleep characterized by prolonged partial upper airway obstruction (hypopnea) and/or intermittent complete obstruction (apnea) that disrupt normal ventilation during sleep and normal sleep patterns. Clinically, obstructive apnea is the lack or diminution of air flow despite the continuation of respiratory efforts. The obstruction can be functional or anatomic. When obstruction is present, respiratory efforts continue and tugging or retraction of the skin can be seen. OSAS accounts for only 10% to 20% of all apneas in preterm infants.[13] It has been estimated that 7% to 9% of children snore regularly, with an estimated prevalence of OSAS of 0.7% in 4- to 5-year-old children. Most affected children breathe normally while awake. However, a minority with marked upper airway obstruction also have noisy, mildly labored breathing while awake.

Obstruction lasting 10 seconds or longer is regarded as significant in adults. For some children,

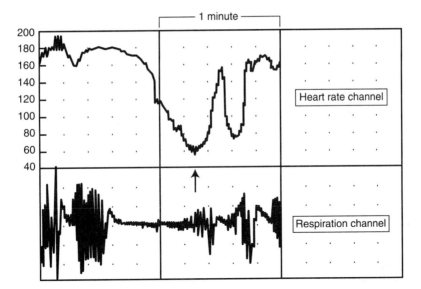

Fig. 32-5

Forty-second central apnea with secondary bradycardia detected and recorded by a Corometrics 500-E memory monitor.

however, durations of obstruction shorter than 10 seconds are important. Thus some physicians have suggested using a criterion of two respiratory cycles in duration, whereas others have suggested 6 or 8 seconds as durations indicating significant upper airway obstruction during childhood. In some infants with clinically significant OSAS, little or no snoring may be heard by the caregiver, unlike the clinical manifestations of OSAS in older children and adults.[2]

Obstructions can be caused by the presence of an anatomic abnormality, neurologic condition, or medical condition. Reduction of the airway size leads to increased respiratory effort, which can create negative airway pressure and paradoxically worsen the obstruction. The most common anatomic factors leading to OSAS include large tonsils or adenoids, obesity, micrognathia (small jaw), or other anatomic anomalies. Muscular hypotonia is one of the most common neurologic factors contributing to OSAS. Normal muscle tone inhibition during REM sleep can change respiratory patterns with more breath-to-breath variability increasing the risk of full or partial airway obstruction. Hypotonia can be commonly seen in Down syndrome, muscular dystrophy, and other genetic disorders. Allergies or even mild upper respiratory tract infections can serve to swell mucous membranes and thereby contribute to obstruction. Some of the less common risk factors include laryngomalacia, pharyngeal flap surgery, sickle cell disease, structural malformations of the brain stem, and certain metabolic and genetic disorders.

COMPLICATIONS

Apneas and hypopneas lead to a drop in oxygen saturations and an increase in blood carbon dioxide and often will cause a full or partial arousal pattern in sleep EEG tracings. When these events occur multiple times at night there are several anticipated effects. The presence of frequent arousals leads to fragmented and inefficient sleep. This can lead to increased daytime sleepiness. In young children, this can result in increased time sleeping. In older children, this sleepiness is often manifested by behavioral changes and poor school performance (in appropriately aged children). All children are at risk for cardiac and pulmonary effects of recurrent hypoxia and hypercarbia. These can lead to *cor pulmonale,* a condition in which the blood pressure in the vessels of the lung is increased and the right side of the heart enlarges in order to compensate. With time, these abnormalities can become irreversible.

TREATMENT

Adenoid and tonsillar enlargement account for most cases of pediatric obstructive sleep apnea. Removal of the adenoids and/or tonsils usually provides a cure in those instances. Older children may also benefit from nasal continuous positive airway pressure (NCPAP), which is also commonly used in adults. NCPAP acts as a splint to prevent collapse of the pharyngeal tissues. Because a range of pressures may be therapeutic, NCPAP must be titrated to the patient. Usually this is done in the setting of an overnight polysomnogram to obtain a precise titration. The major drawbacks to NCPAP are poor patient tolerance and poor compliance. Children will often benefit from the opportunity to become acclimated to the mask, and behavioral support may improve compliance. If the obstruction is severe and unresponsive to other interventions, tracheostomy may be necessary.

Mixed sleep apnea is the combination of central and obstructive apnea, with the central component usually followed by obstruction (see Fig. 32-4). Because of this, therapies that are effective for central apnea are also effective in treating mixed apnea. For example, during infancy, medications can be used to treat both forms of apnea.

In the normal neonate, particularly the premature infant, breathing can be irregular. Periodic breathing is defined as episodic pauses in respiratory movements each lasting 4 to 10 seconds alternating with several appropriate breaths. Apnea is considered a more serious condition because the respiratory pause is longer lasting and is frequently associated with more significant decreases in heart rate below 80 beats per minute and declining oxyhemoglobin values. Although periodic breathing is usually considered benign, for very small infants even short apneic pauses can cause significant bradycardia and oxygen desaturations.

Periodic breathing can occur during wakefulness, active sleep (REM), and quiet sleep (NREM), but its prevalence is increased in active sleep. In quiet sleep, periodic breathing becomes regular, that is, breathing and apneic intervals are of similar duration. In active sleep, the frequency of respirations and subsequently periodic breathing becomes irregular. The most well-defined periodic breathing observable in small infants is in quiet sleep during the EEG pattern known as tracé alternant, commonly seen in infants younger than 44 weeks' conceptional age.[19] Tracé alternant is an episodic EEG pattern in which complex bursts of moderate- to high-amplitude slow waves are superimposed on a continuous background of polymorphic theta and faster rhythms.[20]

All types of apnea are seen in the neonatal intensive care unit (NICU) and at home in the first year of life, although obstructive apnea is less common in infants. The causes of apnea in the NICU are numerous. The most important include apnea of prematurity (idiopathic), gastroesophageal reflux, hypoxia, anemia, and intraventricular hemorrhage. Sedative drugs passed to the infant during labor and delivery, or later through breast milk, can also lead to apnea.

Apnea during infancy at home can be a component of an ALTE. These episodes were often referred to as "near miss" SIDS in the past. Those that require vigorous stimulation or CPR are severe ALTEs and demand special attention because there is an increased risk of subsequent death. Episodes that occur while the infant is awake are more likely to be associated with gastroesophageal reflux, seizures, incoordination of swallowing and breathing during feedings, and crying with breath-holding.[21] In contrast to the neonate in the NICU and the infant at home, the older child is predominately affected by OSAS.

HOME CARDIORESPIRATORY MONITORS

Because apnea and/or respiratory instability have been the most prominent hypotheses for several decades, cardiorespiratory monitors (also called apnea monitors) are frequently prescribed for high-risk infants. Recordings of a small number of SIDS deaths, however, show that bradycardia is present for several minutes before the advent of central apnea.[22] The cause of this bradycardia then becomes the crucial issue. It may be secondary to hypoxemia after apnea.

One of the consequences of our uncertainty about the cause or causes of SIDS is that a rational approach to prevention is difficult. Cardiorespiratory monitors theoretically should be useful in prevention of either cardiac or respiratory death, but the efficacy of these devices has not been scientifically proved or disproved, and monitored infants have died despite quick parental response to the alarm.[22] Conversely, there are hundreds of anecdotal reports that infants have been saved after a caregiver is alerted by a monitor alarm.

Cardiorespiratory monitors for use at home have two immediate purposes: they alert the caregiver to a cardiorespiratory abnormality, and they are diagnostic devices.[23] Ultimately, they are intended to prevent death. The standard monitor in the United States is an impedance-type monitor that detects chest movements and ECG tracings through electrodes placed on the chest. The monitors contain alarms for conditions such as apnea, tachypnea, bradycardia, tachycardia, and sometimes oxygen desaturation. The settings at which each alarm may ring are typically adjustable. Because the monitors detect chest wall movement, they are not as sensitive for obstructive apneas, since chest wall movements may continue through the apnea.[24]

Many alarms can record data in memory for later downloading and analysis. In this manner, the conditions leading up to an alarm can be evaluated for clinical significance and "false alarms" eliminated. Often, alarms will be programmed to save data recorded just before, during, and after an alarm (Fig. 32-6). However, the alarm memory will also indicate the total recording time, which is a useful gauge of parental compliance with monitoring. Ensuring compliance may be important because some studies suggest that the majority of infant deaths with prescribed monitors occur during periods of noncompliance or inappropriate use.[25,26] Hence, encouraging parents to use the monitor is vital.

False alarms are often apnea alarms for which the monitor fails to detect the breathing movements that are actually present. Inspection of the recorded waveforms may show a complete lack of breathing movements but without any associated change in the heart rate or oxygen saturation. The presence of the ECG allows confirmation of bradycardia and

recognition of some arrhythmias. This is how the monitor functions as a diagnostic device.

Several studies have shown that false apnea alarms and loose lead alarms can be frequent and can substantially outnumber true alarms.[25,26] False alarms can be reduced by attention to electrode placement so that the electrodes "see" maximal chest or abdominal wall movements. This often means that parents must be properly trained in lead placement. However, there will always be some false alarms. Appropriate attention to the monitor settings can help eliminate false alarms set off by patient crying or movement.

It is essential that parents and other caretakers be fully trained in how to respond to an alarm. This includes being able to distinguish a false alarm

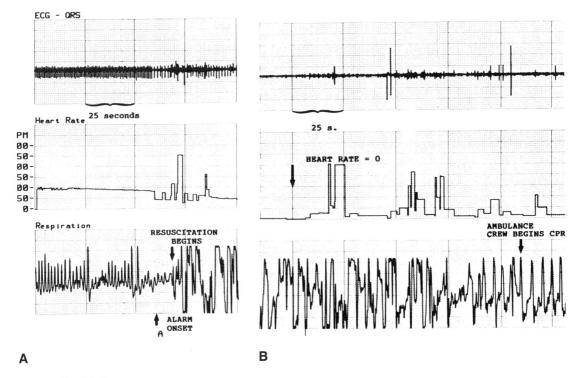

Fig. 32-6

A, Recording from patient over 100 seconds, including 62 seconds of prealarm data. At the beginning of the prealarm phase, the heart rate is already low at 100 beats per minute. Subsequently, there is a slow but steady drop in heart rate to 80 beats per minute, followed by an abrupt drop to 40 beats per minute 2 seconds before the bradycardia alarm. A resuscitation artifact can be seen 6.5 seconds after alarm onset. **B,** Recording over 150 seconds shows the heart rate falling to 0 beats per minute as parental resuscitation efforts continue. The heart rate then increases to an apparent rate of 250 beats per minute, but the ECG channel *(top panel)* shows artifact. Toward the end of this tracing, resuscitation becomes much more rhythmic after the arrival of the ambulance crew. No central apnea is seen in either **A** or **B,** because the resuscitation efforts would obscure this. *ECG,* Electrocardiogram; *CPR,* cardiopulmonary resuscitation. (From Kelly DH, Pathak A, Meny RG: Sudden severe bradycardia in infancy. *Pediatr Pulmonol* 1991; 10:203. Copyright 1991, John Wiley & Sons, Inc. Reprinted by permission of Wiley-Liss, Inc., a subsidiary of John Wiley & Sons, Inc.)

from a true event and to be prepared to administer CPR if necessary. CPR is a complex skill that we expect parents to be able to perform effectively at a time when they are worried or panicked. In fact, there is evidence that parents forget CPR training within a matter of weeks.[27] Affording the parents the opportunity to have repeated CPR training sessions may be lifesaving because many repeat ALTEs occur within weeks after discharge from the hospital on a home monitor.

Monitors are traditionally intended only for infants in various high-risk groups, which include those with severe ALTEs and preterm infants who continue to have apneas and bradycardias as discharge from the NICU approaches. As monitoring is begun it is often helpful to have clear clinical criteria for the discontinuation of monitoring at a later date. Monitoring is often perceived by families as an important safety net, and it can often be difficult to stop monitoring even when the clinical indications for monitoring are no longer present. Because parents are understandably often incorrect in their assessment of alarms, it follows that discontinuation is much easier and surer when the infant is on a memory-equipped monitor.

The time of hospital discharge is an emotionally taxing time for parents. The anxiety produced by having a child on a monitor at home is magnified by the likelihood that parents' sleep will be more disrupted to attend to false alarms during the night. A support system composed of personnel from the monitor supply company and medical professionals responsible for the infant's care can lessen this burden.[28] The most important criterion for the discontinuation of a home apnea monitor is the absence of any significant events for 2 consecutive months. A significant real event is a real alarm for which the infant, in the judgment of the clinician, required stimulation.

REFERENCES

1. Tildon JT, Meny RG, O'Brien J: Sudden infant death syndrome. In Dulbecco R, editor: *Encyclopedia of human biology*. San Diego. Academic Press, 1991; pp 315-322.
2. Loughlin GL et al: Standards and indications for cardiopulmonary sleep studies in children: official statement of the American Thoracic Society adopted by the ATS board of directors, July 1995. *Am J Respir Care Med* 1996; 153:866-878.
3. National Commission on Sleep Disorders Research: *Report of the National Commission on Sleep Disorders*. Department of Health and Human Services publication. No. 92-XXXX. Vol. 1. Washington, DC. US Government Printing Office, 1992.
4. Glotzbach S, Ariagno R, Harper R: Sleep and the sudden infant death syndrome. In Ferber R, Kryger M, editors: *Principles and practice of sleep medicine in the child*. Philadelphia. WB Saunders, 1995; p 231.
5. Skadberg BT, Morild I, Markstad T: Abandoning prone sleeping: effect on the risk of sudden infant death syndrome. *J Pediatr* 1998; 132(2):340-343.
6. Mitchell EA et al for the New Zealand Cot Death Study: Changing infant's sleep position increases risk of sudden infant death syndrome. *Arch Pediatr Adolesc Med* 1999; 153:1136-1141.
7. Oyen N, Markestad T, Skaerven R: Combined effects of sleeping position and prenatal risk factors in sudden infant death syndrome: the Nordic Epidemiological SIDS Study. *Pediatrics* 1997; 100:613-621.
8. Kemp JS et al: Positional ventilatory impairment in a serial study of 23 SIDS cases. *Pediatr Res* 1992; 31:360A.
9. Carroll JL, Siska ES: SIDS: counseling parents to reduce the risk. *Am Fam Physician* 1998; 57:1566-1572.
10. Haglund B, Cnattingius S: Cigarette smoking as a risk factor for sudden infant death syndrome: a population-based study. *Am J Public Health* 1990; 80:29-32
11. Kinney HC et al: Reactive gliosis in the medulla oblongata of victims of the sudden infant death syndrome. *Pediatrics* 1983; 72:181-187.
12. Panigrahy A et al: Decreased kainate receptor binding in the arcuate nucleus of the sudden infant death syndrome. *J Neuropathol Exp Neurol* 1997; 56:1253-1261.
13. Miller MJ, Martin RJ: Pathophysiology of apnea of prematurity. In Polin RA, Fox WW, editors: *Fetal and neonatal physiology*. Philadelphia. WB Saunders, 1998; pp 1129-1143.
14. National Institutes of Health: Consensus development conference on infantile apnea and home monitoring, 1986. *Pediatrics* 1987; 79:292-299.
15. Anders T: Developmental course of nighttime sleep-wake patterns in full-term and premature infants during the first year of life. *Sleep* 1985; 8:173-192.
16. Parks JD: *Sleep and its disorders*. London. WB Saunders, 1985; pp 4-70.
17. Hauri PJ: *Current concepts: Sleep disorders*. Kalamazoo, Mich. The Upjohn Company, 1992.
18. Kleitman N: *Sleep and wakefulness*. Chicago: University of Chicago Press, 1963. (Original work published in 1939) (Midway reprint edition, pp 122-127).
19. Rigatto H: Control of breathing during sleep in the fetus and neonate. In Ferber R, Kryger M, editors: *Principles and practice of sleep medicine in the child*. Philadelphia. WB Saunders, 1995; p 35.
20. Pedley TA, Lombroso C, Hanley R: Introduction to neonatal electroencephalography: interpretation. *Am J EEG Technol* 1981; 21:15-29.
21. Spitzer AR et al: Awake apnea associated with gastroesophageal reflux: a specific clinical syndrome. *J Pediatr* 1984; 104:200-205.
22. Kelly DH, Pathak A, Meny R: Sudden severe bradycardia in infancy. *Pediatr Pulmonol* 1991; 10:199-204.
23. Meny RG et al: Sudden infant death and home monitors. *Am J Dis Child* 1988; 142:1037-1040.
24. Ward SLD et al: Sudden infant death syndrome in infants evaluated by apnea programs in California. *Pediatrics* 1986; 77:451-458.
25. Weese-Mayer DE et al: Assessing validity of infant monitor alarms with event recording. *J Pediatr* 1989; 115:701-708.
26. Nathanson I, O'Donnell J, Commins MF: Cardiorespiratory patterns during alarms in infants using apnea/bradycardia monitors. *Am J Dis Child* 1989; 143:476-480.
27. Berardi C et al: CPR skill retention in caregivers of high risk home monitored infants. *Pediatr Pulmonol* 1991; 11:369.
28. Ahmann E, Wulff L, Meny RG: Home apnea monitoring and disruptions in family life: a multidimensional controlled study. *Am J Public Health* 1992; 82:719-722.

CHAPTER 33

Pediatric Airway Disorders and Parenchymal Lung Diseases

Loren A. Bauman
Douglas R. Hansell

THE PEDIATRIC AIRWAY

Airway disorders may cause severe and at times sudden threats to a child's life. The special susceptibility of children to disorders of the airways stems from several factors. Congenital abnormalities of airway structures tend to cause difficulties early in life. Even when normal anatomy is present, the relatively small size of the pediatric airway puts children at a distinct disadvantage. The inherently narrow trachea, bronchi, and bronchioles can become critically compromised by minimal swelling of the respiratory mucosal lining or by the presence of foreign objects. Children are at increased risk for such narrowing or obstruction because of their susceptibility to respiratory infections and their tendency to engage in risky behaviors, such as placing small objects in their mouths.

In comparison to the adult, once a child's airway does become narrowed or obstructed, the pediatric respiratory system is less able to cope with the resulting ventilation abnormality. In the event of complete airway obstruction, children undergo rapid onset of hypoxia, with its resultant neurologic damage or death. The rapidity of this oxygen desaturation is in part caused by the child's small functional residual capacity combined with an overall increased metabolic rate. Essentially there is minimal oxygen reserve available to supply the child's oxygen requirement. This combination of increased susceptibility to and decreased ability to cope with airway compromise helps explain why children suffer so frequently from airway disorders.

UPPER AIRWAY

Many unique aspects of anatomy must be understood to appropriately support and intervene on behalf of a child during respiratory illness. The upper airway consists of all structures connecting the mouth and nose with the glottis. This includes the nose, nasal choanae, nasopharynx, mouth, oropharynx, and structures of the larynx (Fig. 33-1). When compared with that of the adult, the anatomy of the infant's airway contains several characteristics and functional limitations.

The epiglottis is long, floppy, and angled away from the tracheal axis. It shrouds the laryngeal opening because of poor support by the surrounding tissues. Structurally, the infant's larynx is positioned higher in the neck (near C3-4) when compared with an adult's larynx (at C4-5). Because of this superior location, the tongue base tends to "hide" the larynx from view during direct laryngoscopy. The cricoid cartilage is a nonexpandable cartilaginous ring that is normally the only complete ring of cartilage in the airway. In the pediatric airway, it is the larynx's narrowest portion. With this reduced and fixed dimension, an endotracheal tube may pass through the vocal cords and yet not proceed to the subglottic

trachea. This already narrowed portion of the airway becomes severely narrowed by even small amounts of edema that develop with diseases such as laryngotracheobronchitis (LTB) or trauma (e.g., endotracheal intubation).

Infants are considered obligate nose breathers until 3 to 6 months of age. Immaturity of coordination between respiration and oropharyngeal motor activity accounts partly for obligate nasal breathing. Also, the infant's tongue is closer to the roof of the mouth and makes mouth breathing difficult. Because the large tongue and small mouth make air passage through the mouth impossible, except when crying, patency of the nasopharynx is critical in an infant.

The upper airway and lung do not complete development until approximately 8 years of age. The immature cartilage found in the infant's trachea and bronchi is soft and highly compressible. When the supporting cartilage is excessively flexible, the diagnosis of laryngomalacia or tracheomalacia is applied.

LOWER AIRWAY

The trachea divides into the mainstem bronchi, which in turn divide into smaller divisions called subsegmental bronchi. This repeated division continues in the adult to 23 generations of smaller and smaller air passages, creating a huge surface area for gas exchange. At birth, however, the infant has only 16 to 17 generations (divisions) of airways. The terminal generation of airways, the respiratory bronchioles, are present in relatively small numbers, resulting in a small transectional area for gas exchange in the infant. Because of the developmentally small airway cross-sectional area, small amounts of inflammation at the level of the respiratory bronchioles can result in severe respiratory embarrassment. In young children, the respiratory bronchioles are commonly attacked by viruses, such as respiratory syncytial virus (RSV), resulting in respiratory failure. The same infection will have little or no respiratory effect on an adult or older child with a larger number of terminal airways.

AIRWAY OBSTRUCTION

Obstruction of the upper or lower airway of a child may lead to life-threatening hypoxia and/or hypercarbia. With the high risk of morbidity comes the need to identify the etiology, recognize the clinical signs and symptoms, and choose the diagnostic methods for and treatment of the many causes of airway obstruction.

Radiographic evaluation of the upper airways includes both frontal anteroposterior and lateral

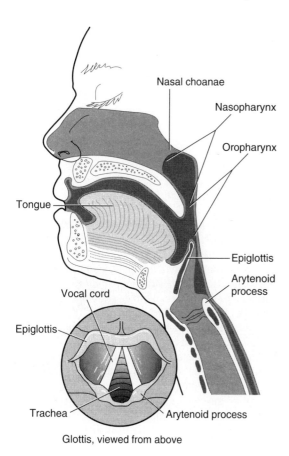

Nasal choanae

Nasopharynx

Oropharynx

Tongue

Epiglottis

Arytenoid process

Vocal cord

Epiglottis

Trachea

Arytenoid process

Glottis, viewed from above

Fig. 33-1

Normal upper airway structures.

views. When performed at the proper angle and exposure, these films are helpful in evaluating the site of upper airway obstruction (Fig. 33-2).

Fearing the unfamiliar surroundings of a hospital or clinic, a child may wiggle and scream, further increasing respiratory effort. To be successful in what could be a very difficult examination, the practitioner must proceed with slow and deliberate movement in a kind and gentle manner. However, this does not guarantee cooperation from a frightened and ill child.

The narrow airway of the child makes even a small obstruction significant, leading to a marked increase in respiratory effort. Obvious clinical signs of impaired respiratory function are cyanosis, retractions, nasal flaring, and a change in mental state, including a reduced level of consciousness or increased agitation. As a rule, tachypnea and nasal flaring alone suggest a less severe obstruction than the presence of deep retractions. However, if obstruction is severe with prolonged respiratory distress, the child may be exhausted and only able to exhibit nasal flaring. The child's mental state may range from fearful and agitated to lethargic or even unconscious. A child with mild hypoxia tends to have increased levels of agitation, whereas the

child with increasing hypoxemia and hypercarbia becomes more lethargic.

Auscultation of the child's upper airway (over the trachea) and the lower airway (over the thorax) is vital to determine the extent of air movement and obstruction. Some sounds, such as stridor, may be so prominent that they are audible from outside the patient's room! Stridor is a coarse, vibrating noise generated by airway soft tissue that typically occurs in the presence of narrowed or obstructed upper airway. Extrathoracic obstruction of the trachea causes stridor during inspiration. The deeply negative intrathoracic pressure causes the pressure inside the trachea to fall and allows the higher atmospheric pressure (outside the trachea) to collapse the trachea or larynx. This results in the "crowing" sound of stridor. During exhalation, the positive intraairway pressure forces the airway open and eliminates the stridor (Fig. 33-3). When airway narrowing is intrathoracic, stridor is present during a forced exhalation. The positive intrathoracic pressure that occurs with exhalation causes the circumferential tracheal cartilage, and hence the trachea, to collapse. During inspiration, stridor from an intrathoracic airway obstruction is minimized by

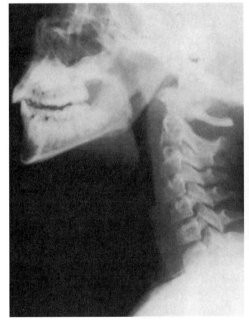
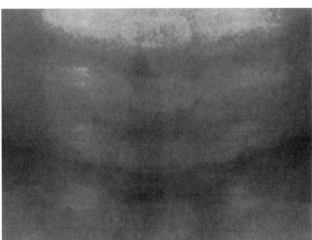

A   **B**

Fig. 33-2

Normal cervical soft tissue radiographs. **A,** Lateral view shows a thin epiglottis. **B,** Anteroposterior view illustrates the "shoulders" appearance of the subglottic trachea.

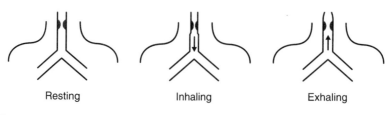

Resting   Inhaling   Exhaling

Fig. 33-3

Obstruction of the upper (extrathoracic) airway. Dynamic motion during the respiratory cycle causes accentuated narrowing during inspiration, resulting in stridor.

the radially outward tracheal traction from negative intrathoracic pressures.

Auscultation of air movement during inspiration and expiration aids in determining the severity and location of the obstruction. The pitch of the stridor can be used to assess improvement or worsening of the obstruction. Low-pitched sounds signify mild obstruction, whereas a higher pitch indicates that the child is in more distress and is attempting to generate a higher air flow rate. Sounds heard on inspiration but not expiration may indicate a "ball valve" obstruction and an accompanying risk for a pneumothorax. Absence of air movement constitutes a true emergency.

UPPER AIRWAY DISORDERS

SUPRALARYNGEAL OBSTRUCTION

Common causes of obstruction above the larynx include congenital lesions, acute inflammatory disorders, and disorders related to abnormal supralaryngeal tissue or airway tone or both (e.g., obstructive apnea).

Choanal Atresia. Choanal atresia, the stenosis or absence of the nasal passages (choanae), typically presents in the immediate postnatal period. The infant presents with severe respiratory distress that appears to lessen with crying, when the infant manages to exchange air through the mouth, and is exacerbated again once the crying stops. Occasionally, the condition is discovered when attempting to nasally suction the infant and the catheter cannot be passed through the nares. Insertion of an oral airway provides temporary relief of the obstruction but does not preclude early surgical intervention.

Pierre Robin Syndrome. Other congenital anomalies that present similarly include masses that obstruct the nasopharynx, such as encephaloceles (an outpouching of the brain into the airway) and dermoid cysts. Infants with Pierre Robin syndrome have extremely small mandibles and a small

oropharynx that causes the tongue to occlude the airway. The respiratory distress is not relieved by crying. Treatment includes temporary insertion of oral or nasal airways, placement of the infant in a prone position, and surgical repair.

Tonsillar Enlargement. The child with an acute illness characterized by fever and sore throat may develop swelling of the oropharyngeal tissues. Inflammation and swelling can progress to airway obstruction. Tonsillitis, or *streptococcal pharyngitis,* presents as exudative pharyngitis and cervical adenopathy. However, the presence of a cough and nasal congestion increases the likelihood that the infection is viral. A throat culture or rapid streptococcal antigen test is obtained to identify the causative organism. Therapy is routinely restricted to antibiotics unless the swelling is severe.

Retropharyngeal Abscess. Retropharyngeal abscess commonly occurs in children younger than 3 years of age and can cause obstruction from forward displacement of the posterior pharyngeal wall. Infectious agents involved are group A *Streptococcus, Staphylococcus aureus,* and, occasionally, anaerobic bacteria. The child often presents with a sore throat, fever, dysphagia, and voice changes. The voice sounds as if the child is attempting to speak without moving the tongue while maximally expanding the oropharyngeal airway. This is described as "hot potato voice." A lateral neck radiograph is obtained to determine the tissue thickness surrounding the abscess. Visualization of the posterior pharynx may reveal a displaced retropharynx. Surgical drainage is the preferred treatment, along with administration of appropriate antibiotics based on culture results of the aspirated material.

Obstructive Apnea. Children with a chronic history of noisy snoring and air flow loss, in spite of active chest wall movement, are likely suffering from obstructive apnea. Abnormally large adenoids or tonsils with or without abnormal positioning of the airway tissues are likely causes of obstruction. During sleep, the airway tone is decreased, resulting in more severe airway obstruction. Typically, the child with a neuromuscular disorder, such as cerebral palsy, enlarged tonsils and adenoids, or morbid obesity, is at risk for developing obstructive apnea. An electrocardiogram is obtained if nocturnal hypoxia with right ventricular hypertrophy is suspected. Sedation is usually avoided because it exacerbates airway obstruction. Surgery may relieve the obstruction in a child who has not "outgrown" the obstruction. Weight loss is often beneficial in obese children. In the interim, nasal continuous positive airway pressure can noninvasively ameliorate the disorder.

PERIGLOTTIC OBSTRUCTION

Obstruction of the airway at or just below the level of the glottis typically presents as high-pitched stridor. This region is relatively fixed in diameter because the noncompliant cartilage surrounding the glottis does not "balloon open" to allow air passage around the obstruction, as easily occurs in the more pliable tissues of the supralaryngeal airway. As a result, progressive obstruction of the periglottic area quickly leads to significant distress with both inspiratory and expiratory compromise. The most common causes of periglottic obstruction in the pediatric age group are infectious, with epiglottitis and LTB representing important causes of respiratory morbidity for this patient population.

Congenital lesions that present as periglottic obstruction are rare and include laryngeal webs and cysts and subglottic hemangioma. Vocal cord paralysis may be congenital or iatrogenic, caused by birth trauma or inadvertent surgical injury to the recurrent laryngeal nerve. Subglottic stenosis may also be congenital or acquired secondary to local trauma after intubation. A more common and benign congenital cause of upper airway obstruction is laryngomalacia. In this condition the epiglottis and arytenoid processes are oversized and floppy, causing collapse into the glottis during vigorous breathing. High-pitched stridor is noted during the neonatal period but tends to disappear by the child's first or second birthday.

EPIGLOTTITIS

Epiglottitis is a life-threatening infection that affects both children and adults.[1] It results from bacterial invasion of the soft tissues of the larynx, causing inflammation of the supraglottic structures. This leads to sudden, marked swelling of the epiglottis and surrounding tissues and may result in complete airway obstruction and death. Historically, epiglottitis has been a disease of childhood, with little prodrome, and rarely recurs. In contrast, adult symptoms are more nonspecific and often clouded by coexistent diseases.

Incidence and Etiology. The most common organism causing epiglottitis has been *Haemophilus influenzae* type B. Before widespread vaccinations with *H. influenzae* type B vaccine, bacterial epiglottitis was a fairly common pediatric illness, seen most often in children younger than 6 years of age. With the advent of widespread vaccination in 1985, the incidence has decreased by over 95%. Despite the vaccinations and reduced incidence, *H. influenzae* type B still causes 75% of epiglottitis episodes.[2] Although the vaccination program has profoundly reduced the incidence of epiglottitis, multiple isolated cases have occurred in patients with a complete vaccination history.[3] With the initiation of the vaccination program, patients with epiglottitis now tend to be older, with non–*H. influenzae* type B, principally group A β-hemolytic *Streptococcus,* being the infecting organism. Primary group A β-hemolytic streptococcal epiglottitis can develop as a rare complication of varicella in an otherwise normal host. Noninfectious causes of epiglottitis in children include thermal epiglottitis from aspiration of hot liquid and traumatic epiglottitis from repeated intubation attempts or a blind finger sweep to remove a foreign body from the airway.

Signs and Symptoms. Onset of bacterial epiglottitis is usually abrupt and associated with high fever; severe sore throat; dysphagia with drooling; cough, progressing rapidly over a few hours to stridor; muffled ("hot potato") voice without hoarseness; air hunger; and cyanosis. Suprasternal, substernal, and intercostal retractions, along with nasal flaring, bradypnea, and dyspnea, are frequently displayed. The child assumes a characteristic position of sitting upright with the chin thrust forward and with the neck hyperextended in a tripod position. The streptococcal variant of epiglottitis may be associated with a longer prodrome lasting more than 24 hours.[4]

Diagnosis. Diagnosis of epiglottitis must be assumed based on the clinical presentation. Table 33-1 lists the clinical characteristics used in the differential diagnoses for epiglottitis and LTB. Because manipulation or agitation of the child with epiglottitis can trigger complete upper airway obstruction, unnecessary diagnostic procedures are avoided (e.g., arterial blood gas analysis, chest radiography) and every attempt made to maintain a nonthreatening atmosphere for the child. Until controlled intubation can be achieved (conducted under general anesthesia with a pediatrician, otolaryngologist, and anesthesiologist present), attempts to directly visualize the

TABLE 33-1	DIFFERENTIAL DIAGNOSIS OF LARYNGOTRACHEOBRONCHITIS AND EPIGLOTTITIS	
	Laryngotracheobronchitis	**Epiglottitis**
Age	3 mo-3 yr	2-6 yr
Cause	Viral (parainfluenza, RSV)	Bacterial (*Haemophilus influenzae,* type B)
History	Gradual onset (2-3 days)	Acute onset (few hours)
	Previous cold symptoms	Complaint of sore throat
Symptoms	Stridor	Stridor
	Barking cough	Minimal cough
	Fever variable	High fever
	Hoarse voice	Muffled voice
	No position preferred	Prefers sitting upright with
	Retractions	chin forward
	Irritable	Retractions
	Does not appear acutely ill	Drooling
		Anxiety
		Appears acutely ill
Radiographic findings	Subglottic narrowing	Swollen epiglottis (thumb sign)

RSV, Respiratory syncytial virus.

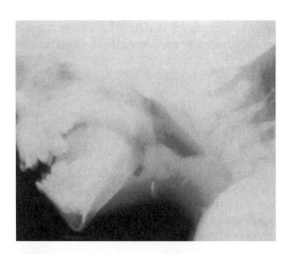

Fig. 33-4

Epiglottitis. The lateral neck radiograph illustrates the distorted, thumb-shaped epiglottic shadow.

epiglottis, draw blood, insert intravenous lines, or lay the child flat for an examination are avoided. Instead, allow the child to assume a position of comfort with "blow-by" oxygen therapy provided if necessary. If the clinical history and physical appearance of the child are only mildly suggestive of epiglottitis, more detailed examination or neck radiographs (Fig. 33-4), or both, are helpful in confirming the diagnosis.

Treatment. Establishment of a stable, artificial airway is the first priority in the treatment of epiglot-

titis. Placement of an endotracheal tube (ETT) under general anesthesia is a safe way to provide a secure, temporary artificial airway. Because there is considerable swelling to the upper airway structures, an ETT one size smaller than the predicted size (based on age) is typically used. Dramatic improvement in respiratory distress is expected after intubation, which bypasses the site of obstruction. Once the ETT is inserted, it must remain in place during the 12 to 48 hours required for the inflamed tissue to shrink in response to therapy.

Treatment of infectious epiglottitis is relatively short, with a 2-day course of ceftriaxone as equally effective as 5 days of chloramphenicol. This may be adjusted based on patient response and on the results of culture and sensitivity reports from blood and epiglottis swab specimens taken at the time of intubation. Close nursing supervision, constant use of arm restraints, along with continuously infused sedatives may suffice to prevent attempts at self-extubation. Mechanical ventilation may be needed for a short time if heavy sedation is required.

Extubation is usually considered within 24 hours when signs of toxicity (e.g., fever) diminish and when an air leak at 20 cm H_2O pressure develops around the ETT. Traumatic epiglottitis often takes several days longer for complete recovery. The physician may choose to directly visualize the epiglottis (by direct laryngoscopy or bronchoscopy) before attempting extubation to ensure adequate tissue shrinkage has occurred. The child is closely monitored for the return of stridor and other signs of respiratory distress for 12 to 24 hours after extubation.

LARYNGOTRACHEOBRONCHITIS

Incidence and Etiology. LTB, also known as croup, is the most common cause of airway obstruction in children between 6 months and 6 years of age. Typically, it presents in the fall and winter. Parainfluenza virus 1 is the most common cause, resulting in biennial epidemics in the United States during October and February of odd-numbered years. Other much less common infectious causes include influenza viruses, RSV, herpes simplex virus, and *Mycoplasma pneumoniae*.

The viral infection causes a mucosal edema and exudate formation in the glottic and subglottic areas, involving the airways from the larynx to the bronchus, hence the name laryngotracheobronchitis. The edema develops over several days, and the resultant airway narrowing becomes severe enough to cause various degrees of airway obstruction. Obstruction is more severe during inspiration, owing to the deeply negative airway pressures needed to inspire against the edematous airway. Average hospital admission rate for LTB is more than 40,000 children per year, resulting in an annual cost of $190 million, with approximately 91% of the children younger than 5 years of age.[1]

Signs and Symptoms. The child with LTB presents with a gradual prodrome of low-grade fever, malaise, rhinorrhea, and hoarse voice. Over several days, the illness progresses to inspiratory stridor and a "barky" cough, often described as sounding like the bark of a seal. Physical examination reveals nasal flaring, nasal congestion, use of accessory muscles, and suprasternal, subcostal, and intercostal retractions that along with the stridor become worse when the child is agitated.

Estimating the severity of the disease can be difficult. The illness usually occurs during cold seasons. Transporting an ill child in moderate distress in an automobile with cold ambient air commonly results in the child being virtually symptom-free on arrival in the emergency department. Inhalation of the cold air reduces the swelling and rapidly reduces the respiratory distress. More recent attempts to quantify LTB severity have centered around the presence of pulsus paradoxus[5] and the Croup Score developed by Westley (Table 33-2).[6]

Diagnosis. A lateral neck radiograph, sometimes obtained to help differentiate the disease from epiglottitis, demonstrates a large retropharyngeal air shadow without epiglottic swelling. The anteroposterior chest radiograph reveals the classic "steeple sign," a sharply sloped, wedge-shaped, linear narrowing of the trachea. This demonstrates the

TABLE 33-2	CROUP SCORING SYSTEM	
Indicators of Severity	**Findings**	**Croup Score**
Inspiratory stridor	None	0
	At rest, with stethoscope	1
	At rest, without stethoscope	2
Retractions	None	0
	Mild	1
	Moderate	2
	Severe	3
Air entry	Normal	0
	Decreased	1
	Severely decreased	2
Cyanosis	None	0
	With agitation	4
	At rest	5
Level of consciousness	Normal	0
	Altered mental status	5

From Westley CR, Cotton EK, Brooks JG: Nebulized racemic epinephrine by IPPB for the treatment of croup: a double-blind study. *Am J Dis Child* 1978; 132:484-487.

subglottic tracheal edema that extends from the larynx to the thoracic trachea (Fig. 33-5).

Treatment. Treatment of mild cases of LTB is largely supportive—ensuring temperature control, adequate hydration, and humidification of inspired air. Techniques to cool the airway have traditionally used humidified air with water particles large enough to "rain out" onto the upper airway and tracheal mucosa. Cool mist tents (croup tents) were designed to provide continuous humidified air to the trachea. Little, if any, proof of effectiveness exists on the use of this form of humidification, although anecdotes about its effectiveness are common.

If increasing respiratory effort, irritability, and inability to engage in play or eating develop, hospitalization may be indicated. Hospital care for the child with LTB is largely symptomatic and centers on careful monitoring for advancing respiratory compromise. Regular assessment of the respiratory rate, degree of retractions, mental status, and air exchange is essential. Oxygen saturation monitoring is useful, but generally desaturation is a late finding. Children requiring an F_{IO_2} of more than 0.35 are watched closely for evidence of impending respiratory failure.

Nebulized racemic epinephrine is used to induce vasoconstriction of the upper airway. With the use

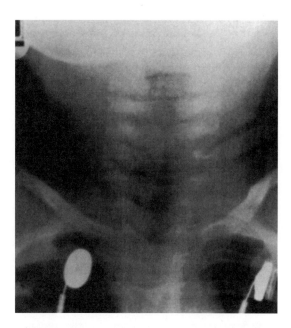

Fig. 33-5

Laryngotracheobronchitis. The anteroposterior neck radiograph reveals steeply angled subglottic walls ("steeple sign").

of a 2.2% solution, 0.5 to 1.0 ml of medication is diluted to a 3.0 ml volume with normal saline and given by inhalation with a face mask over a period of approximately 10 minutes. The aerosols are often begun in an emergency department and the child evaluated for their effectiveness. A reduction in airway edema usually occurs within 10 to 20 minutes, with a gradual reduction of its effect over 2 hours. Although the aerosols may be given as frequently as every 30 minutes, the potential side effects from cardiovascular stimulation and the implied severity of respiratory distress should limit such use to an intensive care unit setting. Reports of a "rebound" effect from persistent use of the racemic epinephrine restricted its use to inpatient settings until recently.[7,8] Today, patients are treated with dexamethasone and racemic epinephrine and discharged from the emergency department to home if they are free of intercostal retractions and stridor after a 2-hour waiting period.[9]

Recommendations for adrenocorticosteroid therapy in patients with LTB have had a long and complicated course. Original proof of effectiveness came with the combined analysis of many studies (meta-analysis) that demonstrated effectiveness of a single dose of dexamethasone at 0.6 mg/kg given intramuscularly. More recent studies have compared inhaled corticosteroids to oral systemic corticosteroids, with and without inhaled racemic epinephrine. Administration of oral dexamethasone at

0.6 mg/kg has been recommended as the least expensive and least invasive means by which to lower hospitalization rates.[7,8]

Endotracheal intubation may be necessary if the child becomes exhausted or severe respiratory distress develops. To avoid traumatizing the inflamed subglottic tissue, the ETT should be at least 1 mm smaller in diameter than that estimated for the child's age. As with epiglottitis, dramatic improvement in respiratory distress is expected after intubation. Attempts at extubation can be made if an air leak develops around the ETT at pressures under 20 to 30 cm H_2O. The child is closely monitored in the 4 to 12 hours after extubation for the return of stridor.

TRAUMATIC AND POSTOPERATIVE LARYNGOTRACHEOBRONCHITIS

Airway obstruction may occur as a sequela of endotracheal intubation. Even the most carefully placed ETT can result in significant injury to the tracheal lining. The cilia in the trachea are easily damaged, especially with aggressive suctioning procedures. Excessively large endotracheal tubes lead to necrosis of the tracheal mucosa. An ETT leak of 20 to 25 cm H_2O is recommended to minimize the pressure the ETT applies against the surface of the trachea near the cricoid ring. The value of this leak has been called into question in studies in which the presence of an ETT leak was found to be less predictive of postextubation LTB than the duration of intubation.[10]

Historically, noncuffed endotracheal tubes have been used in children younger than 8 years of age. This practice began several decades ago when low-volume, high-pressure endotracheal tubes used during anesthesia became overdistended when nitrous oxide diffused into the ETT cuff, resulting in pressure-related injury to the trachea. The safety of cuffed endotracheal tubes has since been reevaluated in several studies. When selecting a cuffed ETT, the following formula is used:

$$\frac{Age \ (years)}{4} + 3$$

In one study when this was done, 99% of the patients had a minimal leak with no increase in the incidence of postextubation LTB when compared with patients using a noncuffed ETT.[11]

Direct airway injury from suctioning induces scar tissue and granuloma development that will result in varying degrees of airway obstruction. Granulomas have developed even after very brief periods of endotracheal intubation in infants.[12]

Children who exhibit postextubation stridor are treated with racemic epinephrine per inhalation, using the same dosage of medication as when treating LTB. Dexamethasone is also given at 0.5 mg/kg intravenously (maximum dose 10 mg), repeated every 6 hours for two doses.

LOWER AIRWAY DISORDERS

BACTERIAL TRACHEITIS

Bacterial tracheitis is a medical emergency that can result in complete airway obstruction and death. Patients typically have an antecedent upper respiratory infection or LTB-like symptoms for several days before presentation with severe airway obstruction. Although the slow progression of the disease closely resembles LTB, the fever, toxic appearance, and elevated white blood cell count with an increased percentage of premature white cell forms (bands) all suggest the likelihood of a bacterial disease. Neck and chest radiographs reveal narrowing of a subglottic airway with irregular mucosal surface, without evidence of epiglottic swelling.[1]

Bacterial tracheitis responds poorly to racemic epinephrine and typically requires the placement of an artificial airway to manage the copious tracheal secretions. Treatment includes antibiotics to cover for *S. aureus, H. influenzae,* and *S. pneumoniae.* The disease resolves more slowly than epiglottitis, requiring nearly a week before extubation is attempted.

OBSTRUCTION OF THE TRACHEA AND MAJOR BRONCHI

Tracheal narrowing produces either expiratory or biphasic (inspiratory and expiratory) wheezing. The degree and flexibility of the airway narrowing will determine the severity of the wheeze. Because the trachea serves as the final conduit for the removal of secretions, lesions in this area may result in pooling of mucus with rhonchi audible during auscultation. The abnormalities are heard radiating throughout the chest but are best appreciated over the sternal area. It is often difficult to discern where the wheezes or rhonchi originate in a small child. Wheezes or rhonchi that remain equal in pitch across all regions of the chest but are heard loudest around the sternum most likely have originated in the trachea. Larger bronchial lesions produce similar manifestations but are more localized to the side of the lesion.

Tracheomalacia. Tracheomalacia is a condition of dynamic tracheal collapse caused by abnormal shape and flexibility of the tracheal cartilage rings. The abnormality can affect either a small section or the entire length of the trachea. Although often idiopathic in origin, there may be identifiable extrinsic causes that have led to tracheal wall softening. Common injurious events include neonatal ventilation with high pressures, chronic trauma to the trachea from a malpositioned ETT or aggressive endotracheal suctioning, and external compressive structures, such as a vascular ring.

In most cases of tracheomalacia the infant or child presents with chronic wheezing that becomes more severe with vigorous breathing. Fortunately, the abnormality tends to improve with time as the child's airway grows, and little intervention is necessary. Severe tracheomalacia may result in complete obstruction and profound episodic hypoxemia, especially during forced exhalation. Repeated airway collapse during exhalation leads to increasingly severe lung hyperinflation. Because exhalation is impaired by airway collapse, once the lung is completely inflated air movement is no longer possible. This scenario is most often seen in older infants with a history of prolonged positive-pressure ventilation and severe bronchopulmonary dysplasia (BPD). During severe agitation, these infants become cyanotic and even bradycardic, with little or no air movement in spite of increased respiratory effort.

Treatment options are few, mostly unsatisfactory, and include prolonged continuous positive airway pressure or ventilatory support with a tracheostomy tube in place to distend or "splint open" the airways. For milder cases, chronic sedation may avoid the episodic agitation that leads to the airway obstruction.

Congenital Tracheal or Bronchial Stenosis. Like tracheomalacia, congenital tracheal or bronchial stenosis may involve extensive or short lengths of the involved airway. The severity of symptoms depends on the degree and length of the stenosis. A common cause of stenosis in the newborn is the formation of a vascular ring. This occurs in infants with congenital malformation of the great vessels of the heart, usually a double aortic arch. With this malformation, the aorta wraps around both the esophagus and trachea. Infants can present with feeding difficulties and uncontrollable wheezing. Surgical correction of the defect can reduce symptoms, although the residual presence of focal tracheomalacia may cause respiratory symptoms to persist postoperatively.

Intraluminal Obstruction. An acquired cause of airway narrowing is the development of intraluminal obstruction. In the child, foreign body obstruction is encountered more frequently than the adult problem of endobronchial tumor. Infectious agents (e.g., *Mycobacterium tuberculosis*) or a neoplasm, classically Hodgkin's lymphoma, may cause lymphadenopathy that compresses the airway. The diffuse, chronic wheeze associated with these disorders is often confused with asthma. Endobronchial compression is suspected in an infant or child with persistent wheezing that does not respond to bronchodilator therapy. Diagnostic studies to differentiate the cause of wheezing in these patients include barium swallow (for evidence of a vascular ring), bronchoscopy, and computerized tomography of the chest. Treatment of intrinsic tracheal and major airway obstruction is frequently surgical and is directed at widening the narrowed area. Additionally, treatment of the primary cause for the lymphadenopathy, such as Hodgkin's lymphoma, is critical.

FOREIGN BODY ASPIRATION

Incidence. A leading cause of accidental death in the toddler is foreign body aspiration. The degree of respiratory sequelae depends on the nature of the material aspirated, whereas the severity of neurologic sequelae depends on the duration of ventilatory compromise. Mobile infants and toddlers are at particularly high risk by virtue of their tendency to place objects in their mouths. Inappropriate toys for a child's age may have loose parts, whereas certain foods (e.g., nuts, Vienna sausages, hot dogs) are just the right size to become lodged in a child's airway.

Signs and Symptoms. Signs and symptoms of foreign body aspiration vary with the location of

impaction and the degree of airway obstruction. They can range from unilateral wheezing or recurrent pneumonia, as when peanuts or popcorn obstruct the smaller airways, to immediate occlusion of the upper airway with complete absence of air movement and rapid death from suffocation, as seen in hot dog or balloon aspiration fatalities.

Diagnosis. The cause of the obstruction and adequacy of ventilation should be quickly determined. A thorough history of the circumstances surrounding the onset of symptoms aids in determining if this is a foreign body aspiration or an infectious process. However, a complete history is frequently difficult to obtain. Examiners must determine, first and foremost, the adequacy of ventilation, followed by the location of the obstruction. Children with sudden onset of wheezing, particularly if wheezing has never occurred before and is unilateral in nature, raise suspicions of foreign body aspiration.

Anteroposterior and lateral neck radiographs are useful if the object is radiopaque. Although the appearance of a radiopaque foreign body on a radiograph is striking, many aspirated materials, such as peanuts and carrots, cannot be detected in this fashion (Fig. 33-6). Foreign body aspiration usually occurs at the laryngeal level. Deviation in the airway

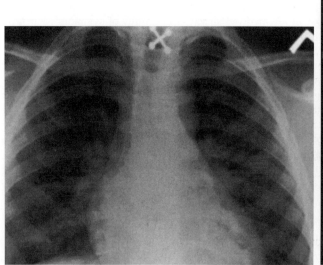

A

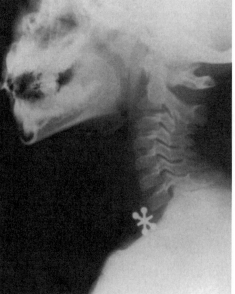

B

Fig. 33-6

Foreign body obstruction. Posteroanterior (**A**) and lateral (**B**) chest radiographs reveal an esophageal foreign body that caused respiratory distress from posterior pressure on the trachea.

shape may indicate a foreign body not otherwise visible. Recurrent pneumonia in the same lobe is also suspicious. Asymmetric lung hyperinflation can result from a ball-valve effect of foreign material localized in a major bronchus. This defect is most often apparent on an expiratory film (Fig. 33-7).[13]

Fiberoptic laryngoscopy or bronchoscopy is helpful in both finding and retrieving the foreign body. Pulse oximetry is used to determine the need for supplemental oxygen. Arterial blood gas analysis is indicated if hypercarbia is suspected in the child with severe obstruction.

Treatment. Therapy employed will vary with the severity of the obstruction. If the child is well oxygenated and ventilated, a controlled therapeutic bronchoscopy or laryngoscopy with appropriate anesthesia is preferred. When foreign body aspiration is suspected and respiratory symptoms are acute, urgent bronchoscopy with removal of the object is necessary. Even if the child appears to be stable, movement of the object to a more critical area can result in sudden clinical deterioration. The child with complete obstruction may require emergent cricothyrotomy to establish a patent airway.

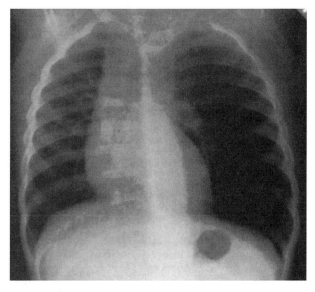

A

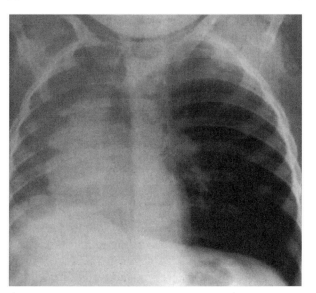

B

Fig. 33-7

Foreign body aspiration. Asymmetric lung volumes **(A),** accentuated during exhalation **(B),** indicate an obstructing ball-valve type of lesion in the left bronchus.

Blind finger sweeps of the pediatric airway may only serve to push the object farther into the airway. Five back blows followed by five chest compressions is the recommended technique for removal of an occluding foreign body in an infant. The Heimlich maneuver is not recommended for infants younger than 1 year of age, owing to the increased likelihood of intraabdominal injury.

Once the obstruction is relieved, some children will be discharged as soon as they recover from anesthesia. In others, resolution of symptoms may be delayed. Airway edema may develop and require corticosteroid therapy along with careful monitoring to ensure that a progressive obstruction does not ensue. Reactive granulation tissue at the site of impaction along with postobstructive infection may take some time to resolve. A second bronchoscopy may be required because of reaccumulation of secretions.

If intubation and mechanical ventilation is indicated, the ventilation strategies often include synchronized intermittent mandatory ventilation (SIMV), pressure support, or volume support. Because these children usually have normal lung function, the F_{IO_2} and minute ventilation requirements are low and are set to obtain normal arterial blood gas values. Once patency of the airway is ensured, mechanical ventilation is weaned. Secondary infection and prolonged intubation are occasional complications.

ATELECTASIS

Etiology and Pathophysiology. Atelectasis is collapsed lung parenchyma and is best compared to a wet sponge that fails to reinflate after being compressed. Many processes can cause atelectasis. Internal or parenchymal disorders that are characterized by an inadequate tidal volume, loss of lung compliance (e.g., acute respiratory distress syndrome), airway obstruction (e.g., mucus plugging), and increased elastance of lung tissue can all result in atelectasis. External forces also lead to compression of lung parenchyma, with the reduction in lung volume resulting in atelectasis. These include chest wall disorders (e.g., kyphosis, flail chest), accumulation of pleural fluid, obesity, and abdominal ascites.

The right middle lobe, which has the poorest collateral air circulation and smallest bronchial opening of the major lung segments, is particularly prone to mucus plugging and collapse. Intubated patients, particularly young infants, have a propensity toward right upper lobe collapse. This is most likely related to their supine positioning and tendency toward obstruction of the right upper lobe bronchus (the most proximal of all the lobar bronchi) by a migrating ETT. Postoperative patients are at particular risk of atelectasis because of an ineffective cough,

impaired mucus transport, and the effect of anesthesia. Surfactant deficiency may occur in the child after smoke inhalation or lung contusion, resulting in various degrees of lung collapse. Tracheobronchial suctioning has also been related to atelectasis in children and is believed to result from the negative pressure that the airway is exposed to during the suctioning process.

Signs and Symptoms. Clinical presentation will vary with the cause and severity of the lung volume loss. Clinical history may reveal slow regression of activity and deterioration of pulmonary function, as may be seen with a slowly growing pleural tumor. Conversely, the patient may experience rapid-onset dyspnea and cyanosis from a foreign body aspiration that occludes a large bronchus, leading to airway collapse.

Patients with enough atelectasis to create a severe ventilation/perfusion ($\dot{V}/\dot{Q}$) mismatch exhibit clinical symptoms of cyanosis, tachypnea, nasal flaring, retractions, and grunting. The patient may complain of chest pain on deep inspiration if the pleura is inflamed or there is accompanying pneumothorax.[14]

Arterial blood gas analysis reveals low oxygen saturations, manifesting low $\dot{V}/\dot{Q}$ ratios. The Pa_{CO_2} levels often remain normal in the presence of atelectasis, owing to the rapid diffusion characteristics of CO_2 and close regulation of the Pa_{CO_2} by an altering respiratory rate.

Diagnosis. Although atelectasis is most often found on a chest radiograph, it may first be suspected during a physical examination. Decreased breath sounds, increased tactile fremitus, tracheal deviation, and an elevated diaphragm may indicate atelectasis; however, many patients with atelectasis are asymptomatic on physical examination. Diagnosis is confirmed with evidence of volume loss on a chest radiograph (Fig. 33-8).

Treatment. Treatment of atelectasis is aimed at removing the cause and depends on the individual patient's clinical course. Drainage of pleural fluid or removal of external compressors will allow the lung to reexpand. If the cause is airway obstruction, bronchoscopy or good pulmonary hygiene, including aerosolized bronchodilators and chest physiotherapy, will facilitate returned airway patency. In the intubated patient, the use of continuous distending pressure may reverse and prevent further lung collapse.[15] Early mobilization and position changes in postoperative patients, along with encouragement in coughing and deep breathing (e.g., incentive spirometry), are techniques used to prevent and often treat atelectasis.

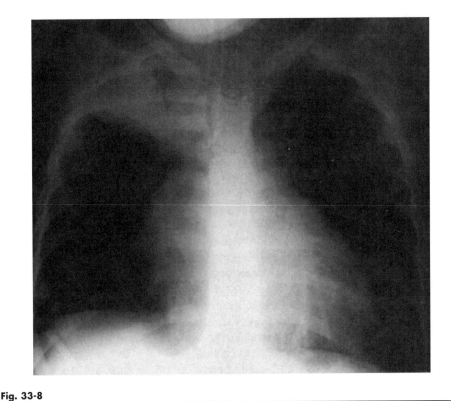

Fig. 33-8

Anteroposterior chest radiograph with right upper lobe atelectasis *(arrow).*

BRONCHIECTASIS

Etiology and Pathophysiology. Bronchiectasis is defined as irreversible dilation of the bronchial tree. Typically, the segmental and subsegmental bronchi become irregularly shaped and dilated, leading to a loss of the typical funnel configuration that allows smooth central flow of secretions. Additionally, ciliary activity in the area of the dilation is inadequate and further contributes to the difficulty in mobilizing secretions. The secretions become infected as they pool. The lower lobes, particularly the left lower lobe, are most frequently involved.

A small number of patients may have congenital bronchiectasis in which there is a defect in the development of bronchial cartilage or there is developmental failure of the elastic and muscular tissues of the trachea and main bronchi. Most patients "acquire" the disease, and bronchiectasis develops as a result of airway obstruction or chronic infection. Causes include bronchial obstruction (e.g., foreign body aspiration, mediastinal mass), infections (e.g., measles, pertussis, pneumonia), Kartagener's syndrome, and cystic fibrosis (CF).

Signs and Symptoms. Bronchiectasis may occur acutely after an infection or have a more insidious onset in patients suffering from chronic pulmonary diseases such as CF. Patients experience chronic cough, often productive of copious amounts of thick purulent sputum, and only occasional hemoptysis. Pulmonary infections are common, with recurrent fever and foul-smelling breath or sputum. Dyspnea on exertion and clubbing of the digits manifest in some cases. The lower lobes, particularly the left lower lobe, are most frequently involved.

Diagnosis. Bronchiectasis may be suspected on the basis of the clinical history and physical examination. Plain chest radiographs are seldom normal but alone are not definitive in diagnosing the disease. The abnormal pattern of bronchiectasis is seen most strikingly during bronchography.[16] However, this is rarely performed today. Instead, computed tomographic scanning is used to confirm the diagnosis (Fig. 33-9). Pulmonary function may be abnormal, with spirometry demonstrating an obstructive pattern. A combined obstructive and restrictive disease pattern may be present in the more severe cases.[17]

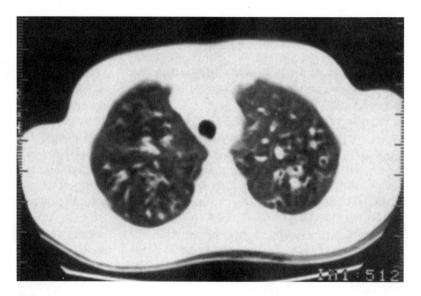

Fig. 33-9

Bronchiectasis. Computed tomographic scan of the chest of a child with cystic fibrosis reveals widened, thick-walled bronchial tubes *(cut in cross section)* in the peripheral lung zones.

Treatment. Medical management depends on the severity of the disease. Chest physiotherapy, including postural drainage and percussion, along with adequate hydration is performed to improve the mobilization of pulmonary secretions.

Antibiotic therapy is given orally, by nebulization (i.e., tobramycin), or by the intravenous route. The choice of antibiotic is based on the results of the individual patient's sputum culture results. Blind use of broad-spectrum antibiotics in this chronic disease may lead to more resistant colonization.[18]

In those cases in which the child suffers severe illness (i.e., failure to thrive, severe hemoptysis) in spite of antibiotic therapy and chest physiotherapy, surgical resection of the bronchiectatic section of lung may be considered. Patients with the disease localized to only one or two lobes are considered better candidates for surgical intervention.[19,20]

ACUTE BRONCHIOLITIS

Etiology and Pathophysiology. The term *acute bronchiolitis* is applied to a condition in infants in which a viral respiratory tract infection results in clinical symptoms of small airway obstruction.[21,22] In the majority of infants with bronchiolitis, the causative organism is respiratory syncytial virus (RSV).[23]

RSV is a highly contagious virus and has its greatest impact on young infants. Infants younger than 6 months of age are at particular risk of severe infection, with the peak incidence for hospitalization

occurring between 2 and 6 months of age.[24] Although most cases are mild and do not require hospital admission, epidemics of the infection occurring between December and March result in nearly 100,000 hospitalizations in the United States each year.[25] Postmortem evaluation of infants with severe bronchiolitis reveals obstructed airway lumina from impacted cellular debris. In vitro studies suggest that an intense inflammatory response occurs in the infant's airways and may contribute to increased mucus secretion and transudation of fluid into the airways and airway walls.[26]

Incidence. Acute bronchiolitis is seen most often in infants who are younger than 1 year of age, have a history of prematurity, live in a crowded environment, attend day-care facilities, and are exposed to passive smoke.[24] Bronchiolitis with RSV infection is particularly devastating to infants with certain at-risk conditions, including premature birth, chronic lung disease (e.g., BPD, CF), congenital heart disease (especially those with pulmonary hypertension), and immunodeficiencies.[27] These infants are at risk of respiratory failure and death.

Signs and Symptoms. Physical findings vary considerably with the patient's age. Infants (younger than 1 year of age) develop coryza, cough, respiratory distress, wheezing, and tachypnea. In contrast, the principal symptoms in children older than 2 years of age are profound nasal congestion and

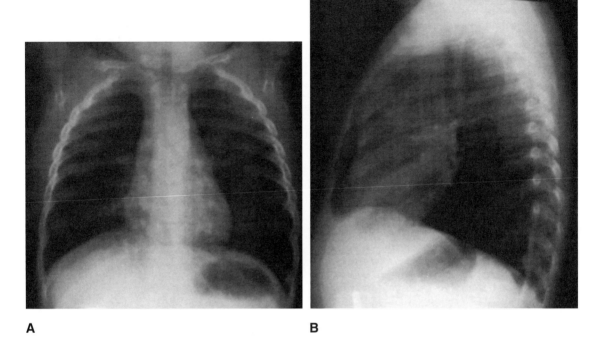

A   B

Fig. 33-10

Severe bronchiolitis. Posterior (**A**) and lateral (**B**) chest radiographs reveal flattening of the diaphragm and widening of the anteroposterior diameter, which is indicative of severe air trapping. Perihilar markings are accentuated.

productive cough. Chest auscultation reveals diffuse coarse, "sticky" rales (Velcro rales), which may be accompanied by wheezes. A chest radiograph typically reveals intense lung hyperinflation with flattened hemidiaphragms, with occasional films showing evidence of collapse or consolidation (Fig. 33-10).

Severe, life-threatening apnea is a common symptom in the very young infant with bronchiolitis, especially in those with cardiorespiratory disease or a history of premature birth or apnea. An infant may also be agitated and have difficulty feeding as a consequence of hypoxia. This may lead to dehydration as well as respiratory failure. Development of cyanosis usually heralds impending respiratory failure.

Diagnosis.   Clinical diagnosis of acute viral bronchiolitis is confirmed by identifying the RSV or other respiratory virus. Nasopharyngeal aspirate or nasal lavage provides samples of the virus. Diagnosis is based on the clinical presentation and the results of viral culture and antigen detection assays (i.e., enzyme-linked immunosorbent assays).[28]

Treatment.   Treatment of bronchiolitis is largely supportive, along with careful monitoring. The infection is self-limiting in many patients, and hospitalization is not necessary if symptoms are mild. The infant is monitored for apnea, hypoxia, and dehydration. Care is taken to provide adequate feedings and prevent further respiratory distress.

The decision to hospitalize a child with bronchiolitis involves a multifactorial assessment of the risk factors, clinical symptoms, age, and familial resources. Supportive care with supplemental oxygen, intravenous hydration if needed, and close clinical monitoring is essential. In most cases, oxygen therapy with a hood at low oxygen concentrations (30% to 40%) is sufficient to reduce the hypoxia and respiratory distress. Patients with recurrent apnea or respiratory failure may need intubation and mechanical ventilation. Continuous monitoring with pulse oximetry is essential, as well as arterial blood gas analysis in those patients whom respiratory failure is suspected.

Infants with tachypnea, agitation, and cough are at risk of dehydration. This is a frequent concern in those patients who experience vomiting with the cough. Intravenous fluids or frequent small-volume feedings are both routes to consider when fluid intake is poor.

Although the role of bronchodilators in the management of bronchiolitis is controversial, there is some evidence that they are effective. In some studies, albuterol brought significant short-term improvement in clinical scores but was not found to reduce admission rates or decrease the length of hospitalization.[29] Ipratropium bromide and theophylline have not proven to be beneficial as bronchodilators in the treatment of bronchiolitis.[30,31] Despite the evidence of airway inflammation, use of systemic or inhaled corticosteroids early in the symptomatic phase of the disease does not tend to improve outcome.[32] However, inhaled corticosteroids are sometimes given to reduce short-term morbidity when there is delayed recovery.

Ribavirin, a broad-spectrum virustatic agent, continues to play a contentious role in the treatment of bronchiolitis. It is administered as an aerosol and delivered to the patient, through either an oxygen hood or a ventilator circuit, for 12 to 18 hours per day. Although early studies proclaimed its benefits, concerns remain about its safety, cost, and efficacy. Reported side effects are uncommon; however, precautions are taken to minimize exposure to hospital personnel and family.[33] Ribavirin is expensive to use, and there is no convincing evidence that its use aids in reducing morbidity or mortality.[34-36] Studies that have concluded that there is a reduction in the morbidity and mortality rate among high-risk patients have been criticized, with many centers suggesting that the improvement was caused by improved supportive care rather than the antiviral therapy.[37] For those who support the use of ribavirin, the majority consider it most beneficial in treating extremely ill patients and those requiring mechanical ventilation. Today the role of ribavirin remains controversial and its use varies significantly among clinicians.

RSV spreads rapidly and is transmitted through touch, with the virus able to survive on hands and other surfaces (e.g., bed rails, toys). RSV prevention is accomplished by strict avoidance of other infected children and careful attention to hand washing. Disease prevention in high-risk patients (e.g., those with BPD or premature birth) can best be accomplished by passive immunization with immune serum globulin (RSV-IGIV). This passive immunity decreases the incidence of RSV hospitalization by 40% to 65% and decreases the number of hospital days by 50% to 60%.[29,38] Strict avoidance of air pollutants, especially cigarette smoke, assists in the long-term recovery from bronchiolitis.

Prognosis.　The mortality rate of infants in high-risk groups is much improved over the past several years. Recurrence of bronchiolitis episodes is seen in some patients; however, subsequent infections are usually much less severe. Studies have indicated that many patients have recurrent cough and wheezing several years after RSV infection. An increase in bronchial responsiveness is often found later in childhood.[23]

PRIMARY CILIARY DYSKINESIA

Etiology and Pathophysiology.　Normal cilia beat in a coordinated fashion, effectively propelling overlying mucus in one direction out of the airway. The upper and lower respiratory tract is cleared of secretions, inhaled particles, and bacteria. Without the forward thrust of the cilia and coordinated ciliary beating, mucus transport is slowed and there is an accumulation of particles, secretions, and bacteria in the dependent portions of the lungs.

In 1933, Kartagener described a unique clinical triad of situs inversus, chronic sinusitis, and bronchiectasis. This became known as Kartagener's syndrome. Subsequent studies found that these patients had defects in the ultrastructure of the cilia that line the mucous membranes of the sinus cavities, lungs, and nose. The syndrome was initially called immotile cilia syndrome. However, further studies have demonstrated that the cilia in patients with this syndrome are not always immotile but often have uncoordinated or ineffective cilia motility.[39] The term *primary ciliary dyskinesia* (PCD) is used increasingly today.

Signs and Symptoms.　Chronic cough, often productive, is the most common presenting feature of PCD. It is most apparent early in the morning and with sleep and exercise. Although the mucopurulent sputum initially clears with antibiotic therapy, with age the patient develops increasingly severe airway obstruction. Physical findings include persistent crackles, although wheezing is relatively uncommon. A chest radiograph may reveal lung hyperinflation and changes consistent with bronchiectasis.

Upper respiratory tract infections are common. Persistent nasal congestion, a common presenting feature, may progress to chronic nasal drainage with radiographic evidence of sinusitis. Chronic otitis media, with or without chronic effusions, frequently occurs and requires prolonged use of transtympanic ventilation tubes.[39]

A right-to-left reversal of the position of the heart and intestinal structures, known as situs inversus, is seen in approximately 50% of the patients with PCD. Isolated dextrocardia may also be found. The accepted explanation for the association of situs inversus with the ciliary defect is that normal rotation of chest and abdominal organs depends on properly functioning embryonic cilia during closure of the thoracic and abdominal cavities. Because similar functional defects are found in both mucosal cilia and sperm flagella, the abnormal cilia motility affects male fertility and males are nearly always sterile.

Diagnosis. Diagnosis can be made rapidly by microscopic evaluation for ciliary motility in specimens taken from paranasal sinuses, nose, or tracheal mucosa. Light and electron microscopy of bronchial mucosal cells reveal abnormal cilia numbers with abnormal ciliary structures. Patients with PCD have defects in the dynein arms, radial spokes, and nexin links. Cilia with an inadequate number of out-dynein arms may be immotile or may have some disorganized rigid movement.[40] Absence of radial spokes and alteration in the figuration of the microtubules in the cilia are other ciliary ultrastructural changes.[41]

Treatment. Treatment of PCD focuses on reducing the volume of pooled respiratory secretions in the lung. Chest physiotherapy for airway clearance is essential and is used with exercise and aerosolized β_2-agonists. Children with PCD have evidence of obstructive pulmonary disease. The obstruction is best minimized by exercise before physiotherapy, instead of relying on β_2-agonist therapy.[42] Because cough is one of the few mechanisms available for removing secretions, antitussive therapy is contraindicated.

Nebulized recombinant human DNase (Pulmozyme) is indicated for treatment of cystic fibrosis. It reduces sputum viscosity, improves pulmonary function, and results in a small reduction in acute respiratory exacerbations. It has been found to be beneficial in the treatment of PCD. Aerosolized or intravenous antibiotics directed by bacterial antibiotic sensitivities, in combination with CPT and Pulmozyme therapy, are believed to reduce the progression of obstructive pulmonary disease. Although rarely necessary, surgical excision of the pulmonary segments is considered when suppurative disease is poorly controlled and localized to a single area.

PNEUMONIA

Lower respiratory tract infections are a leading cause of morbidity and mortality in the pediatric population. They most often affect children younger than 2 years of age. These children typically experience the greatest number of complications. At the University of North Carolina at Chapel Hill, Denny and Clyde monitored the number of patients treated for pneumonia in their outpatient clinic.[43] Their results trace the incidence and cause of pneumonia in specific age groups (Fig. 33-11).

Gram-positive cocci, particularly group B *Streptococcus* and *S. aureus,* along with gram-negative enteric bacilli, are the source of most neonatal pneumonias. Children between 1 month and 5 years of

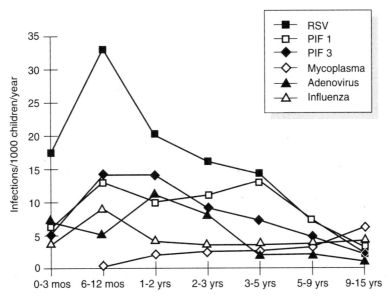

Fig. 33-11

Etiology of pediatric lower respiratory tract infection in Chapel Hill, NC by age during an 11-year period. (Modified from Denny FW, Clyde WA: Acute lower respiratory tract infections in nonhospitalized children. *J Pediatr* 1986; 108:635.)

INFECTIOUS CAUSES OF PNEUMONIA

VIRUSES
Respiratory syncytial virus
Parainfluenza types 1, 2, and 3
Influenza virus
Adenovirus
Rhinovirus
Cytomegalovirus
Epstein-Barr virus
Herpes simplex virus

MYCOPLASMA
Mycoplasma pneumoniae
Ureaplasma urealyticum

BACTERIA
Streptococcus pneumoniae
Haemophilus influenzae
Staphylococcus aureus
Streptococcus agalactiae
Legionella pneumophila
Mycobacterium tuberculosis

PROTOZOA
Pneumocystis carinii

FUNGI
Histoplasma capsulatum
Coccidioides immitis
Candida spp.
Blastomyces dermatitidis
Cryptococcus neoformans

RICKETTSIAE
Coxiella burnetii (Q fever)

CHLAMYDIA
Chlamydia pneumoniae
Chlamydia trachomatis
Chlamydia psittaci

PARASITES
Ascaris lumbricoides

---

age are the most frequent victims of viral pneumonia. RSV and parainfluenza viruses types 1, 2, and 3, along with adenovirus, are the most common infectious viral agents. However, *Chlamydia pneumoniae, H. influenzae, S. pneumoniae,* and *S. aureus* are occasional bacterial agents in this age group. *S. pneumoniae* is the major cause of bacterial pneumonia in children older than 5 years, whereas *M. pneumoniae* and *C. pneumoniae* are more common in school-age children and young adults. Box 33-1 lists the infectious causes of pneumonia in the pediatric population.

VIRAL PNEUMONIA

Respiratory Syncytial Virus. Nearly 80% of all pneumonias in the pediatric population have a viral etiology, with RSV occurring most often. RSV commonly affects children younger than 2 years old, although it has been found in older immunocompromised children or in children with chronic lung disease. Outbreaks occur annually during the winter and are rarely seen during the spring and summer. RSV often causes bronchiolitis, but pneumonia can develop.[44]

The first symptoms noted are usually coryza and nasal congestion, followed by cough, fever, and malaise. Retractions, nasal flaring, tachypnea, wheezes, and rhonchi are common. The chest radiograph typically shows hyperinflated lungs with patchy infiltrates and/or atelectasis (most often involving the right upper lobe). Dehydration can develop as a result of tachypnea, cough, and decreased feeding.

Diagnosis is confirmed with rapid immunofluorescent detection of RSV antigen in nasal washings or enzyme-linked immunosorbent assays of nasal secretions. Test methods are relatively inexpensive.

Aerosolized ribavirin is an antiviral agent that may be used to treat the infection; however, its use remains controversial. Hypoxemia and hypercarbia are complications of RSV pneumonia and may mandate supplemental oxygen for an extended period. Supportive care is aimed at monitoring the severity with pulse oximetry and arterial blood gas analysis. Patients may experience progressive hypoxemia and respiratory failure, necessitating intubation and mechanical ventilation. There may be further progression to advanced respiratory failure, in spite of maximal ventilatory support. Those patients may require extracorporeal membrane oxygenation (ECMO). Patients thought to have a less than 20% chance of survival without ECMO have a nearly 60% chance of survival with ECMO.[45]

Parainfluenza Virus Types 1, 2, and 3. The parainfluenza viruses are the second most common cause of LTB and pneumonia. Type 3 is the most common cause in children younger than 5 years of age and occurs year round with no seasonal peak. Clinical presentation is similar to that described for RSV. Chest radiographs typically reveal patchy or interstitial infiltrates. Diagnosis is confirmed with rapid antigen testing or viral isolation from a nasal washing. Therapy is supportive, with supplemental oxygen and additional hydration provided as needed. Parainfluenza virus is not to be confused with influenza virus, which has a very narrow seasonal peak.

Influenza Virus. Although influenza virus may cause pneumonia, it occurs predominantly in the very young and very old patient. Yearly epidemics occur during the late winter and early spring. Clinical symptoms consist of rapidly developing fever, malaise, and myalgia. Duration of the illness is usually shorter than that of RSV and the parainfluenza viruses. Although rarely occurring, a rapid pneumonia may result in death within 2 days of onset. Diagnosis and treatment are similar to that of RSV and parainfluenza virus infections. Vaccines are provided annually and are recommended for those high-risk children with chronic cardiopulmonary and immunologic disorders. Chest radiographs typically reveal interstitial or patchy alveolar infiltrates.

Adenovirus. Although it occurs year round, adenoviral pneumonia is most often seen in the late summer and early fall. It occurs most often in children younger than 2 years of age. It is easily confused with bacterial illnesses because it mimics their symptomatology: rapid onset, high fever, leukocytosis, and chest radiograph consistent with pneumonia. Additional findings may include lymphadenopathy and conjunctivitis. A chest radiograph reveals patchy or interstitial infiltrates.

Certain adenoviral types (i.e., 3, 7, 21) are associated with a high mortality rate owing to the overwhelming sepsis and cardiovascular collapse that occurs. Diagnosis is confirmed with rapid antigen testing or viral isolation from a nasal washing. Therapy is supportive, and no specific treatment is available. Close monitoring for bacterial superinfection is suggested.

BACTERIAL PNEUMONIA

Incidence. Although the incidence of bacterial pneumonia is less than that of viral pneumonia, it has a higher mortality rate. It may occur as a secondary problem to a primary viral pneumonia, as is often seen with pneumonia from influenza virus. Certain other factors known to increase the risk of bacterial pneumonia include compromised immune function, recurrent aspiration from gastroesophageal reflux, malnutrition, day-care attendance, exposure to passive cigarette smoke, and congenital abnormalities of the airway (e.g., tracheoesophageal fistula). Bacterial pneumonia is seen throughout the year, with a peak incidence in the winter and early spring.

Etiology. Bacterial agents that cause pneumonia vary considerably throughout the pediatric age group. In the neonatal patient, the offending bacteria are most often contaminates from the mother's genital tract and include group B *Streptococcus*, *Escherichia coli*, *Listeria monocytogenes*, and *C. trachomatis*.[46] Infants older than 4 to 6 weeks of age tend to develop pneumonia from *S. pneumoniae*, *H. influenzae*, and *S. aureus*. Less likely organisms include *Bordetella pertussis*, *M. pneumoniae*, and *C. pneumoniae*.

Bacterial pneumonia develops when the intrinsic host defenses are decreased, either by another disease process (e.g., viral infection) or when the anatomic protective mechanisms are destroyed (e.g., primary ciliary dyskinesia). Therefore, any microorganism colonizing the upper respiratory tract has the potential to cause pneumonia if it evades these defenses.

Signs and Symptoms. There are no symptoms that distinguish a bacterial pneumonia from a viral pneumonia in children, although children with bacterial pneumonia tend to present with more severe symptoms of fever and distress. Prodromal symptoms are often nonpulmonary in nature and include headache, fever, malaise, and abdominal pain. Productive cough, with sputum often swallowed, and chest pain during inspiration (pleuritic pain) are common complaints. Physical examination usually reveals nasal flaring, accessory muscle use, intercostal and subcostal retractions, tachypnea, and shallow breathing. Crackles, decreased breath sounds, increased fremitus, and dullness to percussion are often found during auscultation and examination of the chest.[47]

Diagnosis. The chest radiograph is an important diagnostic tool when evaluating a child with suspected bacterial pneumonia. Although bacterial pneumonia is commonly manifested as an alveolar consolidation, lobar and interstitial infiltrates are often found as well as pleural effusion. It has been suggested that certain radiographic findings vary among the various bacterial agents involved and may help determine the etiology.[48,49]

An elevated total band count (>1500 total bands) is common in the presence of bacterial pneumonia. Increased C-reactive protein levels and erythrocyte sedimentation rates provide supporting, albeit not specific, evidence of inflammation. Blood culture is the most helpful test to give absolute confirmation of bacterial disease, but it is only positive in 25% of patients with *S. pneumoniae* pneumonia and 33% of patients with *S. aureus* pneumonia. Similarly, the latex particle agglutination and countercurrent immunoelectrophoresis studies are insensitive in most cases of pneumonia. When pleural fluid is present in significant quantities, sampling for Gram's stain and culture will yield specific bacterial diagnosis in 65% to 80% of the patients. Bronchoalveolar lavage fluid obtained during a bronchoscopy can be used for atypical presentations. Lung tissue may be obtained for culture through an open-lung biopsy, transthoracic needle aspiration biopsy, or percutaneous lung puncture.

Precise microbiologic diagnosis is not always obtained even though bacterial pneumonia is suspected. There are several reasons why clinicians may take an empirical approach to treatment. Many of the diagnostic procedures are much too invasive for any but the sickest patients. Some procedures use instruments (e.g., bronchoscope, suction catheter) that pass through the contaminated pharynx or upper airway. Although it is difficult to obtain a sputum specimen in children younger than 8 years of age, when it is obtained the flora in the upper airway contaminates the sputum, making the etiologic diagnosis questionable.

Treatment. Standard initial treatment of bacterial pneumonia varies considerably according to the patient's age and immunologic status, time of year, and local antibiotic sensitivity patterns. The need for hospitalization is often determined by the severity of the symptoms. When the cause is identified, antimicrobial therapy is determined and is usually given for 7 to 14 days by the parenteral route, although the clinical symptoms and history of underlying disease often guide empirical therapy. Neonatal pneumonia is routinely treated with intravenous antibiotics. The patient is monitored with pulse oximetry and arterial blood gas analysis when indicated. Supplemental oxygen is provided if hypoxia occurs and mechanical ventilation is provided if there is respiratory failure. The role of chest physiotherapy in the treatment of pneumonia is debated, with some clinicians doubting its efficacy.

Streptococcus pneumoniae. The most common cause of bacterial pneumonia is the pneumococcus.[50] The clinical picture differs with age. The infant presents initially with a sudden fever and diarrhea or vomiting. Signs of respiratory distress, including nasal flaring, tachypnea, grunting, and retractions, appear along with restlessness and cyanosis. The classic clinical presentation of the older child is that of rapid-onset respiratory distress, high fever, shaking chills, headache, pleuritic pain, and cough with rust-colored sputum. The chest radiograph usually reveals lobar or segmental alveolar consolidation, which may be accompanied by a pleural effusion or empyema. Sputum reveals sheets of gram-positive diplococci and many white blood cells. The clinical diagnosis can be made based on these findings. However, in reality the clinical presentation is rarely this clear and treatment of suspected bacterial pneumonia includes pneumococcal coverage.

Pneumococcal pneumonia can be rapidly fatal without appropriate therapy. Penicillin is the antibiotic of choice; erythromycin is used in the penicillin-allergic individual. Although penicillin resistance in the United States is rare, it is increasingly common in Europe and Africa. Therefore, treatment should be guided by antibiotic susceptibilities when an organism is recovered. Other antibiotics that have successful activity against *S. pneumoniae* include cephalosporins, chloramphenicol, clindamycin, and vancomycin.

Haemophilus influenzae. Before the use of vaccination against serotype b, this gram-negative rod was a frequent cause of pneumonia in children. Infection occurs most often in children younger than 5 years of age. The chest radiograph is highly variable and can exhibit any pattern from a bronchiolitic-type picture with hyperinflation to patchy infiltrates to segmental or lobar consolidation. Pleural effusion is present in about one third of the patients. Positive blood culture results or positive results on urine antigen screens confirm diagnosis. Empirical therapy is usually with a cephalosporin. Other potentially therapeutic drugs effective against all *H. influenzae* isolates include trimethoprim-sulfamethoxazole, clarithromycin, azithromycin, chloramphenicol, and amoxicillin/clavulanate.

Staphylococcus aureus. Pneumonia caused by *S. aureus* ("staph") is a virulent, aggressive disease that can be rapidly fatal, particularly in infants younger than 1 year of age. This organism is commonly found on the skin and mucosa, with 20% to 30% of the population carrying bacteria in the nose. Pneumonia is frequently seen in debilitated patients who often have associated skin infections. It is common to have a history of an antecedent viral infection, particularly influenza.[50]

The severity of clinical symptoms varies, with the typical presentation being an upper respiratory tract infection, fever, cough, and respiratory distress. The clinical course in the neonate is often rapidly progressive and is associated with a high mortality rate shortly after the onset of symptoms. The chest radiograph usually reveals large consolidation that can progress rapidly to a "whiteout" of the lung. Pleural effusion and empyema as well as a pneumothorax often complicate the clinical picture. While resolving, areas of consolidation often progress to pneumatoceles, which are round, air-filled areas of lung destruction that are easily visible on the radiograph. The pneumatoceles may contain fluid and change rapidly in number and size, leading to a mediastinal shift.

Diagnosis is by positive blood, skin abscess, or pleural fluid culture results. Therapy is with antistaphylococcal penicillins such as nafcillin and oxacillin. Susceptibility testing is imperative to exclude the possibility of methicillin-resistant *S. aureus,* which requires treatment with vancomycin.

ATYPICAL PNEUMONIA

The major pathogens of pneumonia that are commonly missed by the tests listed previously cause "atypical" pneumonia. In the neonate, those agents include the uncommon viral diseases of rubella, varicella-zoster, and cytomegalovirus and the even rarer nonbacterial agents of *Toxoplasma, Treponema pallidum,* and *C. trachomatis.* In the older child, *M. pneumoniae, C. pneumoniae,* and *M. tuberculosis* cause atypical pneumonia.

Mycoplasma pneumoniae. *M. pneumoniae* commonly causes a community-acquired pneumonia that is seen year-round but peaks in the late summer and early fall. Although it occurs in all age groups, it is most often a disease of school-aged children and young adults.[51]

The incubation period is 2 to 3 weeks, and it presents as a viral upper respiratory infection. Clinical onset is insidious, with a gradual development of malaise, fever, and cough, which are the most prominent symptoms. Cough is nonproductive or productive with blood-tinged sputum. Chills, pharyngitis, headache, nausea, vomiting, diarrhea, and chest pain are also associated with this infection. Crackles are heard most often during auscultation, with occasional wheezing, although there may be no abnormal findings at the beginning of the illness. The clinical and radiographic findings are often out of proportion with the clinical severity, hence the common lay description of "walking pneumonia" is often applied to this infection. The chest radiograph usually reveals bronchopneumonia with patchy infiltrates.[52,53] The complete blood cell count is usually normal; however, a cold hemagglutinin assay with titers of 1:64 is highly suggestive of infection with *M. pneumoniae.*

Without treatment, the illness resolves in 2 to 4 weeks. Oral erythromycin for 10 to 14 days provides optimal therapy and the patient usually becomes afebrile within 48 hours. Azithromycin has also shown efficacy.[54]

Chlamydia pneumoniae. Infected respiratory droplets most likely transmit *C. pneumoniae.* Primary infection occurs most often in school-aged children and young adults.[55] Only a small portion of patients infected are clinically symptomatic, yet some patients experience severe illness leading to death. Most infections with *C. pneumoniae* are mild and are commonly coincidental with other bacterial pathogens. Illness is characterized by pharyngitis, followed several days later with cough. Fever is often present early in the illness but does not persist. Wheezing is frequently heard on auscultation. In fact, this infection has a strong correlation with recent-onset asthma.[56,57]

Host factors appear to influence the severity of this illness. Immunocompromised patients with the acquired immunodeficiency syndrome, malignancy, primary immune deficits, and sickle cell disease may have severe or frequent infections. *C. pneumoniae* is a frequent cause of acute chest syndrome in children with sickle cell disease and may also act as a trigger for acute asthma.[58]

C. pneumoniae is difficult to isolate, even in tissue culture, and requires special handling of the culture sample. Because of long delay in serologic diagnosis, empirical antibiotic therapy is commonly employed. Infection with *C. pneumoniae* is treated with tetracycline or erythromycin for 10 to 14 days, although a prolonged course of 21 days is not uncommon.

VENTILATOR-ASSOCIATED PNEUMONIA

A patient who is receiving mechanical ventilatory support is at risk of developing pneumonia. New onset of pulmonary infiltrates can occur, stemming from a multitude of causes including atelectasis, infection, spontaneous or catheter-related pulmonary emboli, or acute lung injury. The pathogenesis appears to involve the microaspiration of oropharyngeal organisms. Clinical and radiographic criteria for diagnosing ventilator-associated pneumonia are unreliable.

The development of ventilator-associated pneumonia increases hospitalization stay by 30% but does not change mortality rates. In pediatric patients undergoing mechanical ventilation, polymicrobial aerobic and anaerobic flora are isolated from pulmonary specimens. Predominant aerobic bacteria are *Pseudomonas aeruginosa* and *Klebsiella pneumoniae,* whereas the predominant anaerobic bacteria are *Prevotella, Porphyromonas, Peptostreptococcus, Fusobacterium,* and *Bacteroides fragilis.*[59]

To better establish the diagnosis of ventilator-associated pneumonia, Gram's stain of bronchoalveolar lavage fluid is obtained through a fiberoptic bronchoscope. Bronchoalveolar lavage fluid is considered positive for ventilator-associated pneumonia when the following conditions occur:

(1) polymorphonuclear neutrophils are greater than 25 per optic field at a magnification times 100; (2) squamous epithelial cells are less than 1%; and (3) one or more microorganisms are seen per optic field at a magnification of 1:1000. Gram's stain of bronchoalveolar lavage fluid is 77% sensitive and 87% specific with a positive predictive value of 71% and a negative predictive value of 90%.[60] Although bronchoalveolar lavage samples acquired through bronchoscopy are used to diagnose ventilator-associated pneumonia, quantitative cultures of endotracheal aspirates are easier and less expensive to obtain. Persistence of significant numbers of pathogens in quantitative cultures of endotracheal aspirates occurred in 82% of the samples. This quantitative culture of endotracheal aspirates is reproducible and may be useful in the diagnosis of ventilator-associated pneumonia.[61]

Multiple forms of therapy have been attempted to minimize the risk of developing ventilator-associated pneumonia, including routine hand washing, closed airway suctioning, frequent humidifier and ventilator tubing changes, heat and moisture exchangers instead of a heated water humidifier, and heated wire circuits. Some studies suggest that the use of heat and moisture exchangers is a cost-effective clinical practice associated with fewer late-onset hospital-acquired ventilator-associated pneumonias and results in improved resource allocation and utilization.[62] However, other studies conclude their use does not affect the frequency of ventilator-associated pneumonia.[63] Decreasing the frequency of ventilator circuit changes from three times per week to once per week had no adverse effect on the overall rate of ventilator-associated pneumonia.[64] Scheduled changes in antibiotic class for empirical treatment of ventilator-associated pneumonia have been demonstrated to lower the incidence of bacteremia associated with antibiotic-resistant gram-negative bacteria.

TUBERCULOSIS

INCIDENCE AND ETIOLOGY

Tuberculosis (TB) is the most frequent infectious cause of death throughout the world. Although the frequency declined in the 1980s and early 1990s, the disease is again increasing in incidence and severity.[65,66] It is a chronic bacterial disease caused by infection with *M. tuberculosis*. This organism is a very hearty and virulent bacteria that resists inactivation by drying, heat, and sunlight. Patients infected with *M. tuberculosis* are usually medically underserved, poverty stricken, or immunocompromised. Most children do not develop clinical disease unless disease resistance declines, owing to malnutrition, fatigue, or chronic illness.[67]

TRANSMISSION

Transmission is airborne, occurring through the inhalation of viable respiratory droplets in an enclosed space (e.g., room, hospital). The pathogen is rapidly killed by ultraviolet light in the outside air. The household contact for an infant or child is usually an adult; rarely is there child-to-child transmission. The incubation period lasts from 2 to 10 weeks, at which time a skin test becomes positive, manifesting a delayed-type hypersensitivity (Box 33-2).

SIGNS AND SYMPTOMS

Most infants and children who become infected with *M. tuberculosis* never develop TB and remain asymptomatic. They may continue with few if any clinical symptoms or may manifest nonspecific signs of fever, weight loss, and failure to thrive. Most patients develop cough and wheezing, with crackles and rhonchi heard in some cases. Chest radiography in these individuals reveals focal or diffuse infiltrates. Many cases of pulmonary infection with *M. tuberculosis* are caused by reactivation and are characterized by focal findings on chest radiography in a patient with chronic respiratory and systemic symptoms.

DIAGNOSIS

Diagnosis in the adult is based on identification of stains of gastric or respiratory washings that have

---

BOX 33-2

CUT-OFF SIZE OF INDURATION FOR POSITIVE MANTOUX TUBERCULIN SKIN TEST

≥5 MM
  Contacts of infectious cases
  Abnormal chest radiograph
  HIV-infected and other immunosuppressed patients

≥10 MM
  Foreign-born persons from areas of high prevalence
  Low-income populations
  Residents of prisons, nursing homes, institutions
  Intravenous drug users
  Other medical risk factors
  Health care workers
  Locally identified high-risk populations
  Infants

≥15 MM
  No risk factors

Modified from Starke JR, Jacobs RF, Jereb J: Resurgence of tuberculosis in children. *J Pediatr* 1992; 120:839.
HIV, Human immunodeficiency virus.

bacteria uniquely resistant to acid decoloration ("acid fast"). In children, owing to the low number of bacilli, 3 consecutive days of gastric washings may increase the sensitivity of this test. More commonly, the diagnosis of TB is based on a positive skin test (Mantoux skin test) in a patient with an appropriate clinical picture and radiographic findings.[67,68] Proper interpretation of these skin tests is critical and is based on the probability of disease using a combination of risk factors, clinical findings, and the size of induration resulting from the skin test (see Box 33-2). Differential diagnosis includes asthma, foreign body aspiration, tumors, sarcoidosis, and all pulmonary pathogens.

TREATMENT

Treatment of TB in children focuses on early diagnosis, identification of the primary case that spread the disease to the child, and long-term antituberculosis medications. For the patient with active disease, multiple medications are indicated for an extended period. These include isoniazid, rifampin, pyrazinamide, and ethambutol. Corticosteroid therapy can be safely used in conjunction with antituberculosis drug therapy to lower the inflammatory response to the infection, reduce the size of enlarged lymph nodes, and accelerate the resorption of fluid when a large pleural effusion has developed

SICKLE CELL DISEASE

INCIDENCE AND ETIOLOGY

Sickle cell disease is an autosomal recessively inherited disorder of the hemoglobin structure and is the most common inherited disease of the African-American population. Defective hemoglobin S converts from a soluble hemoglobin molecule contained in the red cells to a gelatinous state in the presence of low oxygen, low pH, rapid temperature changes, or hypernatremic dehydration. This gelatinous state causes the red cells to "sickle," resulting in a variety of complications including acute chest syndrome, cardiomegaly and left ventricular failure, splenectomy, and renal disease. Pulmonary complications are the primary cause of illness and death in patients with sickle cell disease.[69,70]

PATHOPHYSIOLOGY

A complex interaction between the abnormal cells and vascular endothelium exists, resulting in a hypercoagulable state. Recent reports of high levels of endothelin-1, an endothelial-derived vasoactive mediator, are present during a vasoactive crisis. An abnormality of the vascular endothelium may contribute to the development of acute chest syndrome. The red blood cells are more rigid, resulting in increased viscosity of blood, which causes plugging of the blood vessels.

The pulmonary effects that occur most often in patients with sickle cell disease include pneumonia, acute chest syndrome, pulmonary vascular injury, pulmonary infarction, and sickle cell chronic lung disease. Bacterial pneumonia is a frequent cause for hospitalization, and pulmonary vascular injury can cause sudden death if the occlusion is in a large vessel.

SIGNS AND SYMPTOMS

Acute chest syndrome is the leading cause of death in sickle cell disease and presents as pleuritic or chest wall pain and dyspnea. The chest radiograph often reveals pulmonary infiltrates, frequently located in the lower lobes, as well as atelectasis and pleural effusion. Young children, aged 2 to 4 years old, who present with acute chest syndrome have fever, cough, and a negative physical examination, with little or no pain. Adults are often afebrile, complaining of severe dyspnea, chills, and severe pain along the ribs, sternum, abdomen, and back.[71]

Reports in the 1970s suggested that sickle cell disease was caused by a bacterial infection; however, more recent studies suggest that bacterial infection is found in only 3% to 14% of patients, whereas *Mycoplasma* and/or *Chlamydia* infections are found in approximately 15%. Children younger than 5 years of age tend to have a milder disease course that is usually triggered by infection. Risk of death is four times higher in adults with acute chest syndrome than in children and most likely related to the higher incidence of fat embolism from bone marrow infarction. Aplastic crisis in young children with sickle cell disease is typically associated with acute human parvovirus B19 infection. Infection with this pathogen may also be related to acute chest syndrome.[72]

Pneumonia and pulmonary infarction can occur simultaneously and are sometimes difficult to differentiate. Fever and chills are seen more often with pneumonia, with fever resolving slowly. Acute pulmonary symptoms with tachypnea and pleuritic chest pain are more suggestive of pulmonary infarction. In some cases, pneumonia causes hypoxemia that leads to pulmonary infarction.[73]

Sickle cell chronic lung disease occurs most often during the teenage years and may develop after multiple episodes of acute chest syndrome. Hypoxemia is present as a result of pulmonary fibrosis and a reduction in diffusion and pulmonary perfusion. Parenchymal lung injury and an increase in pulmonary vascular resistance cause progressive dyspnea and cor pulmonale. Diffuse interstitial markings and edema are common findings on the chest radiograph.[70,72,74]

TREATMENT

Empirical therapy includes antibiotics for gram-positive encapsulated organisms of *Streptococcus, Staphylococcus,* and *Salmonella.* Erythromycin is used to provide coverage for the pathogens *M. pneumoniae* and *C. pneumoniae.* Antibiotics are quickly instituted because the infections, especially a pneumococcal pneumonia, can become life threatening.[73]

Adequate hydration is an essential therapeutic modality and is used cautiously to avoid pulmonary edema. Red blood cell transfusions are provided to improve the hemoglobin's ability to transport oxygen and reduce the incidence of acute chest syndrome, myocardial ischemia, and sickle cell chronic lung disease. Aerosolized bronchodilators and adequate pain control are also important adjuvants. Supplemental oxygen is used when indicated. In cases of impending respiratory failure, mechanical ventilation is instituted.[75,76] Successful treatment of acute chest syndrome with venovenous ECMO is reported in patients experiencing life-threatening acute chest syndrome despite maximum conventional ventilation support.[77]

RECURRENT ASPIRATION SYNDROME

ETIOLOGY

Neurologically impaired patients, those with abnormal anatomy of the gastrointestinal tract or airways, and patients with gastroesophageal reflux are often diagnosed with recurrent aspiration syndrome. The patient aspirates respiratory secretions and/or stomach contents. The low pH of the stomach contents results in a chemical pneumonitis and inflammatory response in the airways. The patients and their families suffer through multiple hospitalizations for pneumonia and airway hyperreactivity. Children who are treated for frequent asthma exacerbations, yet have negative responses to allergens, benefit from evaluation for recurrent aspiration. Infants with gastroesophageal reflux are at particular risk for pneumonia.[78]

DIAGNOSIS

Diagnosis is based on clinical and radiographic findings. Barium swallow may reveal a tracheoesophageal fistula or other malformation that requires surgical intervention. Bronchoscopy with bronchoalveolar lavage can reveal pathogens normally found in the gastrointestinal tract as well as provide visual confirmation of inflamed airways.[79]

TREATMENT

The cause and severity of the disease determine treatment. Fundoplication, a surgical tightening of the gastroesophageal junction, may alleviate gastroesophageal reflux. Appropriate antibiotic coverage is necessary to control infection. Inhaled corticosteroids are indicated to control and reduce the airway damage that occurs from chronic inflammation. Prevention of recurrent aspiration is paramount to obtaining a long-term, positive outcome. Prognosis in uncontrolled recurrent aspiration syndrome is guarded, owing to the chronic reinjury of the respiratory parenchyma.[80] Respiratory and cardiac insufficiency may develop over time. Accurate and early diagnosis, prevention, and prophylaxis may reduce the severity of the injury and improve the patient's quality of life.

REFERENCES

1. Grad R: Acute infections producing upper airway obstruction. In Chernick V, Boat TF, Kendig EL, editors: *Disorders of the respiratory tract in children.* Philadelphia. WB Saunders, 1998; pp 447-461.
2. Frantz TD, Rasgon BM: Acute epiglottitis: changing epidemiologic patterns. *Otolaryngol Head Neck Surg* 1993; 109:457-460.
3. Breukels MA et al: Invasive infection with *Haemophilus influenzae* type B in spite of complete vaccination. *Ned Tijdschr Geneeskd* 1998; 142:586-589.
4. Lacroix J et al: Group A streptococcal supraglottitis. *J Pediatr* 1986; 109:20-24.
5. Steele DW et al: Pulsus paradoxus: an objective measure of severity in croup. *Am J Respir Crit Care Med* 1998; 157: 331-334.
6. Westley CR, Cotton EK, Brooks JG: Nebulized racemic epinephrine by IPPB for the treatment of croup: a double-blind study. *Am J Dis Child* 1978; 132:484-487.
7. Super DM et al: A prospective randomized double-blind study to evaluate the effect of dexamethasone in acute laryngotracheitis. *J Pediatr* 1989; 115:323-329.
8. Kairys SW, Olmstead EM, O'Connor GT: Steroid treatment of laryngotracheitis: a meta-analysis of the evidence from randomized trials. *Pediatrics* 1989; 83:683-693.
9. Rizos JD et al: The disposition of children with croup treated with racemic epinephrine and dexamethasone in the emergency department. *J Emerg Med* 1998; 16: 535-539.
10. Khalil SN et al: Absence or presence of a leak around tracheal tube may not affect postoperative croup in children. *Paediatr Anaesth* 1998; 8:393-396.
11. Khine HH et al: Comparison of cuffed and uncuffed endotracheal tubes in young children during general anesthesia. *Anesthesiology* 1997; 86:627-631.
12. Kelly SM, April MM, Tunkel DE: Obstructing laryngeal granuloma after brief endotracheal intubation in neonates. *Otolaryngol Head Neck Surg* 1996; 115:138-140.
13. Kenna MA, Bluestone CD: Foreign bodies in the air and food passages. *Pediatr Rev* 1988; 10:25-31.
14. Johnson NT, Pierson DJ: The spectrum of pulmonary atelectasis: pathophysiology, diagnosis, and therapy. *Respir Care* 1986; 31:1107-1119.
15. Duncan SR et al: Nasal continuous positive airway pressure in atelectasis. *Chest* 1987; 92:621-624.
16. Westcott JL: Bronchiectasis. *Radiol Clin North Am* 1991; 29:1031-1042.

17. Ferkol TW, Davis PB: Bronchiectasis and bronchiolitis obliterans. In Taussig LM, Landau LI, editors: *Pediatric respiratory medicine.* St Louis. Mosby, 1999; pp 784-792.
18. Barker AF, Bardana EJ: Bronchiectasis: update of an orphan disease. *Am Rev Respir Dis* 1988; 137:969-978.
19. Wilson JF, Decker AM: The surgical management of childhood bronchiectasis: a review of 96 consecutive pulmonary resections in children with nontuberculous bronchiectasis. *Ann Surg* 1982; 195:354-363.
20. Annest LS, Kratz JM, Crawford FA: Current results of treatment of bronchiectasis. *J Thorac Cardiovasc Surg* 1982; 83:546-550.
21. Balck-Payne C: Bronchiolitis. In Hilman BC, editor: *Pediatric respiratory disease, diagnosis and treatment.* Philadelphia. WB Saunders, 1993; pp 205-217.
22. Wohl MEB: Bronchiolitis. In Chernick V, Boat TF, Kendig EL, editors: *Disorders of the respiratory tract in children.* Philadelphia. WB Saunders, 1998; pp 473-484.
23. Everard ML: Acute bronchiolitis and pneumonia in infancy resulting from the respiratory syncytial virus. In Taussig LM, Landau LI, editors: *Pediatric respiratory medicine.* St Louis. Mosby, 1999; pp 580-595.
24. Sandritter TL, Kraus DM: Respiratory syncytial virus-immunoglobulin intravenous (RSV-IGIV) for respiratory syncytial viral infections: I. *J Pediatr Health Care* 1997; 11:284-291.
25. Levy BT, Graber MA: Respiratory syncytial virus infection in infants and young children. *J Fam Pract* 1997; 45:473-481.
26. Everard ML et al: Analysis of cells obtained by bronchial lavage of infants with respiratory syncytial virus infection. *Arch Dis Child* 1994; 71:428-432.
27. American Academy of Pediatrics Committee on Infectious Disease: Use of ribavirin in the treatment of respiratory syncytial virus infection. *Pediatrics* 1993; 92:501-504.
28. Hughes JH, Mann DR, Hamparian VV: Detection of respiratory syncytial virus in clinical specimens by viral culture, direct and indirect immunofluorescence and enzyme immunoassay. *J Clin Microbiol* 1988; 26:588-591.
29. Klassen TP: Recent advances in the treatment of bronchiolitis and laryngitis. *Pediatr Clin North Am* 1997; 44:249-261.
30. Wang EEL et al: Bronchodilators for treatment of mild bronchiolitis: a factorial randomized trial. *Arch Dis Child* 1992; 67:289-293.
31. Schena JA, Crone RK, Thompson JE: Theophylline therapy in bronchiolitis. *Crit Care Med* 1984; 12:225.
32. Roosevelt G et al: Dexamethasone in bronchiolitis: a randomised controlled trial. *Lancet* 1996; 348:292-295.
33. Fackler JC et al: Precautions in the use of ribavirin at the Children's Hospital. *N Engl J Med* 1990; 322:634.
34. Moler FW et al: Effectiveness of ribavirin in otherwise well infants with respiratory syncytial virus-associated respiratory failure. *J Pediatr* 1996; 128:422-428.
35. De Boeck K, Moens M, Schuddinck L: Early ribavirin treatment did not prevent disease in high-risk bronchopulmonary dysplasia patients with respiratory syncytial virus infection. *Pediatr Pulmonol* 1996; 21:343.
36. Randolph AG, Wang EE: Ribavirin for respiratory syncytial virus lowers respiratory tract infection. *Arch Pediatr Adolesc Med* 1996; 150:942-947.
37. Groothuis JR et al: Early ribavirin treatment of respiratory syncytial viral infection in high-risk children. *J Pediatr* 1990; 117:792-798.
38. Wandstrat TL: Respiratory syncytial virus immune globulin intravenous. *Ann Pharmacother* 1997; 31:83-88.
39. Leigh MW: Primary ciliary dyskinesia. In Chernick V, Boat TF, Kendig EL, editors: *Disorders of the respiratory tract in children.* Philadelphia. WB Saunders, 1998; pp 819-826.
40. Pedersen M, Mygind N: Ciliary motility in the "immotile cilia syndrome." *Br J Dis Chest* 1980; 74:239-244.
41. Boat TF, Carson JL: Ciliary dysmorphology and dysfunction—primary or acquired? *N Engl J Med* 1990; 323: 1681-1684.
42. Phillips GE et al: Airway response of children with primary ciliary dyskinesia to exercise and beta$_2$-agonist challenge. *Eur Respir J* 1998; 11:1389-1391.
43. Denny FW, Clyde WA: Acute lower respiratory tract infections in nonhospitalized children. *J Pediatr* 1986; 108:635-646.
44. Glezen WP: Viral pneumonia. In Chernick V, Boat TF, Kendig EL, editors: *Disorders of the respiratory tract in children.* Philadelphia. WB Saunders, 1998; pp 518-525.
45. ECMO Registry of the Extracorporeal Life Support Organization (ELSO), Ann Arbor, Mich, July 1998.
46. Correa AG, Starke JR: Bacterial pneumonias. In Chernick V, Boat TF, Kendig EL, editors: *Disorders of the respiratory tract in children.* Philadelphia. WB Saunders, 1998; pp 485-502.
47. Chin TW, Nussbaum E, Marks M: Bacterial pneumonia. In Hilman BC, editor: *Pediatric respiratory disease, diagnosis, and treatment.* Philadelphia. WB Saunders, 1993; pp 271-281.
48. Swischuk LE, Hayden CK Jr: Viral vs. bacterial pulmonary infections in children (is roentgenographic differentiation possible?). *Pediatr Radiol* 1986; 16:278-284.
49. Overall J: Is it bacterial or viral? Laboratory differentiation. *Pediatr Rev* 1993; 14:251-261.
50. Miller MA, Ben-Ami T, Daum RS: Bacterial pneumonia in neonates and older children. In Taussig LM, Landau LI, editors: *Pediatric respiratory medicine.* St Louis. Mosby, 1999; pp 595-664.
51. Murphy SM, Florman AL: Lung defenses against infection: a clinical correlation. *Pediatrics* 1983; 72:1-15.
52. Fernaldl GW: Infections of the respiratory tract due to *Mycoplasma pneumoniae.* In Chernick V, Boat TF, Kendig EL, editors: *Disorders of the respiratory tract in children.* Philadelphia. WB Saunders, 1998; pp 526-531.
53. Hailen M: *Mycoplasma pneumoniae* infections. In Hilman BC, editor: *Pediatric respiratory disease, diagnosis, and treatment.* Philadelphia. WB Saunders, 1993; pp 282-284.
54. Shehab Z: *Mycoplasma* infections. In Taussig LM, Landau LI, editors: *Pediatric respiratory medicine.* St Louis. Mosby, 1999; pp 737-742.
55. Thom DH et al: *Chlamydia pneumoniae* strain TWAR, *Mycoplasma pneumoniae,* and viral infections in acute respiratory disease in a university student health clinic population. *Am J Epidemiol* 1990; 132:248-256.
56. Atmar RL, Greenberg SB: Pneumonia caused by *Mycoplasma pneumoniae* and the TWAR agent. *Semin Respir Infect* 1989; 4:19-31.
57. Hahn DL, Dodge RW, Golubjatnikov R: Association of *Chlamydia pneumoniae* (strain TWAR) infection with wheezing, asthmatic bronchitis, and adult-onset asthma. *JAMA* 1991; 266:225-230.
58. Hammerschlag MR: *Chlamydia trachomatis* and *Chlamydia pneumoniae* infections. In Chernick V, Boat TF, Kendig EL, editors: *Disorders of the respiratory tract in children.* Philadelphia. WB Saunders, 1998; pp 978-987.
59. Brook I: Pneumonia in mechanically ventilated children. *Scand J Infect Dis* 1995; 27:619-622.
60. Prekates A et al: The diagnostic value of Gram stain of bronchoalveolar lavage samples in patients with suspected ventilator-associated pneumonia. *Scand J Infect Dis* 1998; 30:43-47.

61. Bergmans DC et al: Reproducibility of quantitative cultures of endotracheal aspirates from mechanically ventilated patients. *J Clin Microbiol* 1997; 35:796-798.

62. Kirton OC et al: A prospective, randomized comparison of an in-line heat moisture exchange filter and heated wire humidifiers: rates of ventilator-associated early-onset (community-acquired) or late-onset (hospital-acquired) pneumonia and incidence of endotracheal tube occlusion. *Chest* 1997; 112:1055-1059.

63. Boots RJ et al: Clinical utility of hygroscopic heat and moisture exchangers in intensive care patients. *Crit Care Med* 1997; 25:1707-1712.

64. Long MN et al: Prospective, randomized study of ventilator-associated pneumonia in patients with one versus three ventilator circuit changes per week. *Infect Control Hosp Epidemiol* 1996; 17:14-19.

65. Centers for Disease Control and Prevention: Tuberculosis morbidity—United States, 1997. *Morb Mortal Wkly Rep* 1998; 47:253-257.

66. Nahmias AJ et al: Older and newer challenges of tuberculosis in children. *Pediatr Pulmonol Suppl* 1995; 11:28-29.

67. Inselman LS, Kendig EL: Tuberculosis. In Chernick V, Boat TF, Kendig EL, editors: *Disorders of the respiratory tract in children.* Philadelphia. WB Saunders, 1998; pp 883-919.

68. American Academy of Pediatrics Committee on Infectious Diseases: Update on tuberculosis skin testing of children. *Pediatrics* 1996; 97:282-284.

69. Nickerson BG: The lung in sickle cell disease. In Chernick V, Boat TF, Kendig EL, editors: *Disorders of the respiratory tract in children.* Philadelphia. WB Saunders, 1998; pp 1117-1122.

70. Smith JA: Cardiopulmonary manifestations of sickle cell disease in childhood. *Semin Roentgenol* 1987; 22:160-167.

71. Sprinkle RH et al: Acute chest syndrome in children with sickle cell disease: a retrospective analysis of 100 hospitalized cases. *Am J Pediatr Hematol Oncol* 1986; 812:105-110.

72. Weil JV et al: Pathogenesis of lung disease in sickle hemoglobinopathies. *Am Rev Respir Dis* 1993; 148:249-256.

73. Barrett-Connor E: Pneumonia and pulmonary infarction in sickle cell anemia. *JAMA* 1973; 224:997-1000.

74. Powars D et al: Sickle cell chronic lung disease: prior morbidity and the risk of pulmonary failure. *Medicine* 1988; 67:66-76.

75. Bunn HF: Pathogenesis and treatment of sickle cell disease. *N Engl J Med* 1997; 337:762-769.

76. Collins FS, Orringer EP: Pulmonary hypertension and cor pulmonale in the sickle hemoglobinopathies. *Am J Med* 1982; 73:814-821.

77. Pelidis MA et al: Successful treatment of life-threatening acute chest syndrome of sickle cell disease with venovenous extracorporeal membrane oxygenation. *J Pediatr Hematol Oncol* 1997; 19:459-461.

78. Orenstein SR, Orenstein DM: Gastroesophageal reflux and respiratory disease in children. *J Pediatr* 1988; 112:847-858.

79. Meyers WF et al: Value of tests for evaluation of gastroesophageal reflux in children. *J Pediatr Surg* 1985; 20:515-520.

80. Blister A, Krespi YP, Oppenheimer RW: Surgical management of aspiration. *Otolaryngol Clin North Am* 1988; 2:743-750.

CHAPTER **34**

Asthma

Thomas Kallstrom

Asthma is the most common chronic childhood disease, affecting an estimated 4.8 million children. Approximately 7.5% of children in the United States have asthma.[1] It is the number one reason for pediatric hospitalizations and the most common cause of absence from school.[2] The prevalence and severity of asthma are increasing worldwide, with the greatest increases among inner-city children and young adults.[3] The morbidity and mortality of asthma continue to rise, in spite of improved understanding of the pathophysiology along with advancements in the quality and variety of medications. Although greater awareness and changing definitions of the disease are thought to be explanations for this increase, many believe the rise is caused by increased exposure to air pollution and indoor allergens, urbanization, poverty, poor accessibility to medical care, and overreliance on β_2-agonists.

There is a great need to reverse this trend in morbidity and mortality and to overcome the shortcomings in diagnosis, treatment, and prevention. In 1991, the National Heart, Lung, and Blood Institute of the National Institutes of Health convened a consensus panel of professionals to develop national guidelines for the management of asthma in children and adults.[4] These guidelines were updated in 1997 and have been widely distributed in an effort to improve asthma care.[5]

PATHOGENESIS OF ASTHMA

DEFINITION

Asthma is most recently defined as a chronic inflammatory process disorder of the airways in which many cells and cellular elements play a role, in particular, mast cells, eosinophils, T lymphocytes, macrophages, neutrophils, and epithelial cells. In susceptible individuals, this inflammation causes recurrent episodes of wheezing, chest tightness, breathlessness, and coughing, especially at night or in the early morning. These episodes are usually associated with widespread but variable air flow obstruction that is often reversible either spontaneously or with treatment. The inflammation also causes an associated increase in the existing bronchial hyperresponsiveness to a variety of stimuli.[5]

PATHOPHYSIOLOGY

Asthma is characterized by airway inflammation, bronchial hyperresponsiveness, and hypersecretion of mucus. Airway obstruction is the consequence of these pathologic mechanisms. Approaches to therapy are directed toward blocking the inflammation as well as preventing and relieving airway obstruction.

Airway Inflammation. The role of inflammation has taken on a more significant role in the definition of asthma, as compared with past years when asthma was considered more of a bronchospastic disease and was treated primarily with bronchodilator medications. We now know that airway inflammation is persistent and that early intervention with antiinflammatory medications may help to slow the course of the disease.[6] This revised interpretation is the basis for the diagnosis, management, and prevention of asthma.

Airway Obstruction. There are four significant components to airway obstruction. These include acute bronchoconstriction, airway edema, mucus plug formation, and airway remodeling.[5] The obstruction can result in increasingly difficult air entry, air trapping, atelectasis, ventilation-perfusion abnormalities, hypoxia, and hypercarbia.

Exposure to certain allergens causes an immunoglobulin E–dependent release of mediators from the mast cell. These mediators include histamine, tryptase, leukotrienes, and prostaglandins. They directly contract airway smooth muscle and result in acute bronchoconstriction, or airway hyperresponsiveness. Airway hyperresponsiveness refers to the tendency of airways to react too easily and too much to a variety of stimuli.[7] Other "triggers" of air flow obstruction include aspirin and nonsteroidal antiinflammatory drugs, exercise, cold air, irritants, gastroesophageal reflux, respiratory infections, and psychologic stress.

Airway edema plays a significant role in the reduction of air flow in the airways and can occur with or without bronchoconstriction. The increase in vascular permeability and leakage causes airway mucosa to thicken and become rigid.

The released mediators stimulate the production of mucus. The excessive mucus secretion and plugging of the airway may act to reduce the diameter of the airway and further limit air flow.

Convincing evidence suggests that asthma associated with chronic airway inflammation may result in permanent structural changes in the airway wall. Alterations in the amount and composition of the extracellular matrix in the wall can lead to airway remodeling and irreversible abnormalities in lung function.

RISK FACTORS FOR DEVELOPMENT OF ASTHMA

Although the etiology of asthma is not well defined, there appear to be risk factors associated with the onset and persistence of asthma. Asthma is more prevalent in prepubescent boys but more common in girls after puberty. It is more frequent among inner-city and African-American and Hispanic children in the United States; however, there is disagreement as to whether racial and ethnic background is a risk factor or if poverty has the greater impact. Currently available data from genetic studies in asthma suggest that there is a strong genetic component to asthma. However, the exact mode of inheritance is unknown. Low-birth-weight infants as well as children born to young mothers tend to have an increased incidence of asthma.

Atopy seems to be the strongest identifiable predisposing factor for developing asthma, with atopic dermatitis often preceding the onset of asthma.[8] Infants who become sensitized to food allergens early in life have an increased risk for developing asthma. The majority of children with asthma are atopic, but not all atopic children develop asthma. Inhaled allergens are thought to be the most important factor in the onset of asthma. Unfortunately, the "energy-efficient" home today tends to increase indoor allergen exposure and provide an ideal setting for dust mites.[9]

Tobacco smoke is the indoor pollutant most closely linked with increased asthma prevalence and morbidity.[10] Other studies have found that children who were both sensitized and exposed to high concentrations of allergens in their homes were more likely to have asthma.[11] It appears that exposure to any environmental allergen, if it is intense and persistent, may lead to sensitization in atopic children and then be associated with chronic asthma.

There has been a great amount of research devoted to the relationship between wheezing illnesses in infants and the development of asthma. Respiratory syncytial virus is the most common viral respiratory tract pathogen isolated from infants who wheeze. Many of these infants with severe infection with respiratory syncytial virus develop recurrent wheezing and asthma later in life.

NATIONAL ASTHMA EDUCATION AND PREVENTION PROGRAM GUIDELINES

PURPOSE

The National Asthma Education and Prevention Program (NAEPP) was formed by the National Institutes of Health in the late 1980s to assist in the promotion of asthma education to the public, the health care professional, and the patient. The most significant undertaking of this organization has been the development and dissemination of the *Expert Panel Report 2: Guidelines for the Diagnosis and Management of Asthma,* also known as "The Asthma Guidelines."[5] The first edition of these guidelines was released in 1991.[4] Because there had been numerous changes in the diagnosis and treatment of asthma, particularly in the pharmacologic care, an updated set of guidelines was developed and published 6 years later. Both sets of guidelines were written by a science-based committee of experts from all medical disciplines, all based in the United States.

The stated purpose of the guidelines is to serve as a comprehensive tool in the diagnosis and management of asthma. The report is not an official regulatory document of any government agency. The NAEPP implicitly states that the guidelines are to serve as a guide and not to be the only method by which to treat the patient with asthma. It is recognized that every patient presents with a different history, and this must be considered when implementing the guidelines. In spite of massive public promotion directed to the medical community, the response has not been unanimous in acceptance and praise of the guidelines. Disagreement by primary care physicians with components of the guidelines is a potential cause for poor compliance, whereas still other physicians remain unfamiliar with the guidelines. Asthma specialists tend to be more familiar with and receptive to using the guidelines in their practice.[12-14]

COMPONENTS

The guidelines are divided into four key components for long-term control of asthma: (1) measures of assessment and monitoring, (2) pharmacologic therapy, (3) control of factors contributing to asthma severity, and (4) patient education for a partnership.[5]

Measures of Assessment and Monitoring. The patient populations are divided into (1) adults and children older than 5 years of age and (2) infants and children younger than 5 years of age. Specific and detailed requirements that must be present to make a diagnosis of asthma are discussed for each population. Directions on estimating the severity of

---

BOX 34-1

GOALS OF ASTHMA MANAGEMENT

1. Prevent chronic asthma symptoms and minimize asthma exacerbations, using the least aggressive therapy that is sufficient.
2. Maintain normal activity levels including exercise and other physical activities; avoid missing school activities.
3. Maintain normal or near-normal pulmonary function.
4. Prevent recurrent asthma exacerbations and minimize the need for emergency department visits or hospitalizations.
5. Provide optimal pharmacotherapy with minimal or no adverse effects.
6. Meet patient's and family's expectations of and satisfaction with asthma care received.

---

chronic asthma are provided. The levels of severity correspond to "steps" of pharmacologic therapy that are discussed later in the guidelines.

Pharmacologic Therapy. Box 34-1 lists six goals of asthma therapy that are suggested as the foundation for the patient's treatment plan. The goals are aimed at minimizing the impact of the disease on a patient's health and quality of life.

Medications used in the management of asthma are categorized as either long-term control medications or quick-relief medications. Long-term control medications are used to achieve and maintain daily control of asthma. The quick-relief medications are used to provide prompt treatment of acute symptoms.

A stepwise approach to gaining control of asthma is recommended for both patient populations. Both a "step-up" approach and a "step-down" approach are provided, with treatment starting at the step most appropriate to the initial severity of symptoms. Step-down therapy has a gradual reduction in long-term control medications, with the last medication added to the regimen being the first one reduced. The other option is to start treatment at the step most appropriate to severity of symptoms and gradually step-up therapy if control is not achieved and maintained.

Control of Factors Contributing to Asthma Severity. A discussion of avoidance and control of factors that contribute to asthma severity is provided. The role of allergens and irritants and the control measures necessary to reduce exposure to them are detailed. Periodic clinical assessment and patient self-monitoring are encouraged, with a focus on assessing achievement of the goals of asthma therapy.

Patient Education for a Partnership. Providing ways to assist patients in taking control of their asthma is the focus of patient and family education. The guidelines discuss ways to improve compliance; develop an "asthma action plan"; address medication regimens; teach the use of inhalers, spacers, and peak flow meters; and assess the influence of the patient's cultural beliefs that may affect asthma care.

DIAGNOSIS

Children who present with chronic or episodic cough, wheezing, difficulty breathing, or chest tightness may have asthma. The diagnosis of asthma cannot be established until there is evidence of air flow obstruction that is at least partially reversible and any alternative diagnoses excluded. The NAEPP guidelines recommend a detailed medical history, physical examination, and spirometry to determine reversible disease.[5]

MEDICAL HISTORY

A detailed medical history is essential in identifying the symptoms, triggers, and severity of asthma. A diagnostic history includes recurrent wheezing, chest tightness, shortness of breath, and cough, with nocturnal symptoms being common. Symptoms that occur or worsen with various stimuli (e.g., allergens, respiratory infections, exercise, weather changes) or follow a seasonal pattern are highly suggestive of asthma.

A thorough history includes descriptions and frequency of previous exacerbations, hospitalizations, number of emergency department visits or unscheduled office visits, amount of school missed because of symptoms, and response to previous therapy. It is also important to determine if symptoms are episodic or persistent. A history of allergic disorders (including family history), premature birth, and sinus and respiratory infections is often linked to asthma.

PHYSICAL EXAMINATION

A physical examination of the upper respiratory tract, chest, and skin is essential for the diagnosis of asthma, as well as to rule out another disorder. However, examinations may be completely normal between acute exacerbations, and the medical history is a stronger factor in supporting a diagnosis of asthma. Symptomatic children may present with audible wheezing and prolonged expiration, cough, retractions, use of accessory muscles, and tachypnea. Examination of the upper airways may show evidence of allergic disease (e.g., allergic shiners, edematous nasal mucosa, postnasal drip). Atopic

dermatitis is typical in the presentation of asthma; however, digital clubbing is rarely found in asthma and raises the suspicion of cystic fibrosis. There are many physical examination findings that lead to consideration of a diagnosis other than asthma.

PULMONARY FUNCTION TESTING

Pulmonary function testing is used to help confirm the diagnosis of asthma, estimate the severity of airway inflammation, and follow the response to changes in therapy.[15] Because essentially all pulmonary function tests are effort dependent, children must be old enough to correctly perform the test and provide maximum effort. Some children can perform an acceptable expiratory maneuver at 4 years of age, and there are others who are unable to accomplish this until they are 7 or 8 years of age. Poor effort and/or technique during the testing is unacceptable.

Typical spirometry measurements in the diagnosis of asthma include the total volume of air exhaled forcefully from a maximal inhalation (forced vital capacity, FVC), the volume of air exhaled during the first second of the FVC (forced expiratory volume in 1 second, FEV_1), and the FEV_1/FVC ratio. Other measurements, including the flow in the middle portion of the FVC (FEF_{25-75}), are often reported. The FEF_{25-75} is also known as the maximum midexpiratory flow. It is sensitive to small changes in airway caliber and also decreases with increasing obstructive disease; however, it is highly variable. Airway obstruction is indicated when there is a reduction in the FEV_1 of less than 80% of predicted and FEV_1/FVC values less than 65%, or below the lower limit of normal.

The diagnosis of asthma requires that the airway obstruction be reversible. Spirometry measurements are performed before and again after inhalation of a short-acting bronchodilator (e.g., albuterol). Significant reversibility is established when there is a greater than 12% increase in the postbronchodilator FEV_1 measurement.[16]

Pulmonary function tests are performed at the time of initial diagnosis, after treatment has been initiated or changed, and to document optimal pulmonary function values. If the patient demonstrates a deterioration in pulmonary status, additional testing is warranted. It is recommended that children who require long-term control medication for asthma, and who are capable of performing the tests, have pulmonary function tests performed at least annually.

BRONCHOPROVOCATIONAL CHALLENGES

Airway responsiveness can be assessed using pharmacologic (histamine, methacholine) and nonpharmacologic (exercise, cold air hyperventilation) challenges. Methacholine and histamine are the most common pharmacologic agents used for bronchoprovocational challenge. The challenge is performed in a medical facility with a physician and resuscitative equipment present.

Methacholine Challenge. During a methacholine challenge, carefully increased doses of methacholine are nebulized and delivered directly to the patient through a face mask or mouthpiece. The patient's FEV_1 is measured after inhalation of each concentration until there is a 20% decrease in the FEV_1 or until all nine concentrations have been delivered. A 20% decrease in the FEV_1 is considered a positive challenge. This demonstrates the presence of bronchial hyperresponsiveness and is highly associated with asthma. When the test is completed, the bronchoconstriction may be relieved with inhalation of a quick-relief bronchodilator.

Methacholine challenge is safe and reproducible in children. However, it is recommended that the patient's FEV_1 be greater than 70% predicted before performing the challenge.[7] Patients with well-documented asthma should not be challenged. A negative bronchoprovocational challenge may be useful in ruling out asthma.

Exercise Challenge. Exercise tolerance tests are performed using a variety of forms of exercise, including treadmill running, free running, and bicycle ergometry. Most children are exercised until their heart rate reaches at least 170 beats per minute or more than 85% of the predicted maximum heart rate for their sex and age for 5 to 8 minutes. The FEV_1 is measured immediately after and at 5-minute intervals for 20 to 30 minutes after exercise has stopped. A decrease in the FEV_1 of 15% or more from the pretest baseline indicates a positive response and exercise-induced bronchospasm (EIB).[7,17] When comparing the results of exercise challenge with the pharmacologic challenges, exercise testing has been observed to be less sensitive and a poorer screening test for bronchial hyperresponsiveness.[18]

DIFFERENTIAL DIAGNOSIS

Asthma is the most common cause of recurrent or persistent wheezing, cough, and dyspnea in children. However, several diseases and conditions produce similar signs and symptoms and may simulate an asthma exacerbation. Whether it is the first exacerbation for the child or further assessment of the "difficult-to-manage" asthmatic, other causes of wheezing and airway obstruction must be considered. This is of particular importance in the infant and young child whose small airways are more easily obstructed.[19] The differential diagnosis of condi-

---

BOX 34-2

RESPIRATORY CONDITIONS THAT MIMIC ASTHMA

UPPER AIRWAY DISORDERS
Allergic rhinitis and sinusitis
Vocal cord dysfunction
Tonsillar/adenoid hypertrophy
Laryngeal web
Laryngeal papillomatosis
Laryngotracheomalacia
Tracheobronchomalacia
Tracheoesophageal fistula
Subglottic stenosis
Tracheal stenosis
Bronchial stenosis
Vascular ring
Enlarged lymph nodes or tumor
Foreign body aspiration

LOWER AIRWAY DISORDERS
Acute viral bronchiolitis
Bronchiolitis obliterans
Bronchopulmonary dysplasia
Cystic fibrosis
Primary ciliary dyskinesia
Mediastinal cysts or tumors
Pulmonary embolism
Aspiration syndromes
  Aspiration bronchitis
  Aspiration pneumonia
Gastroesophageal reflux
Hypersensitivity pneumonitis
Allergic bronchopulmonary aspergillosis

CARDIAC DISEASE
Large left-to-right shunts
Congestive heart failure
Cardiomyopathy
Myocarditis

HYSTERICAL SYMPTOMS
Psychogenic cough
Hyperventilation syndrome

---

tions that cause wheezing and airway obstruction varies with the age of the child. A thorough history, including response to prior treatment, physical examination, and data from additional tests can help differentiate other disorders. Box 34-2 lists respiratory conditions that can present with asthma-like symptoms.

MANAGEMENT OF ASTHMA

After the diagnosis of asthma has been made, the NAEPP guidelines suggest a stepwise approach to classification of the severity of asthma (Table 34-1) and then initiation of treatment.[5] Children with

TABLE 34-1	CLASSIFICATION OF ASTHMA SEVERITY			
	Mild Intermittent	**Mild Persistent**	**Moderate Persistent**	**Severe Persistent**
Symptoms	≤2/week	≥2/week	Daily symptoms	Continual symptoms
Nighttime symptoms	≤2/month	≥2/month	>1/week	Frequent
FEV₁/PEF	≥80% predicted	≥80% predicted	60%-80%	<60%
PEF variability	<20%	20%-30%	>30%	>30%

FEV₁, Forced expiratory volume in 1 second; *PEF,* peak expiratory flow.

TABLE 34-2	STEPWISE APPROACH TO MANAGING ASTHMA SYMPTOMS FOR INFANTS AND CHILDREN 5 YEARS OF AGE OR YOUNGER		
	Clinical Features Before Treatment		
	Days with Symptoms	**Nights with Symptoms**	**Long-term-control Daily Medications**
Step 4 (severe persistent)	Continual	Frequent	High-dose inhaled steroid. Add systemic steroid (2 mg/kg/day) if needed. Reduce to lowest or alternate-day dose that stabilizes symptoms. Leukotriene modifier may be considered for children ≥4 years of age.
Step 3 (moderate persistent)	Daily	≥5/month	Medium-dose inhaled steroid. Once control has been established for 2 to 3 months, consider: Lower-dose inhaled steroid and nedocromil **OR** lower medium-dose inhaled steroid and theophylline at 10 mg/kg/day up to 16 mg/kg/day for children ≥1 year of age. Leukotriene modifier may be considered for children ≥4 years of age.
Step 2 (mild persistent)	3 to 6/week	3 to 4/month	1 ampule cromolyn by nebulizer or 1 to 2 puffs TID to QID **OR** 2 puffs nedocromil BID to QID **OR** low-dose inhaled steroid. Leukotriene modifier may be considered in children ≥4 years old.
Step 1 (mild intermittent)	≤2/week	≤2/month	No daily long-term-control medications needed.

mild intermittent asthma are the only ones in whom daily treatment is not recommended. For all other classifications of asthma, daily control medication is recommended and the amount of medication is increased, described as a "step up," as the need for treatment increases. When the asthma is under control, the amount of medication is decreased and described as a "step down." The treatment prescribed is determined by classification of disease severity. Tables 34-2 and 34-3 illustrate the step-

wise treatment approaches for infants and children. Although there is an increase in asthma morbidity and mortality in the United States, for most children with asthma proper disease management helps to provide a normal lifestyle.

The pharmacologic management of asthma requires the use of long-term control and short-term relief medications. Identification, avoidance, and control of factors that worsen asthma symptoms are as essential components of asthma management as

TABLE 34-3	STEPWISE APPROACH TO MANAGING ASTHMA SYMPTOMS FOR CHILDREN OLDER THAN 5 YEARS OF AGE				
	Clinical Features Before Treatment				
	Days with Symptoms	**Nights with Symptoms**	**PEF or FEV$_1$**	**PEF Variability**	**Long-term-control Daily Medications**
Step 4 (severe persistent)	Continual	Frequent	≤60%	>30%	High-dose inhaled steroid **PLUS** 1 to 2 puffs long-acting β$_2$-agonist BID or sustained-release theophylline or long-acting β$_2$-agonist tablets **PLUS** systemic steroid. (Make repeated attempts to reduce systemic steroid.) Leukotriene modifier may be considered.
Step 3 (moderate persistent)	Daily	≥5/month	60%-80%	>30%	Low- to high-dose inhaled steroid **PLUS** 1 to 2 puffs long-acting β$_2$-agonist BID, or sustained-release theophylline, or long-acting β$_2$-agonist tablets. Leukotriene modifier may be considered.
Step 2 (mild persistent)	3-6/week	3-4/month	≥80%	20%-30%	Low-dose inhaled steroid **OR** 1 to 2 puffs cromolyn TID to QID **OR** 1 to 2 puffs nedocromil BID to QID. Leukotriene modifier may be considered.
Step 1 (mild intermittent)	≤2/week	≤2/month	≥80%	<20%	No daily long-term-control medication needed.

the use of medication. The regular monitoring and assessment of asthma severity have been proven to aid in control of the disease. Finally, management of a chronic illness such as asthma requires patient and family involvement in developing a treatment plan and in understanding the illness.

PHARMACOLOGIC THERAPY

Long-term Control Medications. Pharmacologic management involves using medications to control and relieve symptoms. Any medication that is taken to provide ongoing control of asthma is classified as a long-term control medication. Long-term control medications are taken daily to achieve and maintain control of persistent asthma.[5] A more detailed discussion of the medications used to treat asthma is presented in Chapter 26.

Antiinflammatory agents. Antiinflammatory agents are still considered the most effective long-term treatment for chronic inflammation in asthma. The inhaled nonsteroidal antiinflammatory agents cromolyn sodium and nedocromil sodium both appear to prevent release of mediators from mast cells and provide control of chronic inflammatory airway changes. They are considered first-line antiinflammatory agents for children with mild to moderate asthma. Although the potency of their antiinflammatory activity is less documented than that of inhaled corticosteroids, they have few adverse effects.[20]

Corticosteroids include inhaled and systemic glucocorticosteroids. Inhaled corticosteroids are the most consistently effective controller medication for asthma and are considered first-line therapy for treatment of persistent asthma. Their advantage over oral corticosteroids is that they are clinically effective without having significant side effects. They are most often used for moderate to severe disease in children who have not had control of symptoms with the nonsteroidal antiinflammatory agents. Oral corticosteroid–dependent patients have been able to decrease or discontinue their use of oral corticosteroids when appropriate inhaled corticosteroid therapy is initiated. Studies have shown that beginning inhaled corticosteroid therapy early in the disease course has resulted in better clinical benefit than when treatment is delayed.[21]

Even though there is much less risk of developing adverse events with inhaled compared with systemic corticosteroids, the potential for side effects remains. Dysphonia, voice change, reflex cough, and oral candidiasis occur most often with higher doses, although these manifestations can occur at any dose. Use of spacers or holding chambers along with rinsing after inhalation may reduce these effects. Questions remain about the clinical significance of all side effects, particularly concern surrounding growth suppression in children. Until more data are obtained, the NAEPP guidelines recommend that children be maintained on the lowest dose of inhaled corticosteroid tolerated with close monitoring of linear growth and development.

Systemic or oral corticosteroids are often required during an asthma exacerbation. However, daily or every-other-day use, along with high doses of an inhaled corticosteroid, is necessary in some patients with very severe disease. The side effects of long-term, regular use of systemic corticosteroids are significant and are listed in Box 34-3. Once asthma control is achieved, efforts are made to wean the patient from oral corticosteroids.

BOX 34-3

SIDE EFFECTS OF LONG-TERM USE OF SYSTEMIC CORTICOSTEROIDS

Adrenal suppression	Osteoporosis
Growth suppression	Peptic ulcer
Muscle myopathy	Cataracts
Aseptic hip necrosis	Acne
Hyperglycemia	Weight gain
Increased risk of infection	Obesity
Skin atrophy and striae	Hirsutism
Psychological disturbances	Glaucoma
Easy bruising	"Moon" facies
Fluid retention	"Buffalo hump"
Hypertension	

Long-acting β₂-agonists. Salmeterol and formoterol are the only long-acting inhaled β₂-agonists available in the United States. Salmeterol is available alone as a metered-dose inhaler or in a dry-powder discus. It is also available in a dry-powder discus in combination with the corticosteroid fluticasone. Formoterol is available in a dry-powder inhaler device. These agents have no antiinflammatory actions and are used only in combination with an antiinflammatory agent, usually an inhaled corticosteroid, in patients with moderate to severe disease. Although both are bronchodilators, they are not used for treatment of acute asthma symptoms.

Methylxanthines. Although theophylline was at one time a prominent component of daily asthma treatment, its role has changed dramatically over the past 10 years. With the current focus on antiinflammatory therapy for asthma, along with its narrow therapeutic window and need for close monitoring of serum levels, theophylline has limited use in the pharmacologic management of asthma in children.

Leukotriene modifiers. Leukotrienes are potent proinflammatory mediators that promote bronchospasm, mucus production, and airway edema. Leukotriene modifiers are the first new class of medicines for asthma treatment in 20 years. Leukotriene action is modified by agents that either inhibit production of the leukotrienes or block their action. These agents are still relatively new, and studies are needed to determine their role in pediatric asthma care.

Zileuton is the only approved agent that inhibits the production of the leukotrienes; however, suggested dosing is four times daily and there have been reports of elevated results of liver function tests in patients taking the medication. Therefore it has a limited role in pediatric asthma care.

Medications that block leukotriene action include zafirlukast and montelukast. Current dosing for zafirlukast is twice daily, 1 hour before or 2 hours after meals. Dosing for montelukast is once daily, given in the evening. It does not need to be taken on an empty stomach.

Quick-relief Medications. Medications in the quick-relief category are short-acting β₂-agonists, anticholinergic agents, and systemic corticosteroids. These medications are used to relieve acute airway obstruction. All patients with asthma need a quick-relief medication, preferably a short-acting β₂-agonist, to take as needed for acute symptoms.

Short-acting β-agonists. With a rapid onset of action of 5 to 15 minutes and a 4- to 6-hour duration of action, these agents are the treatment of choice for acute episodes of bronchospasm. They are often referred to as "rescue" medications and are most effective when inhaled. They are used only on an as-needed basis and not as part of the regularly scheduled medication regimen. Increased use of these agents, particularly using more than one canister per month, is an indication of inadequate asthma control and increasing severity. The most common side effects are tremor, palpitations, and tachycardia. Although acute respiratory symptoms are relieved, short-acting β_2-agonists have no anti-inflammatory action. They are used to prevent EIB.

Anticholinergics. Ipratropium bromide is the anticholinergic agent approved for use in the United States. It is available alone in a metered-dose inhaler and nebulizer formulation. Given alone it is a less potent bronchodilator than short-acting β_2-agonists. However, current data show additive bronchodilatation of ipratropium when given in combination with the short-acting β_2-agonist albuterol.[22] The combination of ipratropium bromide and albuterol is marketed in a metered-dose inhaler and a nebulizer unit-dose preparation.

Systemic corticosteroids. Patients with acute exacerbations often receive 3- to 10-day bursts of prednisone or methylprednisolone. The bursts are primarily used to hasten recovery and prevent recurrence of symptoms. The dose of corticosteroid is tapered as symptoms resolve. However, if the symptoms return within 1 month or if the bursts are frequently required, changes are likely required in the long-term control medication regimen.

Delivery Systems. Asthma medications are usually given through inhalation in an aerosol form. The medications are administered by a metered-dose inhaler, by a dry-powder inhaler, or by nebulization. The majority of propellants that power the metered-dose inhalers utilize chlorofluorocarbons, chemicals that have been found to contribute to depletion of the ozone. Manufacturers of metered-dose inhalers are investigating replacement propellants. Recently, a nonchlorofluorocarbon propellant, HFA-134A, has been shown to improve delivery of medication.

Spacers and valved holding chambers are simple, inexpensive tools that have been developed to use with metered-dose inhalers. Their purpose is threefold: (1) to slow aerosol velocity, (2) to minimize particle impaction in the oropharynx, and (3) to enhance deposition in the lower respiratory tract. Their use in children is recommended to reduce the problem of coordinating actuation of the metered-dose inhaler with the inhalation. Studies have demonstrated that the decrease in pharyngeal deposition results in improved drug efficacy and a reduction in local side effects. It is imperative that patients along with parents or caregivers are instructed in the proper use of all inhalers, nebulizers, masks, and spacers or valved holding chambers.

CONTROL OF ASTHMA TRIGGERS

Most children with asthma have an allergic component to their disease. If asthma is to be managed adequately, then the allergens and irritants that worsen symptoms must be identified and controlled. The most common allergens implicated in chronic asthma are listed in Box 34-4. Exposure to allergens and irritants may significantly increase bronchial hyperresponsiveness, whereas reduced exposure to allergens can decrease asthma symptoms.

Identification of Allergens. Because childhood asthma is often exacerbated by allergen exposure, it is helpful to identify the allergens. Allergy skin testing, along with a thorough history and physical examination, is one test that an allergist uses to determine which allergens may be aggravating a child's asthma. Another common test used to determine what allergens are responsible for allergic disease is the radioallergosorbent (RAST) test.

Avoidance and Control Measures. It is nearly impossible for a child with asthma to avoid exposure to all offending allergens and irritants. But it is possible to minimize exposure to them. This begins with teaching the child and family to recognize the triggers and using measures to control and avoid them. Box 34-5 lists control measures for environmental factors that often exacerbate asthma in children.

BOX 34-4

ALLERGENS ASSOCIATED WITH ASTHMA

House dust mite
Pet allergen
   Cat
   Dog
   Guinea pig
   Rabbit
Rodent
   Rat
   Mouse
Cockroach
Indoor mold
   Aspergillus
   Penicillium
Outdoor mold
   Alternaria
   Cladosporium

BOX 34-5

ENVIRONMENTAL CONTROL MEASURES

HOUSE DUST MITE
- Kill with hot water (>130° F) and dry cleaning
- Enforce bedroom dust control
- Encase pillows, mattresses, and box springs in zippered allergen-impermeable covers
- Wash sheets and blankets weekly in hot water
- Replace wool bedding with cotton or synthetics
- Avoid feather or down bedding
- Remove stuffed toys, wall hangings, and other "dust-catchers"
- Hot-water wash or freeze stuffed toys weekly
- Vacuum/dust weekly wearing mask; vacuum with double-thick bag and HEPA filter
- Keep heat, ventilation, and air conditioner filters clean
- Remove carpeting; wash rugs; avoid heavy curtains and blinds
- Keep clothing in closets with doors closed
- Clean with damp cloths
- Reduce indoor humidity
- Replace upholstered furniture with wood, vinyl, or leather

ANIMAL DANDER
- Remove animal from house or restrict animal to washable area (may take 4 to 6 months to remove cat allergen)
- Banish animal from bedroom
- Close bedroom door and vents
- Use HEPA or electrostatic filter in bedroom
- Remove carpets and minimize upholstered furniture and other allergen reservoirs

COCKROACH
- Hire professional exterminator
- Use poison baits
- Store food and garbage in sealed containers
- Perform meticulous regular cleaning
- Eat only in kitchen/dining room
- Wrap plumbing to eliminate condensation

INDOOR MOLD
- Kitchen, bathroom, and basement are most common sites
- Leaky pipes, shower curtains, refrigerator drip pans, garbage pails, and window edgings are major sources
- Use commercial fungicides and bleach solution
- Reduce humidity to less than 45% with dehumidifiers, air conditioning, and increased ventilation
- Avoid humidifiers and vaporizers
- Close windows, especially in bedroom
- Remove moldy items
- Repair water leaks
- Dry clothing/shoes before placing in closet
- Limit houseplants and remove them from bedroom
- Avoid live Christmas trees

NONALLERGEN IRRITANTS
- Avoid tobacco smoke and passive smoke in the home and closed car
- Avoid wood stoves, kerosene heaters, cleaning products, and perfumes

---

Role of Immunotherapy. Allergen avoidance can produce changes in asthma disease activity and bronchial hyperresponsiveness, but often there are no practical means for avoiding exposure to all allergens. The NAEPP guidelines recommend that allergen immunotherapy, or "allergy shots," may be considered for asthma patients when (1) there is clear evidence of a relationship between asthma symptoms and allergen exposure, (2) the patient is symptomatic during a major portion of the year, and (3) symptoms are difficult to control with pharmacologic therapy.

The value of immunotherapy in children with asthma remains controversial.[23-25] Evidence suggests that it can be safely given to children with asthma and that life-threatening reactions are uncommon when the process is prescribed and supervised by an appropriately trained physician. However, the risk of anaphylaxis remains and the injections must be administered in a health care facility where personnel, medication, and emergency equipment are immediately available to treat a systemic reaction.[26] The patient waits 20 to 30 minutes after each injection because this is the interval of highest risk for a systemic reaction. It is also suggested that the immunotherapy be delayed when the child has an acute illness or asthma exacerbation. Allergen immunotherapy is typically given every 7 to 28 days for 3 to 5 years, with a positive effect often seen within 1 year of therapy.

PEAK FLOW MONITORING

Using a peak flow meter to monitor peak expiratory flow rates (PEFR) is an important tool in asthma management. It is easily performed in children as young as 3 to 4 years old. Monitoring assists children and parents or caregivers in recognizing changes in respiratory status, affording them the

BOX 34-6

USES FOR PEAK EXPIRATORY FLOW MONITORING

- Monitor progress in treatment
- Evaluate asthma severity
- Determine when physician intervention is needed
- Check response to treatment during an acute exacerbation
- Provide feedback for patients with poor perception of illness severity
- Assess exercise-induced bronchospasm
- Assess diurnal variability
- Identify specific triggers

chance to make necessary interventions. Box 34-6 lists the various uses for peak flow monitoring.[27]

Peak Flow Meter. The peak flow meter is a comparatively inexpensive monitoring tool that measures the PEFR (Fig. 34-1). It is used only for ongoing monitoring and not to diagnose asthma. Different brands of peak flow meters are available, and it is possible to get a slightly different peak flow value when using a different meter. Because there is variation between different brands, it is important to use the same peak flow meter or model for long-term monitoring.[28] Box 34-7 lists the steps in performing a peak flow maneuver. Patients are asked to bring their peak flow meter to their physician's office to check the accuracy of the meter as well as to recheck for proper technique. When a quick-relief medication is taken because of an increase in asthma symptoms, it is suggested that a peak flow reading be obtained before and after taking the medication.

Peak Flow Diary. The NAEPP guidelines recommend once-daily monitoring of the PEFR, preferably in the morning. Keeping a diary or chart of the readings is for many patients an important part of their treatment plan. Graphs for plotting peak flows are often included with the peak flow meter and can be photocopied for additional use. With daily peak flow monitoring, a patient may see a drop in the peak flow before severe symptoms are felt and may begin early treatment or seek medical help. This may prevent asthma exacerbations from occurring or lessen the seriousness of an episode by medicating at the first sign of low peak flow readings. The physician reviews the peak flow diary at each office visit.

Personal Best Reading. There are predicted "normal" peak flow values that are determined by height, age, gender, and race. However, it is neces-

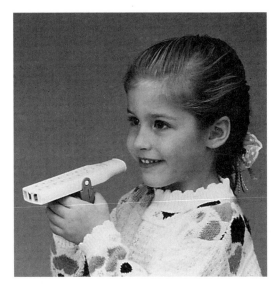

Fig. 34-1

Child with peak flow meter. (Courtesy Respironics HealthScan Asthma & Allergy Products, Cedar Grove, NJ.)

BOX 34-7

HOW TO USE A PEAK FLOW METER

1. Make sure the meter reads zero or the indicator is at the bottom of the numbered scale.
2. Stand up (unless there is a physical disability). Remove any food or gum from your mouth.
3. Take as deep a breath as possible, filling your lungs completely.
4. Place the meter in your mouth, behind your teeth, and close your lips around the mouthpiece. Do not let your tongue block the mouthpiece.
5. Blow out as hard and as fast as you can in a single blow. Do not cough into the meter.
6. The force of your breath moves the indicator on the peak flow meter. The number opposite the indicator is your peak flow.
7. Write down the peak flow number obtained.
8. Repeat the steps two additional times. Record the highest of the three attempts (not the average) in your diary or on your peak flow chart.

sary to determine a child's "personal best" peak flow reading. This is defined as simply the highest or best measurement obtained when the patient is free of symptoms and asthma is under control. To determine the personal best reading, the patient records peak flow readings at least once a day for

---

BOX 34-8

TRAFFIC LIGHT ZONE SYSTEM

GREEN ZONE: PEAK EXPIRATORY FLOW IS GREATER THAN 80% OF PERSONAL BEST NUMBER
- Good control of asthma is indicated.
- Patient is relatively symptom-free.
- Quick-relief medication is not indicated.
- Long-term-control medication is only medication indicated.
- If peak flow is constantly in the Green Zone with minimal variation, the physician may consider changing or decreasing daily medication.

YELLOW ZONE: PEAK EXPIRATORY FLOW IS 50% TO 80% OF PERSONAL BEST NUMBER
- "Cautious" zone; asthma is worsening.
- There is less than optimal control of asthma.
- Asthma symptoms may be increased, with awakening at night.
- Quick-relief medication is needed (usually a short-acting β_2-agonist).
- Increase in daily maintenance therapy may be needed.

RED ZONE: PEAK EXPIRATORY FLOW IS LESS THAN 50% OF PERSONAL BEST NUMBER
- "Danger" zone; exacerbation is severe.
- Asthma is poorly controlled.
- Asthma symptoms are serious and possibly life threatening.
- Immediate intervention is required (usually a short-acting β_2-agonist).
- Depending on physician's direction and patient's response to quick-relief medication, patient may be directed to seek emergency care.

---

2 to 3 weeks. The best peak flow reading will usually occur in the early afternoon.

Peak Flow Zone System. Once a patient's personal best peak flow has been established, every effort is made to maintain the peak flow values within 80% of this number. One peak flow monitoring system uses a zone system to indicate asthma severity and to guide a patient to an appropriate response. As illustrated in Box 34-8, green, yellow, and red zones are established. The zones are broad guidelines designed to simplify asthma management.

ASTHMA ACTION PLAN

The physician provides a written management plan, or action plan (Fig. 34-2), with information that the patient can immediately refer to should the patient

become symptomatic. No action plan should be developed without the physician's input. Based on the patient's current peak flow reading and the personal best number, the plan provides the patient with appropriate actions to take when the peak flow values drop. Included are detailed instructions specifying when to begin quick-relief medications, when to increase daily medications, and when to contact a physician or seek emergency care. Also identified are the specific medications to be given, the route of administration, the dose to be administered, and the frequency of dosing. Reminders to recheck the peak flow reading are included. It is helpful to have the physician's name and phone number on the plan along with the phone number of a close relative or neighbor.

Patients are instructed to take the action plan and peak flow meter with them when traveling. If the patient attends school, a copy of the plan is provided for the school to be used by the teacher or school nurse in the event of an exacerbation or to prevent EIB while at school.

PATIENT AND FAMILY EDUCATION

For any asthma disease management program to be successful, there must be development of an active partnership between patients, their families, and health care providers. This partnership is critical when the patient has a chronic disease such as asthma. Patient and family education begins at diagnosis and is a continual process, with the ultimate goal being to improve self-management.

It is unlikely that the patient's physician has the time to devote to a complete regimen of education; therefore all members of the health care team need to work together to reinforce the same message. It is recommended that clinicians teach patients and families the essential information concerning the disease process, medication skills, self-monitoring techniques, and environmental controls.[5]

A successful partnership keeps the lines of communication open. Asking open-ended questions can lead to the patient and family being more free in discussing concerns, fears, and expectations regarding asthma care. Perception of the disease and beliefs about treatment are influenced by earlier experience with the disease, education, personality characteristics, socioeconomic and cultural background, and the available support systems.[29] It is important to be sensitive to the cultural background of the patient and family. Ethnic beliefs can often affect the way the patient and family view asthma and its treatment. For example, some cultures view an illness as either a "hot" or a "cold" disease. Many in the Hispanic population believe that asthma should be treated with a "hot" remedy

Name: _____ No. _____
Date: _____

ASTHMA ACTION PLAN USING YOUR PEAK FLOW READINGS

Know your zone. Measure your peak flow every _____ and anytime you need to know your zone.

GREEN ZONE: You are in the **GREEN** zone if your reading is at least _____ (>80% personal best).
Green zone means GO. No sign of cough, wheeze, or chest tightness.

Take these medications daily: How much   When to take

1. _____   _____   _____
2. _____   _____   _____
3. _____   _____   _____
4. _____   _____   _____
5. _____   _____   _____

Take ___ puffs of _____ before you exercise, if needed for exercise-induced asthma.

YELLOW ZONES: (50-80% of personal best). You may have increased asthma symptoms,
awakening at night with asthma, or inability to do your normal activities.
  HIGH YELLOW ZONE: Your peak flow is between _____ and _____.
  • Take _____ puffs of _____ (quick relief medicine) or an updraft treatment. * Repeat
    every _____ hours until in the Green zone.
  • Take _____ puffs of _____ (anti-inflammatory medicine). Repeat every _____ hours
    until in the Green zone. Then return to your Green zone dose.

  LOW YELLOW ZONE: Your peak flow is between _____ and _____. Follow this plan if the peak
  flow does not reach **High** Yellow Zone within 15 minutes after taking inhaled quick-relief medicine or
  updraft treatment, or drops back into Low Yellow Zone within 4 hours.
        • Continue _____ puffs of _____ (quick relief medicine) or an updraft
          treatment every _____ hours.*
        • Add oral steroids** _____. Continue _____ mg/day for _____ days or
          till in Green Zone for 24 hours.
        • Contact your doctor to report persistent low readings or use of oral steroids.
  **If your condition does not improve within 2 days after starting oral steroids, contact your doctor again.

RED ZONE: Your peak flow reading is below _____. (< 50% personal best).
Red zone means STOP. Your asthma symptoms are serious.
  • Take _____ puffs of _____ (quick relief medicine) or an updraft
    treatment.*
  • Take oral steroids _____ mg immediately
  • If your peak flow does **not** reach the **low yellow zone** in 15 minutes after taking your
    quick-relief medicine or drops back into the Red zone in four hours, contact your doctor
    or go to the emergency room.

*Always measure your peak flow 15 minutes after taking your quick-relief medicine.

Fig. 34-2

Example of an asthma action plan.

such as hot tea. Often there is no harm in the belief; however, there may be times when the clinician must intercede in the interest of patient safety.

Asthma Disease Process.   Key points concerning the disease process include a basic understanding of what asthma is and what can trigger asthma episodes. Often drawings of a normal airway con-

trasted to that of one with asthma helps patients visualize what is occurring in their own lungs.

Medication Skills.   It is imperative that patients (depending on age) and families understand the names of their medication, proper dosing, when and how to take each medication, and the side effects of each. Providing written instructions for each medication assists in understanding and adherence to the treatment regimen. Proper inhaler technique is instructed and then reviewed at each subsequent physician visit. It is stressed that the long-term control medications are preventive in nature and are to be taken even if the patient is symptom free. Patients often discontinue use of their controller medications, only to develop an asthma exacerbation within 3 to 4 weeks.

Identification and Control of Triggers. Patients and their families need information to discern what triggers their asthma as well as ways to avoid the triggers. Although all triggers may not be totally avoidable, the patient and family are urged to take all necessary measures and learn to monitor which variables influence their symptoms.

Self-monitoring Techniques. Patients must learn to monitor and recognize signs and symptoms of worsening asthma. Education in the proper use of a peak flow meter and how to follow an asthma action plan is an essential component of asthma education. Reinforcing appropriate behavior includes reviewing peak flow monitoring, inhaler technique, and implementation of the action plan. Review of the action plan at each visit has been shown to improve patient compliance and decrease the chance for confusion.

MANAGING ASTHMA EXACERBATIONS IN THE EMERGENCY DEPARTMENT

Approximately 570,000 patients younger than 15 years of age are treated for acute asthma in emergency departments annually. Patients presenting to the emergency department have often had previous emergency admissions and hospitalizations for treatment of severe asthma. Often these patients have no primary care physician and rely on symptomatic control and emergency departments as their primary source of medical care. Along with inadequate use of corticosteroids, these characteristics are associated with an increased risk for fatal asthma.[30]

ASSESSMENT

The intensity and progression of the asthma exacerbation can vary and will determine the intensity of treatment in the emergency department. On admission, a physical examination is performed along with measurement of oxygenation and air flow. A pulse oximeter is used to measure oxygen saturation. Oxygen saturation is maintained at more than 95% using a nasal cannula or mask. Continuous monitoring of oxygen with a pulse oximeter is crucial.

A peak flow meter or spirometer can provide assessment of the severity of airway obstruction from inflammation and bronchospasm. If a child who normally uses a peak flow meter is unable to perform the maneuver during an attack, severe air flow obstruction is considered and intensive medical therapy is indicated. Peak flow measurements are taken before and 5 to 15 minutes after β_2-agonist therapy.

β_2-AGONISTS

One of the first lines of therapy is with β_2-agonist agents, such as albuterol or levalbuterol. The NAEPP guidelines recommend that the patient receive three treatments given every 20 to 30 minutes by either nebulization or MDI. If there is an inadequate response to this, continuous nebulization of albuterol may be initiated.[31]

Continuous or frequent nebulization of β_2-agonists does not present without some risks. The preservative benzalkonium chloride (BAC) is contained in some commercially available β_2-agonists and acts to prevent bacterial contamination in the solution. BAC is a potent bronchoconstrictor and can produce paradoxical bronchospasm and may be of concern during frequent or continuous nebulizer treatments.[34] Not all formulations of albuterol contain BAC. It is currently contained in the "screw-cap" unit-dose bottles and in the multi-dose mixtures. The amount of BAC per 2.5 mg of albuterol dose is sixfold higher with the unit-dose mixture than with the multi-dose dropper.

A concern faced with continuous or frequent dosing of albuterol is the potential for serum electrolyte alterations.[35] After two to five albuterol treatments, potassium levels have been documented to have decreased as a direct result of therapy.[36] Adverse effects typically seen with the use of β_2-agonists, such as tremor, tachycardia, and nervousness, are often pronounced, and some patients may not want to take the treatment because of this.[37] Levalbuterol has been shown to have fewer side effects, including a significant reduction in the serum potassium alterations.[38]

ANTICHOLINERGICS

Recently, the anticholinergic agent ipratropium bromide has been demonstrated to provide additional bronchodilation and improvement in peak flow values when given with albuterol.[22] Administering ipratropium bromide in combination with albuterol in the emergency department has been associated with a significant reduction in hospital admissions in children.[39] It is recommended that 500 µg (2.5 ml) of ipratropium bromide be given with the second and third doses of 0.25 to 0.5 mg albuterol, every 20 to 30 minutes for three doses and then every 6 hours as needed.[5,32]

CORTICOSTEROIDS

It is critical that corticosteroids be given to treat the inflammation that occurs during an acute exacerbation. Early treatment, which may include the use of intravenous corticosteroids, is effective in preventing an increase in the severity of symptoms and may avoid hospitalization and relapses.[40] Because intravenous lines are uncomfortable and can be difficult to place in a child, studies have investigated the use of oral corticosteroids in the emergency setting.[41,42] Data suggest that giving oral corticosteroids early is helpful in decreasing hospitalization and may be equivalent to intravenous steroids in children who are moderately ill. The suggested dose of oral prednisone is 1 to 2 mg/kg/day.

HOSPITALIZATION AND RESPIRATORY FAILURE

Regardless of the care given in the emergency department, some children will not respond adequately and will require hospitalization. Criteria for hospitalization vary; however, continuing deterioration or failure to improve with therapy is an indication for intensive monitoring and treatment. Box 34-9 lists criteria considered for hospitalization.

INTUBATION

If all attempts to reverse bronchospasm and improve air flow are futile, careful consideration is given to intubation and mechanical ventilation. Diligent patient monitoring is essential, and immediate steps are taken once the patient demonstrates respiratory muscle fatigue or failure.

It is best to intubate on a semi-elective basis rather than in an emergent situation, and it should be per-

---

BOX 34-9

CRITERIA FOR HOSPITALIZATION

- Poor response to 4 hours of bronchodilator therapy
- Previous visit to emergency department within 24 hours
- Hospitalization with asthma within the past year
- Previous hospitalization with admission to intensive care unit
- History of mechanical ventilation for asthma
- Poor access to medical care
- Recent increase in need for oral corticosteroids

---

formed by the clinician most experienced in managing pediatric airways. Intubation is attempted only under controlled settings with continuous cardiorespiratory monitoring and resuscitation equipment and medication available. Sedation before intubation is accomplished usually with ketamine; however, propofol may be a useful sedative because it appears to cause bronchodilation, sedation, and amnesia.[32,43] Once intubated and stabilized, the patient is monitored in a pediatric intensive care unit, which may mean transporting the child to another medical facility.

MECHANICAL VENTILATION

After intubation, the child is mechanically ventilated with low tidal volumes without positive end-expiratory pressure (PEEP) because the lungs are hyperinflated and there is a degree of auto-PEEP present. The mode of ventilation and set respiratory rate is determined according to the patient's degree of sedation, peak inspiratory pressures generated, oxygenation, and acceptable levels of $Paco_2$. Initially the Fio_2 is 1.0, with the goal to decrease the level to 0.5 or less when able. Ventilation with permissive hypercapnia is allowed with an inspiratory to expiratory ratio that allows for adequate exhalation.

All patients receiving mechanical ventilation are at risk of complications, including auto-PEEP, air trapping, pneumothorax, hypotension, adult respiratory distress syndrome, and death. The child with asthma is especially prone to such problems because of the high degree of airway resistance and the need for high inspiratory pressures.

HELIOX

A combination of helium and oxygen may improve ventilation and can be given through a non-rebreather mask or a ventilator. Its effect may decrease the work of breathing and respiratory muscle fatigue, allowing time for the bronchodilator and corticosteroid therapy to reverse airway obstruction and inflammation.

EXERCISE-INDUCED BRONCHOSPASM

Sometimes referred to as exercise-induced asthma, EIB begins during exercise and tends to reach its peak 5 to 10 minutes after the child has ceased activity. It may take another 20 to 30 minutes for symptoms to spontaneously resolve. EIB is caused by a loss of heat and/or water from the child's airway during exercise. This is often caused by hyperventilation of cool or dry air.

The prevalence of EIB has been reported to vary from 40% to 90% in children with asthma, with greater prevalence in those children with severe asthma. Absenteeism from school and poverty have been associated with findings of EIB. Early detection of EIB in school-aged children through screening could facilitate early treatment, enhance exercise-related activities, and possibly decrease the number of school absences. Notifying day-care personnel, schoolteachers, and coaches that a child has EIB can alert them to monitor symptoms and may elicit a more effective response should symptoms occur.

The diagnosis of EIB is based on a history that is compatible with asthma symptoms that occur with or directly after exercise. An exercise challenge can be performed to confirm the diagnosis.

The management of these episodes is generally of a preventive nature. Recommended treatment is inhalation of a β_2-agonist, cromolyn sodium, nedocromil, or salmeterol, given 5 to 60 minutes before exercise, preferably closer to the start of exercise if possible. Providing a 5- to 10-minute "warm-up" period before any exercise is recommended as well. An increase or change in long-term control medications may be appropriate in some children with EIB. Outdoor activities may need to be adjusted if conditions are unfavorable. This is particularly important if the pollen, weed, or mold count is elevated. Extreme cold and windy weather are also circumstances that may call for more caution to be taken to ensure that asthma symptoms do not develop during the activities. Efforts to prevent EIB require open communication with the schoolteacher and coach to allow premedication by the student athlete under a physician's guidance.

ASTHMA AT SCHOOL

One third of those with asthma in the United States are younger than 18 years of age. Dealing with asthma while at school can present problems for the child, the parent, and the school personnel. Asthma symptoms can interfere with many activities that the school-aged child desires to pursue. It is the leading cause of school absences, with an average of more than 10 days per year missed. The child with severe asthma may miss more than 30 days per year. An obvious conclusion drawn from these statistics is that missing school may result in poor academic achievement, inability to participate in school activities, and low self-esteem. The goal of the school-aged child with asthma is to keep symptoms under control and participate fully in the physical and extracurricular activities the school system may offer.

Various organizations provide resources to aid in the care of children with asthma in the school systems. The American Association for Respiratory Care offers a program that involves direct education of school administrators, teachers, and students.

The educational interventions can address each particular school because not all schools have similar needs or programs. Another similar school intervention is available through the American Lung Association. A child-centered asthma school-based education program has been associated with an increase in knowledge of asthma, improvement in skills for peak flow meter and inhaler use, and a reduction in the severity of asthma symptoms.[44] One program directed at inner-city African-American schoolchildren demonstrated a 15% improvement in mean peak flow rates and a 66% decrease in quick-relief medication use.[45]

School personnel, including teachers, coaches, and nurses, need to be familiar with the early warning signs of an impending asthma attack and what to do if the symptoms are present. It is recommended

---

BOX 34-10

IS YOUR SCHOOL ASTHMA FRIENDLY?

- Does the school have a "NO SMOKING" policy for all personnel, including teachers and custodial staff?
- Does the school maintain clean indoor air quality? How is this ensured?
- Is there a school nurse available at the school at all times? If not, how often is she/he there? Is she/he trained in pediatric asthma care?
- Can children with asthma take prescribed medications at school? Can they carry their rescue medications on their person? Must the medications be kept in a locked location?
- Does the school have an emergency plan for treating a child with a severe asthma episode?
- Does the school staff know the early warning signs of an asthma episode? Do they know the possible side effects of asthma medications and how they may impact the student's performance at school?
- Are students encouraged to participate in school activities and sports, regardless of having asthma? Are less strenuous activities provided if a recent exacerbation precludes full participation?
- Do teachers and coaches understand that exercise, especially that in cold air, can trigger asthma?
- Is the school staff provided opportunities to learn about asthma and allergies?
- Is there a copy of the asthma action plan in each student's classroom?
- Do school personnel understand that asthma is *not* an emotional or psychological disease but that strong emotions can trigger an acute episode?

that a copy of the child's asthma action plan be kept at the school and that the teacher and school nurse be familiar with the plan. It is unfortunate, but many school systems do not employ a school nurse dedicated to each individual school. Therefore there are occasions when the nurse is not available and other school personnel may need to provide care for the child. It is essential that the asthma action plan, peak flow meter, and rescue medications be readily accessible to school staff.

Parents can take a proactive role by determining how "asthma friendly" the school's environment is for their child. Some key questions to ask are listed in Box 34-10. The school building can present a hostile environment for children with asthma. There are numerous potential triggers found in most schools, including dust mites, mold, cockroaches, chalk dust, birds, rodents, animal dander, and strong odors (e.g., paint, chemicals, perfumes, pesticides). Therefore it is essential that these irritants be minimized or eliminated so that the child with asthma can attend school without risking further complications.

ASTHMA CAMPS

In recent years we have seen a growth in the number of asthma camps for children. These camps offer children with asthma the opportunity to spend time with other children who have the same disorder. This type of experience can be priceless. The camps are structured to assist children in recognizing symptoms and how to respond to them, with particular attention given to use of an asthma action plan. Identification of triggers and avoidance techniques are discussed as well. The proper use of medication delivery devices and peak flow meters is also reinforced.

Positive effects from attending camp include a reduction in the rate of postcamp hospitalizations, school absenteeism, and emergency department visits.[46,47] An improvement in peak flow technique and an increase in spacer and peak flow meter use have been demonstrated in minority children who participate in summer asthma camps.[48,49] The camps are usually operated with a team approach that includes physicians, respiratory therapists, social workers, and nurses.

REFERENCES

1. Mannino DM et al: Surveillance for asthma—United States, 1960-1995. *Mor Mortal Wkly Rep CDC Surveill Summ* 1998; 47(1):1-27.
2. Gergen PJ, Weiss KB: Changing patterns of asthma hospitalization among children: 1979-1987. *JAMA* 1990; 264:1688-1692.
3. Eggleston P et al: The environment and asthma in U.S. inner cities. *Environ Health Perspect* 1999; 107:S439-450.
4. National Asthma Education Program; National Heart, Lung, and Blood Institute: *Guidelines for the diagnosis and management of asthma: expert panel report.* NIH publication No. 91-3642. Bethesda, Md. National Institutes of Health, 1991.
5. National Asthma Education and Prevention Program; National Heart, Lung, and Blood Institute: *Guidelines for the diagnosis and management of asthma: expert panel report 2.* NIH publication No. 97-4051. Bethesda, Md. National Institutes of Health, 1997.
6. Wenzel SE: Asthma as an inflammatory disease. *Ann Allergy* 1994; 72:261-271.
7. Williams PV: Inhalation bronchoprovocation in children. *Immunol Allergy Clin North Am* 1998; 18:149-164.
8. Sporik R et al: Exposure to house-dust mite allergen and the development of asthma in childhood. A prospective study. *N Engl J Med* 1990; 323:502-507.
9. Pongracic J, Evans R: Environmental and socioeconomic risk factors in asthma. *Immunol Allergy Clin North Am* 2001; 21:413-426.
10. Chilmonczyk BA et al: Association between exposure to environmental tobacco smoke and exacerbations of asthma in children. *N Engl J Med* 1993; 328:1665.
11. Eggleston PA: Urban children and asthma. *Immunol Allergy Clin North Am* 1998; 18:75-84.
12. Doerschug KC et al: Asthma guidelines: an assessment of physician understanding and practice. *Am J Respir Crit Care Med* 1999; 159:1735-1741.
13. Picken HA et al: Effect of local standards on the implementation of national guidelines for asthma: primary care agreement with national asthma standards. *J Gen Intern Med* 1998; 13:659-663.
14. Wolff M et al: U.S. family physicians' experiences with practice guidelines. *Fam Med* 1998; 30:117-121.
15. Voter KZ, McBride JT: Pulmonary function testing in childhood asthma. *Immunol Allergy Clin North Am* 1998; 18:133-147.
16. American Thoracic Society: Standardization of spirometry—1994 update. *Am J Respir Crit Care Med* 1995; 152:1107-1136.
17. Custovic A et al: Exercise testing revisited: the response to exercise in normal and atopic children. *Chest* 1994; 105:1127-1132.
18. Zwiebel AH: Bronchoprovocation testing. *Immunol Allergy Clin North Am* 1999; 19:63-74.
19. Milgrom H, Wood RP, Ingram D: Respiratory conditions that mimic asthma. *Immunol Allergy Clin North Am* 1998; 18:113-132.
20. Shapiro GG: Management of pediatric asthma: care by the specialist. *Immunol Allergy Clin North Am* 1998; 18:1-23.
21. Agertoft L, Pedersen S: Effects of long-term treatment with an inhaled corticosteroid on growth and pulmonary function in asthmatic children. *Respir Med* 1994; 88:371-381.
22. Schuh S et al: Efficacy of frequent nebulized ipratropium bromide added to frequent high-dose albuterol therapy in severe childhood asthma. *J Pediatr* 1995; 126:639-645.
23. Johnstone ED, Dutton A: The value of hyposensitization therapy for bronchial asthma in children: a 14-year study. *Pediatrics* 1968; 42:793-802.
24. Giovane AL et al: A three-year double-blind placebo-controlled study with specific oral immunotherapy to *Dermatophagoides*: evidence of safety and efficacy in paediatric patients. *Clin Exp Allergy* 1994; 24:53-59.
25. Adkinson NF Jr et al: A controlled trial of immunotherapy for asthma in allergic children. *N Engl J Med* 1997; 336:324-331.

26. Ownby DR: The role of immunotherapy in childhood asthma. *Immunol Allergy Clin North Am* 1998; 18:199-209.

27. Spahn JD, Szefler SJ: Pharmacologic management of pediatric asthma. *Immunol Allergy Clin North Am* 1998; 18:165-181.

28. Jackson AC: Accuracy, reproducibility, and variability of portable peak flow meters. *Chest* 1995; 107:648-651.

29. Ponte CM: Education of the patient with asthma. *Immunol Allergy Clin North Am* 1999; 19:161-169.

30. Dales RE et al: Asthma management preceding an emergency department visit. *Arch Intern Med* 1995; 152: 2041-2044.

31. Lin RY et al: Continuous versus intermittent albuterol nebulization in the treatment of acute asthma. *Ann Emerg Med* 1993; 33:1847-1853.

32. van der Jagt EW: Contemporary issues in the emergency care of children with asthma. *Immunol Allergy Clin North Am* 1998; 18:211-240.

33. DiGiulio GA, Ruddy RM: Asthma: emergent and hospital care. In Dozor AJ, editor: *Primary pediatric pulmonology.* Armonk, NY. Futura, 2001; pp 121-136.

34. Asmus M, Sherman J, Hendeles L: Bronchoconstrictor additives in bronchodilator solutions. *J Allergy Clin Immunol* 1999; 104:S53-60.

35. Katz RW et al: Safety of continuous nebulized albuterol for bronchospasm in infants and children. *Pediatrics* 1992; 92:666-669.

36. Bodenhamer J et al: Frequently nebulized beta$_2$-agonists for asthma: effects on serum electrolytes. *Ann Emerg Med* 1992; 21:1337-1342.

37. White M, Sander N: Asthma from the perspective of the patient. *J Allergy Clin Immunol* 1999; 104:S47-52.

38. Gawchick SM et al: The safety and efficacy of nebulized levalbuterol compared to racemic albuterol and placebo in the treatment of asthma in pediatric populations. *J Allergy Clin Immunol* 1999; 103:615-621.

39. Qureshi F et al: Effect of nebulized ipratropium on the hospitalization rates of children with asthma. *N Engl J Med* 1998; 339:1030-1038.

40. Tal A, Levy N, Bearman JE: Methylprednisolone therapy for acute asthma in infants and toddlers: a controlled clinical trial. *Pediatrics* 1990; 86:350-356.

41. Barnett PL, Caputo GL, Baskin M: Intravenous vs. oral corticosteroids in the management of acute asthma in children. *Ann Emerg Med* 1997; 29:212-217.

42. Scarfone RJ et al: Controlled trial of oral prednisone in the emergency department treatment of children with acute asthma. *Pediatrics* 1993; 92:513-518.

43. Parmar M, Sansome A: Propofol induced bronchodilation in status asthmaticus. *Anesthesia* 1995; 50:1003-1005.

44. Christianson S et al: Evaluation of a school-based asthma education program for inner-city children. *J Allergy Clin Immunol* 1997; 100:613-617.

45. McEwen M et al: School-based management of chronic asthma among inner-city African-American schoolchildren in Dallas, Texas. *J School Health* 1998; 68:196-201.

46. Kelly CS et al: Outcomes analysis of a summer camp. *J Asthma* 1998; 35:165-171.

47. Menng A et al: Asthma day camp. *MCN Am J Matern Child Nurs* 1998; 23:300-306.

48. Sorrells VD, Chung W, Schlumpberger JM: The impact of a summer camp experience on asthma education and morbidity in children. *J Fam Pract* 1995; 41:465-468.

49. Fitzpatrick SB, Coughlin SS, Chamberlin J: A novel asthma camp intervention for childhood asthma among urban blacks. The Pediatric Lung Committee of the American Lung Association of the District of Columbia (ALADC) Washington DC. *J Natl Med Assoc* 1992; 84:233-237.

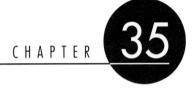

CHAPTER 35

Cystic Fibrosis

Bruce Schnapf
Scott Kirley

Cystic fibrosis (CF) is the most common lethal genetic disorder seen in Caucasian Americans. It is a chronic disorder with primary manifestations in the respiratory, digestive, and reproductive systems. Other complications of CF include diabetes mellitus, cirrhosis, sinusitis, and nasal polyposis. The disease was referred to in German folklore over 1000 years ago; it was in 1938, however, that Anderson first described the fibrocystic changes seen in the pancreas and used the term *cystic fibrosis of the pancreas.*[1]

The disease is characterized primarily by (1) chronic obstruction and infection of the airways; (2) exocrine pancreatic insufficiency, with its consequences of maldigestion and small bowel obstruction; and (3) elevated sweat chloride concentration. CF has an incidence of 1 in 3200 newborns in the United States.[2] It is less common in Hispanics (1 in 9500), African-Americans (1 in 15,000), and Asians (1 in 31,000).[3]

CF is marked by wide variability in the frequency and severity of clinical manifestations and complications. Some children die in infancy, whereas others with CF live beyond their 40s and 50s. The median survival age remains steady at 31 years.[4] In the United States, 36% of all patients with CF are older than 18 years of age, of which 90% are high school (or equivalent) graduates and 30% have attained a 4-year college degree. In nearly 70% of cases, the diagnosis is established before 1 year of age, usually within the first several months of life.[5] Approximately 7.1% of newly diagnosed patients are adults.

GENETICS

The cause of CF is a defect in a single gene on chromosome 7. The gene, which was cloned in 1989, encodes a membrane protein called the cystic fibrosis transmembrane conductance regulator (CFTR).[6] CFTR functions as a cyclic adenosine monophosphate–regulated chloride channel. It normally helps control the flow of ions and substrates across the apical surface of cell membranes lining the airways, intestines, vas deferens, biliary tree, sweat ducts, and pancreatic ducts.[7] CFTR dysfunction alters ion permeability of the cell membrane and creates an imbalance of ions and water in the intracellular areas.[3] When the chloride ion cannot be transported by CFTR, there is an insufficient secretion of fluid and inadequate hydration, which, in turn, alters the physical and chemical properties of secretions. The dehydration results in thickened secretions that plug the airways and ducts, impaired mucociliary clearance, and dysfunction of several organs, including the pancreas, liver, gallbladder, reproductive organs, and sweat glands.[6]

It has recently been suggested that the CFTR defect may reduce the resistance of epithelial cells to bacterial pathogens.[8] This concept provides an explanation for the chronic bacterial colonization observed in the lungs of CF patients. The combination of airway obstruction caused by mucus plugging and persistent infection results in recurrent episodes of lung damage, including bronchiectasis.

CF is inherited as an autosomal recessive disease with mutations in the CFTR gene.[6] Both parents of a child with CF are carriers of the CFTR gene; they carry both a normal CFTR allele and a mutated CFTR allele. These couples have a 1 in 4 chance of having a child with CF who inherits the mutated CFTR allele from both parents. There are 2 chances in 4 that their child will inherit one normal and one mutated CFTR allele and be a carrier. And there is 1 chance in 4 that they will have a normal child. Siblings of an individual with CF have about a 7 in 10 chance of being a carrier, whereas first cousins of a patient with CF have about a 1 in 120 chance of having the disease.[9] There is a family history in only 17% of newly diagnosed patients.

Based on incidence figures, it is estimated that 4% of Caucasians in the United States are carriers (heterozygotes) of the CFTR gene. Heterozygotes have no recognizable clinical symptoms, although an increased incidence of airway reactivity has been reported in CF carriers, suggesting a subtle abnormality of autonomic function.[10]

DIAGNOSIS

Nearly 1000 individuals are diagnosed with CF in the United States each year, with the median age at diagnosis being 6 months old.[4] The diagnosis of CF is suspected based on the presence of one or more distinguishing phenotypic features or a family history of the disease. Box 35-1 lists clinical presentations that are reasons to consider an evaluation for CF. Even though the disease occurs most often in

the Caucasian population, it is considered in the differential diagnosis of patients with diverse racial backgrounds who present with these features. A diagnosis of CF requires positive laboratory testing along with a history or clinical conditions consistent with CF (Box 35-2).[11]

SWEAT TEST

The standard for diagnosis of CF is the sweat test. Normal secretion and resorption of chloride in the sweat gland are dependent on CFTR. In CF, there is production of hypertonic sweat containing high

---

BOX 35-1

CLINICAL PRESENTATIONS INDICATING EVALUATION FOR CYSTIC FIBROSIS

RESPIRATORY
  Persistent wheezing
  Chronic cough
  Frequent thick sputum production
  Recurrent respiratory infections (colds, bronchitis, pneumonia)
  Respiratory infection with pathogens common to cystic fibrosis (*Staphylococcus aureus, Pseudomonas aeruginosa, Haemophilus influenzae, Burkholderia cepacia*)
  Persistent abnormal chest radiograph
  Nasal polyps
  Parasinusitis
  Clubbing of nailbeds

GASTROINTESTINAL
  Failure to thrive
  Frequent, greasy, foul-smelling stools
  Voracious appetite
  Formula/milk intolerance
  Rectal prolapse
  Meconium ileus
  Meconium peritonitis
  Distal intestinal obstruction syndrome
  Pancreatic insufficiency
  Pancreatitis

HEPATOBILIARY
  Hepatomegaly
  Focal biliary cirrhosis
  Prolonged neonatal jaundice
  Cholelithiasis

REPRODUCTIVE
  Obstructive azoospermia

NUTRITIONAL DEFICITS
  Fat-soluble vitamin deficiency (vitamins A, D, E, K)
  Hypoproteinemia, with or without edema
  Hypochloremic metabolic alkalosis

concentrations of sodium and chloride. A sweat chloride concentration greater than 60 mEq/L on two separate occasions confirms the diagnosis of CF. A concentration between 40 and 60 mEq/L is considered a borderline range, and the diagnosis is supported by having other evidence of CFTR dysfunction or clinical symptoms consistent with CF. Normal adults occasionally have elevated sweat chloride concentrations.

It is imperative that sweat testing be performed by experienced personnel at a laboratory certified as a Cystic Fibrosis Foundation–accredited center. Proper

---

BOX 35-2

Diagnosis of Cystic Fibrosis

At least one item from each of the following categories must be present:

Laboratory Testing
Sweat chloride level >60 mEq/L
or
Two CFTR mutations identified
or
Abnormal ion transport across nasal epithelia

History or Condition
Clinical evidence of cystic fibrosis
or
Sibling with cystic fibrosis
or
Positive newborn screening for cystic fibrosis

---

testing uses the Gibson-Cooke method, which involves the quantitative analysis of the chloride content of sweat. The sweat is obtained by stimulating the skin on the forearm with pilocarpine iontophoresis (Fig. 35-1).[12] A pre-weighed gauze or filter paper is used to collect the sweat for 30 minutes, after which the sweat is weighed and the chloride concentration determined. At least 50 mg of sweat must be collected during the 30 minutes to ensure an adequate sample. This amount may be hard to acquire in newborns younger than 3 months of age. Newer systems are requiring a smaller sample size.

False-negative results (i.e., normal sweat chloride level in a child with CF) have occurred when an inadequate amount of sweat is obtained for testing and also when malnutrition, edema, or hypoalbuminemia is present.[13] Conditions that can produce false-positive results (i.e., elevated sweat chloride level in a child without CF) include malnutrition, evaporation, adrenal insufficiency, and hypothyroidism.[14] Because technical errors tend to result in high sweat chloride values, a second test is performed whenever a positive result has been obtained.

CFTR Gene Analysis

A diagnosis of CF can be confirmed when there is evidence of two mutated CFTR alleles. Although over 700 mutations have been identified, current genotyping is generally able to identify fewer than 100 mutated alleles. The most common mutation in CF is the ΔF508.[15] There are individuals who possess the CFTR mutations but do not have the typical clinical presentations of CF. There are also

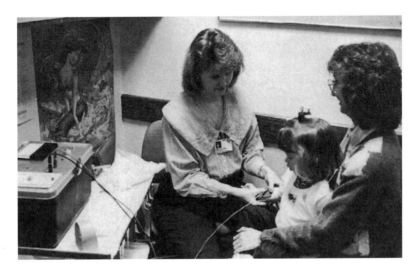

Fig. 35-1

Sweat test being performed. The child is held in her mother's lap while electrodes are positioned on her forearm to stimulate the skin to produce sweat.

individuals with two CFTR mutations, but the mutations are not identifiable through the commercially available screening tests. With these limitations in mind, genetic testing is used to make the diagnosis of CF but not to rule it out completely on the basis of a negative genetic test.

NASAL ELECTRICAL POTENTIAL DIFFERENCE

Measuring the difference in voltage potentials across the nasal epithelium is a newer method used in the diagnosis of CF. Certain alterations in the nasal potential differences are characteristic of CF and can be used to identify some patients with CF.[16] The availability of this analysis remains limited.

NEWBORN SCREENING

Although not done routinely, there are a number of centers that provide newborn screening for CF.[17] The most common method is measurement of serum immunoreactive trypsinogen obtained from a heel-stick blood sample. Elevated levels of serum trypsinogen are associated with pancreatic insufficiency and CF. There is increasing evidence of the benefit of early diagnosis of CF, which may lead to an increase in the use of such screening programs.

PULMONARY DISEASE

Although CF is a disorder involving multiple organs, pulmonary disease accounts for much of the morbidity and is the cause of death in more than 90% of all cases.[4] As a result of CFTR dysfunction, there is abnormal water and electrolyte transport across the respiratory epithelium. This in turn leads to the typical features of CF: thick tenacious mucus, impaired secretion clearance, mucus plugging of the airways, chronic bacterial infection, and airway inflammation. Severity of lung disease varies. Some patients have little or no respiratory compromise and slow progression of symptoms over time, whereas others have severe lung disease with a rapid change in lung function and infection.

MUCUS PRODUCTION AND AIRWAY OBSTRUCTION

The lungs of a newborn with CF are histologically normal at birth.[18] However, airway dysfunction begins during the first year of life, with the earliest pathologic change being thickened mucus and plugging of the submucosal gland ducts in the large airways.[19] These changes appear to precede infection and inflammation.[20]

Goblet cells and submucosal glands are the predominant secretory structures of normal airways. In the CF patient, there is an increased number of goblet cells and hypertrophy of submucosal glands, which leads to an increase in secretions and sputum production. Airway secretions are relatively dehydrated and viscous. Thick and viscid mucus is such a common feature that at one time the disease was referred to as "mucoviscidosis."

Mucociliary clearance is variable in CF, with some patients having severe impairment whereas others have normal clearance. The reduction in clearance is believed to be caused by the increased volume of respiratory secretions and the abnormally thick mucus. Studies have shown the cilia from CF patients to be normal, although chronic inflammation may result in a loss of ciliated cells.[21]

BACTERIAL INFECTION

In time there is colonization of CF airways with various bacteria. Initially, *Staphylococcus aureus* and *Haemophilus influenzae* appear, with *S. aureus* reaching maximum prevalence at ages 6 to 17 years and *H. influenzae* peaking at 2 to 5 years of age.[9]

A distinctive feature of cystic fibrosis is the increased susceptibility to respiratory infection with *Pseudomonas aeruginosa*.[22] By 18 years of age, most patients with CF have inevitably developed a *Pseudomonas* infection.[9] Initial colonization is with nonmucoid strains of *Pseudomonas,* often occurring during a staphylococcal infection. However, more than 80% of patients with advanced lung disease shelter mucoid strains of *Pseudomonas* that are heavy slime producers.[23] The mucoid strains are rarely found in other diseases and prompt investigation for CF when discovered. Once there is colonization of the airways, *Pseudomonas* is virtually impossible to eradicate, in spite of aggressive antibiotic therapy.[24] However, it does tend to remain localized to the respiratory tract.

Infection with *Burkholderia cepacia* (formerly known as *Pseudomonas cepacia*) occurs in about 4% of CF patients.[4] This hardy organism is resistant to aminoglycosides and possibly all antibiotics. Infection may result in an acute necrotizing pneumonia and septic shock. Once colonization occurs, there is the possibility of catastrophic deterioration and a poorer prognosis for survival. It is often transmitted either directly or indirectly by person-to-person transmission, with risk factors including hospitalization and having a colonized sibling.[25] The emergence of *B. cepacia* has profoundly affected infection control policies and has caused a change in activities and visitation among CF patients. Total segregation of colonized patients to different hospital floors or rooms is practiced in some hospitals. Stringent measures are also being taken by many CF care providers who coordinate camps and educational meetings in which there is interaction between individuals with CF.

Patients with CF who do not respond to antimicrobial agents may have colonization of other organisms. These include viruses, atypical mycobacteria, *Klebsiella* organisms, *Aspergillus* species, and *Stenotrophomonas maltophilia.*

The bacterial load, accompanied by the destructive attempts of the immune system to eradicate the infection, results in progressive damage to the airway wall and accumulation of thicker, more caustic sputum within the scarred airways. Severe obstruction of the airway results, and the CF patient eventually develops bronchiectasis and respiratory failure.

AIRWAY INFLAMMATION

Inflammation of the airways is a major component of CF and may occur early in the disease process. Recent studies of bronchoalveolar lavage fluid from infants suggest that airway inflammation is present in those as young as 4 weeks old, possibly occurring before infection.[26] An abundance of neutrophils and the enzyme neutrophil elastase may be responsible for the airway destruction and inflammatory response found in the lungs of CF patients.[27]

CLINICAL PRESENTATION

Nearly half of all patients with CF are diagnosed as a result of pulmonary symptoms.[28] The diagnosis of CF should be considered in every patient who presents with chronic or recurrent lower respiratory tract disorders, including bronchitis, bronchiectasis, pneumonia, and refractory asthma. Children with CF have frequent pulmonary exacerbations, with the most consistent feature being a chronic cough. The cough may be dry and hacking, or it can be paroxysmal with the patient gagging, choking, or even vomiting during coughing episodes. Sputum often becomes mucopurulent and difficult to expectorate. Other symptoms include tachypnea, retractions, dyspnea, and use of accessory muscles. Occasionally, patients will present with hemoptysis and fever. Wheezing, crackles, rhonchi, and decreased air exchange are common findings during auscultation of the chest.

The chest radiograph initially shows hyperinflation with flattened diaphragms secondary to air trapping (Fig. 35-2). Mucus plugging and bronchial wall thickening are also seen. Diffuse fibrosis and bronchiectasis are found predominantly in the upper

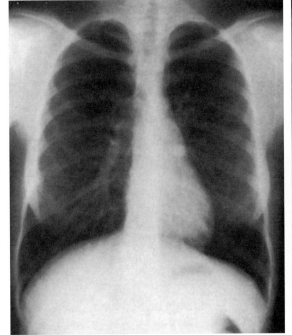
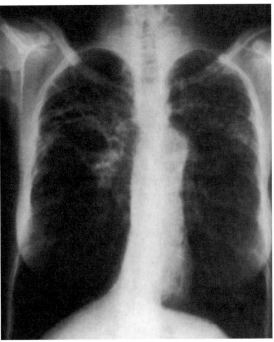

A   B

Fig. 35-2

Cystic fibrosis. Chest radiographs from a patient at ages 14 years (**A**) and 22 years (**B**) illustrating the changes of advancing disease.

BOX 35-3

SIGNS AND SYMPTOMS OF A PULMONARY EXACERBATION IN CYSTIC FIBROSIS

Increased cough
Increased sputum production
Change in sputum appearance
Hemoptysis
Dyspnea
Tachypnea
Increased chest congestion
Change in findings of chest physical
    examination
Decrease in oxygen saturation
Change in chest radiograph
Deterioration in pulmonary function
Fever
Weight loss
Decreased appetite
Increased fatigue
Decreased exercise tolerance

---

lobes. However, over time all lung fields are involved. Pneumothorax occurs most often in older patients with more advanced disease and is a result of rupture of subpleural blebs. The recurrence rate is high at 50% to 70%.[29] The progressive lung disease and chronic hypoxemia lead to an increase in pulmonary vascular resistance, pulmonary hypertension, and cor pulmonale. As cor pulmonale progresses, the electrocardiogram shows thickening in the wall and enlargement of the right ventricle.

Pulmonary function testing initially demonstrates air flow obstruction. As the disease progresses, both a restrictive and an obstructive pattern can be seen, along with a decrease in air flow. About 50% of patients with CF have a positive methacholine challenge test, which indicates airway hyperreactivity. Digital clubbing and pulmonary hypertrophic osteoarthropathy are universal findings in CF patients with advanced pulmonary disease. Pulmonary exacerbations of CF vary in severity and are usually defined by subjective symptoms. Although there is no clear definition of a CF exacerbation, most are associated with the characteristics found in Box 35-3.

TREATMENT OF PULMONARY DISEASE

Treatment of the pulmonary manifestations of CF focuses on routine therapy aimed at physically removing thickened mucus from the airways and pharmacologic control of infection with the aggressive use of antibiotics.

SECRETION CLEARANCE

Airway clearance techniques are used to assist in the removal of bronchial secretions and are recommended at the first indication of lung involvement. Patients with minimal symptoms may only require one treatment session per day, whereas others with a greater volume of thick secretions may need three or more sessions per day. For over 30 years, postural drainage, manual or mechanical percussion, vibration, and assisted coughing have proven to be beneficial in removing secretions. Physical activity and exercise programs have been shown to augment airway clearance.

Several alternative methods have been developed. These include active cycle breathing, forced expiratory technique, positive expiratory pressure (PEP) therapy, autogenic drainage, the ThAIRapy Vest, the Flutter device, and the intrapulmonary percussive device. A detailed discussion of the techniques and devices is provided in Chapter 14. Studies have compared various outcomes, including peak flow rates, sputum production, pulmonary function values, and oximetry, among different airway clearance techniques.[30-36] However, controversy remains concerning the advantage of one form over another. The addition of these new modalities has provided patients with more options when developing a program that best fits their lifestyle. This may improve treatment adherence and be more efficacious overall.

AEROSOL THERAPY

Aerosol therapy in CF patients includes bronchodilators, mucolytic agents, antiinflammatory agents, hydrating agents, proteolytic agents, and antibiotics. Administration is through various devices, depending on the patient's clinical status and the specific agent being used.

Bronchodilators. Airway hyperreactivity is common in the majority of patients with CF.[37] Inhalation of a bronchodilator followed with an airway clearance technique is the most common treatment regimen used routinely between exacerbations. Medications used most often include β_2-agonists and the anticholinergic agent ipratropium bromide. The medication is delivered with either a metered-dose inhaler or a nebulizer. Although bronchodilators are routinely used, their responsiveness has been shown to be variable in CF patients.[38,39] Most patients with CF demonstrate an improvement in lung function after inhalation of a bronchodilator.[40] Occasionally, a patient worsens after bronchodilator therapy.[41] Air flow may decrease or hyperinflation may increase as a result of smooth muscle relaxation and a decrease in airway elasticity. Treatment with ipratropium bromide has resulted in significant improvement in pulmonary function, especially in adult patients.[42] Some patients respond better to combination therapy using albuterol and ipratropium bromide.[43]

Mucolytic Agents. The sputum of CF patients is not only more abundant but also has abnormal viscosity. This is believed to be caused by increased glycoprotein sulfation and the high concentrations of DNA released from dead neutrophils.[44] Although used for many years, most mucolytic agents, including *N*-acetylcysteine, are not effective in the treatment of CF.

Recombinant DNase (rhDNase) has been developed to reduce the viscosity of purulent CF sputum.[45] The synthetically produced rhDNase breaks up the thickened mucus by disrupting the long, sticky DNA molecules. Studies have demonstrated that the lung function of CF patients with mild to moderate pulmonary disease improved after they received aerosolized rhDNase. A reduction in the use of antibiotics for respiratory infections has also occurred after treatment.[46] Voice alteration is the only significant side effect and resolves when the medication is discontinued.

Although not yet established, there has been a renewed interest in the use of nebulized hypertonic saline to facilitate airway clearance.[47] Because hypertonic saline causes bronchospasm in some patients, it may be necessary to premedicate with a bronchodilator.

Antiinflammatory Agents. Because inflammation of the airways is responsible for a large part of the pulmonary symptoms in CF, it seems logical to consider antiinflammatory agents as part of the treatment regimen. Systemic corticosteroids have been shown in clinical trials to improve lung function; however, side effects are serious and include growth suppression and increased susceptibility to osteoporosis and cataracts.[48] Studies have reported using inhaled corticosteroids in CF with improvement in lung function and respiratory symptoms, but the studies had small sample sizes.[49,50]

Amiloride. A characteristic of CF airways is an excessive absorption of sodium and water across the epithelium. It is believed that this abnormality is linked to the CFTR gene mutation. Amiloride is a sodium channel blocker normally used as a diuretic. It is given as an aerosol to CF patients in an attempt to improve sputum viscosity and increase secretion clearance by inhibiting the abnormal sodium absorption.[51] A large multicenter study is currently underway in the United States. Early studies suggest that it reduces the rate of deterioration of lung function and improves mucociliary and cough clearance.

ANTIBIOTIC THERAPY

Except in the case of acute respiratory illness or exacerbation, there are no well-established guidelines for the prophylactic use of antibiotics in CF patients.[52] However, the main focus in the treatment of pulmonary symptoms continues to be secretion removal and antibiotic therapy. Because the airway infection cannot be eradicated, the goal of antibiotic therapy in the treatment of CF is suppression of the infecting organism to a level in which clinical symptoms are minimal.[9] There is currently no consensus regarding the prophylactic use of oral antibiotics.

Antibiotic Selection. Antibiotic therapy is usually given for 2 weeks during pulmonary exacerbations. Antibiotics can be administered orally, by nebulization, or intravenously. The choice of antibiotic is based on results of the individual patient's sputum or throat culture and the sensitivity profile of the specific organisms. If handled properly, the sputum culture accurately reflects infection in the lungs. Agents known to be particularly effective against *S. aureus* and *Pseudomonas* species are usually chosen. For patients infected with *P. aeruginosa,* combination therapy with a β-lactam and an aminoglycoside is administered. Ciprofloxacin is a common choice for an oral antibiotic. Therapy can be extended to cover *S. aureus* if it is also present in the sputum. Because of abnormal pharmacokinetics of most antibiotics in CF patients, a higher than normal dose is usually required to achieve therapeutic levels.[9]

Hospitalization. Advances in providing stable venous access have allowed the intravenous administration of antibiotics at home, with the patient continuing school or work activities.[53] Criteria for proceeding with hospitalization and intravenous therapy include severe illness but also moderate illness that is unresponsive to home therapy, or even mild illness complicated by growth failure. If a patient does not respond to outpatient management, hospitalization is recommended with a 10- to 21-day course of intensive antibiotic therapy. Hospitalization for a pulmonary exacerbation also includes aggressive treatment to remove secretions.

Aerosolized Antibiotics. In spite of questions concerning deposition and efficacy, aerosolized antibiotics have long been used. Inhalation of antibiotics for the treatment of CF began with penicillin in the 1940s. Since then, several other antibiotics have been aerosolized in an attempt to treat the disease. Studies of aerosolized tobramycin have reported improved pulmonary function, fewer hospitalizations, and decreased *P. aeruginosa* sputum density.[54,55] There is growing evidence that inhaled antibiotics are beneficial in reducing the number of pulmonary exacerbations in patients with CF and improving pulmonary function.[56,57]

Oxygen Therapy

With disease progression, CF patients often develop hypoxemia, especially at night and with exercise. Oxygen saturations initially drop to less than 90% during acute exacerbations, then chronically during sleep, and then throughout the day. Supplemental oxygen is provided to reduce the hypoxemia and pulmonary hypertension, which can lead to development of cor pulmonale.

Unlike other pediatric patients, CF patients with advanced disease, particularly those with a baseline $Paco_2$ elevation, may convert from the normal CO_2-driven respiratory pattern to one triggered primarily by hypoxia. Supplemental oxygen, given in excess, can result in significant respiratory drive suppression. Therefore, in CF patients with more severe disease, oxygen flow rates and Fio_2 levels are initially targeted to maintain saturation in the 90% to 95% range only.

Lung Transplantation

Patients with severe CF, who are at significant risk of dying from their disease within 2 years, are increasingly being considered for lung transplantation. There has been no evidence of the redevelopment of CF in the transplanted lungs, but new problems related to lung rejection and opportunistic infection in patients receiving immunosuppressive agents can occur. Although more than 100 CF patients undergo a lung or heart-lung transplant each year, each year patients succumb to the disease while waiting for donor organs. Chapter 27 provides a thorough discussion of lung transplantation.

OTHER CLINICAL MANIFESTATIONS

Although pulmonary compromise is the main factor that limits longevity in CF patients, there are a number of other systems affected by the disease. Certain conditions can prompt consideration of the diagnosis of CF. The more common conditions include meconium ileus, prolonged neonatal jaundice, rectal prolapse, and failure to thrive.

Upper Airway Disorders

Nearly all patients with CF have sinusitis, most often involving the maxillary and ethmoidal sinuses. It is often difficult to control in spite of oral and intravenous antibiotic therapy. The abnormally thick mucus that is characteristic of CF occludes the sinus passages and prevents drainage.[58] These patients also have a high incidence of nasal polyps, occurring most often in the older child and adolescent.[59] Over half of the patients who require surgical removal of the polyps experience a recurrence. A diagnosis of CF is suspected in children who present with sinusitis and nasal polyposis.

Gastrointestinal Disorders

Pancreatic Insufficiency. Nearly all patients with CF have pancreatic insufficiency. CFTR dysfunction results in insufficient secretion of pancreatic fluid, which causes plugging and obstruction of the pancreatic ducts. Siblings with CF often share similar degrees of pancreatic insufficiency.[60] Symptoms are controlled with supplementation of pancreatic enzymes. A small number of CF patients have pancreatic sufficiency and do not require pancreatic enzyme supplements. These patients often have lower sweat chloride values, better lung function, and lower incidence of *Pseudomonas* colonization and are often diagnosed with CF at an older age. Overall prognosis is usually better, but occasional episodes of pancreatitis occur and there is continued risk of the development of pancreatic insufficiency. Therapy is individualized and supplements are taken each time the patient eats. Infants require supplements with any type of milk, including breast milk, and children require them with all snacks and meals.

Failure of the pancreas to produce sufficient enzymes results in malabsorption of fat and protein. The presence of steatorrhea, which is excessive loss of fat in the stool, is often the first indication of CF. These children frequently produce bulky, foul-smelling, oily stools and may experience rectal prolapse. Complaints of constipation or stomach cramps, especially after eating, can lead to a decrease in appetite and oral intake. Infants often present with failure to thrive, failing to gain weight in spite of a voracious appetite. Other clinical consequences include hypoproteinemia with or without edema and deficiency of vitamins A, D, E, and K.

The incidence of diabetes mellitus is much greater in children with CF than in the general pediatric population.[61] As fibrosis of the pancreas progresses, endocrine function is affected and diabetes mellitus develops. Weight loss is usually the first symptom.

Meconium Ileus and Distal Intestinal Obstruction Syndrome. Failure to secrete water into the gut is a result of CFTR dysfunction. Abnormal intestinal electrolyte and water transport can lead to a number of disorders. The earliest clinical manifestation of CF may be meconium ileus.[5] Occurring at birth, nearly every full-term infant who has meconium ileus is considered to have CF until proven otherwise. Presentation includes abdominal distention, vomiting, and abdominal radiograph showing distended loops of bowel with gas bubbles trapped among meconium, giving a ground-glass appearance. With an incidence higher in older patients, distal intestinal obstruction syndrome occurs when the thick, sticky stool of the CF patient adheres to the bowel wall and obstructs the small intestine and colon. Only rarely is this seen in a patient with pancreatic sufficiency.

Rectal Prolapse. Episodes of rectal prolapse are related to malnutrition, abnormal stool (e.g., diarrhea, constipation), and paroxysmal coughing. Onset rarely occurs after 5 years of age.[62] The association with CF is so common that a sweat test is indicated in any child presenting with rectal prolapse.

Gastroesophageal Reflux Disease. Patients with CF often experience heartburn and gastric reflux, especially those with advanced pulmonary disease.[63] This may be the result of frequent coughing, obstructive lung disease with hyperinflation, and increased abdominal pressure. Treatment includes dietary restrictions and medication with antacids and histamine-2 blockers.

HEPATOBILIARY DISORDERS

The hepatobiliary manifestations of CF occur less frequently than the gastrointestinal disorders. Serious complications are uncommon before adolescence. Cirrhosis and portal hypertension are the most common hepatic disorders that occur in CF patients, although only 2% to 4% of patients with CF develop any apparent liver disease.[64] Prolonged neonatal jaundice may occur in neonates with CF and raises the suspicion of a diagnosis of CF.

Gallbladder abnormalities are quite common in CF patients.[65] Microgallbladder is the most common biliary tract disorder. It is believed that mucus obstruction of the cystic duct results in atrophy of the gallbladder. Most patients are asymptomatic. The incidence of abnormalities increases with age, with gallstones occurring quite frequently in patients with pancreatic insufficiency. Cholecystectomy is considered in patients who are symptomatic.

PROGNOSIS

Advances in the management of CF, especially the pulmonary manifestations, have led to a more favorable prognosis. Today the median survival is over 30 years.[5] This is a long stride from the life expectancy of less than 1 year when CF was described by Anderson in the late 1930s.[1] Even though patients with CF continue to survive longer, some children still succumb to the disease before reaching adulthood, in spite of advances in diagnostic techniques and treatment. We know that various factors influence a patient's prognosis, including the progression of pulmonary disease, the involvement of other organ systems, nutritional status, and environment. Investigations and projects that affect these factors will make a difference in the lives of many children.

REFERENCES

1. Anderson DH: Cystic fibrosis of the pancreas and its relation to celiac disease: a clinical and pathological study. *Am J Dis Child* 1938; 56:344-399.
2. Hamosh A et al: Comparison of the clinical manifestations of cystic fibrosis in African-Americans and Caucasians. *J Pediatr* 1998; 132:255-259.
3. Welsh MJ et al: Cystic fibrosis. In Scriver CR et al, editors: *The metabolic and molecular basis of inherited disease,* ed 7. New York. McGraw-Hill, 1995; pp 3799-3879.
4. Cystic Fibrosis Foundation: *Cystic Fibrosis Foundation patient registry 1997 annual data report.* Bethesda, Md, 1998.
5. FitzSimmons SC: The changing epidemiology of cystic fibrosis. *J Pediatr* 1993; 122:1-7.
6. Riordan JR et al: Identification of the cystic fibrosis gene: Cloning and characterization of complementary DNA. *Science* 1989; 245:1066-1073.
7. Cutting GR: Cystic fibrosis. In Rimoin DL, Connor JM, Pyeritz RD, editors: *Emery and Rimoin's principles and practice of medical genetics.* London. Churchill Livingstone, 1997; p 2685.
8. Smith JJ et al: Cystic fibrosis airway epithelia fail to kill bacteria because of abnormal airway surface fluid. *Cell* 1996; 85:229-236.
9. Davis PB: Cystic fibrosis. *Pediatr Rev* 2001; 22:257-264.
10. Davis PB: Autonomic and airway reactivity in obligate heterozygotes for cystic fibrosis. *Am Rev Respir Dis* 1984; 129:911-914.
11. Rosenstein B, Cutting GR: Diagnosis of cystic fibrosis: a consensus statement. *J Pediatr* 1998; 132:589-595.
12. LeGrys VA: Sweat testing for the diagnosis of cystic fibrosis: practical consideration. *J Pediatr* 1996; 129:892-897.
13. MacLean W, Tripp R: Cystic fibrosis with edema and falsely negative sweat test. *J Pediatr* 1973; 83:85-89.
14. Wood RE, Boat TF, Doershuk CF: Cystic fibrosis. *Am Rev Respir Dis* 1996; 833-838.
15. Worldwide survey of the delta F508 mutation—report from the cystic fibrosis genetic analysis consortium. *Am J Hum Genet* 1990; 47:354-359.
16. Boat TF et al: *The diagnosis of cystic fibrosis.* Bethesda, Md. Cystic Fibrosis Foundation, 1998.

17. Wilcken B: Newborn screening for cystic fibrosis: its evolution and a review of the current situation. *Screening* 1993; 2:43-62.

18. Chow C, Landau L, Taussig L: Bronchial mucous glands in the newborn with cystic fibrosis. *Eur J Pediatr* 1982; 139:240-243.

19. Lamb D, Reid L: The tracheobronchial submucosal glands in cystic fibrosis: a qualitative and quantitative histochemical study. *Br J Dis Chest* 1972; 66:240-247.

20. Zuelzer W, Newton W: The pathogenesis of fibrocystic disease of the pancreas: a study of 36 cases with special reference to the pulmonary lesions. *Pediatrics* 1949; 4: 53-69.

21. Katz SM, Holsclaw DS Jr: Ultrastructural features of respiratory cilia in cystic fibrosis. *Am J Clin Pathol* 1980; 73:682-685.

22. Thomassen MJ, Demko CA, Doershuk CF: Cystic fibrosis: a review of pulmonary infections and interventions. *Pediatr Pulmonol* 1987; 3:334-351.

23. Kerem E et al: Pulmonary function and clinical course in patients with cystic fibrosis after pulmonary colonization with *Pseudomonas aeruginosa*. *J Pediatr* 1990; 116: 714-719.

24. Goldman DA, Klinger JD: *Pseudomonas aeruginosa*: biology, mechanisms of virulence, epidemiology. *J Pediatr* 1986; 108:806-808.

25. Tablan OC et al: Colonization of the respiratory tract with *Pseudomonas cepacia* in cystic fibrosis: risk factors and outcomes. *Chest* 1987; 91:527-531.

26. Khan T et al: Early pulmonary inflammation in infants with cystic fibrosis. *Am J Respir Crit Care Med* 1995; 151:1075-1082.

27. Suter S et al: Granulocyte neutral proteases and *Pseudomonas* elastase as possible causes of airway damage in patients with cystic fibrosis. *J Infect Dis* 1984; 149:523-531.

28. Wistrak BJ, Meyer CM, Cotton RT: Cystic fibrosis presenting with sinus disease in children. *Am J Dis Child* 1993; 147:258-261.

29. Spector M, Stern R: Pneumothorax in cystic fibrosis: a 26-year experience. *Ann Thorac Surg* 1989; 47:204-207.

30. Desmond K et al: Immediate and long-term effects of chest physiotherapy in patients with cystic fibrosis. *J Pediatr* 1983; 103:538-542.

31. deBoeck C, Zinman R: Cough versus chest physiotherapy: a comparison of the acute effects on pulmonary function in patients with cystic fibrosis. *Am Rev Respir Dis* 1984; 129:182-184.

32. vanderSchans C et al: Effect of positive expiratory pressure breathing in patients with cystic fibrosis. *Thorax* 1991; 46:252-256.

33. Burnett M et al: Comparative efficacy of manual chest physiotherapy and a high frequency chest compression vest in inpatient treatment of cystic fibrosis. *Am Rev Respir Dis* 1993; 147:A30.

34. Warwick W, Hansen L: The long-term effect of high-frequency chest compression therapy on pulmonary complications of cystic fibrosis. *Pediatr Pulmonol* 1991; 11: 265-271.

35. Konstan M, Stern R, Doershuk C: Efficacy of the Flutter device for airway mucus clearance in patients with cystic fibrosis. *J Pediatr* 1994; 124:689-693.

36. Zach M, Purrer B, Oberwaldner B: Effect of swimming on forced expiration and sputum clearance in cystic fibrosis. *Lancet* 1981; 2:1201-1203.

37. Eggleston P et al: Airway hyperreactivity in cystic fibrosis: clinical correlates and possible effects on the course of disease. *Chest* 1988; 94:360-365.

38. Pattishall EN: Longitudinal response of pulmonary function to bronchodilators in cystic fibrosis. *Pediatr Pulmonol* 1990; 9:80-85.

39. Kattan M et al: Response to aerosol salbutamol, SCH 1000, and placebo in cystic fibrosis. *Thorax* 1980; 35: 531-535.

40. Hordvik NL et al: The effects of albuterol on the lung function of hospitalized patients with cystic fibrosis. *Am J Respir Crit Care Med* 1996; 154:156-160.

41. Zach MS et al: Bronchodilators increase airway instability in cystic fibrosis. *Am Rev Respir Dis* 1985; 131:537-543.

42. Weintraub SJ, Eschenbacher WL: The inhaled bronchodilators ipratropium bromide and metaproterenol in adults with CF. *Chest* 1989; 95:861-864.

43. Sanchez I, Holbrow J, Chernick V: Acute bronchodilator response to a combination of beta-adrenergic and anticholinergic agents in patients with cystic fibrosis. *J Pediatr* 1992; 120:486-488.

44. Lethem MI et al: The origin of DNA associated with mucus glycoproteins in cystic fibrosis sputum. *Eur Respir J* 1990; 3:19-23.

45. Shak S et al: Recombinant human DNase I (rhDnase) greatly reduces the viscosity of cystic fibrosis sputum. *Pediatr Pulmonol* 1990; 5:S173.

46. Fuchs H et al: Effect of aerosolized recombinant DNase on exacerbations of respiratory symptoms and on pulmonary function in patients with cystic fibrosis. *N Engl J Med* 1994; 331:637-642.

47. Robinson M et al: Effect of hypertonic saline, amiloride, and cough on mucociliary clearance in patients with cystic fibrosis. *Am J Respir Crit Care Med* 1996; 153:1503-1509.

48. Eigen H et al, CF Foundation Prednisone Trial Group: a multicenter study of alternate-day prednisone therapy in patients with cystic fibrosis. *J Pediatr* 1995; 126:515-523.

49. vanHaren E et al: The effects of inhaled corticosteroid budesonide on lung function and bronchial hyperresponsiveness in adult patients with cystic fibrosis. *Am Rev Respir Dis* 1994; 149:A667.

50. Nikolaizik W, Schonl M: Pilot study to assess the effect of inhaled corticosteroids on lung function in patients with cystic fibrosis. *J Pediatr* 1996; 128:271-274.

51. Knowles MR et al: A pilot study of aerosolized amiloride for the treatment of lung disease in cystic fibrosis. *N Engl J Med* 1990; 322:1189-1194.

52. Ramsey B: Management of pulmonary disease in patients with cystic fibrosis. *N Engl J Med* 1996; 335:179-188.

53. Donati MA, Guenette G, Auerbach H: Prospective controlled study of home and hospital therapy of cystic fibrosis pulmonary disease. *J Pediatr* 1987; 111:28-33.

54. Steinkamp G et al: Long term tobramycin aerosol therapy in cystic fibrosis. *Pediatr Pulmonol* 1989; 6:91-98.

55. Ramsey BW et al: Efficacy of aerosolized tobramycin in patients with cystic fibrosis. *N Engl J Med* 1993; 328: 1740-1746.

56. Jensen T et al: Colistin inhalation therapy in cystic fibrosis patients with chronic *Pseudomonas aeruginosa* lung infection. *J Antimicrob Chemother* 1987; 19:831-838.

57. Ramsey B, Burns J, Smith A: Safety and efficacy of tobramycin solution for inhalation in patients with cystic fibrosis: the results of two phase III placebo-controlled trials. *Pediatr Pulmonol* 1997; 14:S137-S138.

58. Ramsey B, Richardson M: Impact of sinusitis in cystic fibrosis. *J Allergy Clin Immunol* 1992; 90:547-552.

59. Drake-Lee A, Morgan D: Nasal polyps and sinusitis in children with cystic fibrosis. *J Laryngol Otol* 1989; 103:753-755.

60. Corey M et al: Familial concordance of pancreatic function in cystic fibrosis. *J Pediatr* 1989; 115:273-277.

61. Moran A et al: Pancreatic endocrine function in cystic fibrosis. *J Pediatr* 1991; 118:15-23.

62. Stern RC et al: Treatment and prognosis of rectal prolapse in cystic fibrosis. *Gastroenterology* 1982; 82:707-710.

63. Scott RB, O'Loughlin EV, Gall DG: Gastroesophageal reflux in patients with cystic fibrosis. *J Pediatr* 1985; 106: 223-227.

64. Scott-Jupp R, Lama M, Tanner MS: Prevalence of liver disease in cystic fibrosis. *Arch Dis Child* 1991; 66:698-701.

65. Stern RC, Rothstein FC, Doershuk CF: Treatment and prognosis of symptomatic gallbladder disease in patients with cystic fibrosis. *J Pediatr Gastroenterol Nutr* 1986; 5:35-40.

CHAPTER 36

Acute Respiratory Distress Syndrome

Adam Schwarz

Acute respiratory distress syndrome (ARDS) is refractory hypoxemia and acute respiratory failure that occurs as a result of significant lung injury. The first description of ARDS as a clinical entity appeared in 1967.[1] The term *adult* respiratory distress syndrome was originally used because the pathologic appearance of the lungs was similar to respiratory distress syndrome in premature newborns.[2] Since that time the term *adult* respiratory distress syndrome has been changed to *acute* respiratory distress syndrome to acknowledge that patients of all ages may be affected by the same pathophysiologic mechanisms.[3] A number of other terms, such as shock lung, noncardiogenic pulmonary edema, and traumatic wet lung, have been used synonymously to describe ARDS.[4] All have the same underlying pathophysiology and result in a similar clinical picture of acute hypoxemic respiratory failure.

The simplest clinical definition of ARDS is diffuse lung injury with atelectasis and hypoxemia. Radiographically, there are bilateral areas of consolidation with air bronchograms that reflect alveolar filling and atelectasis (Fig. 36-1).[5,6] Clinically, the patient has moderate to severe respiratory failure, hypoxemia, and stiff, noncompliant lungs. For the purposes of academic studies, several objective definitions of ARDS have been offered.[7,8] The American-European Consensus Conference on ARDS defines ARDS as follows[3]:

1. Acute onset of respiratory symptoms
2. Frontal chest radiograph with bilateral infiltrates
3. Pao_2/Fio_2 less than 200 mm Hg
4. No clinical evidence of left atrial hypertension, with a pulmonary capillary wedge pressure less than 18 mm Hg, if measured

Another objective scoring system that has been utilized in pediatrics is the oxygenation index (OI). The OI is a unitless number defined as:

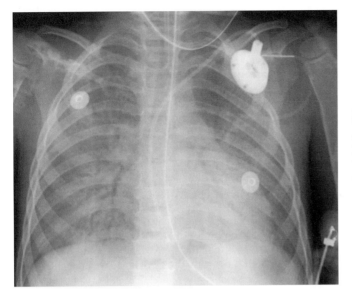

Fig. 36-1

Chest radiograph of a patient with ARDS. Note the infiltrates in all five lobes, the air bronchograms that appear due to areas of consolidation, and the loss of lung volume.

$$OI = \frac{(\overline{Paw} \times FIO_2)}{Pao_2} \times 100$$

where $\overline{Paw}$ is the mean airway pressure while on a ventilator, FIO_2 is the fraction of inspired oxygen, and Pao_2 is the arterial oxygen tension. The OI takes into account not only the ratio of administered FIO_2 to arterial oxygenation but also the degree of ventilator pressure administered, which helps reflect the degree of overall lung "stiffness" or decreased compliance. The OI has been correlated with outcome and used to help determine entry or response criteria for various studies, or for more highly invasive therapies such as extracorporeal membrane oxygenation (ECMO).[9,10]

ETIOLOGY

ARDS is caused by lung injury. Any pulmonary insult, direct or indirect, that disrupts the capillary-alveolar endothelium may cause a proteinaceous noncardiogenic pulmonary edema that results in ARDS (Box 36-1). Primary lung injury refers to a direct insult such as pneumonia, aspiration, or smoke inhalation. Secondary lung injury may be the result of generalized systemic conditions such as sepsis, head injury, or hemorrhagic shock. The most common published causes of ARDS in the pediatric population have been shock, sepsis, and near-drowning.[11,12]

The lack of universally accepted diagnostic criteria and the diversity of underlying causes make it difficult to determine the true incidence of ARDS. Depending on the diagnostic criteria, there may be as many as 150,000 cases of adult ARDS per year in the

BOX 36-1

CONDITIONS ASSOCIATED WITH ARDS

PRIMARY (DIRECT) INJURY
Pneumonia
Aspiration
    Gastric acid
    Near-drowning
    Hydrocarbon
Inhalation
    Smoke
    Oxygen toxicity
    Toxic gases
Emboli
    Air
    Fat
    Amniotic fluid
Pulmonary contusion
Radiation pneumonitis

SECONDARY INJURY
Shock
Sepsis
Trauma
Disseminated intravascular coagulation
Transfusion
Drugs
Increased intracranial pressure
Metabolic disorders
Cardiopulmonary bypass
Cardioversion
Hemodialysis

Data from Royall JA, Levin DL: Adult respiratory distress syndrome in pediatric patients. *J Pediatr* 1988; 112:169-180.

United States.[13] One published single-institution study reported that ARDS was present in 2.7% of pediatric intensive care unit admissions and accounted for 8% of patient-days.[14] Mortality is classically described as between 40% and 80%.[4] The largest description of pediatric ARDS was reported by the Pediatric Critical Care Study Group utilizing data from 41 institutions, in which 679 cases of pediatric ARDS in 1991 had an overall mortality rate of 52%.[15] More recent studies, however, suggest mortality from ARDS has declined, perhaps as a result of modern ventilator strategies and options. One report described 133 pediatric patients with severe hypoxic respiratory failure who had a mortality rate of only 13%.[16]

CLINICAL COURSE

The clinical course of ARDS has several different stages: acute stage, latent period, acute respiratory failure, and severe physiologic abnormalities.[17] The first stage is the actual injury to the lung. The second stage is the latent period, during which the patient could remain quite stable. The patient then develops early signs of pulmonary injury or insufficiency manifested by hyperventilation with hypocarbia and a respiratory alkalosis. The chest radiograph may remain clear, or it may demonstrate a fine reticular pattern owing to the development of pulmonary interstitial fluid.[5,6] The latent period may last for only minutes or persist for several days.

Acute respiratory failure, characterized by refractory hypoxemia caused by the large amount of intrapulmonary shunting and atelectasis, often occurs suddenly. The patient may develop rapid and shallow tachypnea, with increased retractions, grunting, and nasal flaring. Further examination usually reveals diffuse crackles heard on auscultation, and the chest radiograph will demonstrate diffuse bilateral regions of consolidation with or without the presence of air bronchograms. Most patients demonstrate a significant decrease in pulmonary compliance and require endotracheal intubation, mechanical ventilation, and PEEP. The pink-tinged secretions often suctioned initially from the endotracheal tube reflect intraalveolar capillary leak and lung injury.

Pathologically, there is an increase in alveolar-capillary permeability, resulting in an influx of interstitial and intraalveolar fluid, which inactivates surfactant. In addition, the pulmonary interstitial injury damages the type II pneumocytes that are responsible for the production and recycling of surfactant. The result is a decrease in surfactant activity and atelectasis (see Chapter 16).[18-22] Injury to lung parenchyma also triggers an inflammatory response that leads to recruitment of neutrophils, release of inflammatory cytokines, fibrin deposition, production of nitric oxide and free radicals, formation of hyaline membranes, and destruction of the type I pneumocytes lining the lung.

If lung injury and inflammation persist, the patient may develop severe physiologic abnormalities and progress to the last stage of ARDS. Not all patients will progress to this final stage. Some may develop such acute hypoxemia that they may die of respiratory failure. Because ARDS is often secondary to systemic disease or injury such as sepsis, trauma, or near-drowning, the patient may die of the complications of multiple system organ failure. Other patients go on to recover completely without developing severe physiologic abnormalities. Pulmonary fibrosis begins to develop if ARDS persists beyond 7 days. This leads to intractable respiratory failure or chronic lung disease requiring prolonged ventilator support. Collagenous tissue remodeling of the acinar architecture of the lung begins when ARDS persists for more than 3 weeks, resulting in cystic lesions with fibrotic scarring and a life-threatening decrease in the amount of functional surface area available for gas exchange.[23] Current treatment strategies seek to avoid this final, intractable, stage of ARDS.

ROLE OF MEDIATORS

Several mediators of inflammation are implicated in the pathogenesis of ARDS (Box 36-2). It is unclear, however, whether some of these mediators directly cause ARDS or are a secondary product of the inflammation resulting from lung injury. Direct lung injury from aspiration or smoke inhalation, for example, may result in inflammation and the release of inflammatory cytokines that augment microvascular permeability. On the other hand, the systemic inflammatory response syndrome triggered by sepsis often involves the development of ARDS. In this case, inflammatory mediators could themselves disrupt the capillary-alveolar membrane. Alternatively, this disruption may result from the microvascular perfusion abnormalities and ischemia of the systemic inflammatory response syndrome with associated breakdown of the alveolar-capillary membrane. Regardless of whether inflammatory mediators are primarily or secondarily involved in the pathogenesis of ARDS, they are clearly complex contributors to its development. Research efforts are concentrating on attempts to modulate the inflammatory response during ARDS.[24,25]

CHANGES IN PULMONARY MECHANICS

ARDS alters pulmonary mechanics in several ways. The loss of surfactant function, coupled with

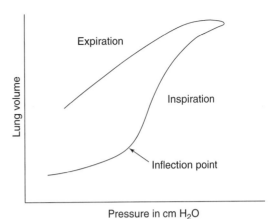

Fig. 36-2

Representation of the pressure-volume (compliance) loop in ARDS. Below the inflection point is the pressure at which the alveoli begin to collapse, leading to loss of lung volume, or FRC.

the development of edema around and within the alveoli, leads to alveolar collapse. The result is a decrease in lung compliance, lung volume, and functional residual capacity. This is associated with a large intrapulmonary shunt fraction $\dot{Q}s/\dot{Q}p$ that contributes to the significant hypoxemia associated with ARDS.

During ARDS, marked hysteresis of the pressure-volume loop occurs, such that much higher transpulmonary pressures are necessary to reach a given lung volume on inspiration than on expiration. The point on the pressure-volume loop where the shape changes from concave to exponential is known as the lower inflection point. It reflects the pressure point at which alveoli begin to collapse and is located above functional residual capacity (Fig. 36-2). This suggests that many gas exchange units will collapse at normal transpulmonary pressures and will need significant PEEP to maintain patency during expiration.

Finally, lung injury and areas of involvement in ARDS are heterogeneous and not uniform through all lung units. Some areas of the lung, typically in the dependent regions, are grossly affected. Other regions of the lung, typically in the nondependent regions, may be relatively unaffected.[26] This creates different areas of compliance within the lung itself. Dependent regions are fluid filled, atelectatic, and noncompliant. Nondependent areas are relatively normal and thus at risk for overdistention and barotrauma or volutrauma during mechanical ventilation.

TREATMENT

The goal in the treatment of ARDS is to treat the underlying disease, achieve adequate tissue oxygenation, and avoid complications. Tissue oxygenation is optimized by ensuring adequate cardiac output and hemoglobin levels. Overhydration could augment pulmonary edema, so fluids should be carefully titrated and monitored to normalize volume and maintain cardiac output. Antibiotics are used to treat pneumonia and sepsis. Adequate nutrition should be provided to optimize caloric intake. Repositioning or placing the patient prone may redistribute perfusion to better-ventilated lung regions and improve oxygenation.[27] Ultimately, however, supplemental oxygen and mechanical ventilation are required.

Every patient with ARDS is hypoxemic by definition. Prolonged administration of high concentrations of oxygen can damage the lungs, owing to the formation of highly reactive oxygen free radicals. Human and animal studies suggest that a prolonged FIO_2 greater than 0.60 should be avoided to prevent oxygen-induced pulmonary damage.[28]

The mainstay in treating ARDS is the administration of PEEP. No gas exchange will occur in atelectatic or fluid-filled alveoli. PEEP helps maintain alveolar patency and restore functional residual capacity. PEEP also maintains the transthoracic pressure above the point at which more alveoli will collapse during expiration. PEEP is typically increased to a level that allows adequate oxygenation, an arterial oxygen saturation (SaO_2) of 85% or greater at an acceptable FIO_2 of 0.60 or less. A PEEP level of 10 to 15 cm H_2O, or even higher, may be required to achieve adequate oxygenation. However, as PEEP levels exceed 12 to 15 cm H_2O, the increase in intrathoracic pressure may adversely affect cardiac output, primarily by decreasing venous return to the heart.[29] As PEEP is increased, the patient is monitored for a decrease in cardiac output or perfusion. In most cases, a fall in cardiac output can be compensated by volume loading and possibly inotropic support.[30,31]

Ventilation is achieved through a combination of respiratory rate and tidal volume. Historically, ventilator volumes between 10 and 15 ml/kg have been used for patients with ARDS. Because the remaining compliant lung volume in a patient with ARDS is significantly reduced, these tidal volumes may require inflation pressures that could result in over-distention and lung injury.[32-37] More recent guidelines recommend limiting the peak end-inspiratory plateau pressure to no more than 30 to 35 cm H_2O. This may require reducing the administered tidal volume to 6 to 8 ml/kg. Limiting the peak inspiratory pressure by reducing the tidal volume may decrease minute ventilation and result in hypercapnia. Recent evidence, however, suggests that low-volume pressure-limited ventilation with permissive hypercapnia may improve outcome in both adults and pediatric patients with ARDS.[16,38] The exact degree of respiratory acidosis that can be safely tolerated remains controversial. However, most undesirable effects are reversible and mostly minor when respiratory acidosis is in a range with the pH greater than 7.15 and the $PaCO_2$ less than 80 mm Hg.[39]

NEW THERAPIES

Some patients are unable to achieve acceptable therapeutic goals while avoiding oxygen toxicity or an intolerably high peak inspiratory pressure with conventional ventilator strategies. Other therapeutic modalities that have been used to treat patients with ARDS include high-frequency ventilation and ECMO (see Chapters 21 and 24).[40,41] Data have not demonstrated convincingly that either therapy ultimately improves outcome when compared with conventional pressure-limited ventilation in ARDS.

Similarly, a recent multicenter trial of perfluorocarbon liquid ventilation in pediatric ARDS was stopped when interim analysis showed that patients in the conventional ventilator group were doing just as well as patients in the liquid ventilation group.[42]

Other adjunct therapies include trials of corticosteroids, inhaled nitric oxide, and surfactant replacement. Although one small study suggests that corticosteroids may improve outcome in patients who progress into the late fibrotic fourth stage, large prospective trials have shown that corticosteroids fail to improve outcome and may be harmful in certain patients.[43-45] Investigations into the use of inhaled nitric oxide and the administration of surfactant are in the early stages.[46,47] Although results are encouraging, it is too early to make any conclusions concerning their role in improving the outcome of severe pediatric ARDS.

REFERENCES

1. Ashbough DG et al: Acute respiratory distress in adults. *Lancet* 1967; 2:319-323
2. Petty TL, Ashbaugh DG: The adult respiratory distress syndrome: clinical features, factors influencing prognosis and principles of management. *Chest* 1971; 60:273-279
3. Bernard GR et al: The American-European Consensus Conference on ARDS. *Am J Respir Crit Care Med* 1994; 149:818.
4. Fackler JC et al: Acute respiratory distress syndrome. In Rogers MC, editor: *Textbook of pediatric intensive care.* Baltimore. Williams & Wilkins, 1996.
5. Aberle DR, Brown K: Radiologic considerations in the adult respiratory distress syndrome. *Clin Chest Med* 1990; 11:737-753.
6. Effman EL et al: Adult respiratory distress syndrome in children. *Radiology* 1985; 157:69-74
7. Petty TL: Adult respiratory distress syndrome: definition and historical perspective. *Clin Chest Med* 1982; 3:3.
8. Murray JF et al: An expanded definition of the adult respiratory distress syndrome. *Am Rev Respir Dis* 1988; 138:720.
9. Rivera RA, Butt W, Shann F: Predictors of mortality in children with respiratory failure: possible indications for ECMO. *Anaesth Intensive Care* 1990; 18:385-389.
10. Durand M et al: Oxygenation index in patients with meconium aspiration: conventional and extracorporeal membrane oxygenation therapy. *Crit Care Med* 1990; 18:373-377.
11. Nussbaum E: Adult type respiratory distress syndrome in children: experience with seven cases. *Clin Pediatr* 1983; 22:401.
12. Holbrook PR et al: Adult respiratory distress syndrome in children. *Pediatr Clin North Am* 1980; 27:677
13. National Heart and Lung Institute, National Institutes of Health: *Respiratory distress syndromes: Task force on problems, research approaches, needs.* DHEW publication No. (NIH) 73-432. Washington, DC. US Government Printing Office, 1972; 165-180.
14. Davis SL, Furman DP, Costarino AJ: Adult respiratory distress syndrome in children: associated diseases, clinical course, and predictors of death. *J Pediatr* 1993; 123:35.
15. Timmons OD, Havens PL, Fackler JC: Predicting death in pediatric patients with acute respiratory failure. *Chest* 1995; 108:789.

16. Fackler JC et al: ECMO for ARDS: Stopping a randomized clinical trial. *Am J Respir Crit Care Med* 1997; 155:A504.

17. Royall JA, Levin DL: Adult respiratory distress syndrome in pediatric patients. *J Pediatr* 1988; 112:169-180.

18. Hallman M et al: Evidence of lung surfactant abnormality in respiratory failure. *J Clin Invest* 1982; 70:673.

19. Holm BA et al: Pulmonary physiological and surfactant changes during injury and recovery from hyperoxia. *J Appl Physiol* 1985; 59:1402.

20. Fuchimukai T et al: Artificial pulmonary surfactant inhibited by proteins. *J Appl Physiol* 1987; 62:429.

21. Holm BA, Notter RH: Effects of hemoglobin and cell membrane lipids on pulmonary surfactant activity. *J Appl Physiol* 1987; 63:1434.

22. Holm BA et al: Type II pneumocyte changes during hyperoxic lung injury and recovery. *J Appl Physiol* 1988; 65: 2672.

23. Tomashefski JF: Pulmonary pathology of the adult respiratory distress syndrome. *Clin Chest Med* 1990; 11:593.

24. Demling RH: The role of mediators in human ARDS. *J Crit Care* 1988; 3:56-72.

25. Rinaldo JE, Christman JW: Mechanisms and mediators of the adult respiratory distress syndrome. *Clin Chest Med* 1990; 11:621-632.

26. Gattinoni L, Pesenti A: ARDS: The nonhomogenous lung: facts and hypothesis. *Intensive Crit Care Dig* 1987; 61:1-3.

27. Murdoch IA, Storman MO: Improved arterial oxygenation in children with the adult respiratory distress syndrome: the prone position. *Acta Paediatr* 1994; 83:1043-1046.

28. Jenkinson SG: Oxygen toxicity. *New Horizons* 1993; 1(4): 504-511.

29. Mitaka C et al: Two-dimensional echocardiographic evaluation of inferior vena cava, right ventricle, and left ventricle during positive-pressure ventilation with varying levels of positive end-expiratory pressure. *Crit Care Med* 1989; 17:205.

30. Mohsenifar Z et al: Relationship between O_2 delivery and O_2 consumption in adult respiratory distress syndrome. *Chest* 1983; 84:267.

31. Pollack MM, Fields AI, Holbrook PR: Cardiopulmonary parameters during high PEEP in children. *Crit Care Med* 1980; 8:372.

32. Tsuno K et al: Histopathologic pulmonary changes from mechanical ventilation at high peak airway pressures. *Am Rev Respir Dis* 1991; 143:1115-1120.

33. Webb HH, Tierney DF: Experimental pulmonary edema due to intermittent positive- pressure ventilation with high inflation pressures: protection by positive end-expiratory pressure. *Am Rev Respir Dis* 1974; 110:556-565.

34. Dreyfuss D et al: Intermittent positive-pressure hyperventilation with high inflation pressures produces pulmonary microvascular injury in rats. *Am Rev Respir Dis* 1985; 132: 880-884.

35. Kolobow T et al: Severe impairment in lung function induced by high peak airway pressure during mechanical ventilation: an experimental study. *Am Rev Respir Dis* 1987; 135:312-315.

36. Corbridge TC et al: Adverse effects of large tidal volume and low PEEP in canine acid aspiration. *Am Rev Respir Dis* 1990; 142:311-315.

37. Parker JC et al: Lung edema caused by high peak inspiratory pressures in dogs: role of increased microvascular filtration pressure and permeability. *Am Rev Respir Dis* 1990; 142:321-328.

38. Hickling KG, Henderson SJ, Jackson R: Low mortality associated with low volume pressure-limited ventilation with permissive hypercapnia in severe adult respiratory distress syndrome. *Intensive Care Med* 1990; 16:372-377.

39. Feihl F, Perret C: Permissive hypercapnia: how permissive should we be? *Am J Respir Crit Care Med* 1994; 150: 1722-1737.

40. Arnold JH et al: Prospective, randomized comparison of high-frequency oscillatory ventilation and conventional ventilation in pediatric respiratory failure. *Crit Care Med* 1994; 22:1530-1539.

41. Green TP et al: The impact of extracorporeal membrane oxygenation on survival in pediatric patients with acute respiratory failure. *Crit Care Med* 1996; 24:323.

42. Furman B et al and LiquiVent Study Group: Multicenter randomized controlled trial (RCT) of LiquiVent partial liquid ventilation (PLV) in pediatric ARDS (abstract). Presented before the 11th Annual Pediatric Critical Care Colloquium, Chicago, 1998.

43. Meduri GU, Chinn A: Fibroproliferation in late adult respiratory distress syndrome: response to corticosteroid rescue treatment. *Chest* 1994; 105(3 suppl):127S-129S.

44. Bernard GR et al: High-dose corticosteroids in patients with the adult respiratory distress syndrome. *N Engl J Med* 1987; 317:1565.

45. Bone RC et al: A controlled clinical trial of high-dose methylprednisolone in the treatment of severe sepsis and septic shock. *N Engl J Med* 1987; 317:653.

46. Abman S et al: Acute effects of inhaled nitric oxide in children with severe hypoxemic respiratory failure. *J Pediatr* 1994; 124:881.

47. Willson DF et al: Calf's lung surfactant extract in acute hypoxemic respiratory failure in children. *Crit Care Med* 1996; 24:1316-1322.

CHAPTER **37**

Shock and Anaphylaxis

Anthony D. Slonim
Heidi J. Dalton

SHOCK

Shock is a syndrome that is associated with an imbalance between the supply of essential nutrients, oxygen, and substrate to the tissues of an organ and the metabolic demand of that organ or organ system. The child's response to the state of shock involves a number of compensatory mechanisms that aim to restore balance to the deranged organ system.[1,2] The clinician's role is to provide early identification of a cause, treat the underlying pathologic process, and provide support that maintains the functioning of the organism throughout the period of treatment and rehabilitation (Fig. 37-1).

PHYSIOLOGIC CHANGES

There are two physiologic levels of analysis to consider when the patient in shock is discussed. The first occurs at the organism level, where the hemodynamic determinants of the cardiac output are considered.[1] The goal is to maintain an adequate cardiac output so that the organism's cells and tissues are continually supplied with an oxygen-rich environment. The supply of essential nutrients to the tissues of an organ depends on the amount of blood the organ receives, the amount of oxygen and nutrients that are contained in the blood, and the ability of the tissues to utilize the substrate that is supplied. Regardless of the type of shock described, the basics of supplying a given tissue bed with nutrients from a systemic point of view are the same.

　The second level of analysis has to do with alterations that occur on the cellular level. The availability of oxygen is intimately linked to the ability of the organism's cells to utilize that oxygen to make energy at the cellular level.[2-4] If the cells do not have an adequate supply of oxygen, the cells will shift to a less-efficient method of providing energy known as anaerobic metabolism. These changes on the cellular level begin to occur well before the organism as a whole begins to elicit signs and symptoms of

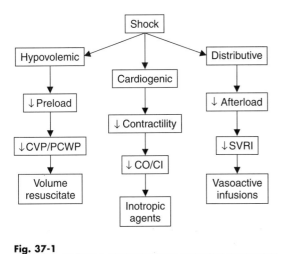

Fig. 37-1

Diagrammatic representation of shock, its classification, clinical measures of altered stroke volume, and treatment strategies. *CVP,* Central venous pressure; *PCWP,* pulmonary capillary wedge pressure; *CI,* cardiac index; *CO,* cardiac output; *SVRI,* systemic vascular resistance index.

shock.[2-7] When these manifestations begin to affect the entire organism, the production of lactic acid and a corresponding acidemia manifest the anaerobic metabolism.

Cardiac Output. In physiologic terms, the cardiac output is the amount of blood that is pumped from the heart to all of the organs and tissues of the body. It is a concept that is expressed mathematically in terms of liters of blood pumped per minute.[8] Because children are different in terms of their size and age, all hemodynamic measurements must be corrected for these differences. When the cardiac output is corrected for size, an expression known as the cardiac index is derived.[9] The cardiac index is the cardiac output divided by the body surface area. In children, normal values for the cardiac index are in the range of 3.6 to 6.0 liters per minute per square meter of body surface area.[10]

The cardiac output represents the amount of blood pumped per minute by the heart to the tissues. It is determined by the heart rate and the stroke volume.[11] The heart rate is simply how fast the heart beats per minute. The stroke volume is the amount of blood that is pumped out of the heart with each mechanical beat. Three components contribute to the stroke volume. They are referred to as preload, inotropy, and afterload.[12]

Preload is a representation of the basal amount of volume present in the heart and great vessels at rest. This volume exerts a pressure against the walls of the blood vessels in the vascular tree. Clinically,

this pressure is measured as the central venous pressure. It increases with increases in the intravascular volume and decreases when the patient has a diminished intravascular volume. The Frank-Starling principle relates this central pressure to the initial stretch on the muscle fibers of the heart.[12] The stretch, and the contractile ability that results, increases as this central pressure increases, up to a limit that is determined by that individual's myocardial compliance. At that point, the contractile ability cannot increase further. *Inotropy* is the term that is applied to this measure of the contractile state of the heart muscle.

Afterload is a measure of the resistance or force against which the heart must pump. It is measured by the systemic vascular resistance, which is the difference of the mean arterial pressure and the central venous pressure divided by the cardiac output and multiplied by a factor of 80. The diastolic blood pressure is a surrogate for the basal level of pressure present within the vascular system. Infants and children have a limited ability to increase stroke volume.[11,13] They will attempt to compensate for a decrease in cardiac output by correspondingly increasing their heart rate.[9] Tachycardia is one of the first signs to be aware of in children with decreased peripheral perfusion. Hypotension is a late finding of shock in children. It occurs when the child's compensatory mechanisms begin to fail. Therefore it is not a reliable indicator of shock.

The shock state can be classified based on whether the inadequate cardiac output is primarily related to a problem with heart rate, preload, inotropy, or afterload.[13] Not only will this schema aid in classification, but it will also target therapeutic interventions to the area of the circulatory system that is experiencing a problem (see Fig. 37-1). In addition, each one of these physiologic parameters is able to be measured clinically in the child with shock, thereby allowing repetitive monitoring and reassessment of the condition in relation to therapeutic strategies.[9,11]

Nutrients and Oxygen in Blood. The cardiac output is responsible for getting blood and nutrients from the heart to the tissues and organs and back again. The nutrients are carried in the blood from one place to another by two physical methods.[14] First, some nutrients and oxygen are dissolved in the blood. This accounts for a relatively small amount of oxygen transport. Second, nutrients and oxygen can be bound to blood cells or macromolecules and "carried" by the cardiac output to the site of utilization. This is the predominant way that oxygen is carried in the blood.[14] The amount of oxygen bound to hemoglobin is

---

FORMULAS USED IN THE CALCULATION OF OXYGEN CONTENT, OXYGEN DELIVERY, AND OXYGEN CONSUMPTION

OXYGEN CONTENT

Cao_2 (ml/dl) = Amount of O_2 dissolved in blood
+ Amount bound to hemoglobin
Amount of O_2 dissolved (ml of O_2/ml of blood)
= 0.003 × Pao_2 (mm Hg)
Amount bound = 1.34 × Hemoglobin (g/dl)
× % Oxygen saturation

OXYGEN DELIVERY

Do_2 = O_2 Content × Cardiac output

OXYGEN CONSUMPTION

$\dot{V}o_2$ (ml/min) = (Arterial − venous) O_2 Content ×
Cardiac output (ml/min)

0.003, A constant that represents the milliliters of oxygen dissolved in 100 ml of blood; *1.34*, a constant that represents the amount of oxygen that can be bound per gram of hemoglobin.

described by the oxyhemoglobin dissociation curve and is affected by physical properties such as temperature and acidosis.[14] The contribution of each of these components is symbolized in a mathematical formula that represents the arterial oxygen content (Box 37-1).[1,3,14] Box 37-2 features an example that demonstrates how the mathematical formulas shown in Box 37-1 may be used to quantify oxygen transport. Once the oxygen content is calculated, it can be considered within the framework of the cardiac output. Oxygen delivery can be thought of as the delivery of substrate to the tissues as it is carried by the cardiac output.

Delivery of Blood to the Tissues. The cardiac output provides the delivery of oxygenated blood to the tissues on a global or systemic level.[12,14-19] Delivery of oxygenated blood, however, is only one part of this complex physiologic process. Once oxygenated and nutrient-rich blood reaches the target organ, the organ must utilize the substrates it receives.[19] For the organ to use the oxygen, there must be uptake in the tissues and cells of the organ.

EXAMPLE OF USE OF OXYGEN CONTENT, OXYGEN DELIVERY, AND OXYGEN CONSUMPTION FORMULAS IN THE CARE OF A 5-YEAR-OLD CHILD IN SHOCK

CASE EXAMPLE

A 5-year-old girl is in septic shock in the pediatric intensive care unit as a result of an overwhelming infection. She has a hemoglobin of 10 g/dl, a cardiac output of 4.0 L/min, and arterial blood gas findings of pH, 7.35; Pco_2, 36 mm Hg; Pao_2, 85 mm Hg; HCO_3^-, 20 mEq/L; and a corresponding oxygen saturation of 95%. A mixed venous blood sample demonstrates pH, 7.32; Pco_2, 34 mm Hg; Pao_2, 37 mm Hg; and an oxygen saturation of 62%. Calculate the oxygen content, delivery, and consumption as follows:

ARTERIAL OXYGEN CONTENT

Cao_2 = Amount dissolved in blood + Amount
bound to hemoglobin (arterial side)
Amount dissolved = 0.003 × Pao_2
Amount dissolved = 0.003 × 85 mm Hg =
0.255 or 0.255 ml of O_2
in 100 ml of blood
Amount bound = 1.34 × Hemoglobin ×
% O_2 saturation
Amount bound = 1.34 × 10 × 0.95 =
12.73 ml of oxygen per
100 ml of blood
Cao_2 = 0.255 + 12.73 = 12.99 ml of O_2 per
100 ml of blood

MIXED VENOUS OXYGEN CONTENT

$C\bar{v}o_2$ = Amount dissolved + Amount bound to
hemoglobin (venous side) = 0.003 ×
$P\bar{v}o_2$
Amount dissolved = 0.003 × $P\bar{v}o_2$
Amount dissolved = 0.003 × 37 mm Hg =
0.115 or 0.115 ml of O_2
in 100 ml of blood
Amount bound = 1.34 × Hemoglobin × %
O_2 saturation
Amount bound = 1.34 × 10 × 0.62 = 8.31 ml
of O_2 per 100 ml of blood
$C\bar{v}o_2$ = 0.115 + 8.31 = 8.425 ml of O_2 per
100 ml of blood

OXYGEN DELIVERY

Do_2 = O_2 content × Cardiac output
Do_2 = 12.99 ml of O_2 per 100 ml of blood ×
4000 ml/min
Arterial Do_2 = 519.6 ml/min

OXYGEN CONSUMPTION

$\dot{V}o_2$ (ml/min) = (Arterial − venous) O_2 content ×
Cardiac output (ml/min)
$\dot{V}o_2$ (ml/min) = (12.99 − 8.425) ml of O_2 per
100 ml of blood ×
4000 ml/min = 182.6

Associated with this uptake of nutrient-rich material is the exchange of organ byproducts that are then transported back to the lungs from that organ. A major component of these byproducts is carbon dioxide, which has a higher solubility in the blood than oxygen.[14]

A measure of how well the tissues are utilizing the substrate supplied to them can be depicted by a concept known as oxygen consumption.[15] Oxygen consumption is a measure of the amount of oxygen utilized by the organs of the body.[14] If one considers the amount of nutrient being supplied to the organs from the arterial circuit and the amount of oxygen remaining in the venous circuit after removal by the organs, one has an estimation of how much oxygen is being consumed.[14,17,20]

The amount of nutrient that is consumed by the organs relative to delivery is referred to as the oxygen extraction.[19] The oxygen extraction is not dependent on supply for patients with shock. As shock worsens, organ tissue perfusion decreases and the organ extracts fewer nutrients from the blood. This is a measure of the severity of shock and has been associated with survival.[9] Regardless of the etiology of the shock, alterations in cell metabolism lead to difficulty with utilization at the cellular level. These changes in cellular oxygen utilization alter the consumption of oxygen in each of the organs. This, in turn, leads to alterations in the functioning of the organs. Organ system dysfunction resulting from shock, if left untreated, ultimately leads to the failure of multiple organ systems. The term *multiorgan dysfunction syndrome* (MODS) has been applied to this disseminated pathologic response.[21]

CLASSIFICATION

There are three major types of shock. Each type of shock can be categorized by the effect that a given derangement in stroke volume has on the cardiac output (see Fig. 37-1). Using this paradigm, health care practitioners are able to identify the potential causes of shock based on the hemodynamic profile that is observed.[11] An understanding of cardiorespiratory interactions is useful not only for the diagnosis and classification of shock but also for the goals of monitoring its progress and the response to treatment.

Hypovolemic Shock. The intravascular volume consists of blood cells, plasma, and fluid.[3] These substances are contained within a potential space that is represented by the venous system and blood vessels that supply the right side of the heart. This intravascular volume is a component of the stroke volume known as preload and contributes directly to the cardiac output of the heart.[3] When there is an

excessive amount of fluid in this space, the patient is referred to as hypervolemic. Those patients with an inadequate amount of body fluid in this space are referred to as hypovolemic. When the decrement in body fluid becomes so severe that there is not enough fluid to supply the most remote cells of the body with necessary nutrients and oxygen, hypovolemic shock is present.[3]

In children, hypovolemic shock is the most common type of shock and arises from many different causes, depending on what component of the intravascular fluid is lost from the vascular space. If red blood cells are lost from the vascular space, a specific subtype of hypovolemic shock known as hemorrhagic shock is present.[3,22] Common examples of hemorrhagic shock include trauma, gastrointestinal bleeding, and bleeding resulting from coagulopathy.

Extracellular fluid is lost from the vascular space when the conditions of vomiting and diarrhea lead to dehydration in patients with gastroenteritis. This is a common cause of hypovolemic shock, especially in infants and younger children.[1,3] Hypovolemia may also occur because of neglecting to provide an adequate fluid intake. Infants who are abused or neglected or who have insufficient replacement to account for losses in warm climates may contribute to this category.

Children with burns and nephrotic syndrome initially lose large amounts of plasma-rich fluid and ultimately experience hypovolemic shock if careful attention to replacement and maintenance fluids is not maintained.[3] Plasma proteins provide a force known as oncotic pressure that helps to maintain the extracellular fluid within the intravascular space. When these proteins are lost, the fluid seeps into the interstitial space and the shock state is perpetuated.

Cardiogenic Shock. The cardiac output is also directly related to the heart rate and two other contributors to the stroke volume: inotropy and afterload (see Fig. 37-1). Inotropy refers to the contractile state of the heart.[12,19] Afterload is a measure of the resistance against which the heart must contract. Cardiogenic shock is present when a lower cardiac output results from a problem related to the heart rate, the contractile state, or the afterload as the heart attempts to supply blood to the tissues of the body.[23,24] In addition, other conditions of the body may indirectly account for a depression of the heart's contractile state.[25-27] For instance, in septic shock, a depression of myocardial contractility can also be seen.[26,27]

An alteration in the heart rate that is outside the normal physiologic range may occur in either a fast or a slow direction and result in a reduction of the cardiac output. A slowing of the heart rate occurs in children who experience hypoxia or heart block.[28] If the hypoxia and its concomitant bradycardia are not corrected in the short term, cardiac output begins to fall and the child manifests poor perfusion and shock. In addition, cardiac rhythms that are faster than the normal physiologic rhythms, such as ventricular or supraventricular tachycardias, may decrease the cardiac output and ultimately affect perfusion of the organs.[23]

When the inotropy of the heart is affected, either because of an inflammatory process, as occurs in a heart with myocarditis, or because of an alteration in contractile state of the muscle, as occurs in cardiomyopathy, the stroke volume and hence the cardiac output are adversely affected.[23] Likewise, there can be increases in the afterload because of valvular or muscular defects or changes in the systemic resistance, such as in hypertensive emergencies that inhibit a full cardiac output by inhibiting stroke volume.[23]

Distributive Shock (Peripheral Vasodilatation). Distributive shock is the classification of shock that results from vasodilatation of the vascular bed (see Fig. 37-1). Vasodilating substances that act directly and indirectly on the cells of the blood vessels create an enlargement of the intravascular potential space such that there is an inadequate amount of fluid to fill the space.[4-7,25-27] The reduced perfusion that results from this increase in intravascular potential space is caused by this comparative hypovolemia.[1]

Distributive shock is a type of shock for which there are many potential causes. Septic shock results from an infectious process.* Neurogenic shock originates from a neurologic insult such as spinal cord contusion or transection. Anaphylactic shock results from antigen exposure and a release of IgE antibody (see later).[31-35] Adrenal insufficiency is also included in this category because of a similar hemodynamic profile. Regardless of the type of distributive shock that is occurring, the physiologic dysfunction is similar. The disturbance is associated with an elevated cardiac output and a reduced afterload.[5,6,20] Because of the vasodilation, the force against which the heart is contracting is lost.

Assessment

The approach to a child in shock begins with an evaluation of vital functions as expounded by the ABCs of resuscitation[28,36,37] (see Chapter 25). A rapid assessment of the airway and whether it is maintained or needs intervention is the first step. Once the

airway is secured, attention can be turned to breathing. Is spontaneous breathing present, and is it effective to promote oxygenation and ventilation? If not, intervention to promote these physiologic processes needs to be performed. Finally, the circulatory system is evaluated by the presence of a pulse. If a pulse is absent, cardiopulmonary resuscitation needs to be performed and cardiotonic medications consistent with advanced life support need to be administered.[28,36,37]

Once the ABCs are evaluated and corrected, attention is directed to measuring vital signs and performing a secondary survey. Normal values for pulse, respiratory rate, and blood pressure are age dependent. Knowledge of these age-related differences is essential to being able to care for any child[38] (see Chapters 5 and 6).

A brief and directed patient history can be obtained at this point. It should include information regarding how long the child has been sick, what interventions have been provided, and how well the child has responded to these interventions. In addition, essential information regarding past medical history, medications, and allergies to medications is obtained.

An examination for fever, skin turgor, bruising, bleeding, or trauma may provide helpful clues that lead to an etiologic diagnosis of shock. After an assessment of vital signs, one's attention can be turned toward the effectiveness of the cardiac output in supplying the perfusion of the organs. Capillary refill, which is the process of blanching the skin for several seconds and timing the return of blood flow to the blanched skin, has been shown to be a quick, useful, and noninvasive test that gives some gross information regarding perfusion in the acute setting.[28] The normal amount of time required to refill the capillary bed after this blanching of the skin should be less than 2 seconds. Prolongation of this refill time is considered as a sign of inadequate tissue perfusion. Assessment of the quality of perfusion to the skin, the kidney, and the brain is often examined next because the data that can be accumulated are readily available after the initial resuscitation is completed. These parameters correlate much better with hemodynamic measurements than does capillary refill.[39]

Evaluation of the skin based on skin color and temperature is easily performed. The skin of children in shock may be pale, cyanotic, or mottled because of poor perfusion. Traditionally, practitioners have described two phases of septic shock.[13] Early septic shock, the so-called warm shock phase, has the skin appearing warm, pink, and well perfused. This is the result of vasodilatation in the setting of an increased cardiac output. Later in the course, however, the

---

*References 4-7, 25-27, 29, 30.

cardiac output begins to fall. The skin examination during this period of "cold shock" is likely to be cool and cyanotic, representing a decrease in the amount of substrate reaching the skin.

Likewise, perfusion to the child's brain can be assessed in the absence of consciousness-altering medications by looking at the child's level of awareness and response to commands. Children in shock may be stuporous or comatose. However, they may also be agitated because of anxiety or the shock state itself. The Glasgow Coma Score adapted for pediatric use is a useful tool to be able to objectively follow neurologic status over time. Perfusion of the child's visceral organs is easily assessed by monitoring the level of urine production. If the child is making adequate urine or more than 1 ml/kg/hr, one can assume that there is adequate renal blood flow and hence adequate circulation to the other visceral components.

MONITORING

Assessment of the child in shock is a continuous and ongoing process that leads to and follows from therapeutic interventions. It occurs so that repetitive attention to the effects of an intervention on vital signs and end organ perfusion can be observed. If the child fails to respond, additional strategies to maintain equilibrium need to be incorporated into the treatment plan. Consistency in measurement, in terms of both what is measured and the responses to care, needs to be considered. If a presumed treatment has not had its intended effect on restoring homeostasis, the underlying etiology of shock needs to be reconsidered.

The available technologies in the pediatric intensive care unit have expanded the assessment and monitoring skills now available to the child with shock.[9,40] These interventions augment the information that is derived from the vital signs and physical examination. The arterial catheter, the central venous pressure (CVP) monitor, and the pulmonary artery catheter are three of the more common strategies employed to detect the physiologic changes and to supplement the clinical assessment, monitoring, and treatment of the child in shock.

Arterial Catheters. The measurement of the blood pressure is vital to an understanding of the condition of the child who presents with shock. As mentioned, however, children maintain their blood pressure until late in the course of shock. Auscultatory methods for the measurement of the blood pressure may be unreliable and cumbersome because of the difficulty of the method and amount of environmental noise. Electronic blood pressure cuff measurements are easier to use, are more reli-

able in children, and have the additional benefit of being able to track the mean arterial blood pressure and the heart rate in addition to the systolic and diastolic measurements.

The placement of a catheter in a peripheral or central artery can also be performed for the monitoring of blood pressure on a continuous basis in the intensive care unit. This procedure also allows for the extraction of blood for arterial blood gas measurements without repetitive arterial punctures. It is a technique whose use is subject to wide disparity based on local practice patterns. The shape and characteristics of the waveform allow one to derive information regarding the characteristics of the cardiac output, including volume, afterload, and contractility.

Central Venous Pressure Measurements. The placement of a catheter in the central venous circulation allows the practitioner to assess the volume status of the child with critical illness. The catheter measures the downstream intravascular pressure in the right atrium. This intravascular pressure represents preload. Preload is one of the three contributors to the stroke volume, which, in turn, contributes to the cardiac output (see Fig. 37-1). Because the left side of the heart receives its blood from the right side of the heart, the measurement of these right-sided heart pressures is accepted as the alternative for the dynamics on the left side of the heart in the patient whose myocardial and pulmonary compliance is normal. This information helps the practitioner to diagnose and treat the patient in shock. In the most basic terms, if the CVP is high in the setting of normal myocardial compliance, then the intravascular volume is adequate and may not be accounting for the reduction in cardiac output. The CVP may also be elevated if the blood is unable to be ejected because of a failing myocardium. If the CVP is low, additional intravenous fluid needs to be given to improve the intravascular volume deficit that is being observed.

Pulmonary Artery Catheter Measurements. The placement of a catheter in the pulmonary artery allows the determination of a number of useful measurements in the diagnosis, monitoring, and treatment of the child in shock. The catheter is inserted into the internal jugular or subclavian venous system of the upper torso or in the femoral vein from the lower torso approach. Placement of the catheter allows one to directly read measurements that represent the contribution to stroke volume and cardiac output. For instance, CVP measurements can also be taken from the pulmonary artery catheter (see Fig. 37-1). In addition, the pulmonary capillary wedge pressure, which measures downstream pressures from the left atrium, and hence the preload to the left ventricle, can also be measured. It is thought to be a more exact measure of preload when the myocardial or pulmonary compliance is not normal.

Inotropy is estimated by measuring the cardiac output and correcting for body surface area (see Fig. 37-1). In addition, pressure measurements from within the pulmonary artery allow the practitioner to identify problems with the pulmonary vasculature or its reactivity as a contribution to shock. If the pulmonary vasculature is constricted, the movement of blood from the right side of the heart to the left side is restricted. Hence, the pulmonary artery catheter provides information regarding the left side of the heart and the interaction between the heart and lungs that is in addition to that provided by the central venous pressure monitor.

In addition to the measurements that are read directly from the catheter, a number of measurements can be derived that will yield information regarding the homeostatic function of the child. For instance, systemic vascular resistance, which is a measure of afterload, can be calculated by measuring the pressure differences across the vascular bed of the heart and dividing by the cardiac output. Similarly, a measure of afterload as it affects only the right ventricle, known as pulmonary vascular resistance, can be calculated by considering only the output of the right ventricle. Oxygen delivery and consumption can be calculated by utilizing the cardiac output measures.[9,10,15-18] Measure oxygen utilization and oxygen extraction by calculating the mixed venous oxygen saturation of blood withdrawn from the pulmonary artery. The normal mixed venous saturation has been shown to be 70% to 75%. Higher measurements of the mixed venous saturation may occur from an inability of the organ to extract oxygen from the blood. This is a bad sign that signifies a more severe stage of shock. From these values, extraction ratios and an analysis of the degree of shock can be calculated. Moreover, a physiologic approach to the treatment and management can be used.

TREATMENT

Respiratory. The goals of treatment of shock are to enhance the delivery of oxygen and nutrients to the organs and tissues of the body. In an attempt to improve oxygen delivery, the practitioner can augment either the cardiac output or the oxygen content. Increasing the oxygen in the blood or increasing the amount of blood available to carry oxygen can increase the delivery of oxygen to an organ.[14,15,17,18] The additional oxygen-carrying

capacity of blood is likely to be beneficial in those patients who are anemic.[40] Additionally, endotracheal intubation with mechanical ventilation may be useful to reduce the work of breathing and optimize oxygen content in the patient in shock.

Vascular Volume. Rapid restoration of an adequate circulating blood volume is essential for a patient in shock regardless of the cause (see Fig. 37-1).[40-43] Keeping in mind that children compensate initially with increases in their heart rate, hypotension is a relatively late sign of shock in the pediatric patient. Normal saline or lactated Ringer's solutions are the fluids of choice for initial resuscitation.[42,43] Some practitioners prefer the use of fluids with macromolecules such as albumin or starch to maintain intravascular volume. Nevertheless, these fluids have not demonstrated a beneficial effect on survival. If there are obvious or suspected losses of blood, however, then the repletion of the intravascular volume with packed red blood cells should be performed.[22,40,41]

Administration of an amount of 20 ml/kg is recommended.[28,41,43] Reassessment of the patient's condition based on vital signs and end-organ perfusion determines the need for additional aliquots of fluid in the same amount. Carcillo and colleagues demonstrated that when the initial amount of volume resuscitation administered within the first hour, the so-called golden hour, was cumulatively greater than 40 ml/kg, the survival rates for these patients with severe cases of shock were improved.[42] Thus the amount of fluid and the rapidity of administration do have outcome benefits. When total volumes reaching 60 ml/kg have been administered, consideration to monitoring of the intravascular volumes by more invasive means should be contemplated. Transportation to a facility capable of these interventions and guiding therapy by the physiologic derangement is important in caring for children in shock.[44]

In the patient with shock originating from a cardiogenic cause, this reassessment is vital. Additional aliquots of fluid may be contraindicated.[23,45] The additional fluid may compromise cardiac function and lead to pulmonary edema because of the relationship to the Frank-Starling principle that was discussed earlier.

Myocardial Function. Once the intravascular volume is optimized, attempts at manipulating other components of the stroke volume to enhance cardiac output should be tried (see Fig. 37-1). If the heart rate is ineffective because it is too slow, such as occurs with heart block or bradycardia, then drugs that can enhance the rate such as atropine should be considered.[28,36,37] It should be noted, again, that brady-cardia may be the primary manifestation of hypoxia in children.[28] Therefore, before primary efforts directed at correcting slow heart rates are undertaken, care must be exercised in ensuring a patent airway, with adequate ventilation and oxygenation.

Abnormalities in heart rate that alter the pumping function of the heart should be addressed in an expedited fashion. If the patient's condition is unstable because of a fast heart rhythm such as supraventricular tachycardia or ventricular tachycardia, then electrical therapy in the form of synchronized cardioversion or defibrillation is indicated.[28] Cardioversion synchronizes the delivery of the shock with the QRS complex on the monitor to prevent deterioration to a more lethal arrhythmia. It should be used in patients who have a palpable pulse. Defibrillation, on the other hand, delivers a shock regardless of the timing of the cardiac cycle. It is indicated to treat rhythms that have resulted in cardiovascular collapse.[28]

Inotropic dysfunction can result from an abnormality in any of the structures of the heart or the abnormal contractility of the heart muscle cells. Initially, adequate preload to maintain stroke volume should be ensured. This may require the judicious use of fluids to augment intravascular volume. This is done to optimize the performance of the myocardium in providing the cardiac output. After preload augmentation, additional fluid may only serve to worsen the ability of the myocardium to maintain its output. Hence, support of the myocardium can then take place with inotropic agents that act by a number of different mechanisms.[23] Drugs that act through the sympathetic nervous system such as dobutamine can enhance contractility.[23,28,36,37]

Alternatively, drugs that belong to a class known as inodilators work through a different mechanism. These drugs enhance inotropy while simultaneously reducing afterload, thereby making it easier for the "weak" heart to eject blood.[23] If the problem with inadequate cardiac function is related to elevations in afterload, consideration to vasodilators should be given.[23] Hydralazine and nitroprusside work to vasodilate the arterial tree and thereby reduce afterload. In addition, a subset of patients may demonstrate pervasive hypotension despite fluid resuscitation.[45] In these circumstances, inotropic agents in combination with vasodilators may be useful.[28,37]

Peripheral Vascular Resistance. The peripheral vascular resistance represents afterload (see Fig. 37-1). Blood pressure is sustained by the interaction of the cardiac output acting in concert with the peripheral vascular resistance. The mean arterial pressure characterizes this relationship.[46] This relationship helps to defend the patient from hypotension. If the problem initiating the shock state causes a reduction in afterload because of vasodilating mediators or inflammatory mediators, such as occurs in sepsis or anaphylaxis, then methods to increase afterload should be considered once adequate preload has been restored. There are a variety of alternatives available to correct this problem.[28,36,37] Drugs that act through the different receptors of the sympathetic nervous system are most often used here. Dopamine works through a dose-dependent response on sympathetic receptors. Epinephrine, norepinephrine, and phenylephrine have differential affinity for sympathetic nervous system receptors. These agents increase vascular tone, peripheral vascular resistance, and afterload. This helps to maintain perfusion to vital organs such as the kidneys and those of the gastrointestinal tract.

Nutritional Status. Nutritional support of the critically ill child has a role in maintaining stability, promoting healing, and improving outcome from acute and chronic illness.[16,47,48] The goals of nutritional support are to promote these end points while simultaneously providing adequate metabolic substrate that will also provide for the growth and development of the child.[47]

Assessment of the nutritional status of critically ill children begins on admission to the intensive care unit. Baseline growth charts and nutritional studies such as measurement of albumin levels will help to allow the practitioner to realize what nutritional state the child is in.[48] For ongoing analysis of the nutritional status, however, these measures are not altered in an acute enough manner to allow them to be helpful. Rather, determination of the level of proteins with rapid turnover such as prealbumin or transferrin helps to identify a child who is experiencing an impairment of nutrition related to an illness.[48] Nitrogen balance is another useful measure that allows one to estimate the adequacy of nutrition.[32] The catabolic state of illness leads to a loss of endogenous protein and places the child at risk of a bad outcome unless the amount of nutrients being supplied offsets the metabolic needs of the body. A child with a negative nitrogen balance is receiving inadequate nutritional supplementation and is at risk for malnutrition because the body is utilizing protein stores for energy.

The method of indirect calorimetry measures the physiologic parameters of oxygen consumption and carbon dioxide production discussed earlier. In this way, an accurate assessment of the resting energy expenditure as it relates to the patient's physiology can be examined.[48] There are difficulties with using each of these methods of measuring nutritional status in children, but approximations that relate caloric needs to the individual's physiology have been shown to be fairly accurate.

When an assessment identifies that the patient is unable to optimize the intake of nutritional materials to meet the metabolic demand, supplementation should take place. The practitioner should encourage an intake provided by the enteral route whenever possible. If this is not possible, supplementation by parenteral methods must then ensue. Substantial work in the area of vitamins, trace elements, and immune-modifying nutritional agents is in progress.

ANAPHYLAXIS

One type of shock that results from peripheral vasodilation is anaphylactic shock. Anaphylactic shock occurs when a foreign antigen interacts with the body and elicits an immediate hypersensitivity reaction that is mediated by antibodies of the immunoglobulin E class.[35] A variety of substances can elicit these reactions.[31-35] Dibs and associates found that latex allergy, foods, drugs, and snake venom were the most common inciting agents in the pediatric population.[31] There are times, however, when a cause of anaphylaxis may not be found despite an exhaustive search.[32,33]

Pathology

After introduction of the antigen into the body, either by an enteral or parenteral route, reaction with the IgE antibody occurs. This evokes the release of a number of chemical mediators from circulating and tissue-based cells that are responsible for the clinical and hemodynamic symptom-complex that is elicited. Histamine is one of the most prominent of the mediators and is in large part responsible for the clinical effects that are observed.[34] A widespread inflammatory reaction occurs that invokes many of the antiinflammatory cascades of the host to modify the response to the antigen.

Presentation

The presentation of the child with anaphylaxis varies depending on the severity of symptoms. Some children with allergies may present with only a skin eruption. Other patients may present with respiratory compromise or cardiovascular collapse and shock that is characteristic of an overt anaphylactic episode.[34,35] The presentation with a respiratory or dermal complaint is much more common than a cardiovascular source of symptoms.[31,33] However, shock can occur without a preceding dermatologic presentation.[34]

The hemodynamic responses of the body to anaphylaxis are similar to those described earlier for distributive shock. A comparative hypovolemia is related to an increase in the ability of the vascular tree to hold more intravascular volume. This occurs related to the vasodilating effects of the chemical mediators, mostly histamine, to which the body is exposed during this insult.[34,35] Because of the decrease in preload and afterload, cardiac output falls.

Treatment

The treatment of anaphylactic shock can be divided into two major phases. First, attention is directed to vital functions. Airway compromise may be present and takes priority over other interventions. Once the airway is secure, attention to the adequacy of breathing can be performed. There is often bronchospasm with concomitant wheezing. The provision of oxygen to ensure adequate oxygenation needs to occur. Efforts to ensure ventilatory competence should also be performed, but the wheezing often abates with the administration of epinephrine for circulatory support. Circulatory dysfunction and shock are the next most pressing issues. For circulatory collapse, large volume infusions, as in other types of shock, help to restore the circulating blood volume. Circulatory support with repeated doses of epinephrine and ultimately an epinephrine infusion help support the patient until the directed therapy can begin.[34,35]

Once the vital functions have been addressed, attention should turn to combating the antigen exposure. If the antigen and route are known, for instance if a blood transfusion is being administered, limitation of the antigen exposure becomes the next priority. Antihistamines should be given to counter the effect of the mediators that were inciting the pathologic response. Corticosteroids may have a role in anaphylaxis based on the analogy to other similar allergic conditions.[34] They improve the inflammatory response associated with these conditions.

SUMMARY

The child with shock experiences a tremendous insult that begins at the cellular level and extends up to the level of the more organized systems of the body. An understanding of the physiology is essential to differentiate from among the different causes of shock and to formulate an approach for its treatment. The oxygen content determines the amount of oxygen and nutrients contained within the blood. The oxygen delivery takes into account how the cardiac output brings those nutrients to the most remote locations of the body. The extraction of oxygen by an organ may represent one measure of the organ's viability.

Shock can be classified based on where the cardiac output is affected. In this way, a targeted therapeutic approach can take place. The problem may be related to a disorder in heart rate or one of the contributors of the stroke volume. If the problem is inadequate preload, additional fluid can be supplied. If the problem is inotropy, agents that enhance the contractile function of the failing heart can be administered. Finally, if the problem is with afterload, agents that increase the vascular tone can be given.

Assessment of the child with shock begins with an appraisal of the ABCs of resuscitation but then moves through to an assessment of individual organs and organ systems. Intensive care unit practitioners have the ability to measure and respond to physiologic changes on a continuous and ongoing basis. This ultimately enhances the outcome of the child with shock regardless of the cause.

REFERENCES

1. Tobin JR, Wetzel RC: Shock and multi-organ system failure. In Rogers MC, Nichols DG, editors: *Textbook of pediatric intensive care,* ed 3. Baltimore. Williams & Wilkins, 1996.
2. Flowers F, Zimmerman JJ: Reactive oxygen species in the cellular pathophysiology of shock. *New Horiz* 1998; 6: 169-180.
3. Thomas NJ, Carcillo JA: Hypovolemic shock in pediatric patients. *New Horiz* 1998; 6:120-129.
4. Murphy K et al: Molecular biology of septic shock. *New Horiz* 1998; 6:181-193.
5. Hollenberg SM, Cunnion RE, Parrillo JE: Effect of septic serum on vascular smooth muscle: *In vitro* studies using rat aortic rings. *Crit Care Med* 1992; 20:993-998.
6. Quezado ZMN, Natanson C: Systemic hemodynamic abnormalities and vasopressor therapy in sepsis and septic shock. *Am J Kidney Dis* 1992; 20:214-222.
7. Suffredini AF et al: Pulmonary and oxygen transport effects of intravenously administered endotoxin in normal humans. *Am Rev Respir Dis* 1992; 145:1398-1403.
8. Ross J, Covell JW: Frameworks for analysis of ventricular and circulatory function: Integrated responses. In West JB, editor: *Best and Taylor's physiological basis of medical practice,* ed 12. Baltimore. Williams & Wilkins, 1990.
9. Pollack MM, Fields AI, Ruttimann UE: Sequential cardiopulmonary variables in infants and children in septic shock. *Crit Care Med* 1984; 12:554-559.
10. Pollack MM, Fields AI, Ruttimann UE: Distributions of cardiopulmonary variables in pediatric survivors and nonsurvivors of septic shock. *Crit Care Med* 1985; 13: 454-459.
11. Hazinski MF: Shock in the pediatric patient. *Crit Care Nurs Clin North Am* 1990; 2:309-324.
12. Ross J, section editor: The cardiac pump. In West JB, editors: *Best and Taylor's physiological basis of medical practice,* ed 12. Baltimore. Williams & Wilkins, 1990.
13. Levy FH, O'Rourke PP: Topics in pediatric critical care. In Czervinske M, Barnhart S, editors: *Perinatal and pediatric respiratory care.* Philadelphia. WB Saunders 1995.
14. West JB, section editor: Gas transport to the periphery. In West JB, editor: *Best and Taylor's physiological basis of medical practice,* ed 12. Baltimore. Williams & Wilkins, 1990.
15. Lucking SE et al: Dependence of oxygen consumption on oxygen delivery in children with hyperdynamic septic shock and low oxygen extraction. *Crit Care Med* 1990; 18:1316-1319.
16. Steinhorn DM, Green TP: Severity of illness correlates with alterations in energy metabolism in the pediatric intensive care unit. *Crit Care Med* 1991; 19:1503-1509.
17. Seear M, Wensley D, MacNab A: Oxygen consumption–oxygen delivery relationship in children. *J Pediatr* 1993; 123:208-214.
18. Hayes MA et al: Elevation of systemic oxygen delivery in the treatment of critically ill patients. *N Engl J Med* 1994; 330:1717-1722.
19. Ross J, section editor: Intracardiac and arterial pressures and the cardiac output: cardiac catheterization. In West JB, editor: *Best and Taylor's physiological basis of medical practice,* ed 12. Baltimore. Williams & Wilkins, 1990.
20. Carcillo JA, Cunnion RE: Septic shock. *Crit Care Clin* 1997; 13:553-573.
21. Proulx F et al: Epidemiology of sepsis and multiple organ dysfunction syndrome in children. *Chest* 1996; 4:1033-1037.
22. Morgan WM, O'Neill JA: Hemorrhagic and obstructive shock in pediatric patients. *New Horiz* 1998; 6:150-154.
23. Bengur AR, Meliones JN: Cardiogenic shock. *New Horiz* 1998; 6:139-149.
24. Feltes TF, Pignatelli R, Kleinert S: Quantitated left ventricular systolic mechanics in children with septic shock utilizing noninvasive wall stress analysis. *Crit Care Med* 1994; 22:1647-1658.
25. Carcillo JA et al: Sequential physiologic interactions in pediatric cardiogenic and septic shock. *Crit Care Med* 1989; 17:12-16.
26. Parker MM: Pathophysiology of cardiovascular dysfunction in septic shock. *New Horiz* 1998; 6:130-138.
27. Parker MM et al: Profound but reversible myocardial depression in patients with septic shock. *Ann Intern Med* 1984; 100:483-490.
28. Chameides L, Hazinski MF, editors: *Pediatric advance life support.* Dallas. American Heart Association and American Academy of Pediatrics, 1997.
29. Mercier JC et al: Hemodynamic patterns of meningococcal shock in children. *Crit Care Med* 1988; 16:27-33.
30. Parker MM et al: Serial cardiovascular variables in survivors and nonsurvivors of human septic shock: Heart rate as an early predictor of prognosis. *Crit Care Med* 1987; 15:923-929.
31. Dibs SD, Baker MD: Anaphylaxis in children: a 5-year experience. *Pediatrics* 1997;99:E7.
32. Ditto AM et al: Idiopathic anaphylaxis: a series of 335 cases. *Ann Allergy Asthma Immunol* 1996; 4:285-291.
33. Novembre E et al: Anaphylaxis in children: Clinical and allergologic features. *Pediatrics* 1998; 101:E8.
34. Lieberman P: Anaphylaxis and anaphylactoid reactions. In Middleton E et al, editors: *Allergy principles and practice,* ed 5., vol II. St Louis. Mosby, 1998; pp 1079-1092.
35. Lieberman P: Specific and idiopathic anaphylaxis: Pathophysiology and treatment. In Bierman CW et al, editors: *Allergy, asthma, and immunology from infancy to adulthood,* ed 3. Philadelphia. WB Saunders, 1996; pp 297-319.
36. Zaritsky AL: Recent advances in pediatric cardiopulmonary resuscitation and advanced life support. *New Horiz* 1998; 6:201-211.
37. Ushay HM, Nottermann DA: Pharmacology of pediatric resuscitation. *Pediatr Clin North Am* 1997; 1:207-233.

38. Behrman RE, Kliegman RM, Arvin AM, editors: *Nelson's textbook of pediatrics,* ed 15. Philadelphia. WB Saunders, 1996.

39. Tibby SM, Hatherill M, Murdoch IA: Capillary refill and core-peripheral temperature gap as indicators of haemodynamic status in paediatric intensive care patients. *Arch Dis Child* 1999; 80:163-166.

40. Pollock MM, Ring JC, Fields AI: Shock in infants and children. *Emerg Med Clin North Am* 1986; 4:841-857.

41. Mink RB, Pollack MM: Effect of blood transfusion on oxygen consumption in pediatric septic shock. *Crit Care Med* 1990; 18:1087-1091.

42. Carcillo JA, Davis AL, Zaritsky A: Role of early fluid resuscitation in pediatric septic shock. *JAMA* 1991; 266: 1242-1245.

43. Kallen RJ, Lonergan JM: Fluid resuscitation of acute hypovolemic hypoperfusion states in pediatrics. *Pediatr Clin North Am* 1990; 37:287-294.

44. Corneli HM: Evaluation, treatment, and transport of pediatric patients with shock. *Pediatr Clin North Am* 1993; 40: 303-319.

45. Ceneviva G et al: Hemodynamic support in fluid refractory pediatric septic shock. *Pediatrics* 1998; 102:E19.

46. Ross J, Schmid-Schoenbein G: Dynamics of the peripheral circulation. In West JB, editor: *Best and Taylor's physiological basis of medical practice,* ed 12. Baltimore. Williams & Wilkins, 1991.

47. Curley MAQ, Castillo L: Nutrition and shock in pediatric patients. *New Horiz* 1998; 6:212-225.

48. Schears GJ, Deutschman CS: Common nutritional issues in pediatric and adult critical care medicine. *Crit Care Clin* 1997; 3:669-689.

CHAPTER 38

Sepsis and Meningitis

Robert L. Hopkins

Sepsis and bacterial meningitis are two situations that the pediatric respiratory care practitioner frequently encounters. Early recognition and aggressive monitoring and support can lead to better outcomes in these potentially devastating clinical scenarios.

SEPSIS

Sepsis was once recognized as severe illness associated with bacteremia. However, as the full spectrum of sepsis was recognized, new nomenclature was needed for clearer clinical descriptions.

Earlier definitions of *sepsis* included the pathophysiologic changes that accompanied the presence of gram-negative or gram-positive organisms in the blood. It is now recognized that many of these changes can occur in the presence of tissue injury and in the absence of active infection. These changes are known as the systemic inflammatory response syndrome.

A recent conference further defined the terms for these changes,[1] and Jafari and McCracken refined them for pediatric patients (Box 38-1).[2]

EPIDEMIOLOGY

There are two peaks in the incidence of pediatric sepsis, one in the neonatal period and another at the age of 2 years. Neonatal sepsis also can be divided into early onset ($<$3 days after delivery) or late onset ($>$3 days after delivery). Early-onset sepsis is associated with several factors, including lack of perinatal care, maternal fever, chorioamnionitis, prolonged rupture of membranes, and maternal colonization with group B *Streptococcus* (GBS).[3]

Organisms that are associated with disease in the early-onset neonatal sepsis period include GBS, *Enterococcus,* and *Escherichia coli.* Later onset of infection is associated with extended hospitalization, invasive devices, and colonization with hospital-acquired organisms. Fungal organisms, gram-negative bacteria, and viruses can all cause late-onset disease, but coagulase-negative

---

BOX 38-1

DEFINITION OF SEPSIS AND SEPSIS SYNDROME IN PEDIATRIC PATIENTS

Bacteremia: Culture-confirmed presence of live bacteria in blood

Sepsis: Evidence of infection with temperature changes, increased heart rate, increased respiratory rate, and leukocytosis or leukopenia

Sepsis syndrome: Sepsis plus at least one of the following: acute mental changes, decreased PaO_2, increased plasma lactate, or decreased urine output

Septic shock: Sepsis syndrome plus hypotension that responds to fluid therapy and/or drug therapy

Refractory septic shock: Sepsis syndrome plus hypotension for more than 1 hour that is not responsive to fluid and/or drug therapy and necessitates use of vasopressors

Multiple organ system failure: Any combination of disseminated intravascular coagulation, acute respiratory distress syndrome, renal failure, and hepatobiliary dysfunction

Modified from Jafari HS, McCracken GH Jr: Sepsis and septic shock: a review for clinicians. *Pediatr Infect Dis J* 1992; 11:739.

Staphylococcus is the most common offending organism.

Causes of sepsis in older infants and children have changed since the introduction of the vaccine for *Haemophilus influenzae* infection and with the emergence of large numbers of children with chronic diseases. *H. influenzae* type b used to be a leading cause of sepsis, meningitis, and epiglottitis. Since the advent of the vaccine, however, epiglottitis has almost disappeared and meningitis due to *H. influenzae* is almost unknown. *S. pneumoniae* and *Neisseria meningitidis* have become the leading causes of sepsis and meningitis in older infants and children.

Toxic shock syndrome, pneumonia with empyema, septic shock, and necrotizing fasciitis are all manifestations of infection by group A β-hemolytic *Streptococcus*. This bacteria, which has been associated with impetigo and pharyngitis, has emerged as an aggressive and invasive pathogen in infants and children. Rapid onset of septic shock, multisystem organ dysfunction, deep soft tissue necrosis, and a generalized erythematous macular rash should alert the physician to the possibility of severe group A β-hemolytic streptococcal infection.

Children with indwelling devices such as vascular catheters or peritoneal dialysis catheters, transplant recipients, and pediatric oncology patients form a

---

BOX 38-2

RISK FACTORS FOR PEDIATRIC SEPSIS

Immunodeficiency
Transplantation
Cancer
Vascular catheters
Peritoneal dialysis catheters
Ventriculoperitoneal catheters

---

newer group of children who are prone to develop sepsis from coagulase-negative *Staphylococcus,* fungi, and gram-negative bacteria (Box 38-2).

PATHOPHYSIOLOGY

The systemic response to infection is complex. It is mediated by proinflammatory and antiinflammatory substances, including cytokines, which are macrophage-derived peptides. Tumor necrosis factor, interleukin-1, and interleukin-8 are proinflammatory.[2] A toxic stimulus such as that from bacteria will trigger a release of cytokines from macrophages. Tumor necrosis factor and interleukin-1 enhance adhesion of leukocytes to endothelial cells with subsequent release of proteases.[4] Both of these substances also stimulate the release of other mediators, including thromboxane, leukotrienes, prostaglandins, and clotting factors.[5]

Modulation of this inflammatory cascade is accomplished through release of antiinflammatory substances. These include interleukin-10, interleukin-4, corticosteroids, catecholamines, and prostaglandin E. This cascade of proinflammatory and antiinflammatory substances has clinically significant expression in organ dysfunction.

Nitric oxide may also be an important mediator of the vasodilation in septic shock.[6] Inflammatory mediators stimulate inducible nitric oxide synthetase. This results in release of nitric oxide from endothelial cells and macrophages. Hypotension, myocardial depression, and increased vascular permeability all ensue.[6,7]

ORGAN SYSTEM DYSFUNCTION AND TREATMENT

Cytokine release and the resulting inflammatory cascade cause vasodilation, increased vascular permeability, edema, ischemia, and eventual capillary occlusion. These microvascular changes lead to dysfunction in multiple organ systems. The number of systems involved and the severity of involvement determine outcome.

Pulmonary. Pulmonary dysfunction is present in all cases of sepsis. Respiratory system compliance is decreased, and airway resistance is increased.

These changes are reflected by hypoxemia and tachypnea. Early intubation and mechanical ventilation will relieve the increased work of breathing and facilitate improved oxygen delivery. Pulmonary edema is commonly seen on a chest roentgenogram, and the clinician must differentiate among respiratory distress syndrome, pneumonia, and cardiac dysfunction.

Mechanical ventilatory strategies in sepsis are not well defined. Current goals are directed toward lower tidal volumes, permissive hypercapnia, and using positive end-expiratory pressure to stabilize small airways and alveoli. This is known as a lung-protection strategy.[8] Studies have not yet validated its use in pediatric patients.

Cardiac System. There are significant negative changes in ventricular contractility associated with sepsis. This decrease in myocardial function coupled with vasodilation and increased vascular permeability leads to the picture of septic shock resulting in inadequate delivery of nutrients (including oxygen) to peripheral tissues. Pediatric shock can occur without hypotension. Decreased mentation, diminished urine output, tachycardia, increased capillary refill time, and diminished peripheral pulses are all signs of shock in the pediatric patient. Decompensated shock includes all these findings plus systemic hypotension.

Renal Dysfunction. Decreased urine output and transient increases in creatinine can occur with sepsis. Volume resuscitation and vasoactive agents can help restore renal perfusion and function. Dialysis is rarely needed; however, renal replacement therapy such as continuous venovenous hemofiltration can assist with fluid balance during the initial resuscitation phase when large volume needs may be coupled with decreased renal function.[9]

Gastrointestinal Dysfunction. Decreased blood flow to the liver and splanchnic bed is common in septic shock. Transiently increased liver enzyme and bilirubin levels are common, but both usually decrease over several days as the patient's condition stabilizes.[10] Hepatic failure is rare. Ileus is often associated with inflammation,[11] and it will usually persist for about 48 hours after the patient is successfully resuscitated. Factors that can extend this period of ileus include narcotics, sedatives, and a delay in enteral feeding.

Differential Diagnosis

The signs and symptoms that alert the clinician to the possibility of sepsis are not specific and may reflect serious diagnoses that need therapy quite dis-

---

BOX 38-3
DIFFERENTIAL DIAGNOSIS OF THE SEPTIC CHILD
Congenital heart disease
Congestive heart failure
Toxic ingestion
Child abuse
Severe anemia
Cerebrospinal fluid shunt dysfunction
Congenital adrenal hyperplasia
Inborn errors of metabolism
Cardiac arrhythmias
Myocardial infarction
Hypoglycemia
Electrolyte disturbances

tinctive from sepsis. These problems are extremely varied, and the clinician needs to keep them in mind, especially if the clinical course is worsening (Box 38-3).

Treatment

Treatment of children with sepsis is multifaceted. The key aspects of this therapy include (1) administration of oxygen, (2) restoration of intravascular volume and replacement of ongoing losses, (3) use of vasoactive drugs to achieve adequate cardiac output and oxygen delivery, (4) administration of antimicrobial agents, and (5) removal of necrotic or purulent material.

Cardiopulmonary Stability. The several goals that must be achieved to restore stability of the cardiopulmonary subsystem include (1) restoration of intravascular volume, (2) decrease in oxygen consumption, and (3) improvement in oxygen delivery. Restoration of intravascular volume is accomplished by aggressive administration of fluid. Initial fluids should be isotonic, and two acceptable choices are normal saline or lactated Ringer's solution. The child who is strongly suspected as having septic shock should initially receive at least 40 ml/kg of isotonic fluids, and further therapy should be directed by changes in heart rate, blood pressure, mentation, perfusion, and quality of peripheral pulses.[12]

Administered fluid volumes during resuscitation may be quite large, owing to the vasodilation and capillary leak associated with sepsis. To monitor fluid therapy, clinical assessment is crucial and intravascular pressure monitoring may be necessary. There is continuing controversy, which is beyond the scope of this discussion, about whether resuscitation fluids should be crystalloids or colloids.[13]

Vasoactive agents may be necessary to achieve adequate cardiac output and acceptable systemic blood pressures. Use of these agents should not replace adequate volume replacement. Dopamine is the usual choice for initial therapy. This drug increases heart rate and contractility at intermediate doses (beta effects) and increases systemic vascular resistance at higher doses (alpha effects). Lower doses may increase renal blood flow (dopaminergic effects).

Other drugs that may help in achieving acceptable perfusion and blood pressure include epinephrine, norepinephrine, and dobutamine. Milrinone, a phosphodiesterase inhibitor, has shown promise in the treatment of pediatric septic shock.[14]

Oxygen consumption can be decreased by treating seizures, controlling body temperature, decreasing pain, and judiciously using sedation. Increased oxygen delivery is accomplished by increasing the cardiac output, administering oxygen, and transfusing packed red blood cells.

The prompt administration of antibiotics is important and must be accomplished early in the resuscitation and stabilization of the septic child. The choice of antibiotics depends on several factors. The age of the patient is the most important factor, followed closely in importance by the patient's immune status and whether the infection is community acquired or nosocomial. Microbial sensitivities in the community and hospital will affect the final choice of antibiotics.

Special Considerations. Table 38-1 outlines initial antibiotic choices based on age. These choices are appropriate for early neonatal infections and community-acquired infections in the older infant and child. Vancomycin should be added to the usual antibiotic regimen used in cases of presumed severe pneumococcal infection, especially meningitis. Pneumococci are becoming increasingly resistant to third-generation cephalosporins and penicillin.

Immunocompromised children suspected of having sepsis should be carefully evaluated by physical examination and by obtaining the appropriate cultures because the usual signs of sepsis such as fever may be altered or absent. Initial antibiotic coverage should include vancomycin and gentamicin or a third-generation cephalosporin.

The drainage of abscesses, excision of necrotic tissues, and removal of large collections of infected fluid such as empyemas are essential for the recovery of septic patients.

The clinician must always be prepared for the transient worsening of a septic patient's condition after antibiotics have been administered. Killing the bacteria releases multiple bacterial components, including cell wall components and toxins. These materials will potentiate the inflammatory reaction and possibly lead to a deterioration in the patient's cardiopulmonary status.[2]

OUTCOME

There has been significant improvement in the outcome of sepsis in children. Survival in neonates is about 75%, but 25% of these survivors have neurologic sequelae and chronic lung disease. Older children have an overall survival of about 60% with less morbidity than neonates.[15-17] Improved survival depends on early diagnosis and well-organized care. Further understanding of the inflammatory response should allow therapeutic manipulation of the response and lead to better survival.

MENINGITIS

Meningitis is the result of invasion and infection of the subarachnoid space and inflammation of the meninges. It is one of the most serious pediatric infections, with a course that can range from complete recovery to serious sequelae or even death.

PATHOPHYSIOLOGY

Bacteria gain access to the meninges usually from the bloodstream. The nasal mucosa of normal children can be colonized by the same pathogens that cause meningitis. Passage from the nasal mucosa to the bloodstream is not clearly understood, but viral respiratory infections may facilitate this event.

A large bacterial inoculum is necessary for the seeding of the central nervous system to lead to meningitis (probably more than 1000 colony-forming units/ml of blood). Bacterial products then elicit an inflammatory process that leads to the production of

TABLE 38-1	INITIAL ANTIBIOTIC REGIMENS FOR SEPSIS	
Age	**Organisms**	**Antibiotics**
Neonatal	Escherichia coli Group B Streptococcus Listeria monocytogenes	Ampicillin and gentamicin or ampicillin and cefotaxime
1-3 months	Group B Streptococcus Neisseria meningitidis Haemophilus influenzae type B	Ampicillin and cefotaxime or ampicillin and ceftriaxone
3 months or older	S. pneumoniae N. meningitidis H. influenzae type B	Cefotaxime or ceftriaxone (Note: add vancomycin for suspected pneumococcus)

tumor necrosis factor and interleukin-1 by macrophages in the central nervous system.[18] These proinflammatory substances provoke production of prostaglandin E_2, which is a stimulus for chemotaxis and leads to a marked increase in neutrophils in the cerebrospinal fluid (CSF) and arachnoid villi.[19]

Bacterial products and the inflammatory process result in endothelial cell damage, which causes (1) disruption of the blood-brain barrier, (2) vasodilation, (3) increased capillary permeability, and (4) cerebral edema with increased intracranial pressure.

ETIOLOGY

Neonatal to 3 Months. Bacterial pathogens that cause meningitis in childhood include both gram-negative and gram-positive organisms. The age of the affected child will help to predict the most likely causative organism.

There are three organisms that commonly cause meningitis in the neonatal through 3-month age group. The most common causative agent is GBS. There is both an early- and a late-onset pattern to illness caused by this organism. Early-onset illness is associated with prematurity and maternal obstetric complications. Maternal prophylaxis for intrapartum GBS has led to a significant decline in the early-onset pattern of GBS sepsis and meningitis. Late-onset GBS sepsis and meningitis occur from 7 days to 3 months of age.

E. coli (K1 serotype) is the next most common cause of meningitis in this age group. Illnesses that are associated with *E. coli* meningitis include galactosemia and urosepsis that resulted in association with malformations of the urinary tract.

In newborns between 10 and 30 days of age, *Listeria monocytogenes* is another cause of meningitis. Resistance to cephalosporin and the possibility of this gram-positive bacillus being dismissed as a contaminant make it imperative for the clinician to think of this unusual organism.

Age 3 Months and Older. In the range of 3 months to 5 years of age, *N. meningitidis* and *S. pneumoniae* are the most common causes of bacterial meningitis. *H. influenzae* used to be the most common cause, but the use of a protein-conjugated vaccine has almost eliminated this organism as a cause of life-threatening disease in children. For school-age children the most common pathogens causing bacterial meningitis in this group are *N. meningitidis* and *S. pneumoniae.*

CLINICAL PRESENTATION

Infants with meningitis often present with less specific signs and symptoms than older children. Upper respiratory tract infection is often a preceding event. Temperature variation, lethargy, vomiting, poor feeding, and a bulging anterior fontanelle are all possible presenting signs. Meningeal signs are not common in this age group.

The older child will present with the more classic signs of bacterial meningitis. These include altered level of consciousness, stiff neck, fever, vomiting, headache, photophobia, and seizures.

In each age range the signs of sepsis and septic shock may be seen. These include poor perfusion, fever, hypotension, decreased urine output, and ileus. Distant infection including septic arthritis, empyema, and purulent pericarditis may also complicate the early presentation of meningitis.

Advanced meningitis will be accompanied by signs of markedly increased intracranial pressure: (1) coma, (2) Cheyne-Stokes breathing, and (3) cranial nerve dysfunction. Focal neurologic findings are indicators of advanced disease and are harbingers of rapid deterioration.

DIAGNOSIS

The first step to diagnosis is suspicion of bacterial meningitis by the clinician. A careful history and close observation of the infant or child can be invaluable. The febrile lethargic infant with a bulging fontanelle describes the typical pediatric patient with probable meningitis. More subtle signs such as poor feeding, vomiting, poor perfusion, loss of interest in surroundings, and lack of response to stimuli should also alert the clinician to the possibility of meningitis.

The actual diagnosis of bacterial meningitis does not vary among age groups. The first step should be lumbar puncture with examination of CSF by the following studies: (1) protein and glucose determination, (2) blood cell count and differential, (3) Gram's stain, and (4) culture and antibiotic sensitivity. Additional studies should include complete blood cell count with differential and urine and blood cultures.

Prior administration of antibiotics may sterilize the CSF. Latex agglutination testing to detect bacteria-specific antigens may be helpful in this circumstance, but it does not take the place of a Gram's stain of the CSF or of culture and sensitivity testing of organisms.

Lumbar puncture is a procedure with few complications; however, there are circumstances that can have catastrophic results. The patient with cardiopulmonary instability should not undergo lumbar puncture until stability is achieved. Positioning of the patient for lumbar puncture could lead to cardiopulmonary collapse in the unstable patient. Stabilization of the airway, fluid resuscitation, and antibiotic administration should precede lumbar puncture in this circumstance.

The patient with focal neurologic signs or posturing should undergo cranial computed tomography to rule out a mass lesion.[20] Lumbar puncture in this circumstance could lead to cerebral herniation. Delaying the lumbar puncture and beginning antibiotics and supportive care may be indicated.

TREATMENT

Treatment of meningitis is divided into general care, antiinflammatory measures, antibiotic therapy, and prophylaxis.

General care consists of supportive measures that are common to the support of any critically ill child. The airway must be maintained either with suctioning and positioning or with endotracheal intubation. Oxygen administration and pulse oximetry should be employed during initial stabilization of all patients. Vascular access is essential for both fluid administration and delivery of medications. This can be challenging in the acutely ill child, and early use of intraosseous access may be necessary. Intravascular volume should be restored with isotonic fluids, and hypoglycemia should be treated. Younger children should have measures to protect their core temperature. These measures can include blankets, increasing treatment room temperature, and careful use of overhead warmers. Control of fever and seizures helps decrease metabolic needs.

A major change in meningitis therapy is the use of dexamethasone. Ideally, dexamethasone is given before antibiotic therapy to decrease the inflammation that occurs with the release of bacterial products after antibiotic therapy. This inflammation can lead to an increased intracranial pressure with decreased cerebral blood flow. Direct neuronal damage also occurs from fluid accumulation, owing to endothelial damage and toxic substances released by activated neutrophils.

Children with meningitis who received dexamethasone before antibiotic therapy had a decreased incidence of ataxia, deafness, seizure disorder, and focal central nervous system deficits. These benefits have been observed mainly in children with *H. influenzae* type B meningitis.[21] Many clinicians recommend dexamethasone for use with pneumococcal and meningococcal meningitis because the inflammatory events are similar in bacterial meningitis caused by these organisms.[22]

Dexamethasone therapy in meningitis should be considered for all infants and children 6 weeks and older. The recommended dosage regimen is 0.6 mg/kg/day in four divided doses given intravenously for the first 2 days of antibiotic therapy. The first dose should be given before institution of

antibiotic therapy or very shortly thereafter. A complete summary of dexamethasone usage is available elsewhere.[22]

Specific antibiotic therapy is determined by the age of the patient, Gram-stained smears of CSF, and CSF culture results. The most common organisms that cause meningitis in the neonate are *E. coli,* group B *Streptococcus,* and *L. monocytogenes.* A regimen of ampicillin plus cefotaxime *or* ampicillin plus an aminoglycoside is acceptable before identification of the causative organism. Selection of antibiotics should *not* be guided only by the result of Gram's staining because these results can vary. Penicillins and cephalosporins should eradicate group B *Streptococcus,* and a cephalosporin (cefotaxime) or an aminoglycoside should have excellent activity against gram-negative organisms causing neonatal meningitis. Ampicillin is the recommended antibiotic for meningitis caused by *L. monocytogenes.* Duration of therapy is 21 days for diseases caused by gram-negative bacteria and 14 to 21 days for meningitis caused by group B *Streptococcus* or *L. monocytogenes.*

The routine use of ampicillin in the neonate for presumed *L. monocytogenes* meningitis has been questioned.[23] The rarity of this infection may not justify routine use of ampicillin in presumed neonatal sepsis without evidence of central nervous system infection.

Treatment of meningitis in the age group 3 months to 5 years should include cefotaxime or ceftriaxone and high doses of vancomycin. There is the possibility of meningitis being caused by pneumococcus that is resistant to both penicillin and third-generation cephalosporins. Choice of antibiotics should not be guided by the Gram-stained appearance of organisms in the CSF.

Early management of antibiotic therapy in the older school-age child and adolescent is identical to that in infants and young children. Associated severe sinusitis should prompt the clinician to add anaerobic coverage and to look for brain abscess or subdural empyema.[24]

Both *H. influenzae* and *N. meningitidis* are highly transmissible, and prophylaxis of close contacts should occur. Rifampin is effective prophylaxis for serious *H. influenzae* disease. Ceftriaxone and rifampin are suitable prophylaxis for invasive meningococcal disease.

COMPLICATIONS

Recognizing the acute complications in the course of bacterial meningitis is essential to avoid serious sequelae and even death (Box 38-4). Pericardial effusion, septic arthritis, pleural empyema, and pneumonia are complications associated with meningitis.

BOX 38-4
COMPLICATIONS OF BACTERIAL MENINGITIS
Septic arthritis Pericardial effusion Pneumonia/empyema Subdural effusion Syndrome of inappropriate secretion of antidiuretic hormone Cerebral edema Subdural empyema Brain abscess

TABLE 38-2	SURVIVORS OF *H. INFLUENZAE* MENINGITIS
Sequelae	Occurrence (%)
Mental retardation	10
Deafness	10
Seizures	8
Impaired vision	3

The clinician must look for these entities to avoid serious additional morbidity or mortality. Poor perfusion and unresponsive shock are hints that a pericardial effusion may be present. Pain on movement or usual positioning of an extremity indicates possible septic arthritis. Pleural effusion and pneumonia will cause persistent fever and increased work of breathing.

Cerebral edema is found in some cases of bacterial meningitis.[25] Severe cerebral edema is associated with increasing coma, fixed eye deviation, bradycardia, hypertension, and respiratory pattern irregularities. Osmotic diuresis with mannitol and tracheal intubation with hyperventilation may acutely decrease the increased intracranial pressure associated with these findings.

Subdural empyema is associated with coma, increased intracranial pressure, recurrent seizures, and decorticate posturing. Diagnosis is confirmed by cranial computed tomography or magnetic resonance imaging. This complication must be carefully excluded in the patient with a history of sinusitis or findings that indicate infection of the sinuses. Surgical evacuation of the empyema is indicated.

The syndrome of inappropriate secretion of antidiuretic hormone (SIADH) is seen in a significant number of patients with bacterial meningitis. The hallmarks are hyponatremia, hyposmolarity, normovolemia, elevated urinary sodium, and no renal disease. Treatment is restriction of fluids to about two-thirds maintenance.

Brain abscess is usually seen as a complication of severe meningitis. It can cause focal neurologic findings and coma. Surgical drainage is the treatment of choice.

Subdural effusion is a common finding in meningitis and requires no treatment. It can be demonstrated by cranial computed tomography. Differentiation from subdural empyema in the severely ill patient may require subdural puncture.

Ventriculitis is a devastating complication that occurs in the neonate or young infant.[26] Necrotic debris blocks the cerebral aqueduct, and infection worsens in the now-isolated lateral ventricles. The clinical picture is an infant recovering from meningitis whose condition worsens with onset of fever, apnea, and bradycardia. Cranial computed tomography will demonstrate enhancement of the ependyma, and ventricular tap will confirm the diagnosis. Prolonged antibiotic therapy and placement of a ventriculostomy may be necessary.

OUTCOME

The outcome of meningitis depends on meticulous attention to detail during diagnosis and therapy. Early diagnosis is important but does not guarantee a good outcome. Long-term sequelae are related to neurologic insults. Most studies of sequelae have been based on survivors of *H. influenzae* meningitis. The findings of young age, seizures, focal neurologic signs, and initial low cerebrospinal glucose concentrations have been predictive of complications and long-term sequelae. These long-term sequelae include hearing deficits, seizures, mental retardation, and impaired vision (Table 38-2).[27] Improved outcomes depend on prompt diagnosis, improved supportive care, new methods to manipulate the inflammatory response, and prevention through vaccines.

SUMMARY

Despite advances in critical care that include improved supportive measures, recognition of the mechanisms of sepsis, and improved antibiotic therapy, the real answer to this terrible disease is vaccination and prophylaxis. The near disappearance of meningitis caused by *H. influenzae* and the ability to administer prophylaxis to close contacts of children with this form of meningitis or with meningococcal meningitis represent important advances in the treatment of this disease.

REFERENCES

1. Rangel-Frausto MS et al: The natural history of the systemic inflammatory response syndrome (SIRS): a prospective study. *JAMA* 1995; 273:117.
2. Jafari HS, McCracken GH Jr: Sepsis and septic shock: a review for clinicians. *Pediatr Infect Dis J* 1992; 11:739.

3. Stoll BJ et al: Early-onset sepsis in very low birth weight neonates: a report from the National Institute of Child Health and Human Development Neonatal Research Network. *J Pediatr* 1996; 129:72.

4. Strieter RM, Kunkel SL: Acute lung injury: the role of cytokines in the elicitation of neutrophils. *J Invest Med* 1994; 42:640.

5. Wheeler AP, Hardie WD, Bernard GR: The role of cyclooxygenase products in lung injury induced by tumor necrosis factor in sheep. *Am Rev Respir Dis* 1992; 145:632.

6. Cobb JP, Danner RL: Nitric oxide and septic shock. *JAMA* 1996; 275:1192.

7. Lorente JA et al: L-Arginine pathway in the sepsis syndrome. *Crit Care Med* 1993; 21:1287.

8. Amato MB et al: Beneficial effects of the "open lung approach" with low distending pressures in acute respiratory distress syndrome: a prospective randomized study on mechanical ventilation. *Am J Respir Crit Care Med* 1995; 152:1835.

9. Zobel G et al: Five years experience with continuous extracorporeal renal support in paediatric intensive care. *Intensive Care Med* 1991; 17:315.

10. Garland JS, Werlin SL, Rice TB: Ischemic hepatitis in children: diagnosis and clinical course. *Crit Care Med* 1988; 16:1209.

11. Frantzides CT et al: Small bowel myoelectric activity in peritonitis. *Am J Surg* 1993; 165:681.

12. Carcillo JA, Davis AL, Zaritsky A: Role of early fluid resuscitation in pediatric septic shock. *JAMA* 1991; 266: 1242.

13. DeBruin WJ, Greenwald BM, Notterman DA: Fluid resuscitation in pediatrics. *Crit Care Clin North Am* 1992; 8:423.

14. Barton P et al: Hemodynamic effects of i.v. milrinone lactate in pediatric patients with septic shock: a prospective, double-blinded, randomized, placebo-controlled, interventional study. *Chest* 1996; 109:1302.

15. Martinot A et al: Sepsis in neonates and children: definitions, epidemiology, and outcome. *Pediatr Emerg Care* 1997; 13:277.

16. Msall ME et al: Multivariate risks among extremely premature infants. *J Perinatol* 1994; 14:41.

17. Rojas MA et al: Changing trends in the epidemiology and pathogenesis of neonatal chronic lung disease. *J Pediatr* 1995; 126:605.

18. Saez-Llorens X et al: Molecular pathophysiology of bacterial meningitis: current concepts and therapeutic implications. *J Pediatr* 1990; 116:671.

19. Mustafa MM et al: Cerebrospinal fluid prostaglandins, interleukin 1B, and tumor necrosis factor in bacterial meningitis: clinical and laboratory correlations in placebo and dexamethasone-treated patients. *Am J Dis Child* 1990; 144:883.

20. Rennick G, Shann F, Campo J: Cerebral herniation during bacterial meningitis in children. *BMJ* 1993; 306:953.

21. Odio CM et al: The beneficial effects of early dexamethasone administration in infants and children with bacterial meningitis. *N Engl J Med* 1991; 324:1525.

22. Saez-Llorens, McCracken GH Jr: Antimicrobial and anti-inflammatory treatment of bacterial meningitis. *Infect Dis Clin North Am* 1999; 13:619.

23. Sadow K, Derr R, Teach SJ: Bacterial infections in infants 60 days and younger: epidemiology, resistance, and implications for treatment. *Arch Pediatr Adolesc Med* 1999; 153:611.

24. Gallagher RM, Gross CW, Phillips CD: Suppurative intracranial complications of sinusitis. *Laryngoscope* 1998; 108:1635.

25. Kline MW, Kaplan SL: Computed tomography in bacterial meningitis of childhood. *Pediatr Infect Dis J* 1988; 7:855.

26. Chang YC et al: Risk factor of complications requiring neurosurgical intervention in infants with bacterial meningitis. *Pediatr Neurol* 1997; 17:144.

27. Arditi M et al: Three-year multicenter surveillance of pneumococcal meningitis in children: Clinical characteristics and outcome related to penicillin susceptibility and dexamethasone use. *Pediatrics* 1998; 102:1087.

CHAPTER **39**

Thermal and Inhalation Injury

Ronald P. Mlcak

THERMAL INJURY

EPIDEMIOLOGY

Modern care for the patient with thermal injury began in 1942, the year of the Coconut Grove Nightclub disaster in Boston in which fire claimed the lives of more than 400 people.[1] Since that time, the successful management of the patient with a severe burn has continued to be a challenge, particularly if the victim is a young child.

In the United States, thermal injury results in 60,000 hospitalizations and approximately 6000 deaths annually. About half of those deaths occur in children, accounting for only approximately 5% of pediatric burn injuries.[2-5] Mortality is highest in very young children and the elderly, with burn injury one of the three leading causes of death in children. Less than 5% of pediatric thermal injuries are the result of chemical or electrical burns. Flame burns account for 10% to 15% of thermal injuries and when associated with smoke inhalation are the cause of most deaths. Scalding burns account for 75% to 80% of the thermal injuries among children.[6,7]

Medical advances have had an impact on reducing the mortality rate and outcome in burn and inhalation injury. However, prevention remains the most important aspect of lowering the risk of these injuries to children. Important measures in preventing pediatric thermal-related injuries are having working smoke detectors, keeping matches out of reach, lowering hot water temperatures, covering electrical outlets, buying flame-resistant children's clothing, and using fire-safe cigarettes.[4,8]

Independently cited as high-mortality risk factors in children are burn injuries exceeding 30% body surface area (Fig. 39-1), associated smoke inhalation, and age younger than 4 years.[9] However, with improved treatment of inhalation injury, advancements in early wound repair techniques, effective antibiotics, precise fluid resuscitation and metabolic control, and avoidance of high pulmonary pressure

Area	Birth 1 yr	1-4 yr	5-9 yr	10-14 yr	15 yr	Adult	2°	3°	Total	Donor areas
Head	19	17	13	11	9	7				
Neck	2	2	2	2	2	2				
Ant. trunk	13	13	13	13	13	13				
Post. trunk	13	13	13	13	13	13				
R. buttock	$2\frac{1}{2}$	$2\frac{1}{2}$	$2\frac{1}{2}$	$2\frac{1}{2}$	$2\frac{1}{2}$	$2\frac{1}{2}$				
L. buttock	$2\frac{1}{2}$	$2\frac{1}{2}$	$2\frac{1}{2}$	$2\frac{1}{2}$	$2\frac{1}{2}$	$2\frac{1}{2}$				
Genitalia	1	1	1	1	1	1				
R. U. arm	4	4	4	4	4	4				
L. U. arm	4	4	4	4	4	4				
R. L. arm	3	3	3	3	3	3				
L. L. arm	3	3	3	3	3	3				
R. hand	$2\frac{1}{2}$	$2\frac{1}{2}$	$2\frac{1}{2}$	$2\frac{1}{2}$	$2\frac{1}{2}$	$2\frac{1}{2}$				
L. hand	$2\frac{1}{2}$	$2\frac{1}{2}$	$2\frac{1}{2}$	$2\frac{1}{2}$	$2\frac{1}{2}$	$2\frac{1}{2}$				
R. thigh	$5\frac{1}{2}$	$6\frac{1}{2}$	8	$8\frac{1}{2}$	9	$9\frac{1}{2}$				
L. thigh	$5\frac{1}{2}$	$6\frac{1}{2}$	8	$8\frac{1}{2}$	9	$9\frac{1}{2}$				
R. leg	5	5	$5\frac{1}{2}$	6	$6\frac{1}{2}$	7				
L. leg	5	5	$5\frac{1}{2}$	6	$6\frac{1}{2}$	7				
R. foot	$3\frac{1}{2}$	$3\frac{1}{2}$	$3\frac{1}{2}$	$3\frac{1}{2}$	$3\frac{1}{2}$	$3\frac{1}{2}$				
L. foot	$3\frac{1}{2}$	$3\frac{1}{2}$	$3\frac{1}{2}$	$3\frac{1}{2}$	$3\frac{1}{2}$	$3\frac{1}{2}$				
						Total				

Cause of burn _____

_____

Time of burn _____

Date of birth _____

Age _____

Sex _____

Weight _____

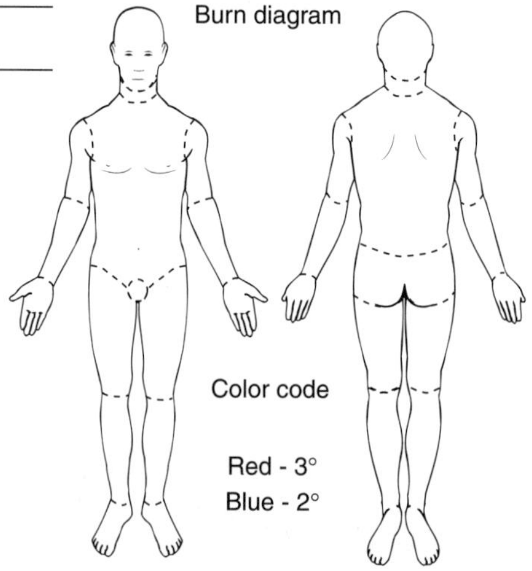

Burn diagram

Color code

Red - 3°

Blue - 2°

Fig. 39-1

Body surface area estimates of burn size based on age. Note the decrease in the surface area of the head and the increase in the areas of the legs from infant to adult. Using this table provides the most accurate percentage for burn size estimates when calculating fluid and nutritional requirements. (From Hess DR et al: *Respiratory care: principles and practice.* Philadelphia. WB Saunders, 2002.)

and oxygen concentrations, the pediatric mortality rate and outcomes continue to improve.[3, 10] With these advances, the mortality rate has dropped 45% over 20 years, and the likelihood is that a child will survive even after burn exposure of up to 60% of the body surface area.[5]

PATHOPHYSIOLOGY

The skin provides four essential functions that are necessary for survival: (1) protecting the body from infection and injury, (2) preventing fluid loss, (3) regulating body temperature, and (4) providing sensory input from the environment.[4] It is composed of two layers: the epidermis and the dermis. The epidermis is the thin, outer layer. Below it is the dermis, which is a deeper, thicker layer. The dermis contains hair follicles, sweat glands, sebaceous glands, and sensory fibers for touch, pain, pressure, and temperature. Beneath the dermis lies the subcutaneous tissue, which is composed of connective tissue and fat.

Classification of Burn Injury. The depth of the burn injury classifies the degree of burn and depends on the temperature and duration of contact with the skin. Contact with flame, heat, chemicals, or electrical current results in varying degrees of tissue destruction. Burn depths also vary as a result of body position and skin thickness. Very young children and elderly patients are especially vulnerable to more severe, full-thickness burns because of their particularly thin skin.

First-degree burns are superficial, involving only the epidermis. The skin appears red without blisters and is hypersensitive and painful.

Second-degree burns are partial-thickness by definition and involve the epidermis and part of the dermis. These burns are usually very painful because nerve endings in the mid and superficial dermal layer survive the injury. Blistering is often present. Healing generally occurs quickly and completely because epithelial cells survive in deeper portions of hair follicles and migrate to the surface.

Third-degree burns are classified as full-thickness burns. They involve injury and necrosis beyond the depths of the hair follicles, through the entire thickness of the skin, and into the subcutaneous tissue. The area swells less rapidly than a second-degree burn and is usually blanched in appearance. Sensory nerves are destroyed, causing local anesthesia.

Percent of Body Surface Area Burn. An estimate of burn size and depth assists in determining the severity, prognosis, and disposition of the patient. Because fluid resuscitation requirements, nutritional support, and surgical interventions are all based on

the size of the burn, an accurate assessment of the percent of body surface area burned is critical. The size of the burn wound is described in terms of the percent of total body surface area.

The "rule of nines" is the method most frequently used to estimate percent body surface area burned. This estimate is based on various anatomic regions representing 9% of body surface area, or a multiple of nine. However, infants and younger children have body proportions different from those of an adult and a modified "rule of nines" may be used. Fig. 39-1 describes the percentages of various anatomic regions as the child ages.[3,9]

MANAGEMENT

First-degree burns heal spontaneously, usually within 2 weeks, and do not require surgical intervention. Excision and grafting of partial- and full-thickness burns, along with topical antimicrobial therapy, have decreased the incidence of burn wound sepsis. Topical agents most commonly used are sulfadiazine (Silvadene), silver nitrate, and mafenide acetate (Sulfamylon).

After burn injury, the area of deepest burn contains cells that are dead without hope of salvage. The dead skin forms an eschar, which is tough and leathery. Because the eschar layer does not expand well, circumferential burns of the limbs often swell and occlude perfusion to peripheral portions of the extremities. In the same manner, circumferential burns of the thorax can restrict ventilation. An escharotomy, which consists of making long incisions into the eschar to allow for wound expansion, relieves the tight, restricting band created by the eschar (Fig. 39-2).[3,9] It is important to prevent both early edema and infection that can destroy dermal remnants and convert a burn wound from partial thickness to full thickness.

A crucial component of burn care is initiating accurate fluid resuscitation as soon as possible after the injury. Several formulas for resuscitation are available, with children younger than 10 years of age requiring a modified formula. Delays in resuscitation often lead to increased fluid requirements. Overaggressive fluid resuscitation may result in increased extravascular hydrostatic pressure, pulmonary edema, and soft tissue swelling. Urine output is the usual indicator of adequate resuscitation. Careful hemodynamic monitoring is required, along with intubation for most patients with severe burns. It is important to view the formulas as simply guidelines to fluid resuscitation and not substitutes for diligent monitoring of urine output, electrolytes, and volume status.[11,12]

The metabolic rate can increase as much as two to three times normal after burn injury and is generally

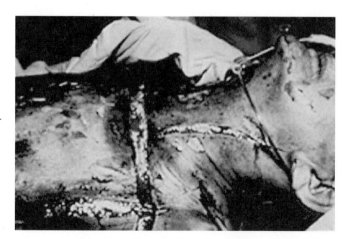

Fig. 39-2

Escharotomy incisions on the chest and neck.

related to the size of the burn. This is accompanied by constant hyperthermia. Nutritional support is extremely important and is best accomplished by calculating caloric needs and correcting electrolyte disturbances that are common to burn patients. Pharmacologic support of the hypermetabolic response consists of using anabolic agents to alleviate muscle wasting and preserve lean body mass and antiadrenergic drugs to decrease myocardial oxygen consumption and cardiac work.[11]

INHALATION INJURY

Over the past decade there have been many advances in the critical care of burn patients. Burn shock, which in the 1930s and 1940s accounted for nearly 20% of burn deaths, is now treated with early, vigorous fluid resuscitation and rarely leads to loss of life.[6,12] Invasive sepsis originating from the burn wound was at one time found to be the major cause of mortality in 80% of autopsies.[13] Aggressive wound excision and grafting, along with the use of topical antibiotics, have dramatically decreased the incidence of burn wound sepsis. Inhalation injury has now emerged as the most frequent cause of death in patients with severe burns.[13-17]

Although the mortality from smoke inhalation alone is low (0% to 11%), smoke inhalation injury in combination with cutaneous burns is fatal in 30% to 90% of patients.[18] Inhalation injury impairs the mucociliary transport mechanism in the lung, predisposing the patient to retained secretions, which leads to pneumonia and atelectasis. The combination of inhalation injury and pneumonia has been shown to carry a mortality rate of 60%.[19,20] Along with burn size and the patient's age, inhalation injury is one of the most significant predictors of burn-related mortality.[21]

BOX 39-1

PHYSIOLOGIC CONSEQUENCES OF INHALATION INJURY

Hypoxemia
Bronchospasm
Airway edema
Airway obstruction
Impaired ciliary activity
Impaired surfactant production
Increased dead space
Increased airway resistance
Increased mucus production
Increased work of breathing
Increased oxygen consumption
Increased intrapulmonary shunting
Increased ventilation/perfusion mismatch
Decreased lung and chest wall compliance

PATHOPHYSIOLOGY

Airway injury after smoke inhalation is complex and can occur at any level of the respiratory system, resulting in impaired ventilation and oxygenation. Box 39-1 lists the physiologic consequences that accompany smoke inhalation.

Upper Airway Injury. Direct thermal trauma is limited to the upper airway and results in obstruction from edema, hemorrhage, and ulceration of the mucosa. In only a few hours, mild pharyngeal edema can rapidly progress to complete upper airway obstruction with asphyxia.[22,23] The worsening of upper airway edema is most prominent in supraglottic structures. Serial nasopharyngoscopic evaluations demonstrate obliteration of the aryepiglottic folds, arytenoid eminences, and interarytenoid areas by edematous tissue that prolapses and occludes the airway.[24,25]

Smoke particles vary in size and most often deposit in the upper airway. The type of gas released during combustion depends on the material burned, the temperature, and the amount of oxygen present. Many of the gases, such as ammonia and hydrogen chloride, are chemical irritants and cause intense coughing, bronchospasm, and upper airway edema.[26]

Lung Parenchyma Injury. Direct thermal trauma after inhalation injury is not responsible for the pathophysiologic changes in the parenchyma of the lung, and the carbonaceous material present in smoke is not directly responsible for parenchymal damage, although it can serve as a carrier for other agents.[27] Only steam, with a heat-carrying capacity many times that of dry air, is capable of overwhelming the extremely efficient heat-dissipatory capabilities of the upper airways and transmitting heat to the subglottic airways.[28]

The damage to the lung parenchyma is caused by inhalation of incomplete products of combustion. There is direct cellular injury to the respiratory epithelium and pulmonary macrophages, resulting in an inflammatory response. The inflammatory mediators cause bronchoconstriction, an increase in tracheobronchial blood flow with edema formation, and leukocyte infiltration. Bronchoscopic study of the airways in the first 24 hours after inhalation injury shows gradual evolution of an edematous tracheobronchial mucosa.[29] As large portions of the respiratory epithelium slough, necrotic cellular debris accumulates in the airways. Progressive separation of the epithelium with formation of pseudomembranous casts causes partial or complete airway obstruction that can be fatal.[30]

The pulmonary parenchyma surrounding injured airways shows varying degrees of congestion, interstitial and alveolar edema, occasional hyaline membranes, and dense atelectasis. Systemic effects of inhalation injury are manifested by (1) an increase in airway resistance, ventilation-perfusion mismatch, and oxygen consumption and (2) a decrease in lung compliance, oxygenation, and surfactant production.[31,32]

Carbon Monoxide Poisoning. Carbon monoxide (CO) is a colorless, odorless, tasteless gas produced by the incomplete combustion of carbon-containing compounds. Smoke inhalation from all types of fires often results in significant CO exposure. The majority of immediate deaths that occur at the scene of building fires are caused by CO poisoning. Every patient received from a fire scene should be evaluated for CO poisoning.

The affinity of CO for the binding sites on the hemoglobin molecule is 200 to 280 times that of

TABLE 39-1	SYMPTOMS OF CARBON MONOXIDE POISONING
Carboxyhemoglobin (%)	**Symptoms**
0-10	None
10-20	Frontal headache, tightness across forehead
20-30	Dyspnea, headache, throbbing temples
30-40	Dizziness, blurred vision, nausea, vomiting, severe headache
40-50	Tachypnea, tachycardia, confusion, collapse
50-70	Depressed consciousness level, seizures, bradycardia
>70	Respiratory failure, death

Modified from Lacey DJ: Neurologic sequelae of acute carbon monoxide intoxication. *Am J Dis Child* 1981; 135:145-147. Copyright 1981, American Medical Association.

oxygen. The formation of carboxyhemoglobin (COHb) leads to a tremendous reduction in the oxygen-carrying capacity of the blood.[33] This shortage of oxygen is made worse by a concomitant shift of the oxyhemoglobin dissociation curve to the left, reducing the ability of hemoglobin to release oxygen to the tissues.[34-36]

Pulse oximetry measurement does not accurately reflect oxygen saturation in the presence of COHb. The pulse oximeter equates COHb with oxygenated hemoglobin and measures the percentage of saturation of available binding sites, regardless of whether the sites are occupied by CO or oxygen. This causes the pulse oximeter to read falsely elevated oxygen saturation values in the presence of COHb.[37] Direct measurement of COHb using co-oximetry is recommended.

The symptoms of CO poisoning correlate roughly with the percentage of COHb in the blood. Table 39-1 lists the expected symptoms based on CO blood concentrations. The major effects are on organs that are most susceptible to anoxia, such as the brain, heart, and central nervous system.

EVALUATION OF INJURY

Clinical Manifestations. The clinical diagnosis of inhalation injury has traditionally rested on various unreliable observations. Smoke inhalation injury is more likely to be present in those with a history of burn injury in an enclosed space, the appearance of facial burns, singed nasal vibrissae and facial hair, erythema of the oropharynx, and the presence of carbonaceous sputum and debris around the nose, mouth, and pharynx.[38] Rhonchi, crackles, wheezes, stridor, dyspnea, cough, and hoarse voice are seldom present on admission, occurring only in persons with the most severe injury and implying an extremely poor prognosis.[39] The admission chest radiograph is often normal and is a very poor indicator of severity of acute lung injury.[40] However, two thirds of patients develop changes of diffuse or focal infiltrates or pulmonary edema within 5 to 10 days of injury.

Bronchoscopy. The current gold standard for the diagnosis of inhalation injury in most burn centers is fiberoptic bronchoscopy.[41] Direct visualization of the upper airway provides information concerning the extent of upper airway injury. The diagnosis of inhalation injury is confirmed in the presence of soot, charring, mucosal erythema and ulceration, hemorrhage, airway edema, and inflammation.[42] The widespread use of bronchoscopy has led to an approximately twofold increase in diagnosis over that based on the traditional clinical signs.

Xenon Scan. The xenon scan is a safe, rapid test used to evaluate parenchymal damage.[43] Requiring minimal patient cooperation, it involves serial chest scintiphotograms after an initial intravenous injection of radioactive xenon gas. It demonstrates areas of decreased alveolar gas washout, which identifies sites of small airway destruction caused by edema or cast formation. Both false-negative and false-positive results are possible, occurring mainly in patients in whom scanning is delayed for 4 or more days or who have preexisting lung disease. The most important limitation is the logistic problem of transporting the unstable patient to the hospital's nuclear medicine department. Although reported in the literature, few burn centers currently use the xenon scan for diagnosis of inhalation injury.

Spirometry. Although not routinely used for the diagnosis of inhalation injury in children, pulmonary function studies are abnormal after inhalation injury. Reductions in the forced expiratory volume in 1 second (FEV_1) and the ratio of FEV_1 to vital capacity (FEV_1/VC) are seen within 24 hours of injury.[44] Over the next several days, vital capacity and peak flow are reduced and pulmonary resistance is increased.[45,46]

Thermal and Dye Dilution. A more recent method of evaluating inhalation injury is the estimation of extravascular lung water by simultaneous thermal and dye dilution measurements. This procedure has been unable to quantify the severity of injury but has proven useful in separating parenchymal injury from upper airway injury.[47]

MANAGEMENT

The management of any patient with an inhalation injury is determined by the degree of hypoxia, airway obstruction and edema, sepsis, and respiratory failure. Current treatment includes oxygen therapy, adequate airway maintenance, aggressive bronchial hygiene therapy, pharmacologic management, and mechanical ventilatory support.

Oxygen Therapy. The goal of oxygen therapy in a patient with inhalation injury is to increase the oxygen content of the blood. All patients should be given 100% oxygen through a non-rebreathing mask immediately after inhalation injury. Oxygenation is monitored by arterial blood gas analysis, and COHb level is analyzed with co-oximetry. The use of hyperbaric oxygen is widely debated.

Airway Maintenance. Acute upper airway obstruction occurs in one fifth to one third of hospitalized burn victims with inhalation injury. Stridor, hoarseness, wheezing, retractions, and tachypnea are all signs of upper airway compromise and mandate prompt intervention. Whenever airway obstruction is suspected, the most experienced clinician should perform endotracheal intubation. It is better to intubate early than to wait and find that the obstruction has progressed to where visualization of the larynx is reduced.

Securing the endotracheal tube can be difficult, owing to burn wounds and the rapid airway swelling that occurs within the first 72 hours after the injury. A nasotracheal tube is often more readily secured than an orotracheal tube. Reintubation after an accidental extubation may be difficult if not impossible if facial and oropharyngeal edema is severe. It is important to secure the tube in a manner that avoids trauma to the skin, especially when the face and neck are burned.[47]

Burns of the neck, especially in children, can cause unyielding eschars that externally compress and obstruct the airway. Escharotomies to the neck may be helpful in reducing the tight eschar and therefore decreasing the pressure exerted on the trachea.

Bronchial Hygiene Therapy. Aggressive bronchial hygiene therapy is an essential component of the respiratory management of patients after inhalation injury. Retained secretions may result in life-threatening airway obstruction. They can also lead to atelectasis and ventilation-perfusion mismatch and, ultimately, contribute to the development of pneumonia, which has been shown to increase mortality after burns and inhalation injury.[48] Early ambulation, therapeutic coughing, chest physiotherapy, airway suctioning, therapeutic bronchoscopy, and pharmacologic agents are used to mobilize and remove retained secretions and fibrin casts.

Early ambulation includes having the patient stand, walk, and sit in a chair. Patients with inhalation injury are routinely gotten out of bed and allowed to sit in a chair to improve lung function. Parents are encouraged to hold and rock their children as a means of therapy and to provide patient comfort.

Tracheobronchial suctioning and lavage are imperative for the removal of secretions and casts in the patient who has an ineffective cough or incapacitated mucociliary apparatus. When secretions or casts become thick and adhere to the airways, bronchial lavage is used as an adjunct to suctioning. Care is taken not to use excessive lavage fluid. Nasotracheal suctioning may be used as a mechanism to stimulate coughing and remove secretions in patients who are not intubated.

Chest physiotherapy, postural drainage, and routine repositioning of the patient every 2 hours have been effective in secretion removal. However, positioning is often limited because of the location of fresh skin grafts and donor sites.

When these techniques fail to remove secretions, the use of fiberoptic bronchoscopy has proven effective. Bronchoscopy allows for visualization of the airway and enables meticulous pulmonary toilet for retained secretions. The presence of inspissated secretions and fibrin casts may require repeated bronchoscopy to maintain airway patency and adequate gas exchange.[42,49]

Pharmacologic Management. Inhalation injury to the lower airways results in a chemical tracheobronchitis that can cause intense bronchospasm and wheezing. This is best managed with β_2-agonists, especially in patients who also have preexisting asthma or reactive airway disease. Aerosolized bronchodilators are effective by providing bronchial smooth muscle relaxation and stimulating mucociliary clearance.

Racemic epinephrine may be used as an aerosolized vasoconstrictor, bronchodilator, and secretion bond breaker. The vasoconstrictive action of racemic epinephrine is useful in reducing mucosal and submucosal edema within the walls of the pulmonary airways. A secondary bronchodilator action serves to reduce potential spasm of the smooth muscle of the terminal bronchioles. Racemic epinephrine has also been used in the treatment of postextubation stridor.

Investigators have suggested that the administration of corticosteroids may be given to decrease mucosal edema and bronchospasm, maintain surfactant function, and decrease the inflammatory response that occurs after inhalation injury. Prospective studies showed no benefit in morbidity and mortality in patients who received intravenous corticosteroids after inhalation injury. Some researchers have suggested that there might be an increase in infection-related complications in patients who receive corticosteroid therapy.[50,51]

N-Acetylcysteine is a powerful mucolytic agent used in respiratory care. It contains a thiol group; the free sulfhydryl radical of this group is a strong reducing agent that ruptures the disulfide bonds that serve to give stability to the mucoprotein network of molecules in mucus. Agents that break down these disulfide bonds produce the most effective mucolysis.[52] *N*-Acetylcysteine has been proven effective in combination with aerosolized heparin for the treatment of inhalation injury in animal studies.[53] Heparin and *N*-acetylcysteine combinations have been used as scavengers for the oxygen-free radicals produced when alveolar macrophages are activated, either directly by chemicals in smoke or by one or more compounds in the arachidonic cascade.[54] Animal studies have shown an increased ratio of Pa_{O_2} to F_{IO_2}, decreased peak inspiratory pressures, and a decreased amount of fibrin cast formation with heparin/*N*-acetylcysteine combinations.[55] Pediatric patients treated with aerosolized heparin/*N*-acetylcysteine combinations showed a reduction in the incidence of atelectasis, number of ventilator days, incidence of reintubation for progressive respiratory failure, and mortality.[56]

Although pneumonia occurs in as many as 50% of children with inhalation injury, the prophylactic use of antibiotics is not recommended. Instead, antibiotic therapy is directed by sputum Gram's stain and blood cultures, with culture specimens obtained when infection or pneumonia is suspected.

Mechanical Ventilatory Support. Despite conservative efforts to support unassisted ventilation, patients with moderate or severe inhalation injury may develop respiratory failure and require mechanical ventilation.[57] Patients with severe inhalation injury are at a substantial risk for iatrogenic, ventilator-induced lung damage. Airway resistance is increased secondary to edema and obstruction caused by cast formation. The increased resistance requires higher airway pressures to maintain sufficient flow to support minute ventilation. Ideally, the optimal treatment of any disease should reverse the pathophysiologic process without causing further injury. When inhalation injury is severe enough to require conventional mechanical ventilation, such an outcome is rarely achieved.

Conventional Mechanical Ventilation. Conventional mechanical ventilation does not reverse the pathologic process, is not characterized by improved clearance of secretions, and may actually compound the existing injury.[58] Conventional volume-limited ventilation in patients with inhalation injury is usually instituted at a tidal volume of 12 to 15 ml/kg. With such a ventilator setting, peak inspiratory pressures are often elevated during the resuscitative and fluid mobilization phase of care.[59] High levels of positive end-expiratory pressure are often maintained, with this type of therapy initiated before hypoxemia occurs.

Over the past 30 years, and especially in the past decade, there has been an increase in new ventilator techniques that present alternatives for the treatment of patients with inhalation injury. Unfortunately, although the number of options available to the clinician has appeared to increase exponentially, well-controlled prospective trials defining the specific role for each mode of ventilation and then comparing them with other modes of ventilation have not been forthcoming, particularly in the pediatric population.

Other ventilator modes have been employed in both animal models and clinical trials of inhalation injury. Pressure-limited ventilation with and without inverse inspiratory:expiratory ratios has been studied in an ovine smoke inhalation model.[60] Although gas exchange was not significantly improved with this mode, adequate ventilation was achieved at lower mean airway pressures, suggesting that ventilator-induced lung injury may be reduced. Excellent results have been reported using pressure-controlled ventilation in a cohort of pediatric burn patients.[61] Their results suggest that the incidences of barotrauma, pneumonia, and deaths were all considerably less than that expected based on historic controls.

High-frequency Percussive Ventilation. High-frequency ventilation has also been employed after inhalation injury. This mode provides oxygenation at lower inspired oxygen concentrations and adequate ventilation at lower peak and mean airway pressures. In addition, a few reports have indicated increased secretion clearance with some forms of high-frequency ventilation.[62]

The terms *high-frequency flow interruption* and *high-frequency percussive ventilation* (HFPV) are used to describe a technique in which ventilation is accomplished by a positive-phase percussion delivered at the proximal airway. In clinical trials, HFPV was found to permit adequate ventilation and oxygenation without increasing barotrauma in a small cohort of patients for whom conventional ventilatory support after inhalation injury had failed.[59,63] Studies in adult patients with burns and inhalation injury reported optimal ventilation, decreases in pneumonia, and improved survival with HFPV when compared with conventional volume-limited ventilation.[64] A retrospective study of the effects of HFPV and conventional ventilation in pediatric patients with inhalation injury found that those patients treated with HFPV showed a decrease in the incidence of pneumonia, a lower peak inspiratory pressure, and improvement in the ratio of PaO_2 to FIO_2.[65]

COMPLICATIONS

The most common complications of inhalation injury that lead to increased mortality are infection and respiratory failure. Patients with inhalation injury have a high incidence of pneumonia. Burn-wound infection and sepsis place the patient at extremely high risk for multiple organ system failure.

Early Complications. The reported early complications of inhalation injury are usually mechanical or infectious. Immediate recognition of these complications is imperative so that appropriate treatment can begin and thus decrease the severity of the injury.

Mechanical complications are usually manifestations of barotrauma. Barotrauma can result from a variety of injuries caused by mechanical ventilation, especially when high peak inspiratory pressures are maintained. Patients with inhalation injury often develop sloughing of the tracheobronchial mucosa, which results in a ball-valve type obstruction. This type of obstruction acts as a one-way valve. The volume from the mechanical ventilator is allowed to enter the lungs; however, expiration is only allowed to partially occur. If this problem is left untreated, further barotrauma may occur and a pneumothorax may result.

Infectious complications may result in tracheobronchitis or pneumonia. The injured trachea is known to be at risk for infections, with respiratory infections being the most common complication after inhalation injury.[66]

The diagnosis of tracheobronchitis or pneumonia can be difficult to establish, owing to the presence of inhalation injury and bacterial colonization of the airways. The diagnosis of tracheobronchitis rests on the presence of fever, leukocytosis, and productive cough, as well as on organisms and white blood cells on Gram's stain of sputum specimens. Additionally, parenchymal infiltrates must be present on the chest radiograph to make the diagnosis of pneumonia.

Late Complications. Late complications of inhalation injury may be related to mechanical damage or to the consequences of an inflammatory response. Mechanical complications occur most often as a result of iatrogenic injury from endotracheal or tracheostomy tube cuffs. This damage may cause erosion of the tracheal cartilage and result in tracheomalacia. Injuries to the tracheal epithelium may result in fibrosis and stenosis of the trachea, which lead to subglottic stenosis. Cuff erosion into adjacent structures (i.e., innominate artery) may result in exsanguinating hemorrhage. The injuries are difficult to diagnose and often develop slowly. Endotracheal tube instability, high cuff pressures (>20 cm H_2O), and duration of intubation all contribute to airway damage. Meticulous attention to detail regarding tube security and cuff pressures can reduce the incidence of mechanical damage that occurs with artificial airways.

Inflammatory complications, such as bronchiectasis and bronchial stenosis, are thought to occur as a result of neutrophil activation at the site of the airway damaged by inhalation injury. Activated neutrophils produce proteases and oxygen radicals, which may cause severe damage to the already injured bronchial mucosa and extracellular matrix. Although most proteases are produced by neutrophils, other cells including alveolar macrophages, mast cells, eosinophils, and fibroblasts all may participate in protease secretion. Normal host defense mechanisms protecting mucosal integrity have been shown to function poorly after inhalation injury.[67] Damage of both smoke-injured and normal tissues by proteases and oxidants may lead to persistent worsening of the inflammatory response, which may prevent healing.

LONG-TERM OUTCOMES

Early reports in the literature indicate that long-term pulmonary parenchyma dysfunction after inhalation injury appears to be uncommon. Patients with inhalation injury alone have significant obstructive defects, whereas those patients with both inhalation and burn injury have a mixed obstructive and restrictive pattern. Although the abnormalities may persist in the early convalescent period, in general most patients have normal lung parenchyma within 5 months of injury.

A study of children with inhalation and burn injury reported pulmonary function changes for up to 8 years after injury. The results indicated that (1) resting lung function studies showed some degree of residual pulmonary pathology; (2) altered lung mechanics, impaired gas exchange, chest wall scarring, and respiratory muscle weakness may have contributed to the decrease in lung function; and (3) children with severe thermal injury and smoke inhalation may not regain normal lung function.[68]

Children evaluated with cardiopulmonary stress testing after thermal and inhalation injury showed an increased ratio of physiologic dead space to tidal volume during exercise as long as 2 years after the injury.[69] The physiologic insults that occur as a result of thermal injury may limit exercise endurance in children.[70] Data from exercise stress testing showed evidence of a respiratory limitation to exercise. This was confirmed by a decrease in maximal heart rate, decreased maximal oxygen consumption, and increased respiratory rate.

Although thermal and inhalation injuries present a challenge to the health care team, an orderly, systematic approach can simplify management. Successful outcome requires careful attention to treatment priorities, protocols, and meticulous attention to details in all areas of care.

REFERENCES

1. Faxon NW, Churchill ED: The Coconut Grove disaster in Boston. *JAMA* 1942; 120:1385-1388.
2. Brigham PA, McLoughlin E: Burn incidence and medical care in the United States: estimates, trends, and data sources. *J Burn Care Rehabil* 1996; 17:95-107.
3. Herndon DN, Spies M: Modern burn care. *Semin Pediatr Surg* 2001; 10:28-31.
4. Joffe MD: Burns. In Fleisher GR, Ludwig S, editors: *Textbook of pediatric emergency medicine,* ed 4. Philadelphia. Lippincott Williams & Wilkins, 2000; p 1427.
5. O'Neill JA: Advances in the management of pediatric trauma. *Am J Surg* 2000; 180:365-369.
6. Cope O, Ruinelander FW: The problem of burn shock complicated by pulmonary damage. *Ann Surg* 1943; 117:915-928.
7. Aub JC, Pittman H: The pulmonary complications: a clinical description. *Ann Surg* 1943; 117:834-840.
8. Barillo DJ et al: The fire-safe cigarette: a burn prevention tool. *J Burn Care Rehabil* 2000; 21:162-164.
9. Finkelstein JL et al: Pediatric burns: an overview. *Pediatr Clin North Am* 1992; 39:1145-1163.
10. Sheridan RL, Schnitzer JJ: Management of the high-risk pediatric burn patient. *J Pediatr Surg* 2001; 36:1308-1312.
11. Ramzy PI, Barret JP, Herndon DN: Thermal injury. *Crit Care Clin* 1999; 15:333-352.
12. Henriques FC Jr: Studies of thermal injury: V. The predictability and significance of thermally induced rate process leading to irreversible epidermal injury. *Arch Pathol* 1947; 43:489-502.
13. Linares HA: A report of 115 consecutive autopsies in burned children: 1966-1980. *Burns* 1982; 8:270-273.
14. Brown JM: Respiratory complications in burned patients. *Physiotherapy* 1977; 63:151-153.
15. Clark WR Jr et al: The pathophysiology of the acute smoke inhalation. *Surg Forum* 1977; 177-178.
16. Foley FD, Moncriff JA, Mason AD Jr: Pathology of the lung in fatally burned patients. *Ann Surg* 1968; 167:251-264.
17. Moylan JA: Inhalation injury: a primary determinant of survival. *J Burn Care Rehabil* 1981; 3:78-84.
18. Haponik EF, Summer WR: Respiratory complications in burned patients: Pathogenesis and spectrum of inhalation injury. *Crit Care* 1987; 2:49-74.

19. Pruitt BA Jr et al: The occurrence and significance of pneumonia and other pulmonary complications in burned patients. *J Trauma* 1970; 10:519-531.

20. Shirani KZ, Pruitt BA Jr, Mason AD Jr: The influence of inhalation injury and pneumonia on burned mortality. *Ann Surg* 1987; 205:82-87.

21. Thompson PB et al: Effects on mortality of inhalation injury. *J Trauma* 1986; 26:163-165.

22. Haponik EF, Lykens MG: Acute upper airway obstruction in burned patients. *Crit Care Rep* 1990; 2:28-49.

23. Waymack JP et al: Acute upper airway obstruction in the post burn period. *Arch Surg* 1985; 120:1042-1044.

24. Haponik EF et al: Upper airway function in burn patients. *Am Rev Respir Dis* 1984; 129:251-257.

25. Haponik EF et al: Acute upper airway injury in burn patients; serial changes of flow volume curves and nasopharyngoscopy. *Am Rev Respir Dis* 1987; 135:360-366.

26. Wald PH, Balmes JR: Respiratory effects of short-term, high-intensity toxic inhalations: smoke, gases, and fumes. *J Intensive Care Med* 1987; 2:260-278.

27. Zirka BA et al: What is clinical smoke poisoning? *Ann Surg* 1975; 181:151-156.

28. Moritiz AR, Henriques FC Jr, McLean R: The effects of inhaled heat on the air passages and lungs: an experimental investigation. *Am J Pathol* 1945; 21:311-331.

29. Head JM: Inhalation injury in burns. *Am J Surg* 1980; 139:508-512.

30. Walker HL, McLeoud CG, McManus WL: Experimental inhalation injury in the goat. *J Trauma* 1981; 21:962-964.

31. Demling RH: Initial effect of smoke inhalation injury on oxygen consumption (response to positive pressure ventilation). *Surgery* 1994; 115:563-569.

32. Liu Z-Y et al: Pulmonary surfactant activity after severe steam inhalation in rabbits. *Burns* 1986; 12:330-336.

33. Rodkey F, O'Neal J, Collison H: Relative affinity of hemoglobin S and hemoglobin A for carbon monoxide and oxygen. *Clin Chem* 1974; 20:83-84

34. Emmans HW: Fire and fire protection. *Sci Am* 1974; 231:21-27.

35. Zirka BA, Ferre JM, Floch HF: The chemical factors contributing to pulmonary damage. *Surgery* 1972; 71: 704-709.

36. Parish RA: Smoke inhalation and carbon monoxide poisoning in children. *Pediatr Emerg Care* 1985; 2:36-39.

37. Barker SJ, Tremper KK, Hyatt J: The effect of carbon monoxide inhalation on pulse oximetry and transcutaneous P_{O_2}. *Anesthesiology* 1987; 66:677-680.

38. Moylan JA, Chan CK: Inhalation injury an increasing problem. *Surgery* 1978; 188:34-37.

39. Stone HH, Martin JD Jr: Pulmonary injury associated with thermal injury. *Surg Gynecol Obstet* 1969; 129:1242-1246.

40. Putman CE et al: Radiological manifestations of acute smoke inhalation. *AJR Am J Roentgenol* 1977; 129: 865-870.

41. Wanner A, Cutchauarece A: Early recognition of upper airway obstruction following smoke inhalation. *Am Rev Respir Dis* 1973; 108:1421-1423.

42. Moylan JA et al: Fiberoptic bronchoscopy following thermal injury. *Surg Gynecol Obstet* 1975; 140:541-543.

43. Moylan JA et al: Early diagnosis of inhalation injury using xenon scan. *Ann Surg* 1972; 176:477-484.

44. Whitener DR et al: Pulmonary function measurements in patients with thermal injury and smoke inhalation. *Am Rev Respir Dis* 1980; 122:731-739.

45. Petroff PA et al: Pulmonary function studies after smoke inhalation. *Am J Surg* 1976; 132:346-351.

46. Garzon AA et al: Respiratory mechanics in patients with inhalation injury. *J Trauma* 1970; 10:57-62.

47. Mlcak RP, Desai MH, Nichols RJ: Respiratory care. In Herndon DA, editor: *Total burn care.* London. WB Saunders, 1996; pp 193-204.

48. Sirani KZ, Pruitt BA, Mason AD: The influence of inhalation injury and pneumonia on burn mortality. *Ann Surg* 1986; 205:82-87.

49. Pruitt BA Jr et al: Evaluation and management of patients with inhalation injury. *J Trauma* 1990; 30:563-568.

50. Levine BA, Petroff PA, Slade CL: Prospective trials of dexamethasone and aerosolized gentamicin in the treatment of inhalation injury. *J Trauma* 1978; 18:118-123.

51. Nieman GF, Clark WR, Hakim T: Methylprednisolone does not protect the lung from inhalation injury. *Burns* 1991; 17:384-390.

52. Hirsh SR, Zastrow JE, Korg RC: Sputum liquification agents: a comprehensive in vitro study. *J Lab Clin Med* 1969; 74:346-350.

53. Brown M et al: Dimethylsulfoxide with heparin in the treatment of smoke inhalation injury. *J Burn Care Rehab* 1988; 9:22-26.

54. Desai MH et al: Reduction of smoke injury with dimethylsulfoxide and heparin treatments. *Surg Forum* 1985; 36:103-106.

55. Desai MH, Brown M, Mlcak RP: Nebulization treatments of inhalation injury in the sheep model with dimethylsulfoxide/heparin combinations and *N*-acetylcysteine. *Crit Care Med* 1986; 14:321-324.

56. Desai MH et al: Reduction in mortality in pediatric patients with inhalation injury with aerosolized heparin/*N*-acetylcysteine therapy. *J Burn Care Rehabil* 1998; 19:210-212.

57. Reynolds EM, Ryan DP, Doody DP: Mortality and respiratory failure in a pediatric burn population. *J Pediatr Surg* 1993; 28:1326-1331.

58. Mammel MC, Boros SJ: Airway damage and mechanical ventilation: a review and commentary. *Pediatr Pulmonol* 1987; 3:443-447.

59. Cioffi WG et al: Prophylactic use of high-frequency ventilation in patients with inhalation injury. *Ann Surg* 1991; 213:575-582.

60. Ogura H, Cioffi WG, Okerberg C: Effects of pressure-controlled, inverse-ratio ventilation on smoke inhalation injury in an animal model. San Antonio TX. US Army Institute of Surgical Research, 1991.

61. Sheridan RL et al: Permissive hypercapnia as a ventilatory strategy in burned children. *J Trauma* 1995; 39:854-859.

62. Arnold JH: High-frequency oscillatory ventilation: theory and practice in paediatric patients. *Paediatr Anaesth* 1996; 6:437-441.

63. Rue LW et al: Improved survival of burned patients with inhalation injury. *Arch Surg* 1993; 128:772-780.

64. Cioffi WG et al: High-frequency percussive ventilation in patients with inhalation injury. *J Trauma* 1989; 29:350-354.

65. Cortiella J, Mlcak RP, Herndon D: High-frequency percussive ventilation in pediatric patients with inhalation injury. *J Burn Care Rehabil* 1999; 20:232-235.

66. Demarst GB, Hudson LD, Altman LC: Impaired alveolar macrophage chemotaxis in patients with acute smoke inhalation. *Am Rev Respir Dis* 1979; 119:279-286.

67. Gadek JE et al: Antielastase of the human alveolar structures. *J Clin Invest* 1981; 68:889-898.

68. Mlcak RP et al: Lung function following thermal injury in children: an 8-year follow-up. *Burns* 1998; 24:213-216.

69. Mlcak RP et al: Increased physiological dead space:tidal volume ratio during exercise in burned children. *Burns* 199; 5:337-339.

70. Desai MH et al: Does inhalation injury limit exercise endurance in children convalescing from thermal injury? *J Burn Care Rehabil* 1993; 14:12-16.

CHAPTER 40

Head Injury and Cerebral Disorders

Paul Mathews
Loretta Mathews

D amage to the brain or skull is among the most potentially serious and handicapping of all traumatic injuries. Head injuries are the primary cause of trauma deaths in both adults and children. A brain injury occurs in the United States every 15 seconds, and more than 1 million people with head injury are seen in emergency departments (EDs) each year. More than 5.3 million Americans are disabled from traumatic brain injury.[1] A substantial percentage of these patients are infants and children. The number of people disabled or killed is even higher when nontraumatic organic causes are factored into the etiologies of brain injury.

Because a child's head is large and heavy in relation to the body, and because balance, coordination, gait, and judgment are immature, children are especially vulnerable to head injury.[2] Children have more frequent falls because of these factors, resulting in a high percentage of head injuries. The size and weight of the head tend to rotate the child's body into a head-down position, leading to headfirst impacts.

Shaking injuries such as shaken baby syndrome (SBS) account for a large number of head and central nervous system (CNS) injuries, especially in infants less than 1 year of age. Because of poorly developed neck muscles, when a baby is shaken, the head moves like a pendulum or church bell, whipping back and forth or side to side, with resulting brain injury as the brain impacts the sides of the skull with each movement. Remember, as a health care professional, you are required by law to report suspected incidents of SBS to legal authorities.

This chapter covers the general causes of brain injury; the anatomic, biophysical, and physiologic factors that influence the type and severity of injury; and the diagnosis and treatment of brain injury. Preventive actions to reduce brain injury and respiratory care procedures to treat and manage head injuries are also discussed.

CAUSES AND ANATOMIC CONSIDERATIONS

Damage to the brain may be classified in many ways. One useful way to classify brain injury is by *general cause*. Brain injury results from one of three general causes: (1) genetic-developmental, (2) toxic-infective, or (3) traumatic (Box 40-1). Although the causal agent may be different in each of these classes, the potential worst-case end results are the same: death or disability. Between the worst-case outcome and a no-harm result lies a continuum of possible outcomes.

The outcome and potential disability caused by each injury may vary in effect and seriousness based on many factors. *Age* is a major factor in some cases, allowing infants and young children to compensate when adults might sustain a permanent injury. Also, repetitive injuries have a cumulative effect, as evidenced by "punch drunk" boxers or football players with multiple concussions.

The brain has functionally specific areas (Fig. 40-1). However, the brains of infants and children apparently have a large degree of *plasticity* in redistributing function from a damaged area to an undamaged area. In adults the ability of the brain

---

BOX 40-1

GENERAL CAUSES OF BRAIN INJURY

GENETIC-DEVELOPMENTAL
  Microcephaly
  Down syndrome
  Hydroencephaly
  Cerebral palsy
  Cerebral aneurysm
  Seizures

TOXIC-INFECTIVE
  Meningitis
  Lead poisoning
  Carbon monoxide poisoning
  Septicemia
  Drug overdose

TRAUMATIC
  Subarachnoid hemorrhage
  Anoxia of childbirth
  Penetrating head wounds
  Falls
  Abuse
  Suffocation, strangulation

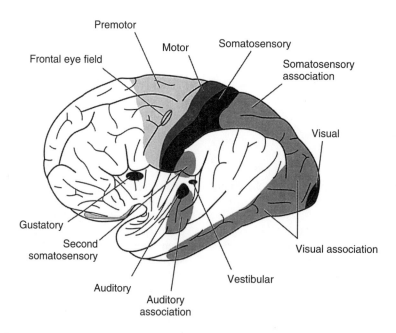

Fig. 40-1

General functional areas of the cerebral cortex. (From Nolte J: *The human brain: an introduction to its functional anatomy.* St Louis, Mosby, 2002; modified from von Economo C: *The cytoarchitectonics of the human cerebral cortex.* Oxford. Oxford University Press, 1929.)

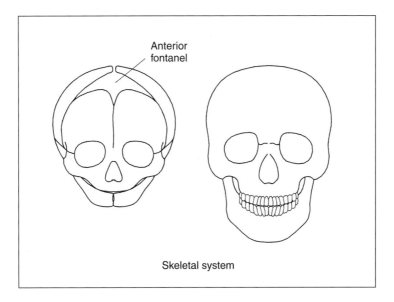

segments to adapt to new functions seems to be rarely, if ever, present. This flexibility of assigned purpose provides protection and enhances rehabilitative potential for infants and children but decreases with age as the maturing brain becomes patterned and locked into its distribution of functional capacity.

Infants and young children have malleable skulls because of the large fontanels ("soft spots") and flat bones of the skull, which have not yet fused and may still be cartilaginous before ossification (Fig. 40-2). These factors allow for elasticity of the cranial vault and prevent both fractures and pressure-related brain injuries during passage through the birth canal. Skull malleability also protects against damage from other sources, such as trauma or illness causing increased pressures in the cranial vault, by allowing expansion of the cranial volume. These normally transitory anatomic features can provide important diagnostic clues as well (see later discussion).

When ill or injured, the body strives to minimize damage, maintain as much function as possible, and maintain or regain homeostasis. Many signs and symptoms are the result of these survival attempts. These clinical features may provide valuable clues as to which part of the brain is injured.

The normal newborn brain and spinal cord are immature and not completely *myelinated* until about 18 months of age (Fig. 40-3). As interbrain connections are completed and the integrative func-

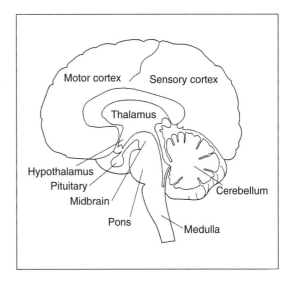

tions of the brain begin to mature, more of the brain becomes active and functional. These conditions are crucial when assessing neurologic status in infants and children; with incomplete CNS development and integration, reactions and responses will change with age and maturity.

INITIAL ASSESSMENT AND DIAGNOSIS

RAPID ASSESSMENT

On arrival at the injury scene by emergency medical services (EMS) personnel and on arrival in the ED, a rapid assessment of the head-injured patient is performed to (1) establish a baseline to measure progress or deterioration and (2) quickly provide information about resources needed to stabilize and treat the patient.

Rapid assessment protocols vary from region to region but generally include certain accepted variables (Box 40-2). On completion of the rapid assessment and initiation of urgent stabilization procedures and therapies, a more detailed assessment should be performed to arrive at a provisional diagnosis. This diagnostic workup includes physical examination, history (previous and causative event specific), and laboratory/radiologic testing.

DIAGNOSTIC ASSESSMENT

As in other conditions, the proper diagnosis of the cause, type, and extent of cerebral injury depends on the subjective and objective data associated with the patient's condition.

Subjective Data. Subjective data cannot be collected by the assessor's senses (e.g., sight, touch, smell) without input from the patient. The presence, extent, and magnitude of pain, fear, and emotional status are examples of subjective data that the patient must be asked to reveal. Because infants and young children often cannot effectively verbalize these factors, the assessor must be alert for clues that suggest a problem.

Parents may be the best sources of information about variations from normal behavior. The exception would be if a high index of suspicion of neglect or abuse exists. Abuse should be suspected if the patient draws away or cringes, suddenly becomes nonverbal, or otherwise shows change in behavior

---

BOX 40-2

RAPID TRAUMA ASSESSMENT IN HEAD INJURY

Airway: clear and patent
Breathing: present with good rate and volume
Circulation: pulses present with adequate perfusion at an acceptable rate
Bleeding: no overt bleeding or abdominal rigidity.
Level of consciousness (AVPU): **a**lert, responds to **v**oice, **p**ain response, **u**nresponsive
Pupillary response: equally reactive and midline bilaterally

---

when the parent or caregiver approaches. In these cases the law requires that health care professionals notify legally designated authorities.

Objective Data. Objective data relate to the mechanism of injury, the patient's medical history (past and present), and the event. The child's past medical history indicates the body's preinjury state. The present medical history may reveal exposure to harmful substances or activities.

Objective data help the clinician track the patient's physiologic response to injury and treatment. Objective data are measurable and allow discovery and recording of trends in the treatment and recovery process. Such data include laboratory studies, radiographs, computed tomography (CT) scans, magnetic resonance imaging (MRI), electrocardiograms (ECGs), electroencephalograms (EEGs), and lumbar puncture (LP). Objective data also include pulse blood pressure, temperature, and respirations.

MECHANISM OF INJURY

Knowledge of the mechanism of injury (MOI) provides the clinician with information on the traumatic external event and the potential internal injuries. MOI includes the object or reason for the injury, the amount of force applied, and the vector or direction of that force. For example, "The patient was the front seat passenger in a two-car motor vehicle accident (MVA). The car in which she was riding was hit on the driver's side at 30 mph while entering an intersection at 5 to 10 mph when the light had just turned green. Both she and the driver were wearing seat belts." This explanation of the mechanism of the patient's injuries provides information concerning potential pathophysiologic impact and helps determine the type and extent of possible injuries.

Head injuries can be classified in several ways according to cause. A primary classification is to distinguish between direct and indirect trauma. *Direct trauma,* such as striking one's head as a result of a fall, is further classified as either a *blunt force* or a *penetrating injury. Indirect trauma* occurs when the head is not the primary site of impact. A further distinction should be made to determine, by radiologic assessment, the presence or absence of *space-occupying lesions.*

Another, complementary, method is to classify the injury by the *direction* or *vector* of impact. For example, *torsion* and *inertial* are terms used to describe the application of force by vector, each with the potential to be either direct or indirect.

Torsion Injuries. Torsion, or *rotational,* CNS injuries occur when the head is rotated or twisted around the vertebral column. If severe, such injuries can result in total paralysis and death. The rotation or torsion may occur not only in the lateral plane but also in the anteroposterior plane. These injuries tend to sever, transect, or partially transect the spinal cord and/or the lower structures of the brainstem, resulting in catastrophic injuries (Fig. 40-4). Less severe twisting may result in muscle strains and tears that are painful but usually limited.

Because of the potential for damage to the spinal cord and brainstem, trauma patients should by moved only by trained and properly prepared individuals unless risk of loss of life is imminent. It is critically important to prevent further damage to the cervical spine (see later discussion).

Inertial Injuries. Inertial injuries are caused by sudden changes in the velocity of the head. When the head stops moving, the brain continues moving until it strikes the inside of the skull in the original direction of movement. In addition to movement-related injuries, assaults can cause significant inertial injuries as the force exerted by the weapon is dissipated on the skull and its contents. The sudden change in acceleration or application of force can result from automobile accidents, sports, falls, or deliberate assaults.

Any blow to the head or sudden change in direction or speed of travel can result in a rebound injury from inertia. This secondary injury is called a *contrecoup injury,* referring to the side opposite the contact (*coup*) side. If there is a bruise on the right side of the skull, the practitioner should exam-ine for trauma on the left side of the brain, because the brain will continue to move at the speed the head was moving before deceleration. The damage may be more severe on the contrecoup, or contra-lateral, side (Fig. 40-5). The degree of damage is related to the magnitude of the abrupt change in force on the skull. The potential damage from a deceleration from 2 to 1 mph is much less than the damage potential when abruptly slowing from 50 to 5 mph.

Volume Displacement Injuries. Volume displace-ment injuries occur when lesions cause an increased volume of tissue to accumulate in the skull, including tumors, spinal fluid, and blood. Cerebral edema secondary to head injury is a major cause of this increased tissue mass in the skull. In these space-occupying lesions, the space that the lesion occupies reduces the space available for other tissues in the skull (see later discussion).

DATA GATHERING

Subjective and objective data are gathered simulta-neously during the patient assessment process. Children are often poor historians because of age, emotional/psychiatric problems, or the injury itself. It is often necessary to rely on eyewitness accounts of the events or reports or educated guesses of accompanying adults to determine cause and mechanism of injury. Trends and alteration from the norm are particularly important in this and other noncommunicative populations.

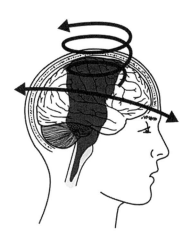

Fig. 40-4

Torsion mechanism of injury. (From McQuillan KA et al: *Trauma nursing: from resuscitation through reha-bilitation,* ed 3. Philadelphia. WB Saunders, 2002.)

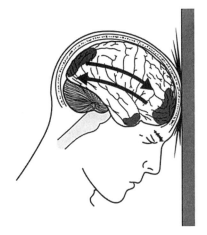

Fig. 40-5

Posterior to anterior coup-contrecoup mechanism of injury. (From McQuillan KA et al: *Trauma nursing: from resuscitation through rehabilitation,* ed 3, Philadel-phia. WB Saunders, 2002.)

STABILIZATION

A complete assessment of the patient from head to toe is desirable but may have to be postponed or abbreviated until the patient's condition is stabilized. For patients of any age, head injuries are often critical, and assessment should at least include the *ABCs plus C:* **a**irway patency, **b**reathing support, adequacy of **c**irculation, and stability of the **c**ervical spine. All children who have injured their upper torso, neck, and head should be assumed to have a cervical spine injury, and precautionary measures should be taken to prevent further spinal cord damage.

Airway Patency

Without a patent airway, other interventions are of little value. A patent airway maintains physiologic integrity, allows intervention to reduce cerebral swelling, and protects the brain from hypoxemia. A patent airway can be initiated by means of a jaw thrust maneuver to open the airway. Maintain the airway with orotracheal intubation, nasotracheal intubation, cricothyrotomy, or tracheostomy. Do not use the head tilt or chin lift maneuvers, since these change the orientation of the spinal column and increase the risk of additional spinal injury.

Avoid nasotracheal intubation, nasotracheal suctioning, or inserting nasogastric tubes because inadvertent cranial intubation may result from open fractures of the cranial vault, especially in patients who may have basilar skull injuries or perinasal fractures. Extreme care should also be taken not to manipulate the head and neck any more than necessary until radiologic tests rule out cervical spine injuries. Caution is necessary when moving or positioning the patient to prevent further displacement of any spinal fractures and additional damage to the spine, spinal cord, and cranial or spinal nerves.

Breathing Support

Breathing support includes providing supplemental oxygen. The patient may require only a nasal cannula or possibly artificial ventilation with bag-valve-mask resuscitators. Breathing support may progress to intubation with bag-valve-tube ventilation and eventually to mechanical ventilation.

Provide for all possible adverse airway events by having the appropriate equipment on hand. Give high concentrations of oxygen, and monitor oxygen saturation with a pulse oximeter and ventilation with a capnometer. Correlate with arterial blood gas (ABG) measurements to determine the adequacy of oxygenation and ventilation. Even with adequate ABG values, continue administering high concentrations of oxygen to maximize cerebral oxygenation. If the patient is breathing without

difficulty and is not likely to vomit and aspirate, a face mask is appropriate.

If the patient's respirations deteriorate or state of consciousness declines, mechanical ventilation should be instituted immediately. Minimize peak inflation pressure (PIP) and mean airway pressure ($P\overline{aw}$), and select inspiratory and expiratory times that favor prolonged expiration if possible. Decreasing $P\overline{aw}$ minimizes outflow tract resistance from the cerebral vasculature, enhancing cerebral perfusion by minimizing effects on intracranial pressure (ICP). Minimize suctioning to prevent coughing and gagging on the tracheal tube or suction catheter, which may increase ICP.

Adequacy of Circulation

Assess pulse rate and pressure at all pulse points and note significant discrepancies. Pulse oximetry is a valuable adjunct for this purpose. Both manual and automatic blood pressure monitors are appropriate for head-injured patients. Blood pressure should be monitored for adequacy and bilateral symmetry. ECG monitoring is mandatory; head injury often results in secondary cardiac and cardiovascular effects. Carefully examine carotid pulses, and force and duration should be equal bilaterally. The practitioner must not take both carotid pluses or obstruct the carotid arteries simultaneously, because this may cut off the blood supply to the brain.

Assessing capillary refill is a quick and specific method of checking the adequacy of peripheral circulation. Normal capillary refill time is less than 2 seconds. Inadequate capillary refill on initial assessment may be caused by regional perfusion problems. To rule out this possibility, repeat the capillary refill test on the opposite hand.

Failure of the patient to maintain blood pressure, heart rate, and rhythm indicates the need for vasopressors, fluid administration, or cardiopulmonary resuscitation (CPR) and consideration of cardiac assist devices such as a pacemaker. It is essential that adequate pulse and perfusion pressures be maintained. A delicate balance may exist between maintaining adequate blood pressures and fluid overload or increasing cerebral vascular and cerebrospinal fluid (CSF) pressure. These procedures are performed only while ensuring that the head and neck orientation is stable and as motion free as possible.

Cervical Spine Precautions

The neck and cervical spine are easily involved in injury when the head is struck or shaken. Injuries to the cervical spine can result in paralysis and loss of sensation. This paralysis and sensory loss can range from limited to profound and may involve the entire body from the neck down. Severe injuries to the first (C1) and second (C2) cervical vertebrae are overwhelmingly fatal. Complete cord transections result in paralysis and sensory loss below the transected area. Partial transections are problematic, with outcomes varying from almost complete recovery to severe residual limitations. Bruising, edema, and hematoma formation may result in damage that is either permanent or completely or partially reversible as the swelling, bruising, and hematoma resolve.

Cervical spine precautions are taught in all life support and first-aid courses in the United States. Basic techniques for spinal immobilization address support for intubation, transportation, and movement during care and transport. If movement of the patient is necessary, keep the head and neck immobilized in a straight line using a cervical collar or sandbags. Do not apply traction to the head and neck because of the high probability of further damage if neck injuries are present.

NEUROLOGIC ASSESSMENT

Keep several factors in mind when diagnosing and caring for neurologically injured individuals. Patients with neurologic damage, at least initially, may react in an exaggerated fashion to outside stimuli. Bright lights, loud sudden sounds, and touching may all evoke hyperreactive responses. Avoid hypothermia because sensitivity to temperature variations is a hallmark of head and spinal injuries. Changes in temperature may result in a cascade of diaphoresis, chills, and shivering. By limiting tactile, auditory, and visual stimuli, the brain is allowed to focus on reintegrating and regaining physiologic balance.

Once the ABC plus C's are under control, the examination and assessment can begin in earnest. Assessment of the patient with probable head injury or brain damage must be thorough, systematic, and repetitive.

The standardized assessment mechanisms are powerful trend and tracking tools for the injured patient. Frequently, altered vital signs and level of consciousness indicate deterioration of cerebral control that demands intervention. Historically, vital signs have included pulse rate, blood pressure, respiratory rate, temperature, and oxygen saturation (SpO_2) using a pulse oximeter. Assessment of the patient's level of pain recently was added to this growing list of vital signs and symptoms.

The six "P"s are another method to assess nervous system function in the injured patient: pain, position, paralysis, paresthesia, ptosis, and priapism.[3] Pupils can be considered a seventh *P*. This assessment system is subject to an individual observer's bias and perception.

PAIN

Pain may be localized or disseminated over large areas. The pain sensations may range from deep, almost unbearable discomfort to a total lack of sensation.

Assessing pain is a difficult task in the infant and pediatric population for several reasons, including the inability to communicate due to age or injury. For children who are responsive and alert, even as young as 2 or 3 years old, a simple *visual analog scale* (VAS) can help assess quantity of pain. For older children, adolescents, and adults the use of the VAS or a modified *Borg scale* can help to quantify and trend pain (Fig. 40-6, *A,* and Table 40-1). Another helpful tool is using a *trend graph of pain* sensations (Fig. 40-6, *B*). Construct this by using a line to indicate the limits of a continuum of pain at either end. Next, instruct patients to mark an "x" at the point on the line that indicates where they feel they are on the line related to how much pain they feel. Then simply measure and record the distance from one end of the line. It is important to use the same length scale every time to record the patient's response.

Each type of scale allows the patient to indicate a level of pain or discomfort for repeated testing and measurement over time, thus providing the ability to track or trend the data as indicated by the patient. In addition to the three previous examples, a fourth method uses a *color bar,* with bright red being the most discomfort and a pale blue the best possible comfort.

POSITION

The position that reproduces the location of pain, or paresthesia, may indicate the level of injury in the cervical spine. With severe brain injury the posture of the body also indicates the section of the brain that is injured. The position that a person's body assumes after head injury can be diagnostic of the level of brain function, with damage to cortical structures forcing one telltale posture while damage to the cerebellum results in a different, but equally specific, position.

Trunk and limb position at rest, spontaneous movements, and response to painful stimuli must be carefully observed. Spontaneous movement of all limbs generally indicates a mild depression of hemispheric function without structural disturbance. Monoplegia or hemiplegia, except in the *postictal* state, suggests a structural disturbance of the *contralateral* hemisphere.

An extensor response to a painful stimulus by the trunk and limbs is termed *decerebrate posturing,* or rigidity. The most severe form is called *opisthotonos,* in which the neck is hyperextended

FACES SCALE

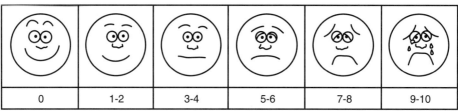

| 0 | 1-2 | 3-4 | 5-6 | 7-8 | 9-10 |

A

NUMERIC PAIN SCALE

No pain   Moderate pain   Worst pain

| 0 | 1 | 2 | 3 | 4 | 5 | 6 | 7 | 8 | 9 | 10 |

B

Fig. 40-6

A, Visual analog pain scale. **B,** Linear pain scale.

TABLE 40-1	MODIFIED BORG SCALE
Scale	**Severity**
0	None
0.5	Extremely slight, just noticeable
1	Very slight
2	Slight
3	Moderate
4	Slightly severe
5	Somewhat severe
6	Moderately severe
7	Severe
8	Very severe
9	Extremely severe, almost maximum
10	Maximum

and the teeth are clenched; the arms are adducted, hyperextended, and hyperpronated; and the legs are extended with the feet plantar flexed. Decerebrate posturing indicates lesions at the level of the cerebrum and is characterized by rigid extension of the limbs, hands turned outward, and head retracted toward the sternum. This rigidity should be considered an ominous sign whether present at rest or in response to painful stimuli. Decerebrate posturing is uncommon in children except after head injury and indicates hemispheric dysfunction with brainstem integrity.

Decorticate posturing indicates lesions at or above the brainstem and is characterized by rigid extended legs, rigid flexed arms, and fists tightly clenched in the middle of the chest.

Rarely, unilateral or mixed presentation of these symptoms is seen, caused by either unilateral trauma or a well-defined disease process. The characteristics of decerebrate and decorticate posturing allow comparison of the various positions associated with specific brain injuries (Fig. 40-7).

PARALYSIS

The inability to move a limb or limbs can be unilateral or bilateral, affecting either the right side, left side, or both. Paralysis can be defined by its vertical extent. *Paraplegia,* for example, refers to paralysis of the lower limbs, whereas paralysis of both upper and lower limbs is called *quadriplegia.* Paralysis may also be complete or may be incomplete, sometimes termed *paresis.* The patient with paresis may either have partial voluntary range of motion in one or more of the affected limbs or have involuntary motions. The location and completeness of paralysis are determined by the location of the CNS lesions or the damage to peripheral nerves in the case of single-limb or partial-limb paralysis.

PARESTHESIA, PTOSIS, AND PRIAPISM

Paresthesia is a sensation of numbness, tingling, "prickly," or heightened sensitivity that is often associated with lesions of the peripheral or central nervous system.

Ptosis is a drooping of a tissue due to paralysis or weakness of a muscle. The term is usually used when referring to the eyelids. Ptosis and a partially contracted pupil is called *Horner's syndrome,*

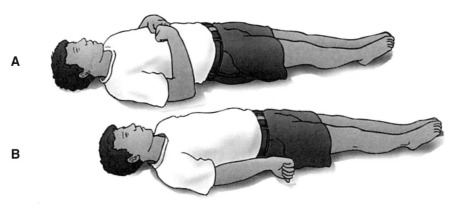

Fig. 40-7

Neurogenic posturing. **A,** Decorticate posturing. **B,** Decerebrate posturing. (From Hess DR et al: *Respiratory care: principles and practice.* Philadelphia. WB Saunders, 2002.)

suggestive of cervical sympathetic nerve trunk injury on the affected side.

Priapism is partial or complete painful erection of the penis that fails to relax. It is not associated with sexual stimulation. This condition may indicate lesions in the supralumbar region.

PUPILS

An additional *P,* the seventh, is pupils. Abnormal pupil size and reactivity are indicative of drug interference or brain injury location (Fig. 40-8). The clinician should be familiar with pupil variation in each type of brain injury.

Metabolic disturbances usually do not affect the pupillary light reflex; its absence in a comatose patient indicates a structural abnormality. The major exception is drug use; fixed, dilated pupils in an alert patient are caused by topical administration of mydriatics. In a comatose patient, hypothalamic damage causes unilateral pupillary constriction. In Horner's syndrome a midbrain lesion or a lateral medullary lesion causes midposition fixed pupils; a pontine lesion causes small but reactive pupils. Tonic lateral deviation of both eyes indicates a seizure originating in the hemisphere opposite the direction of gaze or a destructive lesion in the hemisphere in the direction of gaze.

GLASGOW COMA SCALE AND OTHER MONITORING

The Glasgow Coma Scale (GCS) is sufficiently accurate for use in adults, older children, and adolescents (Box 40-3). Coma scales for younger chil-

dren have proven to be unreliable when compared to vital signs and neurologic assessment trending (Box 40-4). The age-specific GCS is a third system that combines the adult and child forms of the GCS (Table 40-2). This scale allows decision making as to coma level regardless of the patient's age.

Intravenous Access. In addition to vital signs and neurologic monitoring, insertion of an intravenous (IV) line for peripheral access is essential. This access allows the clinician to give the patient fluids, blood, and medications. The encephalic patient is often ventilator dependent. IV medications are administered to sedate the patient, reduce swelling in the brain, reduce cellular damage to the brain, and promote healing. Preexisting IV access also permits blood sampling without causing painful stimuli as well as rapid infusion of resuscitation drugs if needed.

Respirations. Respiratory pattern also helps reveal the location of brain injury as well as helps assist the body's attempt to compensate for physiologic change. In some patients the abnormal respiratory patterns are the body's attempt to alter cerebral perfusion pressure and distribution. In other patients these changes in respiration are the direct result of injury to respiratory control centers in the brain and pons.

Physical Signs. Some classic "signs" are associated with certain head injuries. These signs indicate fractures of the basilar skull. Traumatic head injury may be highlighted by the presence of Battle's sign

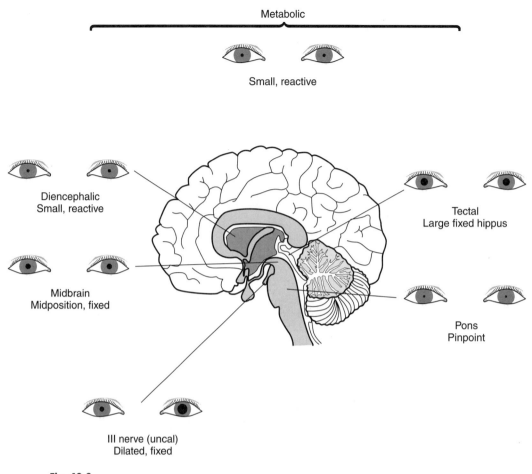

Fig. 40-8

Abnormal pupil response.

or "raccoon eyes." *Battle's sign* represents ecchymosis or bruised areas behind the ear that indicate basilar skull fractures. The self-explanatory term *raccoon eyes* represents bruising discolorations around the orbits. Both Battle's sign and raccoon eyes are the body's attempts to show internal injury with as simple a sign as a small bruise.

TREATMENT PLAN

After assessment and stabilization, a plan is developed for definitive treatment and evaluation. Before and through treatment, a comprehensive plan should be in place that includes goals and evaluation criteria. Preferably these plans are developed by an interdisciplinary team of acute care and rehabilitation professionals and will be reviewed with the patient's family as care progresses.

As previously discussed, protection of the airway and cervical spine, protection from further injury,

and progress toward recovery goals set the plan of care for the brain injury patient into motion. The plan encompasses three major goals, as follows:

1. Determine the correct diagnosis.
2. Treat the injuries and sequelae in an appropriate, caring, and resource-sparing manner.
3. Develop and implement a rehabilitation plan that is timely, centers on increasing quality of life, and employs strategies that maximize the patient's control of and autonomy in the rehabilitation process.

Evaluation of any plan of care is based on the outcome. This evaluation should result in improvements and should be adaptable to make the assessment and the plan a dynamic process. Outcomes are revised as the clinical situation changes with the patient's response to treatment. The evaluation process should be based on achievable and measurable therapeutic goals and objectives. For example, a goal in the brain-injured patient might be to

BOX 40-3

GLASGOW COMA SCALE*

I. BEST MOTOR RESPONSE
  5 = Obeys
  4 = Localizes
  3 = Withdraws (flexion)
  2 = Abnormal flexion
  1 = Extensor response

II. VERBAL RESPONSE
  4 = Oriented
  3 = Confused conversation
  2 = Inappropriate words
  1 = Incomprehensible sounds

III. EYE OPENING
  4 = Spontaneous
  3 = To speech
  2 = To pain
  1 = Nil

From Ghajar J, Hariri RJ: Management of pediatric head injury. *Pediatr Clin North Am* 1992; 39:1093-1126.
*Score = I + II + III. Maximum score = 13; minimum score = 3.

BOX 40-4

CHILDREN'S COMA SCALE*

I. OCULAR RESPONSE
  4 = Pursuit
  3 = Extraocular movement intact, reactive pupils
  2 = Fixed pupils or extraocular movement impaired
  1 = Fixed pupil and extraocular movement paralyzed

II. VERBAL RESPONSE
  3 = Cries
  2 = Spontaneous respirations
  1 = Apneic

III. MOTOR RESPONSE
  4 = Flexes and extends
  3 = Withdraws from painful stimuli
  2 = Hypertonic
  1 = Flaccid

*Score = I + II + III. Maximum score = 11; minimum score = 3.

TABLE 40-2	AGE-SPECIFIC GLASGOW COMA SCALE*	
Points	**Infant/ Preverbal Child**	**Verbal Child/ Adult**
EYE OPENING (E)		
4	Spontaneous	Spontaneous
3	To speech	To speech
2	To pain	To pain
1	None	None
VERBAL RESPONSE (V)		
5	Coos, babbles	Oriented
4	Irritable cries	Confused
3	Cries to pain	Inappropriate words
2	Moans to pain	Incomprehensible sounds
1	None	None
MOTOR RESPONSE (M)		
6	Normal, spontaneous	Obeys commands
5	Withdraws to touch	Localizes pain
4	Withdraws to pain	Withdraws to pain
3	Abnormal flexion	Abnormal flexion
2	Abnormal extension	Abnormal extension
1	None	None

Modified from Laskowsi-Jones L, Salati DS: Responding to pediatric trauma. *Nursing* 2001; 31(9):37-42.
*Score = E + V + M. *Normal,* 15 or 16 points; *mildly impaired consciousness,* 13 or 14 points; *moderate impairment,* 9 to 12 points; *severe impairment,* 3 to 8 points.

reduce positional hypertension or hypotension. The associated objective might be to reduce blood pressure swings to 10 mm Hg with position changes.

Clearly, all members of the care team, the patient, and family should be aware of the plan, its goals and objectives, and the progress toward fulfillment of the goals. This requires open and honest communications beginning early in the process and maintained throughout the stabilization and rehabilitation phases.

OTHER BODY SYSTEMS

In addition to neurologic care, the incapacitated patient needs care for the eyes, gastrointestinal tract, urinary tract, pulmonary system, and cardiovascular system. Keep the head of the bed elevated to control cerebral edema. Hyperventilation or hypoventilation assists in controlling edema as well as maintaining body integrity. Nutritionally, caloric demands need to be met. Preventing skin and muscle deterioration helps to prevent further injury. All these systems must be functional when the patient's brain recovers.

CEREBRAL DISORDERS

Cerebral disorders are the result of trauma, altered cellular function secondary to drugs, metabolic problems, anoxia, or genetic-developmental disorders. Cerebral disorders range from inconsequential to profoundly debilitating, from not being able to remember a distant relative's phone number to being in a persistent vegetative state (PVS).

The term *encephalopathy* is used to describe a diffuse disorder of the brain with many causes. The prominent features of encephalopathy are a decreased state of consciousness, abnormal response to external stimulus, and seizures. An encephalopathy is called *encephalitis* when inflammatory cells are found in the CSF. These altered states of consciousness and rationality may be constant or transitory in nature; they may be temporary disabilities or permanent life altering conditions.

The goal of management of head injury in children is to prevent secondary injury to the brain. Prevention of hypoxia, ischemia, and increased intracranial pressure is essential.[3]

LETHARGY AND COMA

A progressive decline in consciousness can be caused by diffuse or multifocal disturbances of the cerebral hemispheres or by focal injury to the brainstem. Specific characteristics are used to describe and delineate various states of decreased consciousness (Table 40-3).

The GCS, although originally designed for trauma cases, is now used to provide clinicians with a standardized system to assess a patient with an altered level of consciousness (see Box 40-3). The Children's Coma Scale was developed to assess infants and toddlers who are unable to speak or follow commands (see Box 40-4). Although pupil diameter and light reactivity are not addressed in the coma scales, they are important indicators of cerebral herniation and should be assessed during a neurologic examination.[4] The combined and age-specific GCS scoring method may be helpful in transitionally aged children or when age is uncertain (see Table 40-2).

The clinical features that localize the anatomic site of disturbed brain function are state of consciousness, pattern of breathing, pupillary size and reactivity, eye movements, and motor responses.[5]

Lethargy and obtundation are generally caused by mild depression of the cerebral hemispheres. Stupor and coma occur when hemispheric dysfunction is more extensive or when the diencephalon or upper brainstem is involved. Abnormalities in the dominant hemisphere have a greater effect on consciousness than those in the nondominant hemisphere.

RESPIRATORY EFFECTS

Hypothalamic and midbrain damage results in rapid, sustained, deep hyperventilation (*central neurogenic hyperventilation*). Injury to the medulla and the pons affects the respiratory centers and produces several different patterns: (1) *apneustic breathing,* with a prolonged pause at full inspiration; (2) *ataxic breathing,* which consists of random, ineffective, haphazard breaths and pauses without a predictable pattern; and (3) *primary alveolar hypoventilation* (Ondine's curse), a failure to breathe while sleeping, which is the failure of automatic breathing centers when asleep.

Cheyne-Stokes respirations, during which periods of hyperpnea alternate with periods of apnea, result from an extensive, usually bilateral, diencephalic disturbance with an intact brainstem.

The most common cerebral causes of respiratory insufficiency are increased ICP and drugs that depress brain function. Barbiturates are often used to put the brain into an inactive state to treat encephalopathies and intractable seizures (status epilepticus). Intubation and mechanical ventilation must be initiated before barbiturates are given.

PERSISTENT VEGETATIVE STATE

The terms *persistent vegetative state* and *neocortical death* are used interchangeably to describe patients who, after recovery from coma, return to a state of wakefulness without cognition. PVS is "a form of eyes-open permanent unconsciousness in which the patient has periods of wakefulness and physiological sleep/wake cycles, but at no time is the patient aware of him- or herself or the environment."[6] Brainstem

TABLE 40-3	CLASSIFICATIONS OF STUPOR AND COMA			
		Responds Appropriately to:		
Grade	State of Awareness	Name	Light Pain	Deep Pain
1	Drowsy, lethargic, indifferent; does not lapse into sleep	Yes	Yes	Yes
2	Stuporous; lapses into sleep; may be disoriented	No	Yes	Yes
3	Deep stupor; responds to deep pain	No	No	Yes
4	Does not respond to appropriate stimuli; possible decorticate and decerebrate posturing; retains deep tendon reflexes	No	No	No
5	Nonresponsive, flaccid, no deep tendon reflexes, apneic	No	No	No

functions such as respiration and circulation are intact, and with good nursing care, survival is indefinite. With intensive and aggressive therapy, patients tend to maintain basic vital signs but are usually technology dependent and have a poor quality of life.

PVS occurs in 12% of adults who survive nontraumatic coma but is probably less common in children. The usual causes, in order of frequency, are anoxia and ischemia, metabolic or encephalitic coma, and head trauma. Recovery is rare when the vegetative state has persisted for 1 month in adults. The prognosis may be better in children, although recovery after 3 months is unlikely.

The American Academy of Neurology has adopted the policy that all medical treatment, including the provision of nutrition and hydration, may be ethically discontinued when (1) a patient's condition has been diagnosed as a PVS, (2) it is clear that the patient would not want to be maintained in this state, and (3) the family agrees to discontinue therapy.[7]

REYE'S SYNDROME

Douglas Reye, an Australian pathologist, defined the clinical and pathologic features of Reye's syndrome in 1963. Reye's syndrome is not a primary neurologic disorder but if left untreated has fatal neurologic consequences. During later stages the neurologic care plan for Reye's syndrome is similar to that for other conditions producing increased ICP. Reye's syndrome involves multiple organ systems and is a combination of fatty infiltrates in the internal organs, especially in the liver, and progressive encephalopathy.[8]

Reye's syndrome is predominantly a pediatric disease occurring in infancy through adolescence, with males and females affected equally. It usually follows a febrile viral illness such as a respiratory tract infection, gastroenteritis, or chickenpox conditions usually caused by influenza B or varicella viruses. Epidemiologic studies have associated Reye's syndrome with the use of aspirin or other salicylates used to control flu-like symptoms during the initial illness.[9]

Stages. Mortality is related to the severity of the disease, which is classified by five stages (Table 40-4). Early diagnosis and treatment may also contribute to a decrease in mortality. Patients who move rapidly from Stage I to Stage III Reye's syndrome have been reported to have a poor prognosis, as have patients with an initial blood ammonia level greater than 300 mg/dl.[10]

Differential Diagnosis. Although it may be difficult to differentiate Reye's syndrome from other types of encephalopathy, it is important to consider this diagnosis when a patient presents with clinical symptoms of encephalopathy, especially when vomiting is present after a viral-type illness. Elevated serum ammonia and elevated liver enzyme levels are hallmarks of Reye's syndrome. Therefore the syndrome should be highly suspected in children who present with acute encephalopathy after a viral illness and who also have evidence of hepatic dysfunction.

Symptoms appear within 1 week after the onset of the viral illness and may initially include sudden onset of vomiting, a rash, and confusion with personality changes. As the encephalopathy becomes more acute, seizures may occur; the patient becomes lethargic, and lethargy frequently progresses to coma. During the first stages, neurologic status may be assessed by behavioral changes; however, coma progresses throughout Stages III to V. Hyperventilation usually occurs when the patient

TABLE 40-4	CLINICAL STAGES OF REYE'S SYNDROME			
Stage	Consciousness	Motor Response	Seizures	Other Features
I	Lethargy; responds to pain	None	None	Vomiting, rash, hepatic dysfunction, hyperventilation
II	Delirium, combativeness	None	None	Hepatic dysfunction, hyperactive reflexes, hyperventilation
III	Coma, decorticate rigidity, sluggish pupils, doll's eye reflex	None	None	Hepatic dysfunction, hyperventilation
IV	Coma, decerebrate rigidity, sluggish large pupils	No OR	Minimal	Hepatic dysfunction
V	Coma, flaccid, fixed pupils	No reflexes	Present	Respiratory arrest; serum ammonia >300 mg/ml

OR, Oculocephalic reflex.

becomes confused or combative, or both, and is reflected in ABG values, but metabolic acidosis may also be present. Staging of Reye's syndrome is accomplished by frequent neurologic examinations and monitoring of laboratory values.[11]

Treatment. Treating Reye's syndrome focuses on individual symptoms and supportive therapy. Patients in an intensive care unit (ICU) have frequent neurologic monitoring, which includes level of consciousness, reflex activity, and reactions to stimuli. Laboratory values include coagulation studies and blood urea nitrogen levels. Patients in Stages III to V require more intensive monitoring and treatment for the increased ICP, including arterial lines, mechanical ventilation with hyperventilation, hypothermia, osmotic diuretics (e.g., mannitol), and pentobarbital coma.[11]

INCREASED INTRACRANIAL PRESSURE

The patient whose condition has progressed to coma requires testing to determine the presence of increased ICP. Normal ICP is 4 to 13 mm Hg (50 to 180 mm H_2O), and normal CSF pressure is 5 mm Hg (100 mm H_2O). CT scan is used to evaluate the brain for evidence of fluid buildup, displacement of the brain, or displacement of the ventricles of the brain. Alternatively, direct pressure measurements may be obtained by LP or insertion of an intercerebral pressure monitor or ventricular catheter. Because these direct methods are invasive and potentially dangerous, CT is preferred, at least as a screening tool.

Increased ICP can be a life-threatening feature of an encephalopathy. CSF and blood acting on the brain and bony structures of the skull generate ICP. In the newborn and infant, measuring the head circumference and palpating the anterior fontanel allow rapid assessment of ICP. Bulging of the fontanels may be a key sign of increased ICP that requires a response by caregivers. Pulsations of the fontanels may occur normally at a frequency equal to the pulse rate. It is unusual for these pulsations to be of bounding force.

ANATOMIC CONSIDERATIONS

The size of a normal infant's skull is determined by its contents. The growing brain causes the skull to increase in size. Normal head growth in the term newborn is 2 cm per month for the first 3 months, 1 cm per month for the second 3 months, and 0.5 cm per month for the next 6 months. Excessive head growth resulting from separation of the cranial sutures is an important feature of increased ICP throughout the first year of life. When the sep-

aration of cranial sutures is no longer sufficient to decompress increased ICP, the infant becomes lethargic, does not take feedings, and vomits.

After infancy the skull can no longer increase in size, and the total pressure within the skull is caused by the size of its contents—the brain, CSF, and blood. The Monro-Kellie doctrine states that in a closed system, such as the skull, an increase in the size of one part requires compression of the other parts to maintain a constant ICP.[12] If the internal volume of the skull is 500 ml, for example, and the brain, blood, and CSF volume is 450 ml, then 50 ml of expansion volume remains in the skull. According to the Monro-Kellie doctrine, if the volume of these three components increases by more than 50 ml, compression of the skull contents occurs.[13] Because CSF and blood are almost incompressible at physiologic pressures, the compression will occur in the brain tissue.

CLINICAL FEATURES

Headache. A common symptom of increased ICP at all ages is headache, primarily caused by traction and displacement of intracranial arteries. When increased ICP is generalized, as from cerebral edema or obstruction of the ventricular system, headache is generalized and is more prominent in the morning on awakening. The pain is constant but varies in intensity. Coughing, sneezing, straining, and other maneuvers that transiently increase ICP exaggerate the headache. The quality of pain is often difficult to describe. Vomiting in the absence of nausea, especially on arising in the morning, is often a concurrent feature. With knowledge of the MOI, the clinician is able to assess the potential pathophysiologic impact on the patient.

Diplopia and Strabismus. Diplopia is characterized by double vision caused by a disruption of the extraocular muscles or the muscle nerves. Strabismus, caused by paralysis of one or both abducens nerves so that the eye cannot turn outward, is a relatively common feature of generalized increased ICP. Strabismus may be a more prominent feature than headache in children with increased ICP.

Papilledema. Papilledema is passive swelling of the optic disc caused by increased ICP. Examining the eye with an ophthalmoscope allows visualization of the disc. The edema is usually bilateral; unilateral edema suggests a mass lesion behind the affected eye. Early papilledema is asymptomatic, and the patient experiences transitory disturbances of vision only with advanced disease. Preservation of visual acuity differentiates papilledema from primary optic nerve disturbances, such as optic neuritis, in which blindness occurs early in the course of disease.[14]

As edema progresses, the optic disc swells and is raised above the plane of the retina, causing the disc margin to be obscured. Tortuosity of the veins also results. If the process continues, the retina surrounding the disc becomes edematous so that the disc appears greatly enlarged, and retinal exudate radiates from the fovea. Eventually the exudate clears; however, optic atrophy ensues and blindness may be permanent. Even if increased ICP is relieved during the early stages of disc edema, 4 to 6 weeks are required before the retina appears normal again.

Herniation.   Increased ICP may cause portions of the brain to shift from the normal location into other compartments, compressing structures already occupying that space. Such shifts may occur under the falx cerebri, through the tentorial notch, and through the foramen magnum.

LP is generally contraindicated in patients with increased ICP because of the concern that a change in fluid dynamics will cause herniation. LP is especially hazardous when pressure between cranial compartments is unequal. This prohibition is relative, and early LP is the rule in infants and children with suspected CNS infections, despite the presence of increased ICP. LP is also used to diagnose and treat increased ICP in pseudotumor cerebri.

MONITORING

Enthusiasm is declining for the continuous monitoring of ICP in children. Despite advances in technology, the effect of pressure monitoring on outcome is questionable. It is not indicated in children with hypoxic-ischemic encephalopathies and has marginal value in children with other types of encephalopathy.[5] The symptoms and prognosis of increased ICP depend more on the *cause* than on the level of pressure attained. Systemic arterial blood pressure should be monitored along with ABG values and oxygen saturation.

TREATMENT

Head Elevation.   Elevating the head of the bed 30 to 45 degrees above horizontal decreases ICP by improving jugular venous drainage. The head should also be kept in the midline position so that the vasculature on each side of the neck is not compressed. Systemic blood pressure is not affected, so the overall result is increased cerebral perfusion.

Hyperventilation.   ICP declines within seconds of beginning hyperventilation. The mechanism is vasoconstriction resulting from hypocarbia. The goal is to lower the partial pressure of arterial carbon dioxide ($PaCO_2$) from 40 to 25 mm Hg. Further reduction can result in cerebral ischemia and is contraindicated. Vasoconstriction is maintained as long as hyperventilation is continued. When hyperventilation is withdrawn, however, the vessels again dilate and blood flow returns to normal. To prevent a rebound effect, in which blood flow increases above baseline, hyperventilation should be withdrawn gradually.

Hyperventilation is achieved by endotracheal intubation or tracheostomy and mechanical ventilation. Use of hyperventilation should be limited to the first few hours of care to protect against rebound vasoconstriction and increased ICP.

Pneumonia.   In addition to the risks of damage to the tracheal mucosa and development of tracheoesophageal fistula, tracheal intubation or tracheostomy carry the risk of *ventilatory-associated pneumonia* (VAP). A strong correlation exists between nosocomial pneumonia and aspiration of oropharyngeal and gastric emesis. These fluids travel down the open airway past the epiglottis, which is propped open by the tracheal tube. In older children with a cuffed tube, these secretions pool between the larynx and the top of the cuff, poised to flow down the airway into the lungs. The use of continuous positive airway pressure (CPAP) may help prevent this type of pneumonia by increasing the pressure gradient between the airway and the oral cavity, thus restraining the fluid flow.[15]

Osmotic Diuretics.   Mannitol and glycerol are the two osmotic diuretics most widely used in the United States. *Mannitol* is given intravenously as a 20% solution. It does not cross the blood-brain barrier and remains in the plasma, creating an osmotic gradient that draws water from the brain into the capillaries. Onset of action is within 30 minutes, with the peak effect generally lasting 1 to 2 hours after administration. The effect is short term, and infusions must be given three to six times each day to keep serum osmolality at less than 320 mOsm/L (320 nmol/L). Repeated infusions of mannitol cause dehydration as well as fluid and electrolyte imbalances. Rebound may occur when mannitol is discontinued.

Glycerol is given intravenously as a 10% solution three to four times per day. The onset of action is within 30 minutes, with the effect usually lasting 24 hours or longer. As with mannitol, dehydration and electrolyte disturbances may follow repeated administration. Rebound is less prominent than with mannitol.

Corticosteroids.   Corticosteroids, such as dexamethasone, are effective in the treatment of vasogenic edema. Onset of action is 12 to 24 hours, and peak action may be delayed even longer. The mechanism is uncertain, but cerebral blood flow (CBF) is not affected. Corticosteroids are most useful for reducing edema surrounding mass lesions. These agents are not beneficial in cytoxic edema, as seen after hypoxic-ischemic injuries.

Hypothermia. Hypothermia decreases CBF and is frequently used concurrently with pentobarbital coma. Body temperature is generally kept between 27° and 30° C. It is not clear how much improvement is gained by hypothermia in addition to other measures that decrease CBF, such as head elevation, hyperventilation, and pentobarbital coma.

In a recent well-designed study in adults, 392 subjects (16 to 65 years of age), all sustaining closed head trauma, were randomly assigned to a control (normothermic) group or an experimental group (hypothermia within 6 hours of injury to 33° C for 48 hours), with the patients in each group having similar injuries by type and severity and mean age. The outcomes were poor in 57% of each group (vegetative state, disability, or death). The death rates were 27% in the normothermic subjects and 28% in the hypothermic group. The hypothermic subjects also had more complications and more hospital days but fewer episodes of increased ICP. The authors concluded that hypothermia was not advantageous in this group of patients.[16]

Although the applicability of this study to neonates and children is not known, it suggests a need to examine practices for safety, efficacy, and cost-benefit considerations. Greater body surface/body mass ratio, heat loss, and temperature control must be considered in the head-injured infant and child. Hypothermia applied early in the course of injury may be protective in that the lower body temperature may prevent or slow production of cellular end products usually released after tissue injury.[17]

Pentobarbital Coma. Barbiturates such as pentobarbital reduce CBF, decrease edema formation, and lower the brain's metabolic rate. These effects do not occur at anticonvulsant plasma concentrations but require brain concentrations sufficient to produce a burst-suppression pattern on the EEG. Pentobarbital coma is particularly useful in patients with increased ICP resulting from disorders of mitochondrial function, such as Reye's syndrome.

Ventilatory Maneuvers. The increase in intrathoracic pressure that occurs during positive-pressure ventilation may impede cerebral venous return and increase ICP. Therefore the patient should be mechanically ventilated with the lowest peak pressures possible, and a minimal level of positive end-expiratory pressure (PEEP) should be used to maintain adequate ventilation. Chest physical therapy may also exaggerate the ICP and should be used with caution. Suctioning may increase the ICP and should be performed minimally and must be preceded with oxygen-supplemented hyperventilation. It is also important to prevent Valsalva maneuvers and coughing.

STATUS EPILEPTICUS

The condition in which seizures are repetitive and do not stop spontaneously is called status epilepticus. Seizures begin with abnormal neurons that discharge repeatedly. Repetitive seizures increase the body's requirements for adenosine triphosphate, which in turn increases metabolic needs for oxygen and glucose. Apnea, hypoxemia, and hypoglycemia may result, along with increased oxygen consumption and lactic acidosis. Anoxic injury to other organs, as well as cardiac arrhythmias and traumatic injuries (e.g., tongue laceration, concussion), may also occur.

Status epilepticus is a medical emergency that requires prompt attention. A controlled airway must be established immediately, and oxygen and mechanical ventilation should be rapidly available. Venous access is established, and blood is withdrawn for measurement of glucose and electrolyte levels. Other tests, such as anticonvulsant concentrations and toxicology screens, are performed as indicated. After blood is withdrawn, an IV infusion of saline solution is started for the administration of anticonvulsant drugs. An IV bolus of a 50% glucose solution is also administered.

The ideal drug for treating status epilepticus is one that acts rapidly, has a long duration of action, and does not produce sedation. Diazepam and lorazepam are widely used for this purpose, but their duration of action is brief. In addition, children who receive IV benzodiazepines after a prior load of barbiturate often experience respiratory depression.

IV *phenytoin* is a preferable drug because of its long duration of action. A slow rate of administration is necessary to avoid causing cardiac arrhythmias. Phenytoin is usually effective unless status epilepticus is caused by severe acute encephalopathy. If phenytoin fails, the patient should be given a loading dose of phenobarbital. This dose may be repeated, but respiratory depression may ensue. If this fails, pentobarbital coma is a reasonable next treatment.

The patient should be intubated and mechanically ventilated in the ED and then transferred to the ICU. After an arterial line is placed, the patient's blood pressure, cardiac rhythm, body temperature, and oxygen saturation should be monitored.

To achieve pentobarbital coma in the patient with status epilepticus, boluses of pentobarbital are infused until a burst-suppression pattern appears on the ECG monitor, which is continuously recording. Hypotension occurs with large doses, and vasopressor support may be necessary. The coma can be safely maintained for 3 days; longer periods may cause pulmonary edema. The EEG should be checked several times each day for the burst-suppression pattern. The coma can be lifted every 48 to 72 hours to see whether the seizures have stopped. Mechanical ventilation should be continued until the patient regains consciousness and can spontaneously support ventilation and until reflexive airway protection is adequate.

REFERENCES

1. Newsbytes. *Case Manager* 2001; 12(1):6.
2. Laskowski-Jones L, Salati DS: Responding to pediatric trauma. *Nursing* 2001; 31(9):37-42.
3. Strange GG et al: *Pediatric emergency medicine.* New York. McGraw-Hill, 1998.
4. Ghajar J, Hariri RJ: Management of pediatric head injury. *Pediatr Clin North Am* 1992; 39:1093-1126.
5. Plum F, Posner JB: *The diagnosis of stupor and coma,* ed 3. Philadelphia. Davis, 1980.
6. American Academy of Neurology: Position of the American Academy of Neurology on certain aspects of the care and management of the persistent vegetative state patient. *Neurology* 1989; 39:125-126.
7. LeRoux PD, Jardine DS, Loeser JD: Pediatric intracranial pressure monitoring in hypoxic and nonhypoxic brain injury. *Child Nerv Syst* 1991; 7:34-39.
8. Reye RDK, Morgan G, Baral J: Encephalopathy and fatty degeneration of the viscera: a disease entity in childhood. *Lancet* 1963; 2:749-752.
9. Surgeon General's advisory on the use of salicylate in Reye's syndrome, 1981: Reye's syndrome and salicylate usage. *MMWR* 1982; 31:51.
10. Corey L, Rubin RJ, Hattwick MAW: Reye's syndrome: clinical progression and evaluation of therapy. *Pediatrics* 1977; 60:708-714.
11. Crocker JFS, Bagnell PC: Reye's syndrome: a clinical review. *CMA J* 1981; 124:375-383.
12. Morki B: The Monro-Kellie hypothesis: applications in CSF volume depletion. *Neurology* 2001; 56(12):1746-1748.
13. Greitz D et al: Pulsatile brain movement and associated hydrodynamics studied by magnetic resonance phase imaging: the Monro-Kellie doctrine revisited. *Neuroradiology* 1992; 34(5):370-380.
14. Fenichel GM: *Clinical pediatric neurology,* ed 3. Philadelphia. Saunders, 1977; pp 93-95.
15. Finder JD, Yellon R, Charron M: Successful management of tracheotomized patients with chronic saliva aspiration by use of constant positive airway pressure. *Pediatrics* 2001; 107(6):1343-1345.
16. Clifton GL et al: Lack of effect of hypothermia after acute brain injury. *N Engl J Med* 2001; 22:556-563.
17. Narayan RK: Hypothermia for traumatic brain injury: a good idea proven ineffective. *N Engl J Med* 2001 (editorial); 344(8): 602-603.

CHAPTER **41**

Submersion Injury in Children

Jerril Green
Debra Fiser

Submersion injury may be defined as the physiologic alterations that result from any submersion event. This definition includes *drowning,* which is generally accepted as resulting in death within 24 hours after submersion, and *near drowning,* which is suffocation with loss of consciousness due to submersion, but with survival for at least 24 hours. *Aspiration of water* during submersion without loss of consciousness is also a submersion injury.[1,2]

INCIDENCE

Drowning claims 6000 to 8000 lives per year in the United States.[3] Children less than 5 years of age account for about 40% of these deaths, and older children, 5 to 20 years, contribute another 20%.[1,4] Near drowning results in another 8000 hospitalizations per year in U.S. children. Submersions result in more than 30,000 emergency department (ED) visits annually. Submersion injury is a worldwide phenomenon with varying frequency in all cultures. The peak incidence for boys and girls is up to age 4 years and usually involves accidental submersion during a lapse in responsible supervision. Males have a second peak incidence at 15 to 19 years related to alcohol use and other risk-taking behavior.[3,5]

Many factors affect the exact nature and circumstances surrounding submersion events. Males are more affected than females at all ages. Black children drown at a rate of 4.5 per 100,000, most frequently in freshwater lakes and ponds, whereas white children are affected at a rate of about 2.5 per 100,000 and more often drown in pools.[4,6] Pool drowning is more common in warm climates. Freshwater lake, pond, and river drowning occurs more frequently in colder climates. Saltwater drowning is obviously a coastal phenomenon, but

90% of all coastal submersions are in freshwater bodies, including pools.

Inadequate or lapsed supervision of infants and toddlers results in accidental submersion in bathtubs and other small amounts of water.[1,6] These incidents should always raise suspicion of child abuse and neglect.[7] Alcohol use is frequently a factor in submersion injury, including intoxicated adult and adolescent victims and intoxicated caregivers of young children.[8] Adolescent submersions have the highest mortality rate at about 70%, despite being witnessed by adolescent peers about 60% of the time.[5,9] Drowning in younger children is witnessed in less than 20% of cases, although 80% to 85% of victims are in the care of responsible supervision.

Efforts to prevent deaths from drowning are focused on improved supervision, proper fencing around pools, and cardiopulmonary resuscitation (CPR) training. As with all accidental injuries, prevention is the only effective means of reducing morbidity and mortality. This is especially true of submersion injury because outcomes are often poor regardless of therapy.[10]

PATHOPHYSIOLOGY

After submersion, conscious humans have a period of voluntary apnea or breath holding. If submersion continues, partial pressure of carbon dioxide (Pco_2) rises sufficiently to produce voluntary or involuntary respiration, or hypoxemia produces loss of consciousness followed by involuntary respiration. In 85% of submersions, aspiration of the liquid medium occurs at this time, whereas in the remaining 15%, sufficient laryngospasm occurs to prevent aspiration. In either case the resulting hypoxia quickly produces unconsciousness, apnea, and finally cardiac arrest. The duration of this hypoxia and cardiac arrest is the primary determinant of outcome after a submersion injury.[3,6,11]

Severe hypoxic brain injury is the cause of death in the vast majority of drownings and results in the most significant morbidity associated with near drowning. Prolonged hypoxia begins a cycle of neuronal death, cerebral edema, increased intracranial pressure (ICP), further neuronal death, worsened cerebral edema, and so forth.[3] Hypoxic brain injury may result in disability across a wide spectrum of severity, from subtle cognitive and motor impairment to persistent vegetative state and brain death.[11]

Lung injury with adult respiratory distress syndrome (ARDS) and pulmonary edema is a common feature of submersion injury, in both saltwater and freshwater submersion. However, the exact mechanisms and evolution of the lung injury may be subtly different. Surfactant is affected in both freshwater and saltwater submersions by alteration of its functional properties, or dilution and washout. Loss of functional surfactant results in atelectasis, decreased lung compliance, and intrapulmonary shunting. Aspiration of a large volume of hypertonic fluid such as seawater may actually draw fluid from the vascular and interstitial spaces along this osmotic gradient, causing an accumulation of fluid in the alveolar space.[3] Foreign material in the lung, including water contaminated with microorganisms, plant matter, sand, and other debris, elicits an inflammatory response. All these insults lead to transudation of proteinaceous material into the alveoli and progression of the pathologic changes consistent with ARDS.

Other factors may contribute to the lung pathology associated with submersion. Aspiration of acidic stomach contents produces a superimposed aspiration pneumonitis. A number of microorganisms have been associated with pneumonia in submersion victims.[6,11-15] *Aeromonas* is the most common organism associated with submersion (Box 41-1). Although the concentration of chlorine in family pools is probably benign when aspirated, higher concentrations of industrial and household chemicals may produce airway swelling and may result in systemic toxicity when absorbed from alveoli. Debris suspended in aspirated fluid can obstruct larger conducting airways and require bronchoscopy for removal. The clinician must always consider what was in the water in which the patient was submersed.

Differences in the fluid and electrolyte changes seen in saltwater submersion and freshwater submersion have been stressed in the past. The hypertonicity of saltwater aspirated into the lung may

---

BOX 41-1

ORGANISMS ASSOCIATED WITH PNEUMONIA IN SUBMERSION VICTIMS

Aeromonas species
Burkholderia pseudomallei
Pseudallescheria boydii
Streptococcus pneumoniae
Pseudomonas aeruginosa
Francisella philomiragia
Legionella species
Chromobacterium violaceum
Klebsiella pneumoniae
Neisseria mucosa
Aspergillus species
Staphylococcus aureus

From Ender PT, Dolan MJ: Pneumonia associated with near-drowning. *Clin Infect Dis* 1997; 25:896-907.

cause an influx of fluid from the vascular space, resulting in intravascular volume depletion and hemoconcentration with hypernatremia. Aspirated freshwater may have the opposite effect on fluid balance, producing volume overload, hyponatremia, and hemolysis due to decreased serum osmolality. This has been demonstrated experimentally, but other studies have shown that the volumes of fluid actually aspirated during human drowning are inadequate to produce these effects. Case series of human drowning have failed to show significant electrolyte abnormalities. Electrolyte disturbances are most likely secondary to large volumes of swallowed water.[1,16,17]

Other organs are affected in submersion injury. Aspiration of water produces a reflex pulmonary vasoconstriction with pulmonary hypertension and impaired cardiac output. Hypoxia and acidosis may lead to cardiac dysrhythmia and impaired myocardial function both at the time of the injury and later as the clinical course progresses. Multiple organ failure is the result of hypoxic-ischemic injury secondary to cardiopulmonary arrest and includes renal and hepatic dysfunction and disseminated intravascular coagulation. Multiple organ failure is uncommon in submersion injury in the absence of significant neurologic injury.

CLINICAL COURSE

The first important point in the clinical course is rescue at the scene. The severity of the victim's injury depends on the duration of submersion, the temperature of the water, and the presence of other injuries or illness. Brief submersion may result in only mild respiratory distress with coughing and vomiting from aspirated and swallowed water. More prolonged submersion results in loss of consciousness, respiratory arrest, and finally cardiac arrest (Fig. 41-1).

Rapid and appropriate response at the scene may result in the return of spontaneous heart rate and respirations; however, resuscitation is likely to be prolonged if hypoxia has been present for several minutes. Even if spontaneous respiration is restored, the need for continued assisted ventilation should be expected. In submersion injury, asystole is the first recorded rhythm in 55% of patients, ventricular tachycardia or fibrillation in 29%, and bradycardia in 16%.[18] The presence of hypothermia, hypoxia, and acidosis makes treatment of dysrhythmia more difficult and their recurrence more likely, until these factors are corrected. Once a perfusing rhythm has been restored, inotrope and pressor therapy may be needed along with volume resuscitation.

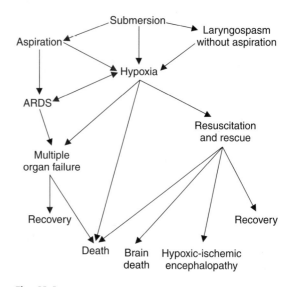

Fig. 41-1

Clinical course of submersion injury.

The presence of other illness or injury should be considered. Diving accidents and falls may result in head and cervical spine injury. Submersion may actually be secondary to a preexisting or unknown medical condition such as seizures, cardiac dysrhythmia, or intoxication. Child abuse should be considered in any household submersion such as bathtubs.[7]

The clinical course in the ED is a continuation of the prehospital resuscitation and stabilization. Victims who are minimally affected with no history of loss of consciousness, no altered mental status, and no respiratory signs and symptoms may be observed for a period of hours in the ED and discharged home if no complications arise. Patients with any degree of respiratory compromise, history of need for rescue breathing, or loss of consciousness should be admitted to the hospital even if stable in the ED, because both neurologic injury and lung injury may progress over the first hours to days. In more severely affected victims, progression of cerebral edema with resultant increased ICP should be anticipated through the first 3 to 5 days. Seizures may occur and should be treated aggressively.

In patients who have a functional recovery, as the cerebral edema resolves, a slow return of neurologic function occurs over weeks to months. Pulmonary edema and ARDS may progress rapidly in the first 24 hours and may be a major management problem, but as with most causes of ARDS, the patient usually responds to careful and aggressive respiratory management. Lung infiltrates, fever, and leukocytosis are common after submersion injury and do not necessarily indicate an infectious pneumonia. If infiltrates worsen and fevers persist, however, pneumonia should be considered. Myocardial dysfunction requiring inotropic support may persist for days after a significant hypoxic insult. Recurrent dysrythmia may also occur but is less likely after the initial hypothermia, acidosis, and hypoxia are corrected. Although it is not especially common in submersion injury, acute renal failure and other organ dysfunction may occur after cardiac arrest from any cause and may require any level of support, including hemodialysis or continuous venovenous hemofiltration and dialysis.

Some degree of hypothermia is almost always present after a significant submersion. When warming is attempted, cardiac dysrhythmia, electrolyte abnormalities, and hypotension due to vasodilation should be anticipated.

TREATMENT

Treatment begins with resuscitation at the scene. Airway management and rescue breathing should begin before the victim is out of the water if possible, and CPR should be started as soon as an adequate surface is available. Care should be taken to stabilize the cervical spine if there is any risk of cervical spine injury. If the airway is not patent, standard maneuvers should be used to clear the airway. The Heimlich maneuver, however, should not be used to remove water from the lung. Any efforts to remove water from the lungs, including the Heimlich maneuver, only delay initiation of effective rescue efforts.[2,19]

As soon as trained emergency personnel are available, more advanced techniques should be used, including endotracheal intubation, positive-pressure ventilation, intravenous (IV) access, and resuscitation drugs if needed. Cardiac monitoring and management of dysrhythmia should be priorities. Hypothermia is difficult to reverse in the field, but every effort should be made to prevent further cooling during the resuscitation.

In the ED, stability of the airway and adequacy of ventilation should be assessed. Arterial blood gas (ABG) sampling gives critical information regarding oxygenation, ventilation, and the severity of acidosis. If ventilation is adequate, treatment of metabolic acidosis with tromethamine (THAM) or sodium bicarbonate is advisable. Cardiac dysrhythmias should be treated but may be refractory in the presence of significant hypothermia. Tissue perfusion and blood pressure should be assessed to determine the adequacy of cardiac output. Intravascular volume expansion may be needed in the presence of postarrest myocardial dysfunction,

and inotrope and vasopressor therapy should be used if needed.

If hypothermia is present, aggressive warming should begin immediately and should proceed as rapidly as possible. Increasing core body temperature is the goal, and simple warming of the skin surface alone should be avoided. Warmed IV fluid and ventilator gases should be used. Irrigation of the stomach, urinary bladder, and peritoneal cavity with warmed saline is effective and relatively low risk. Irrigation of the pleural space with warmed saline has the advantage of warming the central circulation but may compromise ventilation and oxygenation. Extracorporeal bypass is the most effective means of increasing body temperature, and in cases of extreme hypothermia this technique should be used early in the course of management.[20]

Once the initial resuscitation and stabilization is complete, intensive care unit (ICU) treatment is primarily supportive. Neurologic injury is the most serious consequence of submersion injury and should be the focus of care. As with any hypoxic brain injury, ICP monitoring and aggressive pressure-directed therapy do not change the outcome in submersion injury and are not recommended. Basic measures to decrease ICP should be employed, as follows:

1. Elevate the head 15 to 30 degrees.
2. Maintain the head in the midline.
3. Avoid hypercarbia.
4. Ensure adequate blood pressure and oxygenation.
5. Provide adequate sedation and analgesia.
6. Avoid volume overload and hypovolemia.
7. Avoid hyperglycemia.

Seizures and fever should be aggressively treated because both will worsen intracranial hypertension. As the patient becomes more stable, early involvement of physical and occupational therapy is appropriate. The need for extensive rehabilitation is common.

Acute respiratory distress in the context of submersion injury is managed as in any other setting. Adequate positive end-expiratory pressure (PEEP) is the key element of the ventilator strategy, along with minimizing tidal volume and peak inspiratory pressure to reduce the risk of secondary lung injury. Use of artificial surfactant is usually not necessary; although providing temporary improvement in lung function, surfactant probably does not change outcome. There is no specific indication for early use of corticosteoids in submersion injury.

Fever and chest radiograph changes should be expected early in the chemical course of submersion injury. However, these changes occur without bacterial pneumonia and should not necessarily be treated as infection. Early treatment or prophylactic treatment with antibiotics increases the likelihood of later infection with resistant organisms. If strong evidence for bacterial pneumonia develops, such as persistent fever, evolving focal infiltrates on chest radiograph, or positive bacterial cultures for likely organisms, antibiotic therapy should be tailored to treat those organisms most likely in this setting or those found in bacterial culture.[3,11,18]

Foreign bodies should be suspected if lung changes are focal or if segmental air trapping is present. Bronchoscopy may be needed to evaluate and remove foreign bodies. Other organ failure must be managed as well. Acute renal failure may require hemodialysis. Inotropic support may be needed for days after the injury, but myocardial dysfunction is usually not the primary concern in these patients.

Attention to the emotional and social needs of the parents is important. Anger and guilt are common because most submersions are preventable accidents. Family dysfunction should be anticipated and appropriate referral made when needed.[18]

OUTCOME

The topic of outcome fits comfortably at the end of most clinical discussions. With submersion injury, however, outcome may have been more appropriately discussed first. As with any condition that includes hypoxic-ischemic brain injury as a primary part of its pathology, submersion injury has a tragically poor prognosis. It is within the context of this poor prognosis that decisions and management plans are made. A frequent question is, "How far should treatment go?" Much of the most recently published literature on submersion injury attempts to answer this difficult question.

Traditionally, all critically ill patients including submersion victims are approached with aggressive resuscitation and life support so that each potential survivor has the best chance of eventual recovery. This minimizes the risk of allowing a potential survivor to die because maximal support has been withdrawn. This approach, however, also ensures that many patients whose best possible outcome is persistent vegetative state (PVS) will also survive. A strategy to fully support only those patients with a high likelihood of intact neurologic recovery decreases the chance of survival in PVS and decreases the associated cost, but potential intact survivors are likely to be lost. PVS and death are generally accepted as undesirable outcomes. Complete and functional recovery are generally considered acceptable outcomes Reliably predicting which patients will experience which outcome

early in the clinical course would be very helpful in counseling families regarding prognosis and in making decisions about initiating or withdrawing expensive or limited therapeutic resources.

Many variables are associated with poor outcome in submersion injury, including duration of submersion, pH less than 7.00, water and body temperature, need for CPR after arrival in the ED, depth of coma, hyperglycemia, and lack of response to resuscitation. Habib et al predicted outcome in a retrospective case series.[21] Patients arriving in the ED comatose and pulseless had a uniformly poor outcome, whereas those with a pulse and blood pressure in the ED completely recovered. In addition, patients who remained comatose longer than 200 minutes had poor outcomes, and those who were not comatose had normal recovery.

In 1995, Graf et al reported that a combination of four variables—presence of coma, absent pupillary light reflex, male gender, and elevated blood glucose concentration—accurately predicted an unfavorable outcome.[22] Another retrospective review by Christensen et al supports the use of a pH of less than 7.00, the need for CPR in the ED, and that apnea and coma in the ED are predictors of poor outcome. Using these predictors, other investigators have shown that a number of patients predicted to have a poor outcome instead had an unexpectedly good outcome, and limitation of support for these patients would have resulted in the loss of potential survivors.[23] A 48-hour period of observation in the pediatric ICU, in addition to the variables seen in the first hours after submersion, may improve our ability to predict outcome. Persistent coma after 48 hours is consistent with poor outcome.

Our understanding of outcome in cold water submersion is largely anecdotal. The likelihood of improved outcome when frigid water is involved, however, should be a factor in decision making for these patients.[2]

REFERENCES

1. DeNicola LK et al: Submersion injuries in children and adults. *Crit Care Clin* 1997; 13:477-502.
2. Golden FS, Tipton MJ, Scott RC: Immersion, near-drowning, and drowning. *Br J Anaesth* 1997; 79:214-225.
3. Weinstein MD, Krieger BP: Near-drowning: epidemiology, pathophysiology, and initial treatment. *J Emerg Med* 1996; 14:461-467.
4. Centers for Disease Control: Fatal injuries to children: United States, 1986. *MMWR* 1990; 39:442-451.
5. Wintemute GJ: Childhood drowning and near-drowning in the United States. *Am J Dis Child* 1990; 144:663-669.
6. Fields AI: Near-drowning in the pediatric population. *Crit Care Clin* 1992; 8:113-129.

7. Lavelle JM et al: Ten-tear review of pediatric bathtub near-drownings: evaluation for child abuse and neglect. *Ann Emerg Med* 1995; 25:344-348.

8. Orlowski JP: Adolescent drownings: swimming, boating, diving and scuba accidents. *Pediatr Ann* 1988; 17:125-132.

9. Quan L et al: Ten-year study of pediatric drownings and near-drownings in King County, Washington, *Pediatrics* 1989; 83:1035-1040.

10. Spack L et al: Failure of aggressive therapy to alter outcome in pediatric near-drowning. *Pediatr Emerg Med* 1997; 13:98-102.

11. Levin DL et al: Drowning and near-drowning. *Pediatr Clin North Am* 1993; 40:321-336.

12. Mangge H et al: Late-onset miliary pneumonitis after near drowning. *Pediatr Pulmonol* 1993; 15:122-124.

13. Wilichowski W et al: Fatal *Pseudallescheria boydii* panencephalids in a child after near-drowning. *Pediatr Infect Dis J* 1996; 15:365-370.

14. Ender PT et al: Near-drowning-associated *Aeromomas* pneumonia. *J Emerg Med* 1996; 14:737-741.

15. Ender PT, Dolan MJ: Pneumonia associated with near-drowning. *Clin Infect Dis* 1997; 25:896-907.

16. Modell JH: Serum electrolyte changes in near-drowning victims. *JAMA* 1985; 253:253-257.

17. Modell JH et al: Clinical course of 91 consecutive near-drowning victims. *Chest* 1976; 70:231.

18. Fiser DH: Near-drowning. *Pediatr Rev* 1993; 14:148-151.

19. Rosen P, Stoto M, Harley J: The use of the Heimlich maneuver in near drowning: Institute of Medicine report. *J Emerg Med* 1995; 13:397-405.

20. Steiner RB et al: Pediatric extracorporeal membrane oxygenation in posttraumatic respiratory failure. *J Pediatr Surg* 1991; 26:1011-1015.

21. Habib DM et al: Near-drowning: morbidity and mortality. *Pediatr Emerg Med* 1996; 12:255-258.

22. Graf WD et al: Predicting outcome in pediatric submersion victims. *Ann Emerg Med* 1995; 26:312-319.

23. Christensen DW, Jansen P, Perkin RM: Outcome and acute care hospital costs after warm water near drowning in children. *Pediatrics* 1997; 99:715-721.

CHAPTER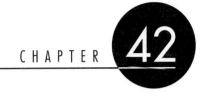

Pediatric Poisoning

Michael P. Czervinske

Since the introduction of child-resistant containers in the early 1970s, there has been a fourfold decrease in mortality from childhood exposure to poisons. Despite this decreased mortality, poisoning continues to be one of the most persistent pediatric medical emergencies and still accounts for 5% of all accidental childhood deaths.[1-3]

There are two classifications of childhood poisoning: accidental and intentional. *Accidental poisoning* accounts for 80% to 85% of cases, most frequently occurs in children 1 to 5 years of age, and is usually a single-substance ingestion.[1] As a general rule, unintentional poisoning victims are brought for medical treatment within 1 hour of the ingestion. *Intentional poisoning* makes up the other 15% to 20% of cases, is more likely to occur in older children or adolescents, and involves multiple substances. In addition, a delay in seeking medical treatment is more likely with intentional poisoning victims, as is the likelihood of hospitalization and intensive care.[3-5]

EPIDEMIOLOGY

Features that make a substance a potential risk for accidental ingestion in the young child age group are (1) bright and colorful, (2) similar appearance to candy or other familiar safe substances, (3) good smell or taste, and (4) easy access, such as storage under the kitchen counter. Fortunately, child-resistant packaging, safety caps, and safety locks help dissuade the child from opening some substances. Additionally, many of the ingestions reported in this age group are of insufficient quantity to cause harmful effects.

The more common substances involved in serious childhood poisoning include acetaminophen, salicylates (e.g., aspirin), theophylline, tricyclic antidepressants, iron, organophosphates, and hydrocarbons. Although there are concerns specific to each substance ingested, the initial stabilization procedure is the same.[6]

TABLE 42-1	TOXIDROMES
Clinical Manifestations	**Possible Toxin**
Agitation, hallucinations, dilated pupils, dry skin, flushed color	Anticholinergics
Slow respirations, pinpoint pupils, coma	Opiates
Salivation, urination, lacrimation, pulmonary congestion	Organophosphates
Coma, convulsions, cardiac arrhythmias	Tricyclic antidepressants
Vomiting, fever, hyperpnea	Salicylates
Sleepiness, slurred speech	Barbiturates
Ataxia (without alcohol on breath)	Tranquilizers

Modified from Mofenson HC, Greensher J: The unknown poison. *Pediatrics* 1974; 54:336.

If possible, it is helpful to determine the identity and quantity of the agent ingested. A detailed history from the parents or guardians may be extremely valuable. If a history does not reveal this information, patterns of physical findings referred to as *toxidromes* may aid in the diagnosis (Table 42-1).[7] Certain screening laboratory values, such as serum electrolytes, glucose, blood urea nitrogen, arterial blood gases, and measured hemoglobin oxygen saturation, can also be helpful in identification of the toxin. The patient's belongings may also hold clues as to the type of ingestion.

GENERAL MANAGEMENT

Clearly, the best treatment is prevention. After the ingestion, however, the mainstay of therapy is stabilization of the respiratory and cardiovascular systems, ranging from simple monitoring to a full resuscitation. Good venous access is necessary for drug and fluid administration in any patient who has ingested a toxic substance.

Once hemodynamic and respiratory stabilization has been achieved, the main goals are to (1) limit further drug absorption, (2) enhance elimination, and (3) directly antagonize drug activity. These maneuvers have variable success; thus the most important therapy remains continued respiratory, cardiovascular, and neurologic support.[8]

Initial *decontamination* consists of removing any remaining agent from the child's skin and mouth. This includes removing all chemical- or toxin-saturated clothing. Further toxin absorption can be limited by gastrointestinal decontamination

through the removal or dilution of gastric contents and the use of gastric adsorptive agents.

Emesis is one of the fastest methods of eliminating poison from the stomach. Administering an emetic agent, such as syrup of ipecac, causes forced vomiting. Contraindications for emesis are patients with a decreased level of consciousness, convulsions, and ingestion of hydrocarbons or other caustic agents. Because of inconsistent results in the amount of poison recovered as a result of emesis, ipecac administration is no longer recommended as a first-line treatment in the emergency department (ED).[1,3] Timing of administration is crucial, and studies show that home administration of ipecac effectively induces emesis and reduces the amount of initial absorption of certain poisons.[9,10] In severe poisoning cases, however, no evidence indicates that emesis improves clinical outcome, and emesis may delay other, more effective decontamination procedures.[3,9,10]

Gastric lavage is the mechanical removal of gastric contents. A large-bore orogastric tube is placed, and large quantities of fluid, usually normal saline, are infused and withdrawn in the hope of removing any remaining poison. The major complication of gastric lavage is aspiration; less common complications include esophageal and gastric perforation. To minimize the risk of aspiration, any patient with a decreased level of consciousness should undergo endotracheal intubation before gastric lavage. Ingestion of a caustic agent is a contraindication to lavage. As with emesis, gastric lavage may delay other, more effective decontamination procedures. Lavage is no longer the standard of care. It is limited in the amount of drug recovery, does not remove solid matter such as undissolved pills, shows little evidence of improved outcomes, and may be psychologically harmful.[11]

Activated charcoal is the most common adsorptive agent. In addition to binding the toxin in the stomach, it is useful in absorbing drugs that undergo enterohepatic recirculation. Charcoal administration is effective without gastric emptying and in single or multiple doses. As such, it is an acceptable alternative for poison first-aid treatment in the home.[3,12] Charcoal is relatively safe, but complications include vomiting, diarrhea, constipation, and aspiration. The main contraindication to its use is the presence of any form of gastrointestinal obstruction. Safer, more concentrated, and smaller dose preparations are beginning to appear on the market for use by emergency services, in hospital departments, and as home first aid, which will help ease administration to small children by panicked parents.

Cathartic agents (e.g., sorbitol, magnesium citrate) are osmotically active agents that cause diarrhea and thus are used to eliminate toxins. The success of these methods is highly variable and depends on the timing between the ingestion and the therapy, the type of toxin, and the amount of toxin ingested. As such, cathartics are no longer recommended in the poison treatment of children.[3]

Whole-bowel irrigation with polyethelene glycol is a potential decontamination procedure targeting the intestinal tract. Bowel irrigation appears helpful with sustained-release medications and metals such as iron, lead, and lithium.[3] Bowel irrigation has the potential to decontaminate substances that resist gastric decontamination and to be effective when charcoal is not, as with these metals.

In some poisoning cases, advanced techniques are necessary to enhance excretion of the toxin. Methods to enhance toxin elimination include forced diuresis, alteration of urinary pH, hemodialysis, peritoneal dialysis, hemoperfusion, and the use of specific drug antagonists that either block the drug at its site of action or enhance its elimination from the circulation.[8,13] Forced diuresis can be effective in the excretion of substances that have primary renal elimination. This is accomplished by administering large volumes of intravenous (IV) fluid and diuretic agents. Contraindications to this include renal failure and cardiovascular instability. Some toxins are more readily soluble and excreted in alkaline solutions (e.g., salicylates, phenobarbital). In these situations, administering sodium bicarbonate alkalinizes the urine to a pH of 7 to 8. Hemodialysis, hemoperfusion, and peritoneal dialysis remove toxins across either a membrane gradient or an adsorptive surface. The effectiveness of these therapies is highly dependent on the specific characteristics of the ingested substance. Drugs that are more amenable to extracorporeal removal have small molecular size, low lipid solubility, small levels of protein binding, and a low volume of distribution.[13]

There are also specific antibodies, antidotes, or other reversal agents for some toxic substances. Examples include naloxone for opioid overdose, digoxin-specific Fab antibody for the treatment of digoxin overdose, flumazenil for benzodiazepine overdose, antivenins for snake and spider bites, and fomepizole for antifreeze ingestion.[8,14-16] These reversal agents do not preclude the need for continued supportive care.

As stated earlier, the best treatment for poisoning is prevention. In fact, the treatment for all ingestions must continue after discharge from the intensive care unit (ICU). Efforts must be made to ensure that poisoning will not recur. Depending on the situation, treatment of any young child who has ingested a toxic substance might also involve a social service evaluation. Any older child or adolescent who has ingested such a substance should receive a psychiatric consultation.

COMMON POISONING AGENTS

ORGANOPHOSPHATES

Organophosphates were originally developed for use in chemical warfare but are now used as insecticides and herbicides. Poisoning can occur through skin exposure or inhalation, but serious injury is usually secondary to ingestion. Organophosphates work by inactivating an important step in neurotransmission: nerve conduction and muscle contraction induced by acetylcholine. *Acetylcholine* activity terminates when it is hydrolyzed by *acetylcholinesterase,* which is found in the neurons, neuromuscular junctions, and red blood cells. Organophosphates inhibit the activity of acetylcholinesterase by bonding to it and forming a stable inactive complex. The resultant lack of acetylcholinesterase causes an initial increase in the availability of acetylcholine and an overstimulation of neurotransmission. With the continued inhibition of acetylcholinesterase, however, the acetylcholine stores become depleted, and neurotransmission ceases. Normal hydrolysis of acetylcholine returns only when new acetylcholinesterase is produced.

Muscarinic signs and symptoms of organophosphate poisoning result from the accumulation of acetylcholine at the receptor. These include bronchoconstriction, increased bronchial secretions, decreased respiratory drive, weakened respiratory muscles, decreased heart rate, confusion, ataxia, seizures, salivation, lacrimation, diarrhea, paralysis, and urination. Most of the fatality and long-term morbidity are from anoxia secondary to respiratory failure.

Decontamination depends on the route of entry. If it is topical, remove all contaminated clothing and place in an impermeable plastic container. Thoroughly scrub the patient using liberal amounts of a soap and water solution. If the organophosphate is ingested, consider gastric lavage, and deliver activated charcoal for decontamination. Use caution because vomited organophosphates can be absorbed through the skin of health care personnel.

Once decontamination is complete, administer *atropine* and anticholinergic agents to antagonize the cholinergic stimuli.[17,18] In patients with severe twitching and muscle weakness, also administer *pralidoxime,* a cholinesterase reactivator, to stimulate the production of new acetylcholinesterase. Give atropine every 10 to 30 minutes until the muscarinic effects abate. Pralidoxime is mixed with saline and infused over a longer period, depending on the patient's age, and repeated in 8-hour intervals as required. Although the symptoms of ingestion can last up to 7 days, therapy is typically required for only 24 to 48 hours.[17,19,20]

One respiratory medication that affects acetylcholine is theophylline. As such, avoid theophylline-containing preparations during the management of symptoms. Additionally, many insecticides are dissolved in a hydrocarbon solution. Treatment for hydrocarbon pneumonitis may be required in addition to organophosphate poison treatment. Other supportive therapy may include treating subsequent pneumonias, treating pulmonary edema, or supporting respiratory efforts with mechanical ventilation.

TRICYCLIC ANTIDEPRESSANTS

Tricyclic antidepressants (TCAs) are among the most widely prescribed drugs in the United States, which increases the child's risk of exposure. TCAs may be used in the treatment of a parent and are increasingly used in the pediatric population for treatment of hyperactivity, sleep disorders, and enuresis. TCAs compose 25% of all serious overdoses, with a mortality rate of 3%. The level of toxicity will correlate with the dose, but in both accidental and intentional ingestions, the dose is rarely known. TCAs are well absorbed orally, and 98% of the drug is bound to glycoproteins and concentrated in the tissues. This binding is highly pH dependent and limits the availability of free drug. TCAs are very lipid–soluble, so methods to eliminate them from the body's water compartment by diuresis and hemofiltration are unsuccessful. Metabolism takes place in the liver, and many metabolites are active.[21]

Patients may be asymptomatic for up to 12 hours after ingestion. Central nervous system (CNS) manifestations include seizures, coma, confusion, ataxia, and central respiratory depression. The cardiovascular derangements account for the majority of the fatal complications. TCAs cause direct myocardial depression with hypotension and conduction abnormalities. Conduction is slowed, with increased PR and QRS intervals and an increase in the refractory period, which causes a decrease in the heart rate. The width of the QRS complex is often used as an indicator of the severity of toxicity, with a QRS width of greater than 160 msec being an indication for concern and an important marker of mortality.[21]

There is no known antidote for TCA poisoning, and support of the cardiorespiratory system takes precedence over all other treatment. Treatment includes immediate decontamination with charcoal administration and other supportive measures. Phenytoin, isoproterenol, and pacemakers have

been used to increase the heart rate, with lidocaine for arrhythmias and norepinephrine or dopamine infusion for severe hypotension. Alkalinization of pH to a range of 7.50 to 7.55 through administration of sodium bicarbonate boluses decreases the amount of free drug and may help reduce the cardiac effects.[13,22,23]

HYDROCARBONS

Hydrocarbons include substances such as the petroleum distillates, gasoline, kerosene, turpentine, lighter fluid, and other products such as pine oil. Many of these products are in the home and are therefore easily available for accidental ingestion. Hydrocarbons are present in products such as lamp oil, spot remover, pine cleaner, furniture polish, nail polish, and glue. Eighty-four percent of hydrocarbon ingestions occur in children younger than 3 years of age. Because these products have a bad taste, large quantities are not usually ingested, with the typical ingestion less than 30 ml of fluid. However, hydrocarbon products may produce gasping, gagging, choking, vomiting, and aspiration as a result of the foul taste.

Very little systemic absorption of hydrocarbons from gastrointestinal exposure occurs, despite severe gastrointestinal irritation. The major toxic exposure is directly to the lungs secondary to aspiration or through vaporization of solvents during ingestion or vomiting. The low surface tension and viscosity of hydrocarbons allow a very small amount in the lung to spread over a large area. Less than 1 ml may produce severe necrotizing pneumonia, pulmonary edema, and even death. Because some of these compounds are highly volatile, vapors may also produce inebriation or alterations in mental status.

The primary symptoms are respiratory distress with dyspnea, tachypnea, intercostal retractions, fever, and cyanosis. Chest auscultation may reveal wheezing and rales. The chest radiograph is consistent with an aspiration pneumonitis with poorly defined patchy infiltrates. Repeat the film in 4 to 6 hours if the initial chest film is negative. The symptoms may appear within 30 minutes of the aspiration or may appear as late as 12 to 24 hours. Symptoms are then usually progressive over the following 24 to 48 hours. They usually peak within 2 to 3 days, after which the patient will either go on to a full pulmonary recovery or experience secondary chronic lung injury by the tenth day after ingestion. CNS findings such as somnolence, coma, and seizures are rare and are secondary to the pulmonary injury with hypoxia and acidosis. Gastrointestinal irritation may produce diarrhea, blood-tinged stools, nausea, and vomiting.

The only treatment is supportive. Airway control and mechanical ventilation may be required due to either respiratory distress or unconsciousness. Additionally, administer oxygen and continuous positive airway pressure (CPAP) for hypoxemia and pulmonary edema. Bronchodilators may be helpful in patients with bronchospasm. Exercise caution with bronchodilator administration because hydrocarbons predispose the myocardium to fibrillation, and catecholamine administration may worsen this effect. Steroids and antibiotics have no proven efficacy. However, antibiotics are administered if fever and leukocytosis increase after 2 to 3 days, indicating a secondary bacterial infection. If conventional supportive measures are ineffective, extracorporeal membrane oxygenation (ECMO) has been used with success in pediatric patients for hydrocarbon pneumonitis.[3]

In the case of hydrocarbon ingestion, gastric emptying is generally contraindicated because it increases the risk of aspiration. However, the procedure may be necessary if very large quantities of the compound are ingested, or if they contain other dangerous products, such as heavy metals or organophosphates. Some of the aromatic hydrocarbons (e.g., toluene, benzene) are toxic to other organ systems and should be removed if possible. Complications found in patients who survive hydrocarbon ingestion include the formation of pneumatoceles and pulmonary function abnormalities.[13,24]

SALICYLATES

The incidence of salicylate ingestion has substantially decreased since the institution of safety packaging and the limitation of the number of tablets allowed per bottle of pediatric flavored aspirin. However, salicylate ingestion continues to be a common cause of poisoning among children and adolescents. Two forms of salicylate poisoning occur, from chronic ingestion and from acute ingestion of large quantities.

Salicylates have a number of toxic effects, including direct stimulation of the respiratory center, uncoupling of oxidative phosphorylation, inhibiting the Krebs cycle, inhibiting lipid and amino acid metabolism, stimulating gluconeogenesis, interfering with normal glucose homeostatic mechanisms, and interfering with hemostatic mechanisms. The result is a respiratory alkalosis, metabolic acidosis from lactate and ketosis, water and electrolyte loss, bleeding disorders, hypoglycemia from chronic ingestion, and hyperglycemia from acute ingestion. Unlike adults, children quickly lose their respiratory drive and may present with both metabolic and respiratory acidosis by the time they reach the hospital.[25]

The clinical signs and symptoms of salicylate poisoning include nausea and vomiting, tachypnea, hyperpnea, hyperpyrexia, dizziness, coma, disorientation, seizures, shock, and pulmonary edema. The vomiting, sweating, pyrexia, and hyperventilation lead to dehydration and electrolyte imbalance. Doses greater than 150 mg/kg are toxic, and doses greater than 500 mg/kg are lethal. Neurologic changes serve as a marker of the severity of toxicity. Nomograms of serum salicylate levels versus the hours since ingestion are available to help estimate the severity of the poisoning. With chronic exposure, many of the symptoms appear at much lower doses. The toxic effects are usually reversible with time. Patients who succumb usually die from CNS injury secondary to hypoglycemia, hypoperfusion, or intractable seizures.[25,26]

Treatment includes replacing fluids and electrolytes, correcting the metabolic acidosis, and administering glucose. Administer activated charcoal, even if medical treatment has been delayed. Lavage may help eliminate some drug but also increases absorption, misses undissolved tablets, and delays activated charcoal administration.[27] With toxic or lethal doses, hemodialysis helps to accelerate elimination and provides a means for rapidly correcting fluid and electrolyte disorders. When severe CNS depression and loss of cardiorespiratory function occur, mechanical ventilation is required.

ACETAMINOPHEN

As acetaminophen has gained acceptance as a substitute for salicylates as the standard pediatric antipyretic and analgesic, more toxic acetaminophen ingestions have been reported. Accidental overdose and intentional overdose occur with similar frequency. Acetaminophen is one of the most common substances used in suicide attempts by adolescents. Intentional overdose ingestion tends to result in a higher toxic serum level than does accidental ingestion.[28] Frequently, multiple agents are ingested during a suicide attempt. Often, with multiple substance ingestions, acetaminophen is overlooked because of its common use and seemingly harmless nature compared with other toxic substances ingested. Serial doses of amounts greater than the recommended dosage may result in overdose. Among children, however, serious complications rarely occur, unless such exposures are from habitual use of large quantities of acetaminophen. Intentional ingestion and delay in treating acetaminophen poisoning after 24 hours are the most frequent causes of severe complications among pediatric patients.[28]

Dissolved acetaminophen rapidly absorbs from the gastrointestinal tract and reaches peak serum concentrations within 60 minutes. Many pediatric overdoses are secondary to the ingestion of the liquid form of acetaminophen, making it readily absorbable after ingestion. The liver rapidly metabolizes acetaminophen, converting a small portion to the toxic metabolite N-acetyl-p-benzoquinonimine. Normally, glutathione conjugates this metabolite in the liver and is excreted in the urine. Toxicity occurs when the available glutathione stores are overwhelmed, and N-acetyl-p-benzoquinonimine accumulates in the liver, causing hepatocellular necrosis. Ingestion of greater than 150 mg/kg in children is considered toxic.

There are four stages of clinical manifestations identified for toxic acetaminophen ingestion.[29] *Stage 1* occurs within 12 to 24 hours of the ingestion. Symptoms include nausea, vomiting, anorexia, diaphoresis, and malaise. Liver function tests are within the normal range. During *Stage 2,* apparently a latent period, the patient's symptoms usually improve. However, serum aspartate (glutamic-oxaloacetic) transaminase, serum alanine (glutamic-pyruvic) transaminase, bilirubin, and prothrombin levels may begin to rise. *Stage 3* occurs 72 to 96 hours after ingestion and is the period of peak hepatotoxicity. Nausea, vomiting, and anorexia reappear. Liver function tests become markedly abnormal, and depending on the degree of hepatic injury, there is evidence of bleeding, jaundice, and encephalopathy. Despite the severity of this stage, less than 2% of all ingestions progress to fulminant and irreversible hepatic failure. Liver transplant may be indicated when this degree of hepatic injury occurs. *Stage 4* is resolution and occurs 7 to 8 days after ingestion. Within 6 months, there is no evidence of chronic hepatic injury.[29]

Treatment includes gastric decontamination and administration of N-*acetylcysteine* (NAC), a glutathione precursor. If NAC is administered within 16 hours of the ingestion, there is a marked decrease in morbidity and mortality. A nomogram plotting serum acetaminophen concentration versus time can be used to identify patients with potentially toxic ingestions who may benefit from NAC therapy.[30] Drug levels must be obtained at least 4 hours after ingestion, to allow serum concentrations to peak, and no more than 24 hours after ingestion, because levels rapidly decrease and toxic effects occur within 24 hours.[13,29,31] In children ages 1 to 5, draw blood levels at 2 hours after ingestion if they ingest the elixir form of acetaminophen. If acetaminophen levels are not readily available, it is recommended that treatment be instituted.[13,30] Oral NAC boluses are required for 3 days or until symptoms abate, whichever is longer. NAC can be mixed with juice or diet cola to offset some of the bad taste. High-dose

IV metoclopramide may alleviate violent emesis episodes if given before administering the loading bolus of NAC.[32] Administering activated charcoal after 1 hour postingestion offers no benefit.[28] In severe overdose or if oral NAC administration becomes impossible, IV NAC is recommended.

THEOPHYLLINE

Formerly, theophylline was the most frequently prescribed medication for the treatment of reactive airway disease. Despite less use than in the past, theophylline is still prescribed and commonly available within the home. Both short-acting and long-acting preparations are rapidly absorbed within the gastrointestinal tract. Metabolism takes place in the liver with excretion in the urine. The therapeutic index for theophylline is very narrow, with little difference between clinically effective drug levels of 10 to 20 µg/dl. Due to its complex pharmacokinetics, changes in diet or interaction with other drugs may accidentally lead to toxic drug levels in children taking theophylline. Children appear to tolerate higher serum levels than do adults, and often, severe complications will not develop until the level is greater than 60 to 70 µg/dl.

Toxicity involves multisystem findings. In pediatrics, gastrointestinal symptoms such as nausea and vomiting usually precede more serious complications. CNS manifestations include confusion, agitation, lethargy, obtundation, and intractable seizures. Although seizures usually occur at higher serum concentrations, their occurrence is determined by the rate of rise of the theophylline level. The most common cardiac complication is supraventricular tachycardia. However, ventricular ectopy may occur with more serious ingestions. Finally, theophylline can result in metabolic derangements such as hypokalemia, hyperglycemia, and metabolic acidosis.

Therapy is largely supportive. First and foremost, airway protection is required if toxic levels are high enough to precipitate seizures. Theophylline is a drug that undergoes enterohepatic recirculation, and thus all ingestions are treated with multiple doses of activated charcoal. Metoclopramide or another antiemetic helps to prevent vomiting after charcoal administration. Bowel irrigation may also be a helpful adjunct if theophylline levels continue to rise after sufficient charcoal administration. Because theophylline has a large volume of distribution throughout the extracellular fluid, it is amenable to removal using hemoperfusion or hemodialysis. Hemoperfusion is much more effective than dialysis, and indications are based on the absolute theophylline level and the presence of serious complications.[34,35]

IRON

The accidental ingestion of iron-containing compounds is one of the 10 most common ingestions in children younger than 5 years of age. Most commercially available tablets contain 20% elemental iron by weight. Ingestion of less than 20 mg/kg of elemental iron is considered *nontoxic,* 20 to 60 mg/kg is *mildly toxic,* greater than 60 mg/kg is *severely toxic,* and greater than 200 mg/kg is *lethal.*[36] Multivitamin ingestion is the most common cause of toxicity. Interestingly, while life-threatening ingestion of iron remains a possibility, most children only develop mildly toxic levels.[37] One of the reasons may be the difference in compounding between the children's chewable multivitamins and adult vitamin supplements.

Iron is readily absorbed from the gastrointestinal tract and binds to transferrin, a carrier protein, in the blood. With acute intoxication the binding capacity of transferrin is exceeded, and free iron circulates in the blood. The gastrointestinal tract, cardiovascular system, liver, and CNS are directly affected by the unbound iron. Most children will begin to show symptoms within 6 hours of ingestion.

Clinical manifestations are grouped into four phases.[36] The *initial phase* is the result of corrosive effects on the gastrointestinal tract and includes nausea, vomiting, abdominal pain, and diarrhea, which can progress to severe hemorrhagic gastroenteritis. In severe poisonings, the cardiac output falls secondary to venous pooling of blood and hypovolemia from an ongoing capillary leak. This in turn results in poor tissue perfusion and a metabolic acidosis. Up to 25% of all deaths from iron ingestion occur in this phase. In less serious ingestions, there is *Phase 2,* which consists of recovery. Some patients will then go on to complete recovery, but for others, Phase 2 is only temporary and they go on to *Phase 3,* which is characterized by the reemergence of severe gastrointestinal symptoms, cardiovascular collapse, and CNS depression. Hepatic dysfunction due to the accumulation of iron in the liver becomes evident and is characterized by abnormal liver function tests, jaundice, hypoglycemia, and coagulopathy. Patients surviving Phase 3 are at risk for the development of *Phase 4,* which is characterized by bowel stenosis secondary to healing gastrointestinal lesions. The chronic sequelae of iron intoxication include hepatic cirrhosis, chronic bowel obstruction, and CNS damage.

Serum levels can predict toxicity, but they must be obtained within 2 to 6 hours after ingestion because iron is rapidly cleared from the plasma. Treatment includes immediate IV hydration, gastric emptying, and chelation therapy. Most children will vomit spontaneously after exposure. Ipecac may be given to initiate gastric emptying only if it can be given within the first 30 minutes after exposure and if there is adequate consciousness for airway protection. Activated charcoal is ineffective, so dilution with gastric lavage may help minimize stomach mucosal lesions.

Intensive whole-bowel irrigation is the treatment of choice.[38] Bowel irrigation decreases iron absorption and reduces the potential for direct mucosal damage in the gastrointestinal tract. Endoscopy and a surgery consult may be required if emptying does not successfully dislodge the iron tablet particles, which could lead to bowel perforation and potentially fatal sepsis.

Desferoxamine, a chelating agent that binds to free and stored iron and is then excreted in the urine, should be administered in any potentially toxic iron ingestion. Administering desferoxamine parenterally accelerates iron excretion, although IV administration is the most effective route to counter the toxic effects of iron. Chelation therapy is continued until measured iron levels return to normal.

ALCOHOLS

Ethyl alcohol ingestion in children presents with a triad of symptoms that differ from adults and adolescents. If ethanol concentration exceeds 50 to 100 mg/kg, the child may present with coma, hypothermia, and hypoglycemia. In children, metabolic acidosis may also be present. Intubation and mechanical ventilation should be instituted if the airway or respirations are compromised. For seizures, which most often result from severe hypoglycemia, treat empirically with IV glucose. Anticonvulsants may also be necessary. Alcohol is absorbed quickly from the gastrointestinal tract, so charcoal is rarely effective. In older children and adolescents, administer charcoal if concomitant ingestion of other toxic agents is likely with an intentional overdose situation. In the event of sustained high blood levels of ethanol, hemodialysis is indicated.

Treatment and symptoms of *isopropyl alcohol* ingestion are similar to those for ethanol. However, isopropyl alcohol is much more intoxicating, and its main toxic effects are myocardial depression and shock. A major metabolite is acetone, which does not produce acidosis. The presence of ketone bodies in the urine without acidosis differentiates isopropyl alcohol ingestion from diabetes. Hemodialysis is indicated with severely toxic isopropyl levels or with any sign of cardiovascular instability. An additional consideration in children is that aggressive topical application of isopropyl alcohol to control fever may lead to toxic levels.[39]

REFERENCES

1. Litovitz TL et al: 1997 Annual report of the American Association of Poison Control Centers Toxic Exposures Surveillance System. *Am J Emerg Med* 1998; 16:443-497.
2. Steinhart CM, Pearson-Shaver AL: Poisoning. *Crit Care Clin* 1988; 4:845-872.
3. Liebelt EL, DeAngelis CD: Evolving trend and treatment advances in pediatric poisoning. *JAMA* 1999; 282:1113-1115.
4. Walton WW: An evaluation of the Poison Prevention Packaging Act. *Pediatrics* 1982; 69:363-370.
5. Frazer LE, Lovejoy FH, Crone RK: Acute poisoning in a children's hospital: a 2-year experience. *Pediatrics* 1986; 77:1441-1451.
6. Kilham HA: Hospital management of severe poisoning. *Pediatr Clin North Am* 1981; 27:603-612.
7. Mafenson HC, Greenshar J: The unknown poison. *Pediatrics* 1984; 54:336-342.
8. Fine JS, Goldfrank LR: Update in medical toxicology. *Pediatr Clin North Am* 1992; 39:1031-1051.
9. American Academy of Clinical Toxicology, European Association of Poison Centres and Clinical Toxicologists: Position statement: ipecac syrup. *Clin Toxicol* 1997; 35:699-709.
10. Bond GR: Home use of syrup of ipecac is associated with a reduction in pediatric emergency department visits. *Ann Emerg Med* 1995; 25:338-343.
11. American Academy of Clinical Toxicology, European Association of Poison Centres and Clinical Toxicologists: Position statement: gastric lavage. *Clin Toxicol* 1997; 35:711-719.
12. American Academy of Clinical Toxicology, European Association of Poison Centres and Clinical Toxicologists: Position statement: single dose charcoal. *Clin Toxicol* 1997; 35:721-741.
13. Steinart CM, Pearson-Shaver AL: Poisoning. *Crit Care Clin* 1998; 4:845-872.
14. Antman EM et al: Treatment of 150 cases of life-threatening digitalis intoxication with digoxin-specific Fab antibody fragments. *Circulation* 1991; 81:1744-1752.
15. Karavokiros KA, Tsipis GB: Flumazenil: a benzodiazepine antagonist. *DICP* 1990; 24:976-981.
16. Brent J et al: Fomepizole for treatment of ethylene glycol poisoning. *N Engl J Med* 1999; 340:832-838.
17. O'Malley M: Clinical evaluation of pesticide exposure and poisonings. *Lancet* 1997; 349:1161-1166.
18. Bardin PG, Van Eeden SF: Organophosphate poisoning: grading severity and comparing treatment between atropine and glycopyrrolate. *Crit Care Med* 1990; 18:956-959.
19. Zwiener RJ, Ginsburg CM: Organophosphate and carbonate poisoning in infants and children. *Pediatrics* 1988; 81:121-126.
20. Farrar HC, Wells TG, Kearns GL: Use of continuous infusion of pralidoxime for treatment of organophosphate poisoning in children. *J Pediatr* 1990; 116:658-661.
21. Henry JA: Epidemiology and relative toxicity of antidepressant drugs in overdose. *Drug Safety* 1997; 16:374-390.
22. Braden NJ, Jackson JE, Walson PD: Tricyclic antidepressant overdose. *Pediatr Clin North Am* 1986; 33:287-297.
23. Liebelt EL: Targeted management strategies for cardiovascular toxicity from tricyclic antidepressant overdose: pivotal role for alkalinization and sodium loading. *Pediatr Emerg Care* 1998; 14:293-298.
24. Klein BL, Simon JE: Hydrocarbon poisonings. *Pediatr Clin North Am* 1986; 33:411-419.
25. Snodgrass WR: Salicylate toxicity. *Pediatr Clin North Am* 1986; 33:381-391.
26. Yip L, Dart RC, Gabow PA: Concepts and controversies in salicylate toxicity. *Emerg Med Clin North Am* 1994; 12:351-364.
27. Vertrees JE, McWilliams BC, Kelly HW: Repeated oral administration of activated charcoal for treating aspirin overdose in young children. *Pediatrics* 1990; 85:594-597.
28. Alander SW et al: Pediatric acetaminophen overdose: risk factors associated with hepatocellular injury. *Arch Pediatr Adolesc Med* 2000; 154:346-350.
29. Rumack BH: Acetaminophen overdose in children and adolescents. *Pediatr Clin North Am* 1986; 33:691-701.
30. Rumack BH, Matthew H: Acetaminophen poisoning and toxicity. *Pediatrics* 1975; 55:871-876.
31. Zed PJ, Krenzelok EP: Treatment of acetaminophen overdose. *Am J Health Syst Pharm* 1999; 56:1081-1091.
32. Wright RO et al: Effect of metoclopramide dose on preventing emesis after oral administration of *N*-acetylcysteine for acetaminophen overdose. *J Toxicol Clin Toxicol* 1999; 37:35-42.
33. Perry HE, Shannon MW: Efficacy of oral versus intravenous *N*-acetylcysteine in acetaminophen overdose: results of an open-label, clinical trial. *J Pediatr* 1998; 132:149-152.
34. Heath A, Knudsen K: Role of extracorporeal drug removal in acute theophylline poisoning. *Med Toxicol Adv Drug Exp* 1987; 2:294-308.
35. Minton NA, Henry JA: Treatment of theophylline overdose. *Am J Emerg Med* 1996; 14:606-612.
36. Banner W, Tong TG: Iron poisoning. *Pediatr Clin North Am* 1986; 33:393-409.
37. Anderson BD et al: Retrospective analysis of ingestions of iron containing products in the United States: are there differences between chewable vitamins and adult preparations? *J Emerg Med* 2000; 19:255-258.
38. Tenenbein M: Whole bowel irrigation in iron poisoning. *J Pediatr* 1987; 111:142-145.
39. Arditi M, Killner MS: Coma following use of rubbing alcohol for fever control. *Am J Dis Child* 1987; 141:237-238.

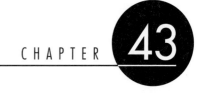

CHAPTER 43

Disorders of the Pleura

Paul C. Stillwell

The pleura surrounds the outer surface of the lungs and the mediastinum as well as the inner surface of the chest wall and the diaphragm. This sliding surface provides minimal resistance between the lung and chest wall during respiratory movements. The pleural "space" is generally only a *potential* space with a normal fluid volume of 1 to 5 ml. The pleural membranes, however, are permeable to both liquid and gas; an estimated 5 to 10 L of fluid per day crosses from the parietal pleura to the visceral pleura in a normal adult.[1]

The pleura lining the chest wall, mediastinum, and diaphragm is called the *parietal pleura.* Its blood supply is from the systemic circulation, and its venous drainage is through the azygos, hemiazygos, and internal mammary veins. The *visceral pleura* covers the surface of the lungs, with its blood supply from the pulmonary arteries or bronchial arteries and its venous drainage through the pulmonary veins. In the healthy subject a *positive* (+) 9 cm H_2O of hydrostatic pressure drives fluid from the parietal pleura capillary bed into the pleural space, and a minus (−) 10 cm H_2O hydrostatic pressure favors absorption of fluid into the visceral pleura capillaries.

Several factors determine the balance of pleural fluid. The *intracapillary* hydrostatic pressures tend to drive fluid out of the capillaries, whereas the *pericapillary* hydrostatic pressures tend to counterbalance this force. The *plasma* colloid osmotic pressures exert a force to retain fluid within the capillaries, whereas the *pericapillary* colloid osmotic pressure tends to favor fluid movement out of the capillaries. Changes in the balance of these forces determine how much fluid is retained within the pleural space. Increased capillary permeability, decreased intravascular colloid osmotic pressure, and increased pulmonary venous pressure are common contributors to accumulation of fluid in the pleural space. Obstructed lymphatic drainage is another factor that favors accumulation of fluid in the pleural space.[1-3] *Chylothorax* is an uncommon cause of pleural effusion in children, except when they have undergone thoracic surgery with interruption of the thoracic duct.[4]

In healthy individuals the chest radiograph seldom demonstrates any pleural fluid. An estimated 4% of normal adults may have minor radiographic evidence of pleural fluid if the films are taken in the decubitus or Trendelenburg's position. A pleural effusion has typical radiographic features (Figs. 43-1 and 43-2). Ultrasound examination or computed tomography (CT) of the chest may be more sensitive in identifying small accumulations of pleural fluid.[5] The CT scan may also provide more information about the underlying lung parenchyma than is available from the plain chest radiograph, especially when large amounts of fluid are present. However, ultrasound and CT usually are not required to identify a clinically significant effusion. Ultrasound may be used to facilitate the thoracentesis.

PLEURAL EFFUSIONS

Pleural effusions may be suspected clinically when there is an area of decreased-intensity breath sounds on chest auscultation with an associated dullness to percussion over the corresponding area.[6,7] Comparison with the contralateral lung can help distinguish the normal boundaries of the thoracic cavity unless the effusion is bilateral. The patient may experience few symptoms from a small pleural effusion but usually has symptoms of respiratory distress with larger accumulations. Chest pain, chest wall tenderness, dyspnea, and pain with coughing or deep breathing are often associated with pleural effusions. In addition to decreased intensity of breath sounds with dullness to percussion, crackles may be appreciated immediately

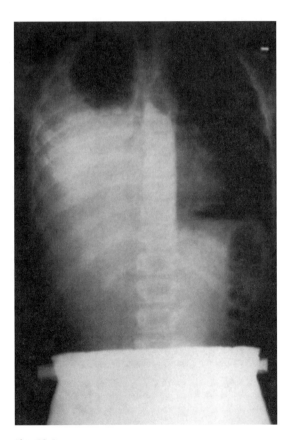

Fig. 43-1

Upright chest radiograph of child with large pleural effusion on the right. The majority of the hemithorax is white with a rounded superior margin (meniscus sign). The diaphragm is obscured, and there are air bronchograms in the right lower lung zone. This parapneumonic effusion was caused by *Haemophilus influenzae* pneumonia.

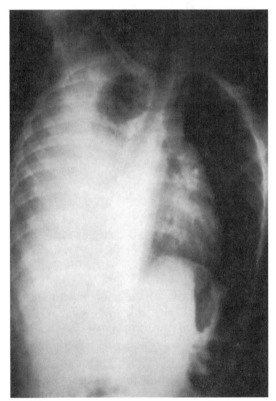

Fig. 43-2

Right-side-down decubitus radiograph of child in Fig. 43-1. The fluid is more prominent on the lateral chest wall margin, indicating free movement of the fluid in the pleural space.

superior to the effusion, where the lung may be involved with underlying pneumonia, or normal lung may be partially compressed by the effusion. The location of these findings may change when the position of the patient is changed if the fluid is flowing free within the pleural space. The respiratory care practitioner may be the first to detect the findings of a pleural effusion during auscultation.

When an effusion is found on a chest radiograph, the initial diagnostic procedure to determine its cause is often a *thoracentesis*.[2,6-8] This procedure consists of placing a needle into the pleural space and withdrawing the pleural fluid for both diagnostic and therapeutic purposes. Occasionally an underlying disease such as overt heart failure or the nephrotic syndrome will leave little doubt as to the cause and nature of the pleural effusion, thereby decreasing the need for thoracentesis.[6-8] When thoracentesis has been performed, the fluid is generally categorized as either a transudate or an exudate based on specific criteria (Table 43-1 and Box 43-1). Certain diagnoses are associated with transudates and exudates in children (Boxes 43-2 and 43-3).[2,6-9]

If a pleural effusion is detected on the chest radiograph, consideration should be given to thoracentesis in all cases. This procedure is usually performed by a physician. In pediatrics, thoracentesis is not usually done without the assistance of nurses or respiratory care practitioners, or both, to provide stabilization, comfort, and reassurance to the patient. They also handle the drained pleural fluid and monitor the child's cardiovascular status during the procedure. The procedure is performed under sterile conditions, so care must be taken that the physician and assistants do not inadvertently contaminate the field or the specimens. The child is usually given parenteral sedation as well as local analgesia to the skin and subcutaneous space. The patient is positioned so that the fluid will be in a dependent position; thus the favored position is either sitting and leaning forward or the lateral decubitus position. The area of dullness should be carefully percussed in an effort to insert the needle in the spot most likely to provide return of fluid.

Ultrasound can be helpful to direct the needle into the area most likely to yield fluid. Care must be taken to pass the needle over the rib to prevent injury to the neurovascular bundle, which generally traverses the inferior margin of the ribs. While the needle is being advanced, gentle suction is applied to the attached syringe so that fluid rapidly flows into the syringe when the effusion is entered. Care must be taken to keep the system closed so that no air is sucked back into the pleural space on

TABLE 43-1	SEPARATING TRANSUDATE FROM EXUDATE	
Measurement	Transudate	Exudate
Protein (g/dl)	<3	>3
Effusion–serum protein	<0.5	>0.5
Lactate dehydrogenase (units/L)	<250	>250
Effusion–serum lactate dehydrogenase	<0.6	>0.6

BOX 43-2

CAUSES OF TRANSUDATIVE PLEURAL EFFUSIONS

Congestive heart failure
Nephrotic syndrome
Cirrhosis or liver failure
Acute glomerulonephritis
Hypoproteinemia
Myxedema
Sarcoidosis
Peritoneal dialysis

BOX 43-1

COMMON PLEURAL FLUID ANALYSES

Total protein
Lactate dehydrogenase
Cell counts and differential cell count
pH
Cytology
Studies for infection
• Gram's stain, bacterial culture
• Acid-fast stain and culture
• Fungal stains and culture
Glucose
Amylase

BOX 43-3

CAUSES OF EXUDATIVE PLEURAL EFFUSIONS

Parapneumonic effusion or empyema
Pulmonary embolism
Neoplasm
Collagen vascular disease
Trauma
Drug hypersensitivity
Lung transplant rejection
Chylothorax
Gastrointestinal diseases
Lymphatic disease
Postcardiac injury syndrome

inspiration. Fluid is withdrawn as long as it drains easily.[8]

Complications of thoracentesis include pneumothorax, hemorrhage, and infection. A *pneumothorax* may be created by nicking the lung with the needle or by not maintaining a closed system and allowing air to enter the chest cavity. *Hemorrhage* may result from nicking a vessel during needle insertion.[8] If sterile technique is not followed, *infection* can be introduced into the pleural space, or the sample sent for microbiology evaluation will be contaminated, or both. Other complications include an allergic reaction to the sedating medicines or hypoventilation resulting from oversedation. It is important for the respiratory care practitioner to be familiar with these complications because he or she is likely to be monitoring the patient's cardiovascular status during the procedure and will be able to auscultate the chest during the procedure without breaking the sterile field. Any deterioration in the patient's clinical status during the procedure should be immediately called to the attention of the physician performing the procedure so that it can be determined whether it is safe to continue.

Several laboratory tests are performed on the pleural fluid to identify the cause of effusion.[2,9] Perhaps the most common cause of pleural effusion in pediatrics is a *parapneumonic effusion*,[10,11] which indicates that the pleural fluid is from an underlying pneumonia. Although typically a bacterial pneumonia, parapneumonic effusion can also result from a virus, fungus, or parasite or from tuberculosis (Box 43-4). If the pneumonia extends to infect the pleural space as well, the effusion is then termed an *empyema*. This entity is diagnosed by the presence of frank pus in the pleural space, by a positive culture of the pleural fluid, by a positive Gram's stain of the pleural fluid,[10] or if the white cell blood count (WBC) is greater than 15,000/mm³.[9,10]

In adult patients the presence of an empyema suggests that a chest tube should be placed to prevent subsequent fibrous entrapment of the lung.[2,12] In children it is less clear that entrapment usually follows empyema, and several physicians elect to perform repeated thoracentesis or to wait for the antibiotic therapy to resolve both the pneumonia and the empyema.[11-13] Regardless of chest tube drainage, prolonged antibiotic therapy is often administered (e.g., 4 to 6 weeks). The availability of long-term indwelling intravenous (IV) catheters allows transition of IV therapy from hospital to home. The duration of combined IV and oral antibiotics necessary for successful resolution is not well defined. Eventual healing with normal lung function and a normal chest radiography is the rule for children, although the chest radiograph may not return to normal for several months. Therefore the decision to place a chest tube or perform a limited thoracotomy in the child with an empyema should be individualized based on the anticipated cause of the empyema and the initial clinical response to aggressive antibiotic therapy.

Other causes besides infectious entities should be considered; malignancy, acute chest syndrome from sickle cell disease, and postsurgical effusions can also create exudative effusions.[10]

In addition to protein and lactate dehydrogenase (LDH) levels, cell counts, and results from special stains, several other evaluations may be helpful. Malignant cells are found in 60% to 90% of effusions caused by malignancy.[14] The respiratory care practitioner may be asked to determine the pleural fluid pH on the blood gas machine. The specimen must be collected anaerobically in a heparinized syringe and kept on ice until it is analyzed. A pH less than 7.0 or less than 0.15 pH units below the arterial pH in a patient with parapneumonic effusion may indicate that the patient is at risk for prolonged effusion and

---

BOX 43-4

CAUSATIVE ORGANISMS IN PLEURAL EFFUSIONS

AEROBIC BACTERIA
Staphylococcus aureus
Haemophilus influenzae
Streptococcus pneumoniae
Streptococcus pyogenes
Group A, β-hemolytic streptococci

ANAEROBIC BACTERIA
Bacteroides species
Peptostreptococcus species
Peptococcus species
Fusobacterium species

TUBERCULOSIS
Mycobacterium tuberculosis

VIRUSES/MYCOPLASMA
Adenoviruses
Parainfluenza viruses
Mycoplasma pneumoniae

FUNGI/FUNGAL ORGANISMS
Coccidioides immitis
Actinomyces species
Nocardia species

PARASITES
Paragonimus species
Cysticercus species
Entamoeba histolytica
Echinococcus multilocularis

subsequent lung entrapment. This has not been extensively studied in children.[9,13,15]

PNEUMOTHORAX

Air in the pleural space is called a pneumothorax. It is termed a *tension pneumothorax* if the pleural air increases with each breath, subsequently pushing the heart and mediastinal structures into the opposite hemithorax. This is generally a life-threatening situation unless the tension is relieved. Sometimes the pleural air is not under tension and causes only minimal or moderate respiratory distress. A small percentage of patients with a pneumothorax are asymptomatic or have only mild and vague symptoms; however, it is much more common for chest pain and shortness of breath to accompany the pneumothorax. The patient with a tension pneumothorax will subsequently go into shock from decreased venous return to the heart and from compromised cardiac output caused by the shift of the mediastinum.[6,7] On examination, breath sounds will have decreased intensity toward the affected side, and the percussion note will be hyperresonant. With a mediastinal shift the location of the heart's point of maximal impulse may change, and the patient is usually cyanotic with severe respiratory distress. Air under the skin is called *subcutaneous emphysema,* which usually indicates a pneumothorax or pneumomediastinum.

A pneumothorax has a characteristic radiographic appearance (Fig. 43-3). Lung markings are lost going toward the peripheral chest wall, with evidence of a collapsed underlying lung. In diseases in which the lung is stiff from underlying illness, such as respiratory distress syndrome of the newborn or cystic fibrosis, the lung may not be completely collapsible and will stay partly expanded (Fig. 43-4). Pneumothorax and pneumoperitoneum may also result from diaphragmatic hernia and barotrauma (Figs. 43-5 and 43-6). Besides the common causes of pneumothorax in neonates and children (Boxes 43-5 and 43-6),[6,7,16-18] other air leakage problems may be associated with pneumothorax, especially with severe barotrauma (Box 43-7).

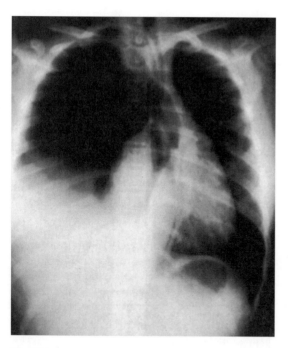

Fig. 43-3

Chest radiograph showing right hydropneumothorax. There are no lung markings in the right chest cavity, and the mediastinal structures are shifted to the left. Fluid fills the lower portion of the right side of the chest cavity. The collapsed right lung is seen as a density to the right of the heart border overlying the spine.

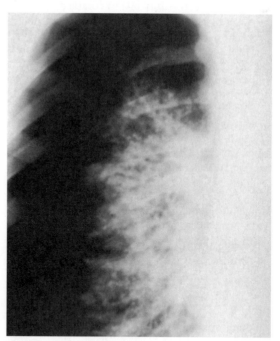

Fig. 43-4

Portion of chest radiograph from young man with cystic fibrosis who has a right-sided pneumothorax. The lung stays partially expanded because it has poor compliance (i.e., it is too stiff to collapse completely). A chest tube has not yet been inserted. The outline of the visceral pleura and lung is clearly seen, and there is a lack of lung markings near the chest wall.

Treatment of the pneumothorax depends on whether it is under tension.[8,16-18] The tension pneumothorax is an emergency and should be relieved as soon as possible. The pleural space is drained with a large-bore needle while awaiting more definitive therapy (see next section). Some small pneumothoraces in patients with chronic lung disease (e.g., cystic fibrosis) might only be observed if there is no clinical deterioration. If the patient is stable, noninvasive therapy with 100% oxygen may be given a brief trial before a more definitive therapy is considered. In rare cases it may be appropriate to withdraw the air by thoracentesis, similar to removing pleural fluid but without resorting to thoracostomy tube drainage.[8,16-18]

THORACOSTOMY DRAINAGE

Tube thoracostomy drainage is the placement of a tube in the pleural space to drain air or fluid, or both, out of the pleural space. Chest tubes are routinely placed after many thoracic surgeries to ensure appropriate drainage of air, fluid, or blood.[8,17-19] Although a chest tube is often placed for an empyema in adults, it does not appear to be mandatory for all empyemas in children.[15,20] The decision to place a chest tube for drainage of a pleural effusion is based on the patient's clinical status and whether the physician thinks that the respiratory system is compromised by the presence of the pleural fluid. Tension pneumothoraces almost always require chest tube drainage.

The insertion of chest tubes outside of the operating room (OR) is generally done in an intensive care unit (ICU) or in a specialized treatment area because of the seriousness of the underlying illness. The duties of the respiratory care practitioner during a thoracostomy are similar to those during a thoracentesis, that is, to monitor the patient's cardiopulmonary status during insertion of the chest tube. The complications of chest tube insertion are similar to those of thoracentesis and may occur more frequently in small premature infants.[8,18,21]

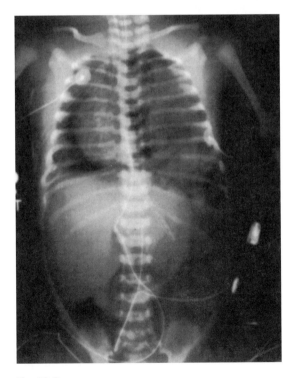

Fig. 43-5

"Whole baby" radiograph of infant with left diaphragmatic hernia and left pneumothorax. Endotracheal and nasogastric tubes are in place. A chest tube is in the right pleural space. Umbilical artery and vein catheters are in place. The abdominal contents are in the left side of the chest with free air evident in the apex. The heart and mediastinum are shifted to the right. There is free air in the abdominal cavity.

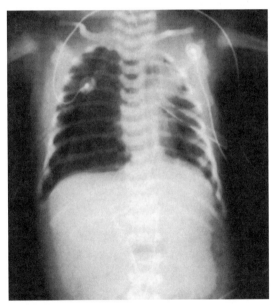

Fig. 43-6

Same infant as in Fig. 43-5 after surgical correction of the diaphragmatic hernia. The density in the left upper lung field is the hypoplastic left lung. There is now a chest tube in the left pleural space as well. There is a persistent pneumothorax on the right despite the chest tube.

BOX 43-5

CAUSES OF PNEUMOTHORAX IN NEONATES

Respiratory distress syndrome
Meconium aspiration
Barotrauma
Spontaneous onset
First breath
Congenital anomaly
• Cystic adenomatoid malformation
• Pulmonary hypoplasia
• Congenital lobar emphysema
Iatrogenic

BOX 43-6

CAUSES OF PNEUMOTHORAX IN CHILDREN

Chronic obstructive lung disease
• Cystic fibrosis
• Bronchopulmonary dysplasia
• Asthma
Trauma
Surgery
Foreign body or ball-valve effect
Tumor
Infection
Pneumatocele
Barotrauma
Spontaneous onset
Congenital anomaly
• Bronchogenic cyst
Iatrogenic

BOX 43-7

CONDITIONS ASSOCIATED WITH AIR LEAKAGE IN PNEUMOTHORAX

Interstitial emphysema
Pneumomediastinum
Pneumopericardium
Pneumoperitoneum
Subcutaneous emphysema

Some patients require more than one chest tube per side, especially if the pleural fluid is very viscous or loculated or if a pneumothorax persists.[18,19]

The patient is given IV or intramuscular (IM) sedation and topical anesthesia. A small incision is made in the skin with a scalpel. Blunt dissection is used to tunnel into the subcutaneous space over one or two ribs to help secure the position of the tube as well as to provide a seal at skin level. The pleural space is then entered just above a rib either by blunt dissection with forceps or with a trocar placed inside the chest tube. When the tube is placed in an appropriate position, there is frequently a gush of air or fluid out of the tube, which is then temporarily clamped to prevent entrance of air into the pleural space with the next inspiration. The tube is then advanced into the desired position and sutured into place at skin level. The end of the tube is connected to commercially available devices that provide both a water seal and a collection chamber (Fig. 43-7). There is a port for wall suction so that continuous negative pressure can be provided to the pleural space to help evacuate its contents. The level of water in the suction control chamber determines the amount of negative pressure applied to the pleural space. Bubbling in the water seal chamber indicates ongoing air leaks, which are usually from the pleural space.[8,18,19]

While caring for the patient, the practitioner must not disrupt the chest tube and its attachments. A change in the patient's clinical status during evaluation by the respiratory care practitioner may indicate either a new problem with the lung or a malfunction of the chest tube system, which demands immediate evaluation. The practitioner should also anticipate patient discomfort at the site of the chest tube and consider this during the manipulation of the patient or surrounding equipment during chest physical therapy or ventilator tubing changes.

The *bronchopleural fistula* presents a difficult management problem. When the integrity of the lung is not reestablished after an air leak or injury, a large portion of the volume of inspired gases may pass directly through the air leak, thus bypassing the gas-exchanging units of the lung. This gas produces hypoventilation in the affected lung and a very large air leak through the chest tube. The bronchopleural fistula may be so severe that hypoventilation occurs despite increasing mechanical ventilatory support and the presence of several chest tubes.[22] Spontaneous healing of a bronchopleural fistula may take several days or even weeks. Surgical intervention may be required to oversew the air leak. In the interim, every attempt is made to reexpand the affected lung and minimize the interference with ventilation. In extreme cases, independent lung ventilation may be required or special valves inserted between the chest tube and wall suction to occlude the chest tube drainage intermittently during the inspiratory cycle of the mechanical ventilator.[22] Special glues and patches have been used to seal the bronchopleural fistula.[23,24]

SURGERY IN THE PLEURAL SPACE

The indications for pleural space surgery in pediatric patients with empyema are less well established than in adults.[25,26] A basic infectious disease tenet is that *pus in a closed space should be drained.* This tenet

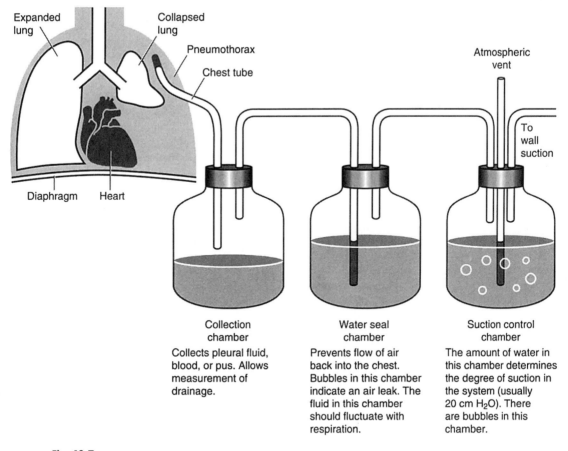

Collection chamber
Collects pleural fluid, blood, or pus. Allows measurement of drainage.

Water seal chamber
Prevents flow of air back into the chest. Bubbles in this chamber indicate an air leak. The fluid in this chamber should fluctuate with respiration.

Suction control chamber
The amount of water in this chamber determines the degree of suction in the system (usually 20 cm H_2O). There are bubbles in this chamber.

Fig. 43-7

Example of the three-bottle system for thoracostomy drainage. Most current systems include all three components in a single plastic container. Not all systems include the three components, and occasionally two components are combined (collection chamber and water seal chamber).

is partly the basis for recommending closed-tube thoracostomy drainage for an empyema. Failure to drain the empyema adequately risks the development of a trapped lung, which subsequently may require pleural decortication.[25] In children the appropriate antibiotic therapy may avoid the need for either chest tube drainage or subsequent decortication.[19] However, the child with an apparent empyema who has had a slow clinical response to broad-spectrum IV antibiotics may benefit from a surgical procedure to evacuate the purulent material and consider a pleural decortication.[26,27]

No clear consensus exists on the most appropriate management of the difficult problem of surgery in the pleural space, so each patient should receive the benefit of an individualized therapeutic plan with flexibility to change depending on therapeutic success.

If a chest tube placed to drain an empyema stops functioning, often the empyema fluid is loculated and the chest tube is in the wrong place.[8,12] Reposi-

tioning the chest tube or adding another may allow better drainage. Injecting streptokinase or urokinase into the pleural cavity may facilitate drainage by liquefying the organizing empyema and dissolving the fibrin septa that are causing loculation.[28-30]

Thoracoscopy is the direct visualization of the pleural space through either rigid or flexible bronchoscopic equipment.[27] This technique has been expanding in the evaluation and management of adult pleural problems, and its use is being extended to pediatric patients.[27,30-32] In 1976 an evaluation of thoracoscopy used to perform lung biopsies in children was reported. Since that time there have been additional reports of its use for (1) biopsy in patients with diffuse lung disease, (2) evaluation and biopsy of mediastinal masses, (3) diagnosis of pleural disease, (4) pleural debridement and irrigation for refractory empyemas, (5) evaluation of pleural effusions, and (6) treatment of spontaneous pneumothorax.[32,33] In larger children, it may even be possible to perform some surgical interventions through the thoracoscope.[34] The major advantage of this approach is the avoidance of a thoracotomy, resulting in less postoperative pain and a shorter recovery period.

The current size limitations of the equipment prevent thoracoscopy from being useful in premature infants and neonates, and some have recommended that it not be used in children less than 6 months of age or in those who weigh less than 8 kg.[34] General anesthesia is usually required, and unilateral ventilation may be used. This may be accomplished by using a double-lumen endotracheal tube in larger patients (adolescents) or by performing mainstem intubation or bronchial blocking with a balloon catheter in the smaller child.[27,34] However, many children younger than 4 years of age cannot tolerate unilateral ventilation and become hypoxic because of their relatively limited functional residual capacity. Pneumothorax, infection, and bleeding are the most often reported complications, although complications often depend on the patient's preoperative condition.[34]

Surgical intervention is seldom needed for persistent pneumothorax or bronchopleural fistula in children. Borrowing from the experience with malignant pleural effusions, *chemical pleurodesis* has been attempted in children who have persistent pneumothorax or recurrent pneumothorax due to cystic fibrosis.[35] This procedure uses agents such as tetracycline or talc to produce a pleural abrasion that results in the adhesion of pleural surfaces.[33] There has been no clear consensus as to whether surgical intervention or chemical pleurodesis is the most appropriate approach to this problem.[36] An individualized patient management plan should be offered, with flexibility to consider alternative options if the initial plan is unsuccessful. The use of chemical or surgical pleurodesis may complicate or prohibit subsequent lung transplantation.

The respiratory care practitioner should be aware of the wide variety of pleural space diseases that might compromise the patient's respiratory function. Familiarity with these diseases will help the practitioner understand the reason for the patient's deterioration or improvement and will contribute to the health care team's management of these problems.

REFERENCES

1. Black LF: The pleural space and pleural fluid. *Mayo Clin Proc* 1972; 47:493-506.
2. Sahn SA: State of the art: the pleura. *Am Rev Respir Dis* 1988; 138:184-234.
3. Yellin A et al: Superior vena cava syndrome with lymphoma. *Am J Dis Child* 1992; 146:1060-1063.
4. Büttiker V, Fanconi S, Burger R: Chylothorax in children: guidelines for diagnosis and management. *Chest* 1999; 116:682-687.
5. Heller RM, Hernanz-Schulman M: Application of new imaging modalities to the evaluation of common pediatric conditions. *J Pediatr* 1999; 135:632-639.
6. Panitch HB, Papastomelos C, Schidlow DV: Abnormalities of the pleural space. In Taussig LM, Landau LI, editors: *Pediatric respiratory medicine*. St Louis, Mosby, 1999; pp 1178-1196.
7. Montgomery M: Air and liquid in the pleural space. In Chernick V, Boat TF, Kendig EL, editors: *Kendig's disorders of the respiratory tract in children*. Philadelphia, WB Saunders, 1998; pp 389-411.
8. Tucker WY: Thoracentesis and tube thoracotomy. In Hilman B, editor: *Pediatric respiratory disease: diagnosis and treatment*. Philadelphia, WB Saunders, 1993; pp 839-844.
9. Heffner JE: Evaluating diagnostic tests in the pleural space: differentiating transudates from exudates as a model. *Clin Chest Med* 1998; 19:277.
10. Hardie W et al: Pneumococcal pleural empyemas in children. *Clin Infect Dis* 1996; 22:1057-1063.
11. Freij BJ et al: Parapneumonic effusions and empyema in hospitalized children: a restrospective review of 227 cases. *Pediatr Infect Dis* 1984; 3:578-591.
12. Sahn S: Management of complicated parapneumonic effusions. *Am Rev Respir Dis* 1993; 148:813-817.
13. Givan DC, Eigen H: Common pleural effusions in children. *Clin Chest Med* 1998; 10:363.
14. McLaughlin FJ et al: Empyema in children: clinical course and long-term follow up. *Pediatrics* 1984; 73:587-593.
15. Redding GJ et al: Lung function in children following empyema. *Am J Dis Child* 1990; 144:337-342.
16. Dickenson CM: Thoracic trauma in children. *Crit Care Nurs Clin North Am* 1991; 3:423-432.
17. Kirby TJ, Ginsberg RJ: Management of the pneumothorax and barotrauma. *Clin Chest Med* 1992; 13:97-112.
18. Miller KS, Sahn SA: Chest tubes: indications, technique, management, and complications. *Chest* 1987; 91:258-264.
19. Cohen S, Stack M: How to work with chest tubes. *Am J Nurs* 1980; April:685-707.
20. Berger HA, Morganroth ML: Immediate drainage is not required for all patients with complicated parapneumonic effusions. *Chest* 1990; 97:731-735.
21. Moessinger AC, Driscoll JM, Wigger HJ: High incidence of lung perforation by chest tube in neonatal pneumothorax. *Pediatrics* 1978; 92:635-637.
22. Baumann MH, Sahn SA: Medical management and therapy of bronchopulmonary fistulas in mechanically ventilated patients. *Chest* 1990; 97:721-728.
23. Dumire R et al: Autologous "blood patch" pleurodesis for persistent pulmonary air leak. *Chest* 1992; 101:64-66.
24. Berger JT, Gilhooly J: Fibrin glue treatment of persistent pneumothorax in a premature infant. *J Pediatr* 1993; 122:958-959.
25. Cassina PC et al: Video-assisted thoracoscopy in the treatment of pleural empyema: stage-based management and outcome. *J Thorac Cardiovasc Surg* 1999; 117:234-238.
26. Khakoo GA et al: Surgical treatment of parapneumonic empyema. *Pediatr Pulmonol* 1996; 22:348-356.
27. Milanez de Campos JR et al: Thorascopy in children and adolescents. *Chest* 1997; 111:494-497.
28. Krishman S et al: Urokinase in the management of complicated parapneumonic effusions in children. *Chest* 1997; 112:1579-1583.
29. Kornecki A, Sivan Y: Treatment of loculated pleural effusions with intrapleural urokinase in children. *J Pediatr Surg* 1997; 32:1473-1475.
30. Kogut KA: Urokinase in the management of complicated parapneumonic effusions in children. *Clin Pediatr* 1999; 38:378-379.

31. Malfroot A et al: Endoscopic diagnosis and closure of a bronchopleural fistula. *Pediatr Pulmonol* 1991; 11:280-282.

32. Merry CM et al: Early definitive intervention by thoracoscopy in pediatric empyema. *J Pediatr Surg* 1999; 34:178-181.

33. Tribble CG, Selden RF, Rodgers BM: Talc poudrage in the treatment of spontaneous pneumothoraces in patients with cystic fibrosis. *Ann Surg* 1986; 204:677-680.

34. Rodgers BM: Pediatric thoracoscopy: where have we come and what have we learned? *Ann Thorac Surg* 1993; 56:704-707.

35. McLaughlin FJ et al: Pneumothorax in cystic fibrosis: management and outcome. *Pediatrics* 1982; 100:863-869.

36. Seddon DJ, Hodson ME: Surgical management of pneumothorax in cystic fibrosis. *Thorax* 1988; 43:739-740.

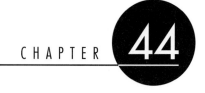

Neurologic and Neuromuscular Disorders

Michael P. Czervinske

C hildren with neurologic and neuromuscular disorders require respiratory support when their respiratory muscles are too weak to expand the chest and when depressed brain function alters respiratory function because of disease or drugs. The muscles that move the chest are primarily the diaphragm, the chest wall, and the abdomen. The sternocleidomastoid and scalene muscles have an accessory role. The respiratory centers in the brainstem integrate the respiratory muscle action and transmit signals through descending pathways in the spinal cord to motor neurons in the cervicothoracic portion of the spinal cord. These motor neurons transmit signals through peripheral nerves and across the neuromuscular junction to muscles of respiration. Dysfunction in any part of this control system, from brainstem to respiratory muscles, can result in respiratory failure. An anatomic approach is useful in determining the causes of respiratory failure and in constructing a treatment plan.

Neuromuscular disorders are diseases of the anterior horn cell *(neuronopathy),* the peripheral nerves *(neuropathy),* the skeletal muscles *(myopathy),* and the junction between the nerves and muscles *(myasthenic syndromes).* Boxes 44-1 and 44-2 summarize the neuromuscular disorders of infancy and childhood, with special reference to those in which respiratory insufficiency may be an early feature. Neuromuscular disorders prevent the chest from expanding by weakening the chest muscles and diaphragm. Neuromuscular disorders that cause respiratory failure immediately after birth are often relentlessly progressive and fatal. Two important exceptions are chronic demyelinating polyneuropathies and myasthenic syndromes. Among older children, the reversible disorders are acute demyelinating polyradiculoneuropathy and myasthenic syndromes.

Weakness and poor muscle tone *(hypotonia)* are usually the initial symptoms of neuromuscular diseases. Many neuromuscular diseases of infancy

<table>
<tr><td>

BOX 44-1

NEUROMUSCULAR DISORDERS OF INFANCY

NEURONOPATHIES
Acute infantile spinal muscular atrophy*
Chronic infantile spinal muscular atrophy

NEUROPATHIES
Congenital hypomyelinating neuropathy*
Hereditary motor sensory neuropathies

MYASTHENIC SYNDROMES
Infantile botulism*
Familial infantile myasthenia*
Transitory neonatal myasthenia gravis

MYOPATHIES
Congenital fiber-type disproportion
myopathies*
Congenital muscular dystrophy
Congenital myotonic dystrophy*
Cytochrome *c* oxidase deficiency*

</td><td>

BOX 44-2

NEUROMUSCULAR DISORDERS OF CHILDHOOD

NEURONOPATHIES
Juvenile amyotrophic lateral sclerosis
Juvenile spinal muscular atrophy

NEUROPATHIES
Acute inflammatory polyradiculoneuropathy
(Guillain-Barré syndrome)*
Hereditary motor sensory neuropathies
Leukodystrophies
Neuropathies with systemic diseases

MYASTHENIC SYNDROMES
Botulism*
Myasthenia gravis*

MYOPATHIES
Dermatomyositis
Endocrine disorders
Hereditary metabolic disorders
Muscular dystrophies
Polymyositis

</td></tr>
</table>

*Conditions in which respiratory failure may be an early feature.

*Conditions in which respiratory failure may be an early feature.

cause generalized hypotonia so that the child is described as "floppy." Brain diseases also cause an infant to look floppy; however, examination of tendon reflexes helps distinguish brain diseases from neuromuscular diseases. Tendon reflexes are usually decreased or lacking in neuromuscular disease and are normal or exaggerated in brain disease. Extreme exaggeration of reflexes causes *clonus,* the repetitive jerking of a limb when the tendon is stretched.

NEURONOPATHIES

Acute paralytic poliomyelitis was once the most common neuronopathy in the United States. Immunization has eliminated all wild infection in the United States; however, the live-attenuated vaccine can cause paralytic poliomyelitis in less than 1 in 1 million vaccinees. Other enteric viruses may cause a polio-like paralytic disease, but never in epidemic proportions. The *spinal muscular atrophies* (SMAs), also known as *Werdnig-Hoffmann disease,* are now the most common cause of anterior horn cell disease in children.

The SMAs are hereditary disorders transmitted by autosomal recessive inheritance and characterized by progressive loss of anterior horn cells. Two forms are recognized: Type I and Type II. Type I is the *acute infantile form,* usually beginning within 3 months of birth, always within 6 months, and often leading to death from respiratory failure within 1 year. Type II is the *chronic childhood form,* with onset after 3 months, often after 6 months, and with a chronic course of motor disability. Both types are

caused by defects at the same site on chromosome 5, and the overlap in clinical features is considerable.[1,2]

ACUTE INFANTILE SPINAL MUSCULAR ATROPHY (TYPE I)

Decreased fetal movements are reported in one third of cases of SMA Type I. The newborn may be limp and have a weak cry or may appear normal. Limb weakness develops rapidly, but facial muscles are less involved, and extraocular muscles are always spared. The result is a child who appears alert and responsive but cannot move. Weakness of sucking and swallowing makes feeding difficult and leads to aspiration. Most infants die of respiratory infection and insufficiency before 1 year of age.

Diagnosis of Type I in the prenatal period is possible through genetic analysis by chorionic villi biopsy. However, the only treatment available for SMA Type I is supportive care. A feeding tube and equipment for suctioning and chest percussion are needed for home care. The use of home ventilator care is controversial. Aspiration often complicates care, and treatment with gastrostomy feeding and mechanical ventilation does little to alter outcome.[3]

CHRONIC CHILDHOOD SPINAL MUSCULAR ATROPHY (TYPE II)

Chronic SMA was once divided into "childhood" and "juvenile" (Type III) forms, depending on the age at onset; however, the two forms are now considered a single disease. The onset and progression of weakness are insidious and may begin as early as 18 months or as late as adolescence. Early motor development is normal, or only mildly delayed, and most children roll over. Some achieve unsupported sitting, but none walk independently, and all will eventually use a wheelchair.

Weakness is greater in the proximal than in the distal muscles, and a fine tremor of the outstretched hands is common. Bulbar weakness that affects speech, swallowing, glottic function, and cough is uncommon, and facial weakness is mild. The development of kyphoscoliosis and joint contractures increases disability. Long intervals without progression of weakness are expected. The course is unpredictable, and survival into adult life is common. As in SMA Type I, electromyographic (EMG) features are diagnostic. The pathologic characteristics of the muscles are consistent with denervation.

Physical therapy helps to prevent deformities that further impair function; however, treatment is not available for the underlying defect. Excessive weight gain further impairs mobility, and dietary counseling is important. Surgery for scoliosis may be required in the second decade of life, usually determined by progressive reductions in *forced vital capacity* (FVC). Inspiratory muscle training may help improve long-term ventilatory function, prevent atelectasis, and overall endurance, but it should not be expected to produce lasting effects.[4] Depending on the severity and progression of the disease, pulmonary complications and death may occur as early as age 3, with a clinical course similar to Type I, or as late as adulthood.

NEUROPATHIES

Diseases of peripheral nerves may start in the nerve fiber *(axonal neuropathies)* or the nerve covering *(demyelinating neuropathies)*. The more common neuropathies of childhood are demyelinating rather than axonal and are reversible despite severe weakness and respiratory paralysis. Ventilator support for such children is often lifesaving.

CONGENITAL HYPOMYELINATING NEUROPATHY

Congenital hypomyelinating neuropathy is a clinical *syndrome* rather than a disease. It encompasses several disorders, some genetic and some immune mediated, with similar clinical and pathologic features.[5] Most cases are sporadic, but advances in genetic research have uncovered the disease-producing genes and are helping to elaborate the molecular processes in this type of disease.[6]

The symptoms in the newborn are indistinguishable from those of SMA Type I. An electromyogram is diagnostic. Fibrillation and fasciculation potentials are present in the muscles, indicating an abnormality of the nerve supply. Motor nerve conduction velocities are slow, indicating that the myelin is affected. The protein concentration of the cerebrospinal fluid (CSF) is always elevated. Nerve biopsy shows that nerve axons are normal but that their myelin covering is lacking. Progressive weakness and skeletal muscle atrophy may present in newborns and rapidly lead to respiratory insufficiency.

Some infants with hypomyelinating neuropathies respond to treatment with corticosteroids, and every affected child should be treated with prednisone.[7] Those who respond become stronger within 4 weeks, and these children should be maintained on alternate-day therapy for at least 1 year.

ACUTE INFLAMMATORY DEMYELINATING POLYRADICULONEUROPATHY (GUILLAIN-BARRÉ SYNDROME)

Guillain-Barré syndrome (GBS) is an acute demyelinating polyneuropathy. More than half the patients have an antecedent infection; respiratory tract infections are the most common, and the remainder are mainly gastrointestinal infections. Enteritis caused by specific strains of *Campylobacter jejuni* stimulates disease in about 18% of patients.[8] It is thought that the myelin is injured by an abnormal immune response to the infection, possibly from activated antiglycosphingolipid antibodies.[9,10]

The clinical features of GBS are so stereotypic that diagnosis can be established without laboratory confirmation.[11] This is especially important because the characteristic laboratory features of GBS may not be present at the onset of clinical symptoms. Two essential features are (1) progressive motor weakness involving more than one limb and (2) loss of tendon reflexes. Weakness is frequently preceded by insidious sensory symptoms: "pins and needles" sensations and muscle tenderness in limbs that soon become weak. Weakness progresses rapidly and will reach a nadir by 2 weeks in approximately 50% of patients, by 3 weeks in 80%, and by 4 weeks in the remainder. The weakness may first affect the arms or the legs but is relatively symmetric. Tendon reflexes are lacking in all weak muscles; their absence can precede the weakness. Bilateral facial weakness occurs in half the cases. Autonomic dysfunction, characterized by dysrhythmias, labile blood pressure, and gastrointestinal dysfunction, may also be present. Respiratory paralysis occurs in 14% to 18% of children with GBS.[12] The concentration of protein in the CSF is elevated after the first week of symptoms. EMG evidence of segmental demyelination is present in 50% of the patients during the first 2 weeks of illness and in 85% during the third week of illness.[13]

Carefully monitor respiratory status, including bedside pulmonary function, especially vital capacity. Intensive care is indicated for children with cardiovascular instability or a declining vital capacity. Elective intubation and mechanical ventilation are required if FVC falls to less than 50% predicted, or 15 ml/kg body weight.[14] Most children who require respiratory support need to be supported for several weeks, possible requiring tracheostomy. Careful mechanical control of respiratory function is an important aspect of patient management in GBS.

Corticosteroids may produce some initial improvement but tend to prolong the disease course. Plasmapheresis has been regarded as the treatment of choice in adults, but its utility in childhood GBS is more limited because of venous access problems and other technical difficulties.[15] Patients too weak to walk without assistance recover more quickly when five doses of intravenous immune globulin (IVIG), 0.4 g/kg/day, are given within 2 weeks of the onset of symptoms.[16-18] However, relapses in adults with GBS treated with IVIG have been reported.[19,20]

If the child is well ventilated during the critical time of profound paralysis, complete recovery can be expected. Improvement begins within 40 days of the onset of disease in more than 80% of patients. Most children fully recover in 6 months, and only 5% to 10% have permanent weakness.

Chronic Inflammatory Demyelinating Polyradiculoneuropathy

Chronic inflammatory demyelinating polyradiculoneuropathy (CIDP) is uncommon in children. It is often thought of as a chronic form of GBS. This condition resembles GBS at its onset, but the progression of weakness is slower. The average duration from onset to peak is 3 months, with a range of 3 weeks to 16 months. Symmetric sensory disturbances and muscle weakness usually start in the legs. Tendon reflexes are decreased or absent. Cranial nerve involvement is uncommon. Weakness is more prominent in distal muscles than in proximal muscles, and respiratory failure is unusual.[21]

The course of CIDP can be characterized by a prolonged progression of weakness and slow recovery or by recurrent relapses and remissions. The average interval between relapses is 10 months. The outcome is more favorable in children than in adults, and full recovery is the rule, although some children have relapses in adult life.[22]

Mandatory clinical criteria for diagnosis include (1) progressive or relapsing motor and sensory dysfunction of more than one limb of a peripheral nerve developing over at least 2 months and (2) are-

flexia or hyporeflexia, usually affecting all four limbs, associated with an elevated CSF protein concentration and EMG evidence of a demyelinating neuropathy.[23]

Treatment for CIDP consists of using high-dose IVIG or prednisone, formerly considered the treatment of choice. However, treatment with IVIG appears to have a more rapid onset, but a follow-up dose of prednisone may be beneficial, especially in treating relapse.[24,25] Plasmapheresis is also beneficial but is technically difficult in smaller children.

DISEASES OF NEUROMUSCULAR TRANSMISSION

The junction between nerve terminals and muscle membrane receptors is bridged by the release of *acetylcholine*. Normal transmission depends on the proper synthesis, storage, release, and breakdown of acetylcholine. Several disease processes interfere with neuromuscular transmission and cause symptoms that range from abnormal fatigability to severe paralysis with respiratory failure.

Infantile Botulism

Human botulism ordinarily results from eating food contaminated by preformed exotoxin of the organism *Clostridium botulinum*. The exotoxin prevents the release of acetylcholine. Infantile botulism is different; the organism, rather than the endotoxin, is ingested. The source of contamination is usually unknown, but honey or corn syrup accounts for 20% of cases. The bacteria colonize the intestinal tract and produce toxin in situ.[26]

The clinical spectrum of infantile botulism includes (1) asymptomatic carriers of organisms; (2) mild hypotonia and failure to thrive; (3) severe, progressive, life-threatening paralysis; and (4) sudden infant death. Infected infants are between 2 and 26 weeks of age and usually live in a dusty environment adjacent to construction or soil disruption from farming. The highest incidence is between March and October. Most infants experience a prodromal syndrome of constipation and poor feeding. Progressive bulbar and skeletal muscle weakness and loss of tendon reflexes develop 4 to 5 days later. Typical features on examination include diffuse hypotonia, ptosis, dysphagia, weak cry, and dilated pupils that react sluggishly to light.

The syndrome is similar to GBS, infantile SMA, and generalized myasthenia gravis. It is difficult to distinguish infantile botulism from GBS by clinical features alone. Infantile botulism differs from infantile SMA by the early appearance of facial and pharyngeal weakness, the presence of ptosis and dilated pupils, and the occurrence of severe constipation.

Infants with generalized myasthenia do not have dilated pupils, absent reflexes, or severe constipation. Repetitive nerve stimulation is diagnostic in 90% of cases. The diagnosis is further confirmed by the isolation of organisms from the stool.

The use of antitoxin and antibiotics does not influence the course of the disease. Intensive care is necessary throughout the period of profound hypotonia. Many infants require ventilator support, especially those with severe paralysis. Sudden apnea and death are a constant danger. Infantile botulism is a self-limiting disease generally lasting 2 to 6 weeks. Recovery is complete, but relapse occurs in as many as 5% of affected infants.[27]

GENETIC MYASTHENIC SYNDROMES

Several genetic defects causing myasthenic syndromes have been identified.[28] Almost all are transmitted by autosomal recessive transmission. Antibodies against the acetylcholine receptor are not detected in any of these syndromes. *Familial infantile myasthenia* and *congenital myasthenia* are terms used to describe the clinical syndromes that are caused by several different genetic defects. Familial infantile myasthenia is the syndrome in which respiratory failure is a prominent feature.

Respiratory insufficiency and feeding difficulty may be present at birth.[29] Many affected newborns require mechanical ventilation. Ptosis and generalized weakness either are present at birth or develop during infancy. Arthrogryposis may also be present. Although facial and skeletal muscles are weak, extraocular motility is usually normal. Within weeks the infants become stronger and no longer need ventilator support. However, episodes of weakness and life-threatening apnea occur repeatedly throughout infancy and childhood and even into adult life in some cases.[30]

The diagnosis is established by the intravenous (IV) or subcutaneous (SC) injection of *edrophonium chloride* (Tensilon). The weakness and respiratory distress reverse almost immediately after IV injection, and within 10 minutes of SC injection. Further confirmation can be accomplished by EMG repetitive stimulation. Long-term treatment with neostigmine or pyridostigmine is needed to prevent sudden episodes of apnea during relapse of the illness. Treatment should be continued throughout childhood.

JUVENILE MYASTHENIA GRAVIS

The term *juvenile myasthenia* is sometimes used to denote myasthenia gravis in children. However, because the nongenetic forms of myasthenia in children are no different from myasthenia in adults, the term should not suggest a separate disorder. It better serves to describe the immune-mediated form of myasthenia that is encountered from late infancy through adult life. Two forms are recognized: (1) *ocular myasthenia,* in which the eye muscles are primarily or exclusively affected, and (2) *generalized myasthenia,* characterized by moderate to severe weakness of the bulbar and limb muscles. Only the generalized form causes respiratory distress.

The first symptoms do not appear until after 6 months of age and do not usually appear until after age 10 years. Prepubertal onset is associated with a slight male bias and ocular symptoms only, whereas postpubertal onset is associated with a strong female bias and generalized myasthenia.[31] The initial features of both the ocular and the generalized forms are usually ptosis or diplopia, or both. Pupillary function is normal.

Between 40% and 50% of patients demonstrate weakness of other bulbar muscles or limb weakness at the onset of myasthenic symptoms. Usually both eyes are affected, but one more than the other. A small number of children with the ocular form of myasthenia develop severe respiratory failure and require intubation and mechanical ventilation. In many patients, however, respiratory muscle weakness can be documented using transdiaphragm or sniffing pressures.[32] Despite limb weakness, tendon reflexes are present, and muscle atrophy does not occur.

Generalized myasthenia is associated with a higher than expected incidence of other autoimmune disorders, especially thyroiditis and collagen vascular diseases. Thymoma is present in 15% of adults with generalized myasthenia but occurs in less than 5% of children.[33] The natural history of myasthenia gravis is marked by exacerbations and remissions, but modern treatment can provide permanent remission.

The Tensilon test has been used as a standard of diagnosis. Tensilon (edrophonium chloride) is a short-acting anticholinesterase administered at an IV dose of 0.15 mg/kg. Repetitive stimulation of the ulnar nerve is abnormal in all patients with generalized myasthenia.[34] The clinical features of myasthenia gravis are attributed to the presence of antibodies against the acetylcholine receptor. Elevated concentrations of the antibody, greater than 10 nmol/L, are detected in the sera of 90% of patients with generalized myasthenia.

Children with generalized myasthenia and increased concentrations of antibody against acetylcholine receptor should undergo thymectomy as quickly as possible after diagnosis; thymectomy should be preceded by plasma exchange if they are extremely weak. Sixty-one percent of these children have remission within 3 years of thymectomy if it is performed early in the disease course. Corticosteroids should be started immediately after surgery. Steroid use may initially increase weakness, so close observation for respiratory deterioration is necessary. Withdrawal of prednisone is attempted after the child has been free of symptoms for 1 year.[3-5]

Anticholinesterase medication is recommended for children with ocular myasthenia who do not have increased blood concentrations of the antibody against acetylcholine receptor. The prognosis for spontaneous recovery in such children is good, even though symptoms are resistant to treatment; immunosuppressive therapy offers no benefit. In refractory cases of myasthenia, high-dose treatment with IVIG has been effective in restoring movement and halting deterioration.[36,37]

TRANSITORY NEONATAL MYASTHENIA

A transitory myasthenic syndrome is observed in 10% to 15% of offspring of myasthenic mothers. The syndrome is believed to be caused by the transfer of antibody from the myasthenic mother to her normal fetus. The severity of symptoms in the newborn correlates with the newborn's antibody concentration but not with the severity or duration of weakness in the mother.[38]

Difficulty feeding and generalized hypotonia are the major clinical features. Neonates with transient myasthenia are eager to feed, but the inability to suck quickly causes fatigue, and nutrition is inadequate. Symptoms usually arise within hours of birth but can be delayed until the third day of life. Some newborns have had intrauterine hypotonia and are born with arthrogryposis.[39] Weakness of cry and facial expression is present in 50% of these infants, but only 15% have limitation of extraocular movement and ptosis. Respiratory insufficiency is uncommon. Weakness becomes progressively worse in the first few days of life and then improves. The mean duration of symptoms is 18 days, with a range of 5 days to 2 months. Recovery is complete, and transitory neonatal myasthenia does not develop into myasthenia later in life.

The diagnosis of transitory neonatal myasthenia is accomplished by demonstrating high serum concentrations of acetylcholine receptor antibody in the newborn and temporary reversal of weakness by SC or IV injection of edrophonium. Treat newborns with severe generalized weakness and respiratory distress with exchange transfusions. For those who are less impaired, an intramuscular (IM) injection of 0.1% neostigmine methylsulfate before feeding sufficiently improves sucking and swallowing to allow adequate nutrition. The dose is progressively reduced as symptoms remit. Neostig-mine may also be administered through a nasogastric tube at a dose 10 times the parenteral level.

MYOPATHIES

Primary muscle disorders may cause respiratory failure either as a terminal event, as in Duchenne's muscular dystrophy, or from birth. Among the disorders presenting in infancy are congenital myotonic dystrophy and acute myotubular myopathy.

CONGENITAL MYOTONIC DYSTROPHY

Congenital myotonic dystrophy is transmitted by autosomal dominant inheritance with variable expressivity. The disease is caused by an unstable DNA region on chromosome 19 that can expand in successive generations and cause a more severe disease in the children than in their parents.[40] In the congenital form, the mother is always the affected parent.

The pregnancy may have been complicated by polyhydramnios. Affected infants are very hypotonic and may require ventilatory support because of muscle weakness and decreased central ventilatory drive. Facial diplegia causes a characteristic tent-shaped mouth, and sucking and swallowing are often impaired. Myotonic dystrophy in adults is a multiorgan disease; in infants, however, the heart generally is not involved. Cardiac involvement, especially conduction defects, often occur by adolescence. Cataracts are also not seen in these infants. Decreased in utero movement may lead to orthopedic abnormalities such as pes equinovarus, hip dislocations, and arthrogryposis. The infants gradually improve and most eventually walk. However, infants requiring mechanical ventilation for more than 4 weeks have a poor prognosis for survival.

Clinical and electrical evidence of myotonia is generally not present in infants. Muscle biopsy changes are diagnostic, but the diagnosis is more easily established by examination of the mother, both clinically and by electromyography. The diagnosis can now be confirmed by genetic analysis of chromosomes.[38] Although no treatment exists, infants do improve with time, although mental and developmental delays are common. Supportive therapy in terms of respiratory support, physical therapy, and bracing should be provided. Fatal complications related to premature labor and intrapartum complications may occur but are less likely in a modern health care facility.[41]

ACUTE MYOTUBULAR MYOPATHY

The abnormal gene that causes acute myotubular myopathy has been mapped to the long arm of the X chromosome (Xq28). Therefore, mothers are carriers, and only boys are affected. The clinical features of this condition in the newborn are generalized hypotonia and respiratory distress. Decreased fetal movement during pregnancy, polyhydramnios, and fetal arrhythmias are common.[42] Sucking, swallowing, and tendon reflexes are depressed or absent. Ptosis and complete ophthalmoplegia may be present. Repeated episodes of apnea, asphyxia, and pneumonia usually lead to death during the neonatal period or in early infancy.

Muscle biopsy is the only diagnostic test, characterized by Type I fiber predominance and hypotrophy, the presence of many internal nuclei, and a central area of increased oxidative enzyme and decreased myosin adenosine triphosphatase activity. No treatment is available for acute myotubular myopathy, and no method exists for prenatal diagnosis.

DUCHENNE'S MUSCULAR DYSTROPHY

Duchenne's muscular dystrophy is caused by a gene defect on the X chromosome. The mean incidence is 1 in 3500 male births. The abnormal gene causes the absence of the structural protein *dystrophin* in skeletal muscle.

Boys with Duchenne's muscular dystrophy have gait disturbances before age 5 years and often before age 3 years. Toe walking and frequent falling are typical initial complaints. Some delay in achieving motor milestones is often elicited in retrospect. Children may not be brought to medical attention until proximal weakness is sufficiently severe to cause difficulty in rising from the floor and an obvious waddling gait. The calf muscles are large and feel rubbery. The Achilles tendon is shortened, and the heels do not quite touch the floor. Tendon reflexes may be present at the ankle and knee but are difficult to obtain.

The decline in motor strength is linear throughout childhood. The severity of weakness may vary widely in children of the same age. Most maintain their ability to walk and climb stairs until 8 years of age. Between ages 3 and 8 years, the child shows progressive contracture of the Achilles tendon and the iliotibial band, increased lordosis, a more pronounced waddling gait, and increased toe walking. The gait is more precarious, and the child falls more often. Tendon reflexes at the knees and ankles are lost, and proximal weakness develops in the arms.

On average, functional ability declines rapidly after 8 years of age because of increasing muscle weakness and contractures.[43] By 9 years of age, some children require a wheelchair, but most can remain ambulatory until 12 year of age and may continue to stand in braces until age 16 years. Scoliosis occurs in some boys; it is not caused by early use of a wheelchair. Deterioration of vital capacity

to less than 20% of normal leads to symptoms of nocturnal hypoventilation, daytime somnolence, headaches, fatigue, and poor concentration.[12] The child frequently awakens and is afraid of sleep.

The immediate cause of death from Duchenne's dystrophy is not always clear; however, respiratory insufficiency is a contributing factor in almost every case. Arrhythmia caused by cardiomyopathy can be documented in some boys. In others with chronic hypoxia, recurrent infection or aspiration produces respiratory arrest.

Although Duchenne's muscular dystrophy is not curable, it is treatable. Prednisone and creatine provide an increase in strength and function that can be maintained for up to 3 years.[44] Treatment goals are to maintain function, prevent contractures, and provide psychological support for the child and family. Every effort should be made to keep children standing and walking as long as possible. This is best accomplished by passive stretching exercises to prevent contractures, a lightweight plastic ankle-foot orthosis to maintain the foot in a neutral position during sleep, and the use of long-leg braces when walking becomes precarious. Orthopedic problems often lead to restrictive lung processes, which further exacerbate the weakened muscles of respiration.

Respiratory monitoring of vital capacity and the rate of change is critical in determining prognosis in patients with Duchenne's dystrophy. A vital capacity less than 1 L is an important predecessor to a terminal event.[45] Inspiratory muscle training and nasal positive-pressure ventilation can help slow the progression of respiratory failure and improve outcome.[4,46] The degree to which improvement is possible depends on the rate of decline in muscle mass and vital capacity.

RESPIRATORY CONSIDERATIONS FOR NEUROMUSCULAR DISORDERS

Not all neuromuscular disorders are treated identically, but some general considerations help to guide the respiratory care of these patients. When evaluating pulmonary function tests, most of these disorders present as restrictive disorders and progress to a severe classification over time. Because muscle tone becomes relatively flaccid, structural integrity of the skeletal system is also affected. As such, skeletal complications such as contractures and severe kyphoscoliosis may also complicate pulmonary function. In select patients, early surgical correction of these problems often results in an improvement in FVC, and more significantly an improvement in functional residual capacity (FRC) and residual volume. Not all patients benefit from surgical correction, and patient selection is an important factor. Late correction generally decreases FRC, probably due to weak diaphragm muscles.[47,48]

Because the main problem in the neuromuscular disease patient is an ineffective ventilatory pump, *hypercapnia* instead of hypoxemia is the primary impairment. As such, treatment plans for severe neuromuscular impairment require ventilation-assist devices, such as noninvasive positive pressure (see Chapter 20), and airway clearance with effective cough support, including mechanical insufflation-exsufflation devices.[49] Management of patients with long-term oxygen therapy may worsen respiratory failure and is generally not indicated.[50]

Inspiratory muscle training exercises may help in the early stages of some neuromuscular disorders. However, the long-term benefit of muscle training exercises is unsubstantiated, considering the primary defect is not the muscle but the nerve or nerve muscle junction.[4] With sufficient bulbar muscle control, glossopharyngeal breathing exercises benefit neuromuscular patients in three ways. First, these exercises provide a method to increase lung volume independently without assistive devices. Second, exercises may help improve respiratory stamina and prevent lung collapse, similar to incentive spirometry. Third, through long-term training, glossopharyngeal breathing in patients with severe neuromuscular impairment may prevent the need for tracheostomy by providing a means for increasing peak flow rates and improving cough flows. *Glossopharyngeal breathing*, or "frog breathing," is accomplished by stacking gulps of air using the glottis to trap the air in the lungs. Such an exercise requires patient motivation, continuous training and conditioning, and minimal airway leaks (e.g., around a tracheostomy tube).

Whereas pulmonary clearance is an important part of managing the patient with a neuromuscular disorder, bronchodilator medications and chest physiotherapy are indicated only if the patient has a reactive airway or secretion problem. Adequate inspiratory capacity and cough flows are usually the key issue, versus mobilizing secretions. Cough-assist devices and manual abdominal thrust techniques help increase the cough flow rate and clearing of secretions. For patients with extreme bulbar muscle weakness, expectoration of secretions is problematic and may require oral suctioning.

In many patients with neuromuscular disorders, *nocturnal hypoventilation* is a common and often unrecognized complication.[12] Using polysomnography to detect obstructive or central apnea is important if the patient has signs of nocturnal hypoventilation, morning headaches, fatigue, and daytime somnolence. Often, children only complain of nightmares and restlessness that wakes them. Frequently, a polysomnogram is not required if it can be demonstrated

that the patient has evidence of (1) frequent fluctuations in nocturnal oxygen saturation less than 90% and (2) evidence of hypoventilation. Noninvasive end-tidal carbon dioxide ($ETCO_2$) monitoring may also be beneficial. Additionally, signs of obstructive episodes normally found on a polysomnogram, such as excessive abdominal movement, may not be present with a neuromuscular disorder. However, treatment for these problems remains the same: nocturnal use of nasal continuous or biphasic positive airway pressure. As daytime hypoventilation ensues, biphasic positive airway pressure or noninvasive mechanical ventilation is indicated.

Monitoring of patients with neuromuscular disorders is critical to determine the proper course of treatment and prognosis. Trend FVC or vital capacity measurements are taken at relatively frequent intervals. The frequency depends on the disorder, but usually 2- to 3-month intervals suffice, with adjustments for periods of remission. Maximal negative inspiratory and positive expiratory pressure measurements must be included in the monitoring. Although not the best measure of cough force, these measurements trend the ability of the respiratory muscles to generate enough pressure to create a forceful cough. Adapting a lip seal device to the mouthpiece is helpful in determining pulmonary function and pressure values if the person exhibits extreme bulbar weakness in which their lips will not seal around the mouthpiece. A sniffing negative pressure may be more helpful because it is an involuntary maneuver, but nasal masks introduce dead space and require adaptation to the manometer.[12]

Noninvasive measurement of $ETCO_2$ helps determine the presence of hypoventilation, and pulse oximetry measurements should also be recorded. Arterial blood gases are of little value and generally not required. Bicarbonate values are easily obtained from electrolyte panels when other laboratory results may be required to assess nutritional status.

The issue of tracheostomy and mechanical ventilation is a very personal decision. The respiratory clinician must make every effort not to let personal bias influence parents' or a patient's decision to undergo a tracheostomy. It is important to provide the facts and answer every question fully and in terms the parents or patient can understand, without frightening technical language. This communication is one of the most difficult tasks in providing care to these patients. It requires tact, skill, empathy, and complete support of the parents or patient once a decision is reached. Most neuromuscular disease foundations and associations offer support groups to help with this and other important decisions.

Neuromuscular disorders predispose a person to respiratory insufficiency, but proper care and monitoring help to minimize the complications associated with respiratory muscle weakness. Attention to pulmonary clearance, augmentation of lung volumes, and patient or caregiver education help many patients achieve some of their normal daily activities, even if they must be assisted by devices or other individuals. Maximizing these efforts also helps to optimize the development of infants and young children who have neuromuscular impairment. Sucking, swallowing, and speech are often impaired and interfere with development. Maximizing these efforts helps to reduce the severity and frequency of complications, despite the ultimate prognosis.[1,4,43,46]

Genetic advances in many of these problems are creating a much better understanding of the molecular mechanisms of these diseases. These advances are improving the chances for a cure or at least are leading to treatments that minimize the impact of complications and optimize the patient's development and normal activities.

REFERENCES

1. Munsat TL et al: Phenotypic heterogeneity of spinal muscular atrophy mapping to chromosome 5q11.2-13.3 (SMA 5q). *Neurology* 1990; 40:1831-1836.
2. Russman BS et al: Spinal muscular atrophy: new thoughts on the pathogenesis and classification schema. *J Child Neurol* 1992; 7:347-353.
3. Birnkrant DJ et al: Treatment of type I spinal muscular atrophy with noninvasive ventilation and gastrostomy feeding. *Pediatr Neurol* 1998; 18:407-410.
4. Koessler W et al: 2 Years' experience with inspiratory muscle training in patients with neuromuscular disorders. *Chest* 2001; 120:765-769.
5. Harati Y, Butler IJ: Congenital hypomyelinating neuropathy. *J Neurol Neurosurg Psychiatry* 1985; 48:1269-1276.
6. Warner LE, Garcia CA, Lupski JR: Hereditary peripheral neuropathies: clinical forms, genetics, and molecular mechanisms. *Annu Rev Med* 1999; 50:263-275.
7. Sladky JT, Brown MJ, Berman PH: Chronic inflammatory demyelinating polyneuropathy of infancy: a corticosteroid-responsive disorder. *Ann Neurol* 1986; 20:76-81.
8. Mishu B et al: *Campylobacter jejuni* infection and Guillain-Barré syndrome. *Ann Intern Med* 1993; 118:947-953.
9. Hartung HP, Pollard JD, Harvey GK: Immunopathogenesis of Guillain-Barré syndrome. *Muscle Nerve* 1995; 18: 137-153.
10. Ariga T, Miyatake T, Yu RK: Recent studies on the roles of antiglycosphingolipids in the pathogenesis of neurological disorders. *J Neurosci Res* 2001; 65:363-370.
11. Kleyweg RP et al: The natural history of the Guillain-Barré syndrome in 18 children and 50 adults. *J Neurol Neurosurg Psychiatry* 1989; 52:853-856.
12. Polkey MI et al: Respiratory aspects of neurologic disease. *J Neurol Neurosurg Psychiatry* 1999; 66:5-15.
13. Albers JW, Kelly JJ Jr: Acquired inflammatory demyelinating polyneuropathies: clinical and electrodiagnostic features. *Muscle Nerve* 1989; 12:435-451.
14. Chevrolet JC, Delamont P: Repeated vital capacity measurements as predictive parameters for mechanical ventilation need and weaning success in Guillain-Barré syndrome. *Am Rev Respir Dis* 1991; 144:814-818.
15. The Guillain-Barré Study Group: Plasmapheresis and acute Guillain-Barré syndrome. *Neurology* 1985; 35:1096-1104.
16. Van der Meche FGA, Scmitz PIM: The Dutch Guillain-Barré Study Group: a randomized trial comparing intravenous immune globulin and plasma exchange in Guillain-Barré syndrome. *N Engl J Med* 1992; 326: 1123-1129.
17. Van der Meche FGA, van Doorn PA: Guillain-Barré syndrome and chronic demyelinating polyneuropathy: immune mechanisms and update on current therapies. *Ann Neurol* 1995; 37(S1):14-31.
18. Kuwabara S et al: Intravenous immunoglobulin therapy for Guillain-Barre syndrome with IgG anti-GM1 antibody. *Muscle Nerve* 2001; 24:54-58.
19. Irani DN et al: Relapse in Guillain-Barré syndrome after treatment with human immune globulin. *Neurology* 1993; 43:872-875.
20. Castro LHM, Ropper AH: Human immune globulin infusion in Guillain-Barré syndrome: worsening during and after treatment. *Neurology* 1993; 43:1034-1035.
21. Ensrud ER, Krivickas LS: Acquired inflammatory demyelinating neuropathies. *Phys Med Rehabil Clin North Am* 2001; 12:321-334.
22. McCombe PA, Pollard JD, McLeod JG: Chronic inflammatory demyelinating polyradiculoneuropathy: a clinical and electrophysiological study of 92 cases. *Brain* 1987; 110:1617-1630.
23. American Academy of Neurology, Ad Hoc Subcommittee of AIDS Task Force: Research criteria for diagnosis of chronic inflammatory demyelinating polyneuropathy (CIDP). *Neurology* 1991; 41:617-618.
24. Van Doorn PA et al: Intravenous immunoglobulin treatment in patients with chronic inflammatory demyelinating polyneuropathy: clinical and laboratory characteristics associated with improvement. *Arch Neurol* 1991; 48: 217-220.
25. Vettaikorumakankav V et al: Chronic demyelinating polyradiculopathy of childhood: treatment with high-dose intravenous immunoglobulin. *Neurology* 1991; 41: 828-830.
26. Spika JC, Shaffer N, Hargrett-Bean N: Risk factors for infant botulism in the United States. *Am J Dis Child* 1989; 143:828-832.
27. Glauser TA, Maguire HC, Sladky JT: Relapse of infant botulism. *Ann Neurol* 1990; 28:187-189.
28. Misulis KE, Fenichel GM: Genetic forms of myasthenia gravis. *Pediatr Neurol* 1989; 5:205-210.
29. Mora M, Lambert EH, Engel A: A synaptic vessel abnormality in familial infantile myasthenia. *Neurology* 1987; 37:206-214.
30. Gieron MA, Korthals JK: Familial infantile myasthenia: report of three patients with follow-up to adulthood. *Arch Neurol* 1985; 42:143-144.
31. Batocchi AP et al: Early-onset myasthenia gravis: clinical characteristics and response to therapy. *Eur J Pediatr* 1990; 150:66-68.
32. Mier-Jedrzejowicz AK, Brophy C, Green M: Respiratory muscle function in myasthenia gravis. *Am Rev Respir Dis* 1988; 138:867-873.
33. Lanska DJ: Diagnosis of thymoma in myasthenics using antistriated muscle antibodies: predictive value and gain in diagnostic certainty. *Neurology* 1991; 41: 520-524.
34. Oh SJ et al: Electrophysiological and clinical correlation in myasthenia gravis. *Ann Neurol* 1982; 12:348-354.

35. Miano MA et al: Factors influencing outcome of prednisone dose reduction in myasthenia gravis. *Neurology* 1991; 41:919-921.

36. Jongen JL, van-Doorn PA, van der Meche FG: High-dose intravenous immunoglobulin therapy for myasthenia gravis. *J Neurol* 1998; 245:26-31.

37. Achiron A et al: Immunoglobulin treatment in refractory myasthenia gravis. *Muscle Nerve* 2000; 23:551-555.

38. Morel E et al: Neonatal myasthenia gravis: a new clinical and immunologic appraisal on 30 cases. *Neurology* 1988; 38:138-142.

39. Belasco C et al: Myasthenie et grossesse: l'atteinte du nouveau-ne peut etre revelatrice [Neonatal myasthenia gravis]. *Arch Pediatr* 2000; 7:263-266.

40. Harley HG et al: Expansion of an unstable DNA region and phenotypic variation in myotonic dystrophy. *Nature* 1992; 355:545-546.

41. Verrijn Stuart AA et al: "Shake hands"; diagnosing a floppy infant—myotonic dystrophy and the congenital subtype: a difficult perinatal diagnosis. *J Perinat Med* 2000; 28:497-501.

42. Tyson RW et al: X-linked myotubular myopathy: a case report of prenatal and perinatal aspects. *Pediatr Pathol* 1992; 12:535-543.

43. Brooke MH et al: Duchenne muscular dystrophy: patterns of clinical progression and effects of supportive therapy. *Neurology* 1989; 39:475-481.

44. Fenichel GM et al: Long-term use of prednisone therapy in the treatment of Duchenne muscular dystrophy. *Neurology* 1991; 41:1874-1877.

45. Phillips MF et al: Changes in spirometry over time as a prognostic marker in patients with Duchenne muscular dystrophy. *Am J Respir Crit Care Med* 2001; 164:2191-2194.

46. Simonds AK et al: Impact of nasal ventilation on survival in hypercapnic Duchenne muscular dystrophy. *Thorax* 1998; 53:949-952.

47. Robinson D et al: Scoliosis and lung function in spinal muscular atrophy. *Eur Spine J* 1995; 4:268-273.

48. Noble-Jamieson CM et al: Effects of posture and spinal bracing on respiratory function in neuromuscular disease. *Arch Dis Child* 1986; 61:178-181.

49. Bach JR: Mechanical insufflation-exsufflation comparison of peak expiratory flows with manually assisted and unassisted coughing techniques. *Chest* 1993; 104:1553-1562.

50. Bach JR et al: Neuromuscular ventilatory insufficiency: effect of home mechanical ventilation use vs oxygen therapy on pneumonia and hospitalization rates. *Am J Phys Med Rehabil* 1998; 77:8-19.

Neonatal and Pediatric Transient and Ambulatory Care

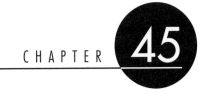

CHAPTER 45

Transport of Infants and Children

John W. Salyer

No element in the continuum of critical care services may be less understood than the transport of patients to hospitals.[1] Few tasks are more challenging to clinicians than transporting critically ill infants and children within and between health care facilities. Respiratory care clinicians must discharge their customary responsibilities of monitoring the status of patients and performing procedures while operating in a changing and often hostile environment, such as a moving ambulance, aircraft, or elevator.

The transport of neonatal and pediatric patients is a broad topic that involves many disciplines within the health care community. The types, ages, sizes, and diagnoses of these transported patients encompass virtually the entire scope of the critically ill population, from the 500-gram infant to the 100-kilogram adolescent. It has now been firmly established that the skilled, rapid transport of patients suffering from serious illness or trauma, including neonatal and pediatric patients, to facilities specializing in the care of these patients results in significantly improved outcomes.[2-31] The importance of these findings should not be overlooked. The skilled transport of critically ill persons is an intervention of the highest value to patients and an activity in which respiratory care practitioners should be proud and enthusiastic to participate.

This chapter details the composition and training of transport teams, describes the necessary equipment, discusses ground versus air transport, describes how to assess patients before and during transport, and describes neonatal and pediatric mechanical ventilation during transport.

USE OF PEDIATRIC AND NEONATAL TRANSPORT SERVICES

The widespread development of tertiary centers for the care of neonates has been an important proving ground for techniques in transporting critically ill infants and children. These centers frequently have a transport team composed of respiratory therapists (RTs), nurses, and physicians from the neonatal intensive care unit (NICU). This type of transport service has been shown effective in reducing neonatal mortality when compared with populations of infants transported by teams who are not specially trained in neonatal transport.[29,32-34]

Transporting high-risk mothers to tertiary neonatal care centers before delivery (prenatal), instead of waiting and transporting the infant after delivery, is now routinely done. The transport of critically ill, low-birth-weight infants is difficult and potentially risky. It should be safer (for the infant) to transport the mother before delivery. Evidence indicates that mortality in postnatally transferred neonates is significantly higher than in those transported prenatally.[23,24,29,35,36] However, prenatal transport will never completely obviate the need for skilled neonatal transport teams because (1) many premature deliveries are precipitous, (2) many neonates who are sick at birth or shortly thereafter are never identified as high risk prenatally, (3) many mothers receive no prenatal care and thus cannot be transported prenatally, and (4) many medical transport programs are adequately prepared for the high-risk obstetrical patient.[37]

The current system of regional tertiary neonatal centers and neonatal transport services has led to overcrowding of some NICUs.[38] The pressure to vacate NICU beds and the extreme cost of this specialized care have led to the practice of "back-transporting" recovering neonates to community hospitals.[38-40] The practice has been shown to result in a significant decrease in total hospital charges.[40] Because these patients, although fairly stable, frequently require oxygen, mechanical ventilation, or both, RTs are often involved in the transport.

The use of air transport services in both adult and pediatric populations is becoming more widespread. About 250 air transport services are in operation in the United States, using more than 280 rotary-wing aircraft.[41-44]

COMPOSITION AND TRAINING OF TRANSPORT TEAM PERSONNEL

The therapeutic goal of any critical care transport system is to provide an extension of an advanced critical care environment to the referring facilities.[45,46] A transport service should model its ability to monitor and support the patient during an acute, life-threatening illness after that of an intensive care unit (ICU).[47] To achieve this, it is mandatory that personnel specially trained in the care of critically ill infants and children compose the transport team.[48] Precise details of team composition are

controversial, and there is no perfect combination of transport personnel for every institution in every situation.[49] Different groupings of personnel who constitute a team include (1) two nurses, (2) nurse and emergency medical technician, (3) nurse and physician, (4) nurse and RT, (5) physician and RT, and (6) nurse, RT, and physician.

More important than the exact credentialing of transport personnel is the training and skills of the team. A qualified neonatal-pediatric transport team should be composed of individuals who (1) have considerable neonatal and pediatric critical care experience, (2) are rigorously trained in the special needs of infants and children during transport, and (3) participate in transport of these patients with sufficient frequency to maintain their expertise. The need for neonatal and pediatric transport teams to have critical care experience is self-evident, and there have been excellent descriptions of the training required.[13,48,50-56] However, pediatric and neonatal patients have unique requirements that make it necessary for personnel to have extensive experience with specialized pediatric and neonatal airway and ventilator management techniques. Adult critical care experience by itself is not sufficient.

In addition to specialized training in neonatal and pediatric patient transport, safety training is required for all personnel who will be working around helicopters.[57] General safety guidelines include (1) stay 100 feet away from the aircraft while the blades are turning; (2) never go near the tail of the aircraft; (3) always approach and leave the aircraft in a crouched position in view of the pilot; (4) never come near the aircraft with anything higher than your head (e.g., intravenous poles); (5) do not handle loose objects around the moving aircraft (e.g., sheets, mattress pads, hats); (6) load and unload patients under the supervision of the flight crew; and (7) no smoking or running within 100 feet of the aircraft.[58]

Another controversy regarding transport team composition involves whether pediatric and neonatal transport teams are unit-based or dedicated teams. *Unit-based teams* are drawn totally or partly from currently assigned ICU staff when interhospital transport is required, whereas *dedicated teams* focus exclusively on patient transport. Both types of teams have strengths and weaknesses. Dedicated teams probably acquire more transport experience (and thus *may* be more skilled, although evidence for this is notably lacking in the literature) but are inherently more inefficient. The actual transport hours as a percentage of total hours paid in such dedicated programs has been reported as low as 33%.[59] When these teams are not actively transporting patients, they are generally not taking patient assignments. Unit-based teams are more efficient because they draw staff who are already being paid for direct patient care and who can return to their patient care assignment when the transport is finished. However, these systems can be a staffing strain on the ICU because patient assignments must be shifted while the transport nurses and therapists are out of the unit. In a survey of 56 centers providing advanced neonatal and pediatric transport services, 68% were dedicated teams, and 32% were unit-based teams.[60]

Whatever the structure of the team, an RT is usually part of the team when an intubated patient is transported or if intubation is anticipated or respiratory instability is suspected.[14]

One study of a pediatric critical care transport service revealed that 45% of all patients transported required the services of an RT in transport.[61] Participation of RTs in the neonatal and pediatric transport team is well established, with surveys indicating that they participate in 50% to 55% of the transports of critically ill infants and children.* RTs' role during transport includes (1) assembly and maintenance of respiratory equipment before departure, (2) immediate assessment of the patient's respiratory condition, (3) airway management, (4) oxygen administration or ventilatory management (or both), (5) patient monitoring, and (6) assistance for other team members. Teams who do not employ RTs should have someone specially trained and highly experienced in airway management and neonatal and pediatric mechanical ventilation.[72,73] RTs have been shown to display better intubation skills than resident physicians on a pediatric transport team.[74] Also, some pediatric transport nurses have significant deficits in some advanced respiratory skills, such as x-ray interpretation, reinforcing the argument for the inclusion of RTs in transport teams.[75] The requisite training for RTs engaged in neonatal and pediatric transport has been well described by the American Academy of Pediatrics (AAP)[48]:

All transport team members should complete a planned formal training program approved by the medical director and supplemented by in-service practical training. The course should be of sufficient duration and content to cover all responsibilities related to the care and monitoring of pediatric patients during transport, technical skills required for emergency management, operation of transport equipment, adaptation to the physical environment of the transport vehicle, and physiologic consequences of the transport on the patient.

The guidelines also advise that RTs should have at least 1 year of experience in pediatric critical care and are either registered respiratory therapists or registry eligible. Many transport systems also require that RTs have completed the AAP's Pediatric Advanced Life Support training as well as the Neonatal Resuscitation Program.

One controversy surrounding the team composition is the inclusion of a physician. Some suggest that a physician must be present during pediatric transport if intensive care is anticipated, whereas others have concluded that a physician's presence may not always be necessary.[46,65,76,77] Much of this controversy centers on whether the severity of the patient's condition can be adequately predicted before the team's departure. Information received over the telephone concerning the condition of a patient before transport can be notoriously inaccurate; thus it might be difficult at times to predict the need for a physician. Most neonatal and pediatric patients can be transported without a physician in immediate attendance, but only if the transport team has highly skilled members and there is radio communication between the team and the physician. Some centers transport critically ill pediatric patients without a physician, and others have an RT and a nurse as the primary team for transporting neonates, adding a physician only for pediatric patients.[52,55,76] The qualifications of physicians on the transport team include critical care experience; the ability to perform endotracheal intubation, chest tube placement, and fluid therapy management; and competency in directing cardiopulmonary resuscitation (CPR) efforts. Knowledge of the management of ventilatory support equipment is also necessary unless an adequately trained RT is in attendance.[14,33,45,48,53]

As with interhospital transport of infants and children, the composition of the transport team is important when selecting personnel for intrahospital transport (Tables 45-1 and 45-2). Intrahospital transport may be regarded rather lightly when, in fact, patients suffer deleterious consequences from intrahospital transport with alarming frequency at times. Studies on mishaps or deterioration in adult patients during intrahospital transport found that the risk to patients increases during transport, no matter how short the distance.[78-85] As with interhospital transport, the goal of moving an ICU patient around the hospital for diagnostic studies is to "take the ICU with the patient."[86] When a dedicated team is used in intrahospital transport, unanticipated problems are encountered less frequently; conversely, when patients are not adequately monitored, major adverse events occur.[87] Properly trained and equipped personnel should help to ensure avoidance of the experience of Dutch investigators, who reported that when untrained personnel were used to transport neonates between hospitals, several patients arrived at the

---

*References 14, 32, 34, 46, 48, 49, 52, 53, 55, 61-71.

TABLE 45-1	CLASSIFICATION OF INTERHOSPITAL TRANSPORT TEAMS ACCORDING TO PATIENT CONDITIONS	
Status Categories*	**Criteria**	**Transport Team**
Status I, II	Infrequent monitoring, no intravenous line, not admitted to ICU, may be ambulatory, no oxygen requirement	RN
Status III	Monitoring every 30 min to 1 hr, has intravenous line, moderate respiratory distress, admitted to intermediate unit, alteration of consciousness	ICU RN
Status IV	Intubated, requires invasive monitoring (arterial line, central line), Foley catheter, more than one intravenous line	ICU RN, RT, MD
Status V	Unstable, requires ongoing therapy during transport	Status IV team†
Status VI	Clinically brain dead before transport	Status IV team

Modified from Dobrin RS et al: The development of a pediatric emergency transport system. *Pediatr Clin North Am* 1980; 27:663.
*Patient status categories used for triage of critically ill children.
†"Disease-related" team (e.g., burn, surgeon)
RN, Registered nurse; *ICU,* intensive care unit; *RT,* respiratory therapist; *MD,* medical physician.

TABLE 45-2	TRANSPORT TEAM COMPOSITION FOR INTRAHOSPITAL TRANSPORT OF INTENSIVE CARE UNIT PATIENTS
Type of Patient	**Staff to Accompany and Remain with Patient**
Stable with only one intravenous line	Determined by head nurse or ICU coordinator
Stable with arterial line	RN
On mechanical ventilator	RN and RT
Pulmonary artery catheter or vasoactive drips or both	RN and resident-MD
Arterial line, mechanical ventilator, pulmonary artery catheter	RN, RT, resident-MD
Unstable patient	RN, RT, resident-MD

Modified from Branson RD: Intrahospital transport of critically ill, mechanically ventilated patients. *Respir Care* 1992; 37:775-795.
ICU, Intensive care unit; *RN,* registered nurse; *RT,* respiratory therapist; *MD,* medical physician.

regional center dead, a fact unknown at that time to the transporting personnel.[88]

RISK TO PATIENTS AND PROVIDERS

Participation in air transport exposes everyone involved to some degree of risk. The National Traffic Safety Board conducted a study of 59 medical rotary-wing aircraft accidents and determined that 68% of all accidents involved pilot error or poor judgment as part of the probable cause.[89,90] Part of the judgment errors involved the decision to fly in marginally acceptable weather conditions; 25% of the accidents and 61% of all fatalities involved reduced visibility. Since the time of this study, weather information available to pilots and their ability to interpret weather reports have improved.

Another aspect of pilot error that is more difficult to quantify is the role of fatigue in decision making.[91] The National Emergency Medical Services Pilots Association recommends that pilots be restricted to a maximum 12-hour shift and that each pilot be on duty no more than 180 hours per month. Civilian medical air transport safety has improved dramatically because of better weather-worthy aircraft and better aircraft training for the medical crew.[92]

Safety concerns continue regarding accidents during ground transport. An 11-year retrospective study (1987 to 1997) analyzed 339 ambulance crashes that resulted in 405 fatalities and 838 injuries.[93] This study verified earlier findings that the most common ambulance accidents occur at intersections, during emergency response, and on clear, dry, newly improved roads.[94]

Clearly, the health care providers who participate in air or ground transport of patients are taking a risk. Controversy surrounds the relative benefit to patients of air versus ground transports.[7,8] Anyone who participates in the transport system will be faced with the question, "Why did we take the helicopter up for this patient, who could easily have been transported on the ground?" Some have suggested little or no benefit to using air transport in urban areas that have well-developed ground transport systems.[95] Other studies failed to demonstrate improved outcomes in patients transported by air versus ground for both interhospital transport and scene transport.[96-99] The benefit of air transport has been clearly demonstrated in the most critically ill patients, but it is estimated that the percentage of air ambulance flights that involve patients receiving advanced life support may be as low as 20%.

TRANSPORT EQUIPMENT

This section discusses only equipment that is directly or indirectly related to the administration of

BOX 45-1
"Golden Rules" of Patient Transport

1. Transports are palliative, not curative.
2. No form of transport is ideal for every patient.
3. Any hospital is a better hospital than an airplane or ambulance.
4. If it is possible for a sick person to become sicker, he or she probably will.
5. Large problems are simply small problems you have not anticipated.
6. Nothing lasts forever (e.g., air, oxygen, battery).

Modified from Kissoon N: Triage and transport of the critically ill child. *Crit Care Med* 1992; 8:37-57.

respiratory care, because many other types of equipment are involved in interhospital and intrahospital patient transport. Ensuring that the transport team has all the equipment necessary to render intensive care during transit and that this equipment is functioning properly is crucial when planning any transport; equipment can and does malfunction. The "golden rules of transport" follow the "five-*P* principle": *proper planning prevents poor performance* (Box 45-1). Specified equipment should be included in the kit of any RT engaging in the transport of a critically ill neonatal or pediatric patient (Box 45-2). A common practice that works well for respiratory supplies is the use of large canvas bags or "fishing tackle" boxes to carry some materials. Any container used must be organized compartmentally in a logical

BOX 45-2
Respiratory Equipment and Supplies for Neonatal and Pediatric Transport

Airway
Stethoscope
Portable suction unit
Suction catheter kits (sizes 6, 8, 10, 14 French)
Yankauer suction apparatus
Suction connection tubing
Laryngoscope handles (small, medium, large)
Straight and curved laryngoscope blades (small [premie], medium, and large)
Laryngoscope bulbs (small and large)
Magill forceps (pediatric and adult)
Sodium chloride for lavage
Endotracheal tubes

Uncuffed	Cuffed
2.5	4.0
3.0	4.5
3.5	5.0
4.0	5.5
4.5	6.0
5.0	6.5
5.5	7.0
6.0	7.5

Stylettes (neonatal, pediatric, adult)
Shiley tracheostomy tubes:
  Neonatal sizes: 00, 0
  Pediatric sizes: 0, 1, 2, 3
Oropharyngeal airways (sizes 00, 0, 1, 2, 3, 4, 5)
Heat-moisture exchangers (neonatal, pediatric, adult)

Oxygen Therapy
Oxygen and compressed air supply
Air-oxygen blender
Aerosol masks (neonatal, pediatric, adult)
Partial rebreathing mask
Nonrebreathing mask

Nasal cannulas (neonatal, pediatric, adult)
Oxygen tubing
Oxygen nipple adaptor
Oxygen hood
Oxygen analyzer
Corrugated tubing

Mechanical Ventilation
Mechanical ventilator
Two ventilator circuits (second one as reserve)
Manual resuscitator
  Neonatal and pediatric
  Must be capable of delivering 100% oxygen with positive end-expiratory pressure (PEEP)
Reserve self-inflating resuscitation bag (neonatal and pediatric)
Resuscitation masks (sizes 0, 1, 2, 3, 4)
Airway pressure manometer

Miscellaneous
Replacement batteries for all battery-powered equipment
Colorimetric exhaled–carbon dioxide monitor
Hand-held nebulizer kit
Feeding tubes (sizes 5, 6, 8, 10 French)
Tincture of benzoin
Cloth adhesive tape ($\frac{1}{2}$ and 1 inch)
10-ml syringe
Various sizes of tubing adaptors
Pulse oximeter
Pulse oximeter probes
Electrocardiograph monitor
Scissors
Hemostats
Screwdrivers
Adjustable wrench
Cold-weather clothing (if conditions warrant)

manner so that needed supplies can be quickly located under stressful adverse conditions. All transport personnel should be familiar with the supply system. A pretransport checklist helps to ensure that all necessary supplies and equipment go with the transport team, and a posttransport checklist should be used for restocking.

MEDICAL GAS SUPPLY

It is essential that the RT ensure that an adequate supply of medical gases is available *before leaving the transport center.* Because many factors could cause a delay during the transport, it is prudent to take at least *twice* the amount of oxygen that the RT anticipates will be needed for a given patient.[100] An alternative to carrying large numbers of cylinders to meet gas needs during transport is the use of liquid systems, which greatly increases the amount of gas that can be carried in a limited space. One liquid system used on a fixed-wing aircraft has an oxygen supply equivalent to 22 E cylinders.[101] Anticipating the amount of oxygen needed can be difficult because the information about the patient's condition before leaving the transport center can be inadequate or inaccurate.

The RT must remember that some equipment uses medical gases at prodigious rates during transport. When used with a flowmeter attached or in certain modes, air-oxygen blenders may have a continuous bleed of gas in addition to the flow rate set on the flowmeter. The Bird 3800 Microblender (Bird Products) bleeds 10 to 12 L/min, whereas the Bird HI/LO flow oxygen blender has a bleed rate of 12 to 14 L/min. Thus, if the Bird HI/LO flow oxygen blender were used in the low-flow setting with auxiliary flow turned on and the flowmeter set at 10 L/min, it would consume a total of 24 L/min. Some types of pneumatically powered, fluidic-controlled transport ventilators, such as the MVP-10 (Bio-Med Devices), also have internal gas consumption besides the flow rate set on the ventilator. Bio-Med includes a chart for the estimation of total gas consumption based on ventilator settings. At a frequency of 50 breaths/min, the MVP-10 has an internal gas consumption of approximately 4 L/min.[102]

MECHANICAL VENTILATORS

One controversy surrounding the equipment used during the transport of pediatric and neonatal patients both within and between hospitals is the use of a ventilator. It is clear that manual ventilation during transport can lead to considerable variation in ventilatory parameters including unintentional hyperventilation.[78,102-104] The use of a transport ventilator is the preferred method of ventilation during transport, but manual ventilation may be acceptable when a skilled

RT is available.[86] Some transport services still rely on manual ventilation during transport, but it is hoped that this practice will continue to diminish.

Controversy also surrounds the optimal type of ventilator to use during transport. The extreme variability in the size and condition of neonatal and pediatric patients makes the use of any single type of transport ventilator for all patients difficult and has led some transport services to develop their own modified devices. Some transport services even have specially modified high-frequency ventilators for use during intrahospital transport.[105]

Because transport services try to "take the ICU to the patient," the same basic guidelines used in the selection of ventilators for ICU patients should be applied during transport, with a few special considerations. A transport ventilator (1) should be able to generate a peak inspiratory pressure (PIP) that is adequate for the patient population being ventilated, possibly up to 120 cm H_2O; (2) should be able to function as a constant inspiratory flow generator; (3) should have an adjustable PIP-limiting valve; and (4) should have minimal compressible gas volume in the breathing circuit.[81,106] Although primarily directed toward the ventilatory requirements of adults, these recommendations have merit for a large portion of transported pediatric ICU patients.[107-111] The neonatal transport ventilator (1) should have continuous flow with a range of 0 to 10 L/min, (2) should be pressure controlled, (3) should have an auxiliary (or backup) pressure relief mechanism in addition to the primary pressure-controlling mechanism, (4) should be capable of cycling frequencies from 0 to 120 breaths/min, and (5) should have low gas consumption. Low gas consumption should be a strong consideration in the selection of transport ventilators for all age groups.

In the extremely noisy transport vehicle, audible ventilator alarms are generally useless because they cannot be heard above the ambient noise, and the patient is visually monitored virtually the entire period of any interhospital transport. During intrahospital transport, however, especially when patients are going for lengthy diagnostic studies, the same monitoring guidelines for ICU patients should be followed.[112,113]

All transport ventilators may not perform according to their reported capabilities. Some volume ventilators do not deliver the set volume when operating against low compliance and high resistance.[106,114] Respiratory care practitioners should not assume that the ventilators operate within the performance specifications provided by manufacturers. Thus it is important to test the performance of all ventilators in use.[115] This caveat applies to all respiratory care equipment. Also during transport, tidal volume should be monitored (if possible) at the initiation of ventilation, when ventilator settings are adjusted, and when the patient's respiratory parameters change, such as PIP or breath sounds.[106]

EQUIPMENT PROBLEMS AND FAILURES

Essential equipment to be taken on every transport includes these basic tools: tank key, screwdriver, pliers, scissors, hemostats, and small flashlight (especially during night transports). If equipment malfunctions, simple repairs may be necessary en route. Plans should be made and implemented on how to deal with equipment failure during transport. For example, if a manual resuscitator malfunctions, a backup device must be available. If the isolette heater fails, chemical-heating packets must be used. When checking equipment in preparation for transport, the clinicians should ask, "What will I do if this piece of equipment fails?"

Another concern about equipment used during transport is the amount of *electromagnetic interference* (EMI) generated by transport equipment. EMI is electromagnetic energy that interrupts, obstructs, or otherwise degrades or limits the effective performance of an electronic device, similar to the interference seen on a television screen, for example, when an electric drill is being operated nearby.[116] This EMI has the potential for affecting the performance of avionics equipment and thus aircraft operation. Nish et al tested the amount of EMI emitted by more than 20 neonatal monitors, incubators, and ventilators and found that approximately 70% of the equipment failed U.S. Air Force testing standards for EMI emissions.[116] The authors concluded that although no aircraft accidents have yet been proved to be caused by excessive EMI, the potential for catastrophe exists. They suggest that transport programs not purchase equipment from manufacturers who refuse to meet EMI standards and that the Federal Aviation Administration develop EMI standards for civilian transport equipment as soon as possible. However, they did admit that military EMI standards may be too strict for the civilian population.

Extreme precautions must be taken during transit to secure all equipment adequately to prevent it from falling while the vehicle is in motion. In describing one accident, a transport team member stated that "things were flying everywhere."[62]

TRANSPORT TEAM ATTIRE

Transport personnel should dress appropriately. Even though aircraft cabins are heated, it is imprudent to depart without suitable cold-weather clothing (when the climate demands). If an aircraft is forced down in a remote area during cold weather, transport crews may have to spend some time exposed to the elements before rescue. An Arizona paramedic spent 12 hours on the side of an 8000-foot mountain during a snowstorm after the crash of an aeromedical helicopter.[117] In another report an Illinois rotary-wing flight team was forced to land in a remote cornfield because of an engine fire. Some members of the flight team (wearing scrubs and sneakers) would have soon succumbed to the −20° F wind-chill factor had they not quickly located a farmhouse.[117] Flying in extreme heat and humidity can also pose problems for the transport teams. Care must be taken to have plenty of oral fluids for the crew to avoid dehydration when transporting in hot-weather conditions.

PATIENT ASSESSMENT AND STABILIZATION

INITIAL ASSESSMENT

Assessment of the transport patient's condition begins before leaving the transport center. The importance of good communication in the process of transporting high-risk pediatric patients cannot be overemphasized.[68,117,118] The basic information required to initiate transport includes (1) the patient's age, weight, and name; (2) a synopsis of the patient's general condition and appearance; (3) the patient's vital signs; (4) any major problems; and (5) the course of events leading to the patient's present status. Current respiratory care interventions and the latest arterial blood gas (ABG) determinations should also be identified. The ideal communication system should allow continuous discussion of the patient's condition between the transport center and the transport team while en route.[13]

Assessment and stabilization of the patient before departure may be the most critical aspects of interhospital care because they minimize the chance for subsequent deterioration in a setting that may not easily permit detection or treatment of problems, such as in a moving ambulance or aircraft.[63,119] Transport team members who remain at the referring hospital for extended periods to assist in stabilizing the patient may improve patient outcome.[71] One study showed that 13% of transported infants and children required at least one major procedure in the period between the arrival of the transport team and departure of the patient.[120]

The initial physical assessment of the patient by the transport team should be performed immediately on arrival at the referring facility (Box 45-3). The initial phase of this assessment involves resuscitation priorities, including airway management and adequate ventilation and circulation, as described in protocols for pediatric advanced life support.[121]

PHYSICAL ASSESSMENT OF PATIENT ON ARRIVAL AT REFERRING FACILITY

OBTAIN A BRIEF HISTORY
    Summary of present illness
    Chronic conditions contributing to present
        illness

EVALUATE LEVEL OF CURRENT RESPIRATORY SUPPORT

PERFORM PHYSICAL INSPECTION OF PATIENT
    General appearance
        Patient position
        Level of consciousness
        Color
    Inspection of chest and lungs
        Thoracic shape
        Retractions, grunting, flaring
        Respiratory rate and rhythm
        Auscultation of breath sounds
    Inspection of airway
        Stridor and patency in nonintubated patients
        Position, security, and patency in intubated
            patients

OBTAIN/REVIEW CLINICAL AND LABORATORY VALUES
    Arterial oxygen saturation
    Temperature
    Blood pressure
    Capillary refill time
    Heart rate
    $Ptcco_2$ or $Ptco_2$, or both
    Arterial blood gas values
    Hemoglobin/hematocrit values
    Most recent radiographs

$Ptcco_2$, Transcutaneous carbon dioxide pressure; $Ptco_2$, transcutaneous oxygen pressure.

Ensuring that the patient has a patent airway should be the first step. If respiratory deterioration is imminent or is considered a possibility, intubation and transport support with 100% oxygen should be accomplished as soon as possible. In the vast majority of acute respiratory emergencies, high fractional concentration of inspired oxygen (FIO_2) levels can be delivered without acute harmful effects.[121] There are occasional exceptions to this rule. It has long been held that patients with chronically elevated arterial carbon dioxide tension ($Paco_2$) levels (as in cystic fibrosis or bronchopulmonary dysplasia) may experience diminished respiratory drives if high FIO_2 levels are administered. However, this theoretic concern has probably been given more credibility historically than it merits scientifically. In addition, because of the short-term nature of interhospital transports, consider-

ation of limiting FIO_2 due to so-called hypoxic drive during transport is inappropriate. Also, low-birthweight neonates are placed at higher risk for the development of retinopathy of prematurity if hyperoxemia is allowed to persist, although hyperoxemia can occur with relatively low FIO_2, and conversely, the patient with very high FIO_2 can still have hypoxemia. Those concerns should not overshadow the need to achieve acceptable oxygenation in the critically ill patient. Instead, the clinician should consider cautious titration of oxygen in these patients once cardiorespiratory stability has been firmly established.

AIRWAY MANAGEMENT

With patients who may have only marginal respiratory difficulties, the temptation to delay intubation at the referring hospital until after the transport should be avoided. Intubation of a neonate or child in a moving ambulance or aircraft cabin is difficult, if not impossible, and the clinician should use any means to avoid this situation.

Some have suggested that if intubation (or reintubation) en route is required, the ambulance should be stopped for the procedure.[49] Securing the endotracheal (ET) tube is crucial because accidental extubation during transport can be catastrophic, especially in small helicopter cabins with insufficient room to perform reintubation. Accidental extubation seems to be more prevalent in the smaller patient and has been reported frequently in NICU patients both in the hospital and during transport.[122,123] Although various taping techniques are used, evidence indicates that the use of elastic tape (e.g., Elastoplast) and tincture of benzoin is a superior method.[123,124] Excellent taping technique alone, however, cannot ensure the prevention of accidental extubation. Manual stabilization of ET tubes by the transport staff may further reduce the movement of even the well-taped ET tubes.[121] The use of extremity restraints in active patients is essential, and sedation and paralysis may become necessary, although this point is controversial.[125]

Venous access must be rapidly established before transport. If attempts at venous access are unsuccessful, a rapid and safe alternative is an intraosseous infusion. Because hypovolemic shock is a common problem in pediatric patients who require emergency care, volume expansion may be required.[121,126-129]

During the secondary phase of patient assessment, the RT should ensure that the following parameters have been considered: (1) temperature, (2) blood pressure, (3) heart rate, (4) respiratory rate and status, (5) color, and (6) radiographic and laboratory results, including hematocrit values and ABG analysis. If the patient has been intubated, ET tube position should be confirmed by radiography, and adequate ventilatory support should be confirmed by ABG analysis before departure. In addition, if noninvasive respiratory monitors are to be used during transport (e.g., transcutaneous monitors, pulse oximetry), their agreement with ABG measurements should be established before departure.

The ongoing evaluation of ET tube position during transport can be difficult. Depending on the mode of transport used, noise in the transport vehicle can make the assessment of breath sounds nearly impossible. The noise level in the workspace of most helicopters exceeds 100 db, making ordinary conversation impossible.[100,130] The noise level in most transport incubators has also been shown to be excessive during transport.[131] Studies have revealed that breath sounds are often impossible to hear during both ground and air transport and may even be difficult to hear with an amplified stethoscope.[132-134] The AAP recommends that aircraft cabin noise levels be less than 85 db.[64]

Vibration is also a concern during the transport of patients, especially in rotary-wing aircraft, although it can also be quite pronounced in some ground ambulances. "Bouncing" of patients can often be so exaggerated that it may be impossible to discern any chest wall movement and thus the adequacy of ventilation.

An alternative method of assessing ET tube position is the use of colorimetric end-tidal carbon dioxide ($ETCO_2$) detectors. These small devices are placed between the patient's ET tube and ventilator circuit and change color in the presence of elevated carbon dioxide levels. In an intubated patient, changes in $ETCO_2$ concentration will occur in the gas passing through the ET tube. If the tube became displaced from the trachea and slipped into the esophagus, the CO_2 concentration in the ET tube would drop, and thus the adapter would not change color. This device was tested on 100 emergency intubations on the ground, in the air, and in emergency departments and correctly identified all tracheal (98) and esophageal (2) intubations.[135] $ETCO_2$ measurement has been reported as a technique for assessing the adequacy of CPR as well.[136] Studies of the accuracy of $ETCO_2$ detectors in identifying intubation are conflicting, with various degrees of success reported.[137,138] Nevertheless, these devices are gaining widespread approval.

TEMPERATURE CONTROL

The humidification of gases delivered to ET tubes is a concern during transport. The risk of secretions occluding ET tubes is progressively more pronounced in smaller tubes and has been reported as an adverse event during pediatric interhospital transport.[122,139] Cold humidification of inspired gases may not be sufficient to avoid this problem

because the absolute humidity of cold gases is considerably less than that of warm gases at the same relative humidity. The use of heated humidifiers during transport is possible but requires heavy, bulky equipment that adds a considerable power drain on battery systems.

One solution is the use of heat and moisture exchangers or hygroscopic condenser humidifiers.[139] These small devices are placed between the ventilator circuit (or bag) and the ET tube and capture exhaled moisture and heat. The inspired gas is then conditioned with this heat and moisture. These exchangers and humidifiers are becoming widely used in neonatal and pediatric transport because of their small size and low cost. Several reports describe the utility of these devices in pediatric and neonatal applications, and in general they seem to be superior to using no humidification system.[140-143] However, these devices are not as effective in conditioning the inspired gas as conventional heated humidifiers and thus may not be suitable for long-term use. Other concerns are that they may add airway resistance and may lead to the development of inspissated secretions, although in neonates the amount of resistance added is probably not clinically significant.[144] Clinicians should be cautious when using these devices on patients who have excessive secretion production, because ET tube occlusion secondary to inadequate airway humidification has been reported when using a heat and moisture exchanger for such patients.[145]

Monitoring and control of the body temperature of transported infants and children are of paramount importance. A significant proportion of morbidity and mortality in small premature infants is related to cold stress, with mortality increasing with each degree of temperature loss.[63] Transport Isolettes should be prewarmed, have fully charged battery packs, and be capable of maintaining the patient's temperature. It is prudent to carry extra battery packs for the isolette.

NONINVASIVE RESPIRATORY MONITORING DURING TRANSPORT

Environmental limitations in the ability to auscultate breath sounds, determine proper ET tube position, and assess the adequacy of ventilation during patient transport have essentially made the use of noninvasive respiratory monitoring a standard of care in transporting critically ill neonatal and pediatric patients.[64] Monitoring techniques during transport include pulse oximetry, transcutaneous gas monitoring, and $ETCO_2$ measurements* (Fig. 45-1).

---

*References 13, 49, 53, 55, 146-151.

PULSE OXIMETRY

Pulse oximetry with cardiorespiratory monitoring is probably the most widely used method of noninvasive monitoring during transport. Its accuracy, convenience, and reliability have been widely tested in a variety of populations and have generally been found acceptable, with an overall degree of inaccuracy of ±2% to 3%. Notable exceptions include the presence of elevated levels of abnormal hemoglobin and profound hypoxemia. Detailed descriptions of the use of pulse oximetry in the neonatal and pediatric critical care populations are available.[152,153]

The usefulness of pulse oximetry is not in guiding initial treatment but in the continuous monitoring of the oxygenation status of patients in adverse transport environments.[154] Pulse oximetry offers vital information about the degree of oxygen saturation of the blood; however, the clinician must be careful not to assume that this is an indication of overall oxygen delivery. The most serious limitation

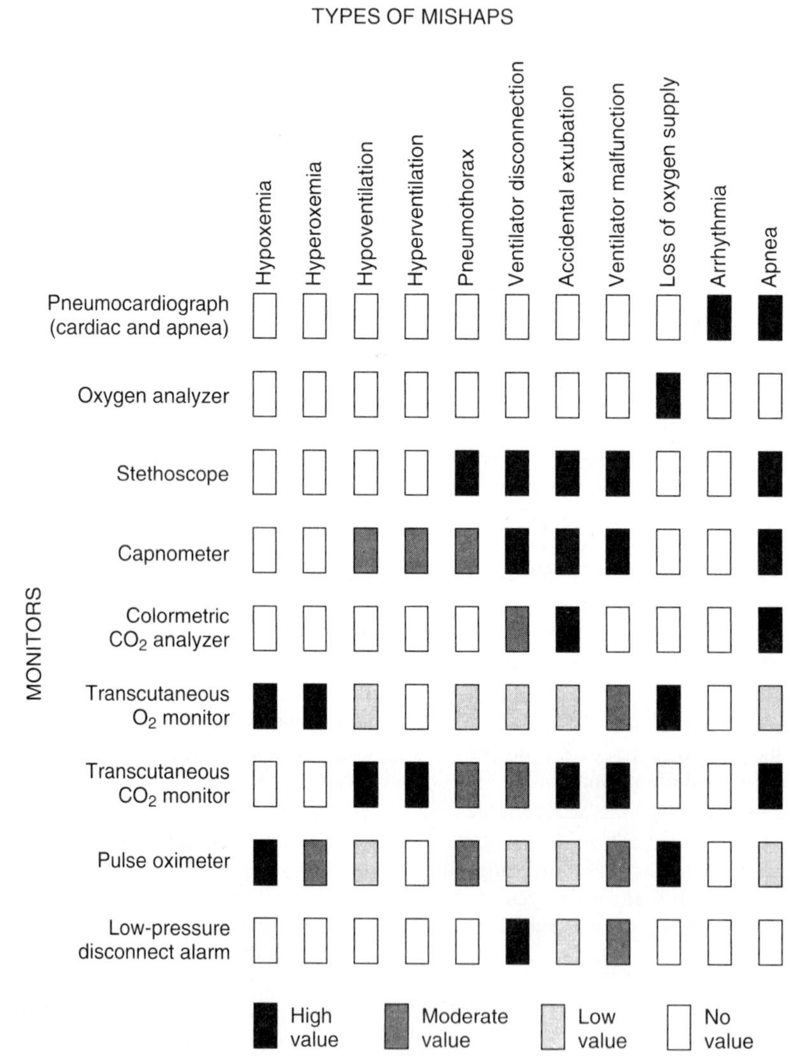

TYPES OF MISHAPS

MONITORS	Hypoxemia	Hyperoxemia	Hypoventilation	Hyperventilation	Pneumothorax	Ventilator disconnection	Accidental extubation	Ventilator malfunction	Loss of oxygen supply	Arrhythmia	Apnea
Pneumocardiograph (cardiac and apnea)	No	No	No	No	No	No	No	No	No	High	High
Oxygen analyzer	No	No	No	No	No	No	No	No	High	No	No
Stethoscope	No	No	No	No	High	High	High	High	No	No	No
Capnometer	No	No	Moderate	High	High	High	High	High	No	No	No
Colormetric CO_2 analyzer	No	No	No	No	No	Moderate	High	No	No	No	High
Transcutaneous O_2 monitor	High	High	Low	No	Low	Low	Low	Moderate	High	No	Low
Transcutaneous CO_2 monitor	No	No	High	High	Moderate	Moderate	High	Moderate	No	No	High
Pulse oximeter	High	Moderate	Low	No	Moderate	Low	Low	Moderate	High	No	Low
Low-pressure disconnect alarm	No	No	No	No	No	High	Moderate	Moderate	No	No	No

Legend: ■ High value ▨ Moderate value ▨ Low value □ No value

Fig. 45-1

Guide to determining the relative value of various monitors to identify mishaps during transport. (Modified from Lake CL: *Clinical monitoring.* Philadelphia. WB Saunders, 1992; adapted from Whitcher C et al: Anesthetic mishaps and the cost of monitoring: a proposed standard for monitoring equipment. *J Clin Monit* 1988; 4:5-15.)

to the use of pulse oximetry during transport is its sensitivity to motion artifact. This may or may not be a problem, depending on how vigorously the patient is moving and how much vibration is present in the transport vehicle.[155]

Pulse oximetry has also been used as a technique for assessing blood pressure in aircraft cabins. This technique involves placing the blood pressure cuff as usual on the patient's upper arm and the pulse oximeter probe on the ipsilateral finger. The cuff is inflated to greater than the systolic blood pressure, as indicated by the disappearance of the plethysmographic waveform on the pulse oximeter, and is then slowly deflated at a rate of 2 to 3 mm Hg per second until the pulse waveform reappears. The pressure at which the waveform reappears is recorded and the systolic blood pressure estimated.[156,157]

TRANSCUTANEOUS MONITORING

Transcutaneous monitoring remains an important tool for the neonatal transport team and has two distinct advantages, as follows:

1. Use of combined oxygen and carbon dioxide electrodes allows the noninvasive monitoring of ventilation as well as oxygenation, a capability not realized with the pulse oximeter.
2. The transcutaneous monitor is generally much less sensitive to motion artifact.

Both pulse oximeters and transcutaneous monitors have been tested in flight and were found to produce data approximately as accurate as that reported in studies on patients in an ICU.[158,159]

END-TIDAL CARBON DIOXIDE MONITORING

$ETCO_2$ monitoring during patient transport is not widely reported but may be useful. In patients without pulmonary disease or serious ventilation-perfusion disturbances, peak $ETCO_2$ values generally correlate well with $PaCO_2$ measurements (gradient less than 2 to 3 mm Hg).[160] Unfortunately, many transported neonatal and pediatric patients have pulmonary disease, ventilation-perfusion disturbances, or both. Thus the utility of $ETCO_2$ monitoring in these patients becomes somewhat reduced and needs further examination.[161]

EFFECT OF ALTITUDE ON TRANSPORT CARE

During air transport of critically ill patients, transport team members must be aware of the physiologic effects of increasing altitude. Barometric pressure is inversely related to altitude; thus, as aircraft ascend in the atmosphere, the barometric pressure rapidly falls (Table 45-3). This decrease has several implications for the respiratory care practitioner.

First, any free gas in various body cavities (e.g., gastric gas, pleural gas with pneumothorax) may not have direct communication with the ambient gas and will remain at the ground-level pressure. This gas will expand as the aircraft climbs; at an altitude of 8000 feet, a 30% expansion occurs. A small pneumothorax might quickly increase in size and impede ventilation. Gastric gas may increase in volume and result in vomiting, aspiration, or bowel rupture. It may also limit the movement of the diaphragm and impede ventilation. Care must be taken to evacuate this increased volume of air with negative pressure to either a chest tube (pneumothorax) or an orogastric tube (gastric insufflation). Air in an ET cuff may also expand as aircraft ascend; frequent cuff pressure measurement should avoid cuff rupture and tracheal injury.

TABLE 45-3	EFFECTS OF ALTITUDE ON INSPIRED OXYGEN TENSION					
Altitude		**Barometric Pressure**		**Inspired Oxygen Tension**		**Equivalent**
(ft)	**(m)**	**(mm Hg)**	**(kPa)**	**(mm Hg)**	**(kPa)**	**FIO_2***
0	0	760	101	149	20	0.21
1000	305	733	97	143	19	0.20
2000	610	707	94	138	18	0.19
3000	914	681	91	133	18	0.19
4000	1210	656	87	127	17	0.18
5000	1524	632	84	122	16	0.17
6000	1829	609	81	117	16	0.16
8000	2438	564	75	108	14	0.15
10,000	3048	523	70	99	13	0.14

From Chatburn RL, Salyer JW: Physiologic monitoring. In Chatburn RL, Lough MD, editors: *Handbook of respiratory care,* ed 2. Chicago. Year Book Medical, 1990; p 98.
*Fractional concentration of inspired oxygen at sea level that would produce the same inspired oxygen tension.

Second, in addition to the expansion of free air in response to reduced atmospheric pressure, the oxygen content of the blood (Po_2) will drop with increasing altitude. As barometric pressure decreases, atmospheric Po_2 will decrease, thereby decreasing alveolar oxygen tension (PAo_2) and thus decreasing arterial oxygen tension (Pao_2), which will result in a lower arterial oxygen saturation (Sao_2). At a cabin pressure equivalent to an altitude of 8000 feet, the barometric pressure would be 564 mm Hg with an atmospheric Po_2 of 119 mm Hg. The resultant PAo_2 would be 65 mm Hg and the Pao_2 would be 56 mm Hg with Sao_2 of 89%. If respiratory disease is present, Pao_2 might be diminished further. Thus Fio_2 levels need to be adjusted to maintain adequate Sao_2. Humans without respiratory disease are rarely affected clinically at altitudes of up to 8000 feet. However, prolonged exposure to altitudes of 6000 to 8000 feet can reduce night vision and decrease the ability of crew members to perform tasks requiring cognitive skills.[162] Fixed-wing aircraft involved in patient transports generally have pressurized cabins, whereas helicopters do not. The clinician must be aware that a pressurized cabin only reduces the impact of altitude on physiology; it does not eliminate it (Table 45-4).

TABLE 45-4	TRACHEAL OXYGEN PRESSURE AND ALVEOLAR OXYGEN AND CARBON DIOXIDE PRESSURE AS A FUNCTION OF ALTITUDE			
Altitude (ft)	Barometric Pressure (mm Hg)	Tracheal Po_2 (mm Hg)	Alveolar Po_2 (mm Hg)	Alveolar Pco_2 (mm Hg)
BREATHING AIR				
Sea level	760	149	103	40
5000	632	122	79	38
10,000	523	100	61	36
15,000	429	80	46	33
20,000	349	63	33	30
22,000	321	57	30	28
BREATHING 100% OXYGEN				
33,000	196	149	109	40
36,000	170	123	85	38
39,000	148	100	64	36
42,000	128	81	48	33
45,000	111	64	34	30
46,000	106	59	30	29

Modified from Fromm RE, Duvall JO: Medical aspects of flight for civilian aeromedical transport. In Fromm RE, editor: *Problems in critical care: critical care transport.* Philadelphia. Lippincott, 1990; pp 495-507.

REFERENCES

1. American Academy of Pediatrics, American College of Obstetricians and Gynecologists: *Guidelines for perinatal care,* ed 2. Elk Grove Village, Ill, American Academy of Pediatrics, Washington, DC, American College of Obstetricians and Gynecologists, 1988; pp 209-222.
2. Clemmer TP et al: Outcome of critically injured patients treated at level I trauma centers versus full service community hospitals. *Crit Care Med* 1985; 13:861.
3. Kissoon N: Triage and transport of the critically ill child. *Crit Care Clin* 1992; 8:37-57.
4. Hulsey TC, Pittard WB, Ebeling M: Regionalized perinatal transport systems: association with changes in location of birth, neonatal transport, and survival of very low birthweight deliveries. *J SC Med Assoc* 1991; 37:581-584.
5. Nugent RR: Perinatal regionalization in North Carolina, 1967-1979: services, programs, referral patterns, and perinatal mortality rate declines for very low birthweight infants. *NC Med J* 1982; 43:513-515.
6. Goldenberg RL et al: Infant mortality: relationship between neonatal and postneonatal mortality during a period of increasing perinatal center utilization. *J Pediatr* 1984; 106:301-303.
7. Boyd CR, Corse KM, Campbell RC: Emergency interhospital transport of major trauma patient: air versus ground. *J Trauma* 1989; 29:789-794.
8. Edge WE et al: Reduction of morbidity in inter-hospital transport by specialized pediatric staff. *Crit Care Med* 1994; 22:1186-1191.
9. Valenzuela TD et al: Critical care air transportation of the severely injured: does long distance transport adversely affect survival? *Ann Emerg Med* 1990; 19:169-172.
10. Pollack MM et al: Improved outcomes from tertiary center pediatric intensive care: a statewide comparison. *Crit Care Med* 1991; 19:150-159.
11. Ramenofsky ML: EMS for pediatrics: optimum treatment or unnecessary delay. *J Pediatr Surg* 1983; 18:498-504.
12. Boyd DR: Comprehensive regional trauma and emergency medical service delivery systems: a goal of the 1980s. *Crit Care Q* 1982; December:1-21.
13. Britten AG, Rogers MC: Transportation of critically ill children. In Rogers MC, editor: *Textbook of pediatric intensive care.* Baltimore, Williams & Wilkins, 1987; pp 1385-1400.
14. Dobrin RS et al: The development of a pediatric emergency transport system. *Pediatr Clin North Am* 1980; 27:633-646.
15. Lam DM: Wings of life and hope: a history of aeromedical evacuation. *Probl Crit Care* 1990; 4:477-494.
16. Fisher GW: Acute arterial injuries treated by the U.S. Army Medical Service in Vietnam. *J Trauma* 1967; 7:844-852.
17. Haller JA et al: Organization and function of a regional pediatric trauma center: does a system of management improve outcome? *J Trauma* 1983; 23:691-696.
18. Frankel LR: The evaluation, stabilization, and transport of the critically ill child. *Int Anesthesiol Clin* 1986; 25:77.
19. Breaux CW, Smith G, Georgeson KE: The first two years' experience with major trauma at a pediatric trauma center. *J Trauma* 1990; 30:37-43.
20. Sweeny DB, Turtle MJ: Paediatric retrievals in south Australia. *Anaesth Intensive Care* 1985; 13:410-414.
21. Colombani PM et al: One-year experience in a regional pediatric trauma center. *J Pediatr Surg* 1985; 20:8-13.
22. Duncan AW et al: A paediatric emergency transport service: one year's experience. *Med J Aust* 1981; 2:673-676.
23. Shlossman PA et al: An analysis of neonatal morbidity and mortality in maternal (in utero) and neonatal transports at 24-34 weeks' gestation. *Am J Perinatol* 1997; 14:449-456.

24. Hauspy J et al: Intrauterine versus postnatal transport of the preterm infant: a short-distance experience. *Early Hum Dev* 2001; 63:1-7.

25. Fallon MJ, Copass M: Southeast Alaska to Seattle emergency medical air transports: demographics, stabilization, and outcomes. *Ann Emerg Med* 1990; 19:914-921.

26. Ohlsson A, Fohlin L: Reproductive medical care in Sweden and the Province of Ontario, Canada: a comparative study. *Acta Paediatr Scand* 1983; 306S:3-15.

27. Black RE et al: Air transport of pediatric emergency cases. *N Engl J Med* 1982; 307:1465-1468.

28. Haller JA: Toward a comprehensive emergency medical system for children. *Pediatrics* 1990; 86:120-122.

29. Saule H, Riegel K, Beltinger C: Effectiveness of neonatal transport systems. *J Perinat Med* 1987; 15:515-521.

30. Downes JJ: The historical evolution, current status, and prospective development of pediatric critical care. *Crit Care Clin* 1992; 81:1-22.

31. Yeh TS: Regionalization of pediatric care. *Crit Care Clin* 1992; 8:23-36.

32. Hood JL et al: Effectiveness of the neonatal transport team. *Crit Care Med* 1983; 11:419-423.

33. Chance GW et al: Neonatal transport: a controlled study of skilled assistance. *J Pediatr* 1978; 93:662-668.

34. Salyer JW, Chatburn RL: Patterns of practice in pediatric respiratory care. *Respir Care* 1990; 35:879-888.

35. Kollee LAA et al: Intra- or extrauterine transport? Comparison of neonatal outcomes using a logistic model. *Eur J Obstet Gynecol* 1985; 20:393-399.

36. Sepkowitz S: Unconvinced of value of prenatal transfer to level 3 intensive care units. *Pediatrics* 1985 (letter); 75:801.

37. Jones AE et al: A national survey of the air medical transport of high-risk obstetric patients. *Air Med J* 2001; 20:17-20.

38. Bose CL, LaPine TR, Jung AL: Neonatal back-transport. *Med Care* 1985; 23:14-19.

39. Jung AL, Bose CL: Back transport of neonates: improved efficiency of tertiary nursery bed utilization. 1983; 71:918-922.

40. Phibbs CS, Mortensen L: Back transporting infants from neonatal intensive care units to community hospitals for recovery care: effect on total hospital charges. *Pediatrics* 1992; 90:22-26.

41. Air transport program directory. *J Air Med Transport* 1990; 9:45-51.

42. Annual transport statistics. *Hosp Aviat* 1989; 8:3.

43. Thomas F et al: A nation-wide survey of civilian air ambulance services. *Aviat Space Environ Med* 1985; 56:547-552.

44. Rinnert KJ et al: A descriptive analysis of air medical directors in the United States. *Air Med J* 1999; 18:6-11.

45. Kissoon N et al: The child requiring transport: lessons and implications for the pediatric emergency physician. *Pediatr Emerg Care* 1988; 4:1-4.

46. Smith DF, Hackel A: Selection criteria for pediatric critical care transport teams. *Crit Care Med* 1983; 11:10-12.

47. Crone RK: Paediatric and neonatal intensive care. *Can J Anaesth* 1988; 35:S30-S33.

48. American Academy of Pediatrics Committee on Hospital Care: Guidelines for air and ground transportation of pediatric patients. *Pediatrics* 1986; 78:943-950.

49. Donn SM, Faix RG, Gates MR: Neonatal transport: current problems. *Pediatrics* 1985; 15:1-65.

50. Pettet G et al: An analysis of air transport results in the sick newborn infant. Part 1. The transport team. *Pediatrics* 1975; 55:774-782.

51. Harris BH: Performance of aeromedical crew members: training or experience? *Am J Emerg Med* 1986; 4:409-411.

52. McCloskey KA, Johnston C: Pediatric critical care transport survey: team composition and training, mobilization time, and mode of transportation. *Pediatr Emerg Care* 1990; 6:1-3.

53. Merenstein GB, Pettett G: Transport of ventilated infants. In Goldsmith JP, Karotkin EH, editors: *Assisted ventilation of the neonate.* Philadelphia, WB Saunders, 1988; pp 376-396.

54. Webster H, Wirth D: Life flight. *Pediatr Nurs* 1983; 10:17-20.

55. Ray LR, Cunningham W: Transport. In Koff PB, Eitzman DV, Neu J, editors: *Neonatal and pediatric respiratory care.* St Louis, Mosby, 1988; pp 318-331.

56. Connolly HV, Fetcho S, Hageman JR: Education of personnel involved in the transport program. *Crit Care Clin* 1992; 8:481-490.

57. Porter B: From the ground up. *Emergency* 1985; 17:26-29.

58. Higgins B, Popil V: Air transport of trauma patients (AACN clinical issue). *Crit Care Nurs* 1990; 1:451-463.

59. Gurland BH, Asensio JA, Kerstein MD: A more cost-effective use of medical air evacuation personnel. *Am Surg* 1995; 61:773-777.

60. Woodring BC, Tidei-Duin J: Who's moving the children? Pediatric transport: selection education and management. *Issues Compr Pediatr Nurs* 1994; 17:93-105.

61. Smith D, Hackel A: Staffing requirements for pediatric critical care transport teams. *Crit Care Med* 1981 (abstract); 9:289.

62. Clews DL: Inter-hospital transport of the critically ill child. *Holist Nurs Pract* 1989; 4:24-29.

63. Mir NA, Javied S: Transport of sick neonates: practical considerations. *Indian Pediatr* 1989; 26:755-764.

64. American Academy of Pediatrics, American College of Obstetricians and Gynecologists: *Guidelines for perinatal care,* ed 2. Elk Grove Village, Ill, American Academy of Pediatrics, Washington, DC, American College of Obstetricians and Gynecologists, 1988; pp 210-222.

65. McCloskey KA, King WD, Byron L: Pediatric critical care transport: is a physician always needed on the team? *Ann Emerg Med* 1989; 18:247-249.

66. Burgess WR, Chernick V: *Respiratory therapy in newborn infants and children,* ed 2. New York, Thieme, 1986; pp 285-286.

67. Jeffs M: Air medical transport in 1991. *Respir Care* 1992; 37:796-806.

68. Gabram SGA, Piacentini L, Jacobs LM: The risk of aeromedical transport for the cardiac patient. *Emerg Care Q* 1990; 5:72-81.

69. Yamamoto LG et al: A one year series of pediatric prehospital care. I. Ambulance runs. II. Prehospital communication. III. Inter-hospital transport services. *Pediatr Emerg Care* 1991; 7:206-214.

70. Beyer AJ, Land G, Zaritsky A: Nonphysician transport of intubated pediatric patients: a system evaluation. *Crit Care Med* 1992; 30:96-98.

71. Krug SE: Staff and equipment for pediatric critical care transport. *Curr Opin Pediatr* 1992; 4:445-450.

72. Rhee KJ, O'Malley RJ: The effect of an airway algorithm on flight nurse behavior. *J Air Med Transport* 1990 (abstract); 9:6-8.

73. Hopkins D, Evans B: A program for certification in airway management and intubation for pediatric transport nurses and respiratory therapists. *J Air Med Transport* 1989 (abstract); 8:63.

74. Adams K et al: Comparison of intubation skills between interfacility transport team members. *Pediatr Emerg Care* 2000; 16:5-8.

75. King BR, Wolfson JB, Geller E: A comparison of the radiographic interpretation skills of pediatric transport

nurses and pediatric residents. *Pediatr Emerg Care* 1999; 15:373-375.

76. Beyer JA, Land G, Zaritsky A: Nonphysician transport of intubated pediatric patients: a system evaluation. *Crit Care Med* 1992; 20:961-966.

77. Strauss RH, Rooney B: Critical care pediatrician-led aeromedical transports: physician interventions and predictiveness of outcome. *Pediatr Emerg Care* 1993; 9:270-274.

78. Braman SS et al: Complications of inter-hospital transport in critically ill patients. *Ann Intern Med* 1987; 107:469-473.

79. Weg JG, Haas CF: Safe intra-hospital transport of critically ill ventilator dependent patients. *Ann Intern Med* 1989; 96:631-635.

80. Taylor JO et al: Monitoring high risk cardiac patients during transportation in hospital. *Lancet* 1970; 2:1205-1208.

81. Waddell G: Movement of critically ill patients within hospital. *Br Med J* 1975; 2:417-419.

82. Ehrenwerth J, Sorbo S, Hacker A: Transport of critically ill adults. *Crit Care Med* 1986; 14:543-547.

83. Insel J et al: Cardiovascular changes during transport of critically ill and postoperative patients. *Crit Care Med* 1986; 14:539-542.

84. Rutherford WF, Fisher CJ: Risks associated with in-house transportation of the critically ill. *Clin Res* 1986 (abstract); 34:414.

85. Venkataraman ST et al: Adverse events during intrahospital transport of critically ill pediatric patients. *Crit Care Med* 1991; 19:571.

86. Branson RD: Intrahospital transport of critically ill, mechanically ventilated patients. *Respir Care* 1992; 37:775-795.

87. Link J et al: Intrahospital transport of critically ill patients. *Crit Care Med* 1990; 18:1427.

88. Srikasibhandha SS, Cats BP: Transport of the newborn. *Z Geburtshilfe Perinatol* 1977; 181:460-464.

89. Frazer R: Air medical accidents: a 20-year search for information. *AIRMED* 1999; 5:34-39.

90. De Lorenzo RA, Freid RL, Villarin AR: Army aeromedical crash rates. *Mil Med* 1999; 164: 116-118.

91. Caldwell JA: The impact of fatigue in air medical and other types of operations: a review of fatigue facts and potential countermeasures. *Air Med J* 2001; 20:25-32.

92. De Lorenzo RA: Military and civilian emergency aeromedical services: common goals and different approaches. *Aviat Space Environ Med* 1997; 68:56-60.

93. Kahn CA, Pirrallo RG, Kuhn EM: Characteristics of fatal ambulance crashes in the United States: an 11-year retrospective analysis. *Prehosp Emerg Care* 2001; 5:261-269.

94. Marsh TO, Templin-Marsh M: Personal risk. *Emergency* 1987; 11:39.

95. Schiller WR et al: Effect of helicopter transport of trauma victims on survival in urban trauma center. *J Trauma* 1988; 28:1127-1134.

96. Argken CL et al: Effectiveness of helicopter versus ground ambulance services for interfacility transport. *J Trauma Injury Infect Crit Care* 1998; 45:785-790.

97. Brathwaite CE et al: A critical analysis of on-scene helicopter transport on survival in a statewide trauma system. *J Trauma Injury Infect Crit Care* 1998; 45:140-144.

98. Koury SI et al: Air vs ground transport and outcomes in trauma patients requiring urgent operative interventions. *Prehosp Emerg Care* 1998; 2:289-292.

99. Cunningham P et al: A comparison of the association of helicopter and ground ambulance transport with the outcome of injury in trauma patients transported from the scene. *J Trauma Injury Infect Crit Care* 1998; 44:1114-1115.

100. Harris BH, Belcher JW: Equipment and planning for neonatal air transport. *Med Instr* 1982; 16:253-255.

101. Demmons LL, McGreevy T: Critical care transport of a cardiac infant: a case study. *Neonatal Network* 1991; 10:39-44.

102. Hurst JM et al: Comparison of blood gases during transport using two methods of ventilatory support. *J Trauma* 1989; 29:1637-1640.

103. Gervais HW et al: Comparison of blood gases of ventilated patients during transport. *Crit Care Med* 1987; 15:761-764.

104. Dockery WK et al: A comparison of manual and mechanical ventilation during pediatric transport. *Crit Care Med* 1999; 27:802-806.

105. Scuderi J, Elton CB, Elton DR: A cart to provide high frequency jet ventilation during transport of neonates. *Respir Care* 1992; 37:129-136.

106. McGough EK, Banner MJ, Melker RJ: Variations in tidal volume with portable transport ventilators. *Respir Care* 1992; 37:233-239.

107. Nolan JP, Baskett PJF: Gas-powered and portable ventilators: an evaluation of six models. *Prehosp Disaster Med* 1992; 7:25-34.

108. Phillips GD, Skowronski GA: Manual resuscitators and portable ventilators. *Anaesth Intensive Care* 1986; 14: 306-313.

109. Park GR, Johnson S: A ventilator for use during mobile intensive care and total intravenous anaesthesia: the Drager Oxylog. *Anaesthesia* 1982; 37:1204-1208.

110. Harber T, Lucas BGB: An evaluation of some mechanical resuscitators for use in the ambulance service. *Ann R Coll Surg Engl* 1980; 62:291-293.

111. Heinrichs W, Mertzlufft F, Dick W: Accuracy of delivered versus preset minute ventilation of portable emergency ventilators. *Crit Care Med* 1989; 17:682-685.

112. Salyer JW: Respiratory monitoring in the neonatal intensive care unit. In Kacmareck R: *Monitoring in respiratory care.* St Louis, Mosby, 1992.

113. Banner MJ, Desuatels DA: Special ventilatory techniques and considerations. In Kirby RJ, Banner MJ, Downs JB, editors: *Clinical applications of ventilatory support.* New York, Churchill Livingstone, 1990; pp 253-254.

114. Branson RD, McGough EK: Transport ventilators. In Banner MF, editor: *Problems in critical care: positive pressure ventilation.* Philadelphia, Lippincott, 1990; pp 254-274.

115. Desautels DA: Ventilator performance evaluation. In Kirby RJ, Banner MJ, Downs JB, editors: *Clinical applications of ventilatory support.* New York, Churchill Livingstone, 1990; pp 121-144.

116. Nish WA, Walsh WF, Swedenburg M: Effect of electromagnetic interference by neonatal transport equipment on aircraft operation. *Aviat Space Environ Med* 1989; 60: 599-600.

117. Gibbons M: Routine Arizona flight ends in disaster. *Adv Respir Care Practitioner* 1992; 5:8.

118. Finsterwald W: Neonatal transport: communication—the essential element. *J Perinatol* 1988; 8:358-360.

119. Holland J: Preparation of the patient for helicopter transport: physiologic and clinical considerations. *Emerg Care Q* 1991; 6:47-54.

120. Beddingfield FC et al: Factors associated with prolongation of transport times of emergency pediatric patients requiring transfer to a tertiary care center. *Pediatr Emerg Care* 1996; 12:416-419.

121. Chameides L, editor: *Textbook of pediatric advanced life support.* Dallas, American Heart Association, American Academy of Pediatrics, 1988.

122. Kanter RK, Tompkins JM: Adverse events during interhospital transport: physiologic deterioration associated with pretransport severity of illness. *Pediatrics* 1989; 84:43-48.

123. Brown MS: Prevention of accidental extubation in newborns. *Am J Dis Child* 1988; 142:1240-1243.

124. Kallstrom TJ et al: A comparison of two different endotracheal-tube taping techniques in the neonate. *Respir Care* 1990 (abstract); 35:1121-1122.

125. Moss JE, Purohit DM: Drug-induced paralysis (muscle relaxant) therapy in the mechanically ventilated neonate. *J Perinatol* 1988; 8:321-324.

126. Kronick JB, Kissoon N, Frewen TC: Guidelines for stabilizing the condition of the critically ill child before transfer to a tertiary care facility. *Can Med Assoc J* 1988; 139:213-220.

127. Rosetti VA et al: Intraosseous infusion: an alternative route of pediatric intravascular access. *Ann Emerg Med* 1985; 14:885-888.

128. Glaeser PW, Losek JD: Intraosseous needles: new and improved. *Pediatr Emerg Care* 1988; 4:135-136.

129. Wagner MB, McCabe JB: A comparison of four techniques to establish intraosseous infusion. *Pediatr Emerg Care* 1988; 4:87-91.

130. Ridenour J et al: Noise exposure to flight crew from the MBB BO-105 and MBB BK-117. *J Air Med Transport* 1990 (abstract); 9:76.

131. Macnab A et al: Vibration and noise in pediatric emergency transport vehicles: a potential cause of morbidity? *Aviat Space Environ Med* 1995; 66:212-219.

132. Hunt RC et al: Inability to assess breath sounds during air transport in a MBB-BO 105 helicopter. *J Air Med Transport* 1989 (abstract); 8:47.

133. Campbell AN et al: Mechanical vibration and sound levels experienced in neonatal transport. *Am J Dis Child* 1983; 138:967-970.

134. Yoder BA: Long-distance neonatal transport. *Am J Perinatol* 1992; 9:75-79.

135. Gerard J et al: Verification of endotracheal intubation using a disposable end-tidal CO_2 detector. *J Air Med Transport* 1989 (abstract); 8:48.

136. Higgins D et al: Effectiveness of using end tidal carbon dioxide concentration to monitor CPR. *Br Med J* 1990; 300:581-582.

137. Bhende M et al: Validity of a disposable end-tidal CO_2 detector in verifying endotracheal tube placement in infants and children. *Ann Emerg Med* 1992; 2:142-145.

138. Ours J et al: Evaluation of the effectiveness and usefulness of a disposable end-tidal CO_2 detector in the prehospital/inter-hospital setting of urban helicopter flight nursing. *J Air Med Transport* 1990; 9:69.

139. Owen J, Duncan AW: Towards safer transport of sick and injured children. *Anaesth Intensive Care* 1983; 11:113-117.

140. Gedeon A, Mebius C, Palmer K: Neonatal hygroscopic condenser humidifier. *Crit Care Med* 1987; 15:51-54.

141. Bissonnette B, Sessler DI, LaFlamme P: Passive and active inspired gas humidification in infants and children. *Anesthesiology* 1989; 71:350-354.

142. Wilkinson KA et al: Assessment of a hygroscopic heat and moisture exchanger for pediatric use. *Anaesthesia* 1991; 46:296-299.

143. Salyer J, Bailey A. Witte M: Three humidification techniques during pediatric ventilation. *Respir Care* 1997; 42:1072.

144. Salyer JW, Butler RB: Resistance in a series of vital signs neonatal hygroscopic condenser humidifiers. *Respir Care* 1992 (abstract); 37:1341.

145. Cohen IL et al: Endotracheal tube occlusion associated with the use of heat and moisture exchangers in the intensive care unit. *Crit Care Med* 1988; 16:277-279.

146. Hankins CT: The use of pulse oximetry during infant transport from outside facilities. *J Perinatol* 1988; 8:346.

147. McGuire TJ, Pointer JE: Evaluation of a pulse oximeter in the prehospital setting. *Ann Emerg Med* 1988; 17: 1058-1062.

148. Giard DA, Ross CS: The use of pulse oximetry in prehospital treatment and transport. Denver, Ohmeda, 1989.

149. Adams KS, Branson RD, Hurst JM: Monitoring oxygenation with oximetry during transport. *Respir Care Manager* 1987; 1(6):1, 3.

150. Peterson C, Budd R, Tjelmeland K: Comparative evaluation of three end-tidal carbon dioxide monitors during flight. *J Air Med Transport* 1990 (abstract); 9:70.

151. Tjelmeland K et al: Evaluation of the accuracy of the end tidal carbon dioxide monitor during altitude changes using the canine model. *J Air Med Transport* 1990 (abstract); 9:71.

152. Kelleher JF: Pulse oximetry. *J Clin Monit* 1989; 5:37-62.

153. Salyer JW, Lewis DD: Pulse oximetry: application in the pediatric and neonatal critical care unit (AACN clinical issue). *Crit Care Nurs* 1990; 1:339-347.

154. Ross C, Rnazi F: Role of pulse oximetry in the initial airway management of helicopter transported victims. *J Air Med Transport* 1990 (abstract); 9:88.

155. Fuchs S, Kompare E: Evaluation of pulse oximetry during pediatric air and ground transports. *J Air Med Transport* 1989 (abstract); 8:75.

156. Talke PO, Nichols RJ, Traber DL: Monitoring patients during helicopter flight. *J Clin Monit* 1990; 6:139-140.

157. Talke PO: Measurement of systolic blood pressure using pulse oximetry during helicopter flight. *Crit Care Med* 1991; 19:934-937.

158. Reimer JM, Schreiber MD, Dimand RJ: Portable transcutaneous O_2 and CO_2 monitors and pulse oximeters during transport of critically ill newborn infants. *J Air Med Transport* 1992; 11: 9-13.

159. O'Connor TA, Grueber R: Transcutaneous measurement of carbon dioxide tension during long-distance transport of neonates receiving mechanical ventilation. *J Perinatol* 1998; 18:189-192.

160. Pascucci RC, Schena JA, Thompson JE: Comparison of a sidestream and mainstream capnometer in infants. *Crit Care Med* 1989; 17:560-562.

161. Bacon CL et al: The use of capnography in the air medical environment. *Air Med J* 2001; 20:27-29.

162. McFarland RA, Evans JN: Alterations in dark adaptions under reduced oxygen tensions. *Am J Physiol* 1939; 127:37.

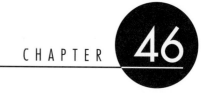
Home Care

Debra Greene

The availability of "high-tech" home care services has greatly increased due to advancements in medical technology and changing attitudes that promote direct participation by parents. The development of monitoring devices and techniques that are easier to operate and more portable has facilitated the ability to provide treatment for an expanding number of children. These new developments enable children to be placed on portable equipment, which allows them to attend school and lead normal social lives.

The following issues need to be addressed before making the decision to provide the home care alternative for the pediatric patient[1]:

1. The pediatrician may not be willing to accept the high risk of discharging the patient into the home environment unless the physician is personally familiar with the quality of the home care agency.
2. Parents must be considered on an individual basis. Many parents do not cope well with an ill child at home. Children are not "little adults," and a family-centered approach to care recognizes the unique strengths and concerns of the patient and family.
3. A highly motivated and well-informed multidisciplinary team is necessary in the care of the pediatric patient. Services and providers must be coordinated to provide one complete discharge plan for the child (Box 46-1).

The pediatric staff should be available 24 hours a day, 7 days a week, for consultation and emergency coverage. The staff and patient must use recommended criteria for selecting a home care company (Box 46-2).

There are clear-cut benefits to home care versus the hospital stay. In the pediatric patient, attention must be given to issues of developmental progress, emotional well-being, and physical growth. The total picture needs to be addressed before the medically fragile child's discharge to the home environment.

BOX 46-1

DISCHARGE PLANNING TEAM: HOSPITAL GROUPS AND HOME CARE AGENCIES

HOSPITAL STAFF	HOME CARE STAFF
Family	Family
Physician	Private pediatrician, clinic physician
Discharge planner	Case manager (funding source)
Primary nurse	Nursing agency
Social worker	Social worker
Physical/occupational/speech therapist	Physical/occupational/speech therapist
Respiratory therapist	Home care provider, RN/RRT
Dietitian	Dietitian

RN, Registered nurse; *RRT,* registered respiratory therapist.

BOX 46-2

CRITERIA FOR SELECTING A HOME CARE PULMONARY EQUIPMENT COMPANY

1. Accreditation by the Joint Commission on Accreditation of Healthcare Organizations (JCAHO)
2. Location: within 1-hour driving radius of home
3. Availability of equipment and supplies required for care
4. Experience with equipment required for care
5. Twenty-four-hour on-call service for emergencies
6. Professional home care clinicians on staff*
7. Record system available to communicate with physician
8. Availability of backup equipment on site
9. Experience with similar clinical situations
10. Accept assignment on insurance benefits

*Some areas may require professional services to be contracted. Contracted professionals must be available on 24-hour on-call basis.

KEY CRITERIA FOR SUCCESS

Five key criteria must be met before a patient is discharged from the hospital: medical stability, family involvement, funding, operational plan, and proper equipment.[1-3]

MEDICAL STABILITY

Pediatric respiratory home care requires that the patient be medically stable and on optimal support.[4] This means a program of optimal ventilation, nutrition, and development stimulation. Optimal support is based on the use of medical technology to augment wellness, not just to sustain life. Medically stable means that the child's level of technical support and clinical course have not changed, and are expected to vary little.

FAMILY INVOLVEMENT

A family-centered program is the foundation for success with a pediatric respiratory patient. Initially, the family must be informed of the implications of home care and be willing to accept the challenge. The family must become involved at the hospital with decision making and providing care for their child. They must be motivated and understand what will be involved, including constant direct care and extensive training by the staff. Some home care companies have drawn up contracts describing mutual responsibilities and accountabilities. Respite care is mandatory for psychological health of the caregiver. The family's involvement is critical to the health and well-being of the child.[2]

FUNDING

Cost and funding of pediatric home care can be the two major obstacles to providing quality home care in today's managed care arena. The funding necessary to provide long-term care to the technology-dependent child varies, depending on the complexity of care required, the level of parental capability, and parental responsibilities such as other children and work outside the home.

Because professional care can be costly, it is essential to establish a solid financial plan to fund this care, as well as the other aspects of home care, long before discharge. A needs assessment identifies the cost and sources of reimbursement for the individual services required to maintain safe care at home. The funding source must cover the cost of equipment, supplies, and professional services, such as skilled nursing and physical, occupational, and speech therapies. In most cases, insurance will fund these needs if the patient meets the criteria of medical stability, and the physician certifies a plan of care and completes a certificate of medical necessity.

The social services representative must know how to access the financial resources required to ensure implementation of the long-term plan of care.

A case manager may also be assigned by the payer to monitor the care in the alternative care setting to ensure it is cost-effective. A case manager should be notified early in the discharge process so that he or she can work directly with the discharge planning team and family to maximize available dollars.

OPERATIONAL PLAN

The operational plan is a "prescription" for home care. The plan outlines all components of the program, defines the responsibilities of all parties involved, and provides for the coordination of care. The discharge-planning group is made up of physicians, nurses, respiratory therapists (RTs), physical therapists, occupational therapists, speech therapists, dietitians, and child life personnel.

The plan should provide an evaluation of the home and community environment and outline all anticipated emergencies and elective procedures. The educational part of the plan includes training not only of the primary caregivers, but also of the family members, nurses, and other individuals who have identified themselves as a support person for the family. Generally, training begins at least 1 month before the patient returns home. Training does not end when the child goes home; it is an ongoing process to reinforce all the skills that the caregivers have been taught.

DISCHARGE PLANNING

The home care therapist plays a primary role in the discharge planning process by coordinating services of the involved health care resources. During this period the therapist needs to clarify the time frame in which training and equipment setup must be done. The home care therapist evaluates the initial planning and notes any problems that may affect the successful discharge of the pediatric patient.

Discharge planning is an ongoing process that begins at admission. The discharge plan evolves from a detailed in-hospital care plan, including medical, nursing, respiratory, and psychosocial needs of the patient. Developing the discharge plan does not necessarily mean that the medical problems have improved or resolved. Children with chronic illness may require supportive care for days, weeks, months, or up to a lifetime. The complexity of care varies significantly depending on the medical needs of the patient.[4]

OXYGEN THERAPY AT HOME

In the home environment the luxury of having oxygen piped into the room through the walls, as in a hospital setting, is not available. The three types of oxygen systems available for the home environment are liquid oxygen, oxygen concentrators, and oxygen cylinders.

LIQUID OXYGEN

The liquid oxygen system is the most common system used in the pediatric population. Liquid oxygen systems are easy to operate, portable, and usually cost-effective. Most liquid oxygen systems are low pressure and operate at 18 to 24 psig. Liquid oxygen is stored in a base unit reservoir that can easily be placed in a corner of the room (Fig. 46-1). The storage container resembles a thermos bottle that keeps oxygen temperature at −297° F through vacuum insulation. The liquid goes into a vaporizer circuit that slowly warms the liquid to room temperature. The increasing temperature allows the liquid to evaporate and become gaseous oxygen, which is then ready for patient use.

The base unit has a flowmeter that can deliver oxygen at low to high flow rates. Most systems have interchangeable flowmeters that range from

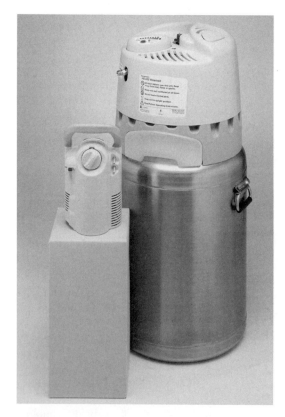

Fig. 46-1

Stationary liquid oxygen (LOX) system with a portable system capable of being refilled by the patient or family. (Courtesy Nellcor Puritan-Bennett, Pleasanton, Calif.)

0.08 to 15 L/min, depending on the child's needs. In some situations, dual-flow systems can be set up to meet the child's continual needs as well as intermediate needs.

Liquid oxygen systems vent continually to prevent pressure from building within the tank. This venting presents a disadvantage for patients who do not require oxygen continually because oxygen is lost whether the system is on or off.

OXYGEN CONCENTRATORS

An oxygen concentrator is a device capable of separating oxygen from nitrogen in room air, collecting the oxygen, and dispensing it through a flowmeter (Fig. 46-2). Two methods are used. The most common method is a process using a molecular sieve material that separates the oxygen from other gases in the air. The other method uses a plastic membrane to separate oxygen and water vapor from room air by the process of absorption. Most concentrators provide greater than 90% oxygen.

Some concentrators can change the flowmeters to low flow rates (Fig. 46-3). The home care provider needs to evaluate each concentrator's specifications before use with pediatric patients. Some manufacturers do not recommend that the equipment be used with low flows. Some concentrators have dual flowmeters to accommodate the varied needs of the pediatric patient (Fig. 46-4).

OXYGEN CYLINDERS

A compressed gas cylinder is usually made of seamless aluminum or fiberglass so that it can be as lightweight as possible. Oxygen cylinders are considered a cost-effective method of providing oxygen. Compressed oxygen can be stored for a long period without leakage. The major disadvantages of cylinders are storage space and potential safety hazards because the gas is contained under high pressure.

Portable cylinders are available in a variety of sizes and are identified by letter designations (Fig. 46-5). At one time, the size E cylinder was the standard portable cylinder, which was one reason that liquid oxygen was a better choice for pediatric patients. Now, with the availability of smaller cylinders and regulators that go down to $\frac{1}{32}$ L/min and the development of custom carrying cases, compressed gas is gaining in popularity. Custom-made

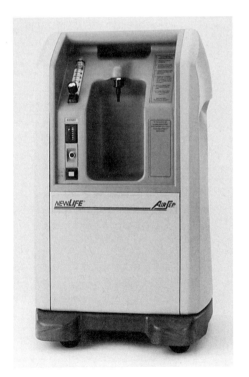

Fig. 46-2

Oxygen concentrator. (Courtesy AirSep, Buffalo, NY.)

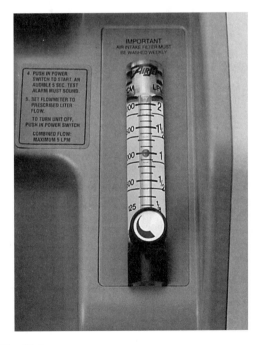

Fig. 46-3

Close-up view of low-range flowmeter on concentrator. (Courtesy AirSep, Buffalo, NY.)

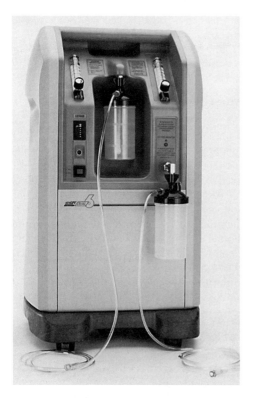

Fig. 46-4

Concentrator with dual flowmeters set at different flow rates. (Courtesy AirSep, Buffalo, NY.)

cases range from backpacks, to waist packs, to over-the-shoulder camera-style bags.

NONINVASIVE MONITORS

Monitoring the pediatric patient noninvasively in the home environment is vital. Various types of monitors are available (Box 46-3).

APNEA-BRADYCARDIA MONITORS

Because the neurologic breathing control mechanisms may not have matured by the time a newborn is discharged, an apnea monitor may be required in the home. An apnea monitor noninvasively monitors an infant during unattended sleep time. The devices are also able to record cardiopulmonary events and compliance with using the monitor. An apnea monitor is indicated when documented episodes of periodic breathing result in prolonged apnea (15 seconds or greater) or bradycardia. Other clinical situations may also indicate using a monitor, for example, an infant who is at risk because a sibling died of sudden infant death syndrome, an infant with bronchopulmonary dysplasia (BPD), or an infant with a neurologic abnormality that causes apnea.

An apnea-bradycardia monitor measures heart rate and respiratory pattern by a method known as

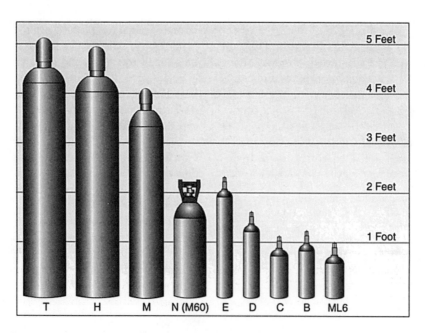

Fig. 46-5

Size and letter designation of medical gas cylinders. (From Hess DR et al: *Respiratory care: principles and practice,* Philadelphia. WB Saunders, 2002.)

impedance pneumography (see Chapter 11). Most monitors have built-in algorithms that differentiate precordial movement from chest wall movement, but false alarm conditions are frequent. The most common causes of false alarms are vigorous infant activity or crying, the Valsalva maneuver, incorrect lead or belt placement, poor skin contact, broken lead wires, and a low battery. Electrical interference from large home appliances, most notably televisions, may also affect proper monitor function.

Changes in heart rate may be the source of annoying intermittent alarms for which a cause is difficult to find. Usually this is from an apneic episode that may not be long enough to alert the parents of apnea but that causes the heart rate to decelerate and briefly activate the bradycardia alarm. A rare infant arrhythmia may also cause a similar situation. Proper settings to minimize false alarms are important because parents become conditioned to most alarms being false alarms. They must be constantly reminded of this phenomenon and encouraged not to delay in responding to the monitor when it alerts them.

Although an apnea-bradycardia monitor may be a helpful adjunct to monitoring an infant requiring mechanical ventilation, the use of this monitor is redundant, and caution should be advised when interpreting alarm conditions. The reverse is also true: as long as heart rate is maintained and minimal chest excursion occurs, the alarm on the monitor will not be activated. However, this does not necessarily indicate that the ventilator is functioning properly.

More importantly, an infant with a tracheostomy is frequently discharged with a monitor. These patients are frequently prone to mucus plugging or decannulation. During these potentially life-threatening events, the apnea alarm will not be activated as long as the infant can struggle against an occlusion in the tracheostomy tube or breathe through an open stoma after accidental decannulation. Likewise, the bradycardia alarm usually becomes activated late during this type of event. When monitoring a child with a tracheostomy, the clinician and parents must be aware of the potential hazards.

PULSE OXIMETERS

The pulse oximeter is used for "spot checks" as well as for continuous monitoring. Oximetry can help identify changes in lung status and can help in early intervention. Potential inaccuracies associated with oximeter readings include poor perfusion and excessive movement of the child.[5]

END-TIDAL CARBON DIOXIDE MONITORS

Monitoring of end-tidal carbon dioxide concentration ($ETCO_2$) helps to establish trends and promote weaning in the ventilator-assisted child. $ETCO_2$ monitoring effectiveness should always be clinically verified before the child goes home with the CO_2 monitor.

New monitors combine both pulse oximetry and $ETCO_2$ monitoring that can be easily used in the home setting. This combined noninvasive technology makes it easier for the clinician and physician to determine the needs of the child quickly.

TRANSCUTANEOUS OXYGEN AND CARBON DIOXIDE MONITORS

Transcutaneous monitoring can provide useful measurements of partial oxygen ($PtcO_2$) and carbon dioxide ($PtcCO_2$) levels. Transcutaneous monitoring can show trends that may be helpful in the ventilator weaning process for the pediatric patient.

COMPRESSORS

Compressors are used for many applications in the home medical setting. Some power small nebulizers used to deliver medication aerosols, whereas others power large-volume nebulizers used to provide humidification. Most smaller compressors are used on an intermittent basis; larger compressors must be capable of continuous use. Most compressors operate off the home electrical power supply, but many portable, lightweight (less than 1 pound), rechargeable battery-operated units are also available (Fig. 46-6).

AIRWAY CLEARANCE DEVICES

SUCTION MACHINES

All children with a tracheostomy should have a stationary and portable suction machine. The portable suction unit must have not only an internal battery that can be charged from AC power, but also a cigarette lighter adapter to charge off the car battery (Fig. 46-7). The caregiver should also carry a Delee suction trap in case both modes fail to power the suction unit. Extra canisters should be placed in the home for emergency backups (see later discussion on suctioning).

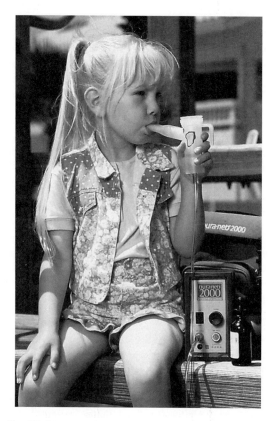

Fig. 46-6

Dura-Neb compressor in use with pediatric patient. (Courtesy PARI Respiratory Equipment, Monterey, Calif.)

COUGH-ASSIST DEVICE

Cough-assist devices aid patients in clearing secretions by gradually applying positive pressure to the airway, then rapidly shifting to negative pressure. The rapid shift in pressure, through a face mask or mouthpiece, produces a high expiratory flow rate from the lungs, simulating a cough. This mode of therapy was originally developed in the 1940s as a mechanical insufflator-exsufflator for patients suffering from exposure to chemical warfare and nerve gas during World War II. Since that time, various portable devices have been manufactured to deliver manual insufflation and exsufflation directly to the airway through a mouthpiece, mask, or endotracheal tube. The Cufflator (OEM) was the best known device.

A modern version of the Cufflator, the Cough Assist Mechanical Insufflator-Exsufflator (J.H. Emerson), has been incorporated into several disease management programs for pediatric patients (Fig. 46-8). Patients with muscular dystrophy, bronchiectasis, asthma, spinal cord paralysis, progressive neuromuscular disease, obesity hypoventi-

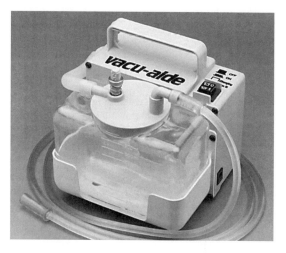

Fig. 46-7

Battery-powered portable suction machine. (Courtesy Sunrise Medical, Longmont, Colo.)

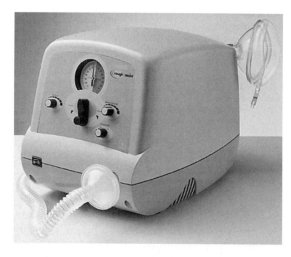

Fig. 46-8

Cough-assist device for mechanical insufflation and exsufflation. (Courtesy JH Emerson, Cambridge, Mass.)

lation syndrome, and central alveolar hypoventilation have benefited from this device.[6-14] Several rehabilitation physicians have created successful home care programs utilizing the insufflator-exsufflator and other noninvasive devices.[15,16]

CLEANING AND DISINFECTING

The potential for transmission of both acute and chronic infections from the child to the caregivers and the caregivers to the child is high. Infection control procedures should be observed as closely as in the hospital and should emphasize good handwashing at all times. The caregivers should avoid crowded public places during the flu seasons. A method to clean and disinfect equipment should be in place at all times and reviewed regularly. The method should also be reviewed if the child is admitted to the hospital with an active respiratory infection.

The choice to use reusable equipment versus disposable equipment must be determined individually. The cost of cleaning and time must be considered. In some cases the cost is not the only benefit of using one over the other. Whatever the choice, there must be a posted schedule for cleaning and changing the equipment.[17]

NONINVASIVE POSITIVE-PRESSURE VENTILATION

Noninvasive positive-pressure ventilation (NPPV) refers to the technique of augmenting alveolar ventilation without an artificial airway (see Chapter 20). NPPV for pediatric patients, in both acute and chronic respiratory failure, is an increasingly popular alternative to mechanical ventilation.[8,18,19]

The benefits of NPPV have encouraged practitioners to explore therapies appropriate for the hospital and home environment. Studies have shown successful NPPV with cystic fibrosis, muscular dystrophy, congenital myopathy, BPD, central hypoventilation syndrome, acute hypoxemic respiratory failure from pneumonia and pulmonary edema, and acute and chronic upper airway obstruction.[18,19]

HOME MECHANICAL VENTILATION

Chronic respiratory failure resulting from chronic pulmonary disease, acquired or congenital neuromuscular impairment, and congenital anomalies are common reasons why an infant or child requires long-term mechanical ventilation, making the patient technology dependent. Even though the number of ventilator-assisted children is relatively small compared with other groups of patients, the cost of care is substantial when specialized equipment and education are required.

The decision to provide care at home must be family centered, not staff generated. Successful home management of the ventilator-assisted pediatric patient depends on the parents' willingness and capacity to meet the needs of their child, because this type of care is time-consuming.[20] The parents must also have the financial resources to fund all aspects of care. As discussed, home care for the technology-dependent patient must be considered a viable alternative to institutional care because of its cost-effectiveness, and the integration of the child into family life can maximize long-term potential. Unlike

adults, many children who are discharged on life support eventually are weaned either completely or to a regimen of nocturnal support. Children who can sustain spontaneous ventilation for periods during the day are more likely to participate in activities of daily living, which will further enhance the outcome.

If the ventilator selected for home mechanical ventilation is not available in the hospital, the home care company may be asked to supply the appropriate machine for a trial period before discharge. Children who require frequent changes in ventilator settings and who need oxygen concentrators greater than 40% are not considered clinically stable and should not be considered for discharge.[20]

SELECTING THE PROPER VENTILATOR

Always consider the child's needs when selecting a suitable ventilator. The factors that need to be considered include, but are not limited to, home vs. public school, distance to the health care provider, and how well it will meet the growing needs of the child.

There is no standard approach for selecting a ventilator for the pediatric patient. The ventilator and the settings chosen must be tailored to meet the needs of each child. The overall goal is to choose a ventilator capable of maintaining clinical stability with arterial blood gas levels as close to physiologic values as possible. Ideally, ventilators chosen for home care should be simple, compact, and portable and operate on a variety of power sources.[1,21] The device should be user-friendly, should incorporate a reliable alarm system, and should be trouble free for extended periods. Home care ventilators should have hidden controls or a locked panel to prevent pediatric patients or siblings from inadvertently altering the settings.

A major advantage of a portable ventilator is the ability to use a variety of power sources, including house current, an internal battery for short periods, and an external battery for extended periods. Some portable ventilators can also operate from a car battery by connecting to the cigarette lighter. An emergency backup system must be available in the event of a ventilator malfunction. Without a backup ventilator in the home, the home care company must assume the responsibility for providing immediate service. Also, a 12-volt battery should be available for use during trips away from home and as an extended backup during an electric power failure. A 12-volt 74-amp/hr, deep-cycle battery can power a ventilator for about 20 hours without recharging. A 12-volt 34-amp/hr, gel-cell battery can power a ventilator for about 10 hours before recharging is required.

Other factors must be considered when selecting a home ventilator. Positive end-expiratory pressure

(PEEP) is usually accomplished by using an external PEEP valve. The ventilator and circuit must be compatible with the PEEP valve. The combination of the PEEP valve and circuit must minimize exhaled resistance. The PEEP valve must be able to function at any angle; this precludes gravity and water columns for home use.

User and clinician manuals should be available from the manufacturer, along with training materials such as videotapes. All educational materials should be well organized and easy to understand. The user information manual and audiovisual material should be left in the home for parents to use as a reference. Various factors must be considered to achieve the goals of pediatric ventilatory support in the home environment (Box 46-4). Practitioners have always been challenged to find the right program for maintaining pediatric patients on assisted ventilation.[22,23]

Once the equipment is placed in the home, problems associated with equipment malfunction are usually minimal (Box 46-5). The source of problems and concerns is usually the ventilated child. Children usually have large leaks associated with uncuffed tubes, so an additional external pressure-limiting device may be used to allow a higher volume setting without the chance of overexpanding the lungs. Studies have shown that 9 of 11 children with uncuffed tubes are inadequately ventilated, with symptoms such as chronic hypercapnia and fatigue.[23-31] The use of pressure control and support ventilation has become an important part of stabilizing and maintaining the pediatric patient on the home ventilator.[22,29]

The major goal for weaning with pressure support is to increase ventilatory muscle endurance and increase the child's threshold to fatigue. To support this goal, the child must be totally supported when on the ventilator. The ventilator is adjusted to maintain carbon dioxide tension between 30 and 35 mm Hg and arterial oxygen saturation greater than 95%. Atelectasis and the development of coexisting lung disease are avoided with optimal ventilator support.

The weaning techniques used in this type of ventilatory management are based on the concept used by athletes. Athletes train for performance by bursts of muscle activity sometimes called "sprints," from which the term *sprint weaning* was derived. With sprint weaning the patient is removed from the ventilator for short periods three times daily. The child is monitored closely for changes in oxygen saturation, heart rate, respiratory rate, and work of breathing. The sprinting times are increased as the child tolerates the time frames. This type of weaning requires that the child receive complete ventilatory support during rest periods to prevent muscle fatigue. Hypercapnia, hypoxia, and acidosis decrease the efficiency of muscle energy production, predisposing the muscle to fatigue.[28,32]

HOME CARE VENTILATORS

T-Bird Legacy. The T-Bird Legacy (Viasys Healthcare, Bird Products) ventilation systems are intended to provide continuous or intermittent mechanical ventilator support for both the pediatric and the adult populations (Fig. 46-9). The T-Bird is a self-contained system that combines an advanced pneumatic system with microprocessor-based technology. The ventilator is suitable for use in institutional and home settings. The compressorless technology allows for uninterrupted ventilation.

The broad range of operating modes includes control, assist/control, synchronized intermittent mandatory ventilation (SIMV), continuous positive airway pressure (CPAP), and pressure-support ventilation. The pressure-supported breaths are available in the SIMV and CPAP modes. The comprehensive monitoring package includes peak inspiratory pressure

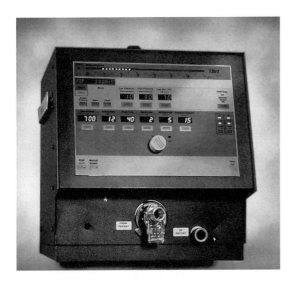

Fig. 46-9

T-Bird Legacy turbine-generated portable ventilator. (Courtesy Viasys, Bird Products Division, Palm Springs, Calif.)

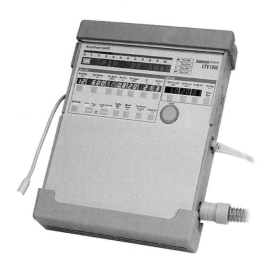

Fig. 46-10

LTV 1000 turbine-generated portable ventilator. (Courtesy Pulmonetic Systems, Colton, Calif.)

(PIP), mean arterial pressure (MAP), breath rate, inspiratory/expiratory (I:E) ratio, tidal volume, minute ventilation, inspiratory time, and PEEP. The T-Bird has an on-off "sigh breath" capability; when the sigh button is turned on, the ventilator delivers one sigh breath every 100 breaths or every 7 minutes, whichever comes first. When delivering a sigh breath, the ventilator increases the tidal volume, breath period, inspiratory time, and high pressure alarm limit by 50%. The T-Bird also has a real-time digital airway pressure manometer with adjustable high-pressure and low-pressure alarms. It has both internal and optional external battery capabilities. The T-Bird Legacy weighs 33 pounds in a $13 \times 11 \times 14\frac{1}{2}$-inch case.

LTV 1000. The main feature of the LTV 1000 (Pulmonetics Systems) is its size. It is a compact, portable ventilator the size of a large laptop computer (Fig. 46-10). The LTV 1000 is microprocessor controlled, using an external exhalation valve of proprietary design with a built-in PEEP valve. It uses turbine technology to provide a range of modes, including SIMV, CPAP, assist/control, pressure control, and pressure support. The ventilator is capable of delivering flow-triggered breaths with tidal volumes ranging from 50 to 2000 ml at pressures up to 99 cm H_2O. Rate is adjustable up to 80 breaths/min. A bias flow of up to 10 L/min is available during exhalation and periods between breaths, with up to 140 L during inflation. The LTV 1000

also provides a terminal flow control to help manage ventilator breaths with large airway leaks. With a high-pressure and a low-pressure source for oxygen, it is capable of delivering 21% to 100% oxygen in the transport, hospital, and home care setting.

The LTV 1000 also incorporates a full complement of digital alarm and monitoring displays on its panel. Alarm and monitor displays include PIP, mean airway pressure, respiratory rate, I:E ratio, tidal volume, minute ventilation, peak flow, and PEEP. The LTV 1000 also has power source indicators to recognize AC, external battery, or internal battery. The ventilator weighs 12.6 pounds in a $12 \times 10 \times 3$-inch case.

LP-6 Plus and LP-10. The LP-6 Plus and LP-10 (Puritan-Bennett) are microprocessor-controlled volume ventilators intended for use in an alternative care setting, at home, or for transport (Fig. 46-11). The LP-6 Plus and the LP-10 are designed to deliver a wide range of volumes, inspiratory times, and breathing rates, which make them suitable for any age. The delivered volume in each machine is adjustable from 100 to 2200 ml, with an inspiratory time setting that adjusts from 0.5 to 5.5 seconds. The rate is adjustable from 1 to 20 breaths/min in increments of 1 breath/min and from 22 to 38 breaths/min in increments of 2 breaths/min. The breathing effort (sensitivity) control establishes the effort needed to trigger an assisted breath. The knob is continuously adjustable from -10 to $+10$ cm H_2O.

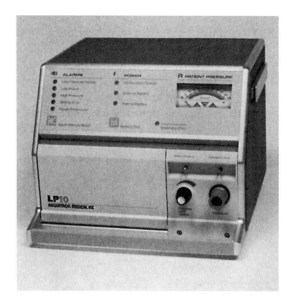

Fig. 46-11

LP-10 portable piston ventilator. (Courtesy Puritan-Bennett, Pleasanton, Calif.)

The difference between the LP-6 Plus and the LP-10 is the pressure-limit feature. The pressure-limit knob is a spring-loaded valve that operates independently of the microprocessor to limit inspiratory pressure in the assist-control or SIMV mode. This function alters the normal waveform by providing a pressure plateau. Activating the pressure-limit control during spontaneous breathing in the assist-control or SIMV mode is an advantage in the pediatric population. The LP-6 Plus and LP-10 both weigh 35 pounds in a $9\frac{3}{4} \times 14\frac{1}{2} \times 13\frac{1}{4}$-inch case.

SUCTIONING THE AIRWAY

Simplicity is an essential component of successful home medical management, especially with suctioning. Several approaches to home suctioning have been recommended. These methods, which are not the same as the aseptic, sterile technique with gloves used in the hospital setting, are referred to as *clean techniques* and include gloved and nongloved procedures.

As long as the infant is not extremely young and is not prone to infection, the parents may prefer to use the simplest and least expensive method, which is the *clean nongloved technique*. When performing suctioning using this technique, the individual washes the hands thoroughly before beginning the procedure. The suction catheter should be sterile and discarded after use; occasionally, however, the catheters may be washed, disinfected, and reused.

If other individuals in the home are ill, a gloved technique should be used temporarily. When providing the care at home, professional clinicians usually choose the clean gloved technique and use the sterile technique only when the infant is ill.

Suctioning is based on respiratory assessment and is performed as needed. Typically the parents are taught to suction when the child wakes up in the morning or after a nap because secretions accumulate in the airway during sleep. They should suction after chest physical therapy and respiratory treatments when indicated and when secretions can be heard in the tube. Suctioning should be performed if the child seems restless or uncomfortable or exhibits signs and symptoms of respiratory distress. If possible, suctioning should be done before meals to prevent vomiting.

The frequency of suctioning depends on the child. If the child has an effective cough, suctioning should be performed infrequently. If the child exhibits copious amounts of secretions or is ill, more frequent suctioning may be required, as often as every 2 to 4 hours. During suctioning the parents should note the amount, color, and consistency of the secretions. Parents must be educated to report significant changes to the physician.

Tissue damage at the level of the carina may result from passing the suction catheter beyond the end of the tube until resistance is met. To prevent injury, the suction catheter is inserted into the tracheostomy tube approximately $\frac{1}{4}$ to $\frac{1}{2}$ inch beyond the tip of the tube.[33] The suction catheter is premeasured by comparing it to another catheter used as a measuring guide.

TRACHEOSTOMY

TUBE CHANGES

The purpose of tracheostomy tube changes in the home environment is to minimize infection and the formation of granulation tissue. As a general rule, the tube is changed once a week or as needed if the tube is obstructed. Parents and all caregivers must be taught to change the tube routinely and during an emergency if the child suddenly experiences signs and symptoms of respiratory distress[34] (Box 46-6).

The tube change should be performed in the early morning before the child eats (Box 46-7). It is ideal for two individuals to be present when changing the tracheostomy tube. The suction machine and a manual, self-inflating resuscitation bag with an appropriate-size mask and oxygen should be available in case of an emergency (Box 46-8). Mask size for the child should be checked periodically by the home care providers. The pediatric patient's needs change continuously, so routine

BOX 46-6

INDICATIONS FOR CHANGING TRACHEOSTOMY TUBE

1. Scheduled change is due.
2. Suction catheter does not pass freely (plugging).
3. Signs of respiratory distress are unresolved by suctioning.
4. Oxygen desaturation episodes are unresolved by suctioning or other interventions.

BOX 46-7

STEPS IN PERFORMING TRACHEOSTOMY CHANGE

1. Wash hands.
2. Gather equipment.
3. Suction patient, then wash hands again.
4. Arrange workspace with adequate lighting.
5. Place obturator in the extra tracheostomy tube, and thread ties or collar through one side of tube.
6. Lightly coat tip with water-soluble lubricant.
7. Place child on back with a rolled towel under the shoulders.
8. Cut and remove old ties and pull tube out with a curved, downward motion.
9. Gently insert tube into the stoma using a downward and forward motion that follows the curve of the tube.
10. Remove the obturator immediately after inserting the tube.
11. Secure the ties.
12. Suction as needed.
13. Assess the child's respiratory status.

BOX 46-8

SUPPLIES REQUIRED FOR TRACHEOSTOMY TUBE CHANGE

- Suction machine with collection chamber, tubing, and catheter
- Manual, self-inflating resuscitation bag (with correct mask size)
- Identical tracheostomy tube (with ties attached)
- Emergency tracheostomy tube (one size smaller)
- Rolled towel
- Scissors
- Water-soluble lubricant (only if required)

---

monitoring is important. Two "trach" tubes should always be available at the bedside, one the same size and one size smaller. The smaller tube should be available in case the appropriate size cannot be replaced.

If resistance is met when replacing the tube, the smaller tube is placed until further medical assistance can be obtained. A child's stoma can close quickly, so placement of a smaller tube will preserve the opening.

HUMIDIFICATION SYSTEMS

Several types of humidification systems can be used in the home care environment. Humidification during mechanical ventilation is necessary to prevent destruction of airway epithelium, hypothermia, atelectasis, and thickening of secretions. The humidification system chosen should provide a minimum of 30 mg H_2O/L of delivered gas at 30° C and meet specifications of the American National Standards Institute. These are especially important in the pediatric population requiring complete ventilation support, such as pressure plateau ventilation, which uses high peak inspiratory flow rates.[20]

A *heat and moisture exchanger* (HME) can be used in the pediatric patient for short periods such as transport. A trial should take place in a controlled setting before the child is discharged home. The caregivers should be taught to observe for signs and symptoms of respiratory distress associated with the lack of humidification. The HME should never be used with another humidification system. The added moisture will wet the exchanger and increase the child's work of breathing through the exchanger. The child with a tracheostomy who does not require mechanical ventilation still requires some form of humidification. Use of a portable, 50-psig air compressor with a large-volume, heated jet nebulizer is required.

If the child requires oxygen, the addition of a T-ring adapter around the tracheostomy tube can reduce the amount of oxygen flow necessary to maintain the child's oxygen saturation levels.

COMMUNICATION AND SPEAKING VALVES

Children begin to communicate from the moment they are born. Communication is an innate component of every human who interacts with the environment. The child with a tracheostomy is limited in the ability to vocalize. Communication research also shows that speech and language development is interdependent and interactive on motor and cognitive development. When one major area is affected, it directly affects development in other areas. Many forms of communication are used with the pediatric tracheostomy patient, including computers, sign language, and speaking valves. The

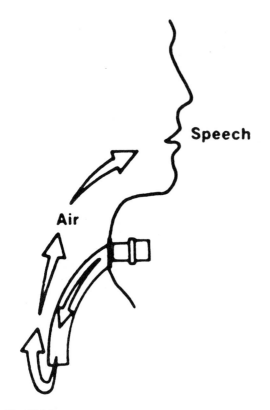

Fig. 46-12

Tracheostomy Speaking Valve enables speech by redirecting exhaled air around the tracheostomy tube and through the larynx and upper airway. (Courtesy of Passy Muir, Irvine, Calif.)

benefits of combining all forms of effective communication are critical to the child's development.

Besides providing a form of communication, use of a *speaking valve* reduces secretions, because airflow is evaporated naturally in the oral and nasal cavities, and enhances the ability to cough effectively (Fig. 46-12). The speaking valve also filters and protects the airway from particles.[35] Before placing the valve, the child must be assessed carefully to ensure a positive experience when the Passy Muir Tracheostomy Speaking Valve (PMV) is first placed. Ideally the PMV should be placed within a few days of the tracheostomy so that the child can consider it as part of the tracheostomy tube. When placing the PMV, successful transitioning techniques include play therapy and distraction techniques such as coloring books, whistles, and stuffed animals. Techniques for training children to exhale include blowing whistles, bubbles, and feathers. Frequently the tracheostomy tube will not allow the child to exhale around the tube, and the tube will need to be downsized.

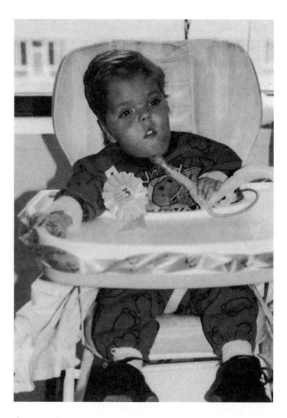

Fig. 46-13

Home ventilation enhances this 3-year-old technology-assisted child's ability to participate in normal daily activities.

ACTIVITIES OF DAILY LIVING

It is important to interact with pediatric tracheostomy patients as normal children (Fig. 46-13). Teaching the parents not to overprotect the child with a tracheostomy is important. A child who is overprotected will feel different than other children and may become demanding. This child is "special" only in the way he or she breathes; helping others to understand this is important.[11] Caregivers must always be prepared when caring for a child with a tracheostomy, and emergency supplies should be available at the bedside (Box 46-9). The child should also never leave home without a "to-go bag" (Box 46-10).

Playing. The pediatric patient with a tracheostomy tube can take part in most play activities suitable for the child's age. With an infant or small child, all small toy parts or objects should be removed from the play area because the child might put these into the tube. Outdoor play is fun, but the caregivers must protect the child's tracheostomy from extreme temperatures and dirt in the air. Extremely cold or hot air may be irritating to the child's lungs. An artificial mask, a disposable mask, or a scarf tied around the neck works well to protect the child's tracheostomy tube. The child should not go swimming unless closely supervised. The pediatric patient may still go to the beach, when it is not windy, as long as the child wears an "artificial nose" (HME) to keep the sand out of the tube.

Bathing. Pediatric patients with a tracheostomy may take a bath in the tub and wash their hair, but water should not be allowed into the tube. To wash an infant's hair, hold the infant on the back over a sink or tub. Wash and rinse the hair using a cup of water and washcloth, or spray carefully. The child can play in the water, but never submerge the child in the water or leave the child alone in the tub. An older child can take a shower as long as the tracheostomy is protected.

Clothing. There is no need to buy special clothes for the pediatric tracheostomy patient. However, instruct parents to buy clothes that do *not* cover the tracheostomy; they should avoid turtlenecks, neck-laces, scarves, or any type of material with fibers that could be released into the tracheostomy opening. The home environment should be kept as free of lint, dust, and animal hairs as possible. Do not smoke, use powders, or spray aerosols around or on the child. Particles and fumes can enter the lungs through the tube and cause breathing problems.

Sleeping. Some children require suctioning at night, so an intercom system is helpful to notify the parent easily. If the child has limited strength, proper positioning and monitoring with an apnea monitor and a pulse oximeter should be done.

"Babysitters." Every caregiver or parent needs a break, so qualified providers must be available to watch over the child in the absence of the primary caregiver. This is a major reason why more than one caregiver should be trained to care for the child. Also, the primary caregiver could become ill and be unable to care for the child for a time.

Transportation. Transporting the pediatric respiratory patient may require extra precautions and planning. Standard restraints may not work for the child. A survey on the methods of transporting technology-dependent children found that the children were restrained well. However, the heavy equipment in two thirds of these patients was not secured.[36]

EDUCATION

Education and orientation of family members in tracheostomy care, ventilator management, respiratory problem solving, and feeding are essential before the pediatric patient's discharge. All education, whether knowledge or skill–based, must be consistent and at the level of understanding of each participant.[34] The teaching of skills requires both material knowledge and practical experience. To be successful, training must be done by an experienced professional who can also recognize unvoiced needs of the primary caregivers. In general, most people obtain more information by actually performing procedures. Providing the caregivers with the opportunity to perform hands-on care with the child in a controlled hospital environment is beneficial.

To aid in consistent training and education of all caregivers involved in the pediatric patient's care, a training book for the specific child's needs should be created. The equipment book should be provided as a resource for professionals and caregivers and should consist of the scope of services provided by the equipment company and emergency phone numbers. This manual provides operational, cleaning, equipment setup, and maintenance guidelines

BOX 46-11

ESSENTIALS OF HOME CARE TRAINING BOOKLET

1. Anatomy and physiology basics
2. Pathophysiology (based on child's specific disease process)
3. Ventilator education topics
4. Tracheostomy education topics
5. Suctioning procedure
6. Use of resuscitation bag
7. Observing clinical signs and symptoms
8. Nutrition and hydration education
9. Administering medications (based on child's specific medication regimen)

BOX 46-12

CHECKLIST FOR NEONATAL/PEDIATRIC HOME CARE ENVIRONMENT

1. Adequacy of wiring
2. Adequacy of electrical power
3. Appropriate heating/cooling
4. Physical space to accommodate the required equipment
   a. Bed/crib
   b. Equipment table
   c. Oxygen system
   d. Wheelchair
   e. Shelving for supplies
5. Adequate lighting
6. Counter space for cleaning equipment
7. Storage space
8. Door sizes
9. Steps or ramps needed
10. Physical space for nurse or caregiver to work

for equipment in the home. In addition to its use for orientation and training of caregivers, the equipment book is also an excellent resource for troubleshooting and reinforcement (Box 46-11).

The primary goal of education is to make the transition from the hospital to home a smooth and safe process for the patient and the family. The family, caregivers, and health care personnel participating in the child's care should become independent and proficient in successfully handling all aspects of home ventilation.[22-24]

ASSESSING THE HOME ENVIRONMENT

The home ventilator company must do a home assessment to address any concerns or problems before the pediatric respiratory patient's discharge. The home evaluation must include the assessment of the electrical capabilities, physical space, heating/cooling system, and the geographic location of the home. Not addressing these issues before discharge could cause problems when the patient arrives home.

The electrical circuitry of the home needs to be evaluated to determine the adequacy for safe operation of equipment. All electrical outlets must be grounded to provide safe operation of the equipment. Because multiple equipment will be running simultaneously, the household electrical circuitry must support the necessary amperage at peak-use periods. Care must be taken to ensure that the circuit can support the total amperage of the equipment to be supplied. If not, another circuit breaker, preferably 20 amp, must be installed.

The patient's room must be assessed to determine ideal placement of the medical equipment. An area for supplies and equipment storage needs to be designated at this time. Counter space is also necessary for cleaning small equipment and reusable items. The room must be draft free and climate controlled with proper ventilation. The amount of medical equipment in the room can cause a small

room to heat up quickly. Certain ventilators will shut down if the temperature exceeds a certain level.

The geographic location of the patient must be considered to plan for backup, transportation systems, and emergency planning (Box 46-12).

PREPARING THE COMMUNITY

The technology-dependent population of children is increasing, and public awareness is a vital part of these patients' acceptance back into the community. The local emergency medical services (EMS) must be notified before the patient's discharge. Some local EMS or volunteer departments have never seen a pediatric tracheostomy patient or ventilator-dependent child. They should have special training and have a plan in place for that child's needs.

If the child is of school age, the schoolteachers and students need to be educated on the patient's special needs and limitations. Such community awareness allows for a smooth transition from the hospital to the home and school environment.

REFERENCES

1. American Association for Respiratory Care: Clinical practice guidelines: discharge planning for the respiratory care patient. *Respir Care* 1995; 40(12):1308-1312.
2. Gilmartin MR: Transition from the intensive care unit to home: patient selection and discharge planning. *Respir Care* 1994; 39(5):456-480.
3. Goldberg AI, Frownfelter D: The ventilator-assisted individuals study. *Chest* 98:428-433, 1990.
4. DeWitt PK et al: Obstacles to discharge of ventilator-assisted children from the hospital to home. *Chest* 1993; 103(5):1560-1565.

5. American Association for Respiratory Care: Clinical practice guidelines: pulse oximetry. *Respir Care* 1991; 36(12): 1406-1409.

6. Bach JR: Respiratory muscle aids for the prevention of pulmonary morbidity and mortality. *Semin Neurol* 1995; 15(3):71-81.

7. Bach JR: Mechanical exsufflation, noninvasive ventilation and new strategies for pulmonary rehabilitation and sleep disordered breathing. *Bull NY Acad Med* 1992; 68:321-340.

8. Bach JR, Alba AS: Management of chronic alveolar hypoventilation by nasal ventilation. *Chest* 1990; 97:S2-S7.

9. Bach JR, Alba AS, Saporito LR: Intermittent positive pressure ventilation via the mouth as an alternative to tracheostomy for 257 ventilator users. *Chest* 1993; 103:174-182.

10. Bach JR et al: Management of end-stage respiratory failure in Duchenne muscular dystrophy. *Muscle Nerve* 1987; 10:177-182.

11. Keen SE et al: Effect of in-home nursing care on distress and coping resources in caregivers of ventilator-assisted children at home. *Am Rev Respir Dis* 1991; 143:A257.

12. Bach JR: Mechanical insufflation-exsufflation: comparison of peak expiratory flows with manually assisted and unassisted coughing techniques. *Chest* 1993; 104:1553-1562.

13. Hardy KA: A review of airway clearance: new techniques, indications and recommendations. *Respir Care* 1994; 39: 440-445.

14. Bach JR: Update and perspectives on noninvasive respiratory muscle aids. Part 2. The expiratory muscle aids. *Chest* 1994; 105:1538-1544.

15. Warren R, Horan S, Stefans V: Respiratory care for children with muscular dystrophy. Arkansas Children's Hospital, April 1997.

16. Lyager S, Steffensen B, Juhl B: Indicators of need for mechanical ventilation in Duchenne muscular dystrophy and spinal muscular atrophy. *Chest* 1995; 108:779-785.

17. Centers for Disease Control: Updates: Universal precautions for prevention of transmission of human immunodeficiency virus, hepatitis B virus, and other blood-borne pathogens in health settings. *MMWR* 1988; 37:377-382, 387-388.

18. Hill NS: Noninvasive ventilation: does it work, for whom, and how? *Am Rev Respir Dis* 1993; 147(4):1050-1055.

19. Teague WG, Fortenberry JD: Noninvasive ventilatory support in pediatric respiratory failure. *Respir Care* 1995; 40(1):86-96.

20. American Association for Respiratory Care Mechanical Ventilation Guidelines Committee: Clinical practice guidelines: humidification during mechanical ventilation. *Respir Care* 1992; 37:887.

21. University of Illinois: *Conference proceedings: Strategies for success in home for medically fragile children.* Springfield, Ill, University of Illinois, Division of Services for Crippled Children, 1989.

22. American Association for Respiratory Care: Clinical practice guidelines: providing patient and caregiver training. *Respir Care* 1996; 41(7):658-663.

23. Glenn KA, Make BJ: Learning objective for positive pressure ventilation in the home. Denver, National Center for Home Mechanical Ventilation and National Jewish Center for Immunology and Respiratory Medicine, 1993.

24. American Medical Association Home Care Advisory Panel: *Physicians and home care: guidelines for the medical management of the home care patient.* Chicago, American Medical Association, 1992.

25. Kacmarek RM et al: Imposed work of breathing during synchronized intermittent mandatory ventilation (SIMV) provided by five home care ventilators. *Respir Care* 1990; 35(5):405-414.

26. Robert P et al: Work of breathing imposed during spontaneous breathing in the SIMV mode of home care ventilators. *Respir Care* 1992 (abstract); 37(11):1358-1360.

27. Gilgoff IS, Peng RC, Keens TG: Hypoventilation and apnea in children during mechanically assisted ventilation. *Chest* 1992; 101:1500-1506.

28. Quint RD et al: Home care for ventilator-dependent children: psychosocial impact on the family. *Am J Dis Child* 1990; 144:1238-1241.

29. Chatburn RL, Volsko TA, El-Khatib M: The effect of airway leak on tidal volume during pressure- or flow-controlled ventilation of the neonate: a model study. *Respir Care* 1996; 41(8):728-734.

30. Keens TG et al: Frequency, causes, and outcomes of home ventilatory failure. *Am Rev Respir Dis* 1993; 147:A408.

31. Bach JR, Alba AS: Tracheostomy ventilation: a study of efficacy with deflated cuffs and cuffless tubes. *Chest* 1998; 978:679-683.

32. Keens TG, Davidson Ward SL: Ventilatory treatment at home. In Beckerman RC, Brouillette RT, Hunt CE, editors: *Respiratory control disorders in infants and children.* Baltimore, Williams & Wilkins, 1992; pp 371-385.

33. Hodge D: Endotracheal suctioning and the infant: a nursing care protocol to decrease complications. *Neonatal Network* 1991; 9(5):7-15.

34. Czervinske MP: Ensuring quality care for infant tracheostomy patients. Part 1. *AARC Times* 1999; 23(9):31-33.

35. Miyasaka K et al: Interactive communication in high-technology home care: video phones for pediatric ventilatory care. *Pediatrics* 1997; 99:1e-6e.

36. Jansen MT et al: Caregiver's safety restraint practices for technology-dependent children during motor vehicle transportation. *Am Rev Respir Dis* 1993; 147:A410.

INDEX